OCCUPATIONAL THERAPY
for Children

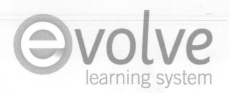

learning system

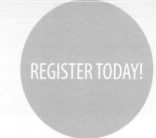

To access your Student Resources, visit:

http://evolve.elsevier.com/Case-Smith/children

Evolve® Student Resources to accompany Case-Smith/O'Brien: Occupational Therapy for Children, 6th edition, offers the following features:

- **Video Clips**

  Case-based video clips are provided for each chapter.

- **Learning Activities**

  Crossword puzzles reinforce key terms.

- **Weblinks**

- **Glossary**

- **Case Studies**

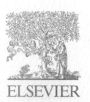

ELSEVIER

OCCUPATIONAL THERAPY
for Children

Sixth Edition

Jane Case-Smith, EdD, OTR/L, FAOTA
Professor
Division of Occupational Therapy
The Ohio State University
School of Allied Medical Professions
Columbus, Ohio

Jane Clifford O'Brien, PhD, OTR/L
Associate Professor
Occupational Therapy Department
University of New England
Westbrook College of Health Professions
Portland, Maine

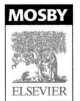

MOSBY

ELSEVIER

3251 Riverport Lane
Maryland Heights, Missouri 63043

Vice President and Publisher: Linda Duncan
Executive Editor: Kathy Falk
Senior Developmental Editor: Melissa Kuster Deutsch
Publishing Services Manager: Julie Eddy
Senior Project Manager: Andrea Campbell
Design Direction: Kim Denando

Printed in the United States of America

Last digit is the print number: 9 8 7 6 5 4 3 2

In memory of First Lt. Keith Heidtman, Sept. 2, 1982 – May 28, 2007, and the men and women of 2nd Squadron, 6th Cavalry Regiment of the 25th Infantry Division.
—JOB

Contributors

LAUREN AMIRAULT, OTR/L
Senior Occupational Therapist
Feeding Disorders Program
Kennedy Krieger Institute
Baltimore, Maryland

REBECCA E ARGABRITE GROVE, MS, OTR/L
Special Education Supervisor
Department of Pupil Services, Office of Special Education
Loudon County Public Schools
Ashburn, Virginia

BETH ANN BALL, MS, OTR/L
Adjunct Clinical Faculty, Board Member
Division of Occupational Therapy
School of Allied Medical Professions
The Ohio State University;
Occupational Therapist
Columbus City Schools
Columbus, Ohio

SUSAN BAZYK, PHD, OTR, FAOTA
Associate Professor
Department of Health Sciences
Occupational Therapy Program
Cleveland State University
Cleveland, Ohio

LAURA CROOKS, OTR/L
Director and Occupational Therapist
Department of Rehabilitation Services
Seattle Children's Hospital, Research and Foundation
Seattle, Washington

DEBORA A. DAVIDSON, PHD, OTR/L
Associate Professor
Department of Occupational Science and
    Occupational Therapy
Saint Louis University
St. Louis, Missouri

BRIAN J. DUDGEON, PHD, OTR, FAOTA
Associate Professor
Department of Rehabilitation Medicine
University of Washington
Seattle, Washington

M. LOUISE DUNN, SCD, OTR/L
Assistant Professor
Division of Occupational Therapy
University of Utah
Salt Lake City, Utah

CHARLOTTE E. EXNER, PHD, OTL, FAOTA
Professor
Occupational Therapy and Occupational Science
Dean
College of Health Professions
Towson University
Towson, Maryland

RUTH HUMPHREY, PHD, OTR/L, FAOTA
Professor
Occupational Science
University of North Carolina at Chapel Hill
Chapel Hill, North Carolina

JAN HUNTER, MA, OTR
Neonatal Clinical Specialist
Infant Special Care Unit;
Assistant Professor
School of Medical Health Professions
University of Texas Medical Branch
Galveston, Texas

LYNN E. JAFFE, SCD, OTR/L
Associate Professor
Department of Occupational Therapy
Schools of Allied Health Science and
    Graduate Studies
Medical College of Georgia
Augusta, Georgia

SUSAN H. KNOX, PHD, OTR/L, FAOTA
Director Emeritus
Therapy in Action
Tarzana, California

MARY LAW, PHD, OT REG (ONT) FCAOT
Professor and Associate Dean
Rehabilitation Science
McMaster University
Hamilton, Ontario, Canada

KATHRYN M. LOUKAS, MS, OTR/L, FAOTA
Associate Clinical Professor
Occupational Therapy Department
University of New England
Westbrook College of Health Professions
Portland, Maine;
Post Professional Doctoral Student
Occupational Therapy Department
Creighton University
Omaha, Nebraska

ZOE MAILLOUX, MA, OTR/L, FAOTA
Executive Director of Administration and Research
Pediatric Therapy Network
Torrance, California

CHERYL MISSIUNA, PHD, OT
Assistant Professor
Occupational Therapy
School of Rehabilitation Science
McMaster University
Hamilton, Ontario, Canada

PATRICIA NAGAISHI, PHD, OTR/L
Occupational Therapy Specialist
Special Education, Birth to 5 Programs, and Clinic Services
Hodges Center, Pasadena Unified School District
Pasadena, California
Part-time Lecturer
Department of Occupational Therapy
College of Health and Human Services
California State University, Dominguez Hills
Carson, California.

L. DIANE PARHAM, PHD, OTR/L, FAOTA
Professor and Director
Occupational Therapy Graduate Program
University of New Mexico
Albuquerque, New Mexico

NANCY POLLOCK, MS, OT
Associate Clinical Professor
Occupational Therapy
School of Rehabilitation Science
McMaster University
Hamilton, Ontario, Canada

PAMELA RICHARDSON, PHD, OTR/L, FAOTA
Professor
Department of Occupational Therapy
San Jose State University
San Jose, California

SANDRA L ROGERS, PHD, OTR
Associate Professor
School of Occupational Therapy
Pacific University
Hillsboro, Oregon

ELIZABETH SNOW RUSSEL, PHD, OTR/L
Program Consultant
Children's Medical Services
California Department of Health Care Services
Los Angeles, California

COLLEEN M. SCHNECK, SCD, OTR/L, FAOTA
Professor and Chair
Department of Occupational Therapy
Eastern Kentucky University
Richmond, Kentucky

JUDITH C. SCHOONOVER, MED, OTR/L, ATP
Assistive Technology Trainer
Office of Special Education
Department of Pupil Services
Loudoun County Public Schools
Ashburn, Virginia

LINDA M. SCHUBERTH, MA, OTR/L, SCFES
Senior Occupational Therapist
Occupational Therapy Department
Kennedy Krieger Institute
Baltimore, Maryland

JAYNE T. SHEPHERD, MS, OTR/L, FAOTA
Associate Professor and Assistant Chairman
Department of Occupational Therapy
Virginia Commonwealth University
Richmond, Virginia

KAREN C. SPENCER, PHD, OTR
Associate Professor
Department of Occupational Therapy
Colorado State University
Fort Collins, Colorado

LINDA C. STEPHENS, MS, OTR/L, FAOTA
Contract Occupational Therapist
Adaptive Learning Center for Infants and Children
Atlanta, Georgia

DEBORAH STEWART, MS, OT
Assistant Professor
Occupational Therapy
School of Rehabilitation Sciences
McMaster University
Hamilton, Ontario, Canada

KATHERINE B. STEWART, MS, OTR/L, FAOTA
Clinical Assistant Professor
Rehabilitation Medicine
Division of Occupational Therapy
University of Washington;
Occupational Therapist and Research Coordinator
Boyer Children's Clinic
Seattle, Washington

YVONNE SWINTH, PHD, OTR/L, FAOTA
Associate Professor
School of Occupational and Physical Therapy
University of Puget Sound
Tacoma, Washington

SUSAN ROODER TAUBER, MED, OTR/L
Founder and Executive Director
Adaptive Learning Center
Atlanta, Georgia

KERRYELLEN VROMAN, PHD, OTR/L
Assistant Professor
Department of Occupational Therapy
University of New Hampshire
Durham, New Hampshire

RENEE WATLING, PHD, OTR/L
Visiting Assistant Professor
School of Occupational Therapy and Physical Therapy
University of Puget Sound
Tacoma, Washington

HARRIET WILLIAMS, PHD
Professor
Department of Exercise Science
School of Public Health
University of South Carolina;
Director
Lifespan Motor Control and Development
    Clinical Laboratories
Columbia, South Carolina

CHRISTINE WRIGHT-OTT, OTR/L, MPA
Private Practice
Adaptive Technology Consultant and Lecturer
Cupertino, California

Preface

ORGANIZATION

The current edition is organized into sections that reflect the knowledge and skills needed to practice occupational therapy with children. The first section describes foundational knowledge and includes chapters on theories and practice models, child development, family centered care and common diagnoses of children who receive occupational therapy services. Chapter 2 reviews established theory of child development and learning, then discusses specific models of practice used in occupational therapy. These theories and models of practice range from those that originated in psychology, education, and basic sciences to ones that were proposed and developed by occupational therapy scholars and practitioners. With this theoretic grounding, children's development of occupations is presented in two chapters: Chapter 3 explains occupational development in infants, toddlers and children and Chapter 4 describes how occupations continue to emerge and mature in youth and young adults. Chapter 5 describes families, illustrates family occupations across the life span, discusses experiences of families who have children with special needs, and explains the importance of family centered care. In Chapter 6, Rogers provides descriptions of common diagnoses of the children who receive occupational therapy, with information on the symptoms, the course of each disorder or disease, and a functional picture of the diagnosis. This foundational knowledge provides a backdrop to the information on evaluation and intervention that follows. This book assumes that the reader has extensive knowledge of human anatomy and physiology, central nervous system function, kinesiology and biomechanics, occupation-based practice, the occupational therapy process, and the evaluation and intervention process.

The second section describes the evaluation process. In Chapter 7, Stewart describes the skills needed in evaluation, the process of evaluation, and considerations for interpreting and documenting evaluation information. Chapter 8 explains the use of standardized tests, including how to administer a standardized test, to score items, interpret test scores, and synthesize the findings. Together these chapters provide essential background on evaluation of children across different settings, using informal and formal tools, and considering a variety of conditions.

In the third and largest section of the book, intervention models of practice and methods are explained. Chapters in this section cover performance areas (e.g., hand skills, visual perception), occupations (e.g. feeding, activities of daily living,

play, social participation), and practice models or approaches (e.g., sensory integration, assistive technology). The chapters explain both the theory and science of occupational therapy practice and discuss practical issues that frequently occur in practice. Together these chapters reflect the breadth and depth of occupational therapy with children.

The fourth section of the book describes practice arenas for occupational therapy practice with children. These chapters illustrate the rich variety of practice opportunities and define how practice differs in medical versus education systems and institutions. Only by understanding the intervention context and the child's environments can occupational therapists select appropriate intervention practices.

DISTINCTIVE FEATURES

Although the chapters contain related information, each chapter stands on its own, such that the chapters do not need to be read in a particular sequence. Case reports exemplify related concepts with the chapter and are designed to help the reader integrate the material. Research literature is cited and used throughout. The goal of the authors is to provide comprehensive, research-based, current information that can guide practitioners in making optimal decisions in their practice with children.

Distinctive features of the book include the following:
* Research Notes boxes
* Evidence-based summary tables
* Case Study boxes

ANCILLARY MATERIALS

The *Occupational Therapy for Children* text is linked to an Evolve website that provides a number of learning aids and tools. The Evolve website provides resources for each chapter, including the following:
* Video clips with case study questions
* Learning activities
* Websites for additional information
* Glossary

The Evolve learning activities and video clip case studies relate directly to the text; it is hoped that readers use the two resources together. In addition, readers are encouraged to access the Evolve website for supplemental information.

Acknowledgments

We would like to thank all the children, who are featured in the video clips and case studies:

Adam	Emily	Luke	Peggy
Ana	Emily	Matt	Samuel
Annabelle	Faith	Micah	Sydney
Camerias	Isabel	Nathan	Teagan
Christian	Jessica	Nathaniel	Tiandra
Christina	Jillian	Nicholas	William
Eily	Katelyn	Paige	Zane
Ema			

A special thank you to the parents who so openly shared their stories with us:

Charlie and Emily Adams	Lori Chirakus	Sandra Jordan	Ann Ramsey
Robert and Carrie Beyer	Joy Cline	Joanna L. McCoy	Teresa Reynolds-Armstrong
Freda Michelle Bowen	Sondra Diop	Maureen P. McGlove	Tuesday A. Ryanhart
Nancy Bowen	Lisa M. Grant	Jill McQuaid	Julana Schutt
Kelly Brandewe	Ivonne Hernandez	Stephanie L. Mills	P. Allen Shroyer
Ernesty Burton	Shawn Holden	David J. Petras	Douglas Warburton
Ruby Burton	Luann Hoover	Theresa A. Philbrick	

We are very appreciative of the siblings and buddies who agreed to help us out:

Aidan	Robert
Lori	Todd and Keith
Megan	Tommy, Owen, and Colin

We thank all the therapists and physicians who allowed us to videotape their sessions and provided us with such wonderful examples:

Chrissy Alex	Katie Finnegan	Dara Krynicki	Ann Ramsey
Sandy Antoszewski	Karen Harpster	Marianne Mayhan	Suellen Sharp
Mary Elizabeth F. Bracy	Terri Heaphy	Taylor Moody	Carrie Taylor
Amanda Cousiko	Katherine Inamura	Julie Potts	
Emily de los Reyes	Lisa A. King		

A special thanks to Matt Meindl, Melissa Hussey, David Stwarka, and Jennifer Cohn for help with videotapes. Thank you to Tracy Whitten for photos. A special thanks to Mariana D'Amico, Peter Goldberg, and Carrie Beyer, for all their expertise with videotaping. Melissa Kuster, Kathy Falk, and Andrea Campbell were instrumental in developing and completing this text. Jane O'Brien would like to thank her family—Mike, Scott, Alison, and Molly for their continual support. She would also like to thank her colleagues and students at the University of New England. Jane Case-Smith thanks her family, Greg, David and Stephen, for their support and patience. She also thanks her colleagues in the Division of Occupational Therapy, The Ohio State University, for their support. We both thank all the authors for their willingness to share their expertise and their labor and time in producing excellent chapters.

Contents

SECTION

I

Foundational Knowledge for Occupational Therapy for Children

CHAPTER

1

An Overview of Occupational Therapy for Children

Jane Case-Smith

KEY TERMS

Child- and family-centered practice
Comprehensive evaluation
Ecologic assessment
Child's active engagement
Just right challenge
Therapeutic relationship
Appropriate intervention intensity

Adaptation and assistive technology
Environmental modification
Inclusion and natural environments
Cross-cultural competence
Evidence-based practice

OBJECTIVES

1. Identify and describe best practices as presented by the chapter authors.
2. Define the rationale for and benefit of child- and family-centered interventions.
3. Identify and explain key elements of an occupational profile and performance analysis.
4. Define and describe components of effective intervention.
5. Describe models for inclusive practice.
6. Identify and discuss elements of cross-cultural competence.
7. Define and illustrate evidence-based practice with children.

Occupational therapists develop interventions based on analysis of the child's behaviors and performance, the occupations in which he or she engages, and the context for those occupations. When evaluating a child's performance, the therapist determines how performance is influenced by impairment and how the environment supports or constrains performance. The therapist also identifies discrepancies between the child's performance and activity demands and interprets the meaning and importance of those discrepancies. Analysis of the interrelationships among environments, occupations, and persons, and the goodness-of-fit of these elements is the basis for sound clinical decisions. At the same time that occupational therapists systematically analyze the child's occupational performance and social participation, they acknowledge that the spirit of the child also determines who he or she is and will become.

This text describes theories, concepts, practice models, and strategies that are used in occupational therapy with children. Its pages present interventions designed to help children and families cope with disability and master occupations that have meaning to them. Although this theoretical and technical information is important to occupational therapy practice with children, it is childhood itself that creates meaning for the practitioner. Childhood is hopeful, joyful, and ever new. The spirit, the playfulness, and the joy of childhood create the context for occupational therapy with children. This chapter describes the primary themes in occupational therapy practice with children that are illustrated throughout the text.

BEST PRACTICES IN OCCUPATIONAL THERAPY FOR CHILDREN

Using the research literature and their own expertise, the book's authors illustrate the role of occupational therapy with children in specific practice areas and settings. Certain themes flow through many, if not most, of the chapters, suggesting that they are important to occupational therapy for children. These are described and illustrated in this chapter. Three themes relate directly to evaluation and intervention:

- Child- and family-centered practice
- Comprehensive evaluation
- Effective interventions

Three additional themes more broadly describe the nature of practice and the environments in which occupational therapists work:

- Inclusion and natural environments
- Cross-cultural competency
- Professional reasoning and evidence-based practice

Child- and Family-Centered Practice

A child is referred to occupational therapy services because he or she has a specific diagnosis (e.g., autism or cerebral palsy) or because he or she exhibits a particular functional problem (e.g., poor fine motor skills or poor attention). Although the diagnosis or problem is the reason for therapy services, the occupational therapist always views the child as a person first. Client-centered intervention has many implications for how the therapist designs intervention. Primary implications of client-centered practice are listed in Table 1-1.

As illustrated in Chapters 7 and 8 and throughout the book, client-centered evaluation involves first identifying concerns and priorities of the child and family. Evaluation also includes learning about the child and family's interests, frustrations, and preferences. What is important to the child and family frames the goals and activities of the intervention. Further, these interests (Figure 1-1) are assessed throughout the

TABLE 1-1   Principles of Client-Centered Intervention

Area of Intervention	Principles
Assessment	Child and family concerns and interests are assessed in a welcoming and open interview.
	The child and family's priorities and concerns guide assessment of the child.
Team interaction	The child and family are valued members of the intervention team.
	Communication among team members is child and family friendly.
	Relationships among team members are valued and nourished.
Intervention	Child and parents guide intervention.
	Families choose the level of participation they wish to have.
	Family and child's interests are considered in developing the intervention strategies.
	When appropriate, the intervention directly involves other family members (e.g., siblings, grandparents).
Lifespan approach	As the child transitions to preadolescence and adolescence, he or she becomes the primary decision maker for intervention goals and activities.

intervention period to ensure that services are meeting child and family priorities. Recent evidence has indicated that, in addition to using adult informants, therapists can invite children to participate more actively in the evaluation process and goal setting if the procedures used are developmentally appropriate.[60] Measures have been developed to assess the child's perspective on his or her ability to participate in desired occupations. The Perceived Efficacy and Goal Setting System (PEGS) is an example of a measure that uses the child as the

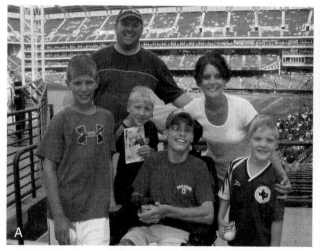
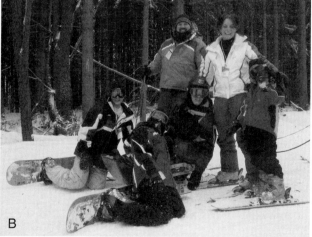

FIGURE 1-1   The family's unique interests determine their priorities for spending time and resources. Occupational therapy services focus on the child's ability to participate in valued family activities.

primary informant.[61] The information gathered from measuring children's thoughts and feelings about their participation in childhood roles can complement results obtained from functional assessments. In addition, occupational therapists may consider gathering information about the child's life satisfaction. Often the best strategy for gathering information about the child is to interview him or her about play interests, favorite activities, best friends, concerns, and worries, using open-ended questions.

In client-centered intervention, building a relationship with the child and family is a priority for the therapist. This relationship is instrumental to the potential effects of intervention. According to Parham et al., a primary feature of sensory integration intervention is "fostering therapeutic alliance" (p. 219).[65] They describe this alliance as one in which the therapist "respects the child's emotions, conveys positive regard toward the child, seems to connect with the child and creates a climate of trust and emotional safety"[65] (see Chapter 11). In a family-centered approach, the therapist is invested in establishing a relationship with the family characterized by open communication, shared decision making, and parental empowerment.[7] An equal partnership with the family is desired; at the same time, parents begin to understand that professionals are there to help them and to provide information and resources that support their child's development.[42,90]

Trust building between professionals and family members is not easily defined, but it appears to be associated with mutual respect, being positive, and maintaining a nonjudgmental position with a family (see Jaffe, Case-Smith, & Humphry, Chapter 5). Trust building can be particularly challenging with certain families— for example, families whose race, ethnicity, culture, or socioeconomic status may differ from that of the occupational therapist. These families may hold strong beliefs about child rearing, health care, and disabilities that are substantially different from those of the occupational therapist. However, establishing a relationship of mutual respect is essential to the therapeutic process. Understanding the family context and respecting the family's perspective are critical to determining the priorities for intervention and the outcomes that are most valued.

Jaffe et al. (Chapter 5) also explain that positive relationships with families seem to develop when open and honest communication is established and when parents are encouraged to participate in their child's program to the extent that they desire. When asked to give advice to therapists, parents stated that they appreciated (1) specific, objective information; (2) flexibility in service delivery; (3) sensitivity and responsiveness to their concerns[55]; (4) positive, optimistic attitudes[16]; and (5) technical expertise and skills.[7]

In Chapter 23, on early intervention services, Meyers, Tauber, and Stephens explain how to collaborate with families. The occupational therapy activities most likely to be implemented by and helpful to the family are those which are most relevant to the family's lifestyle and routines. When interventions make a family's daily routine easier or more comfortable, the intervention has meaning and purpose and will likely have a positive effect on child and family.

Comprehensive Evaluation

The chapter authors advocate and illustrate a *top-down* approach[1] to assessment: the occupational therapist begins the evaluation process by gaining an understanding of the child's level of participation in daily occupations and routines with family, other caregiving adults, and peers. Initially, the therapist surveys multiple sources to acquire a sense of the child's ability to participate and to form a picture of the child that includes his or her interests and priorities. With this picture in mind, the therapist further assesses specific performance areas and analyzes performance to determine the reasons for the child's limitations. Table 1-2 lists attributes of occupational therapy evaluation of children.

Assessing Participation and Analyzing Performance

The child's occupational profile defines the priority functional and developmental issues that are targeted in the intervention goals. With the priorities identified, the therapist completes a performance analysis to gain insight into the reasons for the child's performance limitations (e.g., neuromuscular, sensory processing, visual perceptual). This analysis allows the therapist to refine the goals and to design intervention strategies likely to improve functional performance. Stewart (Chapter 7) and Richardson (Chapter 8) describe the use of standardized assessments in analyzing performance. Assessment of multiple performance areas is critical to understanding a functional problem and to developing a focused intervention likely to improve performance. Many of the chapters describe the evaluation process and identify valid tools that help to analyze a child's performance and behavior.

TABLE 1-2   Description of Comprehensive Evaluation of Children

Evaluation Component	Description of the Occupational Therapist's Role	Tools, Informants
Occupational profile	Obtains information about the child's developmental and functional strengths and limitations. Emphasis on child's participation across environments.	Interview with parents, teachers, and other caregivers. Informal interview and observation.
Assessment of performance	Carefully assesses multiple areas of developmental performance and functional behaviors and underlying reasons for limitations.	Standardized evaluations, structured observation, focused questions to parents and caregivers.
Analysis of performance	Analyzes underlying reasons for limitations in performance and behavior.	In-depth structured observations, focused standardized evaluations.
Environment	Assessment and observation of the environment, focused on supports and constraints of the child's performance.	Focused observations, interview of teachers and parents.

Ecologic Assessment

Several chapters describe and advocate ecologic assessment—i.e., evaluation in the child's natural environment. Ecological assessment allows the therapist to consider how the environment influences performance and to design interventions easily implemented in the child's natural environment. By considering the child's performance in the context of physical and social demands, ecologic assessment helps to determine the discrepancy between the child's performance and expected performance (Figure 1-2). Stewart (Chapter 7) explains that an ecologic assessment considers cultural influences, resources, and value systems of the setting. Two examples of standardized ecologic assessments are the School Function Assessment[22] and the Sensory Processing Measure.[59,66] Both are comprehensive measures of children's functioning in the context of school and/or home. Figure 1-3 shows an example of an activity observed to complete the School Function Assessment.

The importance of ecologic assessment for youth preparing to transition into work and community environments is emphasized by Spencer (Chapter 27). To support adolescents preparing for employment, assessment must occur in the community and the worksite. Through in-depth task analysis and performance analysis, the therapist identifies the skills required for the job tasks and the discrepancy between the task requirements and the youth's performance. If the team seeks to

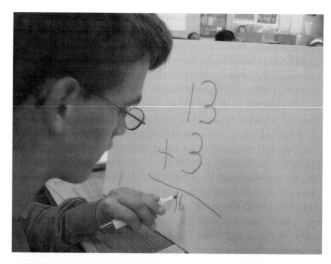

FIGURE 1-3 Through observation of a writing activity at school, the occupational therapist gains an understanding of the accommodations and supports needed as well as the child's performance level.

identify the student's interests and abilities as they relate to future community living, an ecologic assessment would take place in the community and the home. Spencer explains that systematic and careful observation of the student's performance during daily activities (e.g., home chores, food shopping, banking, using transportation, bill paying) enables therapists to target what skills need to be practiced, what tasks modified, and what environmental adaptations made. Ecologic approaches consider the characteristics of the individual and the physical, social, cultural, and temporal demands the individual faces (Spencer, Chapter 27).

Evaluating Context

Occupational therapists also evaluate the contexts in which the child learns, plays, and interacts. Evaluating performance in multiple contexts (e.g., home, school, daycare, other relevant community settings) allows the therapist to appreciate how different contexts affect the child's performance and participation.

Contexts important to consider when evaluating children include *physical, social,* and *cultural factors*. The physical space available to the child can facilitate or constrain exploration and play. Family is the primary social context for the young child, and peers become important aspects of the social context at preschool and school ages. The occupational therapist evaluates physical and social contextual factors using the following questions:

- Does the environment allow physical access?
- Are materials to promote development available?
- Does the environment provide an optimal amount of supervision?
- Is the environment safe?
- Are a variety of spaces and sensory experiences available?
- Is the environment conducive to social interaction?
- Are opportunities for exploration, play, and learning available?
- Is positive adult support available and developmentally appropriate?

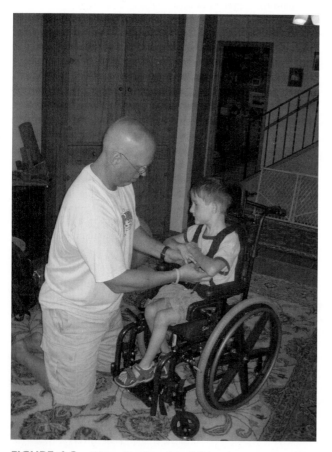

FIGURE 1-2 By evaluating the child at home, the therapist gathers information about how the family uses the child's technology and how the child accesses home environments and participates in activities of daily living.

The occupational therapist evaluates how the environmental and activity demands facilitate or constrain the child's performance. An understanding and appreciation of the family's culture, lifestyle, parenting style, and values have profound influence on the child's development and form a foundation for intervention planning.

Through comprehensive evaluation, the therapist analyzes the discrepancies between performance, expectations for performance, and activity demands. She or he identifies potential outcomes that fit the child and family's story. By moving from assessment of participation to analysis of performance and contexts, the therapist gains a solid understanding of the strengths, concerns, and problems of the individuals involved (e.g., child, parent, or caregiver; family members; teachers). The occupational therapist also understands how to interact with the child to build a trusting and a positive relationship.

Effective Interventions

Much of this book describes interventions for children. Occupational therapists improve children's performance and participation by (1) providing interventions to enhance performance, (2) adapting activities and modifying the environment, and (3) consulting, educating, and advocating. These intervention strategies complement each other and in best practice are applied together to support optimal growth and function in the child.

Providing Interventions to Enhance Performance

This section defines and illustrates the chapter themes that explain how the occupational therapist interacts with, challenges, and supports the child and develops interventions that promote and reinforce the child's participation. The following elements appear to be core to the therapeutic process. The therapist designs and implements intervention activities with the child that:

1. Optimize the child's active engagement
2. Provide a just right challenge
3. Establish a therapeutic relationship
4. Provide adequate and appropriate intensity and reinforcement

Optimize Child's Engagement

Parham and Mailloux (Chapter 11) propose that active participation and tapping the child's inner drive are key features of the sensory integration *intervention*. Engagement is essential because the child's brain responds differently and learns more effectively when he or she is actively involved in a task rather than merely receiving passive stimulation. These authors cite the original work of Ayres, who theorized that children experience a greater degree of sensory integration when actively, rather than passively, participating in an activity (see Chapter 11).[3]

The child's engagement in an activity or a social interaction is an essential component of a therapy session. This engagement funnels the child's energy into the activity, helps him or her sustain full attention, and implies that the child has adopted a goal and purpose that fuels his performance in the activity. Engagement can be difficult to obtain when the child has an autism spectrum disorder. Spitzer suggests that a therapist can engage a child with autism by beginning with his or her immediate interest, even if it appears as meaningless (e.g.,

spinning a wheel, lining up toy letters, lying upside down on a ball).[84] The therapist may begin with the child's obsessive interest (i.e., trains, letters, or balls) and create a more playful, social interaction using these objects. By engaging in the child's preferred activity, the therapist can foster and sustain social interaction, at the same time making the activity more playful and purposeful.

In Chapter 9, O'Brien and Williams explain that the child's engagement in an activity is essential to its therapeutic value in promoting motor control. These authors recommend that the child select and help design the activity to increase his or her engagement in it. The therapist can engage an older child in a task by presenting a problem to be solved. Posing a dilemma in the child's area of interest can help the child focus on the problem, adopt a potential solution as a goal, and stay engaged until the problem is solved. For example, the therapist can explain to a child with poor balance that the therapy room floor has become steamy hot and the child must jump from one stone (plastic disk) to another to avoid the heat. This same therapy floor may turn into ice, and the child has to skate across the floor on pieces of paper. Children learn and retain motor skills more from intrinsically problem-solving a motor action than from receiving external feedback during an action (such as hand-over-hand assistance).

Whole activities with multiple steps and a meaningful goal (versus repetition of activity components) elicit the child's full engagement and participation. Repeating a single component (e.g., squeeze the Play-Doh or place pennies in a can) has minimal therapeutic value. Functional magnetic resonance imaging (fMRI) studies indicate that more areas of the brain are activated when individuals engage in meaningful whole tasks versus parts of the tasks (O'Brien & Williams, Chapter 9).[48] By engaging in an activity with a meaningful goal (e.g., cooking or an art project), children use multiple systems and organize their performance around that goal. This is usually a functional organization that can generalize to other activities. For example, if a game requires that a preschool child attend to a peer, wait for his turn, and correctly place a game piece, the child is developing the joint attention that he or she needs to participate in circle time or a family meal.

Provide a Just Right Challenge

Maximal active involvement generally takes place when therapeutic activities are at just the right level of complexity, where the child not only feels comfortable and nonthreatened but also experiences some challenge that requires effort. An activity that is a child's "just right" challenge has the following elements: the activity (1) matches the child's developmental skills and interests, (2) provides a reasonable challenge to current performance level, (3) engages and motivates the child, and (4) can be mastered with the child's focused effort.

Based on careful analysis of performance and behavior, the occupational therapist selects an activity that matches the child's strengths and limitations across performance domains. The analysis allows the therapist to individualize the difficulty, the pace, and the supports needed for a child to accomplish a task. Generally, the therapist selects highly adaptable activities that can be modified to raise or lower the difficulty level based on the child's performance. To promote change in the child, the activity must be challenging and create a degree of stress. Figure 1-4 provides an example of an activity challenging to a child with sensory integration problems. The stress is meant to elicit a higher level of

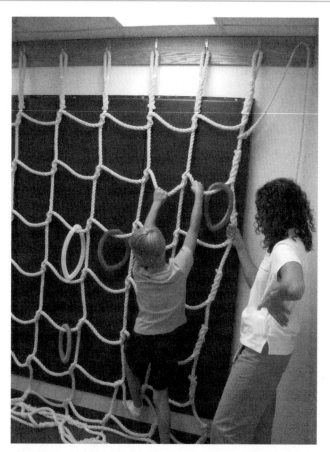

FIGURE 1-4   A climbing wall activity challenged this child's motor planning, bilateral coordination, strength, and postural stability.

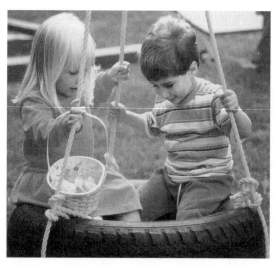

FIGURE 1-5   Applying a sensory integration approach, the therapist gradually introduced the child with gravitational insecurity to unstable surfaces and higher levels of vestibular input.

response. The therapist's and the child's interactions are like a dance: The therapist poses a problem or challenge to the child, who is then motivated by that challenge and responds. The therapist facilitates or supports the action in order to prompt the child to respond at a higher level. The therapist then gives feedback regarding the action and presents another problem of greater or lesser difficulty, based on the success of the child's response. Cognitive, sensory, motor, perceptual, or social aspects of the activity may be made easier or more difficult (Case Study 1-1). By precisely assessing the adequacy of the child's response, the occupational therapist finds the just right challenge.

Parham and Mailloux (Chapter 11) explain that therapy sessions typically begin with activities that the child can engage in comfortably and competently and then move toward increasing challenges. They provide an example of a child with gravitational insecurity (i.e., fear of and aversion to being on unstable surfaces or heights with immature postural balance). Therapy activities begin close to the ground, and the therapist provides close physical support to help the child feel secure. Gradually, in subsequent sessions, the therapist designs activities that require the child to walk on unstable surfaces and to swing with his or her whole body suspended (Figure 1-5). These graded activities pose a just right level of challenge while respecting the child's need to feel secure and in control. This gradual approach is key to maximizing the child's active involvement in therapy.

Meyers, Stephens, and Tauber (Chapter 23) suggest that therapists design and employ play activities that engage and challenge the child across domains (for example, activities that are slightly higher than the child's development level in motor, cognitive, and social domains). When a task challenges both cognitive and motor skills, the young child becomes fully engaged and the activity has high therapeutic potential for improving the child's developmental level of performance.

CASE STUDY 1-1   Grading an Activity: Challenging and Eliciting Full Participation

Aaron, a 10-year-old child with autism, participated in a cooking activity with the occupational therapist and three peers. The children were proceeding in an organized manner—sharing cooking supplies and verbalizing each step of the activity. As they proceeded, Aaron had great difficulty participating in the task; the materials were messy, and the social interaction was frequent and unpredictable. He performed best when the activity was highly structured, the instructions were very clear, and the social interaction was kept at a minimum. To help him participate at a comfortable level, the occupational therapist suggested

that his contribution to the activity be to put away supplies and retrieve new ones. The other children were asked to give him specific visual and verbal instructions as to what they needed and what should be replaced in the refrigerator or cupboard. With this new rule in place, the children gave simple and concrete instructions that Aaron could follow. An important element of this strategy was that it included the support of his peers to elicit an optimal level of participation and could be generalized to other small-group activities involving Aaron and his peers.

Establish a Therapeutic Relationship

The occupational therapist establishes a relationship with the child that encourages and motivates. The therapist first establishes a relationship of trust (Figure 1-6).[9,15,89] The therapist becomes invested in the child's success and reinforces the importance of the child's efforts. Although the therapist presents challenges and asks the child to take risks, the therapist also supports and facilitates the performance so that the child succeeds or feels okay when he or she fails. This trust enables the child to feel safe and willing to take risks. The occupational therapist shows interest in the child, makes efforts to enjoy his or her personality, and values his or her preferences and goals. The child's unique traits and behaviors become the basis for designing activities that will engage the child and provide the just right challenge.

To establish a therapeutic relationship, therapists select an activity of interest that motivates the child and gives the child choices.[36,84] Fostering a therapeutic relationship involves respecting the child's emotions, conveying positive regard toward the child, attempting to connect with the child, and creating a climate of trust and emotional safety.[65] The therapist encourages positive affect by attending to and imitating the child's actions and communication attempts, waiting for the child's response, establishing eye contact, using gentle touch, and making nonevaluative comments. By choosing activities that allow the child to feel important and by grading the activity to match the child's abilities, the therapist gives the child the opportunity to achieve mastery and a sense of accomplishment. Generally, the intrinsic sense of mastery is a stronger reinforcement to the child than external rewards, such as verbal praise or other contingent reward systems. The occupational therapist vigilantly attends to the child's performance during an activity to provide precise levels of support that enable the child to succeed. A child's self-esteem and self-image are influenced by skill achievement and by success in mastering tasks.

The occupational therapist remains highly sensitive to the child's emerging self-actualization and helps the team and family provide activities and environments that support the child's sense of self as an efficacious person. Self-actualization, as defined by Fidler and Fidler,[31] occurs through successful coping with problems in the everyday environment. It implies more than the ability to respond to others: self-actualization means that the child initiates play activities, investigates problems, and initiates social interactions. A child with a positive sense of self seeks experiences that are challenging, responds to play opportunities, masters developmentally appropriate tasks, and forms and sustains relationships with peers and adults. Vroman (Chapter 4) defines self-esteem, self–image, and self-worth and explains how teenagers' self-concept influences health and activity. In Chapter 17, Loukas and Dunn discuss the importance of therapeutic relationships for fostering self-determination in adolescents with significant disabilities.

Research evidence suggests that interventions in which the therapist establishes a relationship with the child and emphasizes playful social interaction within the therapy session have positive effects on children's development.[38,97] Studies of the effectiveness of relationship-based interventions have found that they promote communication and play,[38] social-emotional function,[39,54] and learning.[98] The practitioner's therapeutic relationship with the child appears to be a consistent feature of efficacious interventions.[14]

Provide Adequate and Appropriate Intensity and Reinforcement

Research evidence cited throughout this book indicates that more intense intervention has greater positive effects on performance. One intervention, constraint-induced movement therapy (CIMT), has been shown to have strong positive effects (Exner, Chapter 10).[25] This intervention uses a specific protocol with a specific population of children. In CIMT, the nonaffected hand and arm of children with hemiparesis cerebral palsy is casted, and the child practices specific skills with the affected hand and arm (Figure 1-7). CIMT also

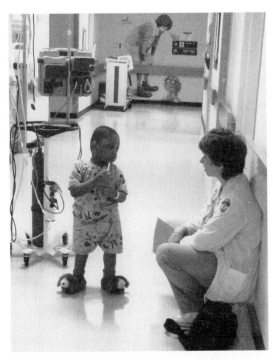

FIGURE 1-6 A hallway conversation helps to establish the therapist's relationship with the child. (Courtesy of Jayne Shepherd and Sheri Michael.)

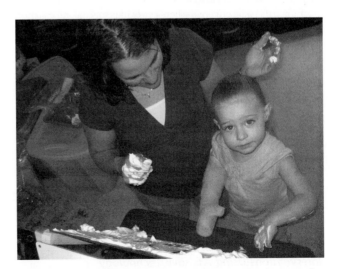

FIGURE 1-7 In constraint-induced movement therapy, the child's less involved arm was casted, and she received intensive therapy to build skills in the involved arm and hand.

provides an intensive dosage of therapy. The "shaping" intervention is provided 6 hours a day for 21 days. The results are unequivocal that the child's movement and function with the involved upper extremity improve.[25,88]

Although this dosage of therapy is not typical and may not be practical in most situations, these research findings suggest that intensive services have clear benefit. Schertz and Gordon conclude that intensive interventions that involve repeated practice and progressive challenge can produce positive changes in functional performance.[79] O'Brien and Williams (Chapter 9) explain the importance of repeated practice in skill attainment. They note that children learn new skills with frequent practice and various types of practice. Motor learning studies have shown that intense (blocked) practice is helpful when first learning a new skill but that the child also needs variable and random practice to generalize and transfer the newly learned skill to a variety of situations.

Although the research evidence demonstrates more positive effects with intensive intervention, for practical reasons the field has not yet embraced this model for providing therapy services. Constrained by resources and systems limited in capacity to deliver intensive therapy, most occupational therapy episodes have limited intensity and duration. The research evidence has created discussion in the field about what model for service delivery is optimal and how children can access the most efficacious interventions.

Research has also demonstrated that interventions in which the child is rewarded for performing well have positive effects.[87,97] Based on a behavioral model, most occupational therapy interventions include reinforcement of the child's efforts. This reinforcement can range from hugs and praises to more tangible objects, such as a prize or piece of candy. Occupational therapists often embed a natural reinforcement within the activity. For example, the therapist designs a session in which a group of four 12-year-olds with Asperger's syndrome bake cookies. The natural reinforcement includes eating cookies and enjoying socialization with others during the activity. Positive reinforcement includes both intrinsic (e.g., feeling competent or sense of success) and extrinsic (e.g., adult praise or a treat) feedback. O'Brien and Williams (Chapter 9) explain that feedback can be most effective when it is given on a variable schedule, with the goal that feedback is faded as the skill is mastered. External feedback appears to be effective when it provides specific information to the child about performance and when it immediately follows performance.[82] In summary, research evidence supports that children's performance improves with intense practice of emerging skills and with a system of rewards for higher level performance.

Occupational therapy interventions are not always focused on the child's performance; at times, the emphasis is on implementing adapted methods or applying assistive technology to increase the child's participation despite performance problems. The following sections explain how occupational therapists use adaptation, assistive technology, and environmental modification to improve a child's participation in home, school, and community activities.

Adapting Activities and Modifying the Environment

Interventions Using Assistive Technology
Occupational therapists often help children with disabilities participate by adapting activities and applying assistive technology (Figure 1-8). Adapted techniques for play activities may

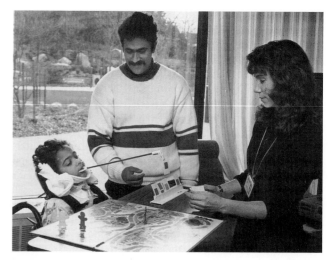

FIGURE 1-8 The occupational therapist designed a mouth stick and game board setup so that the child could play the game with his father.

include switch toys, battery-powered toys, enlarged handles on puzzle pieces, or magnetic pieces that can easily fit together. In activities of daily living, adapted techniques can be used to increase independence and reduce caregiver assistance in eating, dressing, or bathing. In Chapter 16, Shepherd offers many examples of adapted techniques to increase a child's independence in self-care and activities of daily living.

Technology is pervasive throughout society, and its increasing versatility makes it easily adaptable to an individual child's needs. Low-technology solutions are often applied to increase the child's participation in play or to increase a child's independence in self-care. Examples include built-up handles on utensils, weighted cups, elastic shoelaces, and electric toothbrushes. High-technology solutions are often used to increase mobility or functional communication. Examples are power wheelchairs, augmentative communication devices, and computers.

High technology is becoming increasingly available and typically involves computer processing and switch or keyboard access (e.g., augmentative communication devices) (see Chapter 20). Occupational therapists frequently support the use of assistive technology by identifying the most appropriate device or system and features of the system. They often help families obtain funding to purchase the device, set up or program the system, train others to use it, and monitor its use. They also make themselves available to problem-solve the inevitable technology issues that arise.

The role of assistive technology with children is not simply to compensate for a missing or delayed function; it is also used to promote development in targeted performance areas. Research has demonstrated that increased mobility with the use of a power wheelchair increases social and perceptual skills (see Chapter 21).[9,10,13,63] The use of an augmentative communication device can enhance language and social skills and may prevent behavioral problems common in children who have limited means of communicating. Therefore, the occupational therapist selects assistive technology not only to enable the child to participate more fully in functional or social activities but also to enhance the development of skills related to a

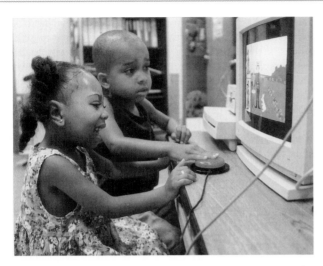

FIGURE 1-9   A switch activates a computer program that simulates a storybook.

specific occupational area. For example, to develop preliteracy skills a child who has a physical disability with severe motor impairments can access a computer program that simulates reading a book; to promote computer skills the child can use an expanded keyboard (Figure 1-9). The computer programs used in schools to promote literacy, writing, and math skills with all children are particularly beneficial to children who have learning and physical disabilities. Because schools have invested in universal design and appropriate accommodations for all learners, many students with disabilities can access computer programs that promote their literacy and writing skills. In Chapter 20, Schoonover, Argabrite Grove, and Swinth describe currently available technologies designed to promote children's functional performance.

Assistive technology solutions continually change as devices become more advanced and more versatile. Although a therapist can extensively train a student to use power mobility, an augmentative communication device, or an adapted computer, the child's skills with the technology will not generalize into everyday routines unless parents, teachers, and aides are sufficiently comfortable with and knowledgeable about the technology. Because it is important that those adults closest to the child be able to implement the technology and troubleshoot when necessary, the occupational therapist must educate them extensively about how to apply the technology—and remain available to problem-solve the issues that inevitably arise. Often, it is necessary to talk through and model each step in the use of the technology. Strategies for integrating the technology into a classroom or home environment (e.g., discussing the ways the device can be used throughout the day) help to achieve the greatest benefit. All team members need to update their skills routinely so that they have a working knowledge of emerging technology.

One trend observed in school systems is that the occupational therapist often serves as an assistive technology consultant or becomes a member of a district-wide assistive technology team. Assistive technology teams have been formed to provide support and expertise to school staff members in applying assistive technology with students. These teams make recommendations to administrators on equipment to order, train students to use computers and devices, troubleshoot technology failures, determine technology needs, and provide ongoing education to staff and families.

Technologic solutions are described throughout this text and are the focus of Chapters 16, 20, and 21. These chapters offer the following themes on the use of assistive technology:

- Assistive technology should be selected according to the child's individual abilities (intrinsic variables), expected or desired activities, and environmental supports and constraints (extrinsic variables).
- Techniques and technology should be adaptable and flexible, so that devices can be used across environments and over time as the child develops.
- Technology should be selected with a future goal in mind and a vision of how the individual and environment will change.
- The strategy and technology should be selected in consultation with caregivers, teachers, and other professionals and all adults who support its use.
- Extensive training and follow-up should accompany the use of assistive technology.

In summary, assistive technologies have significantly improved the quality of life for persons with disabilities. Computers, power mobility, augmentative communication devices, and environmental control units make it possible for children to participate in roles previously closed to them.

In addition to assistive technology designed specifically for children with impairments, children with disabilities also have more access to technology through universal access. The concept of universal access, now widespread, refers to the movement to develop devices and design environments that are accessible to everyone. When schools invest in universal access for their learning technology, all students can access any or most of the school's computers, and adaptations for visual, hearing, motor, or cognitive impairment can be made on all or most of the school's computers. Universal access means that the system platforms can support software with accessibility options and that a range of keyboards, "mice" (tracking devices), and switches are available for alternative access.

Environmental Modification

To succeed in a specific setting, a child with disabilities often benefits from modifications to the environment. Goals include not only enhancing a child's participation but also increasing safety (e.g., reducing barriers on the playground) and improving comfort (e.g., improving ease of wheelchair use by reducing the incline of the ramp). Children with physical disabilities may require specific environmental adaptations to increase accessibility or safety. For example, although a school's bathroom may be accessible to a child in a wheelchair, the therapist may recommend the installation of a handlebar beside the toilet so that the child can safely perform a standing pivot transfer. Desks and table heights may need to be adjusted for a child in a wheelchair.

Environmental adaptations, such as modifying a classroom or a home space to accommodate a specific child with a disability, can be accomplished only through consultation with the adults who manage the environment. High levels of collaboration are needed to create optimal environments for the child to attend and learn at school and at home. Environmental modifications often affect everyone in that space, so they must be appropriate for all children in that environment. The therapist articulates the rationale for the modification and negotiates the changes to be made by considering what is most appropriate for all, including the teacher and other students. Through discussion, the occupational therapist and teacher reach agreement as to what the problems are. With consensus regarding the problems and desired outcomes, often the needed environmental modification logically follows. It is essential that the therapist follow through by evaluating the impact of the modification on the targeted child and others. The Americans with Disabilities Act provides guidelines for improving school and community facility accessibility.

Often the role of the occupational therapist is to recommend adaptations to the sensory environment that accommodate children with sensory processing problems.[26] Preschool and elementary school classrooms usually have high levels of auditory and visual input. Classrooms with high noise levels may be overwhelmingly disorganizing to a child who is hypersensitive to auditory stimulation. Young children who need deep pressure or quiet times during the day may need a bean-bag chair placed in a pup tent in the corner of the room. The therapist may suggest that a preschool teacher implement a quiet time with lights off to provide a period to calm children. Meyers, Stephens, and Tauber (Chapter 23), Watling (Chapter 14), and Parham and Mailloux (Chapter 11) describe contextual modifications to accommodate a child who has sensory processing problems.

Other environmental modifications can improve children's arousal and attention. Sitting on movable surfaces (e.g., liquid-filled cushions) can improve a child's posture and attention to classroom instruction.[80] The intent of recommendations regarding the classroom environment is often to maintain a child's arousal and level of alertness without overstimulating or distracting him or her. Modifications should enhance the child's performance, make life easier for the parent or teachers, and have a neutral or positive effect on siblings, peers, and others in the environment. Due to the dynamic nature of the child and the environment, adaptations to the environment may require ongoing assessment to evaluate the goodness of fit between the child and the modified environment and determine when adjustments need to be made.

Consulting, Educating, and Advocating

Consultation Services

Services on behalf of children include consultation with and education of teachers, parents, assistants, childcare providers, and any adults who spend a significant amount of time with the child. Through these models of service delivery, the occupational therapist helps to develop solutions that fit into the child's natural environment and promotes the child's transfer of new skills into a variety of environments.

In Chapter 11, Parham and Mailloux explain that a first step in consultation is "demystifying" the child's disorder. By explaining the child's behaviors as a sensory processing problem to teachers and parents, therapists foster a better understanding of the reasons for the child's behavior (e.g., constant bouncing in a chair or chewing on a pencil), which gives adults new tools for helping the child change behavior. Reframing the problem for caregivers and teachers enables them to identify new and different solutions to the problem and often makes them more open to the therapist's

intervention recommendations.[8] For a situation in which a highly specific, technical activity is needed to elicit a targeted response in the child, teaching others may not be appropriate, and a less complex and less risky strategy should be transferred to the caregivers to implement. To routinely implement a strategy recommended by the therapist, teachers and caregivers need to feel confident that they can apply it successfully.

A major role for school-based occupational therapists is to support teachers in providing optimal instruction to students and helping children succeed in school.[35] Therapists accomplish this role by promoting the teacher's understanding of the physiologic and health-related issues that affect the child's behavior and helping teachers apply strategies to promote the child's school-related performance. Therapists also support teachers in adapting instructional activities that enable the child's participation, and collaborate with teachers to collect data on the child's performance. This focus suggests that, in the role of consultant, the therapist sees the teacher's needs as a priority and focuses on supporting his or her effectiveness in the classroom.[42] Consultation is most likely to be effective when therapists understand the curriculum, academic expectations, and the classroom environment.

Effective consultation also requires that the teacher or caregiver be able to assimilate and adapt the strategies offered by the therapist and make them work in the classroom or the home. The therapist asks the teacher how he or she learns best and accommodates that learning style.[42] Teachers need to be comfortable with suggested interventions, and therapists should offer strategies that fit easily in the classroom routine. The therapist and teacher can work together to determine what interventions will benefit the child and be least intrusive to the other students.

Education and Advocacy

Therapists also function as advocates, educating role players about the need to improve accessibility to recreational, school, or community activities; modify curriculum materials; develop educational materials; and improve attitudes toward disabilities. By participating in curriculum revision or course material selection, therapists can help establish a curriculum with sufficient flexibility to meet the needs of children with disabilities. Often a system problem that negatively affects one child is problematic to others as well. The occupational therapist needs to recognize which system problems can be changed and how these changes can be encouraged. For example, if a child has difficulty reading and writing in the morning, he or she may benefit from physical activity before attempting to focus on deskwork. The occupational therapist cannot change the daily schedule and move recess or physical education to the beginning of the day, but she or he may convince the teacher to begin the first period of the day with warm-up activities. The therapist can advocate for a simplified, continuous stroke handwriting curriculum, which can benefit children with motor-planning problems but also benefits all children beginning to write. Accessible playgrounds can be safer and enable all children, regardless of skill level, to access the equipment.

Ecologic models of child development recognize the powerful influence of home, school, and community environments on child and youth outcomes (Spencer, Chapter 27).[51] Occupational therapists should advocate for environments that are both physically accessible and welcoming to children with disabilities. With an extensive background on what elements create a supportive environment, therapists can help to design physical and social environments that facilitate every child's participation. To change the system on behalf of all children, including those with disabilities, requires communication with stakeholders or persons who are invested in the change. The occupational therapist needs to confidently share the rationale for change, appreciate the views of others invested in the system, and change and negotiate when needed.

A system change is most accepted when the benefits appear high and the costs are low. Can all children benefit? Which children are affected? If administrators and teachers in a child-care center are reluctant to enroll an infant with a disability, the occupational therapist can advocate for accepting the child by explaining specifically the care that the child would need, the resources available, behaviors and issues to expect, and the benefits to other families.

Convincing a school to build an accessible playground is one example of how a focused education effort can create system change. Occupational therapists are frequently involved in designing playgrounds that are accessible to all and promote the development of sensory motor skills. Another example is helping school administrators select computer programs that are accessible to children with disabilities (see Chapter 19). The occupational therapist can serve on the school committee that selects computer software for the curriculum and advocate for software that is easily adaptable for children with physical or sensory disabilities. A third example is helping administrators and teachers select a handwriting curriculum to be used by regular and special education students. The occupational therapist may advocate for a curriculum that emphasizes prewriting skills or one that takes a multisensory approach to teaching handwriting (see Chapter 18). The occupational therapist may also advocate for adding sensory-motor-perceptual activities to an early childhood curriculum. In Chapter 24, Bazyk and Case-Smith describe the role of occupational therapists in promoting positive behavioral supports to improve school mental health outcomes. These examples of system change suggest that occupational therapists become involved in helping educational systems, as well as medical and community systems, enable participation of all children, prevent disability among children at risk, and promote healthy environments where all children can learn and grow.

Occupational Therapy Services That Support Inclusion

Legal mandates and best practice guidelines require that services to children with disabilities be provided in environments with children who do not have disabilities. The Individuals with Disabilities Education Act requires that services to infants and toddlers be provided in "natural environments" and that services to preschool and school-aged children be provided in the "least restrictive environment." The infant's natural environment is most often his or her home, but it may include a childcare center or a care provider's home. The family defines the child's natural environment. This requirement shifts when the child reaches school age, not in its intent but with recognition that community schools and regular education classrooms are the most natural and least restrictive environments for services to children with disabilities. Inclusion in natural environments or regular education classrooms succeeds only when specific supports and accommodations are provided to children with disabilities. Occupational therapists are often important team members in making inclusion successful for children with disabilities. (This concept is further discussed in Chapters 23 and 24.)

Early Intervention Services in the Child's Natural Environment

The Division of Early Childhood of the Council for Exceptional Children supports the philosophy of inclusion in natural environments with the following statement: "Inclusion, as a value, supports the right of all children, regardless of their diverse abilities, to participate actively in natural settings within their communities. A natural setting is one in which the child would spend time if he or she had not had a disability" (p. 4).[23]

As explained by Meyers, Stephens, and Tauber (Chapter 23), the philosophy of inclusion extends beyond physical inclusion to mean social and emotional inclusion of the child and family.[18,92] The implications for occupational therapists are that they provide opportunities for expanded and enriched natural learning with typically developing peers. Natural environments can be any setting that is part of the child and family's everyday routine where incidental learning experiences occur.[27] Therefore, intervention and consultation services can occur in a childcare center, at a grandmother's house, or in another place that is part of a family's routine. Social, play, and self-care learning opportunities in these environments are plentiful. Figure 1-10 shows an example of a child's natural environment in which the therapist could intervene.

When occupational therapy occurs in a natural environment such as the home, the intervention activities are embedded in naturally occurring interactions and situations. In incidental learning opportunities, the therapist challenges the child to

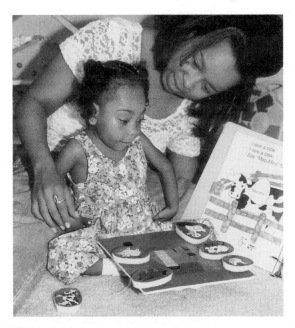

FIGURE 1-10 The occupational therapist coaches the child's mother to facilitate the child's perceptual motor skills.

try a slightly different approach or to practice an emerging skill during typical activities. The therapist follows the young child's lead and uses natural consequences, (e.g., a smile or frown, a pat or tickle) to motivate learning. Research has shown that intervention strategies that occur in real-life settings produce greater developmental change than those that take place in more contrived, clinic-based settings.[12,27] In addition, generalization of skills and behaviors occurs more readily when the intervention setting is the same as the child's natural environment(s).[44,45]

Early intervention therapy services in natural environments require the occupational therapist to be creative, flexible, and spontaneous. The therapist must think through many alternative ways to reach the established goals and then adapt those strategies to whatever situation presents.[41] Recognizing and accepting the family's uniqueness in cultural and child-rearing practices, therapists are able to facilitate the child's ability to generalize new skills to a variety of settings.

Inclusive Services in Schools

In the school-based services, inclusion refers to integration of the child with disabilities into the regular classroom with support to accomplish the regular curriculum. See Box 1-1 for a list of the desired outcomes of inclusive school environments. In schools with well-designed inclusion, every student's competence in diversity and tolerance for differences increases. Related service practitioners provide interventions in multiple environments (e.g., within the classroom, on the playground, in the cafeteria, on and off the school bus), emphasizing nonintrusive methods. The therapist's presence in the classroom benefits the instructional staff members, who observe the occupational therapy intervention. As explained by Bazyk and colleagues (Chapter 24), integrated therapy ensures that the therapist's focus has high relevance to the performance expected within the classroom. It also increases the likelihood that adaptations and therapeutic techniques will be carried over into classroom activities,[100] and it ensures that the occupational therapist's goals and activities link to the curriculum and the classroom priorities (Figure 1-11).

Flexible Service Delivery Models

Children with disabilities benefit when therapy is provided as both direct and consultative services. Even when consultation is the primary service delivery model for a particular child, frequent one-on-one interaction between the therapist and

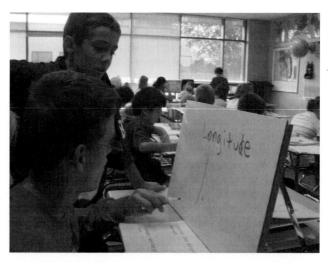

FIGURE 1-11 Writing adaptations and peer support in the classroom promote the child's writing performance.

the child is needed to inform it. Because children constantly change and the environment is dynamic, monitoring the child's performance through opportunities for direct interaction is necessary. With opportunities to directly interact with the child and experience the classroom environment, the occupational therapist can best support the child's participation and guide the support of other adults.

In a fluid service delivery model, therapy services increase when naturally occurring events create a need—for example, when the child obtains a new adapted device, has surgery or casting, or even when a new baby brother creates added stress for a family. Similarly, therapy services should be reduced when the child has learned new skills that primarily need to be repeated and practiced in his daily routine or the child has reached a plateau on her therapy-related goals.

Recently developed models for school-based service delivery offer the possibility for greater flexibility.[15] Block scheduling[68] and the 3-in-1 model[2] are two examples of flexible scheduling that allow therapists to move fluidly between direct and consultative services. In block scheduling, therapists spend 2 to 3 hours in the early childhood classroom working with the children with special needs one on one and in small groups, while supporting the teaching staff (Meyers, Stephens, & Tauber, Chapter 23).[64] Block scheduling allows therapists to learn about the classroom, develop relationships with the teachers, and understand the curriculum so that they can design interventions that easily integrate into the classroom. By being present in the classroom for an entire morning or afternoon, the therapist can find natural learning opportunities to work on a specific child's goals. Using the child's self-selected play activity, the therapist employs strategies that are meaningful to the child, fit into his or her preferred activities, and are likely to be practiced. During the blocked time, the therapist can run small groups (using a coteaching role[21]), coach the teacher and assistants,[76] evaluate the child's performance, and monitor the child's participation in classroom activities.

Another approach that allows more flexible services delivery is the 3-and-1 model.[2] In this model, the therapist dedicates one week a month to consultation and collaboration with the teacher, providing services on behalf of the child rather than

BOX 1-1 Desired Inclusion Outcomes

- Children with disabilities are full participants in school, preschool, and childcare center activities.
- Children with disabilities have friends and relationships with their peers.
- Children with disabilities learn and achieve within the general educational curriculum to the best of their abilities.
- All children learn to appreciate individual differences in people.
- All children learn tolerance and respect for others.
- Children with disabilities participate to the fullest extent possible in their communities.

directly to the child. When the Individualized Education Program (IEP) document states that a 3-and-1 therapy model will be used to support the child's IEP goals, the parents, teacher, and administrators are informed that one quarter of the therapist's time and effort for that child is dedicated to planning, collaborating, and consulting for him or her. Stating that a 3-and-1 model will be used removes the expectation that the therapist will provide one-on-one services for a set number of minutes each week. It facilitates meeting and planning time and establishes that consultation time is as important to the child's progress as one-on-one services. For example, the week of indirect service can also be spent creating new materials and adapted devices for the child (e.g., an Intellikeys overlay to use with the curricular theme of the month). Therapists can write "social stories" for the child or program new vocabulary into the child's augmentative communication device.[37]

Cross-Cultural Competence

Cross-cultural competence can be defined as "the ability to think, feel, and act in ways that acknowledge, respect, and build upon ethnic, [socio]cultural, and linguistic diversity" (p. 50).[52] Cultural competence in health care refers to behaviors and attitudes that enable an individual to function effectively with culturally diverse clients.[74] Occupational therapists with cultural competence can respond optimally to all children in all sociocultural contexts. Chan identified its three essential elements: self-awareness, knowledge of information specific to each culture, and interaction skills sensitive to cultural differences.[19] The following factors, described in this section, support the importance of cross-cultural competence to occupational therapists:

- Cultural diversity of the United States continues to increase.
- A child's development of occupations is embedded in the cultural practices of his family and community.

Cultural Diversity in the United States

The diversity and heterogeneity of American families continue to increase each year. In 2006, the number of immigrants totaled 37.5 million. A total of 1,266,264 immigrants became legal permanent residents of the United States, more than double the number in 1987 (601,516). Most of the immigrants were from Mexico (173,753); however, a substantial number were from China and India.[56] The Census Bureau projects that, by 2050, one quarter of the population will be of Hispanic descent.[56,93]

In 2008, the United States was home to 74 million children. Of these, 15.4 million (~21%) were Hispanic and 10.8 million (~15%) were African American.[20] Children in minority groups are increasing in number at a much faster rate than increases in the general population. Diversity of ethnicity and race can be viewed as a risk or as a resource to child development.[34] Low birthrate, preterm delivery, and infant mortality are higher in African American families, suggesting that these families frequently need early childhood intervention programs. Race can also be a resource; for example, African American families are well supported by their communities and focused on their children (Figure 1-12). Parents often perceive discipline and politeness as positive attributes and instill these in their children.[99] Occupational therapists who work

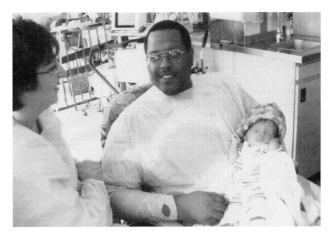

FIGURE 1-12 A father bonds with his just-born son. (Courtesy of Jayne Shepherd and Patti Cooper.)

with African American and Hispanic families find many positive attributes in their family interactions and parenting styles.

Poverty has a pervasive effect on children's developmental and health outcomes.[20] Despite overall prosperity in the United States, a significant number of children and families live in poverty. In 2008, the number of poor children was over 13 million (18%), and the number of children in extreme poverty was almost 6 million (8%). Families in poverty often have great need for, yet limited access to, health care and educational services. Many families who are served by early intervention and special education systems are of low socioeconomic status. When families lack resources (e.g., transportation, food, shelter), their priorities and concerns orient to these basic needs. Responsive therapists provide resources to assist with these basic needs, making appropriate referrals to community agencies. They also demonstrate understanding of the family's priorities, which may not include their children's occupational performance goals.

Influence of Cultural Practices on a Child's Development of Occupations

To impact a child's occupational development, it is critical for the therapist to understand how cultural practices influence skill development. Table 1-3 lists the cultural values that may influence the child's development of occupations. Goals for independence may not be appropriate at certain ages for children of certain cultures. For example, Middle Eastern families often do not emphasize early independence in self-care; therefore, skills such as self-feeding may not be a family priority until ages well beyond the normative expectations.[81] In Hispanic cultures, holding and cuddling are highly valued, even in older children.[101] Mothers hold and carry their preschool children. Recommending a wheelchair for a young child may be unacceptable to families who value close physical contact and holding.

In some cultures (e.g., Polynesian), parents delegate child-care responsibilities to older siblings. Therefore, in established families, siblings care for the infants. Young children in Polynesian cultures tend to rely on their older siblings rather than their parents for structure, assistance, and support. Being responsible for a younger sibling helps the older sibling mature

TABLE 1-3 Cultural Values and Styles That Influence Children's Development of Occupations

Value or Style	Guiding Questions
Family composition	Who are the members of the family? How many family members live in the same house? Is there a hierarchy in the family based on gender or age?
Decision making	Who makes the decisions for the family?
Primary caregiver	Who is the primary caregiver? Is this role shared?
Independence/ interdependence	Do family members value independence? Is reliance on each other more important than independence?
Feeding practices	Who feeds the infant or child? What are the cultural rules or norms about breast feeding, mealtime, self-feeding, eating certain foods? When is independence in feeding expected?
Sleeping patterns	Do children sleep with parents? How do parents respond to the infant during the night? What are appropriate responses to crying?
Discipline	Is disobedience tolerated? How strict are the rules governing behavior? Who disciplines the child? How do the parents discipline their child?
Perception of disability	Do the parents believe that a disability can improve? Do they feel responsible for the disability? Do family members feel that they can make a difference in improving the disability? Are spiritual forms of healing valued?
Help seeking	From whom does the family seek help? Does the family actively seek help, or do the family members expect help to come to them?
Communication and interaction	Does the family use a direct or an indirect style of communication? Do family members share emotional feelings? Is most communication direct or indirect? Does the family value socializing?

Adapted from Wayman, K. I., Lynch, E. W., & Hanson, M. J. (1990). Home-based early childhood services: Cultural sensitivity in a family systems approach. *Topics in Early Childhood Special Education, 10,* 65-66.

quickly by learning responsibility and problem solving.[72] Sibling care may present as a problem when the young child has a disability and needs additional or prolonged care. The literature is replete with examples of the influence of culture on children's occupations.[24,47,72,73] The occupational therapist's appreciation of the influence of culture on children's occupations facilitates the development of appropriate priorities and the use of strategies that are congruent with the family's values and lifestyle.

Because the focus of occupational therapy is to enhance a child's ability to participate in his or her natural environment and everyday routines, the therapist must appreciate, value, and understand those environments and routines. Recommendations that run counter to a family's cultural values probably will not be implemented by family members and may be harmful to the professional–family relationships. The home environment and the family members' interactions help to reveal their cultural values. By asking open-ended questions, therapists can elicit information about the family's routines, rituals, and traditions to provide an understanding of the cultural context. The culturally competent therapist demonstrates an interest in understanding the family's culture, an acceptance of diversity, and a willingness to participate in traditions or cultural patterns of the family. In home-based services, cultural competence may mean removing shoes at the home's entryway, accepting foods when offered, scheduling therapy sessions around holidays, and accommodating language differences. In center-based services, cultural sensitivity remains important, although a family's cultural values may be more difficult to ascertain outside the home. A culturally competent therapist inquires about family routines, cultural practices, traditions, and priorities; demonstrates a willingness to accommodate to these cultural values; and integrates her or his intervention recommendations into the family's cultural practices.

The family's cultural background has a multitude of implications for evaluation and intervention. Cultural values that are important to the occupational therapy perspective include how the family (1) values independent versus interdependent performance; (2) has a sense of time and future versus past orientation; (3) is forward thinking versus lives for the moment; (4) makes decisions that influence family members; (5) defines health, wellness, disability, and illness; and (6) practices customs related to dress, food, traditions, and religion.[53] Often these values vary by cultural group; they also vary in individuals within a cultural group, depending on level of acculturation—that is, the degree to which a family has assimilated into the dominant culture.[34]

Scientific Reasoning and Evidence-Based Practice

With the goal of providing efficacious interventions, occupational therapists and other health care professionals seek and apply practices that have research evidence of effectiveness. In evidence-based practice, occupational therapists emphasize using research evidence to make decisions about interventions. Sackett, Rosenberg, Muir Gray, Haynes, and Richardson defined evidence-based medicine as "the conscientious, explicit, and judicious use of current best evidence in making decisions about the care of individual patients" (p. 71).[77] Therefore, evidence-based practice does not mean that intervention is based solely on research findings. However, it does mean that occupational therapists search for and apply the research evidence, along with their own experiences and family priorities, when making intervention decisions.

The body of research literature supporting occupational therapy with children remains limited when compared with other disciplines (e.g., psychology); however, often research studies and clinical trials in other disciplines have relevance to occupational therapy practice. Research evidence is readily available and accessible through Internet sources. A list of links to health care research databases can be found on the Evolve website. The steps in applying evidence-based practice are listed in Box 1-2.

Using evidence is part of the occupational therapist's scientific reasoning. In scientific reasoning,[78] the occupational therapist uses research evidence, science-based knowledge about the diagnosis, and past experience in all steps of the assessment and intervention process. For example, in the case of Rebecca, a 5-year-old with autism, the occupational therapist noted that developmental play-based approaches that incorporate peers have evidence for moderate treatment effects,[49,50] and that social interactive strategies[46] have been found to be effective. Because Rebecca attends a preschool in which application of these interventions is supported by the team, the occupational therapist decided to use a developmental play-based, interactive approach.

In another example, Aaron, who has arthrogryposis, has limited upper extremity range of motion and difficulty holding utensils or opening packages. He is unable to carry his books during school transitions. Armed with research about arthrogryposis demonstrating that range of motion and strength do not significantly improve over time,[85] the therapist selects a compensatory/adaptation approach to increase Aaron's independence in activities of daily living. In the case of Claire, who has a diagnosis of developmental coordination disorder and poor handwriting, the occupational therapist accessed research by Sullivan, Kantuk, and Burtner.[87] Based on this evidence and her past success in using motor learning strategies with children with developmental coordination disorder, the therapist selected a motor learning approach to increase Claire's

handwriting performance. The therapist reasoned that Claire would need 100% feedback about her performance until new skills were learned.[87] Because the therapist found making holiday cards to be engaging for other girls Claire's age, she selected this activity to practice and reinforce correct letter formation.

In searching for research to inform a clinical decision, the occupational therapist weighs the strength or importance of each study. Studies that provide the most important research evidence are meta-analyses or systematic reviews of clinical trials. The findings of these studies generally have good applicability to practice because they combine the findings of studies that have met a rigorous standard established by the authors. Findings from a rigorous randomized clinical trial also provide strong evidence for practice, followed by results from studies using quasi-experimental designs. Cohort studies and descriptive designs can provide information relevant to clinical decision making; however, their findings are not as strong and should be applied with caution. Outcome research can help practitioners establish benchmarks or standards for performance and client programs; however, descriptive outcome studies do not provide strong evidence for the effectiveness of a specific intervention. The parts summarized next describe some of the evidence for specific occupational therapy interventions or models of practice used in occupational therapy. Examples of interventions and models that have growing evidence of positive effects on children and families are presented.

Sensory Integration

The original studies that compared sensory integration intervention with no treatment[3,4] demonstrated significant positive effects. These studies used samples of children with learning disabilities and compared sensory integration intervention with a control group. Although the effect sizes in Ayres' original studies were high, the sample sizes were small.

Recent studies have found that the effects of intervention using a sensory integration approach are equivalent to the effects of alternative treatment approaches. Polatajko, Kaplan, and Wilson analyzed seven randomized clinical trials of sensory integration treatment that used two or more groups and included a comparison or control group.[67] All studies were of children with learning disabilities between the ages of 4.8 and 13 years. The outcome variables in seven clinical trials did not provide any statistical evidence that sensory integration intervention improved academic performance. Several of the studies found that sensory and motor performance improved with sensory integration intervention. Most of the findings for children who received sensory integration intervention were similar to the findings for the children who received a perceptual motor intervention. A limitation cited by Polatajko et al. was that sensory integration intervention in a research context is quite different from sensory integration intervention in a clinic, where therapists can individualize each session to the needs of the child.[67]

A meta-analysis of sensory integration intervention by Vargas and Camilli showed small treatment effects,[96] substantiating the earlier findings of Polatajko et al.[67] Using a criterion-based selection process, Vargas and Camilli found 14 studies of sensory integration compared with no intervention and 11 of sensory integration compared with an alternative intervention (usually perceptual motor activities).[96] Effect sizes were calculated and weighted for sample size. For comparisons

---

BOX 1-2 Steps in Evidence-Based Practice

STEP 1
- Convert the need for information (about intervention effects, prognosis, therapy methods) into an answerable question.

STEP 2
- Search the research databases using the terms in the research question.
- Track down the best evidence to answer that question.

STEP 3
- Critically appraise the evidence for its:
  - validity (truthfulness)
  - impact (level of effect)
  - clinical meaningfulness

STEP 4
- Critically appraise the evidence for its applicability and usefulness to your practice.

STEP 5
- Implement the practice or apply the information.
- Evaluate the process.

of sensory integration with no treatment, the average effect size was .29, which is a low effect size. When sensory integration is compared with an alternative treatment, the effect size was .09, which means that the effects of sensory integration were not significantly different from those of other treatments. The authors reported that the average effect size for earlier studies (before 1982) was higher (.60) than the average effect size for studies after 1982 (.03). The skill areas that improved were psychoeducational and motor performance areas. Although the effects of sensory integration appear to be small, findings of significant improvement in motor performance following sensory integration intervention are consistent.

Recent studies of sensory integration intervention have shown positive effects. In a randomized clinical trial, Miller, Coll, and Schoen examined the effects of occupational therapy using a sensory integration approach on children's attention, cognitive/social performance, and sensory processing and behavior.[57] Children with sensory modulation disorders and co-occurring diagnoses such as attention deficit hyperactivity disorder (ADHD) and learning disabilities were randomized into three groups, occupational therapy (n=7), activity protocol (n=10), and no treatment (n=7). Children in the occupational therapy group received 10 weeks of two-a-day sensory integration intervention sessions using the protocol developed by these authors.[58] Following the 10-week intervention, the children who received occupational therapy sensory integration made gains greater than those in the other two groups in intervention goals (using Goal Attainment Scaling) and on the Cognitive/Social composite of the Leiter International Performance Scale. The occupational therapy group also made gains in sensory processing and child behavior, but these were not statistically significant when compared with the other two groups. It is probable that the gains in sensory processing behaviors would have been significant if a larger sample size had been used. Although this trial provides evidence for sensory integration intervention effects, the strength of the findings is limited by the small sample size.

An important step in enhancing the rigor of sensory integration trials is the development of a fidelity measure[65] and a manual of procedures for sensory integration intervention.[57,58] Use of standardized intervention protocols will improve the fidelity of sensory integration intervention when administered in future trials and will improve both internal and external validity of the findings. Parham and Mailloux (Chapter 11) further discuss fidelity issues in sensory integration intervention trials.

Sensory Modalities

Application of sensory modalities has also been studied, generally in small samples and with positive results. These studies investigate the application of a specific sensory modality to achieve specific behavioral/performance outcomes in a group of children with the same diagnosis or similar problems. The efficacy of using touch pressure to gain behavioral changes in children with autism or ADHD has been researched.[28,30,94] Edelson and his colleagues investigated the efficacy of the Hug Machine, a device that provides touch pressure through the sides of the body. Using a sample of children with autism, participants who received the Hug Machine treatment twice a week were compared with a control group. The participants who used the Hug Machine exhibited a significant reduction

in tension and a slight change in anxiety. Physiologic measures were not significantly different between groups.

Two studies have examined the effect of pressure through wearing a weighted vest. Fertel-Daly and colleagues investigated the effects of a weighted vest on five preschool children with pervasive developmental disorders.[30] Using an ABA single-subject design, vests were worn for 2 hours per day, 3 days a week, for 5 weeks, with baseline (wearing no vest) data collected before and after the intervention. Attention, number of distractions, and duration of self-stimulation behaviors were measured. All participants demonstrated increased attention and decreased distractibility, and four of five showed decreased self-stimulation behaviors. VandenBerg also examined the effects of a weighted vest on four children diagnosed with ADHD.[94] The children demonstrated greater on-task behaviors when wearing the vests. The summary of the studies using small samples found that touch pressure and deep pressure, applied intermittently, can decrease tension and anxiety, improve attention, and increase on-task behavior.

Another study of sensory modalities examined the effects from children sitting on therapy balls on in-seat behavior and legible word productivity.[80] Occupational therapists sometimes recommend that students sit on therapy balls in the classroom to give them additional vestibular and proprioceptive input while sitting. The children can bounce to stay attentive and alert and receive additional vestibular/proprioceptive feedback when they shift their weight through the ball's movement. Using a multiple-baseline single-subject design, all participants (n=3) improved in in-seat behavior and legible word productivity.[80] The balls seemed to help in sensory modulation with the participants, and they represent a nonintrusive method to promote academic-related outcomes, staying in one's seat, and legible word productivity.

Randomized clinical trials of touch-based interventions, such as massage, have shown positive effects on attention and behavior. In two randomized clinical trials, Field and colleagues completed two trials with children with autism.[29,32] In each the children were massaged (circular application of deep touch on trunk and extremities 1 to 2 times per day) by either parents or therapists. The children who received the month-long treatment demonstrated decreased aversion to touch, off task behaviors, stereotypical behaviors, and impulsivity. Interventions that involve intensive tactile input applied in systematic ways may reduce impulsive, hyperactive, or nonpurposeful behaviors.

Sound-based interventions have been applied to children with autism. Occupational therapists sometimes use modulated music through head phones as an adjunct modality (e.g., Therapeutic Listening®).[33] Research of auditory integration training, generally a 10-day program in which children listen to modulated music through headphones twice a day, shows mixed evidence of benefit.[83] It appears that auditory integration training can improve behavior (decrease aberrant behaviors), but it does not improve auditory reception, language, or adaptive behaviors.[6,62] Hall and Case-Smith used a single-group design to study the effects of Therapeutic Listening[33] in conjunction with a sensory diet.[40] Ten children received a sensory diet for 1 month and then received the Therapeutic Listening program with a sensory diet for 8 weeks. Measures of sensory processing, visual motor skills, and handwriting were used to compare the control and treatment phases. Children's gains in sensory processing included a decrease in irritability, fewer temper tantrums, and less hyper-activity and improvement in affect, interaction, and emotional responding (as measured by the Sensory Profile).

In summary, studies have demonstrated that sensory-based interventions can improve behavior, attention, and activity levels in children with autism, sensory processing disorders, and ADHD. However, these studies were generally of brief intervention duration and did not follow the participants long term. Baranek[5] and Parham and Mailloux (Chapter 11) recommend that therapists pair sensory-based interventions with more holistic and comprehensive interventions. The evidence suggests that when sensory modalities are paired with functional or play-based interventions, children are likely to demonstrate gains in performance and improved adaptive behaviors.[14]

Play-Based, Relationship-Focused Interventions

Occupational therapists often implement a play-based interactive intervention with a goal of engaging the child in a just right challenge to his or her skill set. When these intervention episodes are repeated, practiced, and generalized, children exhibit increased social interaction and cognitive skills. Play-based relationship–focused interventions are frequently implemented with children with autism, who universally have delays in social participation and communication.[38] These interventions allow children to choose activities, provide them with multiple examples of behavior, and systematically reward the child using natural reinforcement. Greenspan and Weider created a relationship-based play intervention similar to occupational therapy play-based interventions.[38] Their floor time intervention emphasizes the child's social-emotional growth and symbolic play as fundamental to learning language and cognitive skills. Greenspan and Weider evaluated the effects of their relationship-based intervention and reported that 58% of the children who had received the intervention (an average of 2 years) had achieved strong positive outcomes (e.g., performance improved to within the normal range).[38] Wieder and Greenspan analyzed 16 of the children whose outcomes immediately after a course of intervention were good to outstanding.[98] These children were evaluated 10 to 15 years after they had participated in the relationship-based intervention. At this follow-up point, the children had become socially competent, responsive, and interactive. Although they exhibited some symptoms of mental illness (depression and anxiety), they did not exhibit the primary characteristics of autism.

Similar interventions focused on encouraging interactions and play have been applied and researched, particularly with children with autism.[69,71] Rogers created comprehensive, interdisciplinary preschool program, the Denver Model, that integrates developmental, relationship-based, and applied behavioral analysis approaches. Components of the Denver Model Intervention for Children with autism are listed in Box 1-3.

Application of the Denver Model with children with autism spectrum disorder has been researched. In a cohort study (one group), Rogers, Herbison, Lewis, Pantone, and Rels measured play and developmental skills before and after a 6-month preschool program.[71] The children who participated (n=26) demonstrated positive change in cognition, communication, and social emotional skills beyond their developmental

---

BOX 1-3   Components of the Denver Model Intervention for Children with Autism

1. A playful environment is established where learning opportunities are plentiful.
2. One-on-one interaction is used.
3. Taking turn in play interaction is emphasized.
4. The activities incorporate children's interests and preferences with learning opportunities.
5. The task sequence is varied and previously mastered tasks are interspersed with not yet mastered tasks.
6. Children are rewarded for attempting new skills as well as performing them successfully.
7. Reinforcers are employed that are directly and inherently related to children's responses.
8. Immediate and contingent reinforcement is given when children demonstrate an appropriate response.

Adapted from Vismara, L. A., & Rogers, S. J. (2008). The Early Start Denver Model: A case study of an innovative practice. *Journal of Early Intervention, 31,* 91-108.

---

trajectory. Rogers and DiLalla completed a retrospective analysis of children's change in developmental rate before and after 8 to 12 months of intervention.[70] Following this intervention period, the children had improved more than was expected in all development areas, making gains comparable to children without autism. This model was applied to a 9-month-old using a version adapted for younger children and combining this approach with behavioral interventions.[97] In this case study, the 9-month-old made substantial gains in social communicative behaviors and attention.

Relationship development intervention (RDI) is a third relationship-based intervention for children with autism similar to occupational therapy play-based interventions.[39] In a recent evaluation of RDI using a one group pre-post design, 16 children (who completed an average of 18 months of treatment) made significant gains, and by the end of the treatment, 10 were functioning in regular education classroom without an aide.

Almost all of the studies of play-based, relationship-focused interventions have used a single group design to analyze the children before and after participation. Therefore, although the results have been universally positive, the findings are weak and the studies need to be replicated to reach definitive conclusions about play-based, relationship-focused interventions. Nevertheless, these studies do provide evidence for positive effects when applying playful interventions focused on social interactions and engaging children in play that targets specific developmental goals. Intervention components that seem to be important to obtaining positive effects include (1) selecting activities of interest to the child, (2) allowing child choice, (3) encouraging or modeling higher level behaviors, (4) promoting engagement, (5) providing natural reinforcers, and (6) encouraging peer interactions.[49,86,97]

Family-Centered Care

Family-centered care is a model advocated in the literature and the legislation for individuals with disabilities. Although it is well described in the literature, efficacy studies investigating the outcomes of family-centered care are few. Rosenbaum, King, Law, King, and Evans reviewed clinical trials of family-centered health care.[75] They identified five clinical trials, published from 1983 to 1995, most of which used a parent education model as part of intervention for chronically ill children. When compared with child-focused models, the positive outcomes of the family-centered interventions included improved child skills, increased parent satisfaction with care, and enhanced child psychological adjustment.

Although clinical trials of family-centered care by occupational therapists have not been published, a number of occupational therapy scholars have examined the outcomes of elements of family-centered care. VanLeit and Crowe investigated the effects of a program designed to help mothers of children with disabilities improve their use of time and the quality of their occupations through an occupational therapy–led support group.[95] Following their participation in the group, the mothers (n=19) reported improved performance and satisfaction as measured by the Canadian Occupational Performance Measure when compared with a control group (n=19). Measures of time use and time perception were no different between the two groups. Investigating the effects of a similar program, qualitative data from the participating mothers were analyzed.[43] This support group program was designed to help mothers cope with difficulties in daily routines with a child with disabilities. The mothers who participated in six weekly small group sessions perceived that their self-image had changed and their coping strategies had increased. This series of studies demonstrated the positive effects of implementing support groups designed to help mothers improve their ability to cope with the daily care of a child with special needs.[43,95] Elements of the intervention that seemed effective were use of small groups of mothers who could support each other, acknowledgement of the stress and challenges inherent in raising a child with special needs, using mothers' accounting of their own routines and activity demands to make recommendations, and allowing mothers to think through their routines and their challenges to develop their own solutions. Family-centered care involves basic elements of good communication and caring, such as listening, demonstrating respect, and providing honest, informative answers to questions; yet these simple elements seem to have important effects on child and family outcomes.

In a qualitative study in which 29 families were interviewed about their experiences in parenting a child with disabilities and working with the intervention systems, four themes emerged.[17] (1) Parents need professionals to recognize that parenting a child with a disability is a 24/7 job with continual and often intensive responsibilities. (2) Both internal (coping and resilience) and external (e.g., extended family) resources are needed to raise a child with a disability; these should be bolstered and encouraged. (3) Parents also ask that professionals respect them as the experts on their child and (4) that they accept their family's values. Although this study's qualitative findings do not constitute rigorous evidence of intervention effects, the findings concur with other descriptive studies of family-centered intervention. When combined, these studies suggest that respecting parents' knowledge of their child, acknowledging their resilience, accepting their values, and facilitating the building of a network of social resources are important components of family-centered intervention.[17,91]

Evidence-based practice means that occupational therapists access research to guide their practice and implement approaches that have known efficacy. Although occupational therapy experimental design research remains limited, the body of interdisciplinary research useful to practice is substantial. Occupational therapists must learn to access, analyze, and apply clinical research to offer the most effective services.

SUMMARY

This chapter introduces the book by describing evidence-based practices with children that are explained and illustrated in the chapters that follow. It concludes by encouraging a commitment from occupational therapists to use research evidence in decision making about interventions for the children and families they serve. Evidence-based practice is achieved when occupational therapists continuously seek new information from research-based sources and thoughtfully apply interventions that reflect (1) their experience and training, (2) the child's and family's priorities, and (3) the research evidence.

Occupational therapy practice with children has matured in recent decades from a profession that relied on basic theory to drive decision making to one that recognizes the complexities and multiple dimensions of professional reasoning. A primary goal of this book is to define and illustrate the application of research evidence in professional reasoning. The remaining chapters expand on the basic concepts presented in this chapter by exploring the breadth of occupational therapy for children, explaining theories that guide practice, illustrating practice models in educational and medical systems, and describing interventions with evidence of effectiveness.

REFERENCES

1. American Occupational Therapy Association. (2008). Occupational therapy practice framework: Domain & process, 2nd ed. *American Journal of Occupational Therapy, 62*(6), 609-639.
2. Annett, M. (2004). Service delivery success: SLPs in Oregon school tackle workload, enhance recruitment. *ASHS Leader, 9*(4), 12-13.
3. Ayres, A. J. (1972). Improving academic scores through sensory integration. *Journal of Learning Disabilities, 5,* 339-343.
4. Ayres, A. J. (1977). Effect of sensory integrative therapy on the coordination of children with choreoathetoid movements. *American Journal of Occupational Therapy, 31,* 291-293.
5. Baranek, G. T. (2002). Efficacy of sensory and motor interventions for children with autism. *Journal of Autism and Developmental Disorders, 32,* 397-422.
6. Bettison, S. (1996). The long-term effects of auditory training on children with autism. *Journal of Autism and Developmental Disorders, 26,* 361-375.
7. Blue-Banning, M., Summers, J. A., Frankland, H. C., Nelson, L. L., & Beegle, G. (2004). Dimensions of family and professional partnerships: Constructive guidelines for collaboration. *Exceptional Children, 70*(2), 167-184.
8. Bundy, A. C. (2002). Play theory and sensory integration. In A. C. Bundy, S. Lane, & E. Murray (Eds.), *Sensory integration: Theory and practice* (2nd ed., pp. 228-240). Philadelphia: Lippincott Williams & Wilkins.
9. Bundy, A., & Koomar, J. A. (2002). Orchestrating intervention: The art of practice. In A. Bundy, S. J. Lane, & E. A. Murray (Eds.), *Sensory integration: Theory and practice* (2nd ed., pp. 242-260). Philadelphia: Lippincott Williams & Wilkins.

10. Butler, C. (1986). Effects of powered mobility on self-initiated behaviors of very young children with locomotor disability. *Developmental Medicine and Child Neurology, 28,* 325-332.

11. Butler, C. (1988). High tech tots: Technology for mobility, manipulation, communication, and learning in early childhood. *Infants and Young Children, 2,* 55-73.

12. Campbell, P. H. (2004). Participation-based services: Promoting children's participation in natural settings. *Young Exceptional Children, 8,* 20-29.

13. Campos, J. J., & Bertenthal, B. I. (1987). Locomotion and psychological development in infancy. In K. M. Jaffe (Ed.), *Childhood powered mobility: Developmental, technical, and clinical perspectives. Proceedings of the RESNA First Northwest Regional Conference* (pp. 11-42). Washington, DC: RESNA Press.

14. Case-Smith, J., & Arbesman, M. (2008). Evidence-based review of interventions for autism used in or of relevance to occupational therapy. *American Journal of Occupational Therapy, 62,* 416-429.

15. Case-Smith, J., & Holland, T. (2009). Making decisions about service delivery in early childhood programs. *Language, Speech, and Hearing Services in Schools, 40*(4), 416-423.

16. Case-Smith, J., & Nastro, M. A. (1993). The effect of occupational therapy intervention on mothers of children with cerebral palsy. *American Journal of Occupational Therapy, 47,* 811-817.

17. Case-Smith, J., Sainato, D., McQuaid, J., Deubler, D., Gottesman, M., & Taber, M. (2007). IMPACTS project: Preparing therapists to provide best practice early intervention services. *Physical & Occupational Therapy in Pediatrics, 27*(3), 73-90.

18. Chai, A. Y., Zhang, C., & Bisberg, M. (2006). Rethinking natural environment practice: Implications from examining various implications and approaches. *Early Childhood Education Journal, 34*(3), 203-208.

19. Chan, S. Q. (1990). Early intervention with culturally diverse families of infants and toddlers with disabilities. *Infants and Young Children, 3*(2), 78-87.

20. Children's Defense Fund. (2009). Children in the United States. Retrieved April 18, 2009, from http://www.childrensdefense.org

21. Cook, L., & Friend, M. (1991). Principles for the practice of collaboration in schools. *Preventing School Failure, 35*(4), 6-9.

22. Coster, W., Deeney, T., Haltiwanger, J., & Haley, S. (1998). *School Function Assessment.* San Antonio: Psychological Corporation.

23. Council for Exceptional Children, Division of Early Childhood. (1993). DEC position statement on inclusion. *DEC Communicator, 19*(4), 4.

24. Deater-Deckard, K., Dodge, K. A., Bates, J. E., & Petit, G. S. (1996). Physical discipline among African American and European American mothers: Links to children's externalizing behaviors. *Developmental Psychology, 6,* 1065-1072.

25. Deluca, S. C., Echols, K., Law, C. R., & Ramey, S. L. (2006). Intensive pediatric constraint-induced therapy for children with cerebral palsy: Randomized, controlled, crossover trial. *Journal of Child Neurology, 21,* 931-938.

26. Dunn, W. (2007). Supporting children to participate successfully in everyday life by using sensory processing knowledge. *Infants and Young Children, 20*(2), 84-101.

27. Dunst, C. J., Trivette, C. M., Humphries, T., Raab, M., & Roper, N. (2001). Contrasting approaches to natural learning environment interventions. *Infants and Young Children, 14,* 48-63.

28. Edelson, S. M., Goldberg, M., Edelson, M. G., Kerr, D. C., & Grandin, T. (1999). Behavioral and physiological effects of deep pressure on children with autism: A pilot study evaluating the efficacy of Grandin's Hug Machine. *American Journal of Occupational Therapy, 53,* 145-152.

29. Escalona, A., Field, T., Singer-Strunck, R., Cullen, C., & Hartshorn, D. (2001). Brief report: Improvements in the behavior of children with autism following massage therapy. *Journal of Autism and Developmental Disorders, 31,* 513-516.

30. Fertel-Daly, D., Bedell, G., & Hinojosa, J. (2001). Effects of a weighted vest on attention to task and self-stimulatory behaviors in preschoolers with pervasive developmental disorders. *American Journal of Occupational Therapy, 55,* 629-640.

31. Fidler, G. S., & Fidler, J. W. (1978). Doing and becoming: Purposeful action and self-actualization. *American Journal of Occupational Therapy, 32,* 305-310.

32. Field, T., Lasko, D., Mundy, P., Henteleff, T., Kabat, S., Talpins, S., et al. (1997). Brief report: Autistic children's attentiveness and responsivity improve after touch therapy. *Journal of Autism and Developmental Disorders, 27,* 333-338.

33. Frick, S. M., & Hacker, C. (2001). *Listening with the whole body.* Madison, WI: Vital Links.

34. Garcia Coll, C., & Magnuson, K. (2000). Cultural differences as sources of developmental vulnerabilities and resources. In S. J. Meisels & J. P. Shonkoff (Eds.), *Handbook of early childhood intervention* (2nd ed., pp. 94-114). Cambridge: Cambridge University Press.

35. Giangreco, M. F., Cloninger, C. J., & Iverson, V. S. (1998). *Choosing outcomes and accommodations for children: A guide to educational planning for students with disabilities.* (2nd ed.). Baltimore: Paul H. Brookes.

36. Girolametto, L., Sussman, F., & Weitzman, E. (2007). Using case study methods to investigate the effects of interactive intervention for children with autism spectrum disorders. *Journal of Communication Disorders, 40,* 470-492.

37. Gray, C. (2000). *The new Social Story book: Illustrated edition.* Arlington, TX: Future Horizons.

38. Greenspan, S. L., & Wieder, S. (1997). Developmental patterns and outcomes in infants and children with disorders in relating and communicating: A chart review of 200 cases of children with autistic spectrum diagnoses. *Journal of Developmental and Learning Disorders, 1,* 87-141.

39. Gutstein, S. E., Burgess, A., & Montfort, K. (2007). Evaluation of the relationship development intervention program. *Autism, 11,* 397-411.

40. Hall, L., & Case-Smith, J. (2007). The effect of sound based intervention on children with sensory processing disorders and visual motor delays. *American Journal of Occupational Therapy, 61,* 209-215.

41. Hanft, B. E., & Piklington, K. O. (2000). Therapy in natural environment: The means or end goal for early intervention? *Infants and Young Children, 12,* 1-13.

42. Hanft, B., Rush, D. D., & Sheldon, M. L. (2004). *Coaching families and colleagues in early childhood.* Baltimore: Paul H. Brookes.

43. Helitzer, D. L., Cunningham-Sabo, L. D., Vanleit, B., & Crowe, T. K. (2002). Perceived changes in self-image and coping strategies of mothers of children with disabilities. *Occupational Therapy Journal of Research, 22,* 25-33.

44. Humphry, R. (2002). Young children's occupations. *American Journal of Occupational Therapy, 56,* 171-179.

45. Humphry, R. & Wakeford, L. (2006). An occupation-centered discussion of development and implications for practice. *American Journal of Occupational Therapy, 60,* 258-267.

46. Hwang, B., & Hughes, C. (2000). The effects of social interactive training on early social communicative skills of children with autism. *Journal of Autism and Developmental Disorders, 30,* 331-343.

47. Jarrett, R. (1996). African American family and parenting strategies in impoverished neighborhoods. *Qualitative Sociology, 20,* 275-288.

48. Klingberg, T., Forssberg, H., & Westerberg, H. (2002). Increased brain activity in frontal and parietal cortex underlies the development of visuospatial working memory capacity during childhood. *Journal of Cognitive Neuroscience, 14*(1), 1-10.

49. Koegel, L. K., Koegel, R. L., Shoshan, T., & McNerney, E. (1999). Pivotal response intervention II: Preliminary long-term outcome data. *Journal of the Association for Persons with Severe Handicaps, 24,* 174-185.
50. Koegel, R. L., Werner, G. A., Vismara, L. A., & Koegel, L. K. (2005). The effectiveness of contextually supported play date interactions between children with autism and typically developing peers. *Research & Practice for Persons with Severe Disabilities, 30,* 95-102.
51. Law, M., Petrenchik, T., Zivinani, J., & King, G. (2006). Participation of children in school and community. In S. Rodger & J. Ziviani (Eds.), *Occupational therapy with children: Understanding children's occupations and enabling participation* (pp. 67-90). Oxford: Blackwell Publishing.
52. Lynch, E., & Hanson, M. (1993). Changing demographics: Implications for training in early intervention. *Infants and Young Children, 6*(1), 50-55.
53. Lynch, E., & Hanson, M. (1997). *Developing cross-cultural competence* (2nd ed.). Baltimore: Brookes.
54. Mahoney, G., & Perales, F. (2005). The impact of relationship focused intervention on young children and children with disabilities. *Topics in Early Childhood Special Education, 18,* 5-17.
55. McWilliam, R. A., Tocci, L., & Harbin, G. L. (1998). Family-centered services: Service providers' discourse and behavior. *Topics in Early Childhood and Special Education, 18*(4), 206-221.
56. Migration Information Source. (2009). *US historical immigration trends.* Retrieved April 18, 2009, from http://www.migrationinformation.org/feature/display.cfm?ID=649
57. Miller, L. J., Coll, J. R., & Schoen, S. A. (2007). A randomized controlled pilot study of the effectiveness of occupational therapy for children with sensory modulation disorder. *American Journal of Occupational Therapy, 61,* 228-238.
58. Miller, L. J., Wilbarger, J., Stackhouse, T., & Trunnell, S. (2002). Use of clinical reasoning in occupational therapy: The TEP-SI model of intervention of sensory modulation dysfunction. In A. C. Bundy, S. J. Lane, & E. A. Murray (Eds.), *Sensory integration: Theory and practice* (2nd ed., pp. 435-452). Philadelphia: F.A. Davis.
59. Miller Kuhaneck, H., Henry, D. A., & Glennon, T. (2007). *Sensory Processing Measure: Main Classroom and School Environments Form.* Los Angeles: Western Psychological Services.
60. Missiuna, C., & Pollock, N. (2000). Perceived efficacy and goal setting in young children. *Canadian Journal of Occupational Therapy, 67,* 101-109.
61. Missiuna, C. Pollock, N. & Law, M. (2004). *The perceived efficacy and goal setting system.* San Antonio, TX: Psychological Corporation.
62. Mudford, O. C., Cross, B. A., Breen, S., Cullen, C., Reeves, D., Gould, J., et al. (2000). Auditory integration training for children with autism: No behavioral benefits detected. *American Journal on Mental Retardation, 105,* 118-129.
63. Nilsson, L., & Nyberg, P. (2003). Driving to learn: A new concept for training children with profound cognitive disabilities in a powered wheelchair. *American Journal of Occupational Therapy, 57*(2), 229-233.
64. Pape, L., & Ryba, K. (2004). *Practical considerations for school-based occupational therapists.* Bethesda, MD: AOTA Press.
65. Parham, L. D., Cohn, E. S., Spitzer, S., Koomar, J., Miller, L. J., Burke, J. P., et al. (2007). Fidelity in sensory integration intervention research. *American Journal of Occupational Therapy, 61,* 216-227.
66. Parham, L. D., & Ecker, C. (2007). *Sensory Processing Measure: Home Form.* Los Angeles: Western Psychological Services.
67. Polatajko, H. J., Kaplan, B., & Wilson, B. (1992). Sensory integration treatment for children with learning disabilities: Its status 20 years later. *Occupational Therapy Journal of Research, 36,* 571-578.
68. Rainforth, B., & York-Barr, J. (1997). *Collaborative teams for students with severe disabilities: Integrating therapy and education* (2nd ed.). Baltimore: Paul H. Brookes.
69. Rogers, S. J., & Dawson, G. (Eds.). (2007). *The Early Start Denver model.* New York: Guilford Press.
70. Rogers, S. J., & DiLalla, D. L. (1991). A comparative study of the effects of a developmental based instructional model on young children with autism and young children with other disorders of be3havior and development. *Topics in Early Childhood Special Education, 11*(2), 29-47.
71. Rogers, S. J., Herbison, J. M., Lewis, H. C., Pantone, J., & Rels, K. (1986). An approach for enhancing the symbolic communicative and interpersonal functioning of young children with autism or sever emotional handicaps. *Journal of the Division for Early Childhood, 10,* 135-148.
72. Rogoff, B. (2003). *The cultural nature of human development.* New York: Oxford University Press.
73. Rogoff, B., & Morelli, G. (1989). Perspectives on children's development for cultural psychology. *American Psychologist, 44,* 343-348.
74. Rorie, J. L., Paine, L. L., & Barger, M. K. (1996). Primary care for women—Cultural competence in primary care services. *Journal of Nurse-Midwifery, 41*(2), 92-100.
75. Rosenbaum, P., King, S., Law, M., King, G., & Evans, J. (1998). Family-centred service: A conceptual framework and research review. *Physical & Occupational Therapy in Pediatrics, 18,* 1-20.
76. Rush, D. D., Shelden, M. L., & Hanft, B. E. (2003). Coaching families and colleagues: A process for collaboration in natural settings. *Infants and Young Children, 16*(1), 33-47.
77. Sackett, D. L., Rosenberg, W. M. C., Muir Gray, J. A., Haynes, R. B., & Richardson, W. S. (1996). Evidence-based medicine: What it is and what it isn't. *British Medical Journal, 312,* 71-72.
78. Schell, B. (2009). Professional reasoning in practice. In E. B. Crepeau, E. S. Cohn, & B. A. B. Schell (Eds.), *Willard & Spackman's occupational therapy* (11th ed., pp. 314-327). Philadelphia: Lippincott Williams & Wilkins.
79. Schertz, & Gordon, W. (2008). Changing the model: A call for a re-examination of intervention approaches and translational research in children with developmental disabilities. *Developmental Medicine & Child Neurology, 51*(1), 6-7.
80. Schilling, D. L., Washington, K., Billingsley, F. F., & Deitz, J. (2003). Classroom seating for children with attention deficit hyperactivity disorder. *American Journal of Occupational Therapy, 57,* 534-541.
81. Sharifzadeh, V. S. (1997). Families with Middle Eastern roots. In E. W. Lynch & M. Hanson (Eds.), *Developing cross-cultural competence* (2nd ed., pp. 441-482). Baltimore: Brookes.
82. Shepherd, J. J. (2008). Using motor learning approaches for treating swallowing and feeding disorders: A review. *Language, Speech, and Hearing Services in Schools, 39,* 227-236.
83. Sinha, Y., Silove, N., Wheeler, D., & Williams, K. (2004). Auditory integration training and other sound therapies for autism spectrum disorders. *Cochrane Database of Systematic Reviews, 1,* CD003681; D01 10.1002/14651858.
84. Spitzer, S. L. (2008). Play in children with autism: Structure and experience. In L. D. Parham & L. S. Fazio (Eds.), *Play in occupational therapy for children* (pp. 351-374). St. Louis, MO: Mosby.
85. Staheli, L. T. (2006). *Practice of pediatric orthopedics* (2nd ed.). Philadelphia: Lippincott Williams & Wilkins.
86. Stahmer, A. C. (1999). Using pivotal response training to facilitate appropriate play in children with autistic spectrum disorders. *Child Language Teaching and Therapy, 15,* 29-40.
87. Sullivan, K. J., Kantak, S. S., & Burtner, P. A. (2008). Motor learning in children: Feedback effects on skill acquisition. *Physical Therapy, 88,* 720-732.
88. Taub, E., Ramey, S. L., DeLuca, S., & Echols, K. (2004). Efficacy of constraint-induced movement therapy for children with cerebral palsy with asymmetric motor impairment. *Pediatrics, 113,* 305-312.
89. Tickle-Degnen, L., & Coster, W. (1995). Therapeutic interaction and the management of challenge during the beginning minutes

of sensory integration treatment. *Occupational Therapy Journal of Research, 15,* 122-141.

90. Trivette, C. M., & Dunst, C. J. (2005). DEC recommended practices: Family-based practices. In S. Sandall, M. L. Hemmeter, B. J. Smith, & M. E. McLean (Eds.), *DEC recommended practices: A comprehensive guide for practical application in early intervention/early childhood special education* (pp. 107-126). Missoula, MT: Division for Early Childhood.

91. Turnbull, A. P., Turbiville, V., & Turnbull, H. R. (2000). Evolution of family-professional partnership models: Collective empowerment as the model for the early 21st century. In S. J. Meisels & J. P. Shonkoff (Eds.), *Handbook of early intervention* (pp. 630-650). New York: Cambridge University Press.

92. Turnbull, A. P., Turnbull, H. R., & Blue-Banning, M. J. (1994). Enhancing inclusion of infants and toddlers with disabilities and their families: A theoretical and programmatic analysis. *Infants & Young Children, 7*(2), 1-14.

93. U. S. Census Bureau. (2009). 2003 American Community Survey Profiles. Retrieved on April 10, 2009, from http://www.census.gov/acs

94. VandenBerg, N. L. (2001). The use of a weighted vest to increase on-task behavior in children with attention difficulties. *American Journal of Occupational Therapy, 55,* 621-628.

95. VanLeit, B., & Crowe, T. K. (2002). Outcomes of an occupational therapy program for mothers of children with disabilities: Impact on satisfaction with time use and occupational performance. *American Journal of Occupational Therapy, 56,* 402-410.

96. Vargas, S., & Camilli, G. (1999). A meta-analysis of research on sensory integration treatment. *American Journal of Occupational Therapy, 53,* 189-198.

97. Vismara, L. A., & Rogers, S. J. (2008). The Early Start Denver model. *Journal of Early Intervention, 31,* 91-108.

98. Wieder, S., & Greenspan, S. (2005). Can children with autism master the core deficits and become empathetic, creative, and reflective? *Journal of Developmental and Learning Disorders, 9,* 1-22.

99. Willis, W. (1997). Families with African American roots. In E. W. Lynch & M. Hanson (Eds.), *Developing cross-cultural competence* (2nd ed., pp. 165-208). Baltimore: Brookes.

100. York, J., Giangreco, M. F., Vandercook, T., & Macdonald, C. (1992). Integrating support personnel in inclusive classrooms. In S. Stainback & W. Stainback (Eds.), *Curriculum considerations in inclusive classrooms: Facilitating learning for all students* (pp. 101-116). Baltimore: Brookes.

101. Zuniga, M. E. (1997). Families with Latino roots. In E. W. Lynch & M. Hanson (Eds.), *Developing cross-cultural competence* (2nd ed., pp. 209-250). Baltimore: Brookes.

2

Foundations for Occupational Therapy Practice with Children

Jane Case-Smith • Mary Law • Cheryl Missiuna
Nancy Pollock • Debra Stewart

KEY TERMS

Foundational theories
Risk and resilience
Family-centered service
World Health
  Organization (WHO)
  International
  Classification system
Developmental theories
Learning and systems
  theories

Person-environment-
  occupation model
Dynamic systems theory
Adaptation approaches
Social skills training
Motor learning
Neurodevelopmental
  theory
Sensory integration
  intervention

OBJECTIVES

1. Explain the history and evolution of theories pertaining to child development.
2. Define the term *occupation* and describe the study of occupation with emphasis placed on the occupations of children.
3. Explain what is meant by person–environment congruence.
4. Articulate the concepts and principles that define family-centered services.
5. Explain the developmental and learning theories of the early and middle 1900s, which provided the foundation for occupational therapy theories.
6. Explain and apply cognitive models of practice.
7. Use a dynamic systems approach to explain how children develop motor skills.
8. Explain how the person-environment-occupation model is used with other specific models of practice in occupational therapy intervention with children.
9. Describe and apply learning theories and approaches.
10. Define and explain the appropriate use of and evidence for neurodevelopmental and sensory integration therapy approaches.
11. Describe strategies that exemplify each practice model using client examples.
12. Compare and contrast intervention activities derived from different theoretical approaches and practice models.

Occupational therapists have developed and used theory as the basis for professional practice for many years. Early developers of occupational therapy focused on the theories of occupation and the use of time.[124,172] As stated by Meyer,

> Our conception of man is that of an organism that maintains and balances itself in the world of reality and actuality by being in active life and active use, i.e., using and living and acting its time in harmony with its own nature and the nature about it. It is the use that we make of ourselves that gives the ultimate stamp to our [being] (p. 64).[124]

Meyer posited that humans maintain rhythms of work, play, rest, and sleep that need to be balanced and that "the only way to attain balance in all this is actual doing, actual practice" (p. 64).[124] Current practices build on many of the original concepts of the profession's founders. Meyer's words are echoed by those of Mandich and Rodger, who explain that through "doing and participation in everyday occupations, children learn and master new skills" (p. 115).[117] Furthermore, social engagement (doing with family and friends) enables children to develop a sense of belonging and self-esteem that contributes to health and well-being. Since the time of Meyer, occupational therapists have continued to develop models of practice based on an understanding of humans as occupational beings. They have also integrated the theories and science of psychologists, neuroscientists, and other disciplines into their practices. This chapter describes current occupational theories, models of practice that reflect those theories, and concepts from other disciplines that support occupational therapy practices.

This chapter begins with a brief overview of the historical and current perspectives on the theories that underlie current service provision: development, occupation, and environment. Foundational theories for occupational therapy practice are discussed next. Then, an overall framework for occupational therapy practice with children, based on a person-environment-occupation (PEO) perspective, is presented, followed by descriptions of current models of practice and the interventions that exemplify those models. Finally, these models of practice are applied to specific practice scenarios, demonstrating the interconnection of theories, models of practice, assessment, and interventions.

OCCUPATIONAL THERAPY PRACTICE WITH CHILDREN

In one version of an ideal childhood, summer is remembered as a time when friends spent the entire day playing outside. Children moved from activity to activity as a group, enjoying one another's company and participating in a variety of play activities. Life was about running with the dog, playing tag in the woods, climbing trees, playing ball in the alley, and pretending to be a superhero or a princess. Adults often have fond memories of their childhood days. As children, however, they did not think about the reasons they engaged in play activities or why particular activities were enjoyable—it was just fun! Occupational therapists, however, have a different perspective on play.

Play is considered a primary occupation of childhood. Multiple, interrelated factors within the child, family, and environment influence a child's ability to engage in play, and a child's play actions become a window for understanding how the child interacts with his environment. Occupational therapists understand that play is essential for development, and they study the concepts and assumptions that underlie the theories of play. It is through play that children learn to adapt to their environments and to develop competencies.[155] By playing, children develop skills that they will later employ in work settings. Children with disabilities face challenges to play. Children with disabilities may exhibit less playfulness (see Chapter 18), demonstrate lower levels of physical play,[151] and require more support to play.[22,175] Play is also a means to the development of other functions (e.g., motor, social, cognitive, and self-care skills).[142] Play activities are generally central to an occupational therapy session because these activities engage and motivate the child, elevating his or her focus and performance.

Parham explains that play "is an active ingredient of a healthy lifestyle" and prepares a person for work.[147,154] As a child undergoes transition to adolescence and adulthood, this primary occupation of play evolves into the occupations of adulthood—work, activities of daily living, and leisure.

Play theories are but one set of theories applied by occupational therapists, who use theories in a variety of ways as a foundation to their reasoning. Therapists make decisions and select strategies using their synthesized knowledge of practice theories, including evidence for those theories, their own experiences, and their perceptions of the client's priorities. Through the use of theory, assessment, and professional reasoning, occupational therapists hypothesize and then develop interventions to improve the occupational performance of children.

For purposes of this chapter, a *theory* is defined as a set of facts, concepts, and assumptions that together are used to describe, explain, or predict phenomena. Using theory, occupational therapists organize knowledge, understand observations, and explain or predict occupational function and dysfunction. Theories, therefore, provide a guide or rationale for occupational therapy intervention. Theories form the foundation for *models of practice* that guide the day-to-day delivery of occupational therapy services. A model of practice (also called a *frame of reference*) is the practical expression of theory and provides therapists with specific methods and guidelines for occupational therapy intervention. Models of practice draw from one or more theories and use concepts and assumptions

to delineate the specific details of an occupational therapy practice, including who receives intervention, what intervention strategies are used, and when and where intervention is provided. The model of practice a practitioner applies can define the evaluations used, the intervention focus and strategies, and expected outcomes. It is the responsibility of the profession to research the theories and models of practice that are core to its practice; this chapter also explains the role of evidence-based practice in the development and application of theory-based models of practice.

Concepts Influencing Occupational Therapy Practice with Children

Development

Perspectives on development and occupation have changed over the past century with changes in our knowledge about children, the factors affecting their development, and their basic need for engagement in purposeful tasks and activities. *Developmental theories* focus on explaining the processes by which infants mature and gain skills to become fully functioning adults. At the core of developmental theories is an explanation of the relationship between human biologic capacity and maturation and the influence of the environment on the behavior and performance of the individual. In fact, developmental theories tend to be distinguished from each other by the relative weight given to these two factors, nature or nurture, or by the emphasis on a particular aspect of human biologic function or environment. The theories of Gesell emphasized the genetic and biologic determinants of development; however, more recent theories (e.g., Piagetian theories) focus on interaction of biologic and environmental determinants of behavior.[70] In current times, developmental theorists generally agree that human development is both the process and the product of biologic maturation and environmental experiences.

Development may be defined as the sequential changes in function that occur with maturation of the individual or species. These sequential changes should be differentiated from the concept of *growth,* which refers to maturational changes that are physically measurable. In the past, different dimensions of development have been emphasized. For example, *longitudinal development* focuses on the stages of development, whereas *hierarchical development* focuses on the prerequisite skills needed for higher-level skills. Evolving views and theories of development place less emphasis on the stages and components of development and more on the person as a whole and his or her development in relation to environment, roles, and occupations.[84] The emerging theories of person–environment relations and complex systems have influenced these changes. Developmental theories are further explained later in the chapter.

Participation in Occupations

Throughout the 1920s and into the 1930s, the focus of occupational therapy was the development of the idea of occupation as a cure for disease and disability. The occupations best suited to cure specific medical problems were identified. Dunton led an effort to analyze occupations systematically.[60] Occupational therapists used the principles of graded, purposeful activity and a balance of work, rest, and play as the basis for treatment methods.[122,172]

In the 1940s, changes in the medical arena (e.g., the discovery of antibiotics and the advancement of specific medical and surgical techniques) had a tremendous influence on the way in which occupational therapists used occupation in treatment. The development of specific techniques increased, and more focus was placed on programs addressing activities of daily living. Occupational therapy treatment focused on the prescription of activities with specific aims.[87] For example, the flexion-extension-pronation-supination (FEPS) loom was developed to ensure that targeted ranges of movement were achieved. As a result of these changes, treatment became "medicalized." In other words, the focus of occupational therapy became a series of technical activities rather than purposeful occupation. The influence of the medical model on the profession dominated for three decades and remains a predominant influence today.

As the 1960s ended, occupational therapists were increasingly uncomfortable with the technical focus of their profession. There was a call for more emphasis on the development of theory and a renewed interest in the roots of the profession: occupation.[203] During this time, Reilly described a theory of occupational behavior in which the individual strives to develop skills and competencies directed toward mastery and achievement.[153,156] Work and play were viewed as the contexts in which these skills and competencies developed. Fidler and Fidler focused on the importance of purposeful activity, or *doing,* in the development of self and the prevention of dysfunction.[65] Kielhofner and Burke, building on Reilly's work, described a model of human occupation that incorporated a systems theoretical view of the nature of occupation.[91] This model expanded the understanding of life roles and the powerful influence they have on daily life and health.

In the past 20 years, a specific academic discipline called *occupational science* became a basis of occupational therapy.[204] Study of the human as an occupational being is essential to an understanding of the complexity of engagement in occupation and the relationship between occupation and human health. As noted by Parham, "A full understanding of occupation requires the integration of knowledge from many disciplines, such as philosophy, biology, psychology, sociology, and anthropology" (p. 25).[142] Wilcock emphasized occupation as purposeful activity and explained that humans need to use time in a purposeful way in order to develop and flourish.[195]

As the study of occupation has developed, occupational therapy scholars have proposed definitions of occupation. Clark and colleagues defined occupations as "chunks of daily activity that can be named in the lexicon of the culture" (p. 301).[36] Christiansen, Clark, Kielhofner, and Rogers defined occupation as the "ordinary and familiar things that people do every day" (p. 1015).[34] The definition adopted by the Canadian Association of Occupational Therapists (CAOT) states that "occupation refers to a group of activities and tasks of everyday life, named, organized, and given value and meaning by individuals and a culture" (p. 34).[30]

Each definition refers to daily activities or "chunks" of activity. Because occupation references daily activity, it is often thought of as simple; that is, the basic activities that people perform each day to look after themselves, to be productive, and to enjoy life. The definition of occupation becomes more complex with the inclusion of its meaning or purpose. The meaning of an occupation for an individual or the value of an occupation determined by a culture begins to show the many layers of occupation and the central relationship of occupation to the human experience.

Participation in occupations meets a basic human need.[30] Dunton expressed his belief that occupation is as necessary to life as food and drink.[60] Occupation also is an important determinant of health. Health can be strongly influenced by a person's engagement in meaningful occupations, and conversely, the absence of meaningful occupation can have dire health consequences.[196] Occupation serves as a means of organizing time, space, and materials. Patterns, habits, and roles evolve through the organization of occupation.[90] Occupations change over the lifespan (as do patterns of time use), representing occupational development.

Play is a key area of occupational focus in practice with children. Chapter 18 describes occupational therapy perspectives on play. Most of the focus in the occupational therapy literature has been on play as a means and an end: as a therapeutic medium (a means to developmental change) and as an indication of developmental level (an outcome of intervention).[142] Therefore, play elicits more than enjoyment; it is also a catalyst to the development of motor or cognitive skills. In their survey of pediatric occupational therapists, Couch, Deitz, and Kanny found that pediatric occupational therapists most often use play in therapy as a medium for developing both the skills underlying function (e.g., understanding cause-and-effect relationships, exploring an object by manipulating it) and an understanding of the rules that guide behavior (e.g., taking turns).[42] Occupational therapists often observe children's play and play with them to determine their level of performance and to analyze their performance (Figure 2-1).[104] Less often, but probably more importantly, therapists view play as a priority outcome of interest, the end rather than the means. Parham suggested that therapists must understand that "play is a legitimate end in itself because it is a critical element of the human experience" (p. 24).[142] Play is therefore a quality-of-life issue that promotes health and well-being.

In a similar way, occupation has a dual role in the profession, as both the focus of intervention and the medium through which occupational therapists often intervene. For example, a child may be struggling at school to successfully fulfill his role as a student because he has Asperger's syndrome. The student struggles with his academic occupations because he is anxious and overaroused. His social participation is limited because he has limited ability to read the social cues of his peers. The occupational therapist evaluates the school activities in which this child is expected to participate and determines the personal and environmental factors that are influencing the child's performance. These occupations become the focus of intervention; for example, the occupational therapist helps the teacher make accommodations to the classroom environment to decrease the student's overarousal and improve his concentration in class. The occupational therapist also helps the student interpret social cues and gestures. The therapist models and instructs the student in appropriate social responses and creates opportunities for him to interact with peers with therapist support. Scaffolding the child's participation in social activities with peers at school is likely to develop skills that generalize to other opportunities

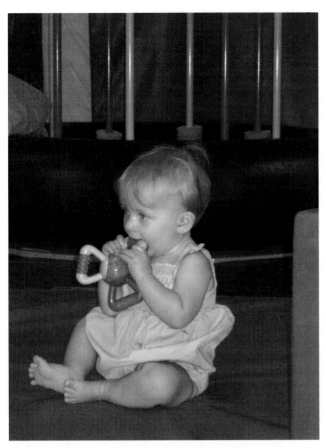

FIGURE 2-1 The infant uses sensory motor play with mouth and hands to explore an object.

for social participation. This brief example illustrates intervention principles that enable children's participation in everyday occupations (Box 2-1).[96]

The goal of an occupation-based model of practice is the child's achievement of optimal occupational performance. What do professionals know about the occupational performance of children with special needs? According to the National Health Interview Survey of 1992 to 1994, 6.5% of

BOX 2-1   Best Practice Principles of Occupational Therapy to Promote Participation in Everyday Life

Occupational therapy:
- Is evidence based and client centered.
- Focuses on occupations important to each person within his or her environment.
- Acknowledges the power of engagement in occupation.
- Recognizes the force of the environment as a means of intervention.
- Has a broad intervention focus.
- Measures outcomes of participation.
- Focuses on occupational important to each person within his or her environment.

From Law, M. (2002). Participation in the occupational of everyday life. *American Journal of Occupational Therapy, 56,* 640-649.

children in the United States with disabilities are limited to some degree in their participation in daily activities.[135] The study investigators reported that children with physical disabilities are "two to three times more likely to be unable to perform their usual activities than children with other conditions (e.g., asthma)" (p. 612).[135] Children with special needs also have lower rates of participation in ordinary daily activities.[173] Researchers have documented that children with disabilities are more restricted in active recreation and community socialization activities.[16] Specifically, Bedell and Dumas found that children with acquired brain injury were most restricted in participating in structured community events, managing daily routines, and socializing with peers and they were least restricted in physical mobility.[17]

Australian studies[113] and Canadian studies[101] have found an inverse relationship in children with disabilities between amount of physical activity and age, with a significant decline in active leisure participation from childhood to adolescence. Although healthy children are less physically active as adolescents, they continue to participate in a wide range of leisure activities. In contrast, adolescents with disabilities engage in fewer leisure and social activities, and their activities tend to be more often home-based than community-based.[168] See Chapter 4 for a discussion of adolescent participation.

In their systematic review of studies of leisure activities in children and youth with physical disabilities, Shikako-Thomas et al. found that children with disabilities participate more in informal activities (e.g., those activities that require little or no planning and are often self-initiated [reading, playing with toys]) than in formal activities (e.g., those with a formally designated coach or instructor [music or art lessons, organized sports]).[168]

Both intrinsic (personal) and environmental (family and community) factors influence the diversity of activities and the intensity of participation. The intrinsic factors include motor function,[140] personality, social skills, age, and gender. Girls tend to participate more in arts and social activities, and boys participate more in group activities involving physical activity and sports.[61,168] Family support can have a positive or negative effect. Children's activities may be restricted by family time constraints, financial burden, and lack of supportive mechanisms (e.g., babysitting).[101] Participation for children with disabilities is positively influenced by high levels of family cohesion, high incomes, strong family coping skills, and low levels of stress.[101,168] Community barriers to children's participation include barriers to physical access, lack of programming, and negative attitudes. Clearly, encouraging participation in the typical activities of childhood needs to be the major focus of pediatric occupational therapy.

Environment

Human ecology is the study of human beings and their relationships with their environments. *Environments* are the contexts and situations that occur outside individuals and elicit responses from them, including personal, social, institutional, and physical factors. Environmental factors can facilitate or limit engagement in occupation. A concept prevalent in the human development literature and more recently in health care is person–environment congruence, or *environmental fit,* which is described as the congruence between individuals and their environments.[176]

Over the past two decades, occupational therapists have stressed the importance of the interaction between individual and environment. Specific models of practice have been developed with a focus on environment.[57,99] Systems theory, emphasizing the interdependent relationship between individual and environment, forms the basis for concepts that define occupational therapy and models of practice. Primary models of practice address the environment in terms of its cultural, social, institutional, and physical dimensions and the transactional relationship between people and the environments in which they live, work, and play.[158,204]

Psychologists who created theories and models about the relationship between humans and their environments that have influenced occupational therapy include Bronfenbrenner,[25] E. Gibson,[71] and J. Gibson.[72] Bronfenbrenner, with a background in developmental psychology, studied how the child's social and cultural environments influenced development.[25] He believed that an interdependent relationship exists between a person and his or her social and cultural environments. Different levels of social support and social interactions surround the individual, including informal (e.g., family and friends) and formal (e.g., occupational therapists and teachers). Levels of the environment are defined by their proximity to the individual; that is, family is most important, then friends and extended family, and then the community and society. Children interact with and are influenced by all levels of the social environment. Changes at any level of the environment influence a person's behavior. Throughout his or her life, a person constantly adapts to and influences changes in his or her social environments.

According to Bronfenbrenner's theories of social development, occupational therapists are part of a person's social environment.[25] These theories help the therapist understand lifespan changes in clients in the context of their social settings. The interdependence between a person and the social environment helps therapists to expand intervention strategies to include families and communities.

Ecologic psychologists E. Gibson and J. Gibson considered the interdependence of a person with his or her environment to be an explanation of *perceptual* development. E. Gibson understood that manipulative play had a key role in the infant's cognitive development.[71] She believed that the child's intrinsically motivated exploratory actions lead to perceptual, motor, and cognitive development through the concept of affordance. An *affordance* is a quality of an object or an environment that allows an individual to perform an action. Action and perception are tightly linked: the child's first actions are to gather new information about the environment and those actions form the basis for perceptual development (the child's understanding of the environment). "As new action systems mature, new affordances open up and new experiments on the world can be undertaken" (p. 7).[71] As explained by E. Gibson:

> The young organism grows up in the environment (both physical and social) in which his species evolved, one that imposes demands on his actions for his individual survival. To accommodate to his world, he must detect the information for these actions—that is, perceive the affordances it holds. How does the infant creature manage this accomplishment? ... I think evolution has provided him with action systems and sensory systems that equip him to discover what the world is all about. He is

"programmed" or motivated to use these systems, first by exploring the accessible surround, then acting on it ... extending his explorations further. The exploratory systems emerge in an orderly way that permits an ever-spiraling path of discovery. The observations made possible via both exploratory and performatory actions provide the material for his knowledge of the world—a knowledge that does not cease expanding, whose end (if there is an end) is understanding (p. 37).[71]

Successful adaptation to the environment occurs when a person matches his or her activities to the affordances of the environment or when the person modifies the environment to ensure successful completion of an activity.

The Gibsons' theories emphasize the importance of understanding a child's development in the context of daily surroundings and activities. Occupational therapists are encouraged to provide activities (based on their understanding of the activity's inherent affordances) that allow a child to explore and learn about the environment, enabling achievement of the child's goals. Figure 2-2 demonstrates an infant's motivation to explore.

Risk and Resilience

Several theories and research programs have been developed to explain the ways the environment influences the developmental outcomes of children and adolescents. Most of this work focuses on the participation of children and youth in everyday activities and on factors that either place children and adolescents at risk for poor outcomes or help them achieve optimal outcomes. For example, psychologist Emmy Werner studied the people of Kauai for more than 40 years. Her research indicated that participation in extracurricular activities plays an important role in the lives of resilient adolescents, especially when they participate in cooperative activities.[192]

Resilience can be defined as the characteristic of an individual who achieves a positive outcome in the context of risk, or factors known to be associated with negative outcomes. Research on risk and resilience has attempted to explain why some children have better outcomes than others who were raised in similar circumstances. The study of resilience has implications for increasing understanding of child development and for

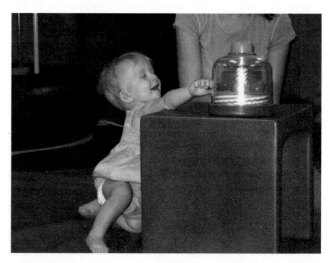

FIGURE 2-2   The infant is motivated to seek and explore a new toy.

developing new interventions to improve outcomes for children at risk. When the concept of resilience was first studied, it was believed to be a stable personality characteristic, such as temperament or IQ. If resilience were an internal, stable characteristic, it would explain why one child did better than another in a particular environment. Currently, researchers understand resilience to be a dynamic process that is refined over time through ongoing transactions between a child and the environment.[110]

What are the risk factors for children who receive occupational therapy? Often the disability is not a primary risk; however, it can add to cumulative risk when the family has socioeconomic disadvantage, negative parental relationships, parental mental illness or physical illness, and lack of extended family support. Emerging evidence indicates that it is the total number of risk factors to which a child is exposed and the resources available to promote resilience for that child that ultimately are predictive of the child's vulnerability to future adverse events and developmental outcomes.[62,163]

Protective factors are defined as characteristics of the child, family, and wider environment that reduce the negative effect of adversity on the child.[120] These protective factors may be specific to the risk factor; for example, having warm and loving parents is a protective factor in early childhood, but may not serve as a protective factor when the child become an adolescent and is more influenced by peers and the teen culture. Researchers such as Rutter[162] and Garmezy[68] have identified general protective factors related to the child, the family milieu, and the social environment. Understanding these general protective factors may be helpful in designing interventions for at-risk children. Child protective factors include strong self-esteem and positive communication skills.[68,192,193] Other child attributes that are associated with positive outcomes include intelligence, emotion regulation, temperament, coping strategies, and attention.[184] Children who can effectively process information and problem-solve can use these abilities in adverse situations. Children who can regulate their emotions can monitor and modify the intensity and duration of their emotional reactions, enabling them to better function at school and in social relationships. An easygoing temperament is also a protective factor because it may evoke more positive attention from adults. Coping skills are also important because children with strong coping skills can moderate the impact of a difficult situation.

Essential resources that lead to resilience in the child are family resources such as love, nurturance, and a sense of safety and security. These must be accompanied by material resources such as nutrition and shelter.[184] Attributes of the family that influence positive outcomes include family cohesion and harmony.[68] Researchers have shown that a high-quality relationship with at least one parent, characterized by high levels of warmth and openness and low levels of conflict, is associated with positive outcomes across level of risk and stages of development.[109]

Protective factors in the community also contribute to the child's development. Neighborhood quality, youth community organizations, quality of school programs and after-school activities can all influence a child's ability to cope with risk factors and overcome adversity.[184] Attributes of the social environment that promote resilience include extended social support and availability of external resources.[68] Environmental factors, such as family-centered service delivery, acceptance of community attitudes, supportive home environments, and mentoring relationships with adults, have been shown to have a positive influence on child development.[157,189,193]

Family-Centered Service

During the past 20 years, families of children with disabilities have increased their role in determining and implementing services for their children. Families have been leaders in promoting family-centered service, a philosophy of service provision that emphasizes the central role of families in making decisions about the care their children receive. Challenged by the changes in the health services field and an increased demand by consumers for involvement in the services they receive, health care providers have made great strides in implementing family-centered service.

The term *family-centered service* arose from early intervention programs. Three important concepts define family-centered service: (1) parents know their children best and want the best for their children; (2) families are different and unique; and (3) optimal child functioning occurs in a supportive family and community context. Chapter 5 explains the rationale for and application of family-centered practice.

In family-centered service the family's right to make autonomous decisions is honored. The relationship between the family and professionals is a partnership in which the family defines the priorities for intervention and, with the service providers, helps direct the intervention process.[59] In working with families, service providers emphasize education to enable parents to make informed choices about the therapeutic needs of their child. Comprehensive education about services and community resources can help families understand the disability, acquire tools to manage behavior, and develop strategies for obtaining community resources. In family-centered practice intervention is based on the family's visions and values; service providers recognize their own values and do not impose them on the family. The family's roles and interests, the environments in which the family members live, and the family's culture make up the context for service provision. Individualization of both the assessment and intervention processes is essential to family centeredness. Intervention is viewed as a dynamic process in which clients and parents work together as partners to define the therapeutic needs of the child with a disability. Services are designed to fit the needs of the family, rather than to force the family to fit the needs of the service providers or the intervention policies already in place. DeGrace explains that occupational therapy intervention needs to fit into a family daily routine because how a family participates in daily routines "defines who that family is and plays a key role in determining its health" (p. 348).[50] Because each family is unique, practitioners need to ask about and learn how each family defines their routines, habits, and values, and to adapt their services to this family-constructed definition.

Research has demonstrated that parents feel more positive about their roles when service providers solicit and value parental participation. Increasing evidence in the literature indicates that interdisciplinary, family-centered service for children with disabilities leads to increased family satisfaction and may lead to greater functional improvement in children with disabilities.[114,161] Parents are less likely to act on behalf of their child when practitioners are unresponsive to the family's needs, are paternalistic, or fail to recognize and accept family decisions.[58]

Family-centered practice is characterized by appreciation and valuing of the family's concerns and priorities, family support, and family education. Therapists who practice family-centered care seek information about how the disability impacts family occupations and what occupations are important to the family.[51] Other examples of family-centered practice include helping families find social supports and network with other families[19] and supporting families in gathering needed resources.[77]

The findings of a recent survey completed by 494 parents and 324 service providers from children's rehabilitation centers indicate that parental satisfaction with service is primarily determined by the family-centered culture of the organization and by parental perceptions of family-centered service.[100] Families' satisfaction with services also decreases feelings of distress and depression and improves feeling of wellbeing.[92] Occupational therapists who work with children enhance the effectiveness of their services when they practice from a family-centered perspective.

World Health Organization International Classification of Functioning, Disability, and Health

The World Health Organization (WHO) International Classification system, which is used in the broad rehabilitation and disability arena, influenced the structure of the Occupational Therapy Practice Framework[2] and has been used to guide the structure of occupational therapy evaluation. The *International Classification of Impairments, Disabilities, and Handicaps* (ICIDH) was first developed and published in 1980.[201] The revised classification system is titled the *International Classification of Functioning, Disability, and Health* (ICF).[202] The ICF views human functioning at three levels: the body (structure and function), the person (activities), and society (participation). It also includes the domain of environmental factors, which can have a significant influence on a person's functioning and health. The ICF model of functioning, disability, and health depicts the dynamic interaction between a person and his or her environment at all levels of functioning. A recent extension of the ICF, the International Classification of Functioning, Disability and Health for Children and Youth (ICF-CY) has been developed to address the unique concerns of developing children.[107] Recently developed measures align with the ICF and enable practitioners to assess children at multiple levels. The School Function Assessment is an example of scale that rates function at two levels, activities and participation.[41] The American Occupational Therapy Association (AOTA) has acknowledged the strong connection between its practice framework and the ICF by establishing the domain of the profession as "supporting health and participation in life through engagement in occupation" (pp. 626-627).[2]

FOUNDATIONAL THEORIES

Foundational theories form the basis of occupational therapy intervention approaches. These theories come from many fields of study, ranging from the biologic sciences to social sciences to humanities. Occupational therapists draw from a wide range of foundational theories to explain occupational performance. Most theories used by occupational therapists who work in pediatrics are concerned with change. Such theoretical perspectives complement the therapist's view of human development as growth that occurs over time in the function of an individual or a species. Considering the complex nature of the PEO perspective and the transactions involved in occupational performance, a number of foundational theories are relevant. This section reviews the theories most commonly used by occupational therapists who work with children and adolescents with disabilities.

Developmental Theories

Developmental theories explain and describe the components of a person as they relate to occupational performance. Different theorists have focused on particular components of the individual in an effort to explain developmental function and dysfunction. The most common theories used by occupational therapists are presented.

Piaget and Cognitive Development

Jean Piaget was concerned with the developmental adaptation of the individual in response to ongoing environmental experiences.[145] He defined *adaptation* as the child's ability to adjust to change to fit into his or her environment, and he examined adaptation through the child's relationships with human and nonhuman objects and through time and space. Piaget[144] introduced the idea that children are intrinsically motivated to learn from their surroundings and that they act on, rather than simply react to, their environment.[95] Piaget used the terms *cognitive structures*, or *schema*, to describe the way in which children represent objects, events, and relationships in their minds. Piaget viewed every interaction as an opportunity either to assimilate new knowledge into existing structures or to adapt existing structures to accommodate new information. Accommodation is new learning, and it is believed to be the way that the cognitive progress is made. Piaget's developmental stages have been the focus of research and critique; however, his descriptions of the gradual accumulation of knowledge in specific content areas remain valid concepts in child development.

Piaget believed the child organizes his experiences into mental schemes (concepts) through mental operations. Operations may be defined as the cognitive methods used by the child to organize his or her schemes and experiences to direct his or her actions. The totality of operational schemes available to the child at any given time constitutes the adapted intelligence, or *cognitive competence*, of the child.

Piaget believed that an invariant, hierarchical development of cognition proceeded from the simple to the complex, from the concrete to the abstract, and from personal to worldly concerns. He specified four maturational levels or periods of cognitive function: sensorimotor, preoperational, concrete operational, and formal operational.[37,67] He believed that this sequence of development leads to the cognitive maturity of adulthood. The culmination of these levels is a person with values, goals, and plans and an understanding of his or her purpose in society. In current times, most child researchers agree that the child is an active learner, but do not view development in discrete stages.

An understanding of Piaget's theory is important to occupational therapists who plan programs for children. Regardless of the therapeutic approach used in treatment, the therapist interacts with a thinking child who is continually learning from his environment. It is essential that the selection and structure of an activity be in accordance with the operational skills and concepts of the child.

The primary focus of Piaget's concept is an explanation of cognitive learning, but Schmidt developed the idea further in the area of motor learning.[167] He proposed that motor schemas are formed as combinations of (1) the initial conditions of the movement, (2) the specific parameters used to create it, (3) the knowledge of the results in the environment, and (4) the sensory consequences of the movement. Through repeated experiences, the child abstracts relationships among these four features and is considered to have learned a new movement.

Vygotsky and the Zone of Proximal Development

Vygotsky viewed human development as historically situated and culturally determined.[194] The child develops by internalizing the social interactions that he experiences. Vygotsky was primarily interested in speech and language development; however, his concepts have important applications to child development across domains. Like his predecessors (e.g., Gesell and Piaget) Vygotsky understood that genetics has unequivocal influence on psychological development. However, he recognized that psychological function could only be explained by considering the role of social interaction. Social interaction has a fundamental influence on the child's development of high mental functions. Vygotsky explained that a child's cognitive processing first requires the assistance of another being within a social interaction before the child can mentally process on his own. Therefore, cognitive processing is a social process before it is an internal process and a child's development and learning are critically dependent on social interaction. Vygotsky defined a "zone of proximal development" to explain how learning occurs through social interaction. The zone of proximal development is "the distance between the actual developmental level as determined by independent problem solving and the level of potential development as determined through problem solving under adult guidance or collaboration with more capable peers" (p. 86).[188] What a child can achieve and learn with the assistance of another is the zone of proximal development and defines the area in which adults can work with the child to promote his development and independence in a particular skill.

When an adult and a child experience an activity together, they interpret the objects and events differently. Adults use language to help the child redefine the situation so that adult and child have a shared definition. When a learning opportunity is created that provides an optimal balance between the child's existing skills and the challenge of the task, the adult can model language and behavior that will help the child progress. Vygotsky's emphasis on the interactions among a child's learning, his environment, the type of instruction provided, and his culture was a precursor to many of the dynamic systems models that influence learning theory today.

Vygotsky's concepts about social learning within the zone of proximal development led to a therapeutic principle called *scaffolding*. Scaffolding is the process by which therapists or adults support or guide a child's actions to improve his or her competence. Appropriate guidance is the just right amount of support that enables the child to perform at a higher level. When using scaffolding to facilitate the child's learning, the adult gradually decreases the amount of support provided such that the child performs more independently. Through this process, actions that are externally supported become internalized. Wertsch makes the point that the child's help-seeking in an activity can be as important to his learning as receiving that assistance.[194] By asking questions and help-seeking, the child becomes more self-directed in his learning; he also develops an understanding about his own learning and how to direct social interactions that can lead to his learning. When the occupational therapist understands a child's zone of proximal development and perceives methods for scaffolding his learning, she or he can design an optimal activity to promote the child's learning. Case Study 2-1 presents an example of applying Vygotsky's theories.

Maslow and the Hierarchy of Basic Needs

Abraham Maslow is generally considered the father of humanistic psychology in the United States.[76] He outlined a hierarchy of basic human needs that is believed to follow a longitudinal sequence.[118,119] An individual's most basic needs, those at the base of this hierarchy, are *physiologic needs*, such as food, water, rest, air, and warmth, that are necessary to basic survival. The next level is characterized by the *need for safety*, broadly defined as the need for both physical and physiologic security. The *need for love and belonging* promotes the individual's search for affection, emotional support, and group affiliation. The *need for a sense of self-esteem*, which is defined as the ability to regard the self as competent and of value to society, is evidenced as an individual grows. The *need for self-actualization*, which represents the highest level, is attained through achievement of personal goals.

Maslow proposed that each of these needs serves as a motivator to achieve a higher level of human potential. Throughout development, individuals must satisfy their most basic needs before they are motivated by or interested in other life goals. Foundational biologic and egocentric needs must be satisfied before an individual has social interests and can fully participate in social relationships. With important social relationships established, an individual becomes interested in the broader community and has a broader sense of commitment and responsibility to others within the community. If the lower level needs are not met, the individual is not able to direct his or her energies toward higher levels. For example, a child who comes to school hungry finds it difficult to concentrate on the classroom learning activities. Recognition of a child's needs and the hierarchy of development of these basic needs helps the occupational therapist understand behaviors that indicate that basic needs are not met and identify needs that should become the focus of goals and interventions.

Learning and Systems Theories

Most important to occupational therapy are theories that integrate concepts about people, their environments, and their occupations. *Development* has been defined as an "evolution of predictable sequences of interactions between a child and the objects in his or her environment" (p. 446).[111] Developmental theories emphasize maturation of the central nervous system as it interacts with the social and physical environment.

CASE STUDY 2-1   Example of Vygotsky: Scaffolding and the Zone of Proximal Development

Sarah is a 4-year-old with an autism spectrum disorder. She demonstrates age-appropriate development in her motor skills; however, she has difficulty with motor planning and sequencing a series of movements. However, her communication, play, and activities of daily living skills appear to be at a 2-year level. She also has difficulty with perceptual skills and often confuses concepts such as up–down, right–left, and spatial awareness. Teresa, an occupational therapist, selected a dress-up activity to promote Sarah's development of visual perception and motor planning in a dressing occupation. Teresa, who has collaborated with the speech language pathologist, also tries to elicit simple questions and use of action verbs in this play scenario.

Teresa sets up the activity by inviting Sarah to come explore the large bin of dress-up clothes in the preschool classroom. As Teresa holds up a fireman's jacket and a doctor's coat, she asks Sarah to identify the top and bottom and to state what part of the body it fits. When Teresa asks Sarah what she wants to be (would you like to be a princess, a nurse, a superhero?), Sarah's pretend skills are not sufficiently developed to choose. Teresa suggests that she be a princess, wearing a gown, princess shoes, and a crown. Teresa asks, "How will you get on your gown?" Sarah is hesitant so Teresa points to the top and bottom, shows the zipper, and indicates that she can step into the gown. Sarah hesitates and Teresa holds her hand to encourage her to step into the gown. She verbally cues her to slide her arms through the sleeves and models the action with an imaginary dress.

Physical assistance is not necessary as Sarah dons the gown with this cueing.

Throughout the activity, Teresa helps Sarah learn and integrate body awareness, saying, "Where are your toes? Let me see your hands and fingers." When Sarah has her gown, shoes, and crown on, Teresa suggests that she dance in front of a mirror to see how the gown flows and to imagine being a princess. They parade through the preschool classroom so that the other children can see her gown. When it is time to go outside and Sarah must take off the gown, Teresa decides to allow Sarah to sequence the undressing activity without verbal or physical cueing. She kneels by Sarah, prepared to help or give guidance, but knowing that undressing is easier, she hopes that Sarah can accomplish it on her own. Although Teresa begins the zipper, Sarah removes her princess clothing independently. Teresa reminds her of top and bottom, right and left during the undressing to reinforce those concepts.

Although this is a simple play scenario, common in preschool classroom, Teresa has applied principles of Vygotsky's theories. She selected an activity within Sarah's proximal zone of development that she could achieve with a minimal amount of support. Teresa was prepared at each step to provide assistance (e.g., physical assistance in donning), but she first observed what support was needed to give the just right amount of support. She reinforced Sarah's learning by making short descriptive comments about the task and by asking about body parts and basic perceptual concepts.

In addition to maturation, the primary process that results in developmental change is learning.

Learning is the acquisition of knowledge, skills, and occupations through experience that leads to a permanent change in behavior and performance. The basis by which humans are able to learn is neuroplasticity (i.e., the ability of the central nervous system to adapt to and assimilate novel information or tasks). Learning theories foundational to occupational therapy practice models include behavioral theories and social cognitive learning. Dynamic system theory provides a comprehensive framework for understanding a child's development in context. Learning principles and system theories foundational to occupational therapy are discussed in the following section.

Behavioral Theories

The past 60 years have witnessed tremendous progress in the field of learning theories. Early learning theorists, such as Thorndike, emphasized the association between a behavior and the resulting reward or punishment as a simple explanation of behavioral change. Skinner described perhaps the best known learning theory from this era. He believed that the environment shapes all human behaviors and that behaviors may be randomly emitted in response to an environmental stimulus.[170] In other words, a person tries a behavior that worked in a previous situation, or an involuntary, reflexive response is elicited by an environmental stimulus. The behavior is then reinforced by the environmental consequences

that follow. This sequence—stimulus situation, behavioral response, and environmental consequence—constitutes a *contingency of behavior,* the mechanism by which the environment shapes behavior.

Skinner stated that through natural occurrences in the environment, a child's adaptive behaviors are reinforced, and behaviors that are not adaptive are ignored or punished.[171] The Skinnerian concept that became fundamental to interventions for children is *instrumental* or *operant learning* or the use of reinforcement to modify behavior. Behavior is strengthened and maintained when it results in positive reinforcement (rather than punishment). If reinforcement is absent (i.e., not given) and therefore is negative, positive behaviors may be extinguished.

Skinner believed that all behavior is a result of the environmental control of the individual, culture, and species. He specified that humans, species, and culture are all part of the environment; therefore, they control as much as they are controlled. Problems arise when an environment changes and becomes inconsistent with prior contingency patterns. For example, children use one set of behaviors with their families and another set with friends. Behaviors that are reinforced by friends may bring complaints from or may be ignored by parents. Critics of this theory cite its failure to explain personality traits (e.g., motivation) and cognitive abilities (e.g., imagination and creativity) and its tendency to generalize across age and gender spectrums with no recognition of developmental differences. Chapter 14 provides further explanation of behavioral interventions.

Extensive research has confirmed that when particular behaviors result in specific, consistent consequences, these behaviors can be modified.[40] Therapists using a behavioral approach can help a child achieve a higher level of performance through a process called *shaping*. Shaping involves breaking down a complex behavior into components and reinforcing each behavior individually and systematically until it approximates the desired behavior (Box 2-2).

In recent years, learning and behavioral theories used with young children have evolved into approaches that can be applied broadly across settings. Applied behavioral interventions primarily use operant conditioning in highly controlled environments in which a therapist or teacher gives the child an instruction and then rewards the child for an appropriate response (reinforcement). Applied behavioral interventions are successful in developing skill; however, skills learned in an isolated setting, as in discrete trial training, do not always generalize into new or higher level behaviors across all settings. Educators have developed behavioral approaches that also use Skinner's framework of instrumental (operant) learning and can be implemented in the child's natural environment to teach children adaptive behaviors that generalize across environments.[94] Educators in early childhood programs have advocated for naturalistic teaching procedures that can be implemented in minimally structured sessions, in a variety of locations and contexts, with a variety of stimuli. Although educators who used naturalistic teaching procedures hold the same developmental goals for children as those who use classical behavioral theory, their procedures are much less structured, incorporate peers, and use naturalistic conditions and reinforcers.[43] Two types of these naturalistic learning procedures, incidental teaching and pivotal response training, are frequently used with young children in early childhood programs.

TABLE 2-1 Comparison of Discrete Trial Training and Incidental Teaching in Early Childhood Programs

Discrete Trial Training	Incidental Teaching
The therapist plans highly structured sessions with planned stimulus and reward.	The therapist plans a loosely structured session with environment designed to elicit specific responses, but directives are not used.
The therapist gives instructions to direct the child's actions.	The child initiates and paces the activity.
The training session is generally one-on-one in a clinic or the home.	The session generally takes place in the classroom, child care center, or home, in the child's natural environment.
The same stimuli are used repeatedly.	A variety of stimuli are used. These stimuli are selected from the natural environment.
The therapist uses artificial reinforcers and often the same reinforcers.	A variety of reinforcers are used and these are selected from the natural environment. The goal is that these reinforcers be available to the child without the presence of the therapist.

Adapted from Cowan, R. J., & Allen, K. D. (2007). Using naturalistic procedures to enhance learning in individuals with autism: A focus on generalized teaching within the school setting. *Psychology in the Schools, 44*, 701-715.

BOX 2-2 Example of Shaping Techniques

Shaping is a systematic process of progressive acquisition of a new behavior through performance of successive acts that collectively represent a more advanced skill. In this process the therapist (1) defines behavior as a series of incremental steps or parts, (2) prompts and cues the child to demonstrate the steps, and (3) rewards each successive approximation of the skill. Shaping is appropriate for multicomponent skills that have a developmental progression in which the skills can be divided into steps and a progression in performance can be elicited.

For example, 5-year-old Anne has left hemiparesis with limited reach and grasp in her left arm. Her therapist initiated building a castle with large Lego pieces. She initially positioned the castle so that Anne used her left hand to place blocks on the left side and at midline. The therapist praised her successful placement of blocks, encouraging her to build a taller and bigger castle. Seeing repeated successes in block placement, the therapist moved the castle to a position that required Anne to reach with her left hand across midline. As the castle grew bigger, Anne had to reach overhead with her left hand, at which time the therapist provided physical support at her left shoulder with continued positive verbal reinforcement. Because overhead movement was an emerging skill, Anne and the therapist practiced this movement repeatedly before moving on to another activity.

In *incidental teaching*, a play environment is created to stimulate the young child's interest and curiosity. It is important that toys used be developmentally appropriate, with both novel and familiar toys. The goal is for the child to select an activity and spontaneously begin to play. The therapist builds on the child's play selection by expanding the play scenario so that it becomes more challenging or creates a problem for the child to solve. The therapist may cue the child to perform a different action and reward the child for attempting more challenging actions. These teaching sessions take a different approach than do behavioral interventions, which use discrete trial training in which the child is given specific directives and rewarded for a specific response. Table 2-1 compares incidental teaching and discrete trial training.

Pivotal response training is also a naturalistic teaching and learning approach used with young children.[93] The goal of pivotal response training is to teach children a set of pivotal behaviors believed to be central to learning. The desired outcomes of pivotal response training include increasing (1) the child's motivation to learn, (2) attention to learning tasks, (3) persistence in tasks, (4) initiation of interactions, and (5) positive affect.[115] Procedures that are used in pivotal behavioral training are similar to those used in incidental teaching with emphasis on methods to promote generalization of learning. When applying pivotal response training, the therapist gives the child a choice in play materials, uses natural reinforcers, intersperses mastered tasks with learned tasks, and reinforces attempts at new learning (Figure 2-3).[43] These

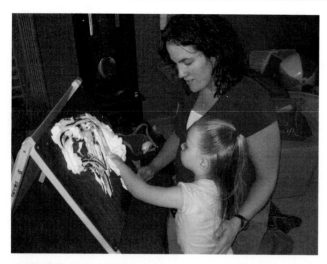

FIGURE 2-3   In this example, the child selected the activity (finger painting) and the medium (shaving cream). The occupational therapist reinforces the child's efforts to reach overhead with praise and touch.

theories are further explained in Chapter 23 on early intervention programs.

Social Cognitive Theories

In general, social cognitive theory explains learning that occurs in a social context. The initial acquisition of highly complex and abstract behaviors was difficult for learning theorists to explain until the advent of the social cognitive theory proposed by Bandura.[11] Bandura[11] and Piaget[144] introduced the idea that children can learn by observing the behavior of others. This learning may not be immediately observed in behavior but becomes part of the child's general understanding of the world. In contrast with the behavioralists, who believe that all learning produces behavioral change, social cognitive theorists believe that learning can occur without observable behavioral changes. A child can learn by observing the behavior of others, such as subtle nonverbal gestures that are used in conversation. These are observed and stored in memory and may not be demonstrated by the child until a much later time, when the child may exhibit similar gestures but with his or her own unique style.

In social cognitive theory, people determine their own learning by seeking certain experiences and focusing on their own goals. Therefore, children do not simply learn random elements from the environment, but they direct their own learning and are goal oriented in what they learn. Social cognitive theorists also believe that children learn indirectly by observing how their peers' behaviors are rewarded or punished. Direct reinforcement is not always needed when learning new behaviors.[138]

Social cognitive learning is often indirect, as when the child learns by observing the consequences of behaviors of those around him or her. Learning that occurs when observing the behaviors of others also depends on the child's goals, interests, and relationship to those observed. Children's learning increases when they are given an incentive to learning (i.e., an anticipated valued outcome or reward). Learning is also promoted when the child establishes his or her own goals, is

given opportunities to work on those goals, and evaluates whether the goal was accomplished. When children set their own goals, they direct their behavior in a specific way, they are more likely to persist in the behavior to achieve the goal, and they are often more satisfied with the outcome.

In this theory, children learn social skills through group experiences. When children have delayed social skills, they can gain an understanding of social gestures and peer interaction by becoming involved in a group where these behaviors are modeled and rewarded. Bandura believed that critical factors in the child influence the learning process, including the child's perception of his or her competencies (i.e., self-efficacy). The ways in which a strong sense of efficacy can enhance personal accomplishment are described next.

The Influence of Motivation and Self-Efficacy on Learning

A number of factors in the child are believed to influence learning, such as cognition, motivation, attitude, and self-perception. The relationship between learning and other affective components is complex. It is widely accepted that children's motivation to perform occupations is influenced by their perceptions of their efficacy, regardless of whether these perceptions are correct.[11] If children experience success in learning situations, it is assumed that they increase their perceived competence and internal control, gain support from significant others, and show pleasure at mastering the task. The assumption is made that children are more likely to seek out optimal challenges if they have experienced success.[13] The corollary of this theory is that children who experience repeated failure begin to avoid challenges and are less likely to seek out new learning situations.[79]

Motivation to learn and to achieve is developed through (1) casual attributions, (2) outcome expectancy, and (3) personal goals. When children feel self-efficacious, they attribute any failure to lack of effort. When children feel inefficacious, they attribute their failure to low ability. The efficacious child remains motivated to try harder and to improve performance; the inefficacious child believes that there is no point in trying harder because he or she is destined to fail. A child self-motivates by setting a personal goal higher than his or her current skill levels. Then the child mobilizes the energy to achieve that goal. With success the child sets a higher goal and become motivated to achieve a higher-level task.

Self-efficacy beliefs contribute to motivation in several ways. They determine the goals people set for themselves, how much effort they expend, how long they persevere in the face of difficulties, and how they respond to failure.[11] All of these decisions contribute to success in a particular goal and contribute to learning. Perceived self-efficacy also contributes to a child's coping ability, which is discussed later in this chapter.

Therapists need to be aware of the importance of providing successful learning opportunities and optimal challenge situations. It is also important to note, however, that when children are young, they may not have the metacognitive awareness required to compare their own performance accurately against that of others. This lack of awareness may actually have an adaptive purpose in childhood. The fact that young children do not evaluate their own performance increases the likelihood that they will put energy and effort into practicing skills in a wide variety of environments with little concern about their actual competency.[21] As children develop, however, their expectation of competence becomes more specific to the type of task and is influenced by their prior experiences with that task, their observations of typically developing peers performing it, and the evaluative feedback provided by credible adults.[12]

Dynamic Systems Theory

Emerging theoretical ideas from systems theory influence today's thinking in many areas of development in children, and these ideas are beginning to lead to creation of alternative models of practice for therapy intervention. In contrast with a hierarchical model of neural organization, systems theory (also called *dynamic systems theory*) proposes a flexible model of neural organization in which the functions of control and coordination are distributed among many elements of the system rather than vested in a single hierarchical level.[186] Work that led to the development of dynamic systems theory includes research by Bernstein,[20] who used concepts from physics related to movement and applied these ideas to motor development. Bernstein proposed that the central nervous system (CNS) controls groups of muscles (not individual muscles) and that these groups can change motor behavior on their own without CNS control. He believed that motor control could emerge spontaneously from relationships among kinematics (muscles) and biomechanics (joints and bones) that naturally limit the degrees of freedom of movement. Therefore the motor system is self-organizing.[169]

Systems theory has its roots in geometric concepts, and at the most basic level, a dynamic system is simply something that changes over time. Dynamic systems theorists emphasize that learning does not occur just in the brain and that the body and environment are all constantly changing and simultaneously influencing each other.[185] In this theoretical approach, instead of viewing behavior (e.g., motor skills) as predetermined in the CNS, systems theory views motor behavior as emerging from the dynamic cooperation of the many subsystems in a task-specific context. It implies that all factors contributing to the motor behavior are important and exert an influence on the outcome by either facilitating performance or constraining it.

In this approach, the therapist looks for periods of stability in learning and watches for signs that a child is ready to shift to a qualitatively different type of behavior. Identification of the system variables that drive the transition from one level to another facilitates learning.[27] These variables can be related to the child, the task, or the environment. Thelen suggested that variables such as physical growth and biomechanics may be more important for motor learning in infancy, whereas factors such as experience, practice, and motivation may be more influential in the learning of motor activities in an older child.[180]

Dynamic systems theory is an ecologic approach that assumes that a child's functional performance depends on the interactions of the child's inherent and emerging skills, the characteristics of the desired task or activity, and the environment in which the activity is performed. Self-organization is optimal in a functional task that has a goal and outcome. Most functional tasks (e.g., eating and drinking) elicit a predictable pattern of movement; therefore, the task itself can organize the movements attempted. These features suggest that dynamic systems theory aligns well with occupational therapy.

Research in dynamic systems theory has focused on explaining the ways new skills are learned.[64,133,181,182] The learning of new movements or ways of completing an activity requires that previously stable movements be broken down or become unstable. New movements and skills emerge when a critical change occurs in any of the components that contribute to motor behavior. These periods of change are called *transitions*. Motor change in young children is envisioned as a series of events during which destabilization and stabilization of movement take place before the transitional phase movement becomes stable and functional.[147]

The period of instability that occurs in a transitional phase is seen as the optimal time to effect changes in movement behavior. Three characteristic situations mark the transitional stage:

1. Variability in motor performance increases. The child experiments with different movement patterns.
2. Through these exploratory movements, the child determines which pattern is the most adaptive.
3. The child selects the movement that is most adaptive, the movement that meets his or her goals given environmental demands and constraints (e.g. which pattern makes it easiest to rise from sit to stand given the effects of gravity and available supports). During this phase, the child repeatedly practices the same movement pattern.

In children with impairments such as cerebral palsy, constraints hinder the emergence of motor functions. Such *constraints* are limitations imposed on motor behaviors by the child's physical, social, cognitive, and neurologic characteristics. The constraint that traditionally has received most attention is the integrity of the CNS; less frequently, other biomechanical constraints are considered, such as biomechanical forces, muscle strength, or a disproportionate trunk-to-limb ratio. *Environmental constraints* include physical, social, and cultural factors not related to a specific task. One example of a physical constraint is a suboptimal surface for the child's activity (e.g., a slippery or inclined surface); a social constraint could be a parent's lack of reinforcement of the acquisition of motor behaviors. *Task constraints* are restrictions on motor behavior imposed by the nature of the task. Established motor behaviors may be altered by specific task requirements. For example, when faced with the task of crawling on rough terrain, infants may alter motor behavior by straightening the knees and "bear walking." When a child reaches for a ball, the ball's size influences the shape of the child's hand and the approach taken (e.g., one hand versus two). The unique features of these tasks have shaped the child's motor behavior. See Table 2-2 for a list of dynamic systems theory principles. Dynamic systems theory has many similarities to the emerging occupational therapy theories that focus on person, environment, and occupation relationships. This theory is further explained in Chapters 3 and 9.

MODELS OF PRACTICE USED BY OCCUPATIONAL THERAPISTS

Occupational therapy practitioners recognize that health is supported and maintained when clients are able to engage in occupations and activities that allow desired or needed participation in home, school, workplace, and community life.[2]

TABLE 2-2   Principles of Dynamic Systems Theory Applied to Motor Development

Dynamic System Theory Principle	Application to Motor Development
Sensory perception and motor systems are coupled. These systems continually interact in learning new motor skills. The infant's perceptions guide his or her movements, which in turn create the infant's perception of the world.	Haptic sense, discrimination of the physical properties of objects through touch, is acquired through object manipulation. Sensory information is gained as the infant's fingers move over the object's surfaces.
Functional synergies are the basis of motor behavior. Movement synergies are based on kinematic (e.g., muscles) and biomechanic (e.g., joints) constraints and are the basic units that control movement. Therefore, the basic units of motor behavior are functional synergies or coordinated structures rather than specific muscle actions. These functional synergies are "soft"—assembled (i.e., they are highly adaptable and highly reliable).	Similar synergies are used for eating and drinking that involve shoulder internal rotation and adduction, elbow extension followed by flexion, forearm pronation followed by slight supination, and a neutral wrist position. This functional synergy is also used, with slight modification in combing one's hair and cleansing face and teeth. This is a stable but flexible synergy.
Transition to new movement patterns involves exploration, selection, and practice phases. The infant or child first explores many different patterns and exhibits high variability in movement. Then the infant selects an optimal pattern to achieve his goal. This pattern is practiced and becomes more adaptable to a variety of environmental demands.	When first learning to eat with a spoon, the infant exhibits a variety of patterns with the spoon, including banging, stabbing, and waving. Then the infant selects a functional pattern that successfully meets the environmental demand (e.g., the toddler learns to supinate the forearm when bringing the spoon to mouth so that the food reaches the mouth rather than spilling down the chest). This adaptive pattern is repeatedly practiced as the toddler insists on always self-feeding.
The infant's unique motor patterns are the result of input from multiple systems that interact in dynamic ways to both facilitate and constrain movement. Behavior is multiply determined and children develop in context. Behavior is determined by an integrated system of perception, action, and cognition. These elements are integrated over time to form a child's unique developmental trajectory.	The pattern an infant uses to reach for an object is determined by many variables. Variables that may influence reaching include biomechanic and kinematic factors such as weight of his or her arm, stiffness of joints, strength, and eye-hand coordination. However, the reaching pattern is also influenced by how successful the child was in previous reach and grasp (did the object move before the child could obtain it?), how motivated the child is to attain the object, general energy level, and curiosity.

Adapted from Case-Smith, J. (1996). Analysis of current motor development theory and recently published infant motor assessments. *Infants and Young Children, 9*(1), 29-41; Spencer, J. P., Corbetta, D., Buchanan, P., Clearfield, M., Ulrich, B., & Schoner, G. (2006). Moving toward a grand theory of development: A memory of Esther Thelen. *Society for Research in Child Development, 77,* 1521-1538.

Thus, occupational therapy practitioners are concerned not only with the child's performance in everyday activities but also the environmental influences that enable a child's engagement and participation in those activities.[197]

This section of the chapter focuses on models of practice developed specifically for occupational therapy assessment and intervention with children. An example of a theoretical framework that focuses on occupation and performance is presented first. Discussion of this overall framework is followed by overviews of specific models of practice used with children and youth. These models of practice are used in conjunction with an overall focus on occupation and occupational performance.

Most occupational therapy practice models explain the interaction of person, occupation, and environment. They recognize the premise that human performance cannot be understood outside of context.[57] In earlier models (e.g., person-environment-performance,[32] person-task-environment[81]), the focus of primary intervention is on the person, with relatively less emphasis on changing environments. Law and colleagues developed the person-environment-occupation (PEO) model, which focuses equally on facilitating change in the person, occupation, and/or environment.[99]

The PEO model was developed using theoretical foundations from the *Canadian Guidelines for Occupational Therapy*, environmental-behavioral theory, and work by Csikszentmihalyi & Csikszentmihalyi[45] on the theory of optimal experience.

The PEO model outlines the concepts of person, environment, and occupation as follows[99]:

- *Person:* A unique being who, across time and space, participates in a variety of roles important to him or her.
- *Environment:* Cultural, socioeconomic, institutional, physical, and social factors outside a person that affect his or her experiences.
- *Occupation:* Any self-directed, functional task or activity in which a person engages over the life span.

The PEO model suggests that occupational performance is the result of the dynamic, transactive relationship involving person, environment, and occupation (Figure 2-4, *A*). Across the lifespan and in different environments, the three major components—person, environment, and occupation—interact continually to determine occupational performance. Increased congruence, or fit, among these components represents more optimal occupational performance (Figure 2-4, *B*).

The PEO model is used as an analytic tool to identify factors in the person, environment, or occupation that facilitate or hinder the performance of occupations chosen by the person. Occupational therapy intervention can then focus on facilitating change in any of these three dimensions to improve occupational performance. Specific models of practice, as outlined next, can be used in conjunction with the PEO model to address specific performance limitations or environmental conditions that impede occupational performance.

OCCUPATIONAL PERFORMANCE

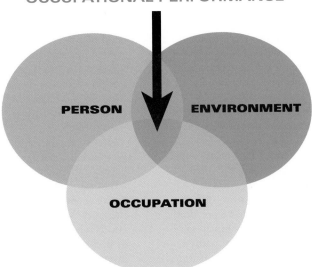

MAXIMIZES FIT
and therefore maximizes occupational performance

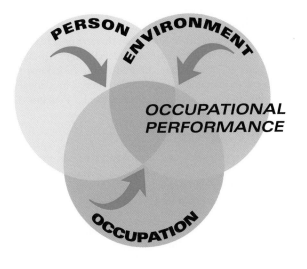

MINIMIZES FIT
and therefore minimizes occupational performance

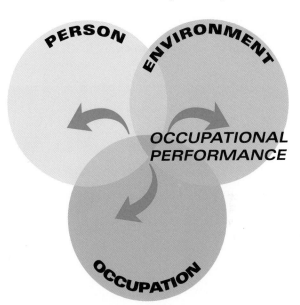

FIGURE 2-4   **A**, Person-environment-occupation model. **B**, Person-environment-occupation analysis.   (From Law, M., Cooper, B., Strong, S., Stewart, D., Rigby, P., & Letts, L. [1996]. The person-environment-occupation model: A transactive approach to occupational performance. *Canadian Journal of Occupational Therapy, 63*[1], 9-23.)

Specific Models of Practice

The models of practice or frames of reference currently used in occupational therapy operate within systems theory, as each considers the interaction of person, environment, and activity or occupation. A discussion of systems theory as it influences occupational therapy interventions is presented first; then specific practice models used by occupational therapists in their work with children are explained.

A Systems Approach

Occupational therapists approach intervention with a child by first gaining an understanding of the environmental, family, and child factors that influence the performance of specific activities. From the literature that discusses the application of systems theory or dynamic systems theory to occupational therapy intervention, the following principles emerge:

- Assessment and intervention strategies must recognize the inherent complexity of task performance. The most useful assessment strategy is to develop a "picture" or "profile" of the ways performance components and environmental and task factors affect performance of the tasks the child wants to accomplish. Assessment of only one or a few components (e.g., balance, mood, strength) is not likely to lead to the most effective identification of constraints.

- The focus of assessment and intervention is on the interaction of the person, the environment, and the occupation. Therapy begins and ends with a focus on the occupational performance tasks a child or youth wants to, needs to, or is expected to perform. When a child shows readiness and motivation to attempt a task or activity, the focus of intervention on that particular activity can effect changes in his or her performance.[97]

- The therapy process focuses on identification and change of child, task, or environmental constraints that prevent the achievement of the desired activity. Some of these factors may be manipulated to enhance the functional motor task or goal; others may be managed by providing the missing component during the execution of the task. Parts of activities can be changed (e.g., different toy sizes, different position for child or activity). Activities should be practiced in a variety of environments that can facilitate completion of the task and promote the flexibility of movement patterns. Activities incorporated into the child's daily routine provide opportunities for finding solutions for functional motor challenges (Figure 2-5).

- When preparing therapeutic activities, the therapist identifies playful activities that would motivate the child, are developmentally appropriate, match the child and family's goals, provide a challenge to current skills levels, and match an expected or hoped for outcome.

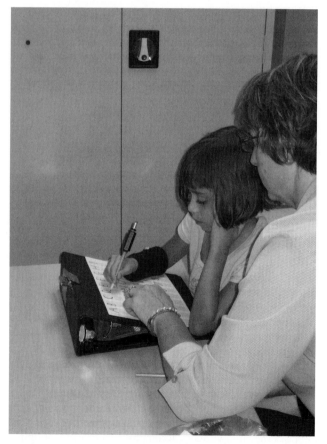

FIGURE 2-5 In this functional activity, a slant board is used to promote improved posture and grasp of the pencil. A weight on the pencil provides added proprioceptive input.

- With intervention through the systems approach, the focus on changing environments and occupations is at least as great as the focus on changing the inherent skills of the child or adolescent. Intervention is best accomplished in natural, realistic environments. The accomplishment of whole occupations, not parts of them, is emphasized. The goal in therapy is to enable a child to accomplish an identified activity, rather than promote change in a developmental sequence or improve the quality of the movement.

- Therapeutic effect and positive outcomes are determined by the child's engagement in the activity, the match between the intervention activities and the child's skill levels, the meaningfulness of the activity, the amount of practice, and the opportunities to transfer and generalize the newly learned skill to a variety of contexts. Positive effects relate to how well the interventions enable the child to perform well across his or her natural environments given age and role expectations.

Models of practice for therapy assessment and intervention, based on dynamic systems theory, are beginning to emerge, although challenges to implementation remain.[31,46] Common among these models is the focus on successful achievement of functional goals rather than on the development of typical patterns of movement.[26,47,169] Ketelaar et al.,[89] in a study of 55 children receiving either functional therapy based on dynamic systems theory or therapy aimed at developing "typical" movement patterns, found that children in the functional therapy group demonstrated significantly more functional skills (mobility and self-care) as measured by the Pediatric Evaluation of Disability Inventory.[89]

Cognitive Approaches

Cognitive approaches are "top down" or occupation-based approaches because the emphasis in therapy is on assisting the child to identify, develop, and use cognitive strategies to perform daily occupations effectively. These models build on Bandura's research[11] supporting the importance of self-efficacy and establishing goals to motivate individual achievement.

In cognitive approaches, the occupational therapist designs interventions to increase a child's repertoire of cognitive strategies and improve the child's ability to select, monitor, and evaluate his or her use of these strategies during the performance of a task. The inherent assumption is that improved performance results from the dynamic interaction of the child's skills with the parameters of the task in the context in which it needs to be performed. Therefore, the child discovers, applies, and evaluates cognitive strategies during task performance in his or her typical environments.[131]

The cognitive model of practice requires that the therapist identify and use a global problem-solving strategy, which provides a consistent framework within which the child discovers specific strategies applicable to tasks that he or she either needs or wants to perform. This global strategy is based on the five-stage problem-solving structure first outlined by Luria.[108] Using occupational therapy terminology, these steps include (1) task analysis, (2) anticipation of the child's difficulties, (3) exploration and selection of task-specific strategies, (4) application of a strategy to the task, and (5) evaluation of the strategy's effectiveness.[130] The child is guided to develop his or her own cognitive strategies based on the problems encountered during tasks. The task-specific strategies a child discovers are unique to him or her.

Using cognitive skills to assess his performance, identifying successful and unsuccessful actions, the child learns to become more efficient in functional activities. The occupational therapist supports the child's goals and self-evaluation. The therapist can also cue, prompt, or model the task, aligning these supports to the child's goals. The atmosphere in the therapy session is one of acceptance and support for taking risks. Although the child guides the selection of activities, the therapist is always aware of the generalization and task-specific strategies that the child needs to learn and creates opportunities for the child to discover these.[131,150]

Because the selection of tasks is critical to the approach, a client-centered tool must be used that allows the child to identify goals for intervention. An appropriate goal-setting instrument for use with children older than 9 years of age is the Canadian Occupational Performance Measure (COPM)[97]; for children 5 to 9 years of age, the Perceived Efficacy and Goal Setting (PEGS) system can be used.[132] The cognitive approach is probably not a suitable model of practice for children under 5 years of age because of its emphasis on the development of metacognitive skill and knowledge.

One of the key features of a cognitive model of practice is the way in which the therapist helps the child explore strategies, make decisions, apply strategies, and evaluate their use. The therapist does not give instructions. Rather, he or she uses questions to help children (1) discover the relevant aspects of the task, (2) examine how they are currently performing the task, (3) identify where they are getting "stuck," (4) creatively think about alternative solutions, and (5) try out these solutions and evaluate them in a supportive environment. Once a strategy is found to be helpful, the therapist uses questions to help the child "bridge" or generalize the strategy, eliciting from the child other times and situations in which that strategy may apply.[150]

In recent years a particular cognitive approach, the cognitive orientation to daily occupational performance (CO-OP),[149] has been researched systematically to determine whether it is an effective model to use with children with developmental coordination disorder. Evidence is accumulating that CO-OP is effective at enabling skill acquisition and that it also results in generalization and transfer of learned skills.[150] A randomized clinical trial comparing CO-OP with an equivalent number of sessions of direct skill training found that, although children in both groups improved and achieved motor goals, the gains in the CO-OP group were greater; long-term maintenance both of the motor goals and of the cognitive strategies was significantly stronger in the CO-OP group, which led parents to report greater satisfaction with this treatment approach.[127] Studies on CO-OP have shown its effectiveness with children with developmental coordination disorder,[127,179] cerebral palsy or acquired brain injury, and Asperger's syndrome.[159,160]

Through research such as this, a variety of cognitive strategies have been identified that seem to be helpful to many different children experiencing occupational performance difficulties. Videotape analysis has been used to systematically identify and describe some of these strategies.[116] It appears that children need to be able to state and apply a global executive strategy, such as "Goal, Plan, Do, Check,"[123] to guide their problem solving. In addition, specific strategies seem to be useful for improving their performance, including verbal self-guidance (child talks himself or herself through the motor sequence); feeling the movement (drawing attention to an aspect of the sensation of movement as it is performed); motor mnemonic (labeling a body position or motor sequence); body position (verbalizing or directing attention to the body position or body parts relative to the task); and task specification (discussing specific parts of the task or actions to change the task).[116]

In summary, occupational therapists who use a cognitive model of practice (1) focus on the occupations a child wishes to perform rather than on foundational skill building; (2) use a general problem-solving framework that guides the child to discover, select, apply, and evaluate the use of specific cognitive strategies; (3) use process questions to increase the child's awareness of the use of strategy during the performance of daily tasks; and (4) plan for transfer and generalization of the strategies that the child has learned.[130,150]

Adaptation and Compensation Interventions

Occupational performance is successful when the demands of the task, the skills of the child, and the features of the environment are congruent. When the skills of the person do not meet the demands of the task in the environment, occupational performance becomes less successful. Most of the models of practice in occupational therapy, particularly with children who are still developing, focus on increasing the child's skills. The adaptation model of practice involves adapting the demands of the task or modifying the environment so that they are congruent with the child's ability level. Adaptations may involve modifying the occupation so that it is easier to perform, using assistive technology devices, or changing the physical or social environment.[44] Often when children have significant impairments, task modification is needed to maximize the child's participation. For example, a child with cerebral palsy may require an adapted spoon and cup to eat dinner with his family. A child with autism may require a picture exchange card system to communicate his need to use the bathroom.

When skills are insufficient to enable performance, task adaptation is used to modify the demands of a task to bring it to the competence level of the child. Task demands are analyzed and functional limitations are identified, and difficulties then are creatively circumvented. An example in school-based practice would be adapting the writing surface by using a slant board so that the child's written work is more easily visualized and the child's hand and arm posture are supported in a posture that promotes writing skill. A child with a learning disability may be able to complete a page of arithmetic problems when the font is enlarged and the paper has a color tint.

Often adaptive equipment or assistive technology (AT) is used to modify or adapt the task. Campbell, Milbourne, and Wilcox view assistive technology as a bridge or mediator between the skills that a child can currently perform and the requirements of the task.[29] Assistive technology may be as simple as adaptive brushes or crayons that allow a preschool child to participate in art activities. A wide variety of assistive technology devices can enable children with significant motor impairments to better access their environment. For example, AT devices can help position the child to perform an activity (e.g., a prone stander) or provide postural support (e.g., wheelchair straps). "High-tech" technology is also available to provide a method for written communication (e.g., a laptop computer) or augmentative communication (e.g., a device for synthesized speech). Chapters 16, 20, and 21 describe assistive technology devices that use this approach to increase children's participation in their natural environments.

With children, the compensatory approach often complements other approaches that focus on skill building. Methods for adapting tasks are selected not only so that the child succeeds at a particular task, but also to promote skills in similar tasks and in other environments. For example, a boy with poor drawing skills can create a picture using peel-off stickers of animals. Although this adaptation allows the boy to create a picture more easily than drawing with markers, peeling off and placing the stickers provide practice of fine motor skills—specifically, bilateral coordination, isolated finger movements, spatial relations, and use of force. Practice in these skills may generalize to other art activities, and the easy success the child achieves when using colorful animal stickers may encourage him to attempt other art activities.

Psychosocial Approaches

Occupational therapists use a variety of psychosocial approaches when working with children and adolescents experiencing problems in occupational performance because of social, emotional, or behavioral issues or difficulties with relationships. Several of these approaches, such as a cognitive approach or the compensatory and environmental approach, are discussed elsewhere in this chapter. These approaches are grounded in theories that focus on the development of self, on family and peer relationships, and on the aspects of the social and cultural environment that influence each of these. Although the number of occupational therapists who work with children with chronic mental health issues is relatively small, all occupational therapists who work in pediatrics use the concepts of psychologic and social development implicitly, because developing the ability to maintain relationships with peers and significant others is an essential part of the occupational performance of childhood and adolescence.

Chapter 13 describes the models of practice that focus on social behavior and the development of self. Personal attributes, such as temperament, self-esteem and self-efficacy, problem-solving ability, and social skills, are considered important determinants of healthy functioning. Environmental influences on behavior and social development suggest the need to consider the expectations and social elements of the home, school, and community environments and to recognize the importance of friends in a young person's life. For the occupational therapist, the critical consideration is the impact of the person's attributes and environmental influences on ability to participate in daily occupations.

Given the complex nature of behavior and social relationships, occupational therapists often draw on a number of intervention approaches in this model of practice. The therapist's knowledge of normal behavior, vulnerabilities associated with particular disabilities, attachment, coping skills, and compatibility of temperaments may guide intervention with a parent–child dyad. Cognitive behavioral strategies may be used by occupational therapists to help young people who are depressed or socially withdrawn develop strategies that encourage participation in social situations (see Chapter 13).

Coping Model

The coping model addresses psychosocial function, uses cognitive behavioral strategies, and is congruent with the PEO model.[199,205] Therapists who use this model emphasize the use of coping resources that enable the child to meet challenges posed by the environment. The goal is to improve the child's ability to cope with stress in personal, social, and other occupational performance areas. When children are successful in coping with their own personal needs and the demands of the environment, they feel good about themselves and their place in the world. Coping strategies are learned, and children build on previous successful experiences in coping with environmental expectations.[205]

All children experience stress when faced with physical, cognitive, and emotional challenges. When these challenges are successfully met by the child's inner resources and caregiving supports, the result is a sense of motivation, learning, and mastery. Stress can evoke negative feelings when the child's resources are poorly matched to the environment's demands. Both internal and external resources assist in the process of coping. Internal coping resources include coping style, beliefs and values, physical and affective states, and developmental skills. External coping resources include human supports and materials and environmental supports.

Internal and External Coping Resources

Children have unique patterns of sensorimotor organization, reactivity, and self-initiation.[206] *Coping style* is the way the child reacts to social interactions and responds to environmental events. Intrinsically motivated and self-initiated behaviors are part of a child's coping style. Examples of these behaviors are the child's exploration of objects and space, initiation of interaction, and persistence in activities. Self-initiated behaviors are particularly important to occupational therapists, because many children with disabilities show limited spontaneous behaviors when exploring the environment, initiating play, and persisting in activity. Physical and affective states influence the child's ability to cope with environmental stress. Energy, endurance, moods, and emotions define the child's ability to respond to, engage in, and persist in activity. Chronic illness, emotional instability, and depression may impair the child's ability to handle the demands of the environment effectively.[148]

Developmental skills and competence are the internal resources a child brings to a task. Often a child with disabilities is placed in situations that match the chronologic age (e.g., a preschooler play group) but not necessarily the developmental age. When expected behaviors do not match developmental skills (e.g., to sit quietly and attend), children experience stress and generally seek external coping supports.

Human supports are people in the child's environment who support the child's coping efforts. Parents and other primary caregivers are the most significant external resources for coping in the child's early years.[199] Parents buffer the child's exposure to stress, make demands, model coping behaviors, encourage and assist the child in coping efforts, and give contingent feedback. They provide material supports and resources, including food, clothing, and shelter. Environmental supports are the spaces and materials available to the child and may include adapted equipment and technology associated with comfort and functional support.

Effective Coping

The child successfully copes with new challenges when (1) he or she has underlying resources that enable a successful response to an environmental demand or new situation; (2) human supports are provided to facilitate his or her performance (e.g., the therapist gives the child a visual or verbal cue); and (3) environmental supports are provided that enable the child to feel safe and comfortable, be attentive and engaged, and feel calm and organized (e.g., a classroom that is quiet and well organized and that has a comfortable lighting level and temperature). The therapist continually evaluates whether the child's skills (internal resources) and environmental supports (external resources) are adequate to meet the demands of the activity. When the child exhibits ineffective coping strategies, the therapist adjusts the task demands and provides more human or environmental support to enable the child to succeed in his or her coping efforts.

To facilitate effective coping, Williamson and Szczepanski defined three postulates[199]:

1. The occupational therapist can grade or modify the environmental demands to ensure that they are congruent with the child's adaptive capabilities. For example, the environment of a child with attention deficit–hyperactivity disorder (ADHD) can be adapted by reorganizing materials to reduce visual demands and enhance visual attention. To enhance the social skills of children with behavioral disorders, a tabletop of materials for an art activity can be provided in insufficient quantity for the number of children, to encourage sharing.

2. The therapist can design intervention activities to enhance the child's internal and external coping resources. Intervention focuses on the child's resources, including coping style, physical and affective states, developmental skills, human supports, and material and environmental supports. The therapist can foster a positive sense of self and can involve the child in activities that promote self-efficacy. For older children, the therapist can facilitate group discussions of personal goals and plans for reaching these goals. Personal social skills may be emphasized by practice of social skills in the context of games with peers. Activities that emphasize group skills, such as problem solving, sharing, and communication, can help older children develop improved personal social skills that can be generalized to school and extracurricular activities.

3. The therapist can provide appropriate, contingent responses to the child's coping efforts. Timely, positive, and explicit feedback to coping efforts helps the child experience a sense of mastery. Feedback that effectively enhances coping efforts emphasizes self-directed, purposeful behaviors. Therefore, the therapist supports child-initiated activity and provides feedback that encourages the extension and elaboration of emerging skills. Because research suggests that children with disabilities tend to assume passive, dependent roles, highly structured and therapist-directed activities should be replaced with child-initiated activities that are specifically and appropriately reinforced and then generalized to other situations (Figure 2-6).

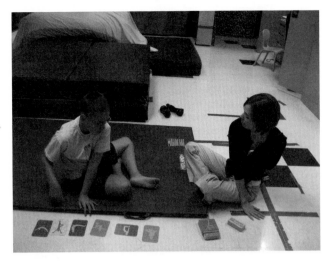

FIGURE 2-6 Teaching yoga to a child with Asperger's gives him a method to improve his coordination, agility, and bilateral integration. It also gives him a method for exercising that can reduce stress.

Social Skills Training

Interventions that develop positive coping strategies in children and adolescents with psychosocial dysfunctions can be essential for promoting the ability to participate in social interactions and relationships. Occupational therapists working with older children and adolescents with mental health problems often use social skills groups to promote coping effectiveness and occupational performance. A group milieu allows young people to master developing skills in a safe and supportive environment. Social skills training groups have shown positive effect with adolescents with autism.[80] Monthly group meetings focused on social skill development resulted in adolescents improving in maintaining and initiating conversation. Broderick, Caswell, Gregory, Marzolini and Wilson evaluated the effect of a social skill group of adolescents with autism spectrum disorder and found that they improved in self esteem and confidence.[24] See Table 2-3 for examples of venues for social skills training.

Social networks have been shown to help a person establish positive attitudes and role behavior, maintain and improve self-esteem, and develop moral and social values.[35,78] Other studies have identified the interactive, protective factors in child, family, and social environment that enable a child to be resilient to the effects of disability. Bedell, Cohn, and Dumas described a "Building Friendship Approach" in which collaborative student-centered school teams (student, school personnel, family, and friends) identify strategies for improving the social opportunities of the student with brain injury.[16] The team helps the student generate his or her own solutions and set goals to improve his or her social opportunities. This approach appears to be effective but the outcomes need to be monitored to ensure that they are maintained.

Research on psychosocial approaches is difficult to review because of its scope and because of the variety of types of practice and their implementation across different disciplines. Evidence in the literature supporting the use of specific approaches is minimal. Studies on the effectiveness of social

TABLE 2-3 Occupational Therapy Interventions Designed to Improve Social Skills

Therapeutic Activity	Targeted Group
Yoga Dyads Children hold hands and cooperate with a partner to perform yoga poses and actions. They experience touch, movement, and mindfulness in a group setting. Emphasis on movement, balance, breathing, meditation.	School-age children with behavioral problems; children at risk who experience increased stress (e.g., disadvantaged homes).
Arts and Crafts Groups These groups work together cooperatively, sharing materials and conversation. Usually they work together to create one product.	School-age children with low social skills; can include Asperger's syndrome, behavioral problems, children at risk.
Social Skills Groups Groups meet to practice conversation skills, social norms, social conventions. These groups generally have themes that can be determined by the group (e.g. sharing information on favorite music bands)	Middle school or high school youth with delayed social skills; can include Asperger's syndrome, high-functioning autism, intellectual impairment.
Cooking Groups These groups often plan a meal, budget the meal, shop for the food items, prepare the meal together, and then eat together.	Middle school or high school youth with delayed social skills; can include high-functioning autism or intellectual impairment. Generally for youth who will require support in employment and community living.
Job Coaching Occupational therapist may help to design the social supports needed for a youth or young adult to succeed at a job.	Youth or young adults with autism, intellectual impairment, or significant behavioral problems.

skills training have been conducted with school-age children with brain injury,[74] depression,[66,152] schizophrenia,[80] and autism.[24,83] Although many of these studies have methodologic limitations, the results seem to offer support for social skills interventions in improving self-esteem, positive affect, problem-solving, and social behaviors.

Motor Learning and Skill Acquisition

Motor learning as a model of practice focuses on helping the child achieve goal-directed functional actions. It may initially appear to be a skill-building approach, because the focus is on the acquisition of skills involved in movement and balance. However, motor learning is actually an occupation-based approach, because it is directed toward the search for a motor solution that emerges from an interaction of the child with the task and the environment.

When a child is learning a new functional task, a general movement structure is brought into place that takes into consideration the relationship involving the child's movement capabilities, the environmental conditions, and the action goal. When the task is performed repeatedly, these correspondences become more refined, and the goal is achieved more successfully. Specific processes, such as muscle contraction patterns, stabilization and positioning of joints, and response to gravity and other forces, are only crudely organized at first. However, with continued practice, these become more organized and finely tuned.[69] These patterns are called *movement synergies*, or *coordinative structures*, and they represent the child's preferred strategy for solving a task in the most energy-efficient way.[180]

Children with motor programming and motor control deficits often have difficulty establishing the timing and sequencing of functional synergies. Task and activity demands may vary, and each of these dimensions is relevant to the way in which tasks are learned. These characteristics of a task determine what motor learning strategies are used to improve performance.

1. *Simple-complex*. Simple tasks, such as reaching for an object, require a decision followed by a sequenced response. Complex tasks, such as handwriting, require the integration of information from a variety of sources and the application of underlying rules that guide performance.

2. *Open loop–closed loop*. In an open-loop task, a motor program is put into place before the action begins and is not modified during the performance of a task. An example of an open-loop task is throwing a ball. In a closed-loop task, the child continues to monitor and respond to feedback that he or she receives intrinsically from the body and extrinsically from the environment. An example of a closed-loop task is cutting out a shape using scissors.[1]

3. *Environment changing–environment stationary*. The difficulty of learning a task is tremendously influenced by the extent to which the task is predictable. When the environment is changeable or variable, the child has to learn the movement and learn to monitor the environment to adapt to change. Running on rough terrain and playing soccer are examples of tasks in which the environment is constantly changing. This concept is not to be confused with the open- and closed-loop features of the task previously described. Brushing the teeth and playing the piano are tasks during which the child must monitor sensory feedback (closed loop), but the environment remains stationary.[177]

4. *Task characteristics*. The ease or difficulty of learning a task depends on the match between the way the task is presented and the preferred learning style of the child. Some children learn best through auditory or visual methods; others prefer movement and touch.

Different types of feedback contribute to the motor learning process. Feedback is *intrinsic* when it is produced by the child's sensory systems and is inherent in a task. An example of intrinsic feedback is information available to the child through vision, proprioception, sensation, or kinesthesia. *Extrinsic* feedback is provided to the child by an external source, such as the therapist, or by observing the results of one's actions.[136,169] *Knowledge of results* is a type of extrinsic feedback in which the therapist provides information to the child about the relationship between the actions and the goal, but only after the fact. For example, a child who is throwing a basketball toward the hoop may be told that the ball is not going high enough and therefore is missing the hoop. *Knowledge of performance* is a type of extrinsic feedback that emphasizes the pattern of movement and its relationship to achievement of the task. In the same example, the child may be told that he is not extending his arms far enough before releasing the ball. In both cases, the therapist's feedback focuses on the outcome of the action, not on the child's effort. These terms are further explained in Chapter 9.

Research on the scheduling, frequency, and amount of feedback that best promote learning has been published.[102,178] Studies have shown that immediate extrinsic feedback may prevent the learner from paying attention to the intrinsic sources of feedback that are always available, such as vision and proprioception. This lack of attention to intrinsic feedback may make the learner dependent on information from the person providing instruction.[167]

Very little research has focused on the effect of different types of feedback on task performance with children experiencing occupational performance difficulties. However, research investigating motor learning principles with children with movement difficulties has suggested that these children may not solve movement problems in a typical way. The research suggests that extrinsic sources of feedback that focus a child's attention on specific aspects of the task and on important sensory cues may be important.[103]

Another important concept in motor learning is the influence of different types of practice on learning and performance. There is no question that practice of a task is beneficial to learning. The difficulty confronting most therapists is the dilemma of whether to practice the *whole* task or only *parts* or components of the task. Study results indicate that the benefits of practicing either the whole task or parts of the task depend on the inherent goals of the task.[169] If coordination or timing of the parts is important to the task, whole-task practice is more effective for learning. Examples of these continuous types of tasks are walking, swinging at a ball, and bicycling. If a task contains distinct parts that can be performed in a serial manner, these can be practiced as parts of the task. A child learning to don his jacket can be taught how to zip it as a first step. Most occupations involving movement are actually a combination of continuous and discrete tasks (Figure 2-7). Consequently, doing the whole task must follow learning its parts. In learning to ride a tricycle, for example, the child can focus on learning to pedal separately from steering, but he or she must then combine them.

Another important consideration in planning practice sessions is the use of random versus blocked practice. During random practice, the environmental conditions vary slightly each time; blocked practice involves drilling the task over and over in the same way. In most cases, random practice produces better learning, because the variable practice allows the child to solve a slightly different movement "problem" every time.[102]

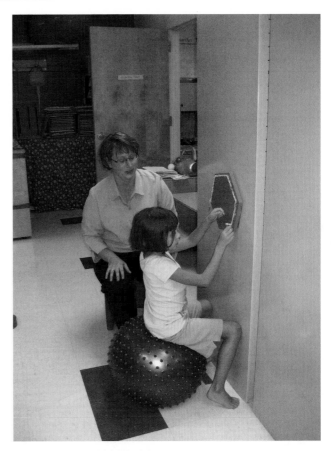

FIGURE 2-7 This activity of threading a string through hooks to create a design involves eye-hand coordination, dexterity, and control of arm in space (strength). It requires multiple steps to achieve a completed product.

Some of the key techniques that therapists use in this model of practice are giving verbal instructions and demonstrating movement strategies. Verbal instructions focus on the relationship between the child and the objects in the environment and emphasize key movement features directly related to achievement of the functional goal.[69] Physical or manual guidance can be helpful during the initial teaching of a movement because it may clarify the goal, guide selective attention, and help the child organize and plan the movement (Figure 2-8). Researchers stress that guidance or facilitation of movement should be removed as soon as possible, arguing that the therapist rapidly becomes part of the environment, which alters the performance context and the intrinsic feedback available to the child.[69]

Motor learning researchers[137,178,200] recognize that learning takes place only when there is evidence of a relatively permanent change in the child's ability to respond to a movement problem or to achieve a movement goal. The learning of a new motor skill needs to be evaluated through tests of retention and transfer, not just immediate changes in performance.[112] Therefore, therapists who use a motor learning model of practice must create opportunities for the child to demonstrate their learning during a subsequent therapy session (retention), on a closely related task (transfer), or in a different setting (generalization). Table 2-4 summarizes motor

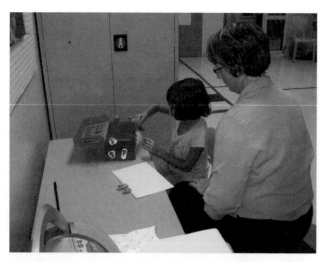

FIGURE 2-8 In this task emphasizing bilateral coordination and hand strength, the therapist suggests an outcome but the child decides what she wants to create.

learning concepts, with examples of application in occupational therapy intervention.

Occupational therapists use theories about motor learning to promote development in areas of function that involve learning complex skills and behaviors. Self-care and handwriting are examples of areas of occupational performance to which occupational therapists have applied a motor learning approach. Handwriting is an area of occupational performance in which a motor learning or acquisitional approach has been advocated (see Chapter 19). Although few studies of the effectiveness of this approach to handwriting have been published, many remedial or practice-based handwriting programs are commercially available. A few published studies have demonstrated that the use of acquisitional principles by therapists and educators in a positive, interesting, and dynamic learning environment promotes the development of handwriting.[15,129] Some handwriting studies provide therapists and educators with strategies for remediation that use some of the concepts previously listed.[18,52] Further research is needed to determine the effectiveness of this approach with different populations of

TABLE 2-4 Application of Motor Learning Concepts

Concept	Definition	Application
Specificity of learning	Practice experiences that result in the fastest learning and best skill retention are those that most closely approximate the entire task in the child's natural context. It is the task, not preexisting practice of components, that assembles the emerging skill.	Child who are learning dressing skills should practice in the context of natural dressing opportunities (e.g., after toileting, when going outside to the playground) rather than practicing components such as a buttoning using a button strip on a table.
Implicit learning	Improvement in performance results from experiences with a task without specific attention to or awareness of a change in performance. Therefore, success is not always necessary for learning.	Children can learn from participating in tasks without explicit reinforcement for their performance and without explicit recognition of the change in their performance. Success in every intervention task is not necessary.
Maximizing opportunity for practice	Repetition is essential for acquisition of motor skills. The most important variable in a training program has been found to be the amount of practice.	Children require guidance and reinforcement to practice a motor skill. It is difficult to dedicate large portions of an intervention session to practice; therefore, it is critical to identify opportunities for the child to practice a new skill across his daily routine.
Blocked and random practice	Blocked practice is repeated practice of the same action many times (e.g., a drill). Random practice is a practice sequence in which the related tasks of a skill are performed in no particular order. Blocked practice may be useful in initial learning, but random practice results in better learning.	When teaching a new skill such as in-hand manipulation, the therapist designs intervention activities so that the child has intermittent but frequent opportunities to rotate or translate objects within the hand (e.g., rotate pencil to erase, game with small pieces, resistive lacing).
Distribution of practice	Learning increases in distributed practice (practice with rest periods) when compared to massed practice.	Competence in a new skill is reached when it is practiced each week for 5-10 minutes rather than spending a 30-minute session practicing a single skill.
Extrinsic feedback	Extrinsic feedback is the information about performance that the therapist gives the child. Extrinsic feedback has been found to improve motivation and to reduce error. Extrinsic feedback is useful to beginners, who may not yet be able to interpret their performance. More frequent feedback is helpful in early learning, and intermittent feedback is better in later learning.	Extrinsic feedback that has been found to improve performance includes information about the adequacy of the child's performance, how long the child will have to persist in the task before the activity ends, and the therapist's pleasure in the child's performance.
Transfer of learning	New learning must be applied consistently in a variety of environments.	Learning transfers optimally to a variety of environments when it is learned and practiced in the child natural routines and environments.

Adapted from Sheppard, J. J. (2008). Using motor learning approaches for treating swallowing and feeding disorders: A review. *Language, Speech, and Hearing Services in Schools, 39,* 227-236.

children across a broad range of skills and areas of occupational performance.

To summarize, a therapist using a motor learning model of practice:

1. Analyzes the movement synergies the child uses to achieve the functional action goal
2. Considers the child's stage of learning and determines how best to facilitate the provision of both extrinsic and intrinsic feedback to improve the efficiency of the movement
3. Provides opportunities for optimal practice of the goal and encourages practice in the natural environment
4. Promotes independent performance and decision making as soon as possible and evaluates whether the motor learning has been acquired, transferred, and generalized

Neurodevelopmental Theory

Historically, the primary concept underpinning a neurodevelopmental therapy (NDT) approach to practice was that normal postural reactions are necessary for normal movement and that these postural reactions are for the most part automatic.[23] Although this intervention approach continues to focus on problems in postural control and motor coordination, as seen in cerebral palsy, the principles underlying the treatment approach have expanded to include motor learning and dynamic systems theories. In addition, NDT principles have shifted to recognize the importance of the environment and to place more emphasis on activities that are clearly functional and meaningful to the child.[82]

When using this approach to evaluate a child, the therapist analyzes the child's movements to identify missing or atypical muscular-skeletal elements that create functional limitations. These missing elements become one focus of intervention and are used to select the developmental level of therapeutic activities. Therapeutic handling is integral to the NDT approach and is used to facilitate postural control and movement synergies and to inhibit or constrain motor patterns that, if practiced, would lead to secondary deformities and dysfunction.[82] A therapist applying NDT strategies focuses on changing movement patterns to achieve the most energy-efficient performance for the individual in the context of age-appropriate tasks.

As the therapist manually guides and handles the child in the context of an activity, these elements are always combined with the child's active participation. With the therapist's guidance, the child practices sequences of movements in slightly different ways to reinforce learning of the task. This practice is important for making a movement strategy functional and automatic. Therapists emphasize quality of movement (e.g., accuracy, quickness, adaptability, and fluency). Although therapeutic handling remains an integral part of NDT, practitioners use many treatment methods, "manipulating the individual task or the environment in order to positively influence function" (p. 63).[82]

Acknowledging that NDT principles have changed over the years to incorporate theories of motor learning and dynamic systems theory, clinical evaluation studies of the neurodevelopmental therapy approach (many of which were completed more than 10 years ago) have raised questions about its efficacy. Comparison studies of this approach for children with cerebral palsy have been conducted over the past 30 years. In these studies, the NDT approach has been compared with functional therapy,[166,174] with infant stimulation,[141] with Vojta therapy,[48] and with differing intensities of therapy.[98,121] The results of these trials have been mixed, with two demonstrating no difference,[99,174] two supporting NDT,[121,166] and two supporting alternate treatments.[48,141] The more rigorous randomized clinical trials have generally produced results that do not support the efficacy of the neurodevelopmental approach.[146]

A recent systematic review of NDT concluded that "the preponderance of results....do not confer any advantage to NDT over alternatives to which it was compared" (p. 789).[28] The only consistent effect of NDT that was statistically significant was an immediate effect on range of motion. In contrast with NDT methods, the motor-based interventions that produce meaningful improvements in functional outcomes for children with disabilities incorporate three essential elements: (1) intensive task repetition, (2) progressive challenges to the learner with increasing difficulty, and (3) the presence of motivators and rewards.[137,165] Despite lack of evidence on efficacy,[165] NDT remains a widely used approach with children who have cerebral palsy and CNS dysfunction affecting motor performance. Because the conceptual basis of NDT has evolved over the past decade, a first step in additional research on its efficacy would be to operationalize the new concepts into treatment protocols that can be measured and replicated for research purposes.

Sensory Integration

The theory of sensory integration, together with the treatment approach derived from that theory, grew from the work of Jean Ayres.[3-5] Ayres developed her theory in an effort to explain behaviors observed in children with learning difficulties based on neural functioning. Specifically, she hypothesized that some children with learning difficulties experience problems in "organizing sensory information for use."[4] She named this neural process *sensory integration*.

Much of Ayres' work, and that of her colleagues, was devoted to the development of evaluation tools that could clearly identify individuals with sensory integrative problems. The Sensory Integration and Praxis Tests (SIPT) are the result of this work.[8] Included in this area of identification and evaluation are a number of studies aimed at describing different subtypes of sensory integrative problems (see Chapter 11 for a summary). Based on current confirmatory studies, these identified subtypes that can be identified by the SIPT include (1) visual and tactile perception with praxis, (2) vestibular and proprioceptive processing with bilateral functions, (3) attention and tactile defensiveness, and (4) visual and tactile discrimination.[134]

In recent years, scholars in sensory integration have further described sensory integration processes[55] and categorized sensory integration disorders.[125] Miller and colleagues proposed three patterns of sensory processing disorder, described in Table 2-5.

Although there is some overlap in these disorders, each suggests a specific type of intervention. Dunn's work identifying children with a sensory modulation disorder has shown that they have patterns of poor registration of sensation, are hypersensitive to stimuli, avoid certain sensations, or seek particular inputs.[53] These sensory processing patterns may be present in children with a variety of developmental disorders, and they are often

TABLE 2-5 Sensory Processing Disorder Categories

Pattern	Subtypes	Definition
Sensory modulation disorder	Overresponsivity Underresponsivity Sensory seeking	Child has difficulty responding to sensory input with behavior that is graded relative to the degree, nature, or intensity of the sensory information. Emotional and attentional responses to sensory input do not match typical adaptive responses.
Sensory discrimination disorder	Visual Auditory Tactile Vestibular Proprioception Taste/smell	Child has difficulty interpreting qualities of sensory stimuli and similarities and differences among stimuli. Emphasis is on discrimination of tactile, proprioceptive, and vestibular systems. Relates to the development of body scheme.
Sensory-based motor disorder	Postural disorder Dyspraxia	Child has poor postural stability, with poor balance and hypotonic muscle tone. Child with dyspraxia has impaired motor planning (i.e., has impaired ability to conceive of, plan, sequence, and execute novel actions).

Adapted from Miller, L., Anzalone, M., Lane, S., Cermak, S., & Osten, B. (2007). Typology and terminology of sensory integration. *American Journal of Occupational Therapy, 61*(2), 135-140.

described in children with pervasive developmental disorders or autism.[14,88,183,191] Dunn and colleagues have developed evaluation tools for identifying sensory processing problems in children and adults.[54,56,63] A number of authors have proposed intervention programs to address sensory modulation disorders.[128,164,198] Although there is significant intuitive appeal for sensory modulation disorders as explanatory models for children's observed behaviors, more research is required to validate these theories and to investigate appropriate interventions.

Ayres also developed interventions that she believed would help to resolve sensory integration problems. She proposed an intervention approach based on assumptions drawn from neuromaturation theory and systems theory.[4,7] Neuromaturation concepts, such as hierarchical organization of cortical and subcortical areas, developmental sequence of learning and skill acquisition, and neural plasticity, are essential to an understanding of the mechanisms of sensory integration. Systems theory also underlies sensory integration because the focus is on the child seeking sensory input and using adaptive behavior as an organizer of the input. Figure 2-9 shows a child's choice of activity. Based on these assumptions, a sensory integration approach seeks to provide the child with enhanced opportunities for controlled sensory input, with a particular emphasis on vestibular, proprioceptive, and tactile input, in the context of meaningful activity. In intervention the therapist facilitates an adaptive response, which requires the child to integrate the sensory information (Figure 2-10). Sensory integration is hypothesized to improve through this process.

Ayres[5,9,10] and Miller[126] have conducted research aimed at evaluating the process of sensory integration and determining the efficacy of sensory integration intervention (see Chapter 11). In a recent study, a group of scholars examined the research literature on sensory integration to develop a fidelity measure for sensory integration intervention.[143] This study involved a comprehensive review of the research literature and produced a definition of the core elements of sensory integration intervention that will be useful to future trials (see Table 2-6).

Early work by Ayres[5,6] and others[9,139] had reported positive changes resulting from sensory integration intervention in such outcomes as motor, academic, and language performance. Studies in the late 1980s and the 1990s evaluated the

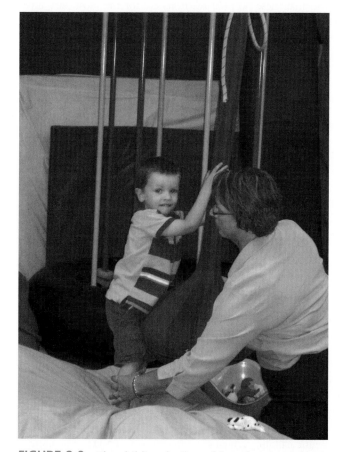

FIGURE 2-9 The child's selection of jumping on an inner tube helps to meet his need for vestibular and proprioceptive input.

efficacy of sensory integration intervention using more rigorous methods, including randomized controlled trials. Using meta-analysis techniques, Vargas and Camilli found that early efficacy studies of sensory integration produced large positive effects, but studies conducted after 1982 did not yield significant positive effects.[187] The more recent studies of sensory

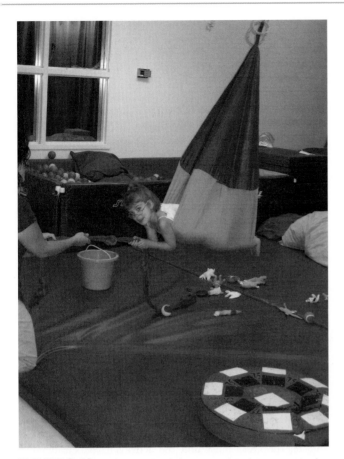

FIGURE 2-10 This child exhibits an adaptive response by pulling on the rope.

integration intervention have demonstrated effects equal to those of alternative treatments in the participants' psychoeducational and motor performance areas, with no improvement noted in sensory perceptual areas.[187]

Recent studies using rigorous methods have shown positive effects of sensory integration interventions. In a randomized trial comparing sensory integration intervention to an activity protocol or no treatment, Miller, Coll, and Schoen assigned 24 children with sensory modulation disorders to one of three groups.[126] The children in the sensory integration group and the activity group received intervention twice a week for 10 weeks, and the control group children were placed on a wait list for intervention. Those in the sensory integration intervention group made significant gains on goal attainment scaling and in attention, cognition, and social performance as measured by the Leiter International Performance Scale. Other measures of child behavior, sensory processing, and electrodermal reactivity improved in the sensory integration group but did not differ when the sensory integration group was compared with the activity and control groups. Miller et al. suggested that a larger sample was needed to detect significant differences in these measures.[126]

Although sensory integration research typically has demonstrated only small positive effects, sensory integration intervention is widely practiced by occupational therapists and is a powerful force in clinical reasoning in the field of pediatrics. In a survey of occupational therapists working with children with autism, fully 99% of the therapists reported using sensory integration techniques with their clients.[190] More recent research has also included parents' perceptions of change in their children and in themselves as a result of occupational therapy that used sensory integration intervention.[38,39] Parents reported positive changes in their children's social participation, perceived competence, and self-regulation. The parents

---

TABLE 2-6 Core Elements of Sensory Integration Intervention

Core Element	Explanation
Provide sensory opportunities	The therapist provides opportunities for the child to experience intense sensory experiences, including tactile, vestibular, and/or proprioceptive input, generally in combination.
Provide "just right" challenges	Activities are developmentally appropriate and challenge the child to exhibit a higher level skill than typical performance. The challenge presented evokes an adaptive response for the child.
Collaborate on activity choice and guide self-organization	Child is an active collaborator in the therapy session. The child selects activities and is encouraged to initiate activities. The therapist supports and guides the child in organizing his or her behavior, making choices, and planning activities.
Support optimal arousal and arrange room to engage child	During the session, the therapist supports the child's optimal arousal and attention, engagement, and comfort. The room is arranged to engage the child's attention and help him or her modulate sensory responses.
Create play context	The therapist creates a play context, building on the child's intrinsic motivation using activities that the child enjoys.
Maximize child's success	The therapist presents and modifies activities so that the child's adaptive response is successful.
Ensure physical safety	The therapist ensures that the child is physically safe by using protective equipment and by maintaining physical proximity to the child.
Foster therapeutic alliance	The therapist conveys positive regard toward the child and makes efforts to build the child's trust.

Adapted from Parham, L. D., Cohn, E. S., Spitzer, S., Koomar, J. A., Miller, L. M., et al. (2007). Fidelity in sensory integration intervention research. *American Journal of Occupational Therapy, 61*, 216-227.

valued the new understanding of the child's behavior and used this perspective to support and advocate for the child more effectively. Ayres' work has had a significant impact on occupational therapy practice with children, and its controversial nature has led to an increased sophistication and rigor in the scholarly work accomplished in the field of occupational therapy.

Developmental Approaches

During the 1960s and 1970s, occupational therapists working with children had a strong developmental perspective. These theories attempted to explain the functioning and growth of children and adolescents from an occupational therapy perspective. Perhaps the best-known occupational therapy theorist of this time was Lela Llorens. She identified a developmental frame of reference that focused on the physical, social, and psychologic aspects of life tasks and relationships.[105,106] Llorens viewed the role of the occupational therapist to be one of facilitating development and assisting in the mastery of life tasks and the ability to cope with life expectations. Chapter 3 explains developmental theories used in occupational therapy.

The section on developmental theories presented earlier in this chapter provides a broad basis for occupational therapy evaluation and intervention. Specifically, the theories of Piaget[145] form a foundation for the spatiotemporal adaptation model of practice.[73] Piaget explained that the adaptation process has four components: assimilation, accommodation, association, and differentiation. *Assimilation* is the reception of sensory stimuli from internal and external environments. *Accommodation* is the motor response to these stimuli. *Association* is the organized process of relating current sensory information with the current motor response and then relating this relationship to past responses. *Differentiation* is the process of identifying the specific elements in a child's situation that are useful and relevant to another situation to refine the responsive pattern. Based on prior experience, the child develops a sense of what is useful and what is not useful to motor activity in the current situation. In this view of development, the child is continually modifying older, more primitive behaviors for effective motor responses, rather than continually acquiring new skills. The spatiotemporal adaptation model of practice[73] views development as a spiraling process, moving from simple to complex. Adaptation is a continuous process of interaction involving the individual, time, and space. This model became central to occupational therapists' view of child development and fostered the development of intervention models.

Recent theories and models of development in the occupational therapy literature incorporate new concepts of PEO relationships, dynamic systems theories, and lifespan changes. Instead of focusing on different components of functioning, such as motor, social, or cognitive development, occupational therapy theorists are addressing the development of occupation across the lifespan.[49,84,86]

Two emerging occupational perspectives on development remain in the conceptual and exploratory stages of theory development and require further research and validation. In one of these proposals, Humphry suggests a dynamic system perspective in a model of developmental processes.[84,85] A child's occupational development is based on complex, reciprocal, and nonlinear relationships involving the child's innate characteristics and environmental factors. Humphry proposes that children learn

through three broad mechanisms. First, communities invest in children by developing programs, places, and opportunities for social engagement that enable them to participate in community life. Examples of community investment in child development include (1) child care centers that allow children with disabilities to attend their programming, (2) play spaces that use universal design allowing all children to use them, and (3) educational programs that encourage the participation of families with young children. Communities that are invested in child development support human resources, child-care centers, educational programs, and spaces that encourage healthy development and learning in children of all abilities. A second mechanism of child development are interpersonal influences (i.e., the social opportunities for children to interact with others). Children learn by observing others perform activity, through play with other children and adults, and through adults teaching and modeling for them. These social mechanisms are the catalyst for much of a child's learning. Humphry noted that vicarious learning through observation of others can be as important as direct teaching.[85] Children also learn through shared occupations such as circle time or group activities in preschool. Occupational therapists need to recognize the complexity of children's learning across domains when children participate in groups.

Although vicarious learning in social situations is important to development, a third mechanism, doing, is equally important. When engaging in a novel activity, the child reorganizes learned skills, adapts skills on the basis of trial and error, and tries new actions to accomplish the activity. Fully engaging in an activity is an important catalyst to learning. To completely engage, the child must find the activity to be meaningful, fun, and challenging. These concepts about development of performance imply that children learn in social contexts and that engagement in activity results in learning. A variety of adult roles are implied by these concepts, including designing group activities, creating learning environments, modeling, encouraging, supporting, and guiding.

Occupational therapy approaches have logically evolved from theories and concepts of psychology, education, neuroscience, and other fields. These practice models guide interventions that consider the child, his or occupations, the environment, and the interactions of these elements. Practitioners recognize that theories are overlapping and complementary. To meet the individual needs of the children they serve, they use theoretical concepts specific to certain problems but also in combination. Occupational therapists seek evidence regarding each practice model's effectiveness in making decisions about which model to implement.

CLINICAL APPLICATION EXAMPLES

In this section, three case studies are used to outline the different assessment and intervention strategies and expected outcomes for the models of practice discussed in the preceding section. The examples include a young child with cerebral palsy (Case Study 2-2), a school-aged child with DCD (Case Study 2-3), and an adolescent with sensory modulation and behavioral problems (Case Study 2-4). For each example, the most commonly used approaches are selected for the clinical situation. These choices do not mean that other approaches cannot be used, but they are applied less often.

CASE STUDY 2-2 Stacey

Stacey is a 4-year-old girl who has cerebral palsy with moderate quadriplegia. She is able to walk short distances using a walker. She has difficulty controlling the movement of her arms and hands. Her parents have set current goals for Stacey that include participation in dressing tasks, drawing and cutting skills in preparation for kindergarten activities, and increased participation with peers in play. In this example, the focus is on the goal of participation in dressing and improved drawing and cutting skills (Table 2-7).

TABLE 2-7 Assessments, Interventions, and Expected Outcomes for Stacey

Practice Model	Assessment Strategy	Professional Reasoning Used to Explain Client Problem	Professional Reasoning Used to Guide Intervention and Predict Outcome	Expected Outcome
Dynamic systems	Stacey's spontaneous posture and movement during functional activities are observed. Physical assessment of muscle tone, postural alignment, balance, coordination, and potential for change is completed. Ability to perform specific tasks, such as dressing and drawing, is assessed. Environment supports and constraints are identified.	Postural and movement impairments are restricting Stacey's ability to perform functional activities and to move efficiently throughout her environment. She appears to have the cognitive skills needed to learn new methods for approaching tasks. Environmental supports include her parents' interest in her learning and development and reasonable expectations.	The therapist selects specific tasks that Stacey performs inconsistently but is interested in doing. In a task such as pulling up pants after toileting, the therapist would use Stacey's cognitive strengths (ability to follow multiple-step directions and motor planning) to facilitate posture and movement to increase balance and weight bearing. Strategies include using an external support (handbar) and giving her extra time after toileting. Intervention included activities for hand strength and coordination to improve her ability to fasten her pants. Repetition and practice reinforce the new learning.	Stacey will pull up and snap her pants after toileting or during dressing. She will problem-solve how to do this in unfamiliar environments.
Motor learning	Observe the motor requirements of various play situations in the preschool. Observe functional skills such as eating and dressing.	Stacey has difficulty controlling the movement of her arms and hands; she also has difficulty using two hands together with coordination. Often the feedback she receives from movement is negative (e.g., she fails in activity). The goals include that Stacey will participate in play situations more easily. She will draw basic shapes (e.g., square and triangle). She will use two hands together to cut with scissors.	Therapist will identify movement positions or transitions necessary for play. Therapist will set up the environment to facilitate practice of these. During practice, therapist will use verbal instruction or physical guidance to improve performance. She will reinforce Stacey's performance with praise and rewards. In a task such as drawing, the therapist provides a glitter marker so that a simple drawing becomes a lovely picture.	Stacey will learn to use intrinsic and extrinsic feedback effectively to guide movement. With the therapist's praise and a completed product, she will practice drawing and cutting often and will be focused in her attempts to improve.

CASE STUDY 2-3 Brian

Brian is a 9-year-old boy with DCD. He is isolated from his peers at school, is clumsy, has difficulty performing any tasks requiring handwriting, is poorly organized, and has trouble staying on task (Table 2-8). A COPM was completed with

Brian, and he identified the following occupational performance issues:
1. Disorganized written work; illegible handwriting
2. Difficulty getting out for recess on time

TABLE 2-8 Assessments, Interventions, and Expected Outcomes for Brian

Practice Model	Assessment Strategy	Professional Reasoning Used to Explain Client Problem	Professional Reasoning Used to Guide Intervention and Predict Outcome	Expected Outcome
Cognitive approaches	Observations and interviewing to analyze Brian's performance. The therapist also interviews him using the Canadian Occupational Performance Measure. The therapist identifies the specific strategies he uses or does not use and notes the points at which he appears to get "stuck."	Brian does not know the strategies he needs to complete each task effectively and/or he is unable to select appropriate strategies to achieve his goal.	Using guided discovery and mediation, it is possible to teach Brian to generalize organizational strategies that will help him organize his desk, his written work, and the sequence in which he dons his outdoor clothing for recess.	Brian will be able to implement task-specific strategies that will help him organize any task that has multiple parts or that requires a sequence of actions. Brian will be able to generalize these strategies to other settings and transfer them to other tasks.
Compensatory/task	Observation of the classroom materials and procedures that are in place for each task. Discussion of options with the teacher for making each task easier for Brian.	Brian currently does not have the skills needed to cope with the demands of the task. Each task needs to be adapted to ensure his success in the classroom.	Brian will be provided with modified materials that will help him organize his desk (e.g., color-coded notebooks to match textbooks; colored schedule on the wall), his written output (e.g., raised lined paper), and his locker (e.g., sequence of instructions posted on locker door.)	With modifications in place, Brian will become more successful at performing these tasks. This will ultimately improve his ability to complete tasks efficiently and to participate with his peers. Over time, other interventions can be used to improve his skills
Sensory integration	Assess Brian, using tools such as the Sensory Integration and Praxis Tests (SIPT) and Clinical Observation of Motor and Postural Skills (COMPS) and observing him in classroom, playground, and home Interview Brian, his teacher, and his parents.	Brian is not integrating sensory input from different sensory systems effectively, leading to maladaptive responses and limiting the development of new skills and the ability to respond effectively to environmental demands.	Provide controlled sensory input—in particular tactile, vestibular, and proprioceptive—to Brian with a demand for an adaptive response through goal-directed, meaningful play activities. This will facilitate sensory integration.	Brian will interact more effectively with his environment; should generalize to all environments as he progresses. Outcome would be a closer relationship between environmental expectations and Brian's performance or response.

TABLE 2-8   Assessments, Interventions, and Expected Outcomes for Brian—Cont'd

Practice Model	Assessment Strategy	Professional Reasoning Used to Explain Client Problem	Professional Reasoning Used to Guide Intervention	Expected Outcome
Sensory processing	Use observation and interview, checklists (e.g., Sensory Profile) to review Brian's behavior and history in different environments; look for patterns of behaviors potentially indicating underlying difficulties processing or modulating sensory input	Brian's behavior and functioning reflect processing/modulation abilities. He is seeking to modulate input to the CNS through various sensory systems.	Modify task and environmental factors to alter sensory experience for Brian, work toward his taking responsibility to do this himself. Increase his awareness of what he needs and how to get it in a functional activity and/or socially acceptable manner. Some believe in use of specific sensory input (e.g., deep pressure) to change the child's CNS state, but there is minimal evidence to support this at present.	Improved modulation of sensory input will prepare Brian for learning and help him to benefit from classroom teaching and participation in school activities.

CASE STUDY 2-4   Chris

Chris is a 15-year-old high school student who is currently struggling to complete grade 10. He has dropped one subject in the current year and has been labeled an underachiever. He has difficulty taking notes in class and reorganizing his work. He has been referred to a community psychiatric service because of problems with low mood, lack of motivation in his academic and social life, poor social adjustment, and disturbed family relations.

His parents complain that Chris regularly lies to them about petty thefts from the home and that hours of confrontation and badgering by them are required to get the truth. They report various other instances of misbehavior. He presents himself as a somewhat disheveled youth who denies any knowledge or insight into his difficulties. His parents are eager in seeking intervention to improve his success in school and his behavior at home (Table 2-9).

TABLE 2-9   Assessments, Interventions, and Expected Outcomes for Chris

Practice Model	Assessment Strategy	Clinical Reasoning Used to Explain Client Problem	Clinical Reasoning Used to Guide Intervention and Predict Outcome	Expected Outcome
Learning/ behavior models	Assessment of school-based "skills" (areas of occupational performance), including handwriting, organization skills.	Chris's acquisitional skills (handwriting, organization) appear to have significant gaps that would benefit from a behavior/learning approach.	Chris's handwriting and organizational skills could improve with an intensive, repetitive program that focuses on the acquisition or learning of these skills. His practice is rewarded with favorite activities after handwriting practice.	Chris identifies a need to improve his handwriting and organization and he is motivated to work on acquiring these skills. He participates in a regular program to improve his handwriting and written productivity.

Continued

TABLE 2-9   Assessments, Interventions, and Expected Outcomes for Chris—Cont'd

Practice Model	Assessment Strategy		Clinical Reasoning Used to Guide	Expected Outcome
Sensory processing	Assessment of Chris's ability to process sensory information (e.g., tactile, vestibular, visual, auditory, proprioceptive). The therapist administers the Adolescent/Adult Sensory Profile.	Chris has difficulty modulating sensory stimuli when the sensory input is intense or combined (i.e., visual and auditory combined). Handwriting skills are affected by poor proprioceptive feedback and low tone in the upper extremities.	If Chris and his teachers develop an awareness of his sensory processing challenges, he will be able to develop cognitive strategies for coping with intense sensory input. A handwriting program that emphasizes enhanced proprioceptive input may improve his speed and automaticity.	Chris and his teachers will develop strategies for modulating sensory stimuli at school that will enable him to focus more on the tasks of schoolwork. Handwriting speed and legibility improve.
Compensatory/ environmental	Assessment of Chris's current environment and the fit of environmental demands with his skill level.	The demands of the school environment are not matched to Chris's skills, resulting in anxiety and behavioral problems. The family is concerned and confused about Chris's behavior	If Chris becomes more aware of his difficulties in the school environment, he can use compensatory strategies to cope with the demands. Environmental adaptation of difficult tasks and people's expectations is needed to create a more supportive environment for Chris.	With the development of compensatory strategies and environmental adaptations, the person-environment fit will improve. Chris will experience increased satisfaction with his school performance. Family and teacher education will help his parents understand his difficulties and will increase use of supportive strategies.

REFERENCES

1. Adams, J. A. (1971). A closed-loop theory of motor learning. *Journal of Motor Behavior, 3,* 111–149.
2. American Occupational Therapy Association. (2008). Occupational therapy practice framework: Domain and process (2nd ed.). *American Journal of Occupational Therapy, 62,* 625–683.
3. Ayres, A. J. (1969). Deficits in sensory integration in educationally handicapped children. *Journal of Learning Disabilities, 2,* 160–168.
4. Ayres, A. J. (1972). *Sensory integration and learning disorders.* Los Angeles: Western Psychological Services.
5. Ayres, A. J. (1972). Improving academic scores through sensory integration. *Journal of Learning Disabilities, 5,* 338–343.
6. Ayres, A. J. (1978). Learning disabilities and the vestibular system. *Journal of Learning Disabilities, 11,* 18–29.
7. Ayres, A. J. (1979). *Sensory integration and the child.* Los Angeles: Western Psychological Services.
8. Ayres, A. J. (1989). *Sensory Integration and Praxis Tests.* Los Angeles: Western Psychological Services.
9. Ayres, A. J., & Mailloux, Z. K. (1981). Influence of sensory integrative procedures on language development. *American Journal of Occupational Therapy, 35,* 383–390.
10. Ayres, A. J., & Tickle, L. (1980). Hyperresponsivity to touch and vestibular stimuli as a predictor of positive response to sensory integration procedures in autistic children. *American Journal of Occupational Therapy, 34,* 375–381.
11. Bandura, A. (1993). Perceived self-efficacy in cognitive development and functioning. *Educational Psychologist, 28,* 117–148.
12. Bandura, A. (1997). *Self-efficacy: The exercise of control.* New York: Freeman.
13. Bandura, A., Barbaranelli, C., Caprara, G. V., & Pasatorelli, C. (1996). Multifaceted impact of self-efficacy beliefs on academic functioning. *Child Development, 67,* 1206–1222.
14. Baranek, G. T., Foster, L. G., & Berkson, G. (1997). Sensory defensiveness in persons with developmental disabilities. *Journal of Autism and Developmental Disorders, 29,* 213–224.
15. Barchers, S. I. (1994). *Teaching language arts: An integrated approach.* Minneapolis: West Publishing.
16. Bedell, G. M., Cohn, E. S., & Dumas, H. M. (2005). Exploring parents' use of strategies to promote social participation of school-age children with acquired brain injuries. *American Journal of Occupational Therapy, 59,* 65–75.
17. Bedell, G. M., & Dumas, H. M. (2004). Social participation of children and youth with acquired brain injuries discharged from

inpatient rehabilitation: A follow-up study. *Brian Injury, 18,* 65–82.

18. Bergman, K. E., & McLaughlin, T. F. (1988). Remediating handwriting difficulties with learning disabled students: A review. *Journal of Special Education, 12,* 101–120.

19. Bernheimer, L. P., & Weisner, T. S. (2007). "Let me just tell you what I do all day...": The family story at the center of intervention research and practice. *Infants & Young Children, 20*(3), 192–201.

20. Bernstein, N. (1967). *Coordination and regulation of movements.* New York: John Wiley & Sons.

21. Bjorklund, D. F., & Green, B. L. (1992). The adaptive nature of cognitive immaturity. *American Psychologist, 47,* 46–54.

22. Blanche, E. I. (2008). Play in children with cerebral palsy: Doing with—not doing to. In D. L. Parham & L. Fazio (Eds.), *Play and occupational therapy* (2nd ed., pp. 375–394). St. Louis: Mosby.

23. Bobath, K. (1980). *A neurophysiological basis for the treatment of cerebral palsy.* London: Heinemann Books.

24. Broderick, C., Caswell, R., Gregory, S., Marzolini, S., & Wilson, O. (2002). "Can I join the club": A social integration scheme for adolescents with Asperger syndrome. *Autism, 5,* 427–431.

25. Bronfenbrenner, U. (1977). Toward an experimental ecology of human development. *American Psychologist, 32,* 513–531.

26. Burton, A. W., & Davis, W. E. (1996). Ecological task analysis: Utilizing intrinsic measures in research and practice. *Human Movement Science, 15,* 285–314.

27. Burton, A. W., & Miller, D. E. (1998). *Movement skill assessment.* Champaign, IL: Human Kinetics.

28. Butler, C., & Darrah, J. (2001). Effects of neurodevelopmental treatment (NDT) for cerebral palsy: An AACPDM evidence report. *Developmental Medicine and Child Neurology, 43*(11), 778–790.

29. Campbell, P. H., Milbourne, S., & Wilcox, M. J. (2008). Adaptation interventions to promote participation in natural settings. *Infants & Young Children, 21,* 94–106.

30. Canadian Association of Occupational Therapists (CAOT). (1997). *Enabling occupation: An occupational therapy perspective.* Ottawa, ON: Canadian Association of Occupational Therapists (CAOT).

31. Case-Smith, J. (1996). Analysis of current motor development theory and recently published infant motor assessments. *Infants and Young Children, 9*(1), 29–41.

32. Deleted in proofs.

33. Christiansen, C., & Baum, C. (1997). *Occupational therapy: Enabling function and well-being.* Thorofare, NJ: Slack.

34. Christiansen, C. H., Clark, F., Kielhofner, G., & Rogers, J. (1995). Position paper: Occupation. *American Journal of Occupational Therapy, 49,* 1015–1018.

35. Christopher, J. S., Nangle, D. W., & Hansen, D. J. (1993). Social skills interventions with adolescents. *Behavior Modification, 17,* 314–338.

36. Clark, F. A., Parham, D., Carlson, M. E., Frank, G., Jackson, J., Pierce, D., et al. (1991). Occupational science: Academic innovation in the service of occupational therapy's future. *American Journal of Occupational Therapy, 45,* 300–310.

37. Cohen, L. B., & Cashon, C. H. (2003). Infant perception and cognition. In R. M. Lerner, M. A. Easterbrooks, & J. Mistry (Eds.), *Handbook of psychology: Developmental psychology* (Vol. 6, pp. 65–90). Hoboken, NJ: John Wiley & Sons, Inc.

38. Cohn, E. S. (2001). Parent perspectives of occupational therapy using a sensory integration approach. *American Journal of Occupational Therapy, 55,* 285–294.

39. Cohn, E., Miller, L. J., & Tickle-Degnen, L. (2000). Parental hopes for therapy outcomes: Children with sensory modulation disorders. *American Journal of Occupational Therapy, 54,* 36–43.

40. Cooper, J. O., Heron, T. E., & Heward, W. L. (2007). *Applied behavior analysis.* Upper Saddle River, NJ: Pearson Merrill Prentice Hall.

41. Coster, W., Deeny, T., Haltiwanger, J., & Haley, S. (1998). *School Function Assessment.* San Antonio, TX: Psychological Corporation.

42. Couch, K. J., Deitz, J. C., & Kanny, E. M. (1998). The role of play in pediatric occupational therapy. *American Journal of Occupational Therapy, 52,* 111–117.

43. Cowan, R. J., & Allen, K. D. (2007). Using naturalistic procedures to enhance learning in individuals with autism: A focus on generalized teaching within the school setting. *Psychology in the Schools, 44,* 701–715.

44. Crepeau, E. B., & Schell, B. A. B. (2008). Analyzing occupations and activity. In E. B. Crepeau, E. S. Cohn, & B. A. B. Schell (Eds.), *Willard & Spackman's occupational therapy* (11th ed., pp. 359–374). Philadelphia: Lippincott Williams & Wilkins.

45. Csikszentmihalyi, M., & Csikszentmihalyi, I. S. (1988). *Optimal experience: Psychological studies in flow in consciousness.* Cambridge, UK: Cambridge University Press.

46. Darrah, J., & Barlett, D. (1995). Dynamic systems theory and management of children with cerebral palsy: unresolved issues. *Infants and Young Children, 8,* 52–59.

47. Darrah, J., Law, M., & Pollock, N. (2001). Innovations in practice: Family-centered functional therapy—a choice for children with motor dysfunction. *Infants and Young Children, 13*(4), 79–87.

48. D'Avignon, M. (1981). Early physiotherapy ad modum Vojta or Bobath in infants with suspected neuromotor disturbance. *Neuropediatrics, 12,* 232–241.

49. Davis, J., & Polatajko, H. (2006). The occupational development of children. In S. Rodger & J. Ziviani (Eds.), *Occupational therapy with children: Understanding children's occupations and enabling participation* (pp. 136–156). Oxford, UK: Blackwell Publishing.

50. DeGrace, B. W. (2003). Occupation-based and family centered care: A challenge for current practice. *American Journal of Occupational Therapy, 57,* 347–350.

51. DeGrace, B. W. (2004). The everyday occupation of families with children with autism. *American Journal of Occupational Therapy, 58,* 543–550.

52. Denton, P., Cope, S., & Moser, C. (2006). Effects of sensorimotor-based intervention versus therapeutic practice on improving handwriting performance in 6-to-11-year-old children. *American Journal of Occupational Therapy, 60,* 16–27.

53. Dunn, W. (1997). The impact of sensory processing abilities on the daily lives of young children and their families: A conceptual model. *Infants and Young Children, 9,* 23–35.

54. Dunn, W. (1999). *The Sensory Profile User's Manual.* San Antonio, TX: Psychological Corporation.

55. Dunn, W. (2001). The sensations of everyday life: Empirical, theoretical, and pragmatic considerations. *American Journal of Occupational Therapy, 66,* 608–620.

56. Dunn, W., & Brown, C. (1997). Factor analysis on the sensory profile from a national sample of children without disabilities. *American Journal of Occupational Therapy, 51,* 490–495.

57. Dunn, W., Brown, C., & McGuigan, A. (1994). The ecology of human performance: A framework for considering the effect of context. *American Journal of Occupational Therapy, 48,* 595–607.

58. Dunst, C. J., Trivette, C. M., Davis, M., & Cornwall, J. (1988). Enabling and empowering families of children with health impairments. *Child Health Care, 17,* 71–81.

59. Dunst, C., Trivette, C., & Deal, A. (1994). *Supporting and strengthening families: Methods, strategies and practices.* Cambridge, MA: Brookline Books.

60. Dunton, W. R. (1919). *Reconstruction therapy.* Philadelphia: W.B. Saunders.

61. Engel-Yeger, B., Jarus, T., Anaby, D., & Law, M. (2009). Differences in patterns of participation between youths with cerebral palsy and typically developing peers. *American Journal of Occupational Therapy, 63,* 96–104.

62. Engle, P. L., Castle, S., & Meno, P. (1996). Child development: Vulnerability and resilience. *Social Science and Medicine, 43*(5), 621–635.

63. Ermer, J., & Dunn, W. (1997). The Sensory Profile: A discriminant analysis of children with and without disabilities. *American Journal of Occupational Therapy, 51,* 283–290.

64. Evans, J. L. (2002). Variability in comprehension strategy use in children with SLI: A dynamical systems account. *International Journal of Language and Communication Disorders, 37*(2), 95–116.

65. Fidler, G. S., & Fidler, J. W. (1978). Doing and becoming: Purposeful action and self-actualization. *American Journal of Occupational Therapy, 32,* 305–310.

66. Fine, S., Forth, A., Gilbert, M., & Haley, G. (1991). Group therapy for adolescent depressive disorder: A comparison of social skills and therapeutic support. *Journal of the American Academy of Child and Adolescent Psychiatry, 30,* 79–85.

67. Flavell, J. (1985). *Cognitive development.* Englewood Cliffs, NJ: Prentice-Hall.

68. Garmezy, N. (1985). Stress-resistant children: The search for protective factors. In J. E. Stevenson (Ed.), *Recent research in developmental psychopathology. Journal of Child Psychology and Psychiatry Book* (Suppl. 4, pp. 213–233). Oxford, UK: Pergamon Press.

69. Gentile, A. M. (1998). Implicit and explicit processes during acquisition of functional skills. *Scandinavian Journal of Occupational Therapy, 5,* 7–16.

70. Gesell (1945). *The embryology of behavior: the beginnings of the human mind.* New York: Harper & Brothers.

71. Gibson, E. (1988). Exploratory behavior in the development of perceiving, acting and acquiring of knowledge. *Annual Review of Psychology, 39,* 1–41.

72. Gibson, J. (1979). *The ecological approach to visual perception.* Boston: Houghton-Mifflin.

73. Gilfoyle, E. M., Grady, A. P., & Moore, J. C. (1990). *Children adapt* (2nd ed.). Thorofare, NJ: Slack.

74. Glang, A., Todis, B., Cooley, E., Wells, J., & Voss, J. (1997). Building social networks for children and adolescents with traumatic brain injury: A school-based intervention. *Journal of Head Trauma Rehabilitation, 12,* 32–47.

75. Haley, S. M., Coster, W. J., Ludlow, L. H., Haltiwanger, J., & Andrellos, P. (1992). *Administrative manual for the Pediatric Evaluation of Disability Inventory.* San Antonio, TX: Psychological Corporation.

76. Hall, C. S., & Lindzey, G. (1978). *Theories of personality* (3rd ed.). New York: John Wiley & Sons.

77. Hanft, B. E., Rush, D. D., & Shelden, M. L. (2004). *Coaching families and colleagues in early intervention.* Baltimore, MD: Brookes Publishing.

78. Hansen, D. J., Watson-Perczel, M., & Christopher, J. S. (1989). Clinical issues in social skills training with adolescents. *Clinical Psychology Review, 9,* 365–391.

79. Harter, S. (1978). Effectance motivation reconsidered: Toward a developmental model. *Human Development, 21,* 34–64.

80. Hayes, R. L., Halford, W. K., & Varghese, F. N. (1991). Generalization of the effects of activity therapy and social skills training on the social behavior of low functioning schizophrenic patients. *Occupational Therapy in Mental Health, 11,* 3–20.

81. Rogers, J. C., & Holm, M. B. (2009). The occupational therapy process. In E. B. Crepeau, E. S. Cohn, & B. A. B. Schell (Eds.), *Willard & Spackman's occupational therapy* (pp. 22–32). Philadelphia: Lippincott Williams & Wilkins.

82. Howle, J. M. (2002). *Neurodevelopmental treatment approach: Theoretical foundations and principles of clinical practice.* Laguna Beach, CA: Neuro-Developmental Treatment Association.

83. Howlin, P., & Yates, P. (1999). The potential effectiveness of social skills group for adults with autism. *Autism, 3,* 299–307.

84. Humphry, R. (2002). Young children's occupations: Explicating the dynamics of developmental processes. *American Journal of Occupational Therapy, 56,* 171–179.

85. Humphry, R. (2009). Occupation and development: A contextual perspective. In E. B. Crepeau, E. S. Cohn, & B. A. B. Schell (Eds.), *Willard & Spackman's occupational therapy* (pp. 22–32). Philadelphia: Lippincott Williams & Wilkins.

86. Humphry, R., & Wakeford, L. (2006). An occupation-centered discussion of development and implications for practice. *American Journal of Occupational Therapy, 60,* 258–267.

87. Hyatt, G. B. (1946). Occupational therapy: Can doses be exact? *Occupational Therapy and Rehabilitation, 25,* 57–61.

88. Keintz, M. A., & Dunn, W. (1997). A comparison of the performance of children with and without autism on the Sensory Profile. *American Journal of Occupational Therapy, 51,* 530–537.

89. Ketelaar, M., Vermeer, A., Hart, H., van, E., & Helders, P. (2001). Effects of a functional therapy program on motor abilities of children with cerebral palsy. *Physical Therapy, 81,* 1534–1545.

90. Kielhofner, G. (2006). *A model of human occupation: Theory and application* (4th ed.). Baltimore, MD: Lippincott Williams & Wilkins.

91. Kielhofner, G., & Burke, J. (1980). A model of human occupation. Part 1. Conceptual framework and content. *American Journal of Occupational Therapy, 34,* 572–581.

92. King, G., King, S., Rosenbaum, P., & Goffin, R. (1999). Family-centred care-giving and wellbeing of parents of children with disabilities: Linking process with outcome. *Journal of Pediatric Psychology, 24,* 41–53.

93. Koegel, R. L., & Koegel, L. K. (Eds.). (2006). *Pivotal response treatment for autism: Communication, social, and academic development.* Baltimore, MD: Brookes.

94. Koegel, R. L., Koegel, L. K., & Carter, C. M. (1999). Pivotal teaching interactions for children with autism. *School Psychology Review, 28,* 576–594.

95. Krantz, M. (1994). *Child development: Risk and opportunity.* Belmont, CA: Wadsworth.

96. Law, M. (2002). Participation in the occupations of everyday life. *American Journal of Occupational Therapy, 56,* 640–649.

97. Deleted in proofs.

98. Law, M., Cadman, D., Rosenbaum, P., DeMatteo, C., Walter, S., & Russell, D. (1991). Neurodevelopmental therapy and upper extremity casting: Results of a clinical trial. *Developmental Medicine and Child Neurology, 33,* 334–340.

99. Law, M., Cooper, B., Strong, S., Stewart, D., Rigby, P., & Letts, L. (1996). The person-environment-occupation model: A transactive approach to occupational performance. *Canadian Journal of Occupational Therapy, 63*(1), 9–23.

100. Law, M., Hanna, S., King, G., Hurley, P., King, S., Kertoy, M., et al. (2003). Factors affecting family-centred service delivery for children with disabilities. *Child Care Health and Development, 29,* 41–53.

101. Law, M., King, G., Kind, S., Kertoy, M., Hurley, P., Rosenbaum, P., et al. (2006). Patterns of participation in recreation and leisure activities among children with complex physical disabilities. *Development Medicine and Child Neurology, 48,* 337–342.

102. Lee, T. D., Swinnen, S. P., & Serrien, D. J. (1994). Cognitive effort and motor learning. *Quest, 46,* 328–344.

103. Lefebvre, C., & Reid, G. (1998). Prediction in ball catching by children with and without a developmental coordination disorder. *Adapted Physical Activity Quarterly, 15,* 299–315.

104. Linder, T. W. (2008). *Transdisciplinary play-based assessment* (2nd ed.). Baltimore, MD: Brookes.
105. Llorens, L. A. (1976). *Application of developmental theory for health and rehabilitation.* Rockville, MD: American Occupational Therapy Association.
106. Llorens, L. A. (1991). Performance tasks and roles throughout the life span. In C. Christiansen & C. Baum (Eds.), *Occupational therapy: Overcoming human performance deficits* (pp. 45–68). Thorofare, NJ: Slack.
107. Lollar, D. J., & Simeonsson, R. J. (2005). Diagnosis to function: Classification for children and youths. *Developmental and Behavioral Pediatrics, 26,* 323–330.
108. Luria, A. (1961). *The role of speech in the regulation of normal and abnormal behaviors.* New York: Liveright.
109. Luthar, S. S. (2006). Resilience in development: A synthesis of research across five decades. In D. Cicchetti & D. Cohen (Eds.), *Developmental psychopathology: Risk, disorder, and adaptation* (2nd ed., Vol. 3, pp. 739–795). Hoboken, NJ: John Wiley & Sons, Inc.
110. Luthar, S. S., & Zelazo, L. M. (2003). Research on resilience: An integrative review. In S. S. Luthar (Ed.), *Resilience and vulnerability: Adaptation in the context of childhood adversities* (pp. 510–549). New York: Cambridge University Press.
111. Lyons, B. G. (1984). Defining a child's zone of proximal development: Evaluation process for treatment planning. *American Journal of Occupational Therapy, 38,* 446–451.
112. Ma, H., Trombly, C. A., & Robinson-Podolski, C. (1999). The effect of context on skill acquisition and transfer. *American Journal of Occupational Therapy, 53,* 138–144.
113. Maher, C. A., Williams, M. T., Olds, T., & Lane, A. E. (2007). Physical and sedentary activity in adolescents with cerebral palsy. *Developmental Medicine & Child Neurology, 29,* 450–457.
114. Mahoney, G., & O'Sullivan, P. (1990). Early intervention practices with families of children with handicaps. *Mental Retardation, 28,* 169–176.
115. Mahoney, G., & Perales, F. (2005). Relationship-focused early intervention with children with pervasive developmental disorders and other disabilities: A comparative study. *Developmental and Behavioral Pediatrics, 26,* 77–85.
116. Mandich, A., Polatajko, H., Missiuna, C., & Miller, L. (2001). Cognitive strategies and motor performance in children with developmental coordination disorder. *Physical and Occupational Therapy in Pediatrics, 20*(2/3), 125–143.
117. Mandich, A., & Roger (2006). Doing, being and becoming: Their importance for children. In S. Rodger & J. Ziviani (Eds.), *Occupational therapy with children: Understanding children's occupations and enabling participation* (pp. 115–135). Oxford, UK: Blackwell Publishing Ltd.
118. Maslow, A. H. (1968). *Toward a psychology of being.* Princeton, NJ: Van Nostrand.
119. Maslow, A. H. (1970). *Motivation and personality.* New York: Harper & Row.
120. Masten, A. S., & Reed, M. G. J. (2002). Resilience in development. In C. R. Snyder & S. J. Lopez (Eds.), *Handbook of positive psychology* (pp. 74–88). New York: Oxford University Press.
121. Mayo, N. E. (1991). The effect of physical therapy for children with motor delay and cerebral palsy. *American Journal of Physical Medicine and Rehabilitation, 70,* 258–267.
122. McColl, M., Law, M., Stewart, D., Doubt, L., Pollock, N., & Krupa, T. (2003). *Theoretical basis of occupational therapy* (2nd ed.). Thorofare, NJ: Slack.
123. Meichenbaum, D. (1977). *Cognitive-behavior modification: An integrative approach.* New York: Plenum Press.
124. Meyer, A. (1922). The philosophy of occupational therapy. *Archives of Occupational Therapy, 1,* 1–10.
125. Miller, L., Anzalone, M., Lane, S., Cermak, S., & Osten, B. (2007). Typology and terminology of sensory integration. *American Journal of Occupational Therapy, 61*(2), 135–140.
126. Miller, L. J., Coll, J. R., & Schoen, S. A. (2007). A randomized controlled pilot study of the effectiveness of occupational therapy for children with sensory modulation disorder. *American Journal of Occupational Therapy, 61,* 228–238.
127. Miller, L., Polatajko, H., Missiuna, C., Mandich, A., Macnab, J., & Malloy-Miller, T. (2001). A pilot trial of a cognitive treatment for children with developmental coordination disorder. *Human Movement Science, 20,* 183–210.
128. Miller, L. J., Wilbarger, J., Stackhouse, T., & Trunnell, S. (2002). Clinical reasoning in occupational therapy: The STEP-SI model of intervention of sensory modulation dysfunction. In A. Bundy, S. Lane, & E. Murray (Eds.), *Sensory integration therapy and practice* (2nd ed., pp. 435–451). Philadelphia: F.A. Davis.
129. Milone, M. N., Jr., & Waslyk, T. M. (1981). Handwriting in special education. *Teaching Exceptional Children, 14,* 58–61.
130. Missiuna, C., Malloy-Miller, T., & Mandich, A. (1998). Mediational techniques: Origins and application to occupational therapy in pediatrics. *Canadian Journal of Occupational Therapy, 65,* 202–209.
131. Missiuna, C., Mandich, A., Polatajko, P., & Malloy-Miller, T. (2001). Cognitive orientation to daily occupational performance (CO-OP). Part 1. Theoretical foundations. *Physical and Occupational Therapy in Pediatrics, 20*(2/3), 69–81.
132. Missiuna, C., & Pollock, N. (2000). Perceived efficacy and goal setting in young children. *Canadian Journal of Occupational Therapy, 67,* 101–109.
133. Mitchell, P. R. (1995). A dynamic interactive developmental view of early speech and language production: Application to clinical practice in motor speech disorders. *Seminars in Speech & Language, 16,* 100–109.
134. Mulligan, S. (1998). Patterns of sensory integration dysfunction: A confirmatory factor analysis. *American Journal of Occupational Therapy, 52,* 819–828.
135. Newacheck, P., & Halfon, N. (1998). Prevalence and impact of disabling chronic conditions in childhood. *American Journal of Public Health, 88*(4), 610–617.
136. Nicholson, D. E. (1996). Motor learning. In C. M. Fredericks & L. K. Saladin (Eds.), *Pathophysiology of the motor systems: Principles and clinical presentations* (pp. 238–254). Philadelphia: F.A. Davis.
137. Nudo, R. J. (2006). Plasticity. *NeuroRx, 3,* 420–427.
138. Ormrod, J. E. (2006). *Educational psychology: Developing learners* (5th ed.). Upper Saddle River, NJ: Prentice Hall.
139. Ottenbacher, K., Short, M. A., & Watson, P. J. (1979). Nystagmus duration changes in learning disabled children during sensory integrative therapy. *Perceptual and Motor Skills, 48,* 1159–1164.
140. Palisano, R. J., Copeland, W. P., & Galuppi, B. E. (2007). Performance of physical activities by adolescents with cerebral palsy. *Physical Therapy, 87,* 77–87.
141. Palmer, F. B., Shapiro, B. K., Wachtal, R. C., Allen, M. C., Hiller, J. E., Harryman, S. E., et al. (1988). The effects of physical therapy on cerebral palsy: A controlled trial in infants with spastic diplegia. *New England Journal of Medicine, 318,* 903–908.
142. Parham, L. D. (2008). Play and occupational therapy. In L. D. Parham & L. Fazio (Eds.), *Play in occupational therapy for children* (2nd ed., pp. 3–42). St. Louis: Elsevier.
143. Parham, L. D., Cohn, E. S., Spitzer, S., Koomar, J. A., Miller, L. M., et al. (2007). Fidelity in sensory integration intervention research. *American Journal of Occupational Therapy, 61,* 216–227.
144. Piaget, J. (1952). *The origins of intelligence in children.* New York: International Universities.
145. Piaget, J. (1971). *Psychology and epistemology: Towards a theory of knowledge.* New York: Viking Press.
146. Piper, M. C. (1990). Efficacy of physical therapy: Rate of motor development in children with cerebral palsy. *Pediatric Physical Therapy, 2,* 126–130.

147. Piper, M. C., & Darrah, J. (1994). *Motor assessment of the developing infant.* Philadelphia: W.B. Saunders.

148. Pless, I. B., Cripps, H. A., Davies, J. M. C., & Wadsworth, M. E. J. (1989). Chronic physical illness in childhood: Psychological and social effects in adolescence and adult life. *Developmental Medicine and Child Neurology, 31,* 746–755.

149. Polatajko, H. J., Mandich, A. D., Miller, L. T., & Macnab, J. J. (2001). Cognitive orientation to daily occupational performance (CO-OP). Part 2. The evidence. *Physical and Occupational Therapy in Pediatrics, 20*(2/3), 83–106.

150. Polatajko, H. J., Mandich, A. D., Missiuna, C., Miller, L. T., Macnab, J., Malloy-Miller, T. (2001). Cognitive orientation to daily occupational performance (CO-OP). Part 3. The protocol in brief. *Physical and Occupational Therapy in Pediatrics, 20*(2/3), 107–123.

151. Poulson, A., & Ziviani, J. (2004). Can I play too? Physical activity engagement patterns of children with developmental coordination disorders. *Canadian Journal of Occupational Therapy, 71,* 100–107.

152. Reed, M. K. (1994). Social skills training to reduce depression in adolescents. *Adolescence, 29,* 293–302.

153. Reilly. (1966). A psychiatric occupational therapy program as a teaching model. *American Journal of Occupational Therapy, 20,* 62–67.

154. Reilly. (1969). The educational process. *American Journal of Occupational Therapy, 23,* 299–307.

155. Reilly. (1974a). *Play as exploratory learning.* Beverly Hills, CA: Sage Publications.

156. Reilly. (1974b). Occupational behavior: A perspective on work and play. *American Journal of Occupational Therapy, 25,* 291–296.

157. Richmond, J. B., & Beardslee, W. R. (1988). Resiliency: Research and practical implications for pediatricians. *Journal of Developmental and Behavioral Pediatrics, 9,* 157–163.

158. Rigby, P., & Letts, L. (2003). Environment and occupational performance: Theoretical considerations. In L. Letts, P. Rigby, & D. Stewart (Eds.), *Using environments to enable occupational performance* (pp. 17–32). Thorofare, NJ: Slack.

159. Rodger, S., & Brandenburg, J. (2009). Cognitive Orientation to (daily) Occupational Performance (CO-OP) with children with Asperger's syndrome who have motor-based occupational performance goals. *Australian Occupational Therapy Journal, 56,* 41–50.

160. Rodger, S., Springfield, E., & Polatajko, H. (2007). Cognitive orientation for daily occupational performance approach for children with Asperger's syndrome: A case report. *Physical and Occupational Therapy in Pediatrics, 27,* 7–22.

161. Rosenbaum, P., King, S., Law, M., King, G., & Evans, J. (1998). Family-centred service: A conceptual framework and research review. *Physical and Occupational Therapy in Pediatrics, 18,* 1–20.

162. Rutter, M. (1990). Psychosocial resilience and protective mechanisms. In J. Rolf, A. S. Masten, D. Cicchetti, K. Nuechterlein, & S. Weintraub (Eds.), *Risk and protective factors in the development of psychopathology* (pp. 181–214). Cambridge, UK: Cambridge University Press.

163. Sandler, I. (2001). Quality and ecology of adversity as common mechanisms of risk and resilience. *American Journal of Community Psychology, 29*(1), 19–61.

164. Schaaf, R. C., & Nightlinger, K. M. (2007). Occupational therapy using a sensory integrative approach: A case study of effectiveness. *American Journal of Occupational Therapy, 61,* 239–246.

165. Schertz, M., & Gordon, A. M. (2009). Changing the model: A call for a re-examination of intervention approaches and translational research in children with developmental disabilities. *Developmental Medicine & Child Neurology, 51,* 6–7.

166. Scherzer, A. L., Mike, V., & Ilson, J. (1976). Physical therapy as a determinant of change in the cerebral palsied infant. *Pediatrics, 53,* 47–52.

167. Schmidt, R. A. (1988). *Motor control and learning: A behavioral emphasis.* Champaign, IL: Human Kinetics.

168. Shikako-Thomas, K., Majnemer, A., Law, M., & Lach, L. (2008). Determinants of participation in leisure activities in children and youth with cerebral palsy: Systematic review. *Physical and Occupational Therapy in Pediatrics, 28,* 155–170.

169. Shumway-Cook, A., & Woollacott, M. H. (2006). *Motor control: Translating research into clinical practice.* Baltimore, MD: Lippincott Williams & Wilkins.

170. Skinner, B. F. (1953). *Science and human behavior.* New York: Free Press.

171. Skinner, B. F. (1976). *Walden two.* New York: Macmillan.

172. Slagle, E. C. (1922). Training aides for mental patients. *Archives of Occupational Therapy, 1,* 11–17.

173. Sloper, P., Turner, S., Knussen, C., & Cunningham, C. (1990). Social life of school children with Down's syndrome. *Child: Care. Health and Development, 16*(4), 235–251.

174. Sommerfeld, D., Fraser, B. A., Hensinger, R. N., & Beresford, C. V. (1981). Evaluation of physical therapy service for severely mentally impaired students with cerebral palsy. *Physical Therapy, 61,* 338–344.

175. Spitzer, S. L. (2008). Play in children with autism: Structure and experience. In L. D. Parham, & L. Fazio (Eds.), *Play in occupational therapy for children* (2nd ed.). St. Louis: Elsevier.

176. Stewart, D., & Law, M. (2003). The environment: Paradigms and practice in health, occupational therapy and inquiry. In L. Letts, P. Rigby, & D. Stewart (Eds.), *Using environments to enable occupational performance* (pp. 3–15). Thorofare, NJ: Slack.

177. Sugden, D. A., & Sugden, L. (1990). *The assessment and management of movement skill problems.* Leeds, UK: School of Education.

178. Sullivan, K. J., Kantak, S. S., & Burtner, P. A. (2008). Motor learning in children: Feedback effects on skills acquisition. *Physical Therapy, 88,* 720–732.

179. Taylor, S., Fayed, N., & Mandrich, A. (2007). CO-OP intervention for young children with developmental coordination disorder. *OTJR: Occupation, Participation and Health, 27,* 124–130.

180. Thelen, E. (1995). Motor development: A new synthesis. *American Psychologist, 50*(2), 79–95.

181. Thelen, E., Schoner, G., Scheier, C., Smith, L. (2001). The dynamics of embodiment: A field theory of infant preservative reaching. *Behavioral and Brain Sciences, 24,* 1–86.

182. Thelen, E., & Spencer, J. P. (1998). Postural control during reaching in young infants: A dynamic systems approach. *Neuroscience and Behavioral Reviews, 22,* 507–514.

183. Tomchek, S. D., & Dunn, W. (2007). Sensory processing in children with and without autism: A comparative study using the Short Sensory Profile. *American Journal of Occupational Therapy, 61,* 190–200.

184. Vanderbilt-Adriance, E., & Shaw, D. S. (2008). Conceptualizing and re-evaluating resilience across levels of risk, time, and domains of competence. *Clinical Child and Family Psychology Review, 11,* 30–58.

185. Van Gelder, T. (1995). What might cognition be, if not computation? *Journal of Philosophy, 91,* 345–381.

186. VanSant, A. F. (1991). Neurodevelopmental treatment and pediatric physical therapy: A commentary. *Pediatric Physical Therapy, 3,* 137–141.

187. Vargas, S., & Camilli, G. (1999). A meta-analysis of research on sensory integration treatment. *American Journal of Occupational Therapy, 53,* 180–198.

188. Vygotsky, L. S. (1978). *Mind in society: The development of higher mental processes. Mind in society: The development of higher mental processes.* Cambridge, MA: Harvard University Press.

189. Wallander, J., & Varni, J. (1989). Social support and adjustment in chronically ill and handicapped children. *American Journal of Community Psychology, 17*(2), 185–201.

190. Watling, R., Deitz, J., Kanny, E. M., & McLaughlin, J. F. (1999). Current practice of occupational therapy for children with autism. *American Journal of Occupational Therapy, 53,* 498–505.

191. Watling, R., Deitz, J., & White, O. (2001). Comparison of sensory profile scores of young children with and without autism spectrum disorders. *American Journal of Occupational Therapy, 55,* 416–423.

192. Werner, E. E. (1989). High-risk children in young adulthood: A longitudinal study from birth to 32 years. *American Journal of Orthopsychiatry, 59,* 72–81.

193. Werner, E. E. (1994). Overcoming the odds. *Developmental and Behavioral Pediatrics, 15,* 131–136.

194. Wertsch, J. V. (2008). From social interaction to higher psychological processes: A clarification and application of Vygotsky's theory. *Human Development, 51,* 66–79.

195. Wilcock, A. (1993). A theory of human need for occupation. *Occupational Science: Australia, 1,* 17–24.

196. Wilcock, A. (1998). Reflections on doing, being, becoming. *Canadian Journal of Occupational Therapy, 65,* 248–256.

197. Wilcock, A., & Townshend, E. (2008). Occupational justice. In E. B. Crepeau, W. S. Cohn, & B. B. Schell (Eds.), *Willard & Spackman's occupational therapy* (11th ed., pp. 192–199). Baltimore, MD: Lippincott Williams & Wilkins.

198. Williams, M. S., & Shellenberger, S. (1994). *How does your engine run? A leader's guide to the alert program for self-regulation.* Albuquerque, NM: Therapy Works.

199. Williamson, G., & Szczepanski, M. (1999). Coping frame of reference. In P. Kramer & J. Hinojosa (Eds.), *Frames of reference in pediatric occupational therapy* (pp. 431–465). Baltimore, MD: Williams & Wilkins.

200. Winstein, C. J., Merians, A. S., & Sullivan, K. J. (1999). Motor learning after unilateral brain damage. *Neuropsychologia, 37,* 975–987.

201. World Health Organization. (1980). *International classification of impairments, disability and handicap.* Geneva, Switzerland: World Health Organization.

202. World Health Organization. (2001). *International classification of disability, functioning and health.* Geneva, Switzerland: World Health Organization.

203. Yerxa, E. J. (1967). Authentic occupational therapy. *American Journal of Occupational Therapy, 21,* 1–9.

204. Yerxa, E. J., Clark, F., Frank, G., Jackson, J., Parham, D., Pierce, D., et al. (1989). Occupational science: The foundation for new models of practice. *Occupational Therapy in Health Care, 6,* 1–17.

205. Zeitlin, S., & Williamson, G. G. (1994). *Coping in young children: Early intervention practices to enhance adaptive behavior and resilience.* Baltimore, MD: Brookes.

206. Zeitlin, S., Williamson, G. G., & Szczepanski, M. (1988). *Early coping inventory.* Bensenville, IL: Scholastic Testing Service.

3

Development of Childhood Occupations

Jane Case-Smith

KEY TERMS

Neuromaturational
  theory
Dynamical systems
  theory
Perceptual-action
  coupling
Functional synergies

Temperament
Risk and resiliency
Cultural practices
Occupations within
  cultural, social, and
  physical contexts
Play development

OBJECTIVES

1. Explain historical and current theories of child development.
2. Define how a child's unique characteristics influence skill development
3. Using an occupational therapy perspective, explain how occupations develop.
4. Explain how individual biological systems and cultural, social, and physical contexts contribute to a child's occupational performance in the first 10 years of life.
5. Describe the development of play and the variables that contribute to the development of play.

An understanding of child development is foundational knowledge for pediatric occupational therapists. Researchers from many disciplines, including medicine, psychology, anthropology, education, sociology, and occupational therapy, have contributed to the literature on human development, and the different perspectives they provide should be woven into a holistic and comprehensive understanding of how children become adults.

Occupational therapists want to know *what* developmental changes occur in children and *how* children develop their unique personhood. The answers to these questions provide essential knowledge for evaluating children and for determining the appropriate materials, activities, and environments to support children's skill development and participation in their communities. They are also interested in how human occupations develop over the life span.

This chapter focuses on child development theories, with emphasis on concepts that have emerged in the past 2 decades. The first section discusses concepts that explain how children develop and what variables and interactions influence developmental outcomes. In the second part of the chapter, a model for the development of childhood occupations is applied to children's development of play in the first 10 years of life. Chapter 4 describes the development of pre-adolescent and adolescent occupations in the second decade of life.

DEVELOPMENTAL THEORIES AND CONCEPTS

Researchers of the 1930s and 1940s identified a sequence of skill maturation that defined the steps of normal development. Gesell and Colleagues[42–44] and McGraw[74] assumed that normal development was revealed through a specific skill sequence that reflected maturation of the central nervous system (CNS). These workers believed that the sequence of motor, cognitive, socioemotional, and language skill development was relatively unaffected by the infant's experiences. The work of these neuromaturational theorists in documenting this developmental sequence has been well respected and has allowed the creation of developmental assessment tools. The sequence of normal development is an important frame of reference for identifying children with disabilities. Gesell and coworkers believed that variations in the normal sequence of development indicate CNS dysfunction. Identifying children with developmental deficits or significant delays remains an important function of physicians, nurses, occupational therapists, and others who provide early intervention services.

Neuromaturation

Neuromaturational theory has been used frequently to explain motor development.[34,76] According to neuromaturational theory, brainstem structures develop first, as evidenced by the reflexive responses of the newborn (e.g., automatic grasp, asymmetric tonic neck reflex), which are controlled by neural pathways originating in the brainstem. Cortical structures appear to develop later, as evidenced by the coordinated and planned actions of the child. The infant's increasing control of action and movement indicates not only development and myelination of the midbrain and cortical structures, but also simultaneous inhibition of brainstem control of movement. Three primary principles of neuromaturational theory are recognized:

1. Movement progresses from primitive reflex patterns to voluntary, controlled movement. In newborn and young infants, motor reflexes provide the first methods of interaction with the environment (e.g., reflexive grasp) and are essential to life (e.g., the sucking and swallowing reflexes).

Because early reflexive movements serve functional needs, the newborn appears surprisingly competent. These reflex patterns subside as balance, postural reactions, and voluntary motor control emerge (i.e., when the infant learns to roll, sit, creep, stand, and walk).

2. The sequence and rate of motor development are consistent among infants and children. The developmental scales of Gesell and Amatruda,[43] Illingworth,[60,61] Bayley,[8,9] and others are based on a typical rate and sequence of development. By assuming that the sequence of milestones (i.e., major motor accomplishments) is constant and predictable, the normative developmental sequence can be used to diagnose neurological impairment and disability.[9]

3. Low-level skills are prerequisites for certain high-level skills. For example, infants develop motor control in a cephalocaudal direction, with head control maturing first, followed by trunk control sufficient for independent sitting, and, finally, pelvic control sufficient for standing and walking.

In assuming a hierarchy of CNS function, the neuro-maturational theory limited the thinking on how a child learns to act in the environment. Using current research models,[47,52,100,102] it has become apparent that multiple variables at different levels influence the child's skill development. The child learns occupations through interaction with his or her environment rather than through the emergence of a predetermined scenario reflecting neuromaturational principles.[57]

Development as an Interplay of Intrinsic and Environmental Factors

Piaget expanded our understanding of a child's maturation by emphasizing that development occurs through the interplay between the environment and the child's innate abilities (see Chapter 2).[83] Piaget emphasized the maturation of cognitive structures that enable the child to understand the environment, language, and social action. Infants develop an understanding of the world by interacting with the environment. The impact of environment on the child's development changes as the child becomes increasingly able to assimilate the complexities of physical and social events. Piaget also believed the development is stagelike and discontinuous. The infant is an active learner who is motivated to learn about the world. Piaget documented the child's maturation through stages to the acquisition of symbolic thought and formal cognitive operations. The developmental stages follow a predictable sequence but vary to the extent that they reflect genetic endowment and the child's experiences. This interplay between the child's abilities and his experience can be appreciated in the early development of tool use. Piaget observed that children at 8 to 10 months manipulate two objects and can move an obstacle to reach an interesting or novel object. By 12 months, infants can relate an object to other objects, in addition to relating the objects to themselves. At this stage, infants use a stick to rake in an object out of reach and place objects into containers. By 18 months, infants begin to use trial and error to solve problems. At 24 months of age, they no longer exclusively need physical manipulation to solve problems and begin to demonstrate use of mental manipulation.[73,83]

Research studies in the 1990s demonstrated that cognitive structures develop at earlier ages than Piaget assumed; they have also demonstrated that child development has more continuity and integration across the stages of development.[13,37] Infants as young as 1 month demonstrate the ability to associate learning from one sensory system with another sensory system. For example, they recognize objects with their eyes that they previously felt in their mouths.[70] Researchers have also found that 9-month-old infants can remember an event 1 week after it happened.[75]

Other research that has updated Piaget's demonstrated that toddlers can manipulate and use tools and can solve problems such as how to grasp and use a spoon. McCarty and colleagues found that children 9 to 14 months of age picked up the spoon using an awkward grasp and then attempted to adjust the spoon's orientation to get the food into the mouth.[73] Children 19 months old planned how to grasp and orient the spoon to get the food before acting, avoiding the use of an awkward grasp that required adjusting. This study showed that children as young as 19 months can solve problems without physical manipulation and trial and error to handle a tool accurately. By this age, the child can scoop food, fill the spoon, and correctly angle it toward the mouth,[56] signifying the early emergence of tool use.

Scholars have critiqued and expanded Piaget's original theories to fully appreciate how the environment influences development. For example, Piaget's theories lack appreciation of the influence of culture, society, and technology on children's development. Current occupational therapy theories consider these variables to have important roles in a child's development.[10,116] In addition, Piaget's theories did not address the development of emotions and did not have a coherent explanation for individual differences, individuality, or variability.[37] The importance of variability has been highlighted in the work of other psychologists[100,103] and by occupational therapy researchers.[59]

The Influence of Social Interaction

Following Piaget, another developmental theorist, Vygotsky, believed that children learn through social interaction.[109] Vygotsky's theories emphasized the importance of culture and shared participation in culturally valued activities to children's development. He demonstrated that children learn when *scaffolding*, or support, is provided by caregivers and teachers. Parents and other family members intuitively provide environmental challenges that encourage the infant to exhibit a higher skill level and then support the infant's efforts to reach that level. Parents and siblings naturally promote the infant's development by modeling actions, assisting the infant's first attempts to perform an action, and reinforcing his or her efforts with praise and expressions of delight.

Vygotsky explains the role of social interaction in children's development by defining a "zone of proximal development" as "the distance between the actual development level as determined by [the child's] independent problem solving and the level of potential development as determined through [his] problem solving under adult guidance or in collaboration with more capable peers" (p. 86).[109] He believed that what children can do with the assistance of others was more indicative of their mental development than what they could do independently. When presented with a *just right* challenge, e.g., a task that is slightly more difficult than the tasks the child has currently mastered, the child generally attempts and succeeds in this challenge, thereby learning the next step in skill development.

Vygotsky and the many subsequent developmental theorists have examined how human development transpires through a dynamic interplay involving the child and the child's cultural, social, and physical environments. Researchers of child development have documented differences in the rate of development in socioeconomic groups, regions, and individuals. For example, rates of development appear different in rural versus urban areas.[106,108] Children's rate of development also differs among cultural groups and generations, in part because of differences in nutrition and child care practices. In human development research, the emphasis currently is on the variations expressed by individual infants and on how human systems and environmental constraints contribute to these variations.

Studies that analyze the uniqueness of individual performance often use longitudinal and qualitative approaches to analyze the performance of children over time and in natural contexts.[11,102] Because these longitudinal studies document the patterns of development over time, they uncover how individual systems are constructed and assembled. Longitudinal approaches make it possible to relate transitions of subsystems to each other and to other dynamic growth parameters.[108] Understanding *how* children acquire qualitative differences in functional performance and *how* they become unique individuals can begin by focusing on the variables that influence a child's developmental course. The following sections examine current theories of development that explain the relationships among a child's biological functions, occupations, and environments.

Dynamical Systems Theory

Dynamical systems theory refers to performance or action patterns that emerge from the interaction and cooperation of many systems, both internal and external to the child.[101] In the context of child development, performance patterns emerge from the interaction of an individual's systems and performance contexts as the child strives to achieve a functional goal.[71,72] The dynamical systems theory is useful in describing how specific motor and process skills develop.

In this model, a child's behaviors and actions are initially highly variable, with many degrees of freedom. The first actions of the infant have been described as random and uncontrolled. Development of skill proceeds by means of constraint of these degrees of freedom as the child gains control of his or her actions. Behavior, therefore, is not prescribed by a hierarchical arrangement of the CNS, but rather emerges from external and internal constraints.[97] These constraints provide information to the brain and body systems that set the boundaries or limits for the child's behavior.[22]

Humans are complex biological systems comprising many subsystems (e.g., motor sensory, perceptual, skeletal, and psychologic subsystems). These subsystems are in constant flux, interacting according to the task at hand and conditions in the environment. The child's actions during the performance of a task, therefore, are the result of the subsystems' interaction with each other and with the environment. These individual systems come together and self-organize in a coordinated way to achieve the child's goal.[97] For example, initially a child is interested in exploring the sensory characteristics of a toy. As he or she reaches for the toy, grasps it, and brings it to midline in hand-to-hand play and then finally to the mouth, the child's attention and cognitive focus are not on planning each of these actions. Instead, they are on assimilating the toy's actions and perceptual features.

Longitudinal studies reveal that children demonstrate unique trajectories of development and that variations in functional performance among children persist into adulthood. Thelen and her colleagues demonstrated the uniqueness of motor development in a study of reaching in 4- and 5-month-old infants.[102] Each 5-month-old infant was able to reach toward an object, but the patterns demonstrated were unique. Some infants demonstrated a slow, cautious first approach to the object, whereas others made ballistic arm movements in an attempt to reach it. Although all first reaches tended to be circuitous, the amount of correction made to obtain the object, the speed at which the attempt was made, and the angle at which arms were held were different. These investigators concluded that the development of reaching did not reflect changes in a single factor, but rather to reach and grasp an object, the infant needed to (1) be motivated, (2) localize the object in space, (3) understand that the object was reachable, (4) plan the trajectory of the reach, (5) correct the movement as the hand approached the toy, (6) lift and stabilize the arm, and (7) grasp the object. How a 5-month-old infant manages all of these components to reach and grasp a toy successfully varies among infants and for different reasons.

In a similar way, between 8 and 10 months, most infants acquire the motivation to be independently mobile. The need to self-initiate movement from place to place emerges as an important task, or goal, to accomplish. This goal reflects the infant's curiosity about the environment, a desire to explore space, and a determination to reach a specific play object. Although mobility becomes a common goal for the infant toward the end of the first year, the method used to achieve that mobility varies greatly. Some infants roll to another space in the room, whereas others scoot on their buttocks in a sitting position. Some infants push backward while lying in a prone position, and others creep forward to explore their environment. How the infant achieves mobility is influenced by many contributing body systems (e.g., strength, coordination, and sense of balance and movement). Conditions in the environment also influence infant mobility (e.g., the surfaces on which the child plays, the encouragement provided by caregivers, and the way in which the task is presented). The child's energy level, motivation, and curiosity about the environment also influence when independent mobility is achieved. In addition to the factors that influence the maturation of mobility skills, becoming mobile influences the development of skills in other performance domains. When an infant achieves mobility, he or she becomes more independent in initiating a social interaction or in seeking help. Therefore, independent mobility contributes to the acquisition of social skills, self-determination, problem solving, and motivation to explore (see Chapter 21). A child learns perceptual skills, spatial relations, form perception, and object relations by moving through the environment.

Perceptual Action Reciprocity

Perception and action are interdependent and inextricably linked. An individual's perception of the environment informs action, and the individual's actions provide feedback about movement, performance, and consequences in the environment. Initially, many of the child's actions are exploratory in nature—that is, the child moves fingers over the surfaces of objects to learn their shape, texture, and consistency. The child waves an object in the air to hear the sounds it makes and feel its weight. These actions help the child perceive sensory and perceptual features (affordances) of objects. *Affordance* is the fit between the child and his or her environment.[46,48,49] The environment and objects in it offer the child opportunities to explore and act. This action is based on what the environment affords, as well as the child's perceptual capability to recognize affordances in that environment. For example, colorful noise-making toys afford manipulation because they have movable parts and rounded surfaces and fit easily into an infant's hand. Learning about affordances entails exploratory activities. Individual finger movements, thumb opposition, hand-to-hand transfer, and eye-hand coordination are facilitated by the physical characteristics of the toy.

Manipulation is guided by visual, tactile, and kinesthetic input.[86,94] Exploration of objects begins with visual exploration and mouthing.[87] By 6 months, infants prefer exploring with their eyes and hands.[86] Fingering and manipulation skills increase substantially between 6 and 12 months, enabling infants to gather more precise information about objects. By 12 months, infants detect object properties with increasing specificity and learn to adjust their exploratory action.[1] For example, to perceive the consistency of a soft, squishy object, a child squeezes it, and to perceive the texture of velvet or corduroy, he or she runs the fingers back and forth over it.

Through object manipulation, the child develops haptic perception (i.e., an understanding of objects' shape, texture, and mass). Bushnell and Boudreau propose that specific motor skills are required to develop haptic perception.[12] They note that infants learn to identify an object's sensory qualities (e.g., texture, consistency, temperature, contour) only when they develop the motor skills to explore each different sensory quality. For example, an infant does not accurately discriminate texture until he or she can explore texture by moving the fingers back and forth (at about 6 months). The child also cannot discriminate hardness until 6 months, when he or she can tighten and lessen the grip while holding an object.[12] Because configural shape requires that two hands be involved in exploring an object's surfaces, children typically cannot accurately perceive shape until 12 months. By 2½ years, children can identify common objects through their haptic sense, and by 5 years, children recognize common objects using active touch (without vision).[16] By 5 years, the child has also fully developed in-hand manipulation skills,[82] suggesting that haptic perception develops in association with the child's development of manipulation skills. Maturation of haptic perception and manipulation underlies the child's ability to use tools for written communication (e.g., handwriting and keyboarding) and activities of daily living.

Functional Performance: Flexible Synergies

As mentioned, the infant begins life with few constraints on performance, which permits the greatest variability in the system for the generation of spontaneous movements. This variability permits flexibility for exploration of the environment and rapid perceptual and cognitive learning. The infant quickly selects functional synergistic movement patterns. For example, from birth the infant demonstrates a pattern of hand-to-mouth

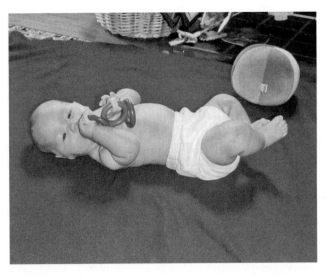

FIGURE 3-1 Hand-to-mouth movement is observed throughout the first year, first for sensory exploration of the mouth and hand and then as a feeding behavior. (From Henderson, A., & Pehoski, C. [2006]. *Hand function in the child: Foundations for remediation* [2nd ed.]. St. Louis: Mosby.)

movement (e.g., for self-calming by sucking on a fist) (Figure 3-1). Only minimal adaptive changes are made in this synergistic pattern (shoulder rotation and horizontal adduction, elbow flexion and forearm pronation, followed by supination and neutral wrist position) as the child learns to self-feed with various utensils (Figure 3-2).

Because synergies that enable tool use are softly assembled around the goal of the task at hand, they are stable but flexible units. Synergies have specific consistent characteristics, such as the sequence of movements and the ratio of joint movement, which can be adjusted to accommodate each new situation. This *adaptable stability* is a hallmark of normal movement.[21] Soft assembly is critical to allow the child to act in changing and variable environments. It also allows the child to explore and select a response to the environment, because his or her response patterns are variable and flexible.[97]

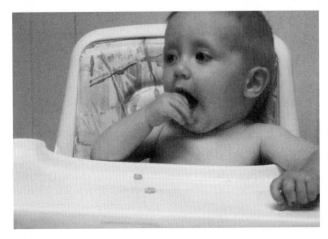

FIGURE 3-2 By 7 to 8 months, an infant finger-feeds, prehending small food pieces and bringing hand to mouth.

The functional synergies that characterize a child's development of occupations are highly adaptable and reliable. The child self-organizes these synergies around tasks and goals, and his or her first goals are embedded in and organized around play (as described later in this chapter).

How Do Children Develop New Performance Skills?

How does a child learn new performance skills? Although learning new skills is not limitless and is constrained by biologic and contextual factors, human development is believed to have relative *plasticity*.[66] This concept has obvious importance to occupational therapists, who provide intervention services designed to change and promote children's performance. Gottlieb defines plasticity as a fusion of the organism (the child) and the environment (including its cultural, physical, and socioeconomic characteristics).[52] Individual development involves the emergence of new structural (e.g., cellular) and functional components (e.g., body systems). The child's experiences produce new neurologic connections (i.e., new associations) and structural changes (e.g., physical growth), and it is the relationships among components, not the components themselves, that are most important to development. Acknowledgment of the system's plasticity places the focus on the child's potential for change and on the contextual features that promote or limit the child's performance.

How does competence develop during childhood? Children generally pass through three stages of learning to acquire a new skill.[48,84,103] The first stage involves *exploratory activity*. The first year of life is primarily a period of sensorimotor exploration. Exploration occurs naturally in all human beings, generally when an individual is presented with a new object or task. Through exploration, a child learns about self and the environment. In this stage, the child experiments with objects and activities using different systems, new combinations of perception and movement, and new sequences of action. In this exploratory stage or when challenged by a new and difficult task, a child tends to demonstrate primitive movement. New challenges tend to elicit lower levels of skills, because these can be accessed more easily than the child's highest-level skills, which demand more energy and effort.[53] By using lower-level skills to address new problems, the child can focus on perceptual learning about the task before beginning to use higher-level skills, which ultimately allow more success in performing the task. Gilfoyle, Grady, and Moore noted that when children are first challenged with a new and difficult performance task (e.g., a first step), they use primitive movement patterns (e.g., balance by stiffening the legs and trunk) before progressing to integrated skill.[50]

In the second stage of learning, *perceptual learning*, the child begins to use the feedback and reinforcement received from his or her exploration. In this transitional stage, the child exhibits more consistency in the movement patterns used to accomplish tasks. Because this second stage is a phase of perceptual learning, certain actions that were tried initially are discarded as ineffective. Interest in the activity remains high as perceptual learning continues and is inherently motivating and meaningful to the child. In this stage, the child appears focused on learning and attempts activities multiple times. The child may fluctuate between higher and lower levels of skill. Connolly and Dalgleish found considerable variability

when toddlers attempted to use a spoon.[26] Greer and Lockman found similar variability when 3-year-olds attempted to use a writing tool.[55] At times, the children grasped the tool using an adult gripping pattern, and at other times, they used a primitive, full-hand grasp. Mature patterns are selected more often as children enter the third stage of skill learning.

In the third stage of learning, *skill achievement*, the child selects the action pattern that works best for achieving a goal. The pattern selected is comfortable and efficient for the child. Selection of a single pattern indicates both perceptual learning and increased self-organization. During this end stage of learning, the child demonstrates flexible consistency in performance. He or she uses the same pattern and approach to the task but easily adapts the pattern according to task requirements. High adaptability is always characteristic of a well-learned task. Another attribute of learned performance is the use of action patterns that are orderly and economical. Children continue to practice performance when given opportunities in the environment. The third stage of learning leads to exploration of new and different activities; therefore, a child's learning continues into new performance arenas, expanding his or her occupations.

For most children, new experiences and new learning are sought and are a source of pleasure. Learning occurs when children seek opportunities for skill development; it also occurs when children adapt to the natural environment and daily activities in which they participate. Ayres explains that children make adaptive responses to the environment.[3,4] An adaptive response is one in which the child responds to an environmental change in "a creative or useful way" (p. 14).[4] These adaptive responses allow skill mastery and help to organize the child's CNS. Therefore, an adaptive response helps to integrate the child's sensory and perceptual systems to respond more skillfully to new challenges to the sensory system. For example, once the infants can pull themselves up to a standing position using a piece of furniture, they have acquired an adaptive skill that enables them to pull up to the mother's lap to ask to be held or explore the objects on a coffee table. This organization of movement patterns was achieved because the vestibular, proprioceptive, and visual systems are innately organized toward achieving upright posture (Figure 3-3).

The Role of Motivation and Self-Efficacy

Children engage in the process of learning with innate motivation and apparent enjoyment. An infant's inner drive motivates her to explore novel objects in the environment, learning their sensory characteristics, their relationships to each other, and their functions. A toddler or young child is motivated to solve problems and to attempt new skills, persevering until it is mastered. The concept of inner drive suggests that children attempt activities that will promote their development without specific teaching by adults. Occupational therapists view this innate drive as the child's inner motivation to engage in occupations (task with meaning and purpose). Learning occurs when the match among child, task, and environment is optimal; hence, this match becomes the occupational therapist's goal.[58] When a child has a disability, motivation to learn and attempt new activities may be lower and the match among child, occupation, and environment may be less than optimal. In this case, a child may not learn independently and adult

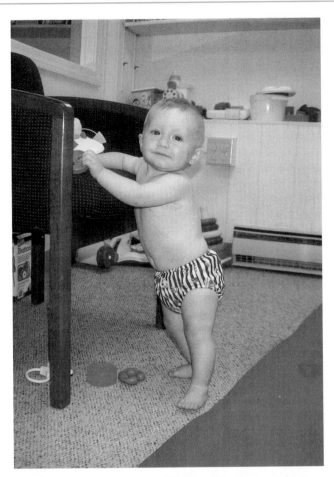

FIGURE 3-3 Infants play in supported standing for extended periods, gaining postural stability and balance when holding onto a stable surface.

support may be needed to motivate, provide a just right challenge, support actions, and reinforce performance.

When a child's inner drive leads to mastery of tasks, he or she develops a sense of self-efficacy.[5-7] Bandura believes that children are inherently self-organizing and goal-directed; they typically have interest in new events and activities, initiate new tasks, and persevere in those tasks. When they succeed, positive self-efficacy is reinforced and they attempt other challenges. When they do not succeed, they are at risk for developing poor self-efficacy and eventually do not attempt new or challenging activities. Therefore, self-efficacy is highly linked to learning and occupational development because it influences levels of motivation, initiative, and perseverance.

Temperament and Emotional Development

The congruence, or *goodness of fit*, between the child and his or her social and physical context determines the quality of development, influencing which occupations are reinforced and which are hindered. *Positive goodness of fit*, meaning that the social and physical environment support the child's skill development, can increase the child's developmental trajectory. Lack of goodness of fit can create disruption of psychologic development and may put the child at risk for behavioral or academic problems.

Chess and Thomas asserted that if a child's characteristics provide a good fit (or match) with the demands of a particular setting, adaptive outcomes result.[19,20] The child's *temperament* is an important determinant in how well a child matches the caregiving environment[67] and is an important attribute in the child's social interaction. According to Thomas and Chess, *temperament* refers to the child's behavioral style, and it is believed to be innate and learned.[104] Nine areas of temperament have been identified: (1) activity level, (2) approach or withdrawal, (3) distractibility, (4) intensity of response, (5) attention span and persistence, (6) quality of mood, (7) rhythmicity, (8) threshold of response, and (9) adaptability. Each of these areas contributes uniquely to the child's ability to form social relationships and respond to the social environment.[104]

Taken together, these areas of temperament have their own continuum: extreme temperament levels are associated with problematic behaviors, and moderate levels are related to easy and appropriate behaviors. Children who exhibit extreme temperament characteristics (e.g., those who are highly active, moody, or irritable) have been identified as *difficult*. The difficult child may not fit with the expectations and schedules of caregivers. Others with happy moods and moderate intensity of response are considered *easy*. A child with an easy temperament may be rhythmic (exhibiting regular sleep/wake cycles) and have positive moods and may have a better fit with caregivers. A match of parent and infant temperament can facilitate strong attachment, just as a mismatch can create difficulties in attachment.

To illustrate how temperament affects goodness of fit, children with arrhythmic, poorly regulated sleep/wake cycles were reported to be difficult to manage by European American families in which the parents worked and needed a consistent routine of sleeping patterns. Puerto Rican parents did not have difficulty in accommodating children with poorly regulated sleep/wake cycles because they molded their schedules around them and allowed their children to sleep when they wanted. In the Puerto Rican families, the incidence of child behavior problems was very low, particularly before school age when a school schedule was imposed.[66] These studies and many others suggest that the child's temperament and behavior affect goodness of fit between the caregiver and the child, which in turn influences developmental outcomes.[20]

Emotions also play an important part in the child's appraisal of his or her experience and in the child's readiness for action in response to contextual change. Emotions relate to how a child evaluates the meaning of an experience in relation to his or her goals. Therefore, if a child engages in an activity with the goal of succeeding but does not, he or she may become disappointed or frustrated. If a child engages in an activity simply to participate and without expectation for success, he or she may experience pleasure irrespective of success. Emotions and temperament (see Chapter 13) influence the child's interest in attempting new activities, the amount of effort demonstrated, and attempts to engage others. These variables influence how a child approaches an activity (e.g., joyfully, reluctantly) and influences its social nature (e.g., whether the child solicits the involvement of others).

Risk and Resiliency

As suggested in the previous section, developmental outcomes have been attributed to the child's personality. Research has shown that certain children attain positive developmental outcomes despite a poor caregiving environment. *Resiliency* refers to a child's internal characteristics that enable him or her to thrive and develop despite high-risk factors in the environment. The concept of resiliency emerged from studies of child development in which the context included risk factors known to have negative effects (e.g., child abuse, parental mental illness or substance abuse, socioeconomic hardship).[107,110] A resilient child has protective factors that enable him or her to develop positive interpersonal skills and general competence despite stressful or traumatic experiences or social environments known to limit developmental potential (e.g., that of an adolescent, single parent). Both child protective factors (e.g., intelligence, prosocial behavior, and social competence) and family protective factors (e.g., material resources, love, nurturance and sense of safety and security, quality of parent-child relationship) are important to positive child outcomes. Researchers have demonstrated that a high-quality relationship with at least one parent, characterized by high levels of warmth and openness and low levels of conflict, is associated with positive outcomes across levels of risk and stages of development.[111]

A child's *resiliency versus vulnerability* also seems to relate to basic physiologic and regulatory characteristics. Children with low cardiovascular reactivity and high immune competence cope better with stressful situations and are less vulnerable to illness when stressed.[110] In middle childhood, well-developed problem solving and communication skills are important to a child's ability to deal with stress. Resilient boys and girls tend to be reflective rather than impulsive, demonstrate an internal locus of control, and use flexible coping strategies in overcoming adversity.[110] Therefore, not only are intelligence and competence important to positive outcomes, but so is emotional regulation, that is, being able to monitor, evaluate, and modify the intensity and duration of emotional reactions.[107]

These concepts suggest that in the interpretation of the influence of environmental factors on a child's development, variables internal to the child can overcome negative contextual variables, including those believed to have a profound influence (e.g., poor caregiving). Although the evidence suggests that children with strong resilience can overcome a high-risk environment (e.g., abusive situations, poverty), a recent research synthesis of risk and resilience studies found that both internal (e.g., child's intelligence, positive affect, emotional regulation) and contextual (e.g., supportive family relationships) protective factors are needed for positive outcomes (e.g., school success, positive relationships).[107] Taken together, the theories that explain how children grow and develop into competent adults and full participants in the community suggest that a child's development of occupations must always be understood as an interaction between the child's biological being and his or her cultural, social, and physical contexts.

AN OCCUPATIONAL THERAPY PERSPECTIVE

Occupations can be defined as the "patterns of action that emerge through transaction between the child and environment and are the things the child wants to do or is expected to do" (p. 22).[58] Although most children accomplish certain occupations and their corresponding tasks in a known sequence, the way these tasks are accomplished is unique for each child. A child learns new occupations based on the facility that she or he brings to the activity. Motor and praxis, sensory-perceptual, emotional regulation, cognitive, and communication and social skills contribute to occupational performance.[2] These skill areas are interdependent; that is, they work together in such a way that the strengths of one system (e.g., visual) can support limitations in others (e.g., kinesthetic). Which systems are recruited for a task varies according to the novelty of the activity and the degree to which the task has become automatic. For example, research has shown that self-feeding using a spoon involves visual-perceptual, kinesthetic, visual-motor, and cognitive systems.[25,45,56] As previously described, grasp of the spoon initially is guided by vision, and the child uses trial and error to hold the spoon so that he or she can scoop the food. With practice and maturation, grasp of the spoon is guided primarily by the kinesthetic system, and correct grasp becomes automatic; vision plays a lesser role. Once food is in the mouth, chewing skills require primarily oral motor skill and somatosensory perception of food texture and food location within the mouth. The skills involved in occupational performance vary not only according to the learning phase but also according to the child's learning preferences and styles.

Development of Occupations

Humphry proposes that three broad mechanisms enable children to develop occupations.[58] These mechanisms, society's investment in children and their participation in the community, interpersonal influences including caregiving adults and peers, and the dynamics of the child's occupational performance, are briefly described next.

The broadest influence on children's occupations is the community in which the child is raised. Communities and society in general have invested in children's occupations by providing playgrounds, preschools, child-oriented music, child-oriented restaurants, and soccer fields. A community's orientation toward children determines available opportunities to play organized sports, learn about art and music, safely play in neighborhoods, and gain friendships with diverse peers. Communities that value organized sports and outdoor activity may have soccer or baseball teams, horseback riding, and swimming specifically designed for children with disabilities (e.g., Special Olympics, Miracle League Baseball, therapeutic horseback riding). Characteristics of the community become barriers or opportunities for the child and family and their desired occupations. As advocates for children with disabilities, occupational therapists can influence the development of programs that are accessible and appropriate for children with a wide range of ability. They can emphasize the importance of supporting the participation of all children in community activities, recognizing the different levels of support and accommodation needed.

Humphry suggests that children learn through both direct and indirect social participation.[58] A young child's first learning about an occupation is often through observing his parents, siblings, and other adults or peers. The first representational pretend play is typically imitation of the mother's actions when cleaning and cooking. Children imitate their parents' gestures and speech without being explicitly taught to do so. They also learn the consequences of actions by observing how their parents respond to each other or to their siblings. They can learn that an action is wrong by observing punishment of a peer for that action. Vicarious learning appears to be particularly important to a child's assuming cultural beliefs and values. Children learn the traditions and rituals of a culture by observing their family's participation in these. Inclusive models of education are believed to be effective learning environments for children with disabilities based on the known benefit of observing and interacting with typical peer models.[31,32] When in a child's presence, therapists should always be conscious that their actions and words influence children's learning and of whether these actions are directed toward the child.

Learning is generally more vigorous when the child actively participates in an occupation. Children's play with each other is an integrated learning experience in which the child acts, observes, and interacts. Play involves most or all performance areas, including affective, sensory, motor, communicative, social, and cognitive. When children play together, they learn from, model for, challenge, and reinforce each other. This flow of interactions occurs in meaningful activities that generally bring pleasure and intrinsic reinforcement and enable learning.

To learn a specific skill, the child must actively practice it. Specific scaffolding, guidance, cueing, prompting, and reinforcement by an occupational therapist can assist the child in learning to perform a skill. This direct support from the therapist (or other adult) can facilitate performance at a higher level or at a more appropriate level so that the fit between the child and desired occupations and context becomes optimal. In the case of a child with disabilities, a more intensive level of direct support and scaffolding may be necessary for learning new skills. Adult guidance and support of the child during play can facilitate a successful strategy, help the child evaluate his or her performance, and encourage and reinforce continued practice. Therapists can also optimize the environment to support and reinforce the child's performance. Participation in play occupations in a natural environment results in integrated learning across performance areas (e.g., including sensory, motor, cognitive, and affective learning).

The child's play and actions are always within a social, cultural, and physical context. To understand the development of occupational performance, the occupational therapist must understand the child's play and actions as coherent occupations within specific contexts.

Contexts for Development

Children develop occupations through participation in family activities and cultural practices. As a child participates in the family's cultural practices, he or she learns occupations and performance skills that enable him or her to become a full participant in the community. Rogoff explains: "People develop as participants in cultural communities. Their development can be understood only in light of the cultural practices and circumstances of their communities" (pp. 3-4).[88] Variations in the child's play activities (e.g., how he or she builds with wooden blocks, draws a picture of himself or herself, or sings a song) reflect the child's biological abilities and the influence of cultural, social, and physical contexts.

A child's cultural, social, and physical contexts change through the course of development and tend to expand as the child matures. The environment surrounds and supports the child's action; it also forces the child to adapt and assists or accommodates that adaptation. As a child perceives the affordances of the environment, he or she learns to act on those affordances, expanding a repertoire of actions. At the same time, the child's understanding of how the world responds to his or her actions increases. Rogoff argued that culture affects every aspect of the child's development, which cannot be understood outside this context.[88] The child is nested in his or her family, culture, and community, which have influenced the child's genetic makeup and continue to provide the learning environment. By recognizing this influence, occupational therapists view each child in his or her cultural context and work as change agents within that context.

Cultural practices are the routine activities common to a people of a culture and may reflect religion, traditions, economic survival, community organization, and regional ideology. The child learns motor and process skills through his or her participation in these cultural practices. Reciprocally, a child's motor and process skills enable participation in the occupations and cultural practices of the child's family and community.

Cultural Contexts

To fully understand how children develop through participation in cultural practices, Rogoff and her colleagues have studied child development in various cultures, including the European American culture. Their findings, as well as the findings of occupational therapists,[10,30] have expanded our understanding of how children develop and have broadened the definition of typical child development.

Cultures vary in many aspects, such as the roles of women and children, values and beliefs about family and religion, family traditions, and the importance of health care and education. The continuum of interdependence versus autonomy of individuals varies in cultural groups and is a significant determinant of childhood occupations. The value a people or community places on interdependence among its members versus individual autonomy creates differences in child-rearing practices and different experiences for developing children.

Most middle-class European Americans value independence as a primary important goal for their children. U.S. parents encourage individuality, self-expression, and independence in their children's actions and thoughts. To foster early independence in children, U.S. parents do not sleep with their infants; instead infants sleep in their own crib and/or room. Yet this practice is unusual within other societies in the world, such as Asia, Africa, and South America, where infants sleep in their parents' bed or room.[77] For example, Japanese parents report that co-sleeping facilitates infants' transformation from separate individuals to persons able to engage in interdependent relationships. Japanese parents are interested in promoting continued reciprocity with their children, encouraging the primacy of family relationships.[88]

One consequence of the early separation of infants from their parents for sleeping is that middle-class U.S. parents often engage in elaborate and time-consuming bedtime routines. In contrast, Mayan parents reported that they do not use bedtime routines (e.g., stories or lullabies) to coax babies to sleep.[89] To encourage interdependence, Mayan parents hold their infants continuously, and they often hold them so that they can orient to the group (i.e., facing other members of the group rather than their mothers). By observing others more than their mother, infants become aware of their adult community. In the Latino culture, which also encourages interdependence, parents are permissive and indulgent with young children. Latino parents do not push developmental skills, in part because they value interdependence with the family as opposed to autonomy of the individual.[117]

In general, cultures that value independence over interdependence also value competition over cooperation. Korean American children have been found to be more cooperative in play than European American children. Mexican children also are more likely to cooperate than European American children.[88] These examples briefly illustrate how cultural beliefs influence the ways parents raise their children and communities support and challenge children.

Social Contexts

Culture influences the social relationships that envelop the child, yet certain aspects of the child's social context appear to be independent of cultural influences and are consistent across cultures. This section defines elements of the social context particularly important to a child's development. The most important relationships formed during infancy are those with parents and/or primary caregivers. When caregivers are sensitive and responsive to the infant, healthy socioemotional development results.[33,68] Infants' interactions with parents serve to enhance the infants' basic physiologic and regulatory systems. When parents attune to the infant's sensory modulation and arousal needs and support these needs, the infant develops secure attachment. Mothers who modulate their behaviors to match their infants' needs for stimulation and comfort also promote the infants' abilities to self-regulate. The child's interaction with a caregiver gives him or her essential information about how self and other are related, which becomes important to engaging in future relationships. Attachment patterns seem to influence the child's style of interaction and engagement in later years. Sensitive responding consolidates the infant's sense of efficacy and provides a foundation of security for confident exploration of the environment.[33]

Csikszentmihalyi and Rathunde describe parenting as a dance between supporting and challenging the child.[29] Supporting the child enables him or her to assimilate or explore the environment—that is, to play. Parental challenge requires a child to accommodate and conform. Parenting provides a combination of these supports and challenges. Rogoff defines the support-challenge combination of guided participation as adults' challenging, constraining, and supporting children in solving problems.[88] All parents use some measure of support to bolster children's attempts to master skills and some degree of challenge to move children toward higher levels of mastery. These elements are subtly provided by parents in the ways they present tasks and select when and how they instruct or intervene. Effective guidance relies on careful observation of the child's cues. Sensitivity and responsivity to the child's needs appear to be among the most important variables in the promotion of child development.[66] The concept of guided participation is similar to Vygotsky's notion of the zone of proximal development. In guided participation, emphasis is placed on parents' sensitivity to the child's skills to determine the level of support or challenge needed.

In typical situations, infants receive care from multiple care providers, including child care providers, grandparents, and other adults. The infant may or may not attach to caregivers other than the parents or primary caregivers; however, these social relationships are important to the infant's emotional development and provide opportunities for the development of social skills. At least 60% of children under 5 years of age participate in non-parent child care, including center-based and family child care.[78] A study for the National Institute of Child Health and Human Development revealed that positive caregiving occurred when children were in smaller groups, child-to-adult ratios were low, caregivers did not use an authoritarian style, and the physical environment was safe, clean, and stimulating.[79] Family factors predicted child outcomes even for children who spent many hours in child care. The family environment appears to have a significantly greater effect on a child's development than the child care environment.[38]

Physical Contexts

The physical environment surrounds and supports the child's action; it forces the child to adapt his or her actions to meet the demands and constraints of the physical surroundings. As a child perceives the affordances of the environment, he or she learns to act on those affordances, thus expanding a repertoire of actions. At the same time, the child's understanding of how the world responds to his or her actions increases. Gibson explained how a child's exploration of physical surfaces and objects allows him or her to develop and practice mobility and manipulation skills.[47] Examples of the interactions of a child and his or her physical environments and the developmental consequences are presented next.

CHILDREN'S OCCUPATIONS, PERFORMANCE SKILLS, AND CONTEXTS

This section describes the child's development of play occupations as enabled by his or her performance skills and cultural, physical, and social contexts. For three age groups—infancy, early childhood, and middle childhood—typical play occupations and activities are described. The contribution of motor, sensory, emotional, cognitive, and social abilities and contexts to the development of play occupations is described. Although children's occupations are similar within a particular age level, the contexts, individual abilities, and activities are varied and diverse, resulting in a unique occupational performance for each child. Recognition of the uniqueness of a child's development and of how these components contribute to performance within individuals is key to analysis of occupational performance.

Although the child learns occupations other than play (e.g., those related to school function), occupational therapists most often use play activities to engage the child in the therapeutic process. Play activities serve as the means to improve performance because they are self-motivating and offer goals around which the child can self-organize.[81] Play also serves as the end or goal of therapy services. Children put effort and energy into play activities because they are inherently interesting and fun. (A more detailed description of play as a goal and modality of therapy can be found in Chapter 18.) Descriptions of a child's development of feeding, self-care, and school function are presented in other chapters (Chapters 15, 16, and 24). The contribution of communication abilities is also important to the development of play and other childhood occupations, but it is not discussed in this chapter because language and communication are not primary concerns for occupational therapists.

Infants: Birth to 2 Years

Play Occupations

The play occupations of infants in the first 12 months are exploratory and social—that is, they are related to bonding with caregivers (Boxes 3-1 and 3-2). As in every stage, these occupations overlap (e.g., bonding occurs during exploratory play with the parent's hair and face, and the parent's holding supports the infant's play with objects). Much of the infant's awake and alert time is spent in exploratory play, often play that occurs in the caregiver's arms or with the caregiver nearby.

Exploratory play is also called *sensorimotor play.* Rubin defined *exploratory play* as an activity performed simply for the enjoyment of the physical sensation it creates.[92] It includes

repetitive movements to create actions in toys for the sensory experiences of hearing, seeing, and feeling. The infant places toys in the mouth, waves them in the air, and explores their surfaces with the hands. These actions allow for intense

---

BOX 3-1 Development of Play Occupations: Infants—Birth to 6 Months

PLAY OCCUPATIONS
Exploratory Play
Sensorimotor play predominates
Social play
Focused on attachment and bonding with parents

PERFORMANCE SKILLS
Regulatory/Sensory Organization
Quiets when picked up
Shows pleasure when touched and handled
Relaxes, smiles, and vocalizes when held
Cuddles
Listens to a voice
Uses hands and mouth for sensory exploration of objects
Fine Motor/Manipulation
Follows moving person with eyes
Develops accurate reach to object
Uses variety of palmar grasping patterns
Secures object with hand and brings to mouth
Transfers objects hand to hand
Examines objects carefully with eyes
Plays with hands at midline
Gross Motor/Mobility
Lifts head (3-4 months) raises trunk when prone (4-6 months)
Kicks reciprocally when supine
Sits propping on hands
Plays (bounces) when standing with support from parents
Rolls from place to place
Cognitive
Repeats actions for pleasurable experiences
Uses hands and mouth to explore objects
Searches with eyes for sound
Bangs object on table
Integrates information from multiple sensory systems
Social
Coos, then squeals
Smiles, laughs out loud
Expresses discomfort by crying
Communicates simple emotions through facial expressions

Data from Parks, S. (2007) *HELP Strands.* Palo Alto, CA: VORT Corp; Gesell, A., & Amatruda, G. (1947). *Developmental diagnosis.* (2nd ed.) New York: Harper & Row.

BOX 3-2 Development of Play Occupations: Infants—6 to 12 Months

PLAY OCCUPATIONS
Exploratory Play
Sensorimotor play evolves into functional play
Functional Play
Begins to use toys according to their functional purpose
Social Play
Attachment to parents and caregivers
Social play with parents and others

PERFORMANCE SKILLS
Regulatory/Sensory Organization
Enjoys being held up in the air and moving rapidly through the air
Listens to speech without being distracted
Finger-feeds self, including a variety of food textures
Cooperates with dressing
Fine Motor/Manipulation
Mouths toys
Uses accurate and direct reach for toys
Plays with toys at midline; transfers hand to hand
Bangs objects together to make sounds
Waves toys in the air
Releases toys into container
Rolls ball to adult
Grasps small objects in fingertips
Points to toys with index finger, uses index finger to explore toys
Crudely uses tool
Gross Motor/Mobility
Sits independently
Rolls from place to place
Independently gets into sitting
Pivots in sitting position
Stands, holding on for support
Plays in standing when leaning on support
Crawls on belly initially, then crawls on all fours (10 months)
Walks with hand held (12 months)
Cognitive
Responds to own name
Recognizes words and family members' names
Responds with appropriate gestures
Listens selectively
Imitates simple gestures
Looks at picture book
Begins to generalize from past experiences
Acts with intention on toys
Takes objects out of container
Social
Shows special dependence on mother
May show stranger anxiety
Lifts arms to be picked up
Plays contentedly when parents are in room
Interacts briefly with other infants
Plays give and take
Responds playfully to mirror (laughs or makes faces)

Data from Park, S. (2007). *HELP Strands.* Palo Alto, CA: VORT Corporation; Linder, T. (2008). *Transdisciplinary play-based assessment* (rev. ed.). Baltimore: Brookes; Gesell, A., & Amatruda, G. (1947). *Developmental diagnosis* (2nd ed). New York: Harper & Row.

perceptual learning and bring delight to the infant (without any more complex purpose).

In the second year of life, the infant engages in *functional*, or *relational*, *play*; that is, an object's function is understood, and that function determines the action (Boxes 3-3 and 3-4). Initially, children use objects on themselves (e.g., pretending to drink from a cup or to comb the hair). These self-directed actions signal the beginning of *pretend play*.[83] The child knows cause and effect and repeatedly makes the toy telephone ring or the battery-powered doll squeal to enjoy the effect of the initial action.

By the end of the second year, play has expanded in two important ways. First, the child begins to combine actions into

---

BOX 3-3   Development of Play Occupations: Infants—12 to 18 Months

PLAY OCCUPATIONS

Relational and Functional Play
Engages in simple pretend play directed toward self (pretend eating, sleeping)
Links 2 or 3 schemes in simple combinations
Demonstrates imitative play from an immediate model
Gross Motor Play
Explores all spaces in the room
Rolls and crawls in play close to the ground
Social Play
Begins peer interactions
Parallel play

PERFORMANCE SKILLS

Regulatory/Sensory Organization
Enjoys messy activities
Reacts to extreme sensations, such as warm, cold, sweet
Fine Motor/Manipulation
Holds crayon and makes marks; scribbles
Holds two toys in hand and toys in both hands
Releases toys inside containers, even small containers
Stacks blocks and fits toys into form space (places pieces in board)
Attempts puzzles
Opens and shuts toy boxes or containers
Points to pictures with index finger
Uses two hands in play, one to hold or stabilize and one to manipulate
Gross Motor/Mobility
Sits in small chair
Plays in standing
Walks well, squats, picks up toys from the floor
Climbs into adult chair
Flings ball
Pulls toys when walking
Begins to run
Walks upstairs with one hand held
Pushes and pulls large toys or boxes on floor
Cognitive
Acts on object using variety of schema
Imitates model
Symbolic play with real props (e.g., pretends to drink with cup)
Understands how objects work
Understands function of objects
Uses trial-and-error in problem-solving
Recognizes names of various body parts
Social
Moves away from parent
Shares toys with parent
Responds to facial expressions of others

Data from Park, S. (2007). *HELP Strands*. Palo Alto, CA: VORT Corporation; Linder, T. (2008). *Transdisciplinary play-based assessment* (rev. ed.). Baltimore: Brookes; Gesell, A., & Amatruda, G. (1947). *Developmental diagnosis* (2nd ed). New York: Harper & Row.

BOX 3-4   Development of Play Occupations: Toddlers—18 to 24 Months

PLAY OCCUPATIONS

Functional Play
Multischeme combinations
Performs multiple related actions together
Gross Motor Play
Enjoys sensory input of gross motor play
Pretend or Symbolic Play
Makes inanimate objects perform actions (dolls dancing, eating, hugging)
Pretends that objects are real or that they symbolize another object
Social Play
Participates in parallel play
Imitates parents and peers in play
Participates in groups of children
Watches other children
Begins to take turns

PERFORMANCE SKILLS

Regulatory/ Sensory Organization
Enjoys solitary play for a few minutes
Uses PlayDoh
Enjoys rough and tumble play
Fine Motor/Manipulation
Completes 4- to 5-piece puzzle
Builds towers (e.g., 4 blocks)
Holds crayon in fingertips and draws simple figures (straight stroke or circular stroke)
Strings beads
Begins to use simple tools (e.g., play hammer)
Participates in multipart tasks
Turns pages of book
Gross Motor/Mobility
Runs, squats, climbs on furniture
Climbs on jungle gym and slides
Moves on ride-on toy without pedals (kiddy car)
Kicks ball forward
Throws ball at large target
Jumps with both feet (in place)
Walks up and down stairs
Cognitive
Links multiple steps together
Has inanimate object perform action
Begins to use nonrealistic objects in pretend play
Continues to use objects according to functional purpose
Object permanence is completely developed
Social
Expresses affection
Shows wide variety of emotions: fear, anger, sympathy, joy
Can feel frustrated
Enjoys solitary play, such as coloring, building
Engages in parallel play
Laughs when someone does something silly

Data from Park, S. (2007). *HELP Strands*. Palo Alto, CA: VORT Corporation; Linder, T. (2008). *Transdisciplinary play-based assessment* (rev. ed.). Baltimore: Brookes.

play sequences (e.g., he or she relates objects to each other by stacking one on the other or by lining up toys beside each other). These combined actions show a play purpose that matches the function of the toy. Second, 2-year-old children now direct actions away from themselves. The objects used in play generally resemble real-life objects.[67] The child places the doll in a toy bed and then covers it. The child pretends to feed a stuffed animal or drives toy cars through a toy garage. At 2 years of age, play remains a very central occupation of the child, who now has an increased attention span and the ability to combine multiple actions in play. The emergence of *symbolic*, or *imaginary*, *play* with toys and objects offers the first opportunities for the child to practice the skills of living.

The child also engages in gross motor play throughout the day. As he or she becomes mobile, exploration of space, surfaces, and large action toys becomes a primary occupation. Movement is also enjoyed simply as movement; the child delights in swinging and running or attempting to run and moving in water or sand. Deep proprioceptive pressure and touch are craved and requested. As in exploratory play, the child's exploration of space involves simple, repeated actions in which the goal appears to be sensation. Often, extremes in sensation seem to be enjoyed and are frequently requested. Repetition of these full-body kinesthetic, vestibular, and tactile experiences appears to be organizing to the CNS. In addition, this repetition is important to the child's development of balance, coordination, and motor planning. Hence, the occupational goal of movement and exploration becomes the means for development of multiple performance areas.

In the first year, the goal of an infant's *social play* is attachment, or bonding, to the parents). As described by Greenspan, this is a period in which the infant falls in love with the parents and learns to trust the environment because of the care and attention provided by the parents or caregivers.[54] These occupations are critical foundations to later occupations that involve social relating and demonstration of emotions. At 1 year of age, infants play social games with parents and others to elicit responses. Although infants at this age engage readily with individuals other than family, they require their parents' presence as an emotional base and return to them for occasional emotional refueling before returning to play.[105]

By the second year, children exhibit social play in which they imitate adults and peers. Imitation of others is a first way to interact and socially relate. Both immediate and deferred imitation of others are important to social play as children enter preschool environments and begin to relate to their peers.

Performance Skills

Sensory and Motor Skills

The newborn can interpret body sensations and respond reflexively. He enjoys and needs a consistent caregiver's physical contact and tactile stimulation. The neonate turns his head when touched on the cheek, relaxes in his mother's arms, and expresses discomfort from a wet diaper. Self-regulation of sleep-wake cycles, feeding, and display of emotions and arousal emerge in early infancy. The infant molds himself to the parents's embrace, clinging to the parent's arms and chest. The newborn's vestibular system is also quite mature as he calms from rocking and enjoys the motion of a parent walking him

about the room. The neonate demonstrates orientation and attention to visual, auditory, and tactile stimuli. An important fact is that the newborn also exhibits *habituation*, or the ability to extinguish incoming sensory information (e.g., ability to sleep by blocking out sound in a noisy nursery).

Gross motor activity begins prenatally in response to vestibular and tactile input inside the womb. The first movements of newborns appear to be reflexive; however, on closer examination, they reveal the ability to process and integrate sensory information. The neonate's motor responses contribute to perceptual development and organization. In the first month of life, the infant moves the head side to side when in a prone position and rights the head when supported in sitting. By 4 months, the prone infant lifts the head to visualize activities in the room. This ability to lift and sustain an erect-head position appears to relate to the infant's interest in watching the activities of others, as well as improved trunk strength and stability. As the infant reaches 6 months, he or she demonstrates increased ability to lift the head and trunk when in a prone position to visualize the environment when prone. The infant can also move side to side on the forearms, then the hands, and can lift an arm to grasp a toy (Figure 3-4). When supine, the child actively kicks and brings the feet to the mouth. Over the next 6 months, this dynamic, postural stability prepares the infant to become mobile.

Rolling is normally the infant's first method of becoming mobile and exploring the environment. Initially, rolling is an automatic reaction of body righting; usually the infant first rolls from the stomach to the side and then from the stomach to the back. By 6 months, the infant rolls sequentially to move across the room. Heavy or large babies may initiate rolling several months later, and infants with hypersensitivity of the vestibular system (i.e., overreactivity to rotary movement) may avoid rolling entirely.

Most infants enjoy supported sitting at a very early age. As their vision improves in the first 4 months, they become more eager to view their environment from a supported sitting position. The newborn sits with a rounded back; the head is erect only momentarily. Head control emerges quickly.

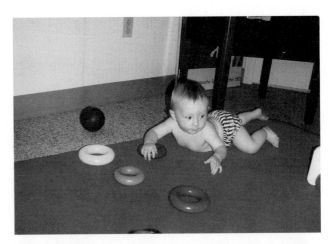

FIGURE 3-4 In prone position, the infant shifts his weight from side to side when playing with toys; later he learns to pivot while prone to expand where he can reach and what he can visualize.

By 4 months, the infant can hold the head upright with control for long periods, moving it side to side with ease. Most 6-month-old infants sit alone by propping forward on the arms, using a wide base of support with the legs flexed. However, this position is precarious, and the infant easily topples when tilted. Many 7-month-old infants sit independently. Often their hands are freed for play with toys, but they struggle to reach beyond arm's length.

By 8 to 9 months, the infant sits erect and unsupported for several minutes. At that time, or within the next couple of months, the infant may rise from a prone posture by rotating (from a side-lying position) into a sitting position. This important skill gives the infant the ability to progress by creeping to a toy and then, after arriving at the toy, to sit and play. By 12 months, the infant can rise to sitting from a supine position, rotate and pivot when sitting, and easily move in between positions of sitting and creeping (Figure 3-5).

After experimenting with pivoting and backward crawling in a prone position, the 7-month-old infant crawls forward. He or she may first attempt belly crawling using both sides of the body together. However, reciprocal arm and leg movements quickly emerge as the most successful method of forward progression. Crawling in a hands-and-knees posture (sometimes called *creeping*) requires more strength and coordination than belly crawling. The two sides of the body move reciprocally. In addition, shoulder and pelvic stability are needed for the infant to hold the body weight over the hands and knees. Mature, reciprocal hands-and-knees crawling also requires slight trunk rotation (Figure 3-6). Through the practice of crawling in the second 6 months of life, the child develops trunk flexibility and rotation. Most 10- to 12-month-old infants crawl rapidly across the room, over various surfaces, and even up and down inclines.

Infants at 5 and 6 months delight in standing, and they gleefully bounce up and down while supported by their parents' arms. The strong vestibular input and practice of patterns of hip and knee flexion and extension are important to the development of full upright posture after 1 year. The young infant also prepares for a full upright posture by standing

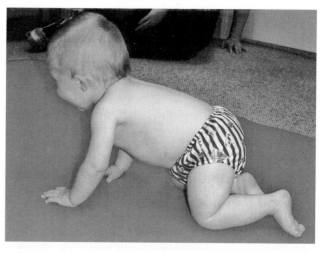

FIGURE 3-6 Crawling on all fours allows the infant to explore new spaces. This form of mobility increases shoulder and pelvic stability for upright stance and promote the rotational patterns needed for ambulation. (From Henderson, A., & Pehoski, C. [2006]. *Hand function in the child: Foundations for remediation* [2nd ed.]. St. Louis: Mosby.)

against furniture or the parent's lap. A 10-month-old infant practices rising and lowering in upright postures while holding onto the furniture. By pulling up on furniture to standing, the infant can reach objects previously unavailable. This new level of exploration and increase in potential play objects motivates infants to practice standing and motivates parents to place breakable objects on higher shelves (Figure 3-7). At 12 months the infant learns to shift the body weight onto one leg and to step to the side with the other leg. The infant soon takes small steps forward while holding onto furniture or the parent's finger.

The infant's first efforts toward unsupported forward movement through walking are often seen in short, erratic steps, a wide-based gait, and arms held in high guard. All these postural and mobility skills contribute to the infant's ability to explore

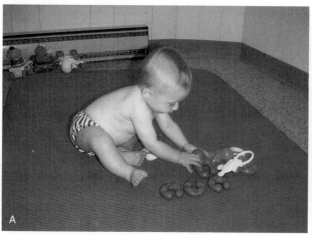
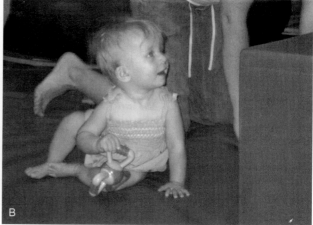

FIGURE 3-5 *A,* In dynamic sitting, the infant has sufficient postural stability to reach in all directions. *B,* By 10 months, the infant easily moves into and out of sitting positions.

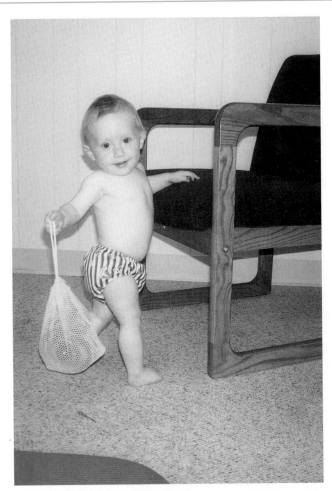

FIGURE 3-7 Supported stance is a favorite play position for infants 8 to 11 months of age.

Grasp changes dramatically in the first 6 months (Figure 3-8, *A* and *B*). Initially, grasping occurs automatically (when anything is placed in the hand) and involves mass flexion of the fingers as a unit. The object is held in the palm rather than distally in the fingers or fingertips. Three- to 4-month-old infants, therefore, squeeze objects within their hands, and the thumb does not appear to be involved in this grasp. At 4 to 5 months, the infant exhibits a palmar grasp in which flexed fingers and an adducted thumb press the object against the palm (Figure 3-8, *C*). At 6 months, the infant uses a radial palmar grasping pattern in which the first two fingers hold the object against the thumb. This grasp enables the infant to orient the object so that it can be easily seen or brought to the mouth (Figure 3-8, *D*). The infant secures small objects using a raking motion of the fingers, with the forearm stabilized on the surface.

Grasp continues to change rapidly between 7 and 12 months.[14,27] A radial digital grasp emerges in which the thumb opposes the index and middle finger pads. At approximately 9 months, wrist stability in extension increases, and the infant is better able to use the fingertips in grasping (e.g., the infant can use fingertips to grasp a small object, such as a cube or cracker). By holding objects distally in the fingers, the infant can move the object while it is in the hand; movement of objects within the hands allows the infant to explore them and use objects for functional purposes. A pincer grasp, with which the infant holds small objects between the thumb and finger pads, develops by 10 to 11 months. The 12-month-old infant uses a variety of grasping patterns, often holding an object in the radial fingers and thumb. The infant may also grasp a raisin or piece of cereal with a mature pincer grasp (i.e., one in which the thumb opposes the index finger).

In the second year of life, grasping patterns continue to be refined. The child holds objects distally in the fingers, where holding is more dynamic. By the end of the second year, a tripod grasp on utensils and other tools may be observed. Other grasping patterns may also be used, depending on the size, shape, and weight of the object held. For example, tools are held in the hand using first a palmar grasp and then a digital grasp. Blended grasping patterns develop toward the end of the second year, allowing the child to hold a tool securely in the ulnar digits while the radial digits guide its use.

Voluntary release of objects develops around 7 and 8 months. The first release is awkward and is characterized by full extension of all fingers. The infant becomes interested in dropping objects and practices release by flinging them from the high chair. By 10 months, objects are purposefully released into a container, one of the first ways the infant relates separate objects. As the infant combines objects in play, release becomes important for stacking and accurate placement. For example, the play of 1-year-old children includes placing objects in containers, dumping them out, and then beginning the activity again.

Between 15 and 18 months, the infant demonstrates release of a raisin into a small bottle and the ability to stack two cubes. Stacking blocks is part of relational play, because the infant now has the needed control of the arm in space, precision grasp without support, controlled release, spatial relations, and depth perception. The infant can also place large, simple puzzle pieces and pegs in the proper areas. At the same time, the infant acquires the ability to discriminate simple forms and shapes. Therefore, the infant's learning of perceptual skills

space and obtain desired play objects. By 18 months, the infant prefers walking to other forms of mobility, but balance remains immature, and the infant falls frequently. He or she continues to use a wide-based gait and has difficulty with stopping and turning. Infants remain highly motivated to practice this new skill, however, because walking brings new avenues of exploration and a sense of autonomy, and the parent must now protect the infant from objects that previously could not be reached and from spaces that have not yet been explored.

The newborn moves the arms in wide ranges, mostly to the side of the body. In the first 3 months, the infant contacts objects with the eyes more than with the hands. By 3 months, he follows his mother's face in a smooth arc, crossing midline. As early as 1 to 2 months, an infant learns to swipe at objects placed at his or her side. This first pattern of reaching is inaccurate, but by 5 months, the accuracy of reaching towards objects increases greatly.[91] The infant struggles to combine grasp with reach and may make several efforts to grasp an object held at a distance. As postural stability increases, the infant also learns to control arm and hand movements as a means of exploring objects and materials in the environment. By the time an infant is 6 months old, direct unilateral and bilateral reaches are observed, and the infant smoothly and accurately extends the arm toward a desired object.[108]

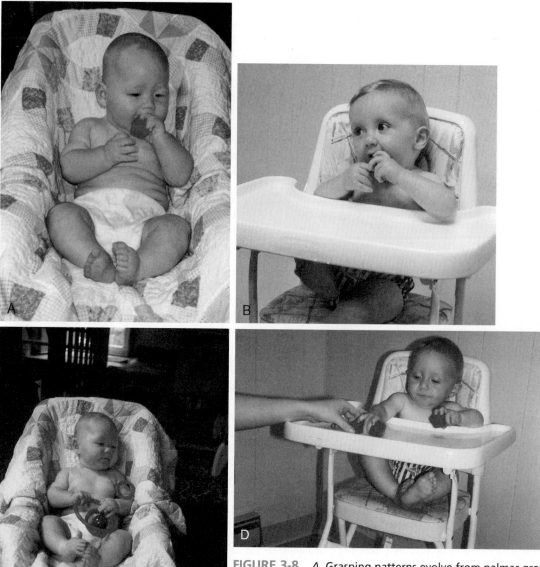

FIGURE 3-8   *A,* Grasping patterns evolve from palmar grasps without active thumb use to radial digital grasps as in *B. C,* At 4 months, the infant holds the object tight against the palm, with all fingers flexing as a unit. *D,* At 8 months, the infant holds objects in the radial digits.   (*A* and *B* from Henderson, A., & Pehoski, C. [2006]. *Hand function in the child: Foundations for remediation* [2nd ed.]. St. Louis: Mosby.)

is supported by improved manipulative abilities, and increased perceptual discrimination promotes the infant's practice of manipulation.[82] Perception of force increases, enabling the infant to hold an object with the just-right amount of pressure (e.g., so cookies are not crushed before eaten).

The complementary use of both hands to play with objects develops between 12 months and 2 years. During this time, one hand is used to hold the object while the other hand manipulates or moves the object. It is not until the third year that children consistently demonstrate use of two hands in simultaneous, coordinated actions (e.g., using both hands to string beads or button a shirt).[36]

Cognitive Skills

In the first 6 months, the infant learns about the body and the effects of its actions. Interests are focused on the actions with objects and the sensory input these actions provide. The infant's learning occurs through the primary senses: looking, tasting, touching, smelling, hearing, and moving. The infant enjoys repeating actions for their own sake, and play is focused on the action that can be performed with an object (e.g., mouthing, banging, shaking), rather than the object itself.[67] By 8 to 9 months, the infant has an attention span of 2 to 3 minutes and combines objects when playing (e.g., placing favorite toy in a container). At this age, children begin to understand object permanence; that is, they know that an object continues to exist even though it is hidden and cannot be seen.[23] They can also find a hidden sound and actively try to locate new sounds.

By 12 months, the infant's understanding of the functional purpose of objects increases. Play behaviors are increasingly determined by the purpose of the toy, and toys are used according to their function. The infant also demonstrates more goal-directed behaviors, performing a particular action with the intent of obtaining a specific result or goal. Tools become important at this time, because the infant uses play tools (e.g., hammers, spoons, shovels) to gain further understanding of how objects work. At the same time, the infant begins to understand how objects work (e.g., how to activate a switch or open a door).

In the second year, the child can put together a sequence of several actions, such as placing small "people" in a toy bus and pushing it across the floor. The sequencing of actions indicates increasing memory and attention span. Some of the first sequential behaviors illustrate the child's imitation of parent or sibling actions; therefore, increased ability to imitate and increased play sequences appear to develop concurrently (Figure 3-9).

Social Skills

The infant's emotional transition from the protective, warm womb to the moment of birth is a dramatic change. The primary purpose of the newborn's system is to maintain body functions (i.e., the cardiovascular, respiratory, and gastrointestinal systems). However, as the infant matures, the focus shifts to increasing competence in interaction with the environment. The sense of basic trust or mistrust becomes a main theme in the infant's affective development and is highly dependent on the relationship with the primary caregivers. According to Erikson, the first demonstration of an infant's social trust is observed in the ease with which he or she feeds and sleeps.[35]

The basic trust relationship has varying degrees of involvement. Parent-infant bonding is not endowed but is developed from experiences shared between parent and child over time. These feelings are seen in the progression of physical contact between parent and infant. The infant shows a differentiated response to the parent's voice, usually quieting and calming. Although infants are capable of crying from birth, they begin to express other emotions by 2 months, such as smiling and laughing.

By 5 to 6 months, the infant becomes very interested in a mirror, indicating a beginning recognition of self. By 4 to 5 months, he or she vocalizes in tones that indicate pleasure and displeasure. In the second year of life, the parents (or caregivers) remain the most important people in the child's life.

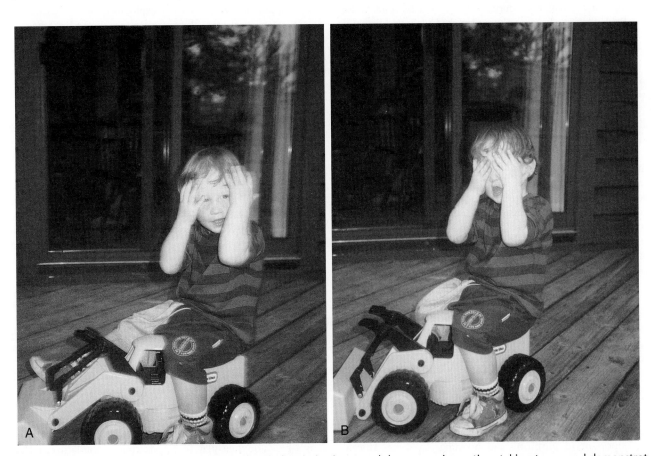

FIGURE 3-9 The 2-year-old boy engages in social play, imitating an adult, sequencing action, taking turns, and demonstrating understanding of object permanence on self.

The 2-year-old infant likes to be in constant sight of the parents and expresses emotions by hugging and kissing them.

Although toddlers practice their autonomy around parents, they have no intention of giving up reliance on them and may become upset or frightened when the parents leave. Two-year-old children are interested in other children, but they tend to watch them rather than verbally or physically interacting with them. In a room of open spaces, these children are likely to play next to each other. Their side-by-side play often involves imitation, with few verbal acknowledgments of each other.

Contexts of Infancy

Cultural Contexts

The family's cultural beliefs and values influence caregiving practices and determine many of the child's earliest experiences. For example, feeding and co-sleeping practices both influence the infant's development. Breast feeding and bottle feeding practices vary in different cultures and ethnic groups. Although practices vary in the United States, European American mothers tend to breast-feed for the first 6 months. Mothers often establish a feeding schedule, separating feedings by longer intervals as the infant matures. African American families expect the infant to make the transition to table food quickly, and infants generally eat only table food by 1 year.[113] In contrast, Chinese and Filipino infants are often breast-fed on demand until 2 to 2½ years of age.[17,18] These parents are often very attentive, carrying and holding their infants throughout the day, even during naps. When the infants are not held, they are kept nearby and picked up immediately if they cry.[18] In many countries, children are fed certain foods as medicine, that is, to improve health or prevent illness. For example, in the Middle East, infants are given tea and herbal mixtures to prevent or cure illness, and a dietary balance of hot and cold foods is believed to be essential to good health.[95]

Children around the world are encouraged to self-feed at different ages using different utensils and methods. In India, toddlers learn to use only the right hand to eat. The left hand is dirty and is used only to clean oneself after defecation. As children learn to self-feed, parents often restrain the left hand.[88] As a result, the right hand develops early advanced skills to manipulate and prehend food without the assistance of the left. These self-feeding practices can contribute to children's rapid maturation of right-hand dexterity. Studies of Japanese child have shown higher-level fine motor skills than those in American children. The greater fine motor skills of Chinese children have been attributed, in part, to their early use of chopsticks as feeding utensils.[114]

In most middle-class U.S. homes, children sleep separated from their parents. For the earliest ages, children are placed in a separate crib and generally a separate room. The parents believe that infants and toddlers need to learn to sleep independently and become independent in self-care skills as soon as possible. In most societies outside the United States, infants sleep with their mothers.[88] Mayan infants and toddlers sleep in the same room with their parents, often in the mother's bed.[77] Asian and Middle Eastern parents tend to sleep with their infants, because they believe that these sleeping arrangements are important to nurturing and bonding. In some African American and Appalachian families, parents sleep with their infants. Close physical contact at night and then into the day can foster interdependence within families, in contrast with the independence that most U.S. parents often foster in their children.

Physical Contexts

Although many infants have a supplemental play area in a child care center, the home provides the infant's first play environment. The crib is often a play environment, providing a place for comforting toys (e.g., music boxes, colorful mobiles). Other early play spaces include the playpen, infant seat, and swing. The infant also spends time playing on the floor's carpeted surface or on a blanket. Because the infant is not yet mobile, safety is not as much of a concern as it will be in the next 2 years of life. Early play also occurs in the parent's or caregiver's arms. Exploratory play and attachment occupations are pursued on the parent's lap, and the infant is fascinated by the parent's face and clothing. At the same time, the infant feels safe and comforted by the parent's presence.

In the second 6 months, the infant requires less support to play, and a major role of the parent becomes one of protector from harm. As the infant becomes more mobile, spaces are closed and objects now within reach are removed. Exploration of all accessible spaces becomes an infant's primary goal.

In the second year of life, the child's environment may expand to the yard, to neighbors' homes and yards, and to previously unexplored spaces in the home. Most children have opportunities for play in their home's yard or in the fenced-in areas of their child care centers. Although the child's increasing interest in visiting outdoor spaces provides important opportunities for sensory exploration, it also creates certain safety concerns. Parents therefore invest in gates and other methods of restricting the child's mobility to safe areas.

Early Childhood: Ages 2 to 5 Years

Play Occupations

The three types of play that predominate in early childhood are (1) *pretend*, or *symbolic, play,* (2) *constructive play,* and (3) *rough-and-tumble,* or *physical, play* (Boxes 3-5 and 3-6). Similar changes are observed in each type of play. First, the child's play becomes more elaborate—that is, the child now combines multiple steps and multiple schema. Short play sequences become long scripts involving several characters or actors in a story.[64,67] Second, play becomes more social. The preschool-age child orients play toward peers, involving one or two peers in the story and taking turns playing various roles. When preschool-age children play with peers, the interaction appears to be as important as the activity's goal. As the child approaches 5 years of age, all play becomes increasingly social, generally involving a small group of peers.[64,99]

Beginning at 2 years of age and continuing through the early childhood years, the child's play is symbolic and imaginative. The child pretends that dolls, figurines, and stuffed animals are real. He or she may also imitate the actions of parents, teachers, and peers. At ages 3 and 4, pretend play becomes more abstract, and objects, such as a block, can be used to represent something else. Pretend play now involves many steps that relate to each other. Children develop scripts as a basis for their play (e.g., one child is the father and one is the mother). They base these scripts on real-life events and play their roles with enthusiasm and imagination, creating their

BOX 3-5 Development of Play Occupations: Preschoolers—24 to 36 Months

PLAY OCCUPATIONS

Symbolic Play
Links multiple scheme combinations into meaningful sequences of pretend play
Uses objects for multiple pretend ideas
Uses toys to represent animals or people
Plays out drama with stuffed animals or imaginary friends
Plays house, assigning roles to other, taking on specific roles

Constructive Play
Participates in drawing and puzzles
Imitates adults using toys

Gross Motor Play
Likes jumping, rough-and-tumble play
Makes messes

Social Play
Associative, parallel play predominates

PERFORMANCE SKILLS

Regulatory/Sensory Organization
Handles fragile items carefully
Enjoys interesting tactile surfaces
Plays with water and sand
May experience difficulty with transitions

Fine Motor/Manipulation
Snips with scissors
Traces form, such as a cross
Colors in large forms
Draws circles accurately
Builds towers and lines up objects
Holds crayon with dexterity
Completes puzzles of 4 to 5 pieces
Plays with toys with moving parts

Gross Motor/Mobility
Rides tricycle
Catches large ball against chest
Jumps from step or small height
Begins to hop on one foot

Cognitive
Combines actions into entire play scenario (e.g., feeding doll, then dressing in nightwear, then putting to bed)
Shows interest in wearing costumes; creates entire scripts of imaginative play
Matches pictures
Sorts shapes and colors
Plays house

Social
Cooperative play, takes turns at times
Shows interest in peers, enjoys having companions
Begins cooperative play and play in small groups
Shy with strangers, especially adults
Engages in dialog of few words
Can be possessive of loved ones

Data from Park, S. (2007). *HELP Strands*. Palo Alto, CA: VORT Corporation; Linder, T. (2008). *Transdisciplinary play-based assessment* (rev. ed.). Baltimore: Brookes.

BOX 3-6 Development of Play Occupations: Preschoolers—3 to 4 Years

PLAY OCCUPATIONS

Complex Imaginary Play
Creates scripts for play in which pretend objects have actions that reflect roles in real or imaginary life
May use complex scripts for pretend sequences; portrays multiple characters with feelings

Constructive Play
Creates art product with adult assistance
Works puzzles and blocks

Rough-and-Tumble Play
Enjoys physical play, swinging, sliding at playground, jumping, running

Social Play
Participates in circle time, games, drawing and art time at preschool
Engages in singing and dancing in groups
Associative play: plays with other children, sharing and talking about play goal

PERFORMANCE SKILLS

Fine Motor/Manipulation
Uses precision (tripod) grasp on pencil or crayon
Colors within lines
Copies simple shapes; begins to copy letters
Uses scissors to cut; cuts simple shapes
Constructs three-dimensional design (e.g., 3-block bridge)
Manipulates objects within the hand

Gross Motor/Mobility
Jumps, climbs, runs
Begins to skip and hop
Rides tricycle
Stands briefly on one foot
Alternates feet walking upstairs
Jumps from step with two feet

Cognitive
Uses imaginary objects in play
Makes dolls and action figures carry out roles and interact with other toys
Categorizes and sorts objects
Shows a sense of humor

Social
Attempts challenging activities
Prefers play with other children; group play replaces parallel play
Follows turn-taking in discourse and is aware of social aspects of conversation
Shows interest in being a friend
Prefers same-sex playmates

Data from Knox, S. (2008). Development and current use of the Knox Preschool Play Scale. In L. D. Parham & L. Fazio (Eds.), *Play in occupational therapy for children* (2nd ed., pp. 55-70). St. Louis: Mosby; Folio, M. R., & Fewell, R. R. (2000). *Peabody Developmental Motor Scales* (rev. ed.). Austin, TX: Pro-Ed.

own stories and enjoying the power of their imaginary roles. Their dramatic play is quite complex at this time. However, when they are in small groups, their interaction with their peers seems to be more important than the play goal, and they can easily turn to new activities suggested by one of the group.

By 5 years of age, this imaginary play is predominantly social, as small groups of two and three join in cooperative play. About one-third of the time, a 5-year-old child engages in pretend play.[93] However, this pretend play is based on imitation of real life and dressing up to play certain roles (e.g., firefighter, police officer, ballerina). Although children of this age demonstrate some understanding of adult roles, they erroneously assume that roles are one-dimensional (e.g., a firefighter has one role, that of putting out fires). Through pretending, children develop creativity, problem solving, and an understanding of another person's point of view (Boxes 3-7 and 3-8).[96]

Play that involves building and construction also teaches the child a variety of skills during early childhood. At first, these skills are demonstrated in the completion of puzzles and toys with fit-together pieces (Figure 3-10). However, with mastery of simple pegs and puzzles, the child becomes more creative in construction. For example, the 4-year-old child can develop a plan to build a structure with blocks and then carry out the steps to complete the project. With instructions and a model, the 5-year-old child can make a simple art project or create a three-dimensional design. A 5-year-old child can also put together a 10-piece puzzle. The final product has become more important, and the child is motivated to complete it and show others the final result. The planning and designing involved in building and construction play helps the child acquire an understanding of spatial perception and object relationships. This activity also appears to be foundational to academic performance in school.

Children from 2 to 5 years of age are extremely active and almost always readily engage in rough-and-tumble play. They continue to delight in movement experiences that provide strong sensory input. Activities such as running, hopping, skipping, and tumbling are performed as play without any particular goal. Although rough-and-tumble play generally involves other children, it is generally noncompetitive and rarely organized. Children enjoy this activity for the simple, simultaneous pleasure of movement as they play together.[15]

In associative physical play, children are generally more interested in being with other children than in the goal of the activity. However, it is important to note that some children enjoy primarily social play, whereas others enjoy solitary play. These differences do not relate to ability as much as they relate to preferences and temperament.[105]

Performance Skills

Sensory and Motor Skills

Young children are amazingly competent individuals, and their repertoire of motor function leaps forward during the preschool years (see Performance Skills in Boxes 3-6, 3-7, and 3-8). By age 2 years, the child walks with an increased length of stride and an efficient, well-coordinated, and well-balanced gait. Although children begin to run by 2 years, they do not exhibit true running (characterized by trunk rotation and arm swing) until 3 to 4 years of age. The 4-year-old child demonstrates a walking pattern similar to that of an adult. By 5 to 6 years of

---

BOX 3-7   Development of Play Occupations: Preschoolers—4 to 5 Years

PLAY OCCUPATIONS

Games with Rules
Begins group games with simple rules
Engages in organized play with prescribed roles
Participates in an organized gross motor games such as kickball or "duck, duck, goose"

Constructive Play
Takes pride in products
Shows interest in the goal of the art activity
Constructs complex structures

Social Play; Dramatic Play
Participates in role play with other children
Participates in "dress" up
Tells stories
Continues with pretend play that involves scripts with imaginary characters

PERFORMANCE SKILLS

Fine Motor/Manipulative
Draws using a dynamic tripod grasp
Copies simple shapes
Completes puzzles of up to 10 pieces
Uses scissors to cut out squares and other simple shapes
Colors within the lines
Uses two hands together well, one stabilizing paper or object and other manipulating object

Draws stick figure or may begin to draw trunk and arms
Copies own name
Strings small beads

Gross Motor/Mobility
Jumps down from high step; jumps forward
Throws ball
Hops for long sequences (4-6 steps)
Climbs on playground equipment, swinging from arms or legs
Throws ball and hits target
Skips for a long distance
Walks up and down stairs reciprocally

Cognitive
Understands rules to a game
Remembers rules with a few reminders
Makes up stories that involve role playing with other children
Participates in goal-oriented, cooperative play with two or three other children
Participates in planning a play activity
Begins abstract problem solving

Social
Enjoys clowning
Sings whole songs
Role plays based on parents' roles

Data from Linder, T. (2008). *Transdisciplinary play-based assessment* (rev. ed.). Baltimore: Brookes.

BOX 3-8   Development of Play Occupation: Kindergartners—5 to 6 Years

PLAY OCCUPATIONS

Games with Rules
Board games
Computer games with rules
Competitive and cooperative games

Dramatic Play
Elaborate imaginary play
Role plays stories and themes related to seasons or occupations
Emphasis is on reality
Reconstructs real world in play

Sports
Participates in ball play

Social Play
Participates in group activities
Organized play in groups
Goal of play (winning) may compete with social interaction at times

PERFORMANCE SKILLS

Fine Motor/Manipulation
Cuts with scissors
Prints name from copy
Copies triangle; traces diamond
Completes puzzles of up to 20 pieces

Traces letters, begins to copy letters
Manipulates tiny objects in fingertips without dropping
Uses two hands together in complementary movements

Gross Motor/Mobility
Hops well for long distances
Skips with good balance
Catches ball with two hands
Kicks with accuracy
Stands on one foot for 8 to 10 seconds

Cognitive
Reasons through simple problems
Bases play more on real life than on imaginary world
Participates in organized games
Uses complex scripts in play
Demonstrates deferred imitation
Sorts objects in different ways
Copies elaborate block structures

Social
Participates in groups of 2 to 4 that play in organized, complex games
Has friends (same sex)
Enjoys singing and dancing; reflects meaning of words and music
Demonstrates understanding of others' feelings

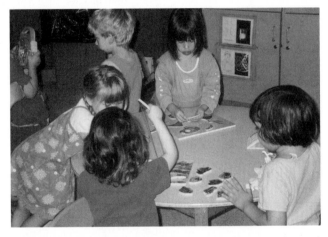

FIGURE 3-10   Four-year-old children complete puzzles and enjoy construction activities in small groups.

age, the mature running pattern has developed, and children test their speed by challenging each other to races.

As mobility develops, children gain access to spaces previously unavailable to them. By 2 years of age, a child walks up stairs without holding onto a parent's hand, and at 2½ years the child can walk down stairs without support. The 3½-year-old child walks up and down stairs by alternating the feet and without needing to hold onto a rail.

Running and stair climbing become possible, in part, because the child's balance and strength increase. Emerging balance can be observed as the 2-year-old child briefly stands on one foot to kick a ball. By 5 years of age, the child can balance on one foot for several seconds and walk on a curb without falling.[40] Between 3 and 5 years, the child may successfully attempt to use skates or roller blades.

Jumping is first observed in the 2-year-old child. This skill requires strength, coordination, and balance. By 3 years of age the child can jump easily from a step. Hopping requires greater strength and balance than jumping and is first observed at 3½ years. Skipping is the more difficult gross motor pattern, because it requires sequencing of a rhythmic pattern that includes a step and a hop. A coordinated skipping pattern is not observed until 5 years of age.[63]

Two-year-old children begin to pedal tricycles and move small riding toys. By 3 years of age they can pedal a tricycle but may run into objects. The 4-year-old child can steer and maneuver the tricycle around obstacles.

By 2½ years, most children can catch a 10-inch ball. This pattern of maturity enables the 4-year-old child to catch a much smaller ball successfully, such as a tennis ball.[40] The first pattern of throwing involves a pushing motion, with the elbow providing the force for the throw. The 4-year-old child demonstrates more forward weight shift with throwing, thereby increasing the force of the ball and the distance thrown. Kicking emerges in the 2- to 3-year-old child, with accurate kicking to a target exhibited by 6 years of age. Ball skills become increasingly important as the child begins participating in organized sports during the primary grades.

Early childhood is a time of rapid improvement in fine motor and manipulation performance. By 4 years of age, children learn to move small objects efficiently within one hand (i.e., in-hand manipulation). The 4-year-old child can hold several small objects in the palm of the hand while moving individual pieces with the radial fingers.[82] In-hand manipulation indicates that isolated finger movement is well controlled and that the thumb easily moves into opposition for pad-o-pad prehension. These skills also indicate that the child can modulate force and that he or she has an accurate perception of the gentle force needed to handle small objects with the fingertips.[82]

With efficient in-hand manipulation, the preschool child also learns the functional use of drawing and cutting tools. Most 3-year-old children hold a pencil with a static tripod grasp (i.e., with the pencil resting between the thumb and first two fingers) and use forearm and wrist movement to draw; however, by 5 years, a child demonstrates a mature, dynamic tripod. In this grasp pattern, the pencil is held in the tips of the radial fingers and is moved using finger movement. By controlling the pencil using individual finger movements, the child can make letters and small forms.

Drawing skills progress from drawing circles to lines that intersect and cross in a diagonal (e.g., an X). The 5-year-old child can draw a person with multiple and recognizable parts. Drawing is often a strong interest at this age and therefore contributes to the child's imaginative play. He or she can also draw detailed figures created in the imagination (i.e., monsters, fairies, and other fanciful creatures).

The development of scissors skills follows the development of controlled pencil use. The first cutting skill, observed at 3 years, is snipping with alternating full-finger extension and flexion. Between 4 and 6 years, bilateral hand coordination, dexterity, and eye-hand coordination improve, enabling the child to cut out simple shapes. Mature use of scissors is not achieved until 5 to 6 years, because it requires isolated finger movements, simultaneous hand control, and well-developed eye-hand coordination for cutting accuracy.[40]

Other fine motor skills acquired during the preschool years are important to the child's constructive and dramatic play. Activities such as putting puzzles together, building towers, stringing small beads, using keys, and cutting out complex designs usually require dexterity, bilateral coordination, and motor planning.

Cognitive Skills

Preschool-age children create symbolic representations of real-life objects and events during play. In addition, they begin to plan pretend scenarios in advance, organizing who and what are needed to complete the activity. Play becomes an elaborate sequence of events that is remembered, acted out, and later described for others. For example, the child may act out the role of an adult, imitating action remembered from an earlier experience. This form of role play demonstrates the child's understanding of how roles relate to actions and how actions relate to each other (e.g., the child may role play a grocery store clerk, displaying items for sale, taking money from the customer, and placing the money in a toy cash register).

Abstract thinking begins in the preschool years as the child pretends that an object is something else. For example, the child may pretend a block is a doll bed; later the same block may become a telephone receiver or a train car.

The motor skills noted in early childhood also reflect cognitive skills. To construct a three-dimensional building, the child must have the ability to discriminate size and shape. Building in three dimensions also requires spatial understanding and problem-solving skills. When building from a set of blocks, the child usually must first categorize and organize the blocks. Next, the child must solve the problem of how to fit them together to replicate a model or create the imagined structure.

In a similar way, the emergence of drawing skills reflects both cognitive abilities and fine motor skills. The 3-year-old child makes crude attempts to represent people and objects in drawings. By 4 years of age, a child can draw a recognizable person, demonstrating the ability to select salient features and represent them on a two-dimensional surface. The 4-year-old child not only identifies the parts of a person but also relates them correctly, although the size of the parts is rarely proportional to real life. At 5 years, the child's drawing is more refined, more realistic, and better proportioned. By this age, pictures begin to tell stories and reflect the child's emotions.[67]

Social Skills

In early childhood, interaction and play with peers take on increasing importance. Children become social beings and identify themselves as individuals (i.e., separate from parents). Autonomy dominates the psychosocial development from 2 to 4 years, as the toddler shows his independence by moving away from the parent. The child is adamant about making personal decisions. The development of trust in the environment and improvements in language bring forth control over self, strengthening the child's autonomous nature.

The discovery of the body and how to control it promotes independence in self-care. Success in acting independently instills a sense of confidence and self-control. The child also begins to perceive that now all of his independent actions meet the approval of adults.

Children need to achieve a balance between initiative to act independently and the responsibility they feel for their own actions. Children 4 to 5 years old explore beyond the environment, discovering new activities. They seek new experiences for the pleasure of learning about the environment and for the opportunities they offer for exploration. If the child's learning experiences are successful and effective and his or her actions meet parental approval, a sense of initiative is developed. Through these activities, the child learns to question, reason, and find solutions to problems.

Adult-child relationships and early home experiences also influence later peer relations. According to research, children whose attachments to their mothers are rated as secure tend to be more responsive to other children in child care settings. They are also more curious and competent.[62,115] Peer play becomes an important avenue for the child's development of social and cognitive abilities. With their peers, they practice social roles, engage in dramatic play, and enjoy rough and tumble play.

The development of autonomy provides a foundation for the child's imagination. Now the young child explores the world not only through the use of his or her senses but also by thinking and reasoning. Although play can be reality based, it usually includes fantasy, wishes, and role play. Words, rhymes, and songs also complement this type of play.

Contexts

Cultural and Social Contexts

The social roles of young children vary across cultures. The following discussion of cultural differences highlights how culture contributes to a child's development. In the United States, the importance of interaction with peers is stressed at young ages. Most American children begin to interact with their peers (same age group) at about 3 years of age. Same-age peers become increasingly important through elementary school and dominate the social life of a teenager. In the United States and much of the world, children are grouped exclusively by age. These age groupings may provide more opportunities for play, but they also diminish opportunities for older children to teach and nurture younger children. Younger children have fewer opportunities to imitate older children.

Children in other parts of the world play and socialize with people of different ages. For example, in Mayan communities, children spend almost all of their time with siblings and other young relatives of a wide range of ages.[10] In Polynesia, children remain with family members, including extended family. They socially participate in mixed-age groups, playing "on the edge" and watching intently until they can join in the play. In Mexican families, toddlers play with children of various ages. Often they play with older siblings. This "enduring social network" remains in place over time to care for, teach, and discipline children to adulthood.[88]

When children spend their days with a variety of ages, they have many opportunities to imitate and learn from older children and adults. Interaction with children of varying ages provides older children the opportunity to practice teaching and nurturance with young children and provides young children with the opportunity to imitate older children.[112]

At very young ages, Mayan children play within their parents' work activities.[10] For example, children engage in play activities while helping their mothers wash clothes. The children's play in the Mayan culture is tolerated during daily work activities but is not specifically encouraged.[10] Bazyk and her colleagues[10] found that children's work was playful, blurring the European American distinction between work and play. When children play in work activities, they are learning skills that will serve them well in adulthood. In contrast, the age-based groupings used in U.S. child care centers and preschools provide children with opportunities to play with same-age peers but reduce their opportunities to play within adult work activities.

Families in the United States specifically design and encourage their children's play and at times become playmates with children. Although play is emphasized as the primary occupation for young children, children demonstrate interest in helping parents accomplish their work. Parents may encourage young children (e.g., 5-6 years) to participate in household tasks, such as picking up their own toys. When children begin school, parents usually expect them to participate more in household tasks such as cleaning and meal preparation.[65]

Physical Contexts

By the age of 5, a child's outdoor environment has expanded beyond the areas around the home and child care center. A variety of outdoor environments offer space for rough-and-tumble play, and expanded social and physical environments give the child new opportunities for learning (and generalizing) the skills he or she has achieved. Although adult supervision remains essential, the entire neighborhood may become the child's playground.

The availability of new indoor environments is also to be expected. Preschool classrooms usually have centers for different types of activities (e.g., creating art, listening to stories, playing games). In addition, community groups often sponsor a variety of indoor activities (e.g., preschool gymnastics, organized play programs) in which the child can take part.

Expanded environments offer children the opportunity to adapt play skills learned at home to the constraints of new spaces. For example, the child who climbs and slides down the stairs at home learns to climb a 6-foot ladder and slide down the slide in the neighborhood park. Parks and playgrounds also provide the child with new surfaces that challenge balance and equipment that offers intense vestibular experiences.

Cultural and socioeconomic differences can influence a child's physical environment. Inner city parents frequently confine their children to the immediate household and forbid them to go outside after school, particularly to play. These protective strategies limit children's exposure to dangerous neighborhood influences, but they also severely restrict the physical context available for play.[41]

Most preschool-aged children also enjoy spending time in quiet spaces. Children, especially those who demonstrate over-reactivity to sensory input, may feel drawn to quiet, enclosed spaces (e.g., a space behind the couch, the safe haven of their bedrooms, a small tent in the corner of the playroom) (Figure 3-11). Quiet spaces can be organizing and calming after a day in a child care center. Other children who may have under-reacting sensory systems may seek stimulating environments that are full of activity, or they may create their own high activity in an otherwise quiet space.

When placed in new environments, children often respond by instinctively exploring the new spaces (e.g., hallways, cupboards, corners, furniture). Exploring the features of an environment can help orient children to the spaces that surround them, promote perceptual learning, and provide an understanding of the play possibilities in that environment.

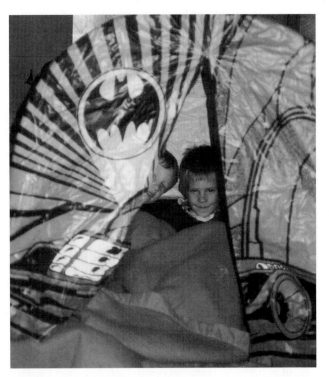

FIGURE 3-11 Special places and favorite play partners have high significance to young children.

Middle Childhood: Ages 6 to 10 Years

Play Occupations

Although 6-year-old children continue to enjoy imaginative play, they begin increasingly to structure and organize their play. By the time a child is 7 or 8 years of age, structured games and organized play predominate (Box 3-9). *Games with rules* are the primary mode for physical and social play. Groups of children organize themselves, assign roles, and explain (or create) rules to guide the game they plan to play. The goal of the game now competes with the reward of interacting with peers, and children become fascinated with the rules that govern the games they play.

At 7 and 8 years of age, children do not understand that rules apply equally to everyone involved in the game, and they are often unable to place the rules of the game above the personal need to win.[39] However, breaking the rules may incur the criticism of peers, who also acknowledge the importance of rules at this time. By 9 and 10 years of age, children are more conscientious about obeying rules. They also learn to negotiate the rules of a game and construct their own rules.

By 8 and 9 years, children become interested in sports, and parents are generally supportive of sports activities. Although a form of play, organized sports can assume a serious nature (i.e., intrinsic motivation and the internal sense of control are overridden by the external demands of practice and serious competition with peers). In addition to organized sports, physical play is a favorite interest, including climbing, rollerblading, skipping rope, and skateboarding (Figure 3-12).

Interest in creating craft and art projects continues into middle childhood. During this time, the child shows an increased ability to organize, solve problems, and create from abstract materials. However, the completion of craft and art projects continues to require the support of adults to organize materials and identify steps. The final product, which is relatively unimportant to younger children, is now valued.

In middle childhood, children play in cooperative groups and value interaction with their peers. When friends come

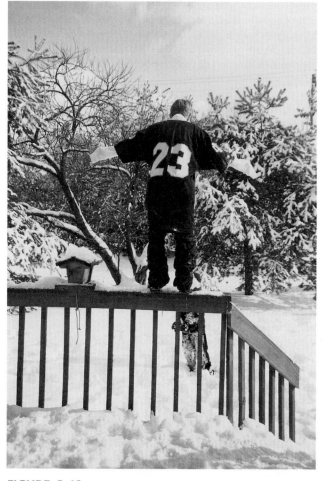

FIGURE 3-12 Children seek opportunities to challenge their balance. By 9 and 10 years, postural stability and strength are sufficiently developed to maintain standing balance on a porch railing.

BOX 3-9 Development of Play Occupations: Middle Childhood—6 to 10 Years

PLAY OCCUPATIONS
Games with Rules
Computer games, card games that require problems solving and abstract thinking
Crafts and Hobbies
Has collections
May have hobbies
Organized Sports
Cooperative and competitive play in groups/teams of children
Winning and skills are emphasized
Social Play
Play includes talking and joking
Peer play predominates at school and home
Plays with consistent friends

PERFORMANCE SKILLS
Fine Motor/Manipulation
Good dexterity for crafts and construction with small objects
Bilateral coordination for building complex structure

Precision and motor planning evident in drawing
Motor planning evident in completion of complex puzzles
Gross Motor/Mobility
Runs with speed and endurance
Jumps, hops, skips
Throws ball well at long distances
Catches ball with accuracy
Cognitive
Abstract reasoning
Performs mental operations without need to physically try
Demonstrates flexible problem solving
Solves complex problems
Social
Cooperative, less egocentric
Tries to please others
Has best friend
Is part of cliques
Is less impulsive, is able to regulate behavior
Has competitive relationships

together, almost all activity is play and fun. Simply talking and joking become playful and entertaining. Children spend more than 40% of their waking hours with peers.[24] In these peer groups, children learn to cooperate but also to compete.[39] They are now interested in *achievement* through play; they recognize and accept an outside standard for success or failure and criteria for winning or losing. With competition in play comes risk taking and strategic thinking. Children who compete in sports and other activities exhibit courage to perform against an outside standard.[85]

Performance Skills

Sensory and Motor Skills

During the elementary school years, motor development continues to focus on the refining of previously acquired skills. With this refinement, hours of repetition of activities to attain mastery of common interests are observed. Children ride bicycles, scale fences, swim, skate, and jump rope (Figure 3-13). Although motor capabilities are highly varied for this age group, balance and coordination improve throughout the middle childhood years, providing children with the agility to dance and play sports with proficiency. Research indicates that children who struggle in physical skills have lower self-esteem and are very socially marginalized.[69] Not only does self-esteem improve as children master physical skills, but peer acceptance improves as well.

Fine motor skills in middle childhood include efficient tool use (e.g., scissors, tweezers) and precise drawing skills. Children handle and manipulate materials (fold, sort, adhere, cut) with competency. The drawing skills of 8- and 9-year-old children demonstrate appropriate proportions and accuracy, and handwriting skills improve in speed and accuracy as children learn manuscript and then cursive writing. These improvements provide evidence of increased dexterity and coordination. Construction skills, manipulation, and abilities to use tools continue to generalize across performance areas, with increases in speed, strength, and precision.

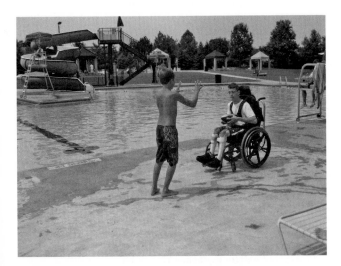

FIGURE 3-13 Favorite play activities for all children include swimming, ball play, and outdoor sports.

Cognitive Skills

In middle childhood, concepts and relationships in the physical world are understood and applied. The child relates past events to future plans and comprehends how situations change over time. Thinking has become more flexible and abstract. The child has become a reasoning individual who can solve problems by understanding variables and weighing pertinent factors before making decisions. They now have a clear understanding of the difference between fantasy and reality and they choose to move from one to the other.

At younger ages, children could apply only one solution, and they often were stuck when the solution of choice did not work. By 8 and 9 years of age, however, they recognize that different solutions can be tried, and they arrive at answers through abstract reasoning rather than through concrete trial and error. At this age, children can also pay attention to more than one physical characteristic at a time and can systematically put elements together.

In play, children order objects by size or shape, demonstrating the ability to discriminate perceptual aspects of objects and to order them accurately. They also understand the relationship of the whole to the parts, and they imagine pieces as parts of a whole. With this understanding, they become more competent in organizing tasks and organizing time. Children 9 and 10 years of age can give instructions to others and tell stories in detail.

By middle childhood, children learn to combine tasks and routines into complex games and competitive sports. Because a number of rules are needed to play sports, such as baseball or hockey, the child understands the need to combine the rules into a complete game. To participate in the activity successfully, he or she also understands when rules apply and when rules can be negotiated.

Social Skills

Children 6 to 10 years of age form close friendships and "belong" to one or more peer groups that greatly influence their decisions, how they spend their time, and what they value. Florey and Greene explain, "In the beginning of middle childhood, friendships are characterized by sharing of interests. Toward the end of this period, children tend to organize around common values, commitment, loyalty, and mutual support" (p. 282).[39]

Children in middle childhood focus on meeting challenges in themselves as well as challenges presented by others. Children appreciate the recognition that comes with successful completion of assignments or projects. Comparison with peers is increasingly important during this time. If a child's schoolwork is compared with the work of a more successful student, a negative evaluation can reduce his or her sense of mastery and may produce feelings of inferiority.

School-aged children seek independence of identity. They are not as egocentric as young children and demonstrate a more objective view of themselves. Children at this age have a definite subculture, or clique, that includes only certain friends. At this age, children are quick to criticize those who do not conform to the group esthetic. Therefore rejection by the child's peers may result from a lack of conformity in dress or physical appearance. Children who have difficulty communicating or who do not know how to initiate relationships are less likely to have close friendships. Children who are socially able and positive are more accepted and have more close friendships.

During middle childhood, children become disinterested in adults, including their parents. The values of peers become significantly more important than those of adults. Data indicate that children between 7 and 10 years of age are highly compliant with and easily shift in the direction of their peers.[28,39]

The child's progression from games with some structure and flexible rules to highly competitive games demonstrates progression in moral development. Early in the child's thinking (before 7 years of age), rules are viewed as absolute, sacred, and unchangeable. Children 7 to 10 years old recognize that rules come from someone in authority, and they accept what this authority says. However, late in the elementary school years, children cast aside their beliefs in the absolute infallibility of rules, because they have gained the knowledge that people are the creators of rules. Questioning of the rules and the authority that makes them begins at this age.[39]

Contexts

Cultural Contexts

Expectations for children to work appear to vary across cultures. These expectations determine the timing and type of occupations children develop and the balance between work and play. In countries other than the United States and those of Europe, the typical age for children to assume work responsibilities is 5 to 7 years. In a study of 50 communities, children at 5 to 7 years are given responsibility for caring for younger children, for tending animals, and for carrying out household chores.[90] In the United States, chores are rarely given to children younger than 8 or 9 years of age. Many American families do not expect children to take responsibility for chores until the age of 10 or 11. In contrast, Polynesian children develop household skills by 3 or 4 years, at which time they gather wood, sweep, or run errands to the store. In West Africa, children have duties and run errands when they are 3 years old. In Kenya, 8-year-old girls perform most of the housework.[88]

Mayan children are continuously at their parents' side during work days. At early ages, they participate in work tasks, such as running errands and helping with cleanup. Bazyk et al. found that although Mayan children began work activities at a very early age, they embedded play in these chores.[10] Children in Central Africa acquire work experience from toddler age, and by age 12 they can trap animals, kill game, make medicines, and garden.[88] Ogunnaike and Houser examined the effects of participation in work activities and errands on cognitive performance in young Yoruban children.[80] In Yoruba, young children are taught to be helpful, responsible, and respectful. Before age 5, Yoruban girls are taught to perform household chores such as washing, sweeping, cooking, and caring for their younger siblings. By middle childhood, the girls take full responsibility for these work roles. The number of errands a child was required to run and cognitive performance were significantly related, indicating that having children participate in work tasks at an early age may enhance cognitive competence.[80]

In the United States, most children and youth have very few opportunities to work with adults. Goldscheider and Waite estimated that children contribute about 15% of all labor in households.[51] Rogoff believes that American children are missing valuable opportunities for learning and gaining self-satisfaction.[88] In comparison with practices in societies outside the United States, the lack of work opportunities for American children limits their practice of skills important to their future and may delay their entry into adult work roles. Through experiences in school and guided participation in household work, children may develop work skills and also learn social rules and cultural values.[65]

Physical Contexts

In middle childhood, the child's play environment is now large and complex; more activities take place in the neighborhood and at school. The school's playground supports both social and physical play of small groups (or pairs) of children. Play occurs on ball fields and in community centers, amusement parks, and sports arenas. Organized activities are often sponsored by churches or by groups such as the Young Men's Christian Association (YMCA). By middle childhood, children have the mobility skills to maneuver through all environments (e.g., rough terrain, busy city streets). The society of school-aged children dominates neighborhood streets and backyards, with bicycle races and spontaneous street hockey games. These children explore the woods and go on adventures in nearby parks to find areas unexplored by others. Although supervision by adults is still needed at times, intermittent supervision usually suffices.

Children spend many of their waking hours in school. Schools offer complex environments (e.g., playgrounds, computer rooms, libraries, classrooms, lunchrooms) with many social and learning opportunities.

SUMMARY

The development of occupational performance is influenced by many systems and variables in the individual child and in the environment. The various patterns observed in children provide insight into how and why a child follows a certain developmental trajectory. Sensory, motor, cognitive, and social skills support the child's performance in play occupations. At the same time, a child's activities are highly influenced by his or her cultural, social, and physical contexts. As an essential occupation of childhood, play provides a means of understanding and appreciating children's performance and a means for enhancing functional performance when development is delayed. The ability to play is also an important outcome of occupational therapy, one that reflects the being of childhood.

REFERENCES

1. Adolf, K. E., Eppler, M. A., & Gibson, E. J. (1993). Development of perception of affordances. In C. Rovee-Collier & L. P. Lipsitt (Eds.), *Advances in infancy research* (Vol. 8, pp. 51–98). Norwood, NJ: Ablex.
2. American Occupational Therapy Association. (2008). Occupational Therapy Practice Framework: Domain and Process (2nd ed.). *American Journal of Occupational Therapy, 62,* 625–683.
3. Ayres, A. J. (1979). *Sensory integration and the child.* Los Angeles: Western Psychological Services.
4. Ayres, A. J. (2005). *Sensory integration and the child: Understanding hidden sensory challenges. 25th anniversary edition.* Los Angeles: Western Psychological Services.
5. Bandura, A. (1978). The self system in reciprocal determinism. *American Psychologist, 33,* 344–358.

6. Bandura, A. (1993). Perceived self-efficacy in cognitive development and functioning. *Educational Psychologist, 28,* 117–148.

7. Bandura, A. (1999). A social cognitive theory of personality. In L. Pervin & O. John (Eds.), *Handbook of personality* (2nd ed., pp. 154–197). New York: Guilford Press.

8. Bayley, N. (1993). *Bayley Scales of Infant Development* (2nd ed.). San Antonio: Psychological Corporation.

9. Bayley, N. (2005). *Bayley Scales of Infant Development* (3rd ed.). San Antonio: Psychological Corporation.

10. Bazyk, S., Stalnaker, D., Llerena, M., Ekelman, B., & Bazyk, J. (2003). Play in Mayan children. *American Journal of Occupational Therapy, 57,* 273–283.

11. Bruner. (1973). Organization of early skilled action. *Child Development, 44,* 1–11.

12. Bushnell, E. W., & Boudreau, J. P. (1993). Motor development and the mind: the potential role of motor abilities as a determinant of aspects of perceptual development. *Child Development, 64,* 1005–1021.

13. Case, R. (1999). Conceptual development in the child and the field: A personal view of the Piagetian legacy. In E. Scholnick, K. Nelson, S. Gelman, & P. Miller (Eds.), *Conceptual development: Piaget's legacy* (pp. 23–51). Mahwah, NJ: Lawrence Erlbaum.

14. Case-Smith, J. (2006). Hand skill development in the context of infants' play: Birth to 2 years. In A. Hendersen & P. Pehoski (Eds.), *Hand function in the child: Foundations for remediation* (pp. 117–142). St. Louis: Mosby.

15. Case-Smith, J., & Kuhaneck, H. (2008). Play preferences of typically developing children and children with developmental delays between ages 3 and 7 years. *OTJR: Occupation, Participation and Health, 28,* 19–29.

16. Cermak, S. (2006). Perceptual functions of the hand. In A. Hendersen & P. Pehoski (Eds.), *Hand function in the child: Foundations for remediation* (pp. 63–88). St. Louis: Mosby.

17. Chan, S. (1998). Families with Asian roots. In E. W. Lynch & M. J. Hanson (Eds.), *Developing cross-cultural competence* (2nd ed., pp. 251–354). Baltimore: Brookes.

18. Chan, S. (1998). Families with Filipino roots. In E. W. Lynch & M. J. Hanson (Eds.), *Developing cross-cultural competence* (2nd ed., pp. 355–408). Baltimore: Brookes.

19. Chess, S., & Thomas, A. (1984). *The origins and evolution of behavior disorders: Infancy to early adult life.* New York: Brunner/Mazel.

20. Chess, S., & Thomas, A. (1999). *Goodness of fit: Clinical applications from infancy through adult life.* New York: Brunner/Mazel.

21. Cioni, G., Ferrari, F., Einspieler, C., Paolicelli, P., Barbiani, T., & Prechtl, H. F. (1997). Comparison between the observation of spontaneous movements and neurologic examination in preterm infants. *Journal of Pediatrics, 130,* 704–711.

22. Clark, J. (1997). A dynamical systems perspective on the development of complex adaptive skill. In C. Dent-Read & P. Zukow-Goldring (Eds.), *Evolving explanations of development: Ecological approaches to organisms-environment systems.* Washington, DC: American Psychological Association.

23. Cohen, L. B., & Cashon, C. H. (2003). Infant perception and cognition. In R. M. Lerner, M. A. Easterbrooks, & J. Mistry (Eds.), *Handbook of psychology: Vol. 6. Developmental psychology* (pp. 65–90). New York: John Wiley & Sons.

24. Cole, M., & Cole, S. (1989). *The development of children.* New York: Scientific American Books.

25. Connolly, K., & Dalgleish, M. (1989). The emergence of a tool-using skill in infancy. *Developmental Psychology, 25,* 894–912.

26. Connolly, K. J., & Dalgleish, M. (1993). Individual patterns of tool use by infants. In A. F. Kalverboer, B. Hopkins, & R. Geuze (Eds.), *Motor development in early and later childhood: Longitudinal approaches* (pp. 174–204). Cambridge: Cambridge University Press.

27. Corbetta, D., & Mounoud, P. (1990). Early development of grasping and manipulation. In C. Bard, M. Fleury, & L. Hay (Eds.), *Development of eye-hand coordination across the life span* Columbia, SC: University of South Carolina Press.

28. Costanzo, P. R., & Shaw, M. E. (1966). Conformity as a function of age level. *Child Development, 37,* 967–975.

29. Csikszentmihalyi, M., & Rathunde, K. (1998). The development of the person: An experiential perspective on the ontogenesis of psychological complexity. In W. Damon (Series Ed.) & R. M. Lerner (Vol. Ed.), *Handbook of child psychology: Vol 1. Theoretical models of human development* (5th ed., pp. 635–684). New York: John Wiley & Sons.

30. Daunhauer, L. A., Coster, W. J., Tickle-Degen, L., & Cermak, S. A. (2007). Effects of caregiver-child interactions on play occupations among young children institutionalized in Eastern Europe. *American Journal of Occupational Therapy, 61,* 429–440.

31. Dunst, C. J. (2001). Participation of young children with disabilities in community learning activities. In M. J. Guralnick (Ed.), *Early childhood inclusion: Focus on change* (pp. 307–333). Baltimore: Paul H. Brookes.

32. Dunst, C. J., Bruder, M. B., Trivette, C. M., Raab, M., & McLean, M. (2001). Natural learning opportunities for infants, toddlers and preschoolers. *Young Exceptional Children, 4,* 18–25.

33. Easterbrooks, M. A., & Biringen, Z. (2000). Mapping the terrain of emotional availability and attachment. *Attachment and Human Development, 2,* 123–129.

34. Ellison, P. H. (1994). *The INFANIB: A reliable method for the neuromotor assessment of infants.* Tucson, AZ: Therapy Skill Builders.

35. Erikson, E. H. (1963). *Childhood and society* (2nd ed.). New York: W.W. Norton.

36. Fagaard, J. (1990). The development of bimanual coordination. In C. Bard, M. Fleury, & L. Hay (Eds.), *Development of eye-hand coordination across the life span.* Columbia, SC: University of South Carolina Press.

37. Feldman, D. H. (2003). Cognitive development in childhood. In R. M. Lerner, M. A. Easterbrooks, & J. Mistry (Eds.), *Handbook of psychology, Vol. 6. Developmental psychology* (pp. 195–210). Hoboken, NJ: John Wiley & Sons, Inc.

38. Fitzgerald, H., Munn, T., Cabrera, N., & Wong, M. M. (2003). Diversity in caregiving contexts. In R. M. Lerner, M. A. Easterbrooks, & J. Mistry (Eds), *Handbook of psychology: Vol. 6. Developmental psychology* (pp. 135–169). New York: John Wiley & Sons.

39. Florey, L. L., & Greene, S. (2008). Play in middle childhood. In L. D. Parham & L. Fazio (Eds.), *Play in occupational therapy for children* (2nd ed., pp. 279–300). St. Louis: Mosby.

40. Folio, M. R., & Fewell, R. R. (2000). *Peabody Developmental Motor Scales* (rev. ed.). Austin, TX: Pro-Ed.

41. Garcia Coll, C., & Magnuson, K. (2000). Cultural differences as sources of developmental vulnerabilities and resources. In J. P. Shonkoff & S. J. Meisels (Eds.), *Handbook of early childhood intervention* (2nd ed., pp. 94–114). Cambridge: Cambridge University Press.

42. Gesell, A. (1945). *The embryology of behavior: The beginnings of the human mind.* New York: Harper & Brothers.

43. Gesell, A., & Amatruda, G. (1947). *Developmental diagnosis* (2nd ed.). New York: Harper & Row.

44. Gesell, A., Halverson, H. M., Thompson, H., Ilg, F. L., Castner, B. M., Ames, L. B., et al. (1940). *The first five years of life.* New York: Harper & Row.

45. Gesell, A., & Ilg, F. (1937). *Feeding behavior of infants.* Philadelphia: Lippincott.

46. Gibson, E. J. (1988). Exploratory behavior in the development of perceiving, acting, and the acquiring of knowledge. *Annual Reviews Psychology, 39,* 1–42.

47. Gibson, E. J. (1995). Exploratory behavior in the development of perceiving, acting, and the acquiring of knowledge. In L. P.

Lipsitt & C. Rovee-Collier (Eds), *Advances in infancy* (pp. xxi–lxi). Norwood, NJ: Ablex.

48. Gibson, E. J. (1997). An ecological psychologist's prolegomena for perceptual development: A functional approach. In C. Dent-Read & P. Zukow-Goldring (Eds.), *Evolving explanations of development: Ecological approaches to organisms-environment systems* Washington, DC: American Psychological Association.

49. Gibson, J. J. (1979). *The ecological approach to visual perception.* Boston: Houghton-Mifflin.

50. Gilfolye, E., Grady, A., & Moore, J. (1990). *Children adapt* (2nd ed.). Thorofare, NJ: Slack.

51. Gottlieb, G. (1997). *Synthesizing nature-nurture: Prenatal roots of instinctive behavior.* Hillsdale, NJ: Lawrence Erlbaum.

52. Goldscheider, F., & Waite, L. (1991). *New families, no families?* Los Angeles: University of California Press.

53. Granott, N. (2002). How microdevelopment creates macrodevelopment: Reiterated sequences, backward transitions, and the zone of current development. In N. Granott & J. Parziale (Eds.), *Microdevelopment: Transition processes in development and learning* (pp. 213–242). Cambridge: Cambridge University Press.

54. Greenspan, G. (1990). *Infancy and early childhood: The practice of clinical assessment and intervention with emotional and developmental challenges.* New York: International Universities Press.

55. Greer, T., & Lockman, J. J. (1998). Using writing instruments: Invariances in young children and adults. *Child Development, 69,* 888–902.

56. Henderson, A. (2006). Self care and hand skill. In A. Henderson & C. Pehoski (Eds.), *Hand function in the child* (2nd ed.). St. Louis: Mosby.

57. Humphry, R. (2002). Young children's occupations: Explicating the dynamics of developmental processes. *American Journal of Occupational Therapy, 56,* 172–179.

58. Humphry, R. (2009). Occupation and development: A contextual perspective. In E. B. Crepeau, E. S. Cohn, & B. A. B. Schell (Eds.), *Willard & Spackman's occupational therapy* (pp. 22–32). Philadelphia: Lippincott Williams & Wilkins.

59. Humphry, R., & Wakeford, L. (2006). An occupation-centered discussion of development and implications for practice. *American Journal of Occupational Therapy, 60,* 258–268.

60. Illingworth, R. S. (1966). The diagnosis of cerebral palsy in the first year of life. *Developmental Medicine and Child Neurology, 8,* 178–194.

61. Illingworth, R. S. (1984). *The development of the infant and young child.* Edinburgh: Churchill Livingstone.

62. Jacobson, S. L., & Wille, D. E. (1986). The influence of attachment pattern on developmental changes in peer interaction from the child to the preschool period. *Child Development, 57,* 338–347.

63. Knobloch, H., & Pasamanick, B. (1974). *Gesell & Amatruda's developmental diagnosis* (3rd ed.). New York: Harper & Row.

64. Knox, S. (2008). Development and current use of the Knox Preschool Play Scale. In L. D. Parham & L. Fazio (Eds.), *Play in occupational therapy for children* (2nd ed., pp. 55–70). St. Louis: Mosby.

65. Larson, E. A. (2004). Children's work: The less-considered childhood occupation. *American Journal of Occupational Therapy, 58,* 369–379.

66. Lerner, R. M., Anderson, P. M., Balsano, A. B., Dowling, E. M., & Bobek, D. L. (2003). In R. M. Lerner, M. A. Easterbrooks, & J. Mistry (Eds.), *Handbook of psychology, Vol. 6. Developmental psychology* (pp. 535–558). New York: John Wiley & Sons.

67. Linder, T. (2008). *Transdisciplinary play-based assessment* (rev. ed.). Baltimore: Brookes.

68. Luthar, S. S., & Latendresse, S. J. (2005). Comparable "risks" at the socioeconomic status extremes: Preadoleescents' perceptions of parenting. *Development and Psychopathology, 17,* 207–230.

69. Mandich, A., Polatajko, H., & Rodger, S. (2003). Rites of passage: Understanding participation of children with developmental coordination disorder. *Human Movement Science, 22,* 583–595.

70. Mandler, J. M. (1990). A new perspective on cognitive development in infancy. *American Scientist, 78,* 236–243.

71. Mathiowetz, V., & Haugen, J. (1994). Motor behavior research: Implications for therapeutic approaches to central nervous system dysfunction. *American Journal of Occupational Therapy, 48,* 733–745.

72. Mathiowetz, V., & Haugen, J. (1995). Evaluation of motor behavior: Traditional and contemporary views. In C. A. Trombly (Ed.), *Occupational therapy for physical dysfunction* (4th ed., pp. 157–186). Baltimore: Williams & Wilkins.

73. McCarty, M. E., Clifton, R. K., & Collard, R. R. (2001). The beginnings of tool use by infants and toddlers. *Infancy, 2,* 233–256.

74. McGraw, M. (1945). *The neuromuscular maturation of the human infant.* New York: Macmillan.

75. Metzoff, A. N., & Moore, M. K. (1992). Early imitation within a functional framework: The importance of person identity, movement, and development. *Infant Behavior and Development, 15,* 470–505.

76. Milani-Comparetti, A., & Gidoni, E. A. (1967). Pattern analysis of motor development and its disorders. *Developmental Medicine and Child Neurology, 9,* 625–630.

77. Morelli, G. A., Rogoff, B., Oppenheim, D., & Goldsmith, D. (1992). Cultural variation in infants' sleeping arrangements: Questions of independence. *Developmental Psychology, 28,* 604–613.

78. Morrissey, T. W., & Banghart, P. (2007). *Family child care in the United States.* Child Care & Early Education Research Connections. Retrieved June 2009 at http://www.childcareresearch.org/location/12036

79. National Institute of Child Health and Human Development (NICHD), Early Child Care Research Network. (2000). Characteristics and quality of child care for toddlers and preschoolers. *Applied Development Science, 4,* 116–135.

80. Ogunnaike, O. A., & Houser, R. F. (2002). Yoruba toddlers' engagement in errands and cognitive performance on the Yoruba Mental Subscale. *International Journal of Behavioral Development, 26,* 145–153.

81. Parham, L. D. (2008). Play and occupational therapy. In L. D. Parham & L. Fazio (Eds.), *Play in occupational therapy for children* (pp. 2–22). St. Louis: Mosby.

82. Pehoski, C. (2006). Object manipulation in infants and children. In A. Henderson & C. Pehoski (Eds.), *Hand function in the child* (pp. 143–160). St. Louis: Mosby.

83. Piaget, J. (1952). *The origins of intelligence in children* (M. Cook, Trans.). New York: International Universities Press.

84. Piper, M. C., & Darrah, J. (1994). *Motor assessment of the developing infant.* Philadelphia: W.B. Saunders.

85. Reilly, M. (Ed.). (1974). *Play as exploratory learning.* Beverly Hills, CA: Sage Publications.

86. Rochat, P. (1989). Object manipulation and exploration in 2- to 5-month-old infants. *Developmental Psychology, 25,* 871–884.

87. Rochat, P., & Gibson, E. J. (1985). Early mouthing and grasping: Development and cross-modal responsiveness to soft and rigid objects in young infants. *Canadian Psychology, 26,* 452.

88. Rogoff, B. (2003). *The cultural nature of human development.* New York: Oxford University Press.

89. Rogoff, B., Mosier, C., Mistry, J., & Goncu, A. (1993). Guided participation in cultural activity by toddlers and caregivers. *Monographs of the Society for Research in Child Development, 58,* 1–179.

90. Rogoff, B., Selless, M. J., Pinotta, S., Fox, N., & White, S. H. (1975). Age of assignment of roles and responsibilities to children: A cross-cultural survey. *Human Development, 18,* 353–369.

91. Rosblad, B. (2006). Reaching and eye-hand coordination. In A. Henderson & C. Pehoski (Eds.), *Hand function in the child* (pp. 89–100). St. Louis: Mosby.

92. Rubin, K. (1984). *The Play Observation Scale.* Ontario, Canada: University of Waterloo Press.

93. Rubin, K., Maioni, T. L., & Hornung, M. (1976). Free play behaviors in middle-class and lower-class children: Parten and Piaget revisited. *Child Development, 47,* 414–419.

94. Ruff, H. A. (1989). The infant's use of visual and haptic information in the perception and recognition of objects. *Canadian Journal of Psychology, 43,* 302–319.

95. Sharifzadeh, V. S. (1998). Families with Middle Eastern roots. In E. W. Lynch & M. J. Hanson (Eds.), *Developing cross-cultural competence* (2nd ed., pp. 409–440). Baltimore: Brookes.

96. Singer, D. G., & Singer, J. L. (1990). *The house of make-believe: Play and the developing imagination.* Cambridge, MA: Harvard University Press.

97. Spencer, J. P., Corbetta, D., Buchanan, P., Clearfield, M., Ulrich, B., & Schoner, G. (2006). Moving toward a grand theory of development: In memory of Esther Thelen. *Child Development, 77,* 1521–1538.

98. Stone, J. L., & Church, J. (1973). *Childhood and adolescence: A psychology of the growing person* (3rd ed.). New York: Random House.

99. Takata, N. (1974). Play as a prescription. In M. Reilly (Ed.), *Play as exploratory learning* (pp. 209–246). Beverly Hills, CA: Sage Publications.

100. Thelen, E. (1995). Motor development: A new synthesis. *American Psychologist, 50,* 79–95.

101. Thelen, E. (2002). Self-organization in developmental processes: Can systems approaches work? In M. Johnson & Y. Munakata (Eds.), *Brain development and cognition: A reader* (2nd ed., pp. 544–557). Malden, MA: Blackwell Publishers.

102. Thelen, E., Corbetta, D., Kamm, K., Spencer, J., Schneider, K., & Zernicke, R. F. (1993). The transition to reaching: Mapping intention and intrinsic dynamics. *Child Development, 64,* 1058–1098.

103. Thelen, E., Corbetta, D., & Spencer, J. P. (1996). The development of reaching during the first year. The role of movement speed. *Journal of Experimental Psychology: Human Perception and Performance, 22,* 1059–1076.

104. Thomas, A., & Chess, S. (1977). *Temperament and development.* New York: Brunner/Mazel.

105. Thompson, R. A., Easterbrooks, M. A., & Padilla-Walker, L. M. (2003). Social and emotional development in infancy. In R. M. Lerner, M. A. Easterbrooks, & J. Mistry (Eds.), *Handbook of psychology: Vol. 6. Developmental psychology* (pp. 91–112). New York: John Wiley & Sons.

106. Touwen, B. C. L. (1979). Examination of the child with minor neurological dysfunction: *Clinics in Development Medicine 71.*

107. Vanderbilt-Adriance, E., & Shaw, D. S. (2008). Conceptualizing and re-evaluating resilience across levels of risk, time, and domains of competence. *Clinical Child and Family Psychology Review, 11,* 30–58.

108. von Hofsten, C. (1993). Studying the development of goal-directed behaviour. In A. F. Kalverboer, B. Hopkins, & R. Geuze (Eds.), *Motor development in early and later childhood: Longitudinal approaches* New York: Cambridge Press.

109. Vygotsky, L. S. (1978). *Mind in society: The development of higher psychological processes.* Cambridge, MA: Harvard University Press.

110. Werner, E. E. (2000). Protective factors and individual resilience. In J. P. Shonkoff & S. J. Meisels (Eds.), *Handbook of early childhood intervention* (pp. 115–134). Cambridge: Cambridge University Press.

111. Werner, E. E., & Smith, R. S. (1992). *Overcoming the odds: High risk children from birth to adulthood.* Ithaca, NY: Cornell University Press.

112. Whiting, B., & Edwards, C. P. (1988). A cross-cultural analysis of sex differences in the behavior of children aged 3 through 11. In G. Handel (Ed.), *Childhood socialization* (pp. 281–297). Cambridge, MA: Harvard University Press.

113. Willis, W. (1998). Families with African American roots. In E. W. Lynch, & M. J. Hanson (Eds.), *Developing cross-cultural competence* (2nd ed., pp. 165–208). Baltimore: Brookes.

114. Wong, S., Chan, K., Wong, V., & Wong, W. (2002). Use of chopsticks in Chinese children. *Child: Care, Health, and Development, 28,* 157–163.

115. Youngblade, L. M., & Belsky, J. (1992). Parent-child antecedents of 5-year-olds' close friendships: A longitudinal analysis. *Development Psychology, 28,* 700–713.

116. Ziviani, J., & Rodger, S. (2006). Environmental influences on children's participation. In S. Rodger & J. Ziviani (Eds.), *Occupational therapy with children: Understanding children's occupations and enabling participation* (pp. 41–66). Oxford, UK: Blackwell Publishing, Inc.

117. Zuniga, M. E. (1998). Families with Latino roots. In E. W. Lynch & M. J. Hanson (Eds.), *Developing cross-cultural competence* (2nd ed., pp. 209–250). Baltimore: Brookes.

4

In Transition to Adulthood: The Occupations and Performance Skills of Adolescents

Kerryellen Vroman

KEY TERMS

KEY TERMS

Adolescents
Psychosocial development
Peer relationships
Body image
Identity

OBJECTIVES

1. Describe the physical, psychological, and social development that occurs in adolescence.
2. Examine the areas of occupation and occupations that promote and support adolescent development.
3. Recognize the interrelationship between health and psychosocial adolescent development.
4. Discuss how developmental issues of adolescents influence and guide the choice of therapeutic activities and interventions.
5. Highlight how parents and practitioners can promote self-determination and opportunities for exploration in adolescence for teens with disabilities.
6. Identify the role and responsibilities of an occupational therapy practitioner in facilitating participation by adolescents with disabilities.

This chapter provides an overview of the physical, cognitive, and psychosocial development that characterizes adolescence. Instead of providing a comprehensive guide to "typical" adolescent development, information that is readily available in human development textbooks, it focuses on the developmental issues that influence adolescents' participation in occupations and occupational performance. In particular, the chapter explores the affect of disabilities and chronic health conditions on adolescents' experiences and participation in age-related occupations. The information in this chapter comes with the caveat that occupational therapy practitioners need to see each adolescent as an individual and apply knowledge of typical development judiciously, cognizant that variability in development is normal. The client's strengths, goals, needs, priorities, context (e.g., socioeconomic, cultural), and current developmental status are all part of a comprehensive evaluation and intervention plan.

ADOLESCENCE

Of all the stages of life adolescence is the most difficult to describe. Any generalization about teenagers immediately calls forth an opposite one. Teenagers are maddeningly self-centered, yet capable of impressive acts of altruism. Their attention wanders like a butterfly, yet they can spend hours concentrating on seemingly pointless involvements. They are lazy and rude, yet when you least expect it they can be loving and helpful (p. xiii).[23]

Adolescents live mostly in the moment. They have moments of joy and pleasure, overwhelming loneliness and isolation, laughter and fun, unbearable emotional pain, anger, frustration, and embarrassment, which are equal to moments of supreme confidence and perceived immortality. They want the security of family, but push boundaries, demanding to be seen as grown up. They desire and experience the closeness of peer friendships; they experience the pleasure and anxiety of exploring intimacy; and they have intense and seemingly eternal passion for clothes, music, sports, or other interests, which for a week, a month, or year are all-absorbing. More than anything, they wish to belong, to fit in, to be seen the same as others, while at the same time wishing to be unique. These are the experiences of *all* American teenagers. In Case Study 4-1, Caroline, whose teenage sister is intellectually developmentally disabled, speaks to the universality of being a teenager.

ADOLESCENT DEVELOPMENT

Adolescence is generally defined as the high school years (between 12 and 18), which are associated with physical maturation and puberty. This intense period of physical and physiologic (biologic) maturation and psychosocial development influences an adolescent's ability to think, relate, and act as a competent adult. Adolescence is also a period of learning, experimentation, and experiences that affect individuals' choice of long-term occupations and their physical and psychological well-being. Box 4-1 lists facts about American teenagers.

In observing the developmental process of adolescence, occupational therapy practitioners observe adolescents' growth and their physical, emotional, and psychological changes; how adolescents perform common age-related tasks; how they choose occupations; and what experiences they seek. The

CASE STUDY 4-1   My Sister Is a Teenager

My younger sister, Corinne, was born with Noonan's syndrome, a genetic disorder that has left her moderately developmentally disabled. Corinne is lucky to have few of the characteristic physical problems of her disorder; however, her speech and cognitive abilities are clearly delayed. Now 17 years old (Figure 4-1), Corinne is meeting many of the same decisions and difficulties that "normal" teenagers face.

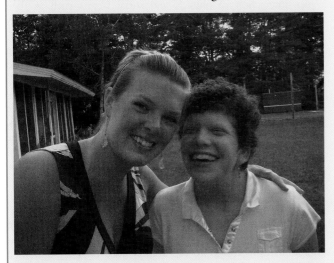

FIGURE 4-1   Sisters Corinne and Caroline

Corinne goes to a public school and takes a mixture of classes. Some are integrated with regular students and others are only with other teenagers with disabilities. High school is a trial for everyone, and my sister is no exception. Seeing people's reactions to Corinne's differences is always interesting, and many times disappointing. She is subject to teasing, bullying, and, perhaps worst of all, pity. Many people do not regularly interact with people who are mentally retarded and do not understand that Corinne wants no special treatment; she simply wants to be like everyone else.

Just like everyone else, Corinne has to tackle the teenage years. As she gets older, she desires more independence, just as I did at her age. When Corinne's disability presents her with situations in which she is forced to accept help, she becomes frustrated and angry. Her mood swings are like those of any other adolescent, easy to trigger and quick to pass. Her adolescence is complicated by the fact that logical explanations do not always satisfy her. Corinne has an incomplete understanding of time and events, which can make it difficult to relate to her way of thinking.

When faced with such daunting challenges, it is easy for Corinne to forget her strengths. Our family tries to remind Corinne of her abilities every day and find that in frustrating situations, it is often helpful to distract her with what she can do, instead of focusing on what she cannot do. Corinne has an incredibly detailed memory and has the ability to locate missing keys or beat anyone in a matching card game. However, her greatest strength is her unwavering ability to love. The kids at school wave to Corinne while passing in the hallway and she responds with unrivaled enthusiasm. In fact, everywhere we go, people recognize her. That's because Corinne is never afraid to say hello to new people, give them a hug, or call them her friend. Even when she is made fun of or excluded, she never judges. As Corinne's older sister, I thought it would be my job to teach her. However, I have come to realize that Corinne has much more to teach me.

Occupational therapy practitioners work with a variety of adolescents. Some are similar to Corinne, who has a stable preexisting condition that limits her functioning. Others have progressive disorders; still others acquire significant physical and/or cognitive disabilities because of trauma or psychosocial disorders that develop during adolescence. Only by thoroughly understanding "typical" adolescent development can an occupational therapy practitioner work with these teens in achieving their optimal abilities and full participation in society.

By Caroline Glass (2008), an English major at Wake Forest University.

BOX 4-1   Facts about American Teenagers

- There are 39.7 million teenagers in the United States: half between 10 and 14 years of age, and half between 15 and 19 years of age.
- Adolescents between 10 and 24 years of age are more racially and ethnically diverse than the general population: 52.2% are White, 16.5% Hispanic, 13.6% Black non-Hispanic, 3.9% Asian/Pacific Islander, and 0.9% American Indian/Alaskan Native.
- Two thirds of teenagers live in suburban areas, with the highest percentage in the South (35.6%) followed by the Midwest (23.5%), West (22.7%), and East (18.1%).
- Two thirds of teenagers between the ages of 12 and 17 years live with both parents (2002 data).

- Approximately 94.6% of teenagers 16 to 17 years of age are enrolled in school (2006 data). More females than are enrolled in school. The high school dropout rate is highest among Hispanics (22.5%), Blacks (10.8%), and Whites (6%) (2005 data). One third of high school students also work.
- Seventeen percent of children and adolescents under the age of 17 live below the Federal Poverty Line. Black and Hispanic adolescents are more likely to experience poverty.
- More than 5 million children and adolescents (8%) between the ages of 5 and 20 years have a disability.

Data from monograph *American adolescents: Are they healthy?* (3rd ed.); and the National Adolescent Health Information Center: Fact Sheet on Demographics: Adolescents (http://www.nahic-ucsf-edu; http://www.census.gov/PressRelease/www/2002/demoprofiles.html).

age-related tasks and experiences are crucial to the process of gaining physical and financial independence from parents and redefining their psychological and emotional relationships with their parent. As they develop, adolescents establish norms and lifestyles congruent with the values and culture of their peers and their families. They accept and explore the physical and sexual development of their bodies. They work to establish their gender, personal, moral, and occupational identity. When successfully navigated, adolescence culminates in an overall state of well-being and the transition to adulthood and adult roles. Failure to integrate and engage in the roles and tasks of adolescence can result in ongoing physical and psychosocial difficulties that will affect future occupational performance and roles.[51]

Effective occupational therapy interventions begin with an evaluation of physical, cognitive, and psychosocial factors associated with adolescents' development and the quality of their occupational performance. This includes standardized criterion-referenced (based on performance expected of an adolescent) or norm-referenced (based on actual performance of other adolescents) assessments that evaluate client factors and performance. Only interventions based on thorough evaluation are likely to be age appropriate and promote performance skills. Therefore, a working knowledge of adolescent development and awareness of occupations that facilitate age-appropriate development are fundamental to effective occupational therapy with adolescents. This chapter provides an overview of adolescent development intended to guide occupational therapy evaluations and interventions with the adolescent population.

PHYSICAL DEVELOPMENT AND MATURATION

Adolescence is characterized by the biologic and physiologic changes of puberty, dramatic increases in height and weight, and changes in body proportion. The age for the onset of puberty is variable and a child may begin to notice these changes from ages 8 to 14 years. The stimulus for this physical growth and physiologic maturation of reproductive systems is a complex interaction of hormones. It involves the hypothalamus and the pituitary gland that releases hormones that control growth and stimulate the release of sex-related hormones from the thyroid, adrenal glands, and the ovaries and testes (collectively referred to as the gonads).[92]

The growth and sex-related hormones initiate a period of rapid physical growth, which varies in intensity, onset, and duration. In this growth phase, people gain approximately 50% of their adult weight and 20% of their adult height. This process, which generally lasts about four years, can start as early as 9 years of age and may continue in some adolescents to age 17. In the United States, the average peak of growth occurs around age 11 for girls and age 13 for boys.

Growth of the skeletal system is not even: head, hands, and feet reach their adult size earliest. Bones become longer and wider. Calcification, which replaces the cartilaginous bone composition of childhood, makes bones denser and stronger. Muscles also become stronger and larger. This process of skeletal growth and muscle development culminates in increased overall strength and endurance for physical activities. Increases in strength are greatest about 12 months after adolescents' height and weight have reached their peak, and is associated with an overall improvement in motor performance, including better coordination and endurance. Increases in muscle mass and heart and lung function are typically greater in boys than in girls. This growth is the basis of the difference in strength and gross motor performance between males and females.[20] Motor performance peaks for males in late adolescence around 17 to 18 years of age.[16] Girls typically show an increase in motor performance, including enhancements in speed, accuracy, and endurance, around the age of 14. However, the changes in motor performance in girls are highly variable and are influenced by a complex interaction of physical and social factors such as their musculoskeletal development, onset of menses, personal interests, motivation, and participation in physical activities.[16]

An adolescent finds security and social confidence in fitting within the "norm" for physical development, and perceived physical competency in activities such as sports builds self-esteem, particularly for young males. Early maturing teens' self-confidence benefits from enhanced physical performance and enhanced social status. However, expectations of coaches, parents, and peers to excel at sport from can add unwelcome pressure and anxiety. These adolescents are more concerned with being liked and are likely to adhere to rules and routines. Adolescents who achieve the "desired standard" for physical appearance and/or level of physical performance (e.g., high school sports teams with high visibility such as football, cheerleading, or basketball) receive validation and approval from their peers and from adults. Hence, during adolescence, early-maturing boys are reportedly more popular, described as better adjusted, more successful in heterosexual relationships, and more likely to be leaders at school. Conversely, late maturing boys are reported to feel self-conscious about their lack of physical development.[42]

Physical Activities and Growth: Teenagers with Disabilities

Physical activity is important for the health of all teens, including those with physical, emotional, or cognitive disabilities. Participation in physical activities maintains functional mobility, enhances well-being and overall health, and provides opportunities for social interaction with peers. However, compared with nondisabled teens, adolescents with disabilities are less likely to engage in regular physical activity.[44] For example, adolescents with cerebral palsy report walking less than they did as children.[2]

Scholars have frequently reported that physical functioning (e.g., mobility) deteriorates in adolescents with congenital physical disabilities because of secondary musculoskeletal impairments associated with adolescent growth.[2,100] These secondary impairments include an inability of muscles to lengthen in proportion to bone growth, deterioration of joint mobility due to contractures, fatigue, overuse syndromes, obesity, and early joint degeneration. However, recent evidence does not support that such deterioration in performance is inevitable.[85] Studies have shown maintenance or improvement in teens with disabilities who engage in physical fitness and/or therapy programs.[3,85] Activity/exercise programs have resulted in adolescents' improving and maintaining gross motor function and walking speed. The achieved independence promotes self-efficacy.[60] For example, Darrah et al. reported that teens with cerebral palsy who participated in a community-based fitness program showed significant gains in strength and reported improved psychosocial skills at school.[24]

Occupational therapy practitioners take an active role in assisting teens to identify opportunities for physical activity within supportive environments (e.g., teams and physical fitness programs that accommodate and welcome adolescents with disabilities). They work with the teen's education team to facilitate inclusion in junior high and high school sports and fitness programs as specified as goals in a teen's individual education program (IEP). Physical activities can also include programs outside of school, such as summer camps and community activities. All such activities strengthen occupational performance skills and promote physical and emotional health.

Physical growth in adolescents with disabilities can lead to performance difficulties that require occupational therapy interventions. For example, changes in height and weight often require reassessment at the level of client factors (e.g., positioning, balance, strength, and coordination) that affect clients' occupational performance and activities of daily living (ADL). Clients may need new or modified assistive devices mobility aids (e.g., a wheelchair); they may also need new adaptive strategies, strengthening, and endurance training to ensure full participation in their occupations. With new environmental and activity demands[1] such as transitioning between classrooms in high school, some teens elect to conserve their energy and use a wheelchair instead of crutches or replace a manual chair with a powered chair.

Teens with progressive disorders (e.g., spinal muscular atrophy, Friedreich's ataxia, and muscular dystrophy) may require ongoing therapy as their functional abilities deteriorate. For example, boys with Duchenne's muscular dystrophy, the most common type of muscular dystrophy, use wheelchairs by early adolescence for functional mobility because of their progressive muscle weakness. Their ability to use their hands and fingers for eating, writing, and keyboarding abilities becomes weaker throughout their adolescence. Respiratory and trunk muscles become progressively weaker, and scoliosis and other skeletal deformities including joint contractures at the ankles, knees, elbows, and hips are common. With these adolescents, occupational therapy practitioners have an active role in facilitating adaptation to the progressive loss of motor function. Often they implement compensatory strategies such as wheelchair seating to maintain skeletal stability, splinting to prevent deformities, and assistive technology (e.g., voice recognition software for computers) to maintain occupational performance.

Primary caregivers must also adjust to the physical growth and physiologic maturation of the adolescent. Adolescence can be challenging, especially for parents/caregivers of adolescents with moderate to severe physical disabilities and/or mental retardation, because of the continued and, at times, increased levels of care required. For example, transferring small children into and out of vehicles, lifting them into the shower, and dressing them are relatively easy. As the adolescent grows and gains weight, these caregiving tasks become more difficult. Significant household modifications may be needed to accommodate the changes, and additional adapted equipment, such as the use of commode chair or hoists for transfers, may be required for basic ADLs.

In other situations, such as when an adolescent is developmentally disabled, the family's challenge is to encourage more autonomy and independence in self-care to prepare for a transition to semi-independent settings such as a group home. This can require that parents reduce supervision and the adolescent develop independence in new self-care routines, such as shaving or managing menses.

Although the occupational therapy practitioner effectively addresses practical needs with adolescents and parents, it is equally important that the practitioner be aware of the emotional adjustment for parents. With each new developmental stage that has a universally recognized marker of progress (e.g., going to junior high school, first date, learning to drive), parents may revisit their grief as they adapt to the realization that their child may not have the opportunity to enjoy many of these activities. Adolescence can heighten parents' awareness of the barriers and limitations that exist for their children.[49] The effective, empathetic practitioner is sensitive to the meaning of adolescence for teens and their families and acknowledges the experience and concerns that this period brings.

PUBERTY

Puberty is the term used to define the maturation of the reproductive system. During puberty, *primary and secondary sex characteristics* develop in conjunction with significant physical growth. This involves both biologic and psychosocial development. A complex interaction/feedback loop involving the pituitary gland, hypothalamus, and the gonads (ovaries in females and testes in males) controls the biologic development. In healthy adolescents, full sexual development may vary as much as 3 years from the average age. The average age at onset of puberty for American girls is between 8 and 13 years, with occurrence of the first period (menarche) between 12 and 13 years of age.[8,81] In boys, puberty generally begins later than it does for girls, on average between 11 and 12 years of age.

Changes in the sex organs involved in reproduction (e.g., menarche in girls and the growth of penis and testicles in males) are the hallmark of puberty. In girls, race, socioeconomic status, heredity, and nutrition influence the time of menarche. Ovulation usually occurs 12 to 18 months after the onset of menarche.[92] Breasts, areolar size, and adult pubic hair patterns develop over a 3- to 4-year period. This is also a period of peak growth in height, and a girl usually reaches her full height two years after she begins menstruating.

Puberty has additional challenges for adolescents already dealing with developmental and physical disabilities. Minimal information about puberty in this population is available to guide these adolescents, their caregivers, or health professionals.[90] Some research suggests that in girls with moderate to severe cerebral palsy, sexual maturation begins earlier or ends much later than it does on average in the general population.[114] A retrospective study involving women with autism spectrum conditions reported menarche either 8 months earlier or somewhat later than is typical (i.e., around the age of 13 years).[62]

In boys, development of the primary sex characteristics, such as an increase in the size of the testicles and the penis (length and circumference), coincides with overall physical growth. Changes include growth of the larynx, causing a deepening of the voice, and the ability to obtain an erection and ejaculate. First ejaculations (spermarche) occur on average between the ages of 12 and 13 years, but the seminal fluid does not contain mature sperm until later (around age 15). In this process, referred to as *adrenarche*, the adrenal glands are largely responsible for the secondary sex characteristic such as the growth of axillary and pubic hair, axillary perspiration, and body odor. Also, many adolescents, especially males (70% to 90%) develop acne because of the effect of testosterone.[39,81]

For adolescents with disabilities, puberty can present additional practical and psychosocial issues. For example, misperceptions exist about the capacity of an adolescent with a disability to be in a sexual relationship, experience sexual desire, and reproduce successfully.[41] Many adolescents with disabilities report that others ignore or avoid their emerging sexuality. Consequently, they receive minimal education about contraception or sexually transmitted diseases or how their disability may affect their sexuality or reproductive.[41,58] Sexual development and the individuation process can be difficult for parents, especially when the child requires extensive caregiving.[58] Adults with disabilities describe the ambivalence and difficulties that their parents had in acknowledging them as sexual beings.[46,104] Mary Stainton poignantly describes the demands associated with managing her menses, the emotional strain this task posed for her mother, and the decisions that denied her womanhood. In the following excerpt, she describes her mother's response to her menses: "Frustration ripped through her as she cleaned between my legs and pulled up the Kotex pad. She felt she constantly needed to be with me when I went to the bathroom. I felt guilty for making a mess: for bleeding at all" (p. 1445).[104] Her menarche was not celebrated as a coming of age as a woman; instead, she writes, "Around the time I was 12 or 13, we started talking about options. She [her mother] took me to doctors. I was put on the pill, then, given shots to stop or at least curtail my menstrual flow. A normal body process was now a huge problem, we had to control" (p. 1445).[104]

A meta-analysis of 36,284 adolescents in the 7th through 12th grades with visible (e.g., physical) and nonvisible (e.g., deafness) disabilities found no differences between adolescents with or without disabilities, with respect to the proportion who have had intercourse, age at first sexual experience, pregnancy, contraceptive use, or sexual orientation.[108] However, a significant number of girls with invisible conditions reported a history of sexual abuse. A similar finding was reported in a study of children and adolescents with mobility impairments in which more girls with visible conditions reported a history of a sexually transmitted disease.[53] The conclusion drawn in these studies is that adolescents with chronic conditions and disabilities are at least as sexually involved as other teens. However, these teens are significantly more likely to be sexually abused.

Occupational therapy practitioners working with adolescents with disabilities and chronic conditions need to be receptive to teen-initiated discussions and open to dialogue with adolescents and their parents on topics ranging from physical development, sexual expression, and contraception. Furthermore, they need to be aware of signs of sexual abuse. Information about sex education as it relates to people with disabilities can be found at websites such as www.sexualhealth.com and the National Information Center for Children and Youth with Disabilities (NICHCY).

Psychosocial Development of Puberty and Physical Maturation

Adolescents regard the physical changes in their bodies and their emerging sexuality with a combination of anxiety and pride.

These changes can cause confusion, excessive anxiety, or emotional turmoil. With changes in physical stature and the development of secondary sex characteristics, physical appearance becomes increasingly important. Sexuality and the development of relationships are critical to positive personal adjustment. Therefore, how an adolescent views his or her own physical and sexual development influences self-esteem.[97] Adolescence involves integrating these significant physical and physiologic changes into a healthy self-concept that includes a positive attitude towards one's body, referred to as *body image* (Table 4-1).

Body image, a dynamic perception of one's body, affects the person's emotions, thoughts, and behaviors and influences both public and intimate relationships.[89] Adolescents need support to learn about their bodies and to understand that their feelings and thoughts about their bodies are universal among their peers. Such support significantly reduces the anxiety associated with physical and sexual development. Support from family and friends and the availability of information positively influence adolescents' adjustment to their bodies' physical and physiologic changes.

Self-esteem, self-worth, and the evaluations of others influence perceptions of and attitudes towards one's body.[22] Teenage girls pepper their conversations with remarks about their appearance (e.g., "Do you think my backside is too big in these jeans?" "I'm too fat," or "I need to lose weight"). Negative body image is associated with both low self-esteem and mental health problems, including anxiety, depression, and eating disorders such as anorexia nervosa. It is estimated that between 50% and 80% of girls, especially in early adolescence, are dissatisfied with two or more aspects of their appearance.[40] Studies show that body dissatisfaction is universal. Girls, regardless of ethnicity, express a desire to be thin.[70] Boys also compare their

TABLE 4-1 Normal Development of Body Image

Stage of Adolescence	Healthy Behaviors and Concerns
Early adolescents	Are preoccupied with self
	Are self-evaluative about their attractiveness
	Make comparisons between their own body and appearance and that of other teens
	Have an interest as well as anxiety about their sexual development
Middle adolescents	Have achieved pubertal changes
	Are developing an acceptance of their bodies
	Are less preoccupied with their physical changes and shift their interest to their appearance, grooming, and "trying to be attractive"
	Are more apt at this age to develop eating disorders and other body image–related disorders (such as anorexia nervosa or body dysmorphic disorder)

Modified from Radizik, M., Sherer, S., & Neinstein, L. (2002) Psychosocial development in normal adolescents. In L. S. Neinstein (Ed.), *Adolescent health: A practical guide* (4th ed.). Philadelphia: Lippincott Williams & Wilkins.

internalized perceptions of masculinity with the image they see of themselves in the mirror. This ideal body image is defined by characteristics such as height, speed, broadness of the upper body, and strength.[121] Boys dissatisfied with their bodies generally want to gain weight and develop muscle mass in their upper body (i.e., shoulders, arms, and chest),[35] and such desires can lead to excessive weight training and use of steroids. However, concerns about being overweight are also becoming prevalent among males.[34] Research shows that, by 18 years of age, boys and girls are more satisfied with their bodies than they were in early and mid-adolescence.[33]

Socially constructed views of femininity and masculinity affect how a teenager develops a body image. One powerful social influence is the media (e.g., advertisements, magazines, music videos, video games, movies, and the fashion industry). The media markets a physical appearance that represents little of the diverse population of American teens. They portray an "ideal" that bears little resemblance to the "average" teen. Therefore, it is not surprising that many adolescents are critical of their bodies.[15] When girls compare themselves with the media's images of slim, perfect skin, large-breasted, small-waisted women or boys try to measure up to the lean, strong, attractive, acne-free men, they inevitability feel inadequate compared with these illusions of perfection. Furthermore, the media's portrayal often includes proximity of equally "perfect" members of the opposite sex, and possessions such as cars and consumer goods equating attractiveness with success.[22]

Since the process of healthy body image development involves comparison with peers and the media's "ideal" image, one might expect that developing a healthy body image would be even more challenging for adolescents with visible disabilities or conditions (e.g., spina bifida, cerebral palsy, Tourette's syndrome, or congenital limb abnormalities). However, the research in this area is contradictory. Stevens et al. (1996) reported no significant differences between disabled adolescents and nondisabled adolescents in self-esteem or satisfaction with physical appearance,[105] and Meeropol (1991) found that a majority of adolescents surveyed with spina bifida and cerebral palsy felt they are attractive to other people.[75] However, other studies report that adolescents with physical disabilities viewed themselves as different from their peers and unattractive to others.[47]

Body image can also be difficult for a teen that develops a disorder or illness (e.g., cancer, diabetes, epilepsy) in adolescence; their previously healthy bodies "fail" them. Research indicates that teens who have long-term effects (e.g., impaired organ function, scars, skeletal deformities) from serious illness have a negative body image and impaired emotional functioning.[14]

As with physical growth and development, sexual maturation has social implications. Adolescents who outwardly appear sexually mature and seem older than their actual age can encounter demands and expectations (including sexual) that they are not psychologically equipped to navigate. Unlike boys, early-maturing girls often demonstrate lower self-esteem and poor self-concept associated with body image, and they engage in more risky behaviors (e.g., unprotected sex).[112] They also experience more psychological difficulties (e.g., eating disorders and depression) than their more slowly developing girlfriends do. They are more likely to have lower grades, engage in substance abuse (alcohol, drugs), and have behavioral issues. Late maturation in boys is associated with such difficulties as inappropriate dependence and insecurity, disruptive behaviors, and substance abuse.[39] Some late maturing boys find validation in academic pursuits and nonphysical competitive activities, especially those from middle and upper socioeconomic status families that value such achievements.[42]

Adolescents use appearance to express their individuality and/or make a statement of belonging (e.g., fashionable clothes similar to those of friends, gang colors and insignia). Since the 1990s, body piercing and tattoos have emerged as forms of self-expression among adolescents. Whatever the "body project" (e.g., clothes, jewelry, hairstyles, make-up, tattoos), these activities related to appearance are within the adolescent's control and are consistent with practices within Western countries.[12] Experimentation with appearance is healthy for most adolescents and is integral to developing self-identity. It promotes a level of satisfaction and connectedness with peers. On the other hand, adolescents with psychological difficulties may abuse their bodies by engaging in activities such as cutting, excessive piercings and tattoos, or extreme weight loss; others will adopt clothing and make-up that marginalizes them. All such actions further alienate vulnerable teens from mainstream society. Piercing and tattooing of minors is regulated in many states and thus the struggle for autonomy can be an act of rebellion, or a public display of "I own my body; I can do to it what I choose."[12]

Adolescents who have a disability may depend on others for their self-care, may not have their own discretionary money from part-time work, and may lack independence in community mobility. Therefore, their opportunities to participate in activities of self-expression, experimentation, and expressing personal control are limited. For example, adolescents with disabilities are not always encouraged or offered opportunities to experiment with appearance (clothes, hairstyles) or interest that differ from those sanctioned by family and caregivers. Furthermore, it is sometimes more comfortable for parents and others to prolong childhood for these teens. Making choices about appearance and experimentation are part of the adolescent experience that contributes to self-identity, self-esteem, and healthy body image; the practitioners can find ways to facilitate experimentation for the adolescent with a disability (developmental or physical).

COGNITIVE DEVELOPMENT

Cognition is the term used to define the mental processes of construction, acquisition, and the use of knowledge, as well as perception, memory, and the use of symbolism and language.[84] Advances in magnetic resonance imaging have enhanced understanding of the neurobiologic processes that enable these higher-level cognitive functions and the changes that occur in the brain during adolescence. For example, the prefrontal lobe matures later than other regions, and its development is reflected in increased abilities in abstract reasoning, as well as processing speed and response inhibition.[119]

Quality of thinking changes in adolescence. Piaget[88] referred to this cognitive development as *logical thinking (formal operations),* which involves functions such as symbolic thought and *hypothetical-deductive* reasoning.[56,121] Adolescents' ability to think becomes more creative, complex, and efficient in both speed and adeptness. Thinking is more thorough, organized, and systematic than it was in late childhood, and problem solving and reasoning become increasingly sophisticated. In developing the capacity to think abstractly, adolescents rely less on concrete examples. Hypothetical-deductive reasoning, for example, does not require actual situations. Instead, a person identifies and explores many imagined possible outcomes to determine the most likely outcome to a particular situation or problem, as well as the relationship between present actions and future consequences. Hypothetical-deductive reasoning is essential for problem solving, and for the process of arguing. Preadolescents have difficulty considering possibilities as generalizations of actual real events, whereas the adolescent appreciates that the actual world is one of many possibilities.[84]

The development of cognitive abilities enables adolescents to achieve independence in thought and action.[19] They develop a perspective of time and become interested in the future. Thus, cognitive development is also central to the development of personal, social, moral, and political values that denote membership in adult society. The development of moral and social reasoning is seen in the adolescent's newly acquired ability to deal with concepts such as justice, truth, identity, and a sense of self.[84]

Because of this cognitive development, teens come to understand the consequences of their actions and the values influencing their decision-making. Furthermore, they become future oriented. They increasingly evaluate their behaviors and decisions in relation to the future they desire. The impulsive behaviors of a middle school or early high school student are replaced by decisions and actions that anticipate the consequences. This emerging self-regulation means that the adolescent gains the ability to control emotions and to moderate behavior appropriately relative to both situation and social cues.

Adolescents with cognitive impairments have difficulties comprehending the consequences of their actions and to moderating their behavior accordingly. Because of the lack of hypothetical-deductive reasoning, problem solving in relation to future, or responsiveness to subtleness of social cues, the self-evaluation that typically informs judgment is lacking. Instead, their impulsive decisions and actions are consistent with a cognitive level arrested at the preformal stage and their occupational performance skills are limited. Adolescents with diagnosed autism-spectrum disorders or teens with developmental disabilities whose abilities are classified in the moderate to higher functioning levels of mental retardation, and teens who have had a traumatic brain injury (TBI) may find at this stage that the academic demands of high school markedly exceed their abilities. Their peers' increasing psychosocial maturity and independence accentuate the long-term implications of their cognitive and social disabilities. At this phase of their education, they often transition into prevocational programs and programs that will facilitate their skills for their optimal level of independence in adulthood.

PSYCHOSOCIAL DEVELOPMENT

It is useful to view adolescent psychosocial development in three phases (Table 4-2). Phase one is early adolescence, which encompasses the middle school years between ages 10 and 13. Phase two is middle adolescence, which occurs during the high school years between ages 14 and 17. Phase three is late adolescence, 17 through 21, which is typically the first years of work or college.[4,91] The middle years of adolescence are the most intense period of psychosocial development. In this phase, peers displace parents as the significant influence in the adolescent's life. Conformity with peer groups is desirable, and the opinions of friends and peers matter.

Late adolescence is a period of consolidation. By this last phase, adolescents ideally are developing into responsible young adults who can make decisions, have a stable and consistent value system, and can successfully take on adult roles, such as an employee or a contributing member of the community. A stable, positive sense of self and self-knowledge of ability enable late adolescents and young adults to establish healthy relationships.

Difficulties navigating psychosocial development can have adverse health and social outcomes such as psychological problems (e.g., eating disorders, depression, substance abuse), and psychopathology with behavioral problems (e.g., oppositional defiance disorder, criminal activity). Psychological problems do not necessarily result in difficulties in adult life, although disorders can increase the vulnerability for further psychological and life challenges. However, some adolescent disorders, such as conduct disorder, are associated with adverse outcomes (e.g., dropping out of school, lower employment rates, substance abuse).[21]

The Search for Identity: Identity Formation

Society permissively tolerates a period of exploration in adolescence as the process that will result in young adults who have defined themselves as individuals, can problem-solve, take responsibility for their actions, self-regulate their emotions and behaviors, and demonstrate commitment to a set of values congruent with the social norms and values of their community.

The adolescent's quest for self-identity is the material for films and literature and the angst that fills the lyrics of popular music.

Self-identity has two elements: an individualistic component (Who am I?) and a contextual component (Where and how do I fit in my world?).[65] The individualistic sense of identity is the internalized, stable self-concept from which a person interacts with the world.[72] The contextual component of self-identity allows a person to understand his/her values, beliefs, interests, and commitments to a job or career and social roles such as daughter or friend.[72] The contextual aspect of a person's identity is visible to others and is shaped by society (Box 4-2).

Erik Erikson (1980) first proposed that acquiring a sense of identity *(identity formation)* is a critical task of adolescence. His theory of how identity develops through recognition of one's abilities, interests, strengths, and weaknesses by the self and others continues to dictate how identity formation is viewed in research and clinical practice.[34] Erikson proposed that identity formation is the optimal outcome of a crisis resolution process in which exploration and experimentation leads to a commitment (i.e., an investment in a set of values, beliefs, interests, and an occupation) to a positive sense of identity.[34] It is a complex process that involves identifying one's spiritual and religious beliefs; intellectual, social, and political interests; and a vocational or career path. It includes relationships and gender orientation (i.e., awareness and acceptance of one's female or male identity and sexual orientation), culture, ethnicity, and perceptions of one's personality traits (e.g., introverted, extroverted, open, conscientious).

TABLE 4-2 Summary of the Typical Characteristics of Psychosocial Development

Stage of Adolescence	Typical Psychosocial Development Characteristics
Early adolescents	Are engrossed with self (e.g., interested in personal appearance)
	Separate from parents emotionally (e.g., reduced participation in family activities)
	Display less overt affection to parents
	Comply less with parents' rules or limits as well as challenge other authority figures (e.g., teachers, coaches)
	Question adults' opinions (e.g., critical of and challenge their parents' opinions, advice, and expectations); begin to see parents as having faults
	Have changeable moods and behavior
	Have mostly same-sex friendships with strong feelings towards these peers
	Demonstrate abstract thinking
	Fantasize idealistically about careers; think about possible future self and roles
	Need privacy (e.g., they have own bedroom with door closed, write in diaries, and have private telephone conversations)
	Become interested in experiences related to personal sexual development and exploration of sexual feelings (e.g., masturbation)
	Self-consciously display modesty (blushing, awkwardness about self and body)
	Display an ability to self-regulate emotional expression and can limit behavior but do not think beyond immediate want or need and therefore are susceptible to peer pressure
	May experiment with drugs (cigarettes, alcohol, and marijuana)
Middle adolescents	Continue to move toward psychological and social independence from parents
	Increase their involvement in peer group culture, displayed by adopting peer value system, codes of behavior, style of dress and appearance, all of which demonstrate in an overt way individualism and separation from family
	Are involved in formal and informal peer group activities, such as sports teams, clubs, gangs
	Accept body development, engage in sexual expression and experiment with sex (e.g., dating, sexual activity with partner)
	Explore and reflect their feelings and those of other people
	Become more realistic in career/vocational aspirations
	Show an increased creative and intellectual ability as well as interest in intellectual activities and capacity to do work (e.g., mentally and emotionally)
	Use risk-taking behaviors to minimize or alleviate feelings of omnipotence (sense of being powerful) and immortality (e.g., reckless driving, unprotected sex, high alcohol consumption, drug use)
	Experiment with drugs (cigarettes, alcohol, marijuana, and other illicit drugs)
Late adolescents	Become more stable as the sense of self becomes stable in opinions, values, and beliefs
	Strengthen relationships with parents (e.g., seek out and value parental advice and assistance)
	Increase their independence in decision making and the ability to express ideas and opinions
	Have increased interest in their future and consider the consequences of current actions and decisions on the future, leading to delayed gratification, setting personal limits, monitoring their own behavior, and reaching compromises
	Resolve their earlier angst regarding puberty, physical appearance, and attractiveness
	Feel diminished peer influence and increased confidence in personal values and sense of self
	Show a preference for one-to-one relationships and start to select an intimate partner
	Become realistic in vocational choice or employment, establishing worker role and financial independence
	Develop a value system (e.g., moral, belief system, religious affiliation and sexual values) that becomes increasingly stable

Data from Radizik, M., Sherer, S., & Neinstein L., (2002). Psychosocial development in normal adolescents. In L. S. Neinstein (Ed.), *Adolescent health care: A practical guide* (4th ed.). Philadelphia: Lippincott Williams & Wilkins; and American Academy of Child and Adolescent Psychiatry website: http://www.aacap.org/publications. Retrieved 9/7/2004.

To achieve a sense of identity, adolescents daydream and fantasize about their real and imagined selves. These images energize and motivate. They actively attempt to make sense of their world and find meaning in what happens to them. To achieve this, they explore different roles, express a variety of opinions and preferences, make choices, and interpret their experiences. They engage in a variety of activities and lifestyles before settling on a viewpoint, set of values, or life goals. Adolescents are reflective and introspective, spending time thinking about themselves, making social comparisons between self and peers, and evaluating how others view them.

They set goals, take actions, learn to resolve conflicts and problems,[65] and, through this process, identify what makes them individual.

Adolescents' behaviors, thoughts, and emotions can seem contradictory, especially between ages 13 and 15. For example, a teen might have body piercings, break parental rules, and attend school erratically, but at the same time they responsibly hold a job and dress appropriately for the work setting. Similarly, adolescents may choose healthy behaviors such as vegetarianism or sports participation, but also experiment with alcohol, drugs, and/or tobacco. Adolescents can be fickle and

---

BOX 4-2   Being Disabled Is Not an Identity

Social acceptance is highly valued and important to identity. Adolescents with disabilities or chronic health disorders have additional challenges. Teens are acutely self-aware and want to be "like everyone else," i.e., like other teens in their social group. However, teens with a disability or health conditions must also constructively integrate their disabilities or health problems into a healthy self-concept, which does not make their disability or health problems their identity.

Adults (e.g., teachers, occupational therapy practitioners) and friends in their lives that refer to them as "disabled teens" or any other label (e.g. autistic, disruptive) reinforce and shape an adolescent identity based on their disability rather than their unique qualities (e.g., personality characteristics, interests, values, and abilities).

The occupational therapy practitioner has a role in:
- Modeling appropriate use of first-person language. For example, rather than "Steve, who has arthrogryposis...," it would be preferable to identify Steve by qualities or characteristics other than his disability, (e.g., "Steve with red hair...").
- Avoiding the use of emotive language that marginalizes and assumes that disability is always a negative experience (e.g., "Lisa who *suffers from* cerebral palsy.")
- Assisting teens to identify abilities, interests, and positive qualities that will be the primary characteristics of their identity

---

contrary; they may be interested in different religions and political systems, arguing passionately with their parents on political views. They express disinterest in relationships with the opposite sex, but spend the following day exclusively with a girlfriend or boyfriend.

Developmental theorist Marcia describes four states of identity: *identity diffusion, moratorium, identity foreclosure,* and successful *identity achievement.*[72] Some developmental theorists claim that describing identity as "states" implies the existence of a final ideal state of identity formation, rather than the reality, which is a complex and ongoing process of negotiation, adaptation, and decision making throughout adulthood. However, describing identity states is common and can be helpful.

Identity diffusion, common in early adolescence, is a state in which a person has an ill-defined sense of identity. In this state, adolescents have little or no interest in exploring their options. They have not made any commitments to choices, interests, or values and are not interested in the question "Who am I?"[9] Adolescents who continue to experience identity diffusion into their middle and late teen years have difficulty meeting the psychosocial demands of adolescence. They may demonstrate an "I don't care" attitude of impulsivity, disorganized thinking, and immature moral reasoning.[20] Identity diffusion is associated with lower self-esteem, a negative attitude, and dissatisfaction with their life, their parents' lifestyle, and school.[20,55] In this state, adolescents seldom anticipate and think about their future and have difficulties meeting day-to-day demands of life such as completing schoolwork or participating in sports or extracurricular activities. Consequently, they may be unhappy and lonely.[8] In later adolescence, because they have not explored their interests or considered their strengths in relation to work, they sometimes have problems finding employment.

Moratorium is a state, common to early and middle adolescence, of actively exploring and developing a sense of identity. While in identity diffusion, adolescents avoid or ignore the task of exploring their identity; in moratorium state, identity is a project that is pursued vigorously. Teens in moratorium openly explore alternatives, striving for autonomy and a sense of individuality. However, later in adolescence, prolonged moratorium becomes problematic. Indecision about life goals, course of study, or future career can cause anxiety, self-consciousness, impulsiveness, and depression.[20]

Identity foreclosure is the state in which an adolescent appears to have achieved a sense of identity but has actually avoided self-exploration and experimentation by making premature decisions about career, relationships, and interests, and thereby committing to an identity.[64] Adolescents demonstrating identity foreclosure commonly accept their parents' values and beliefs and follow family expectations regarding career choices without considering other possibilities. Such adolescents are conventional in their moral reasoning, less autonomous than their peers, less flexible in their thinking regarding opinions about what is "right," and more comfortable with a structured environment.[64] Research has found foreclosure is associated with approval-seeking behaviors, avoidance of new experiences, and a high respect for authority. These teens are less self-reflective, less intimate in personal relationships, and less open to experiences than peers, but foreclosure on identity makes these adolescents less anxious than many of their peers (see Box 4-2).[20]

Successful achievement of a sense of identity through the healthy resolution of experimentation and exploration is coherence between a person's identity and his/her self-expression and behaviors.[64,97] It is characteristic of adolescents in later years of high school or in college or those in the work force. It follows a state of moratorium and represents commitment to interests, values, gender orientation, political views, career or job, and includes a moral stance after exploring the possibilities. Research shows that identity achievement is associated with autonomy and independence, especially in decision making.[64]

Adolescents who have resolved their identity issues are able to adapt and respond to personal and social demands without undue anxiety. A relatively stable sense of self gives adolescents self-esteem and efficacy in their abilities. These adolescents are less self-absorbed, less self-conscious, and less susceptible to pressure from peers. They are open and creative in their thinking and have a capacity for intimacy. They are able to self-regulate emotions, and they demonstrate mature (postconventional) moral reasoning.

Adolescents who are unable to develop a stable and distinct sense of self may have difficulties, such as a lack of confidence and lower self-esteem. As adults, they may have problems with work, establishing and maintaining intimate relationships, and meeting the responsibilities of life, such as parenting or being a contributing member of their community. Identity formation enables adolescents and young adults to integrate contradictory aspects of the self into a global self-concept, which enables them to present differently to meet different situational (contextual) demands.

The study of identity development continues to expand interdisciplinary perspectives, including the effect of external barriers and culture on adolescents' exploration and commitment to identity.[117] Occupational therapy practitioners observe identity exploration in the activities adolescents choose, the roles they take on, and the desires they express about their futures. Practitioners promote psychosocial development, including identity formation, by emotionally supporting adolescents, working with them to develop abilities in their chosen activities and roles, and offering opportunities for self-directed exploration through participation in age-related activities. Occupational therapy sessions should develop and explore work and leisure activities, promote the acquisition of social and life skills, promote participation and self-determinism, as well as address barriers to community access. In short, they should create an environment that supports identity achievement.

Sexual Orientation: Gender Identity

Sexual orientation refers to an individual's pattern of physical and emotional arousal towards other persons of either the opposite or the same sex.[37] Awareness of sexual orientation generally occurs during adolescence, a time of sexual exploration, dating, and romance. Most adolescents identify their sexual orientation as heterosexual, although about 15% of teens in mid-adolescence experience an emotional and/or sexual attraction to their own gender. Approximately 5 percent of teens will identify their sexual orientation as gay or lesbian,[93] although they often delay openly identifying their sexual

orientation until late adolescence or early adulthood. Reasons include a lack of support among their peers and experiences of verbal and physical harassment in high school.[37,55] Openness and a willingness to discuss emerging sexuality with all adolescents is important for all practitioners working with them. Practitioners need to use gender-neutral language (e.g., *partner* rather than *boyfriend* or *girlfriend*; *protection* rather than *birth control*), inquire if they suspect violence in intimate relations, and provide nonjudgmental support to adolescents as they develop their sexuality and sexual orientation.[37]

Self-Concept and Self-Esteem

As adolescents define their identity, their *self-concept* (the feelings and perception of one's identity consisting of stable values, beliefs, and abilities) becomes differentiated.[92] Self-concept is multifaceted. It includes self-acceptance, which is associated with many areas of the adolescent's life (e.g., sports and athletic competence, parent and peer relationships, academic competence, social acceptance, and physical appearance). In adolescence, self-concept develops from a self-absorbed description based on social roles and personality characteristics in early adolescence to an integrated self-concept that reflects development in cognition, moral reasoning, and social awareness.

A significant aspect of self-concept is *self-esteem*, the global self-evaluation of values and positive and negative qualities (i.e., how a person feels about oneself). In early adolescence, self-esteem tends to decline, partly because of an increased self-awareness and a tendency to compare one's self with the ideal and thus realize a discrepancy between one's actual self and desired ideal self.[92] However, self-esteem usually improves throughout adolescence. Table 4-3 provides an outline of the behavioral characteristics of positive and negative self-esteem

TABLE 4-3   Behavioral Indicators of Self-Esteem

Self-Esteem	Behavioral Indicators
The teen with positive self-esteem	Expresses opinions Mixes with other teens (e.g., interacts socially with groups of teens) Initiates friendly interactions with others Makes eye contact easily when speaking Faces others when speaking to them Observes comfortable, socially determined space between self and others Speaks fluently in first language without pauses or visible discomfort Participates in group activities Assumes leadership role among peers Works collaboratively with others Gives directions or instructions to others Volunteers for tasks and activities
The teen with negative self-esteem	Avoids eye contact Appears overly confident (e.g., brags about achievements or skills to mask a lack of self-efficacy in performance skills) Expresses self-criticism, makes self-deprecating comments; makes fun of self as a form of humor Speaks loudly or dogmatically to avoid others responding Is submissive and overly agreeable to others' requests or demands, even if he or she does not wish to do them Gives opinions or views reluctantly, especially if it will draw attention to himself or herself Monitors behaviors (e.g., hypervigilant of surroundings and other people) Makes excuses for performance, seldom evaluates personal performance as satisfactory or good Engages in putting others down, name calling, gossiping, and, at worst, bullying Reports a lack of emotional support from parents and friends

Modified from Santrock, J. W. (2003). *Adolescence.* New York: McGraw-Hill.

throughout adolescence. Persistent low self-esteem is associated with serious psychological difficulties (e.g., depression; anxiety disorders such as social phobia, bulimia, and self-abuse). Self-abuse may take the form of cutting or harming one's self, excessive use of alcohol and drugs, or engaging in risky behaviors such as promiscuity and unprotected sex. Behaviors such as frequently making negative self-critical statements, fears of anticipated failure, and difficulty coping with perceived failure also indicate poor self-esteem. Teens with poor self-esteem are hypersensitive to negative comments from peers and adults alike, and to lack of responsiveness or over-reaction from others, and can be defensive to constructive criticism. In a desire to belong or "fit in" by seeking social approval, they are more susceptible to peer-group influence.

Factors contributing to self-esteem of adolescents with disabilities are similar to those of nondisabled teens, especially the value-laden self-assessment of one's own attributes and limitations. A stereotypical view of adolescents with disabilities infers that self-esteem is low. However, the research data on this topic do not support this view. A meta-analysis of studies examining self-esteem in teens with minor physical disabilities reported that, compared with their nondisabled peers, they had lower self-esteem about physical competencies, but the effect on their general, social, and physical appearance self-esteem was only moderate.[76] This analysis did find a relationship between the severity of physical disability and level of general self-esteem. However, Miyahara and Register found that this low self-esteem was related to misunderstanding by peers and adults and poor performance that reflected lack of effort rather than disability.[77] A study of self-esteem and self-consciousness among adolescents with spina bifida found that their perception of being treated by parents in an age-appropriate manner and parents' tolerance of social participation contributed positively to self-esteem, whereas school problems and the perceptions of disability by others contributed negatively.[113] Occupational therapy practitioners who work with students who are "clumsy" or have poor motor planning or learning disabilities need to recognize these potential obstacles to positive self-esteem and incorporate strategies and experiences that validate and facilitate self-recognition of one's strengths and abilities as part of the therapeutic process.

Adolescence and Mental Health

Mental health is defined as the "successful performance of mental functions, resulting in productive activities, fulfilling relationships with others, and the ability to change and cope with adversity."[107] Adolescents who have good mental health generally have better physical health than peers who have poor mental health; they demonstrate positive social behaviors and are less likely to participate in risky behaviors (Box 4-3).[63] However, adolescents are vulnerable to mental health disorders. Most diagnosable disorders associated with altered thinking, mood, or changes in behavior causing distress and/or impaired cognitive functioning begin in adolescence, many before the age of 14. Adolescents who have mental health

---

BOX 4-3   Critical Health Behaviors of American Adolescents

ALCOHOL & DRUG USE
- Alcohol is the most widely used substance by adolescents (more than tobacco or illicit drugs). Typical initial drug use for boys is alcohol. Among teens surveyed (*Monitoring the Future Study* 2000 [MFS]), 22% of 8th graders and 41% of 10th to 12th graders drank alcohol in the previous month.
- Rural teens have equal access to drugs as urban teens.
- Alcohol is a factor in approximately 41% of all deaths from motor vehicle accidents.

TOBACCO USE
- Every day, approximately 4,000 adolescents aged 12-17 try their first cigarette. Typically, initial drug use for girls is cigarettes. 4.5% of 8th graders, 8.9% of 10th graders and 15.8% of 12th graders report daily cigarette use in the past 30 days. This is a decrease compared with levels reported in surveys.

INJURY & VIOLENCE (INCLUDING SUICIDE)
- Injury and violence is the leading cause of death among youth aged 10-24 years: motor vehicle crashes (30% of all deaths), all other unintentional injuries (15%), homicide (15%), and suicide (12%).

NUTRITION
- Healthy eating is associated with reduced risk for many diseases, including the three leading causes of death: heart disease, cancer, and stroke. In 2007, only 21.4% of high school students reported eating fruits and vegetables five or more times daily (excluding fried potatoes and potato chips) during the past 7 days.

PHYSICAL ACTIVITY
- Between 16% and 22% of adolescents are obese or overweight.
- Overall, in 2007, 35% of 9th to 12th graders had participated in at least 60 minutes per day of physical activity.
- Approximately half of American adolescents (aged 12-21 years) are vigorously active on a regular basis. Inactivity is more common among females (14%) than males (7%) and among black females (21%) than white females (12%).

SEXUAL BEHAVIORS
- Approximately 50% of high school students are sexually active; by graduation, 2/3 will have had sexual intercourse.
- Approximately half of the 19 million new STD infections in the United States are among adolescents aged 15 to 24. In 2007, 39% of sexually active high school students did not use a condom during last sexual intercourse.
- Teenage pregnancy rate is dropping. Between 1991 and 1998 birth age for teens 15-19 declined by 18%.

Data from Monitoring the Future Study (2001-2003). http://www.nida.nih.gov/Infofax/HSYouthtrends.html; National Center for Chronic Disease Prevention and Health Promotion Healthy Youth, YRBSS Youth Online: Comprehensive Results. Available at: http://apps.nccd.cdc.gov/yrbss/QuestYearTable.asp?path=byHT&ByVar=CI&cat=5&quest=508&year=2007&loc=XX and Neinstein, L. S. (2002). *Adolescent healthcare: A practical guide*, (4th ed.). Philadelphia: Lippincott Williams & Wilkins.

disorders (e.g., depression, substance abuse) are likely to have difficulties learning and developing social and life skills, and are likely to engage in risky health behaviors.

The *Mental Health of Adolescents: A National Profile Report* estimates that 1 in 5 adolescents experience symptoms of emotional distress and that 1 in 10 are emotionally impaired.[63] The most common disorders are depression, anxiety disorders, substance use/abuse, and attention deficit disorder (with and without hyperactivity). The Youth Risk Behavior Surveillance study reported that 37% of female and 20% of male high school students answered "yes" to the question "Have you ever felt so sad or hopeless every day for two weeks in a row that you couldn't do some of your usual activities?"[17] This depression in young people (15 to 20 years of age) is often comorbid with other mental health disorders, such as addictions, anxiety disorders, and conduct disorder. Furthermore, suicide, the third leading cause of death in adolescents, is significantly associated with depression. In 2005, 8.4% of high school students attempted suicide. Although suicide attempts were more frequent among female students, especially in the ninth grade, the number of deaths from suicide among males between the ages of 10 and 14 was 2.5% higher than females and 3.5% higher in the 15- to 19-year-old age range.[30]

Other mental health disorders include eating disorders (e.g., anorexia nervosa or bulimia), learning disorders, and behavioral disorders (e.g., conduct disorder and oppositional defiance disorder). Schizophrenia and bipolar disorder are serious, but less common disorders. The onset of schizophrenia (excluding paranoid schizophrenia) in males is typically in late adolescence. Both schizophrenia and bipolar disorder have significant implications for teens because they disrupt participation in typical developmental activities, and these lost opportunities can contribute to lifelong disability.

Occupational therapy practitioners can assist with early identification of children and adolescents with mental health disorders because initially (e.g., in early adolescence) they may receive services for related difficulties such as learning and behavioral problems. Occupational therapy practitioners also are among the professionals involved in interdisciplinary teams providing early detection and intervention for teens with mental health disorders such as schizophrenia and bipolar disorder.

AREAS OF OCCUPATION: PERFORMANCE SKILLS AND PATTERNS

In the American Occupational Therapy Association (AOTA) Practice Framework activities that humans in engage in are categorized into domains. These are ADLs, instrumental activities of daily living (IADLs), rest and sleep, education, work, play, leisure, and social participation.[1] Participation in all of these areas develops self-efficacy (confidence in one's abilities to achieve desired outcomes), peer acceptance, and promotion of social status and self-esteem. Furthermore, adolescents are likely to adopt the values that are associated with the work, play, leisure, and social activities that they participate in.[31] This section describes adolescent development and participation in four domains (work, IADL, play and leisure, and social participation).

Work: Paid Employment and Volunteer Activities

Work is a general term associated with a job (work undertaken as a means of earning money) or a career (an organized life path that often involves a formal occupation or vocation). Studies of working patterns in American teenagers report that approximately 70% of adolescents older than age 16 work while also attending school.[6] Fourteen years is the age at which teens may work; however, the hours they may work are regulated. Beyond the age of 16, teens attending school cannot work more than 4 hours on a day that they attend school and are restricted on the evening hours they may work. Although working can be beneficial for adolescents, excessive working (i.e., more than 20 hours a week) for high school students can be detrimental. It is associated with emotional distress, early onset of sexual activity, and substance abuse.[108] Work takes time away from schoolwork, recreational activities, social activities, and participation in sports, and it may expose teens to work-related injuries.[94] Despite these adverse consequences, approximately 18% of high school students work 20 hours or more per week.[83]

The occupational domain of work also includes unpaid work, namely volunteerism. The 2000 edition of "America's Children: Key National Indicators of Well-being" reported that 55% of high school students participated in volunteer activities. Community service is encouraged by schools and organizations such as sports teams and church groups. Similar to adults, the reasons teens cited for participating in volunteer activities are a desire to help others, social interaction, and recognition of contributions.[99] The motivation for volunteerism is also influenced by adolescents' personal future goals. Students with higher grade point averages and higher academic self-esteem who have plans for higher education volunteer in their communities.[54]

Work (both paid and unpaid) significantly contributes to healthy adolescent development. In work settings, adolescents interact with adults on a more equal level, have opportunities to assume responsibilities and learn social behaviors, shape values, and develop knowledge of their possible preferences for adult career/work.[61] Participating in paid employment and volunteerism also develops life and social skills beyond the work environment, such as managing money, organizing time, developing routines, developing skills in collaboration, and negotiating relationships with other people. It also provides opportunities to learn from and communicate with more diverse social and racial groups than their family and school contexts.[94] The disposable income earned from paid employment gives some adolescents discretionary spending and a sense of economic independence, whereas others need to work to support themselves financially or contribute to their families. Whatever the circumstances, work helps adolescents assume adult-like responsibilities.

Occupational therapy programs for adolescents focus on strategies that develop work skills and behaviors that will assist in their transition from school to work. These skills and behaviors constitute the performance dimension of work required for adult employment. In addition to these skills and behaviors, another significant aspect of engaging in work is the development of an occupational identity.

Occupational identity combines interests, values, and abilities into a realistic choice of a job or career path. It begins in early adolescence with the development of abstract thinking and a capacity for future-oriented thinking. Adolescents start to fantasize about their future work occupations. Initially, these daydreams are idealistic aspirations about a possible adult self. By mid-adolescence, such fantasies become more realistic, and by late adolescence, their aspirations have a realism based on interests, values, and a match between their performance abilities and actual job demands. Pursuing postsecondary education (college or university) delays the transition to full-time work, and settling on an occupational identity may be deferred. Professional academic programs of study that begin with undergraduate degrees (e.g., nursing, occupational therapy, and engineering) proactively facilitate and shape occupational identity generally earlier than postsecondary degrees in the science or liberal arts.

In summary, full-time employment is a tangible marker of the transition from adolescent to adult. The worker role with the accompanying financial independence replaces the student role. The successful transition to the worker role involves a choice of occupation that integrates personal identity and interests with individual occupational performance skills and job requirements. Hence, occupational therapy programs start to explore occupational identity early in adolescence and combine this process with skill development, ensuring future work options.

Work Opportunities for Adolescents with Disabilities

Opportunities for inclusion in paid employment have increased for teens with disabilities. Hence, the transition from school to work is frequently the focus of occupational therapy. These transition programs are most effective when based on students' strengths, interests, and needs. Successful work experiences for teens with disabilities are contingent on strong social networks, formal and informal support within the work setting, support of supervisors, and a workplace culture that positively supports inclusion and diversity in hiring practices.[13]

Instrumental Activities of Daily Living

IADLs support daily life within the home and the community and, although the tasks can appear mundane, competency in the performance skills associated with everyday living is essential. Developing independence and interdependence in IADLs establishes the foundation of physical and financial independence.

Adolescents take on more responsibility for IADLs; for example, the chores and simple routines of childhood increase from cleaning one's room to tasks that contribute to the household (e.g., mowing lawns, doing laundry, cleaning the car, cooking). As autonomy increases, teens gain experience with most IADLs. They learn to drive and/or use public transport so they can move about the community without adult supervision. Although still receiving parental oversight, they take on their own health management, such as taking medications, learning about health risks, and making decisions about health behaviors (e.g., smoking, having protected sex, nutrition, and personal hygiene routines). They learn money management associated with IADLs, such as shopping, planning how and when to spend money, saving for the future, and managing a credit card and bank account.

By middle adolescence, teens may also take on responsibilities of caring for children by babysitting and assisting with

coaching or lifeguarding. With these tasks, they develop a knowledge and awareness of safety and emergency procedures. These roles and associated responsibilities further extend their repertoire of skills. Positive role models such as adult family members and other significant adults facilitate the gradual development of multiple and complex IADLs.

Adolescents initiate communication and use a wide variety of communication technologies to interact with peers. Eighty-seven percent of adolescents between the ages of 12 and 17 interact through online social networks.[68] Consequently, they have almost 24-hour connection with peers through text messaging, cell phones, instant messaging, and increased contact with adults such as teachers and coaches via email. This is particularly true of girls, and their contact increases with age. These social networks are equally available to teens with and without disabilities. Adolescents' use of the Internet has intensified and broadened: they log on more often and do more things when they are online. They shop online, play games, and research information for school assignments. Girls dominate most content-created online by teens; 35% of girls blog, whereas only 20% of boys blog; 54% of girls post photos compared with 40% of boys; but more boys post video content.[69] In a Canadian study, adolescents' reported use of technologies could be seen as a continuum from highly interactive to fixed information sources that fell within one of four domains. These were personal communication (telephone, cell phone, and pager), social communication (e-mail, instant messaging, chat, and bulletin boards), interactive environments (websites, search engines, and computers), and unidirectional sources (television, radio, and print).[102] Consequently, teens have access to a vast amount of information and connect with people beyond their known social network and geographic location.

The enjoyment of creating and social networking on sites such as Myspace and Facebook is tempered with risks. Teens are making moral decisions about the information accessed and people interacted with, often outside of parental/adult oversight. Discerning use of technology integrates cognitive skills, values and interests, and knowledge of the need to protect personal identity and privacy, all at an age when risk taking is more likely, the anticipation of consequences is underdeveloped, and problem-solving skills are inconsistent. The Internet and communication technologies, which provide a complex virtual, social, and physical world for children and adolescents, are increasingly becoming an area of research in child and adolescent development.[43] The future of this research will expand the understanding of how these technologies influence and facilitate cognitive, psychological and social development.

Achieving Competencies in IADLs with a Disability

Adolescents with disabilities and their families face an array of challenges in the area of IADLs. They deal with the paradox of achieving emotional and psychological independence and developing identity as a self-determining individual (which in society is represented overtly by work and autonomy in IADLs) while still physically dependent on their parents or caregivers. These teens may always require the assistance or oversight of other people for many IADLs. Although teens with developmental delays eventually learn skills to optimize their autonomy, most have semi-dependent relationships with their care providers, who will make executive life decisions with them. However, it is a different scenario for cognitively able teens with physical disabilities. To enter adult life, these teens must learn to apply their executive cognitive skills and emotional self-regulation to IADLs. They need opportunities to develop decision-making and problem-solving skills applicable to IADLs such as health management, money management, and community access (maybe driving an adapted vehicle), all decisions previously undertaken by parents. They need these experiences because eventually as adults they will instruct and oversee attendant caregivers. Thus it is the responsibility of the adults in their lives (occupational therapy practitioners, family members, and other caregivers) to augment this learning. As caregivers gradually transfer such responsibilities to the teens, they are simultaneously changing their roles in relation to their children.

Parents as primary caregivers have different demands and new emotional strains as their child enters adolescence. Similar to parents of nondisabled teens, they are seeking the balance of "letting go" while still being supportive. Yet they and their adolescent are dealing with many additional life challenges that are psychologically and socially demanding. This transition is difficult for parents, and retrospective studies report that adults with disabilities say that, as adolescents, their parents tended to be overprotective.[79]

Although adolescents with physical and developmental disabilities may struggle to become autonomous self-determining individuals, at-risk, emotionally troubled teens often find themselves prematurely independent. Although they still need the support and nurturing of a stable family, these teens, because of personal and socioeconomic circumstances, have a pseudo independence that they are not developmentally ready to manage. They may lack adequate cognitive development and performance skills to meet their IADL and ADL needs. Sometimes, they are even caregivers of their own children. Adolescents in such circumstances often deal with issues such as violence, poverty, homelessness, school failure, and discrimination, while struggling through normal developmental processes.[119]

Leisure and Play

Leisure and play activities are the discretionary, spontaneous, and organized activities that provide enjoyment, entertainment, or diversion in social environments that may be different to school and work settings.[86,115] These activities account for more than 50% of American adolescents' waking hours.[66] In an occupational therapy study, teens reported that leisure provided enjoyment, freedom of choice, and "time-out."[87] The use of this free time may seem like "time-out," but it can have a significant role in development. In this free time, teens can explore and engage in new behaviors and roles, be exposed to different interests, establish likes and dislikes, and socialize with an array of social groups, thereby developing skills, patterns of behavior, and self-identity.

Unstructured use of time, in particular passive activities such as watching television and playing computer games, have few positive benefits. The main criticism of passive activities is that they contribute to boredom, which is associated with a greater risk of dropping out of school, drug use, and antisocial/delinquent activities.[111] Alternatively, constructive use of nonschool hours in nonacademic extracurricular and leisure activities such as sports is linked with positive adolescent health and well-being and development of physical, intellectual, and social skills.[32] These extracurricular school programs

(e.g., sport teams, school band or orchestra, drama club) and community-based activities such as scouts, music, or dance classes typically include goal-directed activities as well as a sense of belonging to a peer group (Figure 4-2).

An additional benefit of these activities is relationships with nonfamilial adults. Positive interactions with coaches, adult leaders, and teachers facilitate problem solving, provide social support (sometimes compensating for a lack of parental validation and support), increase teens' self-esteem, and promote skill acquisition and competency.[32] Participation in these extracurricular activities is also associated with higher academic performance and occupational achievement such as the likelihood of attending college.[10] Male students with lower academic achievement and/or those from lower socioeconomic backgrounds who play sports are more likely to finish high school, be involved in the community, and have better interpersonal skills. They also have lower rates of alcohol and drug use or antisocial behaviors.[32,45,73]

An area of concern is the decline of physical extracurricular and leisure activities, which is linked to an increased risk for poor health among adolescents, including obesity and chronic health conditions such as diabetes.[57] The national public health initiatives to promote adolescents' participation in physical extracurricular and leisure activities, which have not been successful, have significant implications. Adolescent physical leisure activity patterns predict adult physical activity levels.[110] Males are more likely to continue to participate in and have a positive attitude toward physical activities than females, perhaps because of the relationship between masculinity and vigorous sport, competition, and sports achievement.[110] The stereotypes of bodily contact, face-to-face opposition, and endurance associated with male sports, and aesthetics or gracefulness with female sports, may explain why some girls drop out of sports and physical activities[47] and why girls are more likely to participate in dance and gymnastics, which do not compromise their femininity. Although stereotypes and other influences such as parents and teachers influence participation in physical activity, the strongest influence is peer participation.[110]

Choosing popular adolescent activities that are transferable beyond the context of occupational therapy develops performance skills and facilitates social behaviors that enhance self-efficacy and autonomy. The outcome of developing leisure skills in occupational therapy can be successful participation in peer activities and increased social inclusion. Having the skills to engage successfully in leisure activities contributes to healthy and perceived quality of life by providing a social network, enjoyment, and constructive use of time. Long-term improvement in performance in leisure skills can have additional value, especially for adolescents who may not gain employment.

Social Participation

Social activities, friendships, and the behaviors associated with these activities and roles that characterize and define individuals within society are salient to adolescents' development of social participation. Social roles and relationships are explored and developed by engaging in a variety of social activities, especially peer group activities.[87] In middle and high school, teens strive to "fit in" and make friends. Peer-focused social interactions and relationships formed in school through

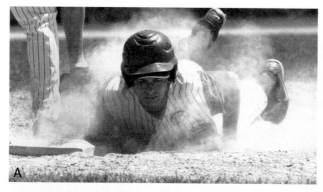

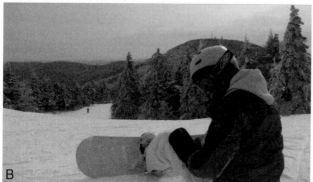

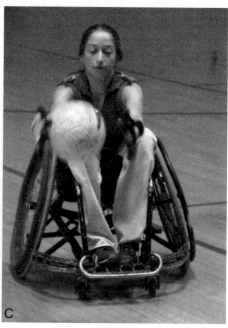

FIGURE 4-2   Examples of goal-directed activities. *A,* Baseball. *B,* Snowboarding. *C,* Basketball.

leisure activities provide social status and develop adolescents' social identity.[50] This emerging identity may differ from the teen's identity in his or her family. The changes represent moving from family members as the primary source of emotional and social support to a reliance on friends, peers, and nonfamily adults.[7,50]

Peer Relationships

Having friends significantly contributes to social and emotional adjustment in adolescents.[118,120] Peer relationships offer social integration and a sense of belonging or acceptance. Initially, these relationships develop around cliques, which are small, cohesive groups of teens that have a somewhat flexible membership, meet personal needs, and share common activities. Participation in peer cliques provides a normative reference for comparison with peers and influences adolescents' developing social attitudes and behaviors, as well as their academic adjustment.[7] Making the shift from middle school to high school can be easier with membership in supportive and peer-recognized cliques. Initially, in early and middle adolescence, membership in cliques develops spontaneously around common interests, school activities, or even neighborhood affiliations. In junior high, cliques are usually same sex; by middle to late adolescence, these groups expand to include the opposite sex. In late adolescence, cliques weaken, and they are replaced by loose associations between groups that consist of couples.[50] Lack of participation in peer groups or exclusion from cliques comes with a cost (e.g., a sense of rejection, a lack of opportunity to participate in peer activities, social isolation, a lack of social status). Adolescents who do not find their niche in cliques

are more likely to be depressed and lonely and have other psychological problems.[19] Exclusion from cliques and the resulting lack of choices are suggested as the reason some adolescents join less constructive peer groups such as gangs or groups who engage in illegal and/or antisocial activities.

Most adolescents also have lasting stable friendships that differ from the relationships within cliques. Initially, they are same-sex friendships that develop around sharing activities and a closeness of mutual understanding. They can be emotionally intense, involve openness and shared confidences, and depend less on social acceptance; however, these same-sex friendships also imply a heightened vulnerability.[19] Girls' friendships are interdependent and reflect a preference of intimacy, whereas boys' friendships are congenial relationships established around shared interests such as sports, music, or computer games. These friendships evolve with social and cognitive development. In middle adolescence, the basis of friendships is shared loyalty and an exchange of ideas; in the latter years, friendships progress to incorporate autonomy and interdependence, and as intimate relationships develop in late adolescence, the salience of these friendships lessens.

Navigating Social Participation with a Disability

Because teens strive for conformity and identification with their peers, making and maintaining friendships can be particularly difficult for teens with disabilities (Case Study 4-2). The data on the social life of adolescents with disabilities provide contradictory information. A national Canadian study found that adolescents with physical disabilities reported

CASE STUDY 4-2   Bullying: Nick's Story

I am a 14-year-old student in eighth grade. I don't like going to school because I have problems with the kids there. Sometimes my classmates yell at me and sometimes they hit me. One time when I was in the locker room a kid punched me and tore my sweatshirt. Another time, I was punched in the face and thrown into a locker. In gym class, people will throw balls at me and hit me with lacrosse sticks. In my class, a girl yells at me and calls me names. She gets other students to join her. Since I've been diagnosed with Tourette's, as well as Asperger's, students call me Tourette's Man and Twitchy. I don't like to go to school because kids don't treat me very nice. I don't feel like I have very many friends. When I'm at school I feel like I'm alone and I feel sad. I wish school was better and I had more friends.

School can become an unhappy place, a daily experience of harassment, alienation, and victimization. Adolescents with Asperger's syndrome are among students who are vulnerable to discrimination. Both teachers and other students can be intolerant toward students with interpersonal and learning challenges, especially when learning and classroom work involve collaboration.[96] Adolescents with disabilities report rejection by other students, bullying, or being ignored and treated negatively when working in groups.[95] Nick's story highlights bullying and the experiences of adolescents who are susceptible to bullying.[18] The passage he wrote for this chapter resonates with the frustration, disappointment, hurt, and isolation that he and other teens experience at the hands of peers.

The level of verbal abuse is consistent across educational levels, whereas physical bullying increases in elementary school, peaks in middle school, and declines in high school.[52] Students subjected to bullying are at risk of mental health problems (e.g., depression). They report being lonely, show deterioration in performance (grades), and avoid school or even drop out.[27] This bullying increases the likelihood that victims will commit acts of violence.[25] Increasingly, bullying is now occurring online. Frequently anonymous, this bullying is cruel, devastating, and has long-term effects because the exposure is wider than the immediate social network. A University of New Hampshire study for the National Center for Missing and Exploited Children reported that online bullying increased by 50% between 2000 and 2005.[116]

Bullying is often underreported, minimized, or unacknowledged in schools. Student surveys have shown that teachers seldom discuss bullying in class or intervene effectively. When adults do intervene, students often see the interventions as ineffective or as worsening the situation.[52] In 2000, the U.S. Department of Education issued an official statement regarding disability harassment in school. That same year, the National Center on Secondary Education and Transition provided advice and strategies on school interventions and educational programs to address and deter bullying (http://www.ncset.org). Specifically targeting the preventing disability harassment, the U.S. Department of Education makes the following recommendations[111]:

- Create a campus environment that is aware of and sensitive to disability concerns and harassment.
- Weave this issue into curriculum or extracurricular programs.
- Encourage parents, students, employees, and community members to discuss disability harassment and report it when they become aware of its occurrence.
- Publicize anti-harassment statements and procedures for addressing discrimination complaints.
- Provide appropriate training for staff and students regarding harassment.
- Counsel both victims and perpetrators of harassment.
- Implement monitoring programs to follow up on resolved issues of disability harassment.
- Assess and modify existing disability harassment policies and procedures to ensure effectiveness.

There are many resources available at: http://www.pacer.org/publications/bullying.asp

Acknowledgment: Nick for writing about his experiences. His frankness about being bullied offers us insight into the experience of being bullied. Thanks also to Nick's mother for her perspective as a parent. This fall, Nick started at a high school that has a zero tolerance policy for bullying that includes consequences for bullies. Nick's grades have improved and he says school is okay.

good self-esteem, strong family relationships, and positive attitudes toward school, teachers, and many close friends.[105] However, other studies have found that because teens with disabilities lack the "qualities" that bestow social status among adolescents (e.g., excellence in sports or physical attractiveness), they often are not included socially in peer groups.[106] Teens with disabilities have reported more loneliness, participation in fewer social activities, fewer intimate relationships, and more social isolation than their peers without disabilities report.[29,106] Even teens with good social relationships in school have less contact with friends outside the school setting than their peers without disabilities.[38,105] Factors that affect social acceptance of teens with physical disabilities include role marginalization (lacking a clear role and the inability to undertake the tasks of typical adolescent roles), lower social achievement, and limited contact with peers.[78] Adolescents without disabilities consider their peers with physical disabilities as less socially attractive and report that they are less likely to interact with them in social settings.[38] An asset for teens with disabilities is academic achievement, because high academic achievement is shown to promote better social acceptance.[78]

Understanding the interaction between adolescents and their environments helps the occupational therapy practitioner facilitate social participation on multiple levels. The World Health Organization's International Classification of Functioning, Disability and Health offers a model to interpret this interaction. It replaced the concepts of disability and handicap with concepts of capacity and performance. The classification defines performance as what an adolescent does (performs) in the environmental context in which he or she actually lives, whereas his/her capacity refers to ability to execute a task or action, usually in a standardized evaluation.[80] Capacity and motivation to engage in an activity produce performance. Teens with disabilities may experience a gap between their capacity and performance because of social and physical environmental barriers that limit their access and opportunities to engage with peers. In other situations, they may lack performance skills for inclusion in age-related social activities. For example, in early and middle adolescence, play and leisure activities frequently involve physical skills, which can exclude adolescents with physical disabilities.[5] Later in adolescence, peers have a driver's license, independently move about the community, and have earned discretionary income to spend on activities. In comparison, teens with disabilities have limited participation because of lack of transportation, limited accessibility, limited opportunities to work, negative peer attitudes, and parental concerns.[58] Exclusion may also occur because of cognitive impairments. However, irrespective of the personal challenges in mobility, communication, and cognitive skills, it is the assumptions of others that most often widen the gap between capacity for friendship and actual ability to form friendships. A resource book by Tashie, Shapiro-Barnard, and Rossetti, *Seeing the Charade: What We Need to Do and Undo to Make Friendships Happen*, provides a user-friendly direct look at friendships for students with disabilities, including how to write goals on friendships in individual education programs (IEPs).[109]

When adolescents with disabilities are with teens without disabilities, they deal with their differences in a variety of ways. Some attempt to mask or make fun of their disabilities, attempting to make their nondisabled peers feel more comfortable. Teens with disabilities' view of themselves (i.e., their self-image and self-esteem) can create barriers to social acceptance and integration. If they internalize the negative societal attitudes, they will limit their social participation and lower their expectations. However, some teens find alternative ways for inclusion that capitalize on their strengths rather than weaknesses and on their ability rather than disability. Doubt and McColl describe one student's approach to forging friendships with his peer group:

> I approached the [hockey team] about being a statistician because I really wanted to get involved in the team. This is probably the closest [to the team] without playing ... that I could [get] ... plus I'm doing work for them too, so I am useful and that's a good way to get involved ... and it really gives me a chance to be one of the guys, finally; a secondary guy but one of the guys nonetheless (p. 149).[29]

The Evolution of Adolescent-Parent Relationships

Adolescents are apt to claim, "Parents don't understand." As increased social participation with peers and close friendships provide intimacy and reflect adolescents' social and emotional adjustment and self-knowledge, the child-parent relationship shifts. Through an almost constant stream of communication among adolescents (being together, e-mailing, and texting), they share their concerns and fears with friends rather than with parents. This reframing of the parent-child relationship and peer friendships facilitates self-identity. It is an important transition because close friendships are associated with better self-esteem and social skills and less anxiety and depression.[20]

Although peer relationships are significant, the stability and security provided by relationships with parents and/or significant adults are equally important. Contrary to popular belief, major conflict between parents and adolescents is not a normal part of adolescence, and if conflicts exist, they are mostly

during early adolescence.[67] When adolescents' relationships with parents are stable, periods of physical and emotional distancing from parents and of questioning parents' values and beliefs eventually evolve into positive adolescent-parent relationships.

THE ENVIRONMENTS OF ADOLESCENCE

The environment is a significant determinant of an adolescent's choice of activities and success.[45] The social (e.g., friends, team members, family, and social groups), cultural (e.g., race, religion), and socioeconomic and physical (e.g., home, school, and community) environments in which the adolescent lives influence his or her development. Environments can encourage positive behaviors and provide opportunities, or conversely fail to provide the adolescent the support and resources needed for healthy development. One example is the influence of membership in social groups. Social groups have cultures, belief systems, and norms that shape values and participation[59] and can offer both social status and privileges. Psychosocial development involves the ability to recognize the expectations of social groups and an ability to develop behaviors and values that are congruent with the norm. In poorer communities, excelling in school sports activities is linked with the identity of "good student," resulting in opportunities and status among peers and within a community. In higher socioeconomic status communities, where academic achievement is highly valued, other types of extracurricular activities such as music, science clubs, theater, and volunteerism are also associated with the "good student" and are positively reinforced.[45]

Environments that are unsafe, lack resources, or are unhealthy can be a barrier to growth and development. Membership in less desirable social groups (e.g., recent immigrants, less popular high school groups, low socioeconomic status) can marginalize teens and make them more susceptible to adverse outcomes and negative influences (e.g., behaviors such as drug use, criminal activity, or dropping out of school or being a victim of bullying). These teens lack opportunities such as access to high-quality education, adequate health care, and the expectation of personal safety. Disenfranchised youth are more likely to seek a sense of belonging in groups such as gangs.

The occupational therapist's understanding of the nuances of an adolescent's social environment and cultural context is vital to the development of an intervention plan.[101] The culturally competent practitioner is cognizant of the norms and expectations of ethnic and sociocultural contexts and how these shape adolescents' perceptions of themselves and the development of constructive self-esteem.[103] These factors influence adolescents' choices of activities, interests, the expectations of their family, and the values they develop. Likewise, the adolescent's social peer context shapes "adaptive social and emotional development" (p. 280).[7]

Context can have adverse consequences on an adolescent's development. Lower socioeconomic status and family disorganization increase the likelihood that a child or adolescent will exhibit deviant and high-risk behaviors leading to adverse outcomes.[73] This is because these environments limit adolescents' (often minority adolescents') access to information and to resources, and limit their opportunities to develop self-esteem, personal mastery, and complex cognitive development.[73] Therefore, experiences in school, therapy, and extracurricular activities can have a compensatory role in meeting a teen's needs and ameliorating the effect of an inadequate social and home environment.

The multidimensional influence of context is considered in all intervention programs. Family contexts that value and facilitate the development of peer partnerships, and participation in extracurricular activities, and mentoring by caring adults promote healthy adolescents. Conversely, school or community contexts that pose barriers to participation, limit positive opportunities, or encourage involvement in unhealthy groups need to be discouraged. For example, in a client-centered approach, the practitioner provides choices, opportunities for decision-making, and autonomy, all of which provide a sense of personal control and efficacy. Similarly, a therapeutic milieu offers the adolescent opportunities for self-directed exploration and experimentation within a safe, supportive environment. Box 4-4 lists some of the characteristics of contexts that support and foster adolescent self-development and acquisition of skills.

OCCUPATIONAL THERAPY TO FACILITATE ADOLESCENT DEVELOPMENT

Improving the quality of life of adolescents with disabilities is a major goal of the national health promotion and prevention initiative Healthy People 2010.[36] The 23% to 35% of American adolescents who have chronic health conditions, disabilities, or special health care needs have the same development needs as other adolescents but, because of their special needs and/or dependence on parents and other caregivers, they have fewer opportunities to explore and develop a sense of their own abilities.[82] Their successful transition from adolescence to adulthood requires that they have the same experiences as teens without disabilities (Case Study 4-3). They need to have opportunities to resolve the psychosocial issues of adjusting to the physical changes of puberty, and to develop psychological, if not physical, independence from parents or caregivers. They need opportunities to build social and intimate relationships with peers to establish a sense of identity and skills that will equip them to navigate adult life. These developmental tasks are prerequisites for choosing a job, completing school, finding meaningful work, and developing adult relationships.[26]

Adolescents with disabilities have fewer opportunities to engage in typical adolescent experiences, to make their own choices, to engage in social relationships, or explore the world of ideas, values, and cultures different from those of their family.[11] As outlined earlier in this chapter, exploration and experimentation provide teens with experiences of success and failure, both of which are required if they are to develop a sense of the boundaries of their competence.[120] Adolescents with disabilities face many additional challenges, including their own and others' negative perceptions and lower expectations of them.[71] They also face barriers such as lack of resources, problems related to mobility and environmental access, discrimination, and the stigma of disability.[29]

Flexibility, a sense of humor, a capacity to see strengths and potential before identifying problems, and the ability to set clear, consistent boundaries are ideal attributes in occupational therapy practitioners working with teens. It is essential that the practitioner integrate typical adolescent developmental needs into the therapy evaluation process and interventions. However, the practitioner needs to keep in mind that most teens, including teens with mental health, developmental, or physical disabilities successfully navigate adolescence.[98] This knowledge means that the practitioner can convey an encouraging attitude grounded in a realistic, yet positive, outcome for most adolescents.

Occupational therapy practitioners provide evaluation and interventions that help adolescents address their difficulties and disabilities, acquiring skills, and fully participating in the social and academic opportunities provided in school and the community. Occupational therapy services within the public school system are available to many adolescents up to the age of 21 years under the Education for All Handicapped Children Act (Box 4-5). The transition from high school to work or other programs is a significant time for students to receive occupational

---

BOX 4-4   Environmental and Contextual Factors of Healthy Adolescent Development

SUPPORT
- Family support that includes positive parent–adolescent communication
- Parental involvement in school activities (e.g., schoolwork, sport activities)
- Constructive relationships with adults (e.g., friends, coaches, teachers)
- Caring, inclusive neighborhood and school environments

EMPOWERMENT
- Community that values youth
- Useful and valued roles in community

- Involvement in community service activities that value their contribution and opinions
- Safe home and community environment

BOUNDARIES AND EXPECTATIONS OF ADOLESCENTS
- Family boundaries that include realistic and fair rules and consequences
- School and neighborhood boundaries that include rules, consequences, and community monitoring of behavior
- Positive and varied adult role models
- Positive peer influences
- High and positive expectations: family, friends, and school personnel expect adolescent to do well

Modified from Search Institute (2009). 40 Developmental assets for adolescents: External assets. Retrieved May 2009 from http://www.search-institute.org/content/40-developmental-assets-adolescents-ages-12-18.

CASE STUDY 4-3   **A Parent's Reflections on Her Daughter's High School and College Experiences**

As an occupational therapy student in the 1970s, never did I think I would be a mother of a young woman who had significant developmental and physical disabilities. Today I cannot imagine life without Brianna (Brie). She is a sweet and joyful person deeply loved by her friends and family. Her smile can lighten up a room.

Brie has a rare condition called Aicardi syndrome; because of her disability, she has many physical and medical challenges. She has seizures, uses a wheelchair, is legally blind, and takes all her liquids and medications through a gastrointestinal tube. She is small and has fragile bones because her body does not produce the necessary growth hormone.

Brie's high school years in a regular school were challenging and fun, for the most part! She took part in the class activities and school community, contributing in creative and unexpected ways. Her education and integration into high school activities were supported in a flexible and community-oriented way. When we were asked how she could participate, we asked, *"What would she do if she didn't have a disability?"* and then we would work out a plan. To help us determine Brie's future and develop a vision for her, we held a large meeting of the people in her life (teachers, occupational therapy practitioners, family) and a skilled facilitator. We wanted to ensure that her late adolescence was also productive. On a daily basis, Brie's circle of support (i.e., an inclusion facilitator hired by the school district, her family, her friends, and other people) had high expectations of her. They created positive volunteer experiences and weaved together her communication, motor, and sensory goals with those opportunities.

Friendships are the best part of her life. Brie's friendships from middle school carried over into high school (Figure 4-3). She had some wonderful times with friends, including birthday parties and sleepovers. However, as these girls aged, they seemed to go their separate ways. Perhaps because Brie had an aide to help her, it was more difficult socially to include a young woman who had an aide tagging along! While some earlier friendships faded, others emerged. Her friends made sure Brie joined in the Prom and got to dance! It is wonderful for Brie when friends are present in her life, for they truly are the best presents.

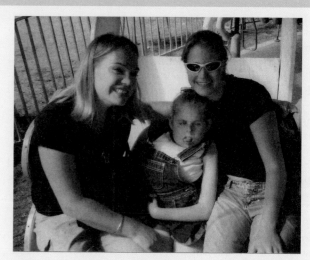

FIGURE 4-3   Brie and friends.

Brie attended graduation ceremonies with her class, who had been with her since kindergarten, and although she did not receive a high school diploma, she continued to be eligible for special education services. These services helped Brie attend the University of New Hampshire. She enrolled in the theater and arts department, took a puppetry course, and with support created fabulous puppets she could touch, feel, and move. Her support person, an energetic "can-do" college student, and her circle of friends included Brie. She ate lunch and hung out with them in the student union building.

Brie volunteers in a preschool and at a community organization supporting families. She has met people who have made her life richer and who notice and call if she does not come in that day. With creativity, Brie delights in contributing to her community.

The best thing I can tell occupational therapy practitioners and students is that every parent and every child has his or her own values and unique story. Ours is one of inclusiveness. We value community participation and relationships. Occupational therapy practitioners can facilitate relationships and friendships, promote full participation in regular classes, and assist in developing a future. As a parent and occupational therapist, I hope each occupational therapist, through his or her actions, is recognized and remembered by the adolescents they work with as "someone who really made a difference in their lives."

Ann Donoghue Dillon, M.Ed., OTR/L.

BOX 4-5   Eligibility for OT Services

- Under the 1975 Public Law 94-142 Education of All Handicapped Children's Act, occupational therapists may evaluate, treat, and recommend services for children and adolescents ages 3 to 21 years.
- In 1997, Public Law 105-17 Individuals with Disabilities Education Act (IDEA-PL105-17) required an Individualized Transition Plan (ITP) be included in the Individualized Education Plan (IEP) of every adolescent with special education before the student reaches age 14.

- By age 16, a statement of needed transition services, goals, objectives, and activities should be included in a student's IEP.
- An amendment to IDEA-PL105-17 expanded the scope of alternative education programs from at-risk students only to all students with disabilities and behaviors that need to be addressed outside the mainstream educational system.

CASE STUDY 4-4   **Understanding that Development Is the Foundation of Effective Occupational Therapy Practice**

Jeremiah, a 15-year-old youth with Down syndrome, is living at home with his parents. His two older siblings have left home to work and attend college. Psychological test scores classify Jeremiah as mildly mentally retarded under the guidelines of the DSM IV-TR. Before high school, Jeremiah had participated in mainstream school activities, with some accommodations within the classroom. He has good social skills and enjoys being with others. However, as the cognitive abilities required to achieve academically in high school have increased, the gap between his functioning and that of his peers has widened. He now spends most of his day in an alternative class that has a vocational emphasis. Jeremiah's recent individual educational program (IEP) prioritized goals to facilitate his transition from high school to the community. His goals are to live in a group home and have a job.

The Individuals with Disabilities Education Act (IDEA) of 1997 recognized the need to facilitate the transition from high school for students with disabilities with an amendment that required an individualized transition plan (ITP). The IDEA requires that the IEP team carefully consider postschool goals when the student is about to enter high school at age 14 because the highest dropout rate occurs in the first two years of high school. Beginning at age 16 (or younger, if appropriate), a statement of transition services needed must be included in a student's IEP. Jeremiah's goals might be that he would achieve semi-independence and a personal sense of autonomy, understand and accept his physical changes, form and maintain friendships, and achieve independence in his community mobility to transition from an educational setting to a community and a work environment. Occupational therapy for adolescents like Jeremiah requires that a practitioner understand the extent to which an adolescent's biologic development (e.g., cognition and motor skills) will support development of social competencies and daily living skills associated with adolescence. Based on the findings of his functional evaluation and specific assessments

of client factors, realistic goal setting and intervention planning can be determined. An occupational therapy practitioner selects evidence-based interventions to help students like Jeremiah acquire the life and social skills they need to live and work in the community with support and/or oversight.

For example, when working with adolescents with cognitive disabilities, the practitioner needs to understand the developmental functional level of their cognitive abilities. This information can identify the types of difficulties the adolescent may have in processing information and how these limitations in understanding and using information will influence the ability to do and acquire everyday skills. This is crucial information in optimizing learning and determining accommodations that will need to be implemented to support functioning. In Jeremiah's case, recognizing that his cognitive assessment scores indicate that he processes information at a pre-formal (i.e., concrete) operational level, the practitioner might use a cognitive disability approach to formulate an intervention plan. He has a stable condition that influences how he learns, how much information he can handle at one time, how well he remembers and recalls information, and the complexity of instructions he can follow. The practitioner may use a direct, skill-teaching approach to ensure that Jeremiah acquires his *ADL, IADL, work,* and *social participation* performance skills. An example would be a visual list to provide the sequence of activities to ensure safety in the kitchen or to improve accessibility. The information about his cognitive abilities and developmental level also helps determine the level of interdependence he will require in his group home; it will also help others understand how to adapt his environment to support his optimal level of independent functioning and, most important, his well-being and life satisfaction. Hence, the skilled practitioner develops expectations *specific to the adolescent* that include just the "right" challenge to meet his goals and to promote his successes.

---

therapy reassessment and interdisciplinary programs that develop life and prevocational skills. Occupational therapy practitioners work collaboratively with students, families, and teachers to identify each student's strengths so that he or she can develop the basic life skills and emotional resources needed to move forward into adulthood. Case Study 4-4 presents an example of occupational therapy that supports adolescents with cognitive deficits; sensory impairments; and physical, communicational, or behavioral disabilities in their school-to-work transition.[28,106]

SUMMARY

Adolescence is a distinct developmental stage characterized by growth and maturation, the refinement of skills, self-determinism, relative individuation, and development of a sense of identity that culminates in a positive self-concept as a healthy adult.

Many of these qualities and skills are achieved through critical tasks in all areas of development. Adolescents' development of critical thinking and reasoning skills is integral to acquiring personal values and beliefs, a sense of accountability, and a burgeoning understanding of one's responsibilities and actions that extends beyond the egocentric concerns for self. These cognitive competencies also support enhanced communication and interpersonal skills, including a capacity for meaningful relationships with peers and adults and, ultimately, intimate adult relationships. The social development of adolescents results in an understanding of their rights and responsibilities as members of society.

In addition to significant cognitive and social development, adolescents experience and adjust to the physical changes and maturation of puberty. Adolescents need to develop a healthy body image that incorporates acceptance of these physical changes. The exploration of physical skills and participation in sports, leisure activities, and work enhances and builds knowledge of one's skills, interests, and performance competency that contribute to identity and occupational choice. An important goal is that healthy lifestyle patterns (e.g., physical fitness and nutrition) become life habits.

The desired outcomes of adolescence are a sense of personal identity, autonomy, independent decision-making, and adequate life skills for adulthood. Occupational therapy practitioners who work with adolescents use clinical reasoning to integrate discipline-specific expertise, knowledge of adolescent development and associated disorders, and occupation-based practice to facilitate healthy development. They forge therapeutic relationships with each teen, his or her family, and interdisciplinary team members to facilitate a successful transition to adulthood.

REFERENCES

1. American Occupational Therapy Association. (2008). Occupational therapy practice framework: Domain and process (2nd ed.). *The American Journal of Occupational Therapy, 62,* 609-639.

2. Anderson, C., & Mattersson, E. (2001). Adults with cerebral palsy: A survey describing problems, needs and resources with special emphasis on locomotion. *Developmental Medicine and Child Neurology, 43,* 76-82.

3. Andrew, M., Penny, P., Simspon, D., Funnell, O., & Mulligan, H. (2004). Functional changes in adolescents with physical disabilities receiving school based physiotherapy over one year. *Journal of Physiotherapy, 32,* 3-9.

4. Arnett, J. J. (2000). Emerging adulthood; A theory of development from the late teens through the twenties. *American Psychologist, 55,* 469-480.

5. Arnold, P., & Chapman, M. (1992). Self-esteem, aspirations and expectations of adolescents with physical disability. *Developmental Medicine and Child Neurology, 34,* 97-102.

6. Bachman, J. G., & Schulenberg, J. (1993). How part-time work intensity relates to drug use, behavior, time use and satisfaction among school seniors: Are these consequences or merely correlates. *Developmental Psychology, 29,* 220-235.

7. Bagwell, C. L., Coie, J. D., Terry, R. A., & Lockman, J. E. (2000). Peer clique participation and social status in preadolescence. *Merrill-Palmer Quarterly, 46,* 280-305.

8. Berger, K. S., & Thompson, R. A. (1998). *The developing person through the life span* (4th ed.). New York: Worth Publishers.

9. Berzonsky, M. D., & Kuk, L. S. (2005). Identity style, psychosocial maturity, and academic performance. *Personality and Individual Differences, 38,* 235-247.

10. Broh, B. A. (2002). Linking extracurricular programming to academic achievement: Who benefits and why? *Sociology of Education, 75,* 69-91.

11. Brollier, C., Shepherd, J., & Markey, K. F. (1994). Transition from school to community living. *American Journal of Occupational Therapy, 48,* 346-354.

12. Brumberg, J. J. (1997). *The body project: An intimate history of American girls.* New York: Vantage Books, Random House.

13. Butterworth, J., Hagner, D., Helm, D. T., & Whelley, T. A. (2000). Workplace culture, social interactions, and supports for transition-age young adults. *Mental Retardation, 38,* 342-353.

14. Calaminus, G., Weinspach, S., Teske, C., & Göbel, U. (2007). Quality of survival in children and adolescents after treatment for childhood cancer: The influence of reported late effects on health related quality of life. *Klinische Pädiatrie, 219,* 152-157.

15. Cash, T. F., & Putzinsky, T. (Eds.). (2002). *Body image.* New York: Guilford.

16. Cech, D. J., & Martin, S. (2002). *Functional movement development across the life span* (2nd ed.). Philadelphia: W. B. Saunders.

17. Centers for Disease Control and Prevention's Adolescent and School Health Division. (2007). *Youth Risk Behavior Surveillance System.* Retrieved from http://www.youthonline.com.

18. Chamberlain, B., Kasari, C., Rotherman-Fuller, E. Involvement or isolation? The social networks of children with autism in the regular classroom. *Journal of Autism & Developmental Disorders, 37,* 230-242.

19. Coleman, J. C., & Hendry, L. (1990). *The nature of adolescence* (2nd ed.). New York: Routledge.

20. Conger, J. J., & Galambos, N. L. (1997). *Adolescence and youth: Psychological development in a changing world* (5th ed.). New York: Longman.

21. Copeland, W. E., Miller-Johnson, S., Keeler, G., Angold, A., Costello, E. J. (2007). Childhood psychiatric disorders and young adult crime: A prospective, population-based study. *The American Journal of Psychiatry, 164,* 1668-1675.

22. Croll, J. (2005). Body image and adolescents. In J. Strang, & M. Story (Eds.), *Guidelines for Adolescent Nutrition Services, Center for Leadership, Education, and Training in Maternal and Child Nutrition, Division of Epidemiology and Community Health, School of Public Health, University of Minnesota.* Retrieved November 2008 from http://www.epi.umn.edu/let/pubs/adol_book.htm.

23. Csikszentmihayli, M., & Larson, R. (1984). *Being adolescent: Conflict and growth in the teenage years.* New York: Basic Books.

24. Darrah, J.Wessel, J., Nearingburg, P., & O'Connor, M. (1999). Evaluation of a community fitness program for adolescents with cerebral palsy. *Pediatric Physical Therapy, 11,* 18-32.

25. Davis, J. L., Nelson, C. S., & Gauger, E. S. (2000). *The Boys Town Model: Safe and effective secondary schools.* Boys Town, NE: Boys Town Press.

26. Davis, S. E. (1985). Developmental tasks and transitions of adolescents with chronic illness and disabilities. *Rehabilitation Counseling Bulletin, 29,* 69-80.

27. Deshler, D., Schumaker, J., Bui, Y., & Vernon, S. (2005). *High schools and adolescents with disabilities: Challenges at every turn.* Retrieved June 2008 from http://www.corwinpress.com/upm-data/10858_Chapter_1.pdf.

28. Dirette, D., & Kolak, L. (2004). Occupational performance needs of adolescents in alternative education programs. *American Journal of Occupational Therapy, 58,* 337-341.

29. Doubt, L., & McColl, M. A. (2003). A secondary guy: Physically disabled teenagers in secondary schools. *Canadian Journal of Occupational Therapy, 70,* 139-150.

30. Eaton, D. K., Kann, L., Kinchen, S., Ross, J., Hawkins, J., Harris, W. A., et al. (2005). *Youth Risk Behavior Surveillance—United States. Division of Adolescent and School Health, National Center for Chronic Disease Prevention and Health Promotion.* http://www.cdc.gov/mmwr/PDF/SS/SS5505.pdf.

31. Eccles, J. S., & Barber, B. L. (1999). Student council, volunteering, basketball or marching band: What kind of extracurricular involvement matters? *Journal of Adolescent Research, 14,* 10-43.

32. Eccles, J. S., Barber, B. L., Stone, M., & Hunt, J. (2003). Extracurricular activities and adolescent development. *Journal of Social Issues, 59,* 865-889.

33. Eisenberg, M., Neumark-Sztainer, D., Haines, J., & Wall, M. (2006). Weight-teasing and emotional well-being in adolescents: Longitudinal findings from Project EAT. *Journal of Adolescent Health, 38,* 675-683.

34. Erickson, E. H. (1980). *Identity and the life cycle.* New York: W. W. Norton and Company.

35. Field, A. E., Austin, B., Camargo, C., Taylor, C. B., Striegel-Moore, R., Loud, K., et al. (2005). Exposure to the mass media, body shape concerns, and use of supplements to improve weight and shape among male and female adolescents and among girls. *Pediatrics, 16,* 214-220.

36. Foundation for Accountability (FACCT), & The Robert Wood Johnson Foundation. (2001). *A portrait of adolescents in America 2001: A report from the Robert Wood Johnson Foundation national strategic indicator surveys.* Portland, OR: The Foundation for Accountability-FACCT.

37. Frankowski, B. L., & Committee on Adolescence. (2004). Sexual orientation and adolescents. *Pediatrics, 113*, 1827-1832.

38. Frederickson, N., & Turner, J. (2002). Utilizing the classroom peer group to address children's social needs: An evaluation of the circle of friends' intervention approach. *Journal of Special Education, 36*, 234-245.

39. Ge, X., Conger, R., & Elder, G. (2001). The relation between puberty and psychological distress in adolescent boys. *Journal of Research on Adolescence, 11*, 49-70.

40. Gilligan, C., Lyons, N. P., & Hanmer, T. J. (Eds.). (1990). *Making connections: The relational worlds of adolescent girls at Emma Willard School.* Cambridge, MA: Harvard University Press.

41. Gordon, P. A., Tschopp, M. K., & Feldman, D. (2004). Addressing issues of sexuality with adolescents with disabilities. *Child and Adolescent Social Work Journal, 21*, 1573-2797.

42. Graber, J., Seeley, J., Brooks-Gunn, J., & Lewinsohn, P. (2004). Is pubertal timing associated with psychopathology in young adulthood. *Journal of the American Academy of Child & Adolescent Psychiatry, 43*, 718-726.

43. Greenfield, P., & Yan, Z. (2006). Children, adolescents, and the internet: A new field of inquiry in developmental psychology. *Developmental Psychology, 42*, 391-394.

44. Grunbaum, J. A., Kann, L., Kinchen, S. A., Williams, B., Ross, J., Lowry, R., et al. (2002). Youth risk behavior surveillance—United States, 2001. *Journal of School Health, 72*, 313-328.

45. Guest, A., & Schneider, B. (2003). Adolescents' extracurricular participation in context: The mediating effects of schools, communities, and identity. *Sociology of Education, 76*, 89-109.

46. Guest, V. (2000). Sex education: A source for promoting character development in young people with physical disabilities. *Sexuality and Disability, 18*, 137-142.

47. Guillet, E., Sarrazin, P., Fontayne, P., & Brustad, R. J. (2006). Understanding female sport attrition in a stereotypical male sport within the framework of Eccles expectancy-value. *Psychology of Women Quarterly, 30*, 358-368.

48. Hallum, A. (1995). Disability and the transition to adulthood: Issues for the disabled child, the family, and the pediatrician. *Current Problems in Pediatric, 25*, 12-50.

49. Harris, S. L., Glasberg, B., Delmino, L. (1998). Families and the developmentally disabled adolescent. In V. B. Van Hasselt, & C. M. Hersen (Eds.), *Handbook of psychological treatment protocols for children and adolescents* (pp. 519-548). Mahwah, NJ: Lawrence Erlbaum Assoc.

50. Heiman, T. (2000). Friendship quality among children in three educational settings. *Journal of Intellectual Disability, 25*, 1-12.

51. Hooker, K. (1991). Developmental tasks. In R. M. Lerner, A. C. Petersen, & T. Brooks-Gunn (Eds.), *Encyclopedia of adolescence* (Vol. 1). London: Garland Publishing.

52. Hoover, J., & Stenhjem, P. (2003). *Bullying and teasing of youth with disabilities: Creating positive school environments for effective inclusion.* Retrieved August 2008 from http://www.ncset.org/publications/issue/NCSETIssueBrief_2.3.pdf.

53. Jemtå L., Fugl-Meyer K. S., Oberg K. (2008). On intimacy, sexual activities and exposure to sexual abuse among children and adolescents with mobility impairment. *Acta Paediatrica, 97*, 641-646.

54. Johnson, M. K., Beebe, T., Mortimer, J. T., & Snyder, M. (1998). Volunteerism in adolescence: A process perspective. *Journal of Research on Adolescence, 8*, 309-332.

55. Kail, R., & Cavanaugh, J. C. (2006). *Human development: A life-span perspective* (4th ed.). Berlmont, CA: Thomson Wadsworth.

56. Keating, D. P. (1991). Cognition, Adolescents. In R. M. Lerner, A. C. Petersen, & T. Brooks-Gunn (Eds.), *Encyclopedia of adolescence* (Vol. 1, pp. 987-991). London: Garland Publishing.

57. Kemper, H. C. G. (2002). The importance of physical activity in childhood and adolescence. In L. Haynan, M. M. Mahon, & J. R. Turner (Eds.). *Health behavior in childhood and adolescence* (pp. 105-142). New York: Springer Publishing.

58. Kewman, D., Warschausky, S., Engel, L., & Warzak, W. (1997). Sexual development of children and adolescents. In M. L. Sipski & C. J. Alexander (Eds.), *Sexual function in people with disabilities and chronic illness: A health professional's guide* (pp. 355-378). Gaithersburg, MD: Aspen Publishers.

59. Kielhofner, G. (2008). *Model of human occupation* (4th ed.). Baltimore: Lippincott Williams & Wilkins.

60. King, G., Schultz, I., Steel, K., et al. (1993). Self-evaluation and self-concept of adolescents with physical disabilities. *American Journal of Occupational Therapy, 47*, 132-140.

61. Kirkpatrick, J. M. (2002). Social origins, adolescents' experiences and work value trajectories during the transition to adulthood. *Social Forces, 80*, 32-37.

62. Knickmeyer, R. C., Wheelwright, S., Hoekstra, R., & Baron-Cohen, S. (2006). Age of menarche in females with autism spectrum conditions. *Developmental Medicine and Child Neurology, 48*, 1007-1008.

63. Knopf, D., Park, M. J., & Muyle, T. P. (2008). The mental health of adolescents: A national profile, 2008. *National Adolescent Health Information Center.* Retrieved August 2008 from http://nahic.ucsf.edu/downloads/MentalHealthBrief.pdf.

64. Kroger, J. (2004). *Identity in adolescence: The balance between self and others.* New York: Routledge.

65. Kunnen, E. S., Bosma, H. A., & VanGeert, P. L. C. (2001). A dynamic systems approach to identity formation: Theoretical background and methodological possibilities. In J. E. Nurmi (Ed.), *Navigating through adolescences: European perspectives* (pp. 251-278). New York: Routledge Falmer.

66. Larson, R., & Verma, S. (1999). How children and adolescents spend time across the world: Work, play and developmental opportunities. *Psychological Bulletin, 125*, 701-735.

67. Laursen, B., Coy, K. C., & Collins, W. A. (1998). Reconsidering changes in parent-child conflict across adolescence: A meta-analysis. *Child Development, 69*, 817-832.

68. Lenhart, M., & Madden, M. (2005). *Teens and technology: Youth are leading the transition to a fully wired and Mobile Nation.* Retrieved November 2008 from http://www.pewinternet.org/report_display.asp?r=162.

69. Lenhart, M., Madden, M., Rankin-MacGill, A., & Smith, A. (2007). *Teens and social media: The use of social media gains a greater foothold in teen life as they embrace the conversational nature of interactive online media.* Retrieved November 2008 from http://www.pewinternet.org/PPF/r/230/report_display.asp.

70. Levine, M. P., & Smolak, L. (2002). Body image development in adolescence. In T. F. Cash & T. Putzinsky (Eds.), *Body image* (pp. 74-82). New York: Guilford.

71. Magill-Evans, J., Darrah, J., Pain, K., Adkins, R., & Kratochvil, M. (2001). Are families with adolescents and young children with cerebral palsy the same as other families? *Developmental Medicine and Child Neurology, 43*, 466-472.

72. Marcia, J. E. (1991). Identity and self-development. In R. M. Lerner, A. C. Petersen, & T. Brooks-Gunn (Eds.), *Encyclopedia of adolescence* (Vol. 1, pp. 529-534). London: Garland Publishing.

73. Marsh, H. W., & Kleitman, S. (2002). Extracurricular school activities: The good, the bad and the nonlinear. *Harvard Educational Review, 72*, 465-515.

74. Mechanic, D. (1991). Adolescents at risk: New directions. *Journal of Adolescent Health, 12*, 638-643.

75. Meeropol E. (1991). One of the gang: Sexual development of adolescents with physical disabilities. *Journal of Pediatric Nursing, 6,* 243-250.

76. Miyahara, M., & Piek, J. (2006). Self-esteem of children and adolescents with physical disabilities: Quantitative evidence from meta-analysis. *Journal of Developmental and Physical Disabilities, 18,* 219-233.

77. Miyahara, M., & Register, C. (2000). Perceptions of three terms to describe physical awkwardness in children. *Research in Developmental Disabilities, 21,* 367-376.

78. Mpofu, E. (2003). Enhancing social acceptance of early adolescents with physical disabilities: Effect of role salience, peer interaction, and academic support interventions. *International Journal of Disability, Development, and Education, 50,* 435-454.

79. Murphy, K., Molnar, G., & Lankasky, K. (2000). Employment and social issues in adults with cerebral palsy. *Archives of Physical Medicine and Rehabilitation, 81,* 807-811.

80. National Disability Authority. (2006). *The WHO's ICF.* Retrieved November 2008 from http://www.nda.ie/cntmgmtnew.nsf/0/6877A99815DA544980257066005369D1?OpenDocument.

81. Neinstein, L. S., & Kaufman, F. R. (2002). Normal physical growth and development. In L. S. Neistein (Ed.), *Adolescent health care: A practical guide* (4th ed., pp. 3-51). Philadelphia: Lippincott Williams & Wilkins.

82. Newacheck, P. W., & Halfon, N. (1998). Prevalence and impact of disabling chronic conditions in childhood. *American Journal of Public Health, 88,* 610-617.

83. National Institute of Occupational Safety and Health. (1997). *Child labor research needs* (NIOSH Publication No. 97-143). Cincinnati, OH: NIOSH.

84. Overton, W. F., & Byrnes, J. P. (1991). Cognitive development. In R. M. Lerner, A. C. Petersen, & T. Brooks-Gunn (Eds.), *Encyclopedia of adolescence* (Vol. 1, pp. 151-156). London: Garland Publishing.

85. Palisano, R., Copeland, W., & Galuppi, B. (2007). Performance of physical activities by adolescents with cerebral palsy. *Physical Therapy, 8,* 77-87.

86. Parham, L. D., & Fazio, L. S. (2008). *Play in occupational therapy for children* (2nd ed.). St Louis: Mosby.

87. Passmore, A., & French, D. (2003). The nature of leisure in adolescence: A focus group. *British Journal of Occupational Therapy, 66,* 419-426.

88. Piaget, J. (1972). Intellectual evoluation from adolescence to adulthood. *Human Development, 15*(1), 1-12.

89. Putzinsky, T., & Cash, T. F. (2002). Understanding body images: Historical and contemporary perspectives. In T. F. Cash, & T. Putzinsky (Eds.), *Body image.* New York: Guilford.

90. Quint, E. (2008). Menstrual Issues in Adolescents with Physical and Developmental Disabilities. *Annals of the New York Academy of Science, 1135,* 230-236.

91. Radzik, M., Sherer, S., & Neinstein, L. S. (2002). Psychosocial development in normal adolescents. In L. S. Neinstein (Ed.), *Adolescent health: A practical guide* (4th ed., pp. 52-58). Philadelphia: Lippincott Williams & Wilkins.

92. Rathus, S. A. (2008). *Child and Adolescent Development, Voyages in Development* (3rd ed.). Belmont, CA: Thomson Wadsworth.

93. Rotherman-Borus, M. J., & Langabeer, K. A. (2001). Developmental trajectories of gay, lesbian, and bisexual youth. In A. R. D'Augelli, & C. Patterson (Eds.), *Lesbian, gay, and bisexual identities among youth: Psychological perspectives* (pp. 97-128). New York: Oxford University Press.

94. Rubenstein, H., Sternabach, M. R., & Pollock, S. H. (1999). Protecting the health and safety of working teenagers. *American Family Physician, 60,* 575-587.

95. Sabornie, E. J. (1994). Social-affective characteristics in early adolescents identified as learning disabled and nondisabled. *Learning Disability Quarterly, 1,* 268-279.

96. Safran, J. (2002). Supporting students with Asperger's syndrome in general education. *Teaching Exceptional Children, 34,* 60-66.

97. Santrock, J. W. (2003). *Adolescence* (9th ed.). New York: McGraw-Hill Higher Education.

98. Scales, P. C., & Leffert, N. (2004). *Developmental assets: A synthesis of the scientific research on adolescent development* (2nd ed.). Minneapolis, MN: Search Institute.

99. Schondel, C. K., & Boehm, K. E. (2000). Motivational needs of adolescent volunteers. *Adolescence, 35,* 335-344.

100. Schwartz, J., Engel, M., & Jensen, L. (1999). Pain in persons with cerebral palsy. *Archives of Physical Medicine and Rehabilitation, 80,* 1243-1246.

101. Schwartz, S. J., & Montgomery, M. J. (2002). Similarities or differences in identity development? The impact of acculturation and gender on identity process and outcome. *Journal of Youth & Adolescence, 31,* 359-372.

102. Skinner, H., Biscope, S., Poland, B., & Goldberg, E. (2003). Adolescents Use Technology for Health Information: Implications for Health Professionals from Focus Group Studies. *Journal of Medical Internet Research, 5,* Retrieved October 2008 from http://www.jmir.org/2003/4/e25/HTML.

103. Spencer, M. B., Dupree, D., & Hartman, T. (1997). A phenomenological variant of ecological systems theory (PVEST): A self-organization perspective of content. *Developmental and Psychopathology, 9,* 817-833.

104. Stainton, M. (2006). Raising a woman. *JAMA, 296,* 1445-1446.

105. Stevens, S. E., Steele, C. A., Jutai, J. W., Kalnins, I. V., Bortolussi, J. A., & Biggar, W. D. (1996). Adolescents with physical disabilities: Some psychosocial aspects of health. *The Journal of Adolescent Health, 19,* 157-164.

106. Stewart, D. A., Law, M. C., Rosenbaum, P., & Willms, D. G. (2001). A qualitative study of the transition to adulthood for youth with physical disabilities. *Physical and Occupational Therapy in Pediatrics, 21,* 3-21.

107. Office of the Surgeon General. (1999). *Surgeon General's Report on Mental Illness.* Retrieved June, 2009, from http://www.surgeongeneral.gov/library/mentalhealth/home.html.

108. Surís, J. C., Resnick, M., Cassuto, N., Blum, R. (1996). Sexual behavior of adolescents with chronic disease and disability. *Journal of Adolescent Health, 19,* 124-131.

109. Tashie, C., Shapiro-Barnard, S., & Rossetti, Z. (2006). *See the charade: What we need to do and undo to make friendships happen.* Nottingham, UK: Inclusive Solutions Inc.

110. Vilhjalmsson, R., & Krisjansdottir, G. (2003). Gender difference in physical activity in older children and adolescents: The central role of organized sport. *Social Science & Medicine, 56,* 363-374.

111. Widmer, M. A., Ellis, G. D., & Trunnell, E. R. (1996). Measurement of ethical behavior in leisure among high and low risk adolescents. *Adolescence, 31,* 397-408.

112. Williams, J., & Currie, C. (2000). Self-esteem and physical development in early adolescence: Pubertal timing and body image. *The Journal of Early Adolescence, 20,* 129-149.

113. Wolman, C., & Basco, D. (1994). Factors influencing self-esteem and self-consciousness in adolescents with spina bifida. *The Journal of Adolescent Health, 15,* 543-548.

114. Worley, G., Houlihan, C. M., Worley, M. E., Houlihan, C. M., & Herman-Giddens, M. E., et al. (2002). Secondary sexual characteristics in children with cerebral palsy and moderate to severe motor impairment: A cross-sectional survey. *Pediatrics, 110,* 897-902.

115. Wynn, J. R. (2003). High school after school: Creating pathways to the future for adolescents. *New Directions for Youth Development, 97,* 59-74.

116. Ybarra, M. L., Mitchell, K. J., Wolak, J., & Finkelhor, D. (2006). Examining characteristics and associated distress related to Internet harassment: Findings from the Second youth Internet Safety survey. *Pediatrics, 118*(4), 1169-1177.

117. Yoder, A. (2000). Barriers to ego identity status formation: A contextual qualification of Marcia's identity status paradigm. *Journal of Adolescence, 23*, 95-106.

118. Youngblood, J., & Spencer, M. B. (2002). Integrating normative identity process and academic support requirements for special needs adolescents: The application of an identity focused cultural ecological (ICE) perspective. *Applied Developmental Science, 6*, 95-108.

119. Yurgelun-Todd, D. (2007). Emotional and cognitive changes in adolescence. *Current Opinion in Neurobiology, 17*, 251-257.

120. Zajicek-Faber, M. L. (1998). Promoting good health in adolescents with disabilities. *Health & Social Work, 23*, 203-214.

121. Zastrow, C. H., & Kirst-Ashman, K. K. (2004). *Understanding human behavior* (6th ed.). Belmont, CA: Brooks/Cole-Thomson Learning.

5

Working with Families

Lynn Jaffe • Ruth Humphry • Jane Case-Smith

KEY TERMS

Family as a dynamic system
Family occupations: routines and rituals
Functions of a family
Family diversity
Family adaptation and resilience
Family-centered services
Parent–professional partnership
Families facing multiple challenges

OBJECTIVES

1. Describe the occupations and functions of families using family systems theory.
2. Appreciate the diversity of families and define methods to learn about a family's culture and background.
3. Explore the implications of having a child with special needs with regard to the co-occupations of family members.
4. Analyze the implications of having a child with special needs with regard to family function.
5. Synthesize information about the family life cycle and transitions to identify times of potential stress for families of children with special needs.
6. Specify the roles of the occupational therapist in collaboration with families.
7. Understand how to establish and maintain partnership with a family.
8. Enact alternative methods of communication that promote family–therapist partnerships.
9. Describe ways families can be empowered to facilitate their children's development.
10. Explain strategies for supporting the strengths of families facing multiple challenges.

This chapter introduces a range of issues related to families, particularly families of children who have special developmental or health care needs. It considers how family members fulfill the functions of a family by collectively engaging in daily or weekly activities and by sharing special events. The chapter explores factors that contribute to the variety of families with whom therapists may work in providing occupational therapy for children.

Having presented this background in the occupations of families and family diversity, the chapter then turns to the ways the special needs of children bring opportunities and challenges to families. This discussion includes the ways that having a child with disabilities can influence how family members organize their time, engage in activities, and interact with one another. Throughout the chapter, the importance of a family-centered philosophy and evidence from the literature are discussed.

REASONS TO STUDY ABOUT FAMILIES

"Why do I need to read a chapter on families? I was raised in a family, I know all about families..."

Families are complex systems. Having a child with a disability or chronic health condition, which can happen in families anywhere on the socioeconomic spectrum, of any educational, ethnic, or genetic background, adds an appreciable degree of stress into this complex system. There is a greater incidence of negative outcomes when the odds are stacked against that family because of low socioeconomic status, poor education, minority status, and difficult genetic structure. Occupational therapists encounter all varieties of families and must be prepared to work with them all. Children cannot be treated as isolated individuals; they are members of families, social units that shape behavior and life experiences. Evidence shows that child outcomes will be shaped by how well therapists communicate with families and how well the partnership between them has been established.[25,52,79] Learning about family systems is important preparation for working in any practice setting.

The development of children's occupations cannot be understood without insight into what shapes their daily activities. Young children first learn about activities, how to perform them, what activities mean, and what to expect as the outcomes of their efforts within the family context.[67] Although children's activities vary from one culture to the next, universally their families play a major role in guiding children in how to spend their time, what to do, and why the things they do are important.[88,135,166] All major health-related disciplines, including but not limited to psychology, sociology, and nursing practice, use the ecological view of children and the family: that each is interconnected with the other and the environments they experience. The more fully occupational therapists understand the influences on the way families operate in their daily routines and their goals for the ways children spend their time, the better prepared they will be to support each family in helping the child engage in activities the family values.

Another reason to study families explicitly is to circumvent the inclination to reference one's own family experiences as a template for the way families operate. Walsh points out that when people speak of "the family," they suggest a socially constructed image of a "normal" family, giving the impression that an ideal family exists in which optimal development occurs.[174] In reality, many different types of families are successfully raising children. In this chapter, two or more people who share an enduring emotional bond, a commitment to pool resources, and carry out the typical family functions can be seen as a family.[39,86,166,175] This chapter focuses on families raising children. One or more parents, grandparents, and stepparents, as well as adoptive or foster parents, can successfully bring up children. The authors refer to the caregiving adult as the "parent" of the child, and focus specifically on the "parent" only when it is germane to the discussion of family diversity (Box 5-1).

A third reason to study families is that the involvement of family members is central to the best practice of occupational therapy. In addition to organizing and enabling daily activities, the family provides the child's most enduring set of relationships throughout childhood, into early adulthood, and possibly beyond. During the course of his or her lifetime, a person with a disability may receive services from people working through health services, educational programs, and social agencies. These relationships exist because professionals bring expertise required by the special needs of the young person. As the type of services needed changes, professionals enter and leave the young person's life. The family represents a source of continuity across this changing pattern of professional involvement. The family forms a unique emotional attachment to their child, and their continuous involvement gives them special insight into the child's needs, abilities, and occupational interests. In light of the family's expertise, occupational therapists strive to collaborate with family members, following their lead and supporting their efforts in promoting the well-being and development of the child with special developmental or health care needs.[14,25,146] Appendix 5-A, which describes the actual experiences of parents raising three children with special needs, provides additional insight into the essential nature of family relationships.

Finally, including families in the process of providing services for children is not just best practice—it is the law. In recognizing the power of families, federal legislation requires service providers and educators to seek the input and permission of a parent or guardian on any assessment, intervention plan, or placement decision. The importance of the family in the early part of the child's life (from birth to 3 years old) is reflected by the emphasis on family-centered services in Part C of the Individuals with Disabilities Education Improvement Act 2004.[69] It requires providers to talk with parents and develop a family-directed Individualized Family Service Plan (IFSP) regarding the resources the family needs to promote the child's optimal development. Later, in the school system, parents are involved in developing the Individualized Educational Program (IEP), which guides special education and related services (see Chapters 23 and 24).

THE FAMILY: A GROUP OF OCCUPATIONAL BEINGS

Family members, individually or together, engage in a variety of activities that are part of home management, caregiving, employed work, education, play, and leisure domains that help them feel connected to each other. A father fulfills one of his family roles by picking up groceries on his way home from work, or a child studies for a test because his parents expect good grades. Family occupations occur when daily activities or special events are shared among family members, such as a parent helping her son study for a test, the whole family going to a movie, or brothers shooting baskets. By engaging in occupations together, families with children fulfill the functions of the family unit expected of them by members of their community. Societies first anticipate that families provide children with a cultural foundation for their development as occupational beings. Family members share and transmit a *cultural model,* a habitual framework for thinking about events, for determining which activities should be done and when, and for deciding on how to interact.[43] By providing a cultural foundation, families ensure that children learn how to approach, perform, and experience activities in a manner consistent with their cultural group. This cultural learning process enables children to acquire the occupations that will make their participation in a variety of contexts possible (Box 5-2). Culture is passed from generation to generation through rituals that include celebrations, traditions, and patterned interactions that give life meaning and construct family identity.[143]

Occupations have meaning because they convey a sense of self, connect us to other people, and link us to place.[54] Routine family occupations give life order and structure the achievement of goals.[143] Routine family occupations and special events also form the basis for repeated interpersonal

---

BOX 5-1   Therapists' Professional Responsibility in Light of Family Diversity

Family diversity is a social construct[39] defined in the eyes of the beholder; families that appear atypical may be defined as "just an average family" in another era or culture. It is not sufficient to strive to treat all families the same because each family has different needs and expectations for how professionals can support them.[172]

Strive to:

- See each family in light of what makes it unique and also how very similar it is to all other families raising children.
- Recognize differences among families by reflecting on one's own cultural model and associated beliefs and critically analyze how knowledge about families is constructed.[1,135]
- Gain an understanding of families with different backgrounds by reading the literature or finding other people who can share an insider perspective because they have been part of a similar family.
- Initiate conversations that solicit a parent's explanation about family membership, the family's cultural model, and the activities valued for and by the child.
- Talk with parents about how they do things together during their daily and weekly routines and the meanings they give these shared activities as a place to start.
- Design interventions that fit into daily routines and are compatible with family traditions.

BOX 5-2 Outcomes of Family Occupations

Family occupations contribute to the following outcomes for children:
1. Establish a cultural foundation for learning occupations that enable children to participate in a variety of contexts.
2. Help shape children's basic sense of identity and emotional well-being.
3. Help children learn to master routines and habits that support physical health and well-being.
4. Foster readiness to learn and participate in educational programs.
5. Foster readiness to assume a place in the community and society.

---

experiences that give family members a sense of support, identity, and emotional well-being.[149] The importance of family occupations is reflected by the fact that families create special activities for the specific purpose of spending time together.[139]

Families are also expected to help their children develop fundamental routines and lifestyle habits that contribute to their physical health and well-being. In the context of receiving care and sharing in family activities children acquire skills that lead to their independence in activities of daily living (ADLs) and learn habits that will influence their health across their life span. For example, in the context of sharing in family dinners and leisure activities after dinner, children establish habits that can reduce or increase future problems with obesity.

A final function of a family is to prepare children for formal or informal educational activities and whatever other practices the community uses to prepare young people to become productive adults.[135] Parents, in the context of their daily routines and through their encouragement, provide children participation experiences that influence how they approach learning.[68] Families of children with certain disabilities have a greater challenge meeting all these expectations, as will be discussed later in this chapter.

Guided by their cultural models, special circumstances, and community opportunities for activities, families use their resources in different ways (Box 5-3). For example, one family

---

BOX 5-3 Family Resources

Family resources: Properties family members use to engage in a balanced pattern of needed and desired activities in a way that enables them to fulfill the family functions.
Financial: Remuneration from productive activities that enable the family to acquire material things such as a place to live, food, and clothing. May also determine what types of community activities are available for family members.
Human: The knowledge and skills family members bring to activities. For example, a teenager who learns to use the Internet at school brings this skill home and can help her parent learn how to pay bills online.
Time: Minutes/hours/days to engage in activities that enable families to fulfill their functional roles.
Emotional energy: Experiencing close interpersonal relationships during shared activities.

---

may choose to pay (using financial resources) to have the yard work done so that time (another asset) on Saturday afternoons can be used for having a picnic together. Another family invests interpersonal energies (an emotional resource) to get everyone to help with the yard work on Saturday afternoon so that money will be available to pay for music lessons. Financial, human, and emotional resources, as well as time, are not limitless, and in healthy families, members negotiate a give and take of their assets. For example, mothers of children with developmental coordination disorder (DCD) or attention deficit–hyperactivity disorder (ADHD) may set aside extra time to help with their children's activities and rely on hired help or assistance from other family members to get household tasks done.[111,142] Typically, families with children have a hierarchical organization in which one or more family members (e.g., a parent) take major responsibility for determining how the resources are distributed, enabling the family to engage in activities that fulfill family functions. Availability of resources varies for many reasons, both within families and within their communities. Challenges for both families and therapists occur when families or the communities they live in have severely limited resources.[147]

SYSTEM PERSPECTIVE OF FAMILY OCCUPATIONS

A family functions as a dynamic system in which its members, comprising subsystems, engage in occupations together to fulfill the functions of a family. As with any system, the activity of one person can influence the activities of other members; this is known as *interdependent influences* that exist among the different parts, much as a change in one piece of a mobile causes movement in every other section. For example, a sixth grader may ask to stay after school with his friend, which means he is not available to watch his sister that afternoon while his mother shops. Consequently, the mother brings her daughter to the grocery store. Shopping with the preschool daughter takes the mother longer than shopping alone. As a result, they do not get home as quickly, and dinner is started late. The interdependent nature of family members' activities is illustrated by the fact that the boy's choice of what he wanted to do in the afternoon altered the activities of his mother and sister and indirectly affected the family's mealtime routine that evening. Recognizing that a family functions as a whole, a therapist who suggests an after-school horseback riding class for a child with cerebral palsy can appreciate that the recommendation must be weighed in light of the family resources and the implications of that activity for the entire family system. As a complex social system, family members have to coordinate what they do and when they do things to share in family routines and rituals (Box 5-4). They accomplish this within subsystems, through their communications and family rules.[28]

With all of the activities a family does and the different members who can carry out these tasks, it would become confusing and draw on family resources if everyone had to negotiate daily who was going to do what, when, and in which way. An effective family system organizes itself into *predictable patterns* of daily and weekly activities and familiar ways with special events. Guided by their cultural models, and often organized through unspoken family rules, families settle into *daily routines* for

1. A family system is composed of individuals who are interdependent and have reciprocal influences on each other's occupations.
2. Within the family, subsystems are defined with their own patterns of interaction and shared occupations.
3. A family must be understood as a whole, and it is more than the sum of the abilities of each member.
4. The family system works to sustain predictable patterns in family occupations and to be part of a larger community.
5. Change and evolution are inherent in a family.
6. A family, as an open system, is influenced by its environment.

various household activities.[26,149] These daily routines include interactive rituals that take on symbolic meaning and seem so matter of course that people do not think of doing them any other way, and they resist changing them.[43,143] Bedtime routines for a child, for example, can have a set sequence of taking a bath, brushing teeth, and the parent reading a book. If routines are interrupted, even by a welcomed event, such as a grandparent coming to visit, family members invest extra family resources reconfiguring their daily routines under the changed circumstances. For example, time is spent making up a bed on the sofa rather than giving the daughter a bath, and emotional energy is expended to help the daughter fall asleep in the living room so that the grandparent can sleep in her bedroom. Families may experience the disruption of their daily routines as unsettling and taxing, and it is not uncommon to hear family members sigh in relief when they can return to predictable patterns, that is, when "things get back to normal."

In addition to routines for daily or weekly activities (Figure 5-1), families also establish predictable patterns for what they do during rituals, such as special events. *Family traditions,* such as cooking special food for birthday celebrations or sharing leisure activities on Sunday afternoons, help families develop a sense of group cohesion and emotional well-being for family members (Figure 5-2). Families may decide to maintain their traditions rather than address an individual member's needs because these customary activities fulfill family functions. For example, a family that traditionally vacations with grandparents for several weeks in the summer may value the way special occupations together reinforce their sense of being a family. Conflict with the occupational therapist could arise if the therapist assumes that the family will shorten the traditional vacation to attend some therapy sessions during the summer. When the occupational therapist offers a range of options and asks the family to set priorities, family members can consider all of their routines and traditions and determine how they want occupational therapy services to fit into their lives.

Celebrations are predictable patterns of doing activities, such as religious rituals, that are shared with members of the community. Therefore, what is done during family celebrations may be similar to what other families that share a similar background do for the same celebration. This link to others gives family members a sense of meaning associated with their special events that connects them to a community of families. Therapists may be asked for assistance so that children can

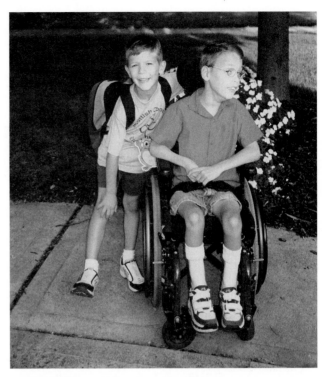

FIGURE 5-1 Matthew and his brother wait for the school bus. (Courtesy Jill and Mark McQuaid, Dublin, Ohio.)

participate in celebrations. For example, a parent may want positioning suggestions so that her daughter with cerebral palsy will be comfortable during Christmas Eve services. The family of a boy with sensory processing problems may need ideas for coping that they can use while attending a Fourth of July fireworks display with the neighbors. By enabling these children's occupational engagement, the entire family participates in community celebrations and confirms their identity as a family like every other family raising children.

Among the researchers who have investigated family routines and practices, Fiese and colleagues[38,99,149] have examined the meaning of routines and related ritual interactions of families' daily activities and religious celebrations. Their studies show that families who reported finding more meaning and commitment to their routines and special activities experienced better health of family members and stronger interpersonal relationships. Occupational therapists who suggest home carryover of interventions must be sure that the activities will fit within the family's values and their existing routines; otherwise the intervention will not be incorporated.[13,144,145]

FAMILY SUBSYSTEMS

Parents

Regardless of the type of family structure (e.g., birth, adoptive, partner, blended, or foster), caregiving adults sharing parental duties need to coordinate their efforts. These adults form the *parent subsystem* of the family, which can be a positive force and can contribute to the child's ability to face developmental challenges. Researchers have found a number of different

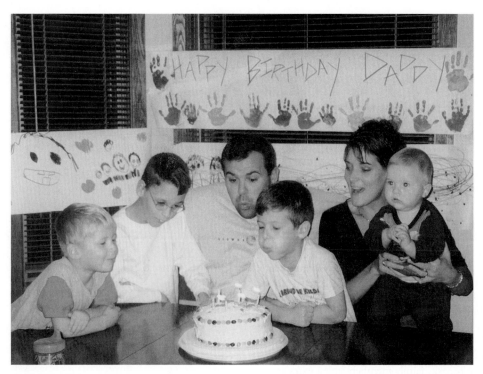

FIGURE 5-2 Matthew's family celebrates Dad's birthday. (Courtesy Jill and Mark McQuaid, Dublin, Ohio.)

solutions in how parents distribute childcare, realizing that the different forms may all be adaptive if they enable the system to operate and meet family functions.[64,176] Studies have found that when a child has a disability, additional time for caregiving co-occupations is required in the mother–child subsystem.[29,30] The type and severity of disability the child will affect the amount of time required; for example, Crowe found that mothers of children with multiple disabilities spent at least 1 hour more per day on child-related activities compared with mothers of children with Down syndrome.[29] Disabilities that seem to create more stress and caregiving effort for the family include autism, severe and multiple disabilities, behavior disorders, and medical problems that require frequent hospitalization and in-home medical care.[23,54,134]

Researchers have reported that mothers experience stress from the increased workload of caring for a child with disabilities.[54,120,149] In addition, mothers may experience more stress than their husbands because they are typically the primary parent working with the intervention team and, as a result, face greater demands on their time and communication skills.[90,93] Mothers often become the conduit for communication, responsible for transferring information and expectations between clinic and family. Therefore, because mothers find themselves caught between the perspectives of both the professionals and family members, the professional must be especially sensitive to the needs of mothers.[30,93,157,170]

Some researchers have found that fathers can be more at risk for stress than mothers because they may feel isolated and helpless compared with the mother, who is more involved. Young and Roopnarine found that fathers spend about one-third the time caring for their children that mothers do.[179] Also, fathers may lack social supports compared with their spouses. Scholars have come to recognize the multidimensional process

influencing what fathers do and why they do it.[126] They have also noted that fathers are more sensitive than mothers to the influence of the ecology of the family and the attitude of others. Other studies have found that mothers and fathers report similar levels of stress related to a child with disabilities.[76,115] Although stress levels were similar,[76] mothers attended 80% of the child's intervention sessions compared with fathers, who attended 33%. The problem that arises from fathers' inability to attend therapy is that information is often conveyed via the mother. Therapists should identify and use more direct methods of communicating with the father to ensure that information is transmitted accurately and to unburden the mother of the responsibility of transmitting information (Figure 5-3).

A child with disabilities can also affect the relationship between husband and wife. Although there is evidence that a child with disabilities can stress the marital relationship and decrease marital satisfaction, some parents have reported that their marriage was strengthened.[134] Differences in marital satisfaction between families of children with disabilities and those of typically developing children tend to be minimal.[20] Stress in dealing with the child may bring parents together for problem solving, and they may rely on each other for emotional support and coping. A strong relationship between husband and wife seems to buffer parenting stress. Britner et al. found that mothers who reported high levels of marital satisfaction also reported less parental distress and found their supports and interventions to be more helpful.[20]

Siblings

As was suggested in the discussion of the system perspective, family members reciprocally influence one another in a dynamic way. Having a brother or sister with special needs

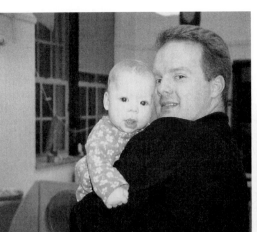
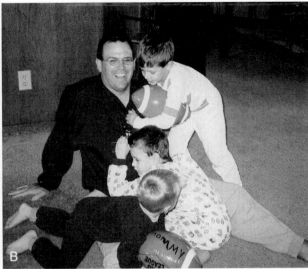

FIGURE 5-3 **A,** Father enjoys holding his child while attending an early intervention program in the evening with his family. **B,** Playtime with Dad before bed.

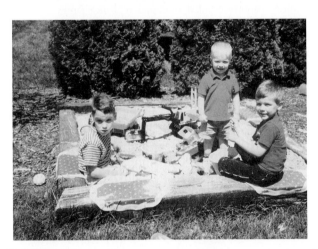

FIGURE 5-4 Matthew and his brothers enjoy backyard play. A sandbox is a fail-proof medium that provides equal opportunity for multiple levels of play. (Courtesy Jill and Mark McQuaid, Dublin, Ohio.)

changes the experiences of other children growing up in that family (Figure 5-4). Williams et al. investigated how having a sibling with special needs influences the typically developing brother or sister.[178] Using a method that allowed them to track direct and indirect effects (structural equation model), they investigated factors that might influence behavioral problems or the self-esteem of children who had a sibling with either a chronic illness (e.g., cancer, diabetes, or cystic fibrosis) or a developmental disability (e.g., autism, cerebral palsy). These workers considered factors that might influence the typical child's experiences, such as how much the child understood

about the disease, the sibling and his or her attitude, and social support. They also asked the mother about the mood and emotional closeness of the family (family cohesion). The researchers reported that the family's socioeconomic status (SES) and cohesion and the siblings' understanding of the disease were related to whether the typically developing sibling had behavioral problems. They also found that when the siblings felt supported, their behavior, mood, and self-esteem were more positive than when they felt unsupported.

Siblings are an important source of support to each other throughout life. In general, the relationships between children with disabilities and their siblings are strong and positive (Figure 5-5).[154] However, the research findings are varied across types of disabilities, sibling place in the family (older or younger), and sibling genders. Conflict among siblings may be more prevalent when a child has a disability such as hyperactivity or behavioral problems. Conflict tends to be less prevalent when a child has Down syndrome or mental retardation.[61,81,154]

Often the roles of siblings are asymmetric, with the typically developing child dominating the child with the disability. Siblings without disability generally engage the child with a disability in play activities they can participate in, such as rough-and-tumble play rather than symbolic play. Siblings may be asked to take on caregiving roles, and assuming caregiving roles can have both positive and negative effects.[154] Siblings learn to relate and interact in the context of a family. Positive and solid marital systems seem to promote more positive sibling relationships, and marital stress has a deleterious effect on sibling relationships. Rivers and Stoneman studied the effects of marital stress and coping on sibling relationships when one child had autism.[134] Using multiple self-report measures of siblings and parents, they found that when marital stress is greater, the sibling relationship is more

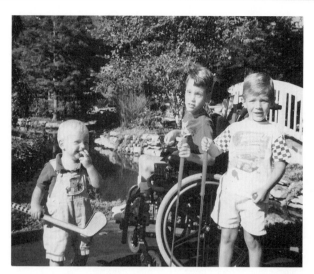

FIGURE 5-5 Although Matthew is the oldest of four boys, his younger brothers already take the initiative to help him participate. A round of miniature golf requires his brothers' assistance, which does not detract from the fun. (Courtesy Jill and Mark McQuaid, Dublin, Ohio.)

negative. This study confirmed the importance of examining sibling relationships in the context of the family, recognizing that all family subsystems affect each other.

As occupational therapists promote engagement in a full range of activities as a way of helping a child participate in family life, the inclusion of siblings is an important step in occupation-centered practice. Peer support groups for the typically developing siblings can also be occupation centered. Therapists can develop a recreational program for brothers and sisters of children with whom they work so that the siblings can meet one another and realize that their family is not the only one that faces challenging behaviors. These groups generally participate in structured activities and have open-ended discussions about what it means to have siblings with disabilities. One formalized support group for siblings is Sibshops, a recreational program that addresses needs and concerns through group activities.[110] Sibshops' primary goals for brothers and sisters of children with special needs are to meet their peers, discuss common joys and concerns, learn how others handle common experiences, and learn more about their siblings with special needs. In addition, parents and professionals are given the opportunity to learn more about the experiences of these typical siblings. When possible, siblings should be involved in occupational therapy sessions. They are likely to be the best playmates and can often elicit maximum effort from their brother or sister. In addition, sibling involvement gives the therapeutic activity additional meaning (play), and siblings can act as models for teaching new skills and providing needed support in a natural context.[82]

Extended Family

In the extended family, the experience of having a child with special needs depends on the meaning family members bring to their relationship with the child. For some grandparents, grandchildren represent a link to the future and an opportunity for vicarious achievement. Researchers find that when children have disabilities, grandparents express both positive and negative feelings and go through a series of adjustments similar to those of the parents.[98,137] Many of the negative feelings, such as anger and confusion, appear to decrease with time. However, some never completely disappear. Positive feelings, such as acceptance and a sense of usefulness, increase over time. A grandparent's educational level and sense of closeness to the child are positively associated with greater involvement with the child. Factors such as the grandparent's age and health and the distance the grandparent lives from the child do not appear to influence involvement (Figure 5-6). Grandparents learn information about their grandchild's condition primarily through the child's parents. However, some seek information from other sources, such as support groups for grandparents of special-needs children. Margetts et al. found that grandparents of children with autism spectrum disorder felt strongly about the caring and support they provided for both their children and grandchildren. These researchers suggested that for professionals to be truly family centered, they need to ask whether the parents want to include the grandparents in the initial assessment of the child.

Patterson, Garwick, Bennett, and Blum interviewed parents of children with chronic conditions about the behavior of extended family members.[130] Family members, such as grandparents, uncles, and aunts of the child, were especially important to fathers and mothers for emotional and practical assistance. When extended family members were not supportive, parents expressed frustration and hurt over their lack of contact. In addition, parents recalled examples of times family members made insensitive comments about the child, ignored the child, or did not want to talk about the child's disability. Parents of children with behavioral problems reported that extended family members tended to blame the child's actions on the parents' inability to discipline correctly.[161] Families may be reluctant to ask relatives for assistance, wishing instead that they might volunteer.[47] With the consent of the parents, occupational

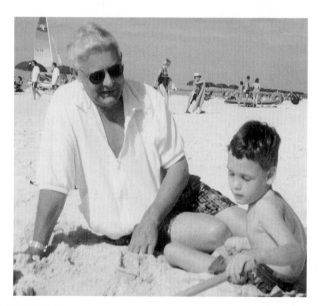

FIGURE 5-6 Matthew's grandparents enjoy their time with him and offer important support to his parents. (Courtesy Jill and Mark McQuaid, Dublin, Ohio.)

therapists can encourage extended family members to become more involved by offering to share information with them and inviting them to therapy sessions. In this way, therapists can help families build on important social and emotional resources.

FAMILY LIFE CYCLE

Family systems undergo metamorphosis and adapt as family members change. Some transitions can be anticipated with developing children and seem to be tied to age more than ability. For example, *normative events* in children that require adjustments in families include the birth of a child, starting kindergarten, transitions between schools, leaving high school, and living outside the home. Other changes in the family are not anticipated. *Non-normative events* may include a grandparent coming to live with the family or a parent accepting a different job in another city. Families that are cohesive and adaptable adjust interactive routines, reorganize daily activities, and return to a sense of "normal" family life. If interactive routines and role designation are too rigidly set, the family may not be able to operate effectively through periods of transition. This is especially true if the family experiences unanticipated, threatening events, such as a job loss or a medical crisis. All families use coping strategies to accommodate periods of transition.

Occupational therapists must understand that all families are unique. Although life-cycle models consist of predictable events, the individuality of each family must be acknowledged. The characteristics and issues at each life stage are highly variable, and each family moves through the stages at different rates. For example, family members may experience and resolve their feelings when they first learn about their child's diagnosis, or they may take months to "come to grips" with the information.[131] In addition, the family may experience cycles of sadness and acceptance later, within and between life stages. Issues that the family seemed to resolve when the child was an infant may occur again when the child reaches school age and an "educational diagnosis" is made or a learning problem is identified. Other life stage–related events, such as the child's ability to develop friendships when first entering grade school, may become an issue again, such as when the child enters high school.[165] Appendix 5-A provides examples of the issues that arise in each of the life stages. Finally, owing to the nature of the family structure, different members of the family may be at different stages at the same time. Therefore, characteristics of the family members and the child's phase of development must be considered. For example, in a skipped-generation family, grandparents frequently have to deal with changes associated with old age at the same time they are parenting their grandchildren. In other families, parents may be taking care of their elderly parents in addition to caring for a child with special needs. Similarly, a young couple may have more energy and resources to cope with the birth of a child with special needs than does an older couple with four other children participating in school activities.

Early Childhood

Identifying a child as being at risk for health or developmental problems is usually a complicated process. Unless the child is born with medical problems, or with congenital problems in a body structure, or has features that suggest a syndrome, many children are not diagnosed until months, and sometimes years, later. Families that describe their experiences in raising a child with a disability frequently recall their journey by looking back to a period when "something was not right."[40] Families of children with pervasive developmental delays recall a sense that they had to search for a diagnosis with repeated testing and visits to several clinics or evaluation centers. Even parents of a child with an unusual physical complaint, such as joint pain that only occurs at night, might have to persevere in finding the cause when professionals initially determine that the child is only seeking attention. After receiving a diagnosis and ending a period of uncertainty, families hope for a period of stability, but as one educated father commented, "No amount of professional or personal preparation trains you for the reality of chronic illness" (p. 243).[63]

Parents' requests for information generally include questions regarding day-to-day childcare, medication management, insurance issues, and support systems available.[65]

Parents whose first child has special needs do not have the same experiences to draw on as those of families with older children.[47] Parents of young children may ask questions such as: "Do you think he can go into a regular classroom?" and "Do you think she will be able to live on her own some day?" Thoughtful responses to these questions recognize the parents' need for optimism and hope. However, the responses must be honest and realistic. Even therapists with years of experience and extensive knowledge about disability and development cannot make definitive statements about the future. Long-range predictions about when the child will achieve a certain milestone or level of independence are always speculative. However, parents feel frustrated when they are told that the future cannot be predicted. Lawlor and Mattingly found that families want to be exposed to anticipatory planning.[90] Parents want to understand that they have reason to expect their child, despite disabilities, will have a place in society and an opportunity to engage in socially valued occupations during adulthood. Therapists can help parents understand the range of possibilities by telling them about the continuum of services for older children and young adults in the community. Talking with parents of older children with a similar condition or hearing the therapist's story of a child with the same characteristics provides some insight into the future.[42,177] Even without knowing the child's developmental course, parents start to develop an understanding that services are in place, and they begin to create new stories about their child's future.

Given information about the system, their rights, and the resources available to them in their communities, parents can solve problems and independently access needed services. The caregiving routines of parents whose young child has a disability are not particularly different from those of all parents of young children. At this time in the child's life, the parent's work consists of managing the child's play environment and introducing new, developmentally appropriate objects and materials. The parent ensures safety and may adjust or arrange the play environment so that the infant can access objects of interest. Feeding, diapering, bathing, and daily care are also natural parenting activities at this time. Only when infants and young children have serious medical conditions or behavioral problems are daily occupations significantly altered.

When children are medically unstable but still at home, a family may have home-based nursing for extended periods (i.e., months to several years). Murphy described the stress created by the constant presence of nurses and professional care providers in the home.[113] Role ambiguity often results when parents feel that they must take on unpaid nursing work and nurses take on parenting roles. Parents also report stress from a lack of privacy and the continual feeling that they are "on duty." Parents of medically fragile children must make tremendous accommodations, which should elicit high levels of sensitivity and responsiveness from professionals. For example, when parents have a medically unstable infant and around-the-clock, in-home nursing care, services such as respite become a priority.

School Age

When a child enters school, all families are excited about the new opportunities for learning and the child's new demonstration of independence. However, school entry is not always a positive event for families of children with disabilities. Families that experienced early intervention services may be disappointed to find fewer family services and less family support offered by the school. Typically, parents are not encouraged to attend classes or school-based therapy sessions. Many parents view the transition to school as an opportunity to be less involved and a sign of their child's maturation. To ease the transition from home to school, the parents of children with special needs should learn about the school's programs, schedules, rules, and policies (Figure 5-7).

For children with mild learning disabilities, entry into school may be the first time that the gap between a child's performance and teachers' expectations for his or her performance is identified. Therefore, this may also be the first time that parents receive information that their child has special needs. When this is the case, parents can experience surprise, disbelief, or relief. School age is a time when children with disabilities may first discover that they have differences. How they make the adjustment to this information depends on the knowledge and sensitivity of the adults and children around them.

To the school-aged child, making friends and maintaining friendships become critically important. Some parents report concern if their children appear lonely, isolated, and friendless. Turnbull and Ruef found that children with behavioral problems frequently have no friends, leaving the parents with the additional responsibility of creating and supervising play opportunities with other children.[161] Teachers and therapists can use different strategies to promote friendships in inclusive environments. Typically developing peers can take turns being a child's "special buddy," and they can offer assistance with projects or tutoring. In situations in which social stigma is an issue, peer relations can be promoted by explaining the disability to the other children and by designing classroom activities that promote cooperation and positive interaction.

Adolescence

Adolescence is a challenging and potentially stressful time for all families, as the development of self-identity, sexuality, and expectations of emotional and economic autonomy herald the transition to adulthood. These issues may pose additional challenges in the lives of children with disabilities as they maneuver through adolescence. Parents need to prepare the young person to handle his or her growing social, financial, and sexual needs, as well as how to avoid substance abuse. (See the review of high-risk behaviors in adolescents with chronic illness by Valencia and Cromer.[169]) In certain cases, parents face decisions about their child's use of birth control and protection from sexually transmitted diseases.[45] With adolescence, new concerns about a son's or daughter's vulnerability increase as that child ventures further into the community and beyond. These decisions will vary significantly depending on the nature of the disability: cognitive, physical, social, visible, or not. They will also be mediated by financial opportunities or constraints.

Although the child usually is well accepted by family members, the social stigma incurred from peers and others may increase during adolescence. As one mother said, "The community accepts our children much more easily when they are small and cute. Babyish mannerisms are no longer acceptable . . . [Our son] has had real problems with his social relationships. He simply does not know how to initiate a friendship. He has difficulty maintaining a sensible conversation with his peers. He doesn't handle teasing well, so he is teased unmercifully" (p. 90).[4]

The cute child with unusual behaviors may become a not-so-cute adolescent with socially unacceptable behaviors. As one parent explained why her son was not invited to a holiday party, "Everyone in the family was invited except Billy. I thought it must be an oversight, but the friend later explained apologetically, 'I thought Billy's presence might make the other guests uncomfortable.' This kind of attitude is difficult to accept, particularly when he had been included very successfully in a similar party. I find myself crying at the unfairness" (p. 16).[140]

Other parents have reported difficulty in caring for their child's growing physical needs. As the child reaches adulthood, parents who are reaching middle age may feel their strength and energy declining. As one parent put it,

The sapping of energy occurs gradually. The isolation it imposes does, too. As I work professionally with young mothers, I see them coping energetically with the demands of everyday life. They are good parents, caring ones, doing everything possible to help their child [with a disability] reach full potential, sometimes doing more than they have to; and if they have other children, they are doing the same for them. Most of these mothers

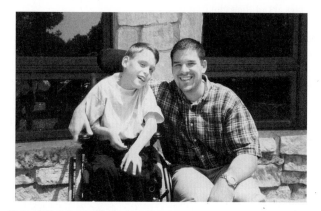

FIGURE 5-7 Matthew has an aide at school who supports his participation in both academic and nonacademic activities. (Courtesy Jill and Mark McQuaid, Dublin, Ohio.)

even get out, see friends, attend meetings, volunteer in the community, and do all the things their friends and families expect them to do. All this is at least possible when one's child is little, although it demands enormous energy. But to look at the mothers of children who have turned into teenagers is to see the beginnings of the ravages. Their lifestyle is changing. They go out less, see fewer people, do less for their children. They are stripping their living to the essentials (p. 144).[112]

Adolescence is the time when most parents must learn to let their children make their way in the world. For parents of children with disabilities, this time may require additional emotional support and financial resources. Magill-Evans, Wiart, Darrah, and Kratochvil conducted a small qualitative study with parents of adolescents with physical disabilities and some of the adolescents themselves that documented the multifaceted needs of each family in balancing the connection of the youth and the parent between the old way of relating and the new acceptance of the autonomy needs of the young adult.[97] They found that both the young person and the parent had issues to be dealt with at this time, ranging from the need of each for emotional support during the transition to the need for financial resources to meet the physical or educational requirements of the young person for care from nonfamily members. Gender differences have also been found to have significant impact during the transition to adulthood. In one survey study of adolescents receiving special education services, the expectations and opportunities regarding work and family for males were perceived to be greater, even though the female respondents placed greater emphasis on having children and going to college. In addition, while both genders were concerned about obtaining health insurance, more of the female respondents rated this as a very important goal.[133] As with all facets of the life cycle, this is a time for a sensitive, collaborative approach between families and service providers so that the right supports and resources are offered to each family.

FAMILY RESOURCES AND THE CHILD WITH SPECIAL NEEDS

Having a child with special needs does not eliminate any of the functions of a family. That is, through their activities, families continue to provide a cultural and psychosocial foundation and guide their children's experiences in activities that will lead to optimal health and participation in the larger community. Understanding how families make choices in light of finite resources and their vision of children's futures puts some of these decisions families make about daily activities and what they want to work on in a different light.[74] For a period, especially when a problem is recently diagnosed or when medical treatment is needed, family resources (e.g., time, money, and emotional energy) may be directed primarily to the needs of the child.[108] For example, a mother who has a full-time job to help pay medical and therapy bills and spends four hours a day feeding her medically fragile child has limited time and emotional energy to devote to helping another child with homework or to sharing in recreational activities. Over time, this allocation of resources can have negative implications for family members, and if the feeding problems are chronic, other choices may need to be made.

Financial Resources

Having a child with special needs has implications for family economics. Parents with children who have disabilities have many hidden and ongoing expenses. When children are hospitalized, many expenses (e.g., days out of work, childcare for siblings, transportation, meals, motel rooms) are incurred, in addition to costs not covered by insurance.[123] Mothers on welfare reported that they faced multiple barriers.[94] Although they wanted to become self-sufficient, they found that employment seemed like a distant dream as they struggled with transportation and finding childcare, particularly for older children.[173] Jinnah and Stoneman offer an excellent review of literature and qualitative study on parents' experiences with finding childcare for their school-age children.[70] Part of their recommendations address the training needs of providers of childcare, as well as the information needs of parents regarding the accessibility requirements of childcare centers under the Americans with Disabilities Act.

Although financial problems create added stress, therapists are often reluctant to discuss finances, especially costs associated with their own services. In a sample of mothers of children with cerebral palsy, Nastro found that insurance coverage was inadequate to meet the families' needs. As one mother reported, "Each piece of equipment has a big price tag. Even the smallest piece has a couple-hundred-dollar price tag. Most insurance companies do not cover it. Medicaid does not cover everything" (p. 52).[116]

Also, many insurance plans have caps on the number of therapy visits allowed per year. Therefore, parents must cut back on services or pay for sessions by finding a way to save somewhere else. Children who require extensive medical treatment can bring economic devastation to a family, especially when insurance coverage is inadequate.[80,124]

Another challenge to financial resources occurs when a parent decides to remain unemployed so that he or she has time to provide extra caregiving. Multiple studies have documented that a parent may need to work fewer hours, if at all, to care for the child.[10,132] With one spouse unable to take on paid employment, these households are at higher risk for problems associated with low income. Financial strain is increased in single-parent homes. Case-Smith found that mothers of children with medical conditions left employment because of the frequency of their children's illness.[23] These children needed specialized medical care (i.e., nursing care) that prohibited their attending community childcare centers. The need to stay home with a child who has multiple medical needs and frequent illness coupled with lack of community childcare for such a child can become a particularly difficult situation for parents to manage. Part of the essence of family-centered care is addressing such needs in a family.[71]

Human Resources

The human resources important to a family in raising children are education, practical knowledge, and problem-solving ability. An understanding of the basis of the child's problems and of possible adaptations is a powerful resource in helping families establish effective patterns of daily activities. As a parent, Marci Greene observed that a comprehensive parent-professional partnership should include ongoing sharing of information with parents.[48] Initially, most parents want additional information about their children's conditions and about accessing services.[82] This is followed by needing information about potential complications, and how to care for their child's physical and psychological needs on a daily basis.[65] However, parents appreciate dialog with professionals beyond informational topics such as the development of feeding skills or behavioral management. Parents want professionals to share conceptual knowledge as well.[48] The timing of parents' ability to use this knowledge and engage in home programs varies appreciably from the time of initial diagnosis of disability through adjustment to their situation, and in qualitative studies having the need for information met is often deemed inadequate.[65,131]

Families who are coping with stress have reported that "the ability to build on personal experience and expertise" (p. 261) is an essential coping strategy.[47] Parents can develop this knowledge through parent-to-parent groups in which families can share strategies with other families who have similar types of issues.[40,177] For therapists, listening to parents and individualizing the information, as well as connecting family members to other resources, helps build the parents' personal resources. The CanChild Centre for Childhood Disability Research has developed a formal, individualized information Keeping It Together™ (KIT) for parents, which has been shown to increase parent "perceptions of their ability and self-confidence in getting, giving and using information to assist their child with a disability" (p. 498).[153] Therapists must remember that many parents are the experts on their own children and often have extensive information or stories to share about what works for them.[11]

Time Resources

Daily and weekly activities, by their very definition, require time investment, and every family at one time or another experiences stress because there are too many things to be done and not enough time. Children with disabilities often depend on caregivers longer than typically developing children, and the extra daily care or supervision needed can extend for many years.[30,40,97] The amount of time spent in shared activities around caregiving can be wearing and frustrating and can reduce the family's time for recreation and social gatherings. In a study of more than 200 families of children with Down syndrome, mothers spent three times as much time in childcare as mothers of typically developing children.[10] The fathers of children with Down syndrome spent twice as much time in childcare as fathers of typically developing children. One commonly used coping strategy of family caregivers is to organize the day into well-established routines.[47] Helitzer and colleagues found that mothers of children with disabilities reported that they used "structure, routine, and organized time management as a way to maintain a sense of control" (p. 28).[57] However, their busy, structured lives often were disrupted by crises, such as trips to the hospital or urgent care department and, as a result, the mothers felt they were "living on the edge" and that every disruption in their routines was experienced as a crisis.

Crowe found that mothers of children with multiple disabilities spent significantly more time in child care activities and less time in socialization than mothers of typical children.[29] In a qualitative study of parents of children with chronic medical conditions and disabilities, parents reported that they had round-the-clock responsibilities in administering medical procedures and performing caregiving tasks.[23] They described the challenges of "always being there" to care for their child's extraordinary medical needs and to engage their very dependent child in developmentally appropriate activities. These parents, whose children were often ill and even hospitalized, were always "on call" and often had to cancel activities outside the home when the child was ill.

Service providers can be a source of threat to the family's time and emotional resources. Providers seeking to implement family-centered practice often expect parents to take on responsibility for implementing therapy.[93,96] Greene described how her family "experienced the burden of home programming" as occupational therapists, physical therapists, and speech and language pathologists made separate recommendations, each requiring a chunk of the day.[93] These home assignments became a source of guilt and marital difficulty as the family struggled to meet the needs both of their daughter and of her typically developing sibling. Less experienced therapists, in their enthusiasm to help, often neglect to consider the family's time commitments when offering suggestions.

Emotional Energy Resources

Families of children with disabilities may experience special forms of stress, social isolation, and less psychological well-being than families with typically developing children.[9,32,102] The idea that parents of children with disabilities experience recurrent grief is pervasive in the literature, yet disputed.[41,166] Fox et al. conducted a qualitative investigation to understand how children with developmental delays and behavioral problems influenced the family's lifestyle.[40] Their parents suggested that dealing with the child's needs required a lot of emotional energy from the different family members. One theme—"It's a 24-hour, 7-day-a-week involvement"—was supported by stories of frustration from responding to challenging behaviors and applying parenting practices that would meet the needs of their children. Parents reported that individuals who offered "a shoulder to lean on" and professional assistance, encouragement, and information were particularly helpful.

Studies have shown that parents of children with disabilities may experience anxiety and depression.[55,120] Mothers appear more vulnerable than fathers. In a large comparison study of families of children with autism, developmental disability, or without disabilities, Olsson and Hwang found that mothers of children with autism were more depressed than mothers of children with mental retardation and that both groups were more depressed than mothers of children without disabilities. The fathers in these families did not exhibit more depression than fathers of typical children. Mothers' self-competence may be more related to the parenting role than that of fathers, and mothers may be more vulnerable when stressful difficulties arise in the parenting domain. Hastings, investigating levels of stress, depression, and anxiety in a cohort of 18 couples with children with autism, found that mothers and fathers felt similar levels of stress; however, mothers were more anxious.[55] Mothers may feel more responsibility for the child[55] and may take on a larger part of the extra care that a child with disabilities requires.[120]

When children have chronic medical problems that require round-the-clock use of technology, parents often find themselves exhausted and sleep deprived. Some of the consequences for parents whose children require routine medical procedures are anxiety and depression because of the risks inherent in the administration of the medical procedures. When parents must administer medical procedures beyond the typical parent–child activities of nurturance, caregiving, and play, they appear to experience stress and anxiety. In addition, they often do not have the time and resources to access energizing and relaxing activities, such as socializing and recreation.[9,80]

Stress level in families with children with chronic diseases or conditions has been found to have a strong relationship with family income and family function, with lower income associated with higher stress, especially as the children become adolescents.[9] Parents with limited resources, whether financial, educational, emotional, or a combination, are at higher risk of experiencing parental stress, which may lead to abusing or neglecting children with disabilities.[150] The added needs of children with chronic health issues or behavioral or intellectual limitations can push the low-resource parent over the edge of reason to a point where maltreatment of the child is the consequence.[58]

SOURCES OF DIVERSITY IN FAMILIES

Families with children who need occupational therapy services come from many different backgrounds and in a variety of forms, and therapists working with these children have the rewarding opportunity to learn from their families. Therapists must find a balance between focusing on the similarities and appreciating the differences among families.[1] Because individuals are inclined to view the world through their own cultural model and to use personal experiences as a point of reference, it takes professional commitment to become skilled at working with a variety of different families.

Family researchers and service providers have focused on understanding how a family's culture and traditions affect child-rearing practices and how these might be adaptive, strengthening a family or bringing about positive developmental outcomes.[83] Families have patterns of different characteristics (e.g., family structure, family income, having a family member with a disability) and the ecology in which families' function varies (e.g., religious opportunity, crime rate in the neighborhood, period in history). Therefore, generalizations of research findings about diverse family groups are rarely accurate, and sensitivity to the unique differences of each family is always needed. Three sources of family diversity discussed next are the family's ethnic background, family structure, and socioeconomic status. A fourth section considers differences in parenting styles and practices.

Ethnic Background

Ethnicity is a term used to describe a common nationality or language shared by certain groups of families. It tends to be a broad concept, and heterogeneity among families within groups described as Latino, African American, Anglo-American, or Asian should be anticipated. Furthermore, people may identify themselves as belonging to more than one ethnic group, making it harder to use the concept to guide the way the therapist works with families. Coll and Pachter offer two reasons for retaining ethnicity as an important variable when working with families raising children.[27] First, families that are not part of the dominant ethnic group experience a discontinuity between their cultural models and the majority culture that shapes the social institutions. Thus a cultural as well as a language gap may exist between health systems and educational programs and the families of minority ethnic groups.[2] In addition, as the proportion of ethnic groups grows in the United States, the sons and daughters of these groups make up a larger proportion of the overall population of children in this country. Occupational therapists who serve children with special needs can anticipate working with an ever-growing, ethnically diverse group of families. The influence of ethnic background on the ways a family fulfills its functions and raises its children is a complex topic that is merely introduced here. Resources on the Evolve website provide further information.

Ethnic groups share cultural practices that can determine who has the authority to allocate family resources and a value system that sets priorities for family routines and special events. Families in an ethnic group may have similar daily activities, ways of interacting, and ways of thinking about events, and may find similar meaning in their routines, traditions, and celebrations. Differences among ethnic groups are expressed in gender role expectations, child-rearing practices, and expectations at certain ages, as well as in definitions of health and views of disability. Cultural practices are not static traits; rather, they change when members of the group adapt to new situations.[53]

Although every family wants their children to be successful members of the community, their vision of what this entails varies among different ethnic groups and influences how children spend their time and what is expected of them.[88] Carlson and Harwood studied the structure and control Anglo-American and Puerto Rican mothers asserted over their infants during ADLs.[22] The researchers observed mothers in their daily routines and found that Puerto Rican mothers controlled their infants' behaviors more than the Anglo-American mothers, who tolerated more off-task behaviors. Carlson and Harwood pointed out that Puerto Rican parents are guided by the anticipation that their children will join a Puerto Rican community that values respectful cooperation. The Anglo-American willingness to follow the child's lead is compatible with valuing individual autonomy. Without insight into ethnic differences, a therapist watching parent–child interaction may mistakenly interpret a Puerto Rican mother's physical control and effort to divert a child's attention to the needs of others as intrusive and insensitive to the toddler's sense of identity and self-efficacy. Therapists avoid this type of error by understanding what a parent hopes to achieve before formulating an opinion about the appropriateness of a family's interactive routines.

The influx of recent immigrants expands the diversity within ethnic groups that therapists will encounter. Within a community, one family may have members who have been in a country for generations, and the family next door may have recently relocated to the country. Migration affects the family and how it functions at multiple levels.[37] First, relocation to another country frequently includes a series of separations and reunions of children and family members. Suarez-Orozco, Todorova, and Louie found that 85% of the 385 youths in their sample of recent immigrants had been separated from a parent and nearly half had lived apart from both of their parents during the process of family migration.[155] Although the length of separation varied, it was not unusual for a child to have been apart from the father for 2 years or longer. In some families, the tradition of having a child live with a grandparent or other relative may buffer the initial separation and help reduce the stress. Yet when the children are brought into the United States to join their immigrant parents, they must leave behind a caregiver and familiar community. Researchers found that reunification could be protracted, because families may not have been able to pay for travel or housing for all family members, meaning that people arrived in stages, months or years apart. In addition, when both parents immigrated ahead of their children, it was not unusual for the children subsequently brought into the country to have to adjust to living not only with their parents again but also possibly with younger siblings born in the new country. Therapists working with immigrant families need to be sensitive to the possibility of family friction, depression, and a sense of uncertainty among family members.

For each immigrant family, the process of *acculturation* varies; this is the process of selectively blending their traditions in how things are done, what activities are important, and interactive styles with the cultural practices of the majority group.[37] Parenting practices might insulate children from exposure to the language, ways, and values of the majority culture until the children go to school. For example, enrolling children in child care programs may seem the equivalent of child abandonment in some cultures, and families may bring a grandparent with them as part of the immigration process so that both parents can find paid employment. This may mean that children entering school have had few experiences beyond their home environment. In school, surrounded by new peers, the children's acculturation process is influenced, creating conflict among family members.[27] Unfortunately, feeling disconnected from home or discriminated against at school leads some youths to drop out of school as a way to ease the tension.[53] When this situation includes a child with disabilities, the occupational therapist has more to consider in addition to the specific needs of the child.[2]

Family Structure

Family features, such as the presence of children in the household, marital status, sexual orientation, and age/generation, are factors described as the *family structure*.[1] It is important to remember in working with families that acceptance of diversity within the family structure and family subsystems is necessary to be effective.

Family structure in combination with its cultural model influences how the family organizes itself to fulfill essential roles, such as caregiving of dependent family members or allocation of family resources. The idea that there is a best family structure in which children are raised is a myth.[174] For example, single-parent families have been portrayed as dysfunctional and as leaving children more vulnerable to having problems[3]; yet single parents have also been found to raise competent, well-adjusted children.[114] One third of the births in the United States are to unmarried women.[117] The majority of single-parent households are headed by women; however, the number of fathers who are single parents has increased.[168] The Fragile Families and Child Wellbeing Study is an attempt

to discard myths and replace them with evidence that will guide intervention and policy making to support low-resource families.[105] Some of their findings demonstrate that "Unwed parents are committed to each other and to their children at the time of birth...Most unmarried mothers are healthy and bear healthy children" (p. 3).[105]

Larson sampled the activities and emotions during activities of employed mothers in two-parent or single-parent homes of adolescents and found that the stereotype of the single-parent home was not necessarily the rule.[87] Single mothers in his study had less stressed, more flexible routines after a day at work, and friendlier relationships with their teenagers than did their counterparts in two-parent homes. Mothers with a husband reported more hassles trying to make and serve dinner by a designated dinnertime and experienced housework as more unpleasant. Larson speculates that the negotiation of responsibilities and trying to live up to expectations of being a "wife" in a two-parent home contributed to these differences. Clearly, every family structure has advantages and risk factors.[87]

Gay, lesbian, and bisexual families reflect one variation of family structure that therapists encounter. Children may be the products of a parent's previous heterosexual relationship or may be born or adopted into families headed by adults who are gay, lesbian, or bisexual.[127] Because parents do not want to expose their children to the prejudice of homophobia, many are reluctant to be identified, and estimates of the number of parents who are not heterosexual range from 1% to 12% of families.[151] Many of the issues and needs of all parents are expressed by gay, lesbian, and bisexual parents.[125]

Because sexual orientation has been the basis for judicial decisions that have denied people parenting rights, recent studies have investigated the issue of whether the sexual orientation of the parent affects the child's behaviors or influences the child's sexual orientation. Studies comparing the psychological adjustment and school performance of children being raised by lesbian or gay parents to those of children with heterosexual parents have generally found no differences.[127]

A final source of stress, divorce, the way many single-parent families are formed, can cause disruption that alters household routines, traditions, and celebrations. Sometimes the stress between the marital partners leads to impaired occupational functioning of the children and the divorce may come as a relief. Factors that contribute to positive developmental outcomes for children after couples break up include the parents' psychological well-being, economic resources, whether the family is part of a larger kinship network, and how parents navigate the separation and dissolution process. For example, Greene, Anderson, Hetherington, Forgatch, and DeGarmo reported contradictory findings regarding how well children adjust after their parents' divorce.[49] Initially, parenting practices were erratic, and the parent–child relationship, especially between custodial mothers and young sons, could be stormy. Yet two years after a divorce, many of the problems had diminished; therefore, some of the consequences of divorce depend on where in the adjustment process researchers conduct their study. Anderson argued that the best way to strengthen single-parent families was to empower parents by recognizing their strengths and encouraging them to reestablish routines.[5] The therapist can be supportive by acknowledging that these parents face considerable challenges in raising children alone and by aiding the parent in identifying resources such as friends, extended family, religious groups, and other single parents.

When birth parents are unable or unavailable to care for children, *kinship care* is a way to preserve family ties that might be lost if children are placed in foster homes.[75] Households in which grandparents are raising their grandchildren are examples of those providing kinship care and are a growing source of differences between families. These families, primarily headed by middle-aged or older women and disproportionately by women of color, are often formed after adverse events, such as child neglect or abandonment, maternal substance abuse, or incarceration or death of the parents.[72,75,85] Much of the research on grandparents raising their children's children explores the issue of caregiver stress. Evidence from both qualitative and quantitative studies suggests that grandparents caring for their grandchildren (or great-grandchildren) find it both rewarding and challenging.[8,75] Grandparents reported satisfaction in being able to "be there" for the child or children and reported that they have had to learn new parenting skills in response to the new generation. However, they also experienced parenting stress, which was exacerbated when they lacked social support, had limited financial resources, or were in poor health. When a child is reported to have behavioral or health problems, the caregiving demands increase the grandparents' sense of emotional distress.[56]

During their childhood, many children experience changes in the family structure. Unwed mothers may marry, or parents in a family may divorce and later one or both may remarry. A child may transition from a two- to a three-generation family when an aging grandparent moves into the home. Therapists should talk with family members in an inclusive manner that does not suggest an assumed family structure. Asking a parent or child, "Can you tell me about your family?" does not suggest any expectations about who is in a family and helps family members openly express their definition of who is in their family.

Socioeconomic Status

The influence of the family's SES on children's occupations and development is complex.[62] SES reflects a composite of different factors, including the social prestige of family members, the educational attainment of the parents, and the family income. These factors influence each other and have various implications for how a family fulfills its functions, by influencing the degree of access families have to activities and experiences for their children. Education influences parenting practices by affecting how an adult incorporates new ideas about a healthy life style and child development into these practices. Factors that influence employment, such as a below-average education, inability to speak English, or disability of a family member, leave families more vulnerable as job opportunities come or go. When employment is found, the job may not pay enough to meet the family's needs, leaving the family with no resources if unexpected events occur.

Researchers have demonstrated that low income or limited education is associated with differences in the quality of parents' interaction with their children.[62,135] In these circumstances, parents may not be as responsive, addressing the child less often, providing fewer learning opportunities, and

not engaging in an interactive teaching process. Parish and Cloud present a compelling review of the literature on the factors that lead children with disabilities to be more likely to live in poverty.[124] These factors include the increased cost of raising such a child and the decreased ability of their mothers to be employed, because of both the needs of the child and the lack of available child care. A recent study in England found the incidence of very preterm birth was much greater among mothers of lower SES, and preterm birth raises risk factors for the child.[148] Suggestions for working with families with low SES are addressed later in the chapter.

Therapists need sensitivity and skill to work with families across the SES continuum. Although this factor has not yet been addressed in the professional literature, having higher SES clearly affords additional opportunities, time, and expectations of parents for those experiences they desire for their children. The concept of "helicopter parents" who hover over every aspect of their child's life tends to extend to their children with special needs. Therapists must draw on their many skills in assisting these parents to find balance between what can be done through direct service, what they can do themselves, and how to allow a child space in which to be a "typical" child.

Parenting Style and Practices

The individual interactive style and parenting practices of an adult raising a child are additional factors that must be considered in gaining an understanding of the diversity of families. Steinberg and Silk distinguish between *parenting style,* the emotional climate between parent and child, and *parenting practices,* goal-directed activities parents do in raising their children.[152] For example, two parents may believe that if they want their children to do well in school, it is their responsibility to spend time with the children reviewing their homework (a parenting practice). However, the interpersonal interactions while they engage in this shared activity (parenting style) can be distinctly different. One parent may discuss the work and help the child find solutions to problems, whereas the other parent may feel he has the emotional energy only to point out errors. There is no test or license for parenting in this country. During the time of extended families, there was mentorship and modeling for parenting practices. In today's nuclear families, stresses run higher and skills may be lacking. When work separates the family, or as the dysfunctional practices of previous generations come to play in the current generation, there is great need to help parents learn parenting skills. Some individual professionals and disciplines, often State Extension Services, are creating programs to teach parenting skills. This is an area in which the holistic occupational therapy knowledge base and framework would prove quite beneficial.

A well-adapted child develops as a result of from complex interactions between parenting style and practice. Regardless of ethnic background, poverty status, and parenting practices, a parenting style that is warm, responsive, and positive and that provides structure and learning opportunities is associated with children who rank higher on many measures of social and cognitive development.[6,152]

Dialog between parents and therapists does not always go smoothly, and the collaborative nature of the relationship is sometimes lost if the parent and therapist hold different ideas about parenting style or parenting practices. This tension increases if the parent worries about the therapist's disapproval.[91] The professional cannot assume greater knowledge than the parent about what the child needs to be able to do or about the interactive style that best accompanies shared activities (Research Note 5-1). Therapists can be supportive and can empower parents by working with them so that family resources such as time and emotional energy are available when shared activities occur.

RESEARCH NOTE 5-1

Kadlec, M. B., Coster, W., Tickle-Degnen, L., & Beeghly, M. (2005). Qualities of caregiver–child interaction during daily activities of children born very low birth weight with and without white matter disorder. American Journal of Occupational Therapy, 59, 57–66.

ABSTRACT

OBJECTIVE/METHOD. This study used expert raters to examine videotapes of daily dressing and snack activities to measure qualities of engagement and directiveness in caregiver–child interactions when the children were 30 months old. Thirty-six pairs were divided into three groups (healthy children born full term, and children born prematurely and very low birth weight with and without white matter disorder) and matched on birth history, maternal education, ethnicity, and child gender.

RESULTS. There were no significant differences between groups for the average caregiver and child ratings, but correlations between caregiver directiveness and positive caregiver engagement ranged across the three groups: parents of full-term infants had higher engagement when they were less directive, whereas parents of children with white matter disorder had high engagement with high directiveness. The correlations between the caregiver and child qualities of positive engagement were small in both very-low-birth-weight groups, suggesting more variability in the responses.

CONCLUSIONS. Results suggest that patterns of caregiver interactions during daily activities may vary according to the child's abilities, as defined here by the level of biological risk. Caregivers of children with the greatest risk were both engaging and directive of their children during the activities, whereas caregivers of full-term children were more positive when less directive, and less positive when the child's behavior required them to be more directive. The findings suggest that caregiver–child interactions vary appreciably according to the level of the children's abilities.

IMPLICATIONS FOR PRACTICE

During activities of daily living (dressing and eating) caregivers appear to adjust their level of social and emotional assistance to the level needed by their young child.

Full-term children who are more capable in these tasks need appreciably less caregiver support.

Daily activities and play activities afford different interactional opportunities; more research is needed in both areas to assist clinicians in working with caregivers and their children.

AN ECOLOGIC PERSPECTIVE

As with any other open system, the social and physical features surrounding the family influence it. Cultural models are partly shaped by values, beliefs, and ways of thinking shared with others who have similar backgrounds.[43] An ecologic and transactional perspective of development and parenting encourages therapists to consider family resources and the adult's psychological background, personal history, and personality, which are in constant interaction with characteristics of the child being parented.[21,84,136] In addition, the occupations of families do not take place just within the home. Many of the resources for family activities that enable families to function effectively are available in the neighborhood and the larger community. Proximity to places of worship, stores, high-quality child care, and friends is part of the family's ecology and influences how family members spend their time. At a slightly more removed level, family functions are supported when social institutions make services available (e.g., a health department that runs an immunization clinic, the volunteer group that helps parents choose the best childcare centers, businesses that raise money for a school system).

The advantage of an ecologic perspective is that it raises awareness of the ways things distant from the family and beyond its control influence how the family fulfills its functions. For example, a large corporation that decides to cut its work force causes job loss in the neighborhood and forces people to leave the area to find employment. Suddenly the parents no longer have a babysitter and have to change leisure time activities. On an even more distant level, shifts in public attitudes during a particular period of time influence the environment and resources for families. For example, families can be affected by the attitudes of voters who determine public policies about the rights of people with disabilities, universal health care coverage, welfare reform, and the rights of undocumented immigrants.[39]

Further illustrating the importance of an ecologic perspective, Stacey and Biblarz noted that child development researchers need to examine not only a family's structure, but also how the family fits into its community.[151] When parents who are gay or lesbian reside in a community accepting of different orientations, the parents may be more likely to engage in open discussion about sexual preferences. Not being part of such a community can be considered a risk factor.[122] Single mothers, especially single adolescent mothers, may be at similar risk for a sense of being disconnected from the community.[92] A family living under these circumstances may be less open to social support offered by people outside the family at times of crisis and thus not as resilient as one living in a community that is accepting of a parent's lifestyle.

For therapists working with children with special needs and their families, it is especially important to take an ecologic perspective and to investigate whether families can access a range of community activities that will enable them to fulfill their functions. For example, in a survey of family-centered services in Ontario, King et al. found that communities vary in how they support the inclusion of families raising children with disabilities.[78] Limited access to recreational resources and lack of social support for parents reduced the participation of children with special needs in leisure activities. Therapists who strive to enable children's occupations that lead to participation in community contexts are no longer focused on the occupation of individual children. Turnbull, Turbiville, and Turnbull propose a collaborative empowerment model in which families draw on their knowledge of their children's abilities and receive support from other families and professionals to make changes at the community level.[163] By joining with families in advocating for children's rights, occupational therapists contribute to a synergistic force that increases the family's access to resources outside their homes and helps them function as a family.

SUPPORTING PARTICIPATION IN FAMILY LIFE

Development of Independence in Self-Care and Health Maintenance Routines

Occupational therapists who understand the nature of family occupations can help parents manage and adapt daily living tasks with their children. The therapist assists the parent in establishing goals about daily routines and tasks that the parent values, and then observes how they are being done. The therapist may engage the parent in a discussion of alternative strategies, or may model techniques that help the child perform daily living activities with greater skill and independence (Figure 5-8). With knowledge of the biomechanics of lifting and moving, the therapist considers whether the task is performed in a way that conserves energy and avoids injury. This consideration is especially important when a physical impairment significantly limits mobility. Strategies to help a 5-year-old bathe, dress, and use the toilet may no longer be safe for the parent's back when the child becomes an adolescent. A therapist's knowledge of adaptive solutions to self-care, such as Velcro fasteners, or, if standing balance is too challenging, dressing while sitting, can be quite helpful to parents, especially first-time parents.[111]

Becoming independent in self-care occupations frequently requires repeated practice until performance becomes a habit.

Occupational therapists who understand principles of behavior management can help parents reinforce a child's efforts at independence. Continuity in frequently repeated self-care occupations, such as using the toilet and eating with utensils, is increased through communication among the occupational therapist, teacher, parents, and others. A notebook that the child carries between school and home may serve this purpose.

Routines that lead to more independence in self-care provide opportunities to enrich the child's learning. During dressing, the child can improve strength by pulling up pants and increase vocabulary by naming colors found on the clothing. Therapists can suggest how to turn tasks into learning situations. However, as with all suggestions, the parent weighs the costs and benefits. Often the occupational therapist hears, "That just won't work for us." When this happens, a decision must be made regarding whether the task can serve two objectives, or whether the simple goal of independent self-care is sufficient.

Any extra time that the therapist asks the parent to spend teaching new steps in self-care should be in response to a parent's identified need. In addition, the effort should be justified by evidence that the altered routine has a good chance of bringing an immediate change. Alternative suggestions should be made quickly when an adapted technique does not work. The goal of occupational therapy recommendations should be to benefit the entire family by increasing the child's independence at minimal cost in time and energy to the parents. As stated by Bernheimer and Keogh, "Successful interventions are the ones that can be woven back into the daily routine; they are the threads that provide professionals with the means to reinforce, rather than fray, the fabric of everyday life" (p. 430) (Figure 5-9).[12]

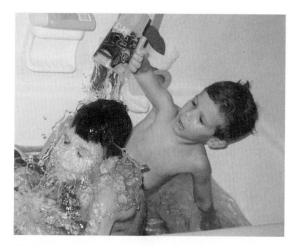

FIGURE 5-8 Matthew's bath time routine allows him to practice a range of skills, including play and social interaction. (Courtesy Jill and Mark McQuaid, Dublin, Ohio.)

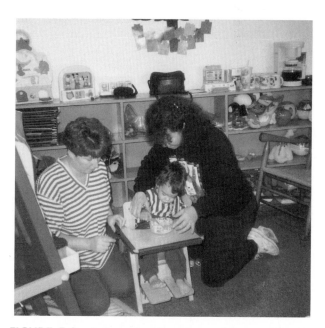

FIGURE 5-9 A therapist gives the mother recommendations for increasing the child's skills in self-feeding. Supportive positioning equipment and adapted feeding utensils make the task easier for the child and the mother.

Participation in Recreation and Leisure Activities

King, Law, Hanna, et al. and King, Law, King, et al. propose that the family's ability to engage family members in recreational and leisure activities is the result of a multidimensional process that includes the community, the family, and the child with a disability (Figure 5-10).[77,78] Their conceptual framework draws on literature in leisure studies and work with families of children with special needs. Some factors can directly influence participation, such as availability of an inclusive program, wherein peers and activity leaders support and believe in the child's ability to participate (Figure 5-11). Other factors, such as the extent to which the parents perceive acceptance from friends and neighbors and how parents view being active, indirectly shape whether families choose to participate in recreational activities in the community. Parents of children with developmental delays and behavioral problems will

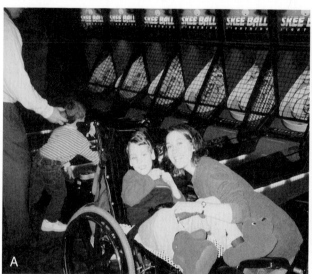
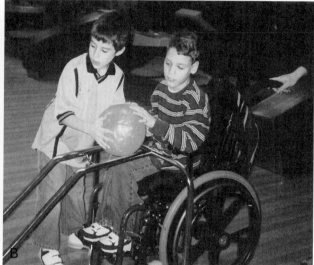

FIGURE 5-10 *A,* Recreational opportunities in the community provide an important family occupation. *B,* Matthew bowls with a friend. (Courtesy Jill and Mark McQuaid, Dublin, Ohio.)

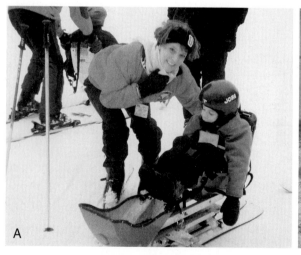
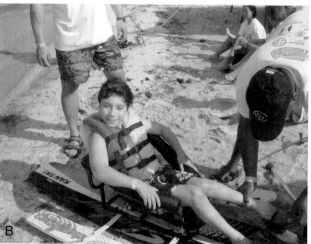

FIGURE 5-11 *A,* Most skiing facilities have equipment for children unable to stand independently. *B,* Wee Can Ski provides equipment for children with a variety of disabilities.

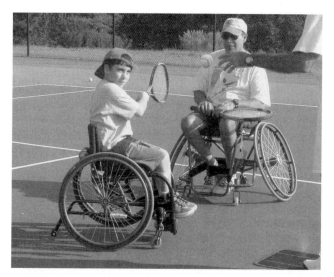

FIGURE 5-12 Keith has a tennis lesson while Dad watches proudly.

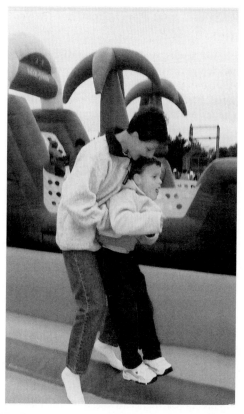

FIGURE 5-14 Activity centers with soft mats, bolsters, balls, and tunnels for tumbling offer safe and accessible environments for children with physical disabilities.

sometimes stop taking their child out in response to negative reactions of other people to their child's noises or tantrums.[41] Parents of children with developmental coordination disorder may need to consider individual rather than team sports as options for their children (Figure 5-12).[111] Resources, such as money to purchase equipment and time to transport children, influence the extent to which a family can participate in recreational activities. If families can afford vacations, many theme parks are now more accommodating to their needs (Figure 5-13).

Occupational therapists can communicate that they respect the value of recreation and leisure by including it in assessment and intervention plans. Therapists can suggest adapted equipment the child can use to make recreational activities possible. With the passage of the Americans with Disabilities Act in 1990, more recreational opportunities became available to individuals with disabilities. Information about community recreational activities is often available in local newsletters or on websites (Figure 5-14). Therapists can note which activities are accessible and appropriate for children with disabilities. They can also suggest strategies for making the family's outings more successful, such as providing headphones for a child with auditory sensitivity. Practitioners can also help parents accomplish caregiving tasks efficiently to make more time available for recreation. Scheduling therapy and education programs to enable families to engage in recreational activities can also support family function.

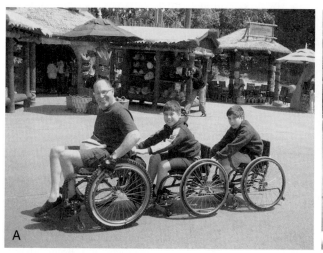

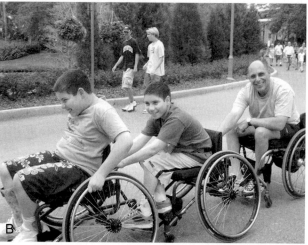

FIGURE 5-13 *A,* Dad pulls his tired children through a theme park. *B,* Years later, Todd returns the favor.

Socialization and Participation in Social Activities

Socialization is needed not only for health; it is an important mechanism for preparing family members to enter their cultural group and participate in community activities. Most families of children with disabilities, particularly those with problem behaviors, report that far too few opportunities exist for participation in the community. Families perceive that they are the only socialization agent for their children because community social activities simply do not accommodate their children.[161] In addition, children with disabilities may interact more frequently with adults than with peers, particularly if they have classroom aides. Constant interaction with adults to the exclusion of peers may exacerbate feelings of incompetence in interactions with peers.

Children with disabilities, particularly those with problem behaviors, face a "glaring void of friendships" (p. 224).[161] Educational and intervention programs should focus more attention on helping friendships to develop and flourish. Although professionals have created more activities and environments that include children with disabilities, they have not necessarily encouraged mutual and reciprocal friendships to develop. Turnbull and Ruef urge professionals to focus on understanding the components of friendship and the connections that form into mutual friendships.[161]

The presence of disability in the child may also create barriers to the parents' opportunities to socialize. Families of children with special needs often feel that they have less time to spend participating in social activities.[30] Because childcare is typically difficult to arrange and must be set up in advance, taking advantage of spontaneous social opportunities is rarely possible.[129] Children who act out or demonstrate disruptive behaviors may be particularly difficult to manage in social situations.

Parents often find it helpful to develop friendships with other parents experiencing similar circumstances. A number of studies have found that increased social supports are associated with healthier family functioning and lower levels of stress.[44,170] Helitzer et al. implemented a program for mothers of children with disabilities to address their concerns and difficulties in daily routines and coping.[57] The mothers were encouraged to provide emotional support to one another and to assist each other in resolving specific dilemmas in daily routines. These mothers perceived that they had changed their self-image and coping strategies through participation in the group sessions. They placed great value on having "a supportive opportunity to discuss their feelings and thoughts in a setting that was nonjudgmental and comfortable" (p. 408).[170] Similar programs offer parents social supports and strategies to help in coping, as well as practical ideas that make everyday life easier, help them adapt to stress, and give them a more positive attitude toward their children.[177] These social supports appear to be of equal or greater importance to families than professional services.[20]

Fostering Readiness for Community Living

Families of children with disabilities express concerns about the future of these children, particularly once they leave school. They worry that these children will not have the life skills needed to live independently.[82,97] As children become adolescents and then young adults, parents need information on possible living arrangements in the community. Often young adults are capable of leaving home but need support persons and arrangements for short- or long-term supervision and monitoring. These young adults may not have many options, and the options either may be overly restrictive (to secure funding) or may not provide sufficient supervision. Parents of young adults with disabilities emphasize the need for information on housing, particularly innovative supported living arrangements. For these young adults to succeed in living in the community with support, families need assistance in finding roommates, other support persons, funding, and arrangements for supervision and monitoring.[97,161]

Young adults with disabilities face many challenges in finding and maintaining employment,[133,161] but there are examples of successful transitions that give hope to families and professionals alike (Appendix 5-A).[97,166] Families and professionals need to work together to advocate for changes in the community to create opportunities for young adults to become employed and productive members of society (see Chapter 27).

FAMILY ADAPTATION, RESILIENCE, AND ACCOMMODATION

Despite the inclination of families to organize their activities into predictable patterns in the form of their routines, traditions, and celebrations, because dynamic systems that exist over time, change is inherent in being a family. Internal or external forces press for family adaptation or changes in what they do and how they interact. Pressures that can alter family activities include daily hassles, such as multiple demands on a parent's time or unpredictable transportation, as well as positive life transitions, such as the birth of a baby or an older son's leaving home to take a job, which alter household routines. Other events requiring that families adapt their routines and traditions may be unexpected, such as job loss, illness, or an event that affects the community (e.g., a natural disaster). When families experience new demands and stresses, they continue to function by creating meaning about the stressful event and by working as a system to adapt and continue their daily activities.

The process of *adaptation* starts when a family recognizes the state of affairs, an interruption in their activities, or a loss of emotional well-being.[46,128] Families use a variety of strategies to make sense of what is happening.[174] For example, they can tell stories about a similar instance or another generation that experienced a comparable event. They can redefine what seems like a catastrophic event by making a comparison with another family in which something they see as more devastating has occurred. For example, finding spiritual meaning in an adverse event is a way of changing how it is experienced. Regardless of the strategy used, by co-constructing their own definitions of events, families diminish the feeling of being out of control and, based on how they define the state of affairs, they can allocate resources to manage the situation.

Families demonstrate resilience when they draw on resources to reconstruct their routines or create new ones that enable them to continue to fulfill family functions. For example, McCubbin, Balling, Possin, Frierdich, and Bryne identified factors that contributed to families' resilience and ability to manage when children were diagnosed with cancer.[101] Based on their interviews of 42 parents, they found *resiliency factors* that made it easier for the family to construct new routines to deal with the situation. These families drew on their own resources, such as religious beliefs and the emotional support of each other, and then reset their definition of how they would live or operate as a family. The parents rearranged their routines so that one parent could be with the child receiving inpatient medical treatment while the other stayed at home with the siblings. Parents reported that they also drew on resources in their community. For example, when neither parent had time to cook, members from their church brought in meals so the family could share meals together. In a longitudinal study of families with a child with developmental delays, Bernheimer and Weisner refer to these changes that maintain daily routines as *accommodations*.[13] They identified 10 accommodation domains (e.g. services, marital roles, social support) that varied in frequency of need over time. When the children were 3 years old, the highest-frequency areas of accommodation were childcare tasks, sources of information, and support. They note, as has been mentioned previously, that family daily routines were strongly influenced by cultural and family values and goals.

The family members' ability to communicate with each other is important to co-construction of meaning and adaptation of daily routines. Families engage in affective and instrumental communication. In *affective communication,* family members express their care for and support of each other. In *instrumental communication,* members give each other role assignments, establish schedules, make decisions, and resolve conflicts. Clear, effective communication is important for establishing meaning for an event or problem and for planning resolution of the crisis. As Patterson put it, "A family's belief in their inherent ability to discover solutions and new resources to manage challenges may be the cornerstone of building protective mechanisms and thereby being resilient" (p. 243).[128]

A child with exceptional health or developmental needs creates new demands on a family system. Families with sufficient resources and flexibility respond by adapting their daily routines and special events so that they can fulfill their family functions. Bernheimer and Keogh illustrated the importance of family resilience in the conclusion of their longitudinal study of families of children with special needs:

The majority of our families are doing quite well. Like the children in our study, they share common characteristics but are strikingly unique in many ways. They are adapting and adjusting within their physical and cultural environments, and are making decisions about the organization of their lives and about their children, consistent with their values and beliefs and with what they think is important (p. 429).[12]

Occupational therapists who recognize the power of daily routines and family traditions are sensitive to disruption of a family's pattern of activities and can assist parents in reestablishing or creating meaningful family routines. For example, the occupational therapist may suggest strategies that enable a child with a gastrostomy tube to participate in the family mealtime (e.g., explaining to the parents what foods the child can safely "taste" at the dinner table). The therapist can also help families find ways to make important traditions possible. If a child with autism has difficulty in a new environment, the therapist can recommend ways to help the child adjust by suggesting that he carry a CD player with his favorite music as preparation for leaving home for the traditional family vacation.

The fact that most families adjust successfully to children's disabilities should not lead occupational therapists to ignore the initial and ongoing challenges that families face. Times of coping and adaptation vary according to whether a family must adjust to an acute traumatic event leading to a disability or the family gains a gradual, unfolding understanding of the child's developmental differences. After the diagnostic period, when the child's problems are identified, the family goes about the process of living. During this period, the demands for adaptation and coping vary. The following sections describe how occupational therapists can offer support, intervention services, and education to families.

PARTNERING WITH FAMILIES

Parent–professional partnership grows from an appreciation that by working together, both the occupational therapist and the parent can share important expertise and knowledge that will make a difference in the child's life. The sustained involvement and special insights families bring have been discussed earlier; this section goes into more specificity regarding the different ways occupational therapists work with families.

Family-centered services refers to a combination of beliefs and practices that define particular ways of working with families that are consumer driven and competency enhancing. Such beliefs and practices are necessary if occupational therapists are to be successful in team development and implementation.[159] Definitions range from acting as service coordinators, to addressing the needs of the family for financial and social resources as part of an intervention program, to empowering family members as part of a team to make decisions relative to their child's program.[96] Three complementary models for family-centered services are (1) family support, (2) direct services, and (3) family collaborative education.

Family support is designed to bolster a network of social support to enhance the family's natural strengths and family functions. DeGrace recommended not being so focused on the child's issues that the therapist does not recognize how the disability impacts family occupations.[32] Social support, such as being able to talk with other parents, decreases the family members' feelings of isolation and stress.[13,102,177] Promoting a family's well-being through emotional support and practical suggestions allows families to engage in responsive interaction with their children. The occupational therapist's role in providing family support is to help the family secure needed resources and capitalize on its existing competencies and strengths.[51]

Direct services are provided when the therapist engages a child in an activity with the goal of promoting the child's skill acquisition and minimizing the consequences of a disability. This is the traditional and, for the therapist and most institutional facilities, the more reimbursable form of interaction. Family members should be present and participating in the therapeutic activity, but the occupational therapist's attention is on promoting the child's engagement in the activity. Unless handled with skill and sensitivity to the family, this type of service may fall outside family-centered practice.

Family collaborative education has a number of purposes and should be individualized to the families' interests, learning styles, and knowledge levels. In parent-mediated therapy, the caregiver is taught how to engage the child in an activity designed to achieve a parent-identified goal or outcome.[7] Strong evidence indicates that the more parents know about development, the more responsive and supportive they are in interacting with that child and the better prepared they are to foster optimal development.[146,153,171] Parents of children with delays are not looking for developmental milestones; their efforts to engage their children in daily activities are not informed by hearing that, typically, children feed themselves with spoons between 15 and 24 months or don simple clothing between 2 and 3 years. Parents want to hear how children with special needs learn things that other typically developing children seem to teach themselves. Kaiser and Hancock reported on an effective, systematic approach to teaching parents new skills.[73] First, the parents identified the outcome or skills they wanted to foster, and the interventionists then guided them in what to do and how to implement child instruction within the natural flow of everyday activities.

Often a variety of methods may be needed to engage the different family members. Ninio and Rinott recommended a number of strategies for encouraging the father's participation.[118] Programs that seem to best support the father's involvement actively attempt to involve the father in planning meetings, offer convenient scheduling for therapy and meetings such as evenings or weekends,[76] focus on providing information about the disability and community resources, and provide opportunities for the father to enjoy activities with his child. When the father is the family's primary decision maker, it is critical that he receive complete information about the decisions that need to be made, including the purchase of assistive technology and accessing resources for the child. Margetts and colleagues focused on the potential of engaging grandparents,[98] whereas Trent-Stainbrook and colleagues researched a successful program in which older siblings were taught how to interact responsively with their younger sibling with Down syndrome.[158]

Sharing information with families is likely to be most effective when the child demonstrates interest in doing the activities the team has targeted. At that point, the therapist becomes a "coach" who facilitates an exchange of ideas that helps the parent discover ways of helping the child learn the activity.[52] This dialogue includes periods of observation and reflection. Coaches bring pragmatic understanding of the intervention strategy and serve as a resource.[73] Unlike in direct therapy, the family is the focus of the therapist's attention, and the parent/family member is the one interacting with the child. Sharing with a family in this way requires a range of skills, including an understanding of development, a well-grounded expertise in how to implement an intervention that has proved effective,[73] and an ability to communicate in an egalitarian way, which the family can choose to follow or not.[93]

Many authors advocate expanding the definition of family education to one in which a collaborative exchange of information occurs among parents, professionals, and people in the community. The therapist wants to empower the family, not engender dependence on a professional's expertise.[7,33,96] If family education focuses on helping the parent minimize the child's disability and optimize developmental gains, the focus is too narrow. Furthermore, if teaching is always a one-way process, it does not necessarily strengthen the family by recognizing the expertise of its members. Involving parents who are knowledgeable about community organizations and activities designed for children with special needs as educators in collaborative teams promotes their expertise. Parents can contribute information, resources, and strategies for caregiving for a child with special needs well beyond the professional's knowledge.[14,160]

Establishing a Partnership

The first interactions of the therapist with a family open the door to the establishment of a partnership. In a family-centered approach, the therapist demonstrates a family orientation that establishes trust and builds rapport through the use of open communication, mutual respect, shared decision making, and parental empowerment.[14] The therapist's initial interview reflects an interest not only in the child's behaviors but also in the family's concerns with managing those behaviors. These first interactions demonstrate that an equal partnership is desired and encourage a give and take of information. At the same time, parents begin to understand that professionals are there to help them and provide information and resources that support the child's development.[7,51,159]

Trust building is not easily defined, and it is associated with nonverbal language, words, and mutual respect. Thinking the best of families is important to the development of this partnership. This may not always be easy, particularly when the family's lifestyle contradicts that of the professional. Being positive and maintaining a nonjudgmental position with a family can be challenging, but it is essential to establish and build a trusting relationship. Parent participants in focus groups defined respect as simple courtesies from professionals, such as being on time to meetings.[15] The professionals who were interviewed linked respect to being nonjudgmental and accepting of families. When professionals are disrespectful to families, parents may become reluctant to access services or may lose their sense of empowerment. Demonstrating respect for families becomes particularly important when they are of different racial, ethnic, cultural, and socioeconomic status. Families from different cultures often have different perspectives on child rearing, health care, and disabilities. Table 5-1 lists cultural characteristics, examples, and the possible consequences for intervention programs.

Qualitative studies have revealed snapshots of actual family experiences with service providers. Blue-Banning and colleagues found families emphasized that partnerships were built on equality and reciprocity.[15] A sense of equality was created when professionals acknowledged the validity of the parents' point of view, and partnerships flourished when there were opportunities for each member to contribute. In contrast, Lea examined the perspectives of teenage mothers and their children's providers of early intervention services and found the perception of a lack of partnering on the part of the providers.[92] These mothers felt that their providers did not know or respect them, and that their concerns were ignored. This in turn led them to have little trust in the providers. Professionals must reflect on their practices and determine whether they are truly valuing the families they are working with and whether their expectations for intervention are aligned with the family's values and goals.[96]

TABLE 5-1 Cultural Considerations in Intervention Services

Cultural Considerations	Examples	May Determine
Meaning of the disability	Disability in a family may be viewed as shameful and disgraceful or as a positive contribution to the family.	Level of acceptance of the disability and the need for services
Attitudes about professionals	Professionals may be viewed as persons of authority or as equals.	Level of family members' participation; may be only minimal if the partnership is based only on respect or fear
Attitudes about children	Children may be highly valued.	Willingness of the family to make many sacrifices on behalf of the child
Attitudes about seeking and receiving help	Problems in the family may be viewed as strictly a family affair or may be shared easily with others.	Level of denial; may work against acknowledging and talking about the problem
Family roles	Roles may be gender-specific and traditional or flexible. Age and gender hierarchies of authority may exist.	Family preference; may exist for the family member who takes the leadership role in the family–professional partnership
Family interactions	Boundaries between family subsystems may be strong and inflexible or relaxed and fluid.	Level of problem sharing/solving in families; family members may keep to themselves and deal with problems in isolation or may problem solve as a unit
Time orientation	Family may be present or future-oriented.	Family's willingness to consider future goals and future planning
Role of the extended family	Extended family members may be close or distant, physically and emotionally.	Who is involved in the family–professional partnership
Support networks	Family may rely solely on nuclear family members, on extended family members, or on unrelated persons. Importance of godparents.	Who can be called on in time of need
Attitude toward achievement	Family may have a relaxed attitude or high expectations for achievement.	Goals and expectations of the family for the member with the disability
Religion	Religion and the religious community may be strong or neutral factors in some aspects of family life.	Family's values, beliefs, and traditions as sources of comfort
Language	Family may be non–English-speaking, bilingual, or English-speaking.	Need for translators
Number of generations removed from country of origin	Family may have just emigrated or may be several generations removed from the country of origin.	Strength and importance of cultural ties
Reasons for leaving country of origin	Family may be immigrants from countries at war.	Family's readiness for involvement with external world

From Turnbull, A. P., & Turnbull, H. R. (1990). *Families, professions and exceptionality: A special partnership* (pp. 156-157). Columbus, OH: Merrill.

Providing Helpful Information

Parents of children with disabilities report that information is a primary need from service providers.[47,65,89,153] The information that therapists provide to families about the intervention system prepares the families to work with existing systems, to use resources available, and to understand their rights as consumers. This information also enables the family members to become informed decision makers and to choose their level of participation in the intervention program.

Child-related information that may be of benefit to parents includes information about the child's development, the disability, the child's health, and assessment results. To provide up-to-date information, therapists must continually engage in reading and other professional development activities. Naturally, families want the most accurate and complete information, which places a responsibility on professionals to obtain current information and continually update their skills. The families in one qualitative study "admired providers who were willing to learn and keep up to date with the technology of their field...[A] competent professional is someone who is not afraid to admit when he or she does not know something, but is willing to find out" (p. 178).[15]

Although parents express that they want information about their child and about the diagnosis, it must be given in a supportive manner. Service providers who focused on the negative aspects of the child's condition or compared the child to typically developing peers were viewed as not supportive.[130] Once a deficit has been identified and the child qualifies for services, hearing the child's developing abilities expressed as delays or deficits can be hurtful for the parents. Describing what the child has accomplished using a criterion-referenced instrument, such as using the Pediatric Evaluation of Disability Inventory,[50] helps parents remain positive and encouraged. Using an occupation-centered approach, the therapist asks what self-care activities the child is attempting or what play skills are emerging. Articulating a therapeutic goal linked to an emerging skill that the parents have identified reduces professional jargon and helps parents understand how the intervention plan relates to their child. Typically, parents hope to receive recommendations for activities that help the child play, for toys that match the child's abilities, and for strategies that lead to independence in self-care. They also look to the therapist for help in managing motor impairments or differences in sensory processing that limit occupational performance.

Providing Flexible, Accessible, and Responsive Services

Because each family is different and has individualized needs, services must be flexible and adaptable. The occupational therapist should continually adapt the intervention activities as the family's interests and priorities change. Families value the commitment of professionals to their work and feel that it is important that professionals view them as "more than a case."[15,52,103] Parents expressed appreciation when professionals exhibited "above and beyond" commitment by meeting with them outside the workday, remembering their child's birthday, or bringing them materials to use.

Although therapists are often flexible and responsive to the child's immediate needs and the parent's concerns, the range of possible services is sometimes limited by the structure of the system. When a parent desires additional services, a change in location (e.g., home-based vs. center-based care), or services to be provided at a different time, the therapist may or may not be able to accommodate the request because of the therapist's schedule. Often the agency or school system enforces policies regarding the therapist's caseloads and scope of services. Practitioners are caught in the middle, between the system's structure and individualized family needs. A ready solution does not always exist for the therapist who is constrained by time limitations, the demands of a large caseload, or institutional policies.

Much of the time, the therapist recognizes that he or she cannot change the structure of the system and must work as efficiently as possible within it. At the same time, the therapist should inform the family of the program's rules and policies so that family members are aware of the constraints of the system. The occupational therapist can also take the initiative to work toward changing the system to allow more flexibility in meeting family needs. There is currently a discussion being carried out among stakeholders regarding what supports and services family-centered practice should encompass, as opposed to the usual focus of how it is carried out.[162] It is necessary for occupational therapists to have a voice in this discussion because it is aimed at policy issues.

Some suggestions for therapists from parents on providing flexible and responsive services include the following[164]:

1. Listen with empathy to understand family concerns and needs.
2. Verbally acknowledge family priorities.
3. Make adaptations to services based on parent input.
4. Explain the constraints of the system when the parents' requests cannot be met.
5. Suggest alternative resources to parents when their requests cannot be met within the system.
6. Discuss parents' suggestions and requests with administrators to increase the possibilities that policies and agency structure can change to benefit families.

Respecting Family Roles in Decision Making

Parents who share in decision making regarding intervention for their child are more satisfied with services.[109] Although professionals tend to acknowledge readily the role of the parents as decision makers, they do not always give parents choices or explain options in ways that enable parents to make good decisions. Too often, plans that should be family-centered are written in professional jargon and do not always address family concerns.[16] Parents are involved in decision making about their child in the following ways:

1. Parents can defer to the therapist in decision making. Deferring to the therapist may reflect confidence in the therapist's judgment and may be an easy way for parents to make a decision about an issue that they do not completely understand.
2. Parents have veto power. It is important that parents know that they have the power to veto any decision made or goal chosen by the team. Awareness of the legitimacy of this role gives parents assurance that they have an important voice on the team and can make changes, should they desire them. This role appears to be quite satisfying to parents.[100]
3. Parents share in decision making. As described in the previous section, when parent–professional partnerships have been established, the parents fully participate in team discussions that lead to decisions about the intervention plan. Service options and alternatives are made clear, and parents have the information needed to make final decisions. Requests of parents are honored (within the limitations of the program).

Families cannot always be given a wide range of choices about who will provide services and when and where these services will be provided. However, their role in decision making should still be emphasized; otherwise, family-centered practice is not occurring.[13,93,96] Families who are empowered to make decisions early in the intervention process will be better prepared for that role throughout the course of the child's development. In most cases, assessment of choices and good decision making are skills that parents promote in their children as they approach adulthood.

COMMUNICATION STRATEGIES

Effective communication is built on trust and respect; it requires honesty and sensitivity to what the parent needs to know at the moment. Therapists have tremendous amounts of information to impart to parents. Effective helping is most likely to occur when the information given is requested or sought by the parent.

Occupational therapists communicate with parents using a variety of methods: formal and informal, written, verbal, and nonverbal. Table 5-2 describes communication strategies consistent with the principles described earlier. The strategies are based primarily on feedback from parents regarding what they have found to be effective help from occupational therapists.[24,52,60]

HOME PROGRAMS: BLENDING THERAPY INTO ROUTINES

Throughout this text, recommendations are given for ways to integrate therapeutic strategies into the daily occupations of children, with the clear recognition that learning occurs best in the child's natural environment. Skills demonstrated in therapy translate into meaningful functional change only when the

TABLE 5-2 Communication Methods between Parents and Professionals

Type of Communication Method	Purpose	Role of Professional
Formal team meeting with the family to develop an IFSP or IEP	To increase the parents' participation and comfort level.	Provide parents with specific information about the purpose, structure, and logistics of the meeting. Information about parental rights must be explained to parents before and during the meeting. Decipher legal terms so that parents have practical knowledge regarding IDEA safeguards. Before meeting, parents should be informed of the questions that the team members may ask (e.g., "What are your visions for your child?") so they can formulate thoughtful responses. Parents should receive assessment results before the meeting so they have an opportunity to think about the assessment and be prepared to discuss their goals for the child in the team meeting. A telephone call before the meeting also gives the therapist an opportunity to ask about the parents' concerns and prepare options for meeting those concerns in the child's educational program or intervention plan. Encourage parents to ask questions, express opinions, or take notes. Use jargon-free language, avoiding technical terms. Plans should be specific and should include dates, tasks, and the names of those who are responsible for the plans.
Informal meetings during or after the child's therapy		The therapist needs to be organized and prepared for parent encounters. Casual or general responses are not adequate. The therapist should give specific examples of recent performance or state when reevaluation will occur and how those results will be reported. Listen to and acknowledge the parent's concerns. Indicate preference to respond after reviewing daily notes and charts on the child. The therapist can later make a telephone call to the parent with the child's chart in hand to avoid giving the parent erroneous or misleading information.
Written and electronic communication	If parents are not physically present, regular communication with family members relies on written strategies or phone calls.	*Notebooks* shared between therapists and parents are a highly valued way to have a regular, reliable method for expressing concerns. Team members may describe a new skill the child demonstrated that day, an action by the child that delighted the class, an upcoming school event, materials requested from the parent, snack information, or the current strategy for working on self-feeding. The parents can share their perceptions of the child's feelings, new accomplishments at home, new concerns, or reminders of appointments that will keep a child out of school. Home-based therapists may initiate a notebook for the parent to record significant child behaviors and for the therapist to make weekly suggestions for activities. In the neonatal intensive care unit, notebooks are sometimes kept at the infant's bedside to provide a method for the parents and therapists to communicate with the nursing staff on successful strategies for feeding and handling the infant. *Handouts* should be individualized and applicable to the family's daily routine. *Handouts* copied from books and manuals are appropriate if they are individualized. Many parents prefer pictures and diagrams. Other parents have remarked that triplicate forms that could be shared between the therapist, parent, and preschool were very useful.[52] Parent perceptions of their ability, confidence, and satisfaction significantly improved after using the Keeping It Together™ information organizer mentioned previously.[153] Photographs are also helpful to serve as a reminder to parents and staff on ways to improve postural alignment.
E-mail and other methods of communication		E-mail has become an easy, end-of-the-day method for noting any particular daily occurrences that would be of interest to the parents. A blog or even a Wiki may be a viable method for regular communication with technology-proficient partners. Regular progress reports are important to parents and are required in most school systems. A simple report covering a few areas of performance may be more meaningful to the parents than a lengthy, complicated report. Child quotes and reports of specific performance send the message that the child is receiving individualized attention. Camcorders with software for sharing have become less expensive and the videos could be uploaded to the Internet or recorded to video cassettes or DVDs. Video can convey information about handling, feeding, and positioning methods. Keep in mind that parents must invest time in watching the tape; short clips of direct relevance to current goals are most efficient. Written materials (and videotapes) are helpful because parents were "not always ready to hear, understand, or accept some information, but that it could be available for later use" (p. 91).[156]

child can generalize the skill to other settings and demonstrate the skill in his or her daily routine. Therapists often recommend home activities for parents to implement with their child, so that he or she can apply new skills at home.

Before making recommendations, the therapist should ask the parents about daily routines and the typical flow of family activities during the week. Understanding which routines and traditions hold special meaning for the family will help therapists focus. The therapist and the parents discuss family occupations during the day and identify naturally occurring opportunities to teach the child new skills by understanding what needs to occur and deciding when it will work for them. The result of this close examination of the typical week enables the therapist and the parents to embed goals and activities in interactive routines, in which the therapeutic process does not diminish the value and pleasure.

The ways mothers use home programs and the characteristics of home programs that parents value and implement have been studied fairly extensively.[24,59,144,157] Hinojosa completed a qualitative study in which eight mothers of preschool children with cerebral palsy (CP) were interviewed.[59] Most of the mothers did not carry out the suggested home programs. Mothers reported that they did not have the time, energy, or confidence to follow the programs effectively. Hinojosa suggested that it is inappropriate to expect mothers to follow a strict home program. Instead, therapists should help mothers find and learn adaptive ways to meet their children's needs with minimal disruption to their lives. Case-Smith and Nastro replicated Hinojosa's study using a sample of mothers from Ohio who had young children with CP.[24] Each had accessed private and publicly funded therapies. Initially, when their children were infants, these mothers had participated extensively in home programs. They indicated that these efforts were self-motivated and did not feel that the specific home programs were "an imposed expectation" on the part of the therapists. As the children reached preschool age, the mothers no longer implemented home programs with their children. Reasons for discontinuing home programs included lack of time and increased resistance on the part of their children. Segal and Beyer examined the use of a specific therapeutic intervention, the Wilbarger Brushing protocol.[145] They found that the factors with the most influence on adherence to the program were the child's response to the intervention, the parent's perception of its benefit, and whether the parent could fit it into daily routines. Tetreault and colleagues found similar results in their study of home activity programs, with the addition of family size as a factor; finding more children in the home tended to led to less adherence, possibly due to the burden on the mother.[157] Lyon expressed a mother's perspective on implementing therapy at home:

> I've come to terms with being "only human." If I could ensure that Zak could go through the day always moving in appropriate ways, flexing when he should flex, straightening when he should straighten, and play and learn and experience and appreciate ... I would; but, that is not possible. I do have a responsibility to help Zachary develop his motor skills, but I also have a responsibility to help him learn about life. So on those days when we have so much fun together or are so busy that bedtime comes before therapy time, I finally feel comfortable that I have given him something just as vital to his development, a real "mom" (p. 4).[95]

Although some mothers tend not to implement specific prescribed strategies, they report appreciating the therapists' suggestions and ideas about home activities that promote child development or make caregiving easier. Case-Smith and Nastro found that the mothers in their sample frequently used the handouts with specific activities and recommendations long after they had been given to them.[24]

Positive relationships with families seem to develop when open and honest communication is established, and when parents are encouraged to participate in their child's program to the extent that they desire. When asked to give advice to therapists, parents stated that they appreciated (1) specific, objective information; (2) flexibility in service delivery; (3) sensitivity and responsiveness to their concerns[106]; (4) positive, optimistic attitudes[24]; and (5) technical expertise and skills.[15] One mother expressed that hope and optimism are always best. "Given a choice, I would want my therapist to be an optimist and perhaps to strive for goals that might be a bit too optimistic, keeping in mind that we might not come to that" (p. 64).[116] McWilliam et al. describe this positive attitude as "a belief in parents' abilities, a nonjudgmental mind-set and optimistic view of children's development, and an enthusiasm for working with families" (p. 213).[106]

WORKING WITH FAMILIES FACING MULTIPLE CHALLENGES

Features that contribute to diversity in families are characteristics that occupational therapists welcome and accommodate in providing individualized services. For example, parents dealing with their own chronic physical illnesses may require help dealing with energy or emotional support as they experience social stigma associated with an illness such as HIV/AIDS (see Research Note 5-2 for a study of parents with physical disabilities).[121] The principles presented in this text remain critically important, but they may be more difficult for therapists to implement when they are working with families facing multiple challenges. Challenges to a family's ability to fulfill its functions (e.g., living in poverty, acute onset of a disability in the parent) increase the vulnerability of children with special needs and add unique challenges to family functions. By identifying protective factors that bolster the child's resilience, the therapist can approach issues from a positive perspective to support strengths, capitalize on family assets, and work to make maximum use of community resources.

The occupational therapist grounded in family systems perspective and committed to empowering families will work effectively with a whole-family system in a family-centered manner, regardless of the type of disability of one or more family members. Understanding and valuing how the family system orchestrates members' occupations to fulfill family function allows the occupational therapist to take a holistic view of the family's needs and priorities. Although parents advocate a positive view, it is important to recognize when an unusual parental behavior reflects family dysfunction (e.g., child abuse, child neglect). Issues in child abuse and child neglect are discussed in Chapter 13. When family dysfunction is pervasive, most occupational therapists need input from colleagues with expertise in counseling and family systems. Services for the child with special needs continue, but the

RESEARCH NOTE 5-2

Prilleltensky, O. (2005). My child is not my carer: Mothers with physical disabilities and the well-being of children. Disability & Society, 19, 209–223.

ABSTRACT

OBJECTIVE. The purpose of this study was to explore the meaning of motherhood and the mothering-related experiences of mothers with physical disabilities.
METHOD. A qualitative study using two focus groups (of mothers with children under eight years old and mothers of older children) plus individualized interviews of eight of the participating mothers were conducted. Most of the mothers were wheelchair users and were well educated.
RESULTS. The categories that emerged were their attempts to ensure the physical and psychological well-being of their children, their child-rearing philosophies and practices that addressed the challenge of setting boundaries and managing their children's behavior when there was a huge reliance on verbal explanations and instructions, and the overall nature of the parent-child relationship.
CONCLUSION. Mothers with disabilities who have access to formal and informal supports (assistance with hiring personal attendants) are better equipped to set boundaries, follow through, and promote cooperative behavior. Consistent parenting practices pave the way for children to be respectful of and feel supported by the parent.

IMPLICATIONS FOR PRACTICE

This article provides another example of working with families comprising parents with special needs. The examples in this study reinforce the need of all parents (and providers) to be consistent in their expectations and communications with their children. Occupational therapists must be aware of community and state resources for their families with special needs.

therapist considers ecologic and family systems factors in collaborating with the team to set priorities and provide services.

Families in Chronic Poverty

Beyond the diversity issues discussed under "Socioeconomic Status," chronic poverty has a pervasive effect on family and child experiences. A majority of families receiving public assistance are children and mothers with poor educational backgrounds, an inconsistent work history, and low-wage jobs. Welfare recipients are often stereotyped as lazy and unmotivated, and as having children "just to make money off the system."[92,141] In current economic circumstances, poverty has any number of causes. The process of "qualifying" for services can be frustrating, depersonalizing, and degrading. Once a family qualifies for help, resources are not always enough to make ends meet. In interviews with hundreds of single mothers living on welfare or working in low-paying jobs, Edin and Lein found that both groups had to engage in a variety of survival strategies to access enough resources to meet their families' needs.[35] Both groups reported sharing apartments and working on the side or having a second job. In addition, both groups relied on financial assistance from their social network, such as the child's father or family and friends.

Seccombe and colleagues conducted an ethnographic study of women receiving welfare and asked about their reasons for needing assistance.[141] Although the participants realized that the U.S. culture tends to emphasize individual responsibility for rising above poverty, many of the women believed that bad luck was a primary reason their families needed assistance. Single parents are particularly vulnerable[35,105]; without family members to help, these mothers lack control over the events in their lives. Unexpected events, such as a car breaking down or special meetings at school about a child, can cause the parent to miss hours at a job and can increase financial strain. Some women have reported that they returned to welfare and Medicaid "for the child."[141] Poverty represents a multidimensional issue, and therapists cannot make assumptions about the reasons a family lives in poverty.

Recognizing that poverty creates a unique cultural worldview enables therapists to consider what it means to provide family-centered services.[66,92] For example, a different world view of time, with the emphasis on the here and now, makes it harder to schedule or keep appointments. Families of low SES are rarely able to follow through with their plans. Therefore, planning for the future has little meaning, and participating in the setting of annual goals at IFSP or IEP meetings may not be considered important.

Further increasing the vulnerability of children with special needs who live in poverty are the multiple challenges that put their parents at greater risk for poor parenting. In one study, almost half (45%) of the mothers struggled with depression, and fewer than half of them reported that they had a family member who could help babysit.[138] Even with incentives such as diapers, toys, and food, low-income mothers got their children to an early intervention program only 40% to 50% of the time, compared with 75% of the time for middle-income mothers.[19] Therapists who are aware that poverty creates special conditions strive to individualize intervention plans and consider how formal support can replicate the positive effects of social support to promote better parenting.[19,34]

It is necessary to look beyond simple associations between poverty and parenting, because some parents do better than others despite a low SES.[114] Occupational therapists need to understand how some parents living in poverty adapt and raise children successfully (Case Study 5-1). For example, single parents who have strict disciplinary standards may seem harsh. However, their parenting practices may be grounded in an anticipation that their children will grow into a world where obedience to people in authority is important for keeping a job. Other parents who restrict their children's community activities may be effective in monitoring who they are with, minimizing the negative influences of poor neighborhoods. When a therapist is sensitive to and deeply understands a family with a low SES, she or he can make recommendations that help the child with special needs while supporting the family in their precarious position.

Parents with Special Needs

Parents themselves may have special needs that require an emphasis on supportive services. Parents who face physical or sensory challenges may need help in solving problems, such

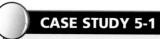

CASE STUDY 5-1   Family with Multiple Challenges

Jason and his mother, Ms. Thorp, lived in a government-subsidized, one-bedroom apartment, and they received food stamps and welfare assistance. Because it was a dangerous neighborhood, Ms. Thorp tried to keep Jason inside as much as possible. At his 4-year-old annual physical, the physician noticed that Jason was not completely toilet trained and that he had limited expressive vocabulary. His mother stated that he did not use a spoon. An interdisciplinary assessment at the Developmental Evaluation Center revealed a short attention span, a below-average self-care standard score on the Pediatric Evaluation of Disabilities Inventory, and 20% delay in expressive language. The occupational therapist also noted that Jason demonstrated poor fine motor skills (i.e., he did not complete puzzles, color with a crayon, or cut along a line). Because Jason had not been exposed to a varied learning environment, the team recommended that he enroll in a childcare program with children his own age. They also recommended that the speech–language pathologist and the occupational therapist consult with his teacher.

In developing an IEP, his mother, with input from the social worker, had selected a childcare program near her home, so she could walk Jason to school. The teachers welcomed him and thought that they could work on toilet training, but they insisted that Jason needed to be able to feed himself lunch before he entered the program.

The therapist discussed Jason's use of a spoon with Ms. Thorp, but she did not instruct her to force Jason to use utensils. The therapist recalled hearing that children living in poverty were less likely to have meals in a particular location or at regular times, and she realized that strategies at different levels would be needed to achieve spoon-feeding.

The therapist decided that she could be supportive and effective in changing mealtime routines by providing services in the home. At the beginning of the home visit, the therapist realized that the family had no kitchen table. In talking about their daily schedule, Ms. Thorp reported that they did not awaken at any specific time. However, Jason was usually up by 11:30 AM to watch his favorite television show. She reported that watching television together was an activity she enjoyed with her son.

Ms. Thorp gave Jason a cheese sandwich sometime in the late morning. She selected cheese sandwiches because the nutritionist said they were good, and Jason did not make a mess when he walked around with them. Ms. Thorp reported that she was not a "morning person," so she frequently did not have breakfast or lunch. Instead, she snacked during the day. For dinner, she frequently made chicken or hamburgers, which she and Jason ate in the living room. The plate was placed on the coffee table, and Jason stood near it and finger fed himself. If she made something like pinto beans, Ms. Thorp fed Jason so that he would not make a mess. She explained, "When we moved in, there were bugs everywhere. I fought hard to kill them because I know they are dirty. I know if he makes a mess with food, the bugs will be right back!"

The therapist brought a cup of pudding as a treat for Jason, and she asked him to spoon it himself. They sat Jason in the corner of the sofa. When he was handed the spoon, he dipped it into the pudding, inverted the spoon as he brought it to his mouth, and sucked the pudding from the spoon. Ms. Thorp became upset when pudding dropped from his spoon onto his shirt. She took the spoon away and fed him the rest of the pudding.

The therapist wanted to understand Jason's weekly routine. She learned that Jason spent every Tuesday night with his father, who would take him out for an ice cream cone. His maternal grandmother occasionally watched Jason on weekends when Ms. Thorp supplemented their income by filling in as a cook's assistant in a coffee shop. The therapist interpreted the family's strengths as the following:

1. Ms. Thorp is a devoted mother who wants her son to be healthy and wants a clean apartment.
2. Ms. Thorp listens to and follows the advice of the nutritionist.
3. The Thorps share an interactive routine around a television show in the morning, which helps create temporal organization.
4. Jason's family includes extended family who see him regularly.

Her concerns about Jason's learning to spoon feed include the following:

1. Jason does not have a place for meals, and he rarely sees anyone using a spoon.
2. Meals are typically foods that can be eaten with the fingers.
3. Jason does not use tools well, and Ms. Thorp does not want him to be messy.
4. Ms. Thorp is easily overwhelmed by details, and she does not seem to solve problems easily.

The next time she visited, the therapist brought a stool from the therapy equipment library. They adjusted the height so that it could be pulled up to the coffee table, creating a place for Jason to sit and eat. She also purchased two place mats with his favorite cartoon hero on them. The therapist brought a container of macaroni and cheese for Jason to eat. Jason loved his "chair" and table. When given the spoon to eat macaroni from a bowl, he scooped but inverted the spoon on the way to his mouth. He looked surprised and then finger fed himself the noodles. Together the therapist and Ms. Thorp planned that Jason would have "noodles" as lunch, and they agreed that lunch would occur immediately before Jason's favorite TV show.

On her third home visit, the therapist arranged to come in the evening when Jason's father came to take him for ice cream. When she arrived, Ms. Thorp returned the stool because her mother had a stool Jason could use. The therapist explained to Jason's father that his son needed more practice using a spoon. He agreed to get cups of ice cream instead of ice cream cones and to eat with Jason.

Within 4 weeks of the therapist's third visit, Ms. Thorp reported that Jason was successfully using a spoon. The team arranged for Jason to begin preschool the next week.

as monitoring the activity of an active child or being alerted to the cry of an infant.[107] Occupational therapists, who work from the perspective that parenting reflects a process of co-occupation, can assist the parent in the modification of tasks. For example, adapting the location of routines, such as diaper changing and infant bathing, can enable parents with physical limitations to participate in caregiving and simple routines that build affection between the parent and child. Therapists can explore the use of adaptive equipment, such as motion detectors or sound-activated alarm systems, to compensate for the parents' sensory deficits and ensure responsiveness to their child's cues. Most parents who have had long-term experiences with a physical limitation independently develop creative solutions for providing care for their children, and they only occasionally seek a therapist's assistance in determining how to perform specific caregiving tasks.

Parents who struggle with drug addiction or mental health conditions may worry whether they are up to caregiving responsibilities.[104] They often require counseling, mental health services, and opportunities to participate in support groups.[119] When parents have special needs that strongly influence their caregiving ability, their needs often become the first emphasis of intervention.

Parents with intellectual disabilities, mental health issues, or drug addiction are at risk for having children with developmental disabilities. Professionals have questioned the competency of parents with intellectual delays, and courts have removed their children in disproportionate numbers.[17] However, with support systems in place, these parents can be surprisingly successful. Parents at risk because of intellectual or mental health impairments appear to be most successful in caring for young children when they are married, have few children, have adequate financial support, and have multiple sources of support.[167]

In providing support to parents with intellectual disabilities, Espe-Sherwindt and Kerlin recommended that professionals focus on the parents' internal and external control, self-esteem, social skills, and problem-solving skills.[36] Therapists can help empower parents to make their own decisions, thereby increasing their sense of self-control. Often individuals with intellectual delay or drug addiction have low self-esteem and lack confidence in their ability to make decisions. Because self-esteem is important in interactions with children, this aspect of interaction should be considered.

Professionals should also focus on helping parents with intellectual or mental health impairments build problem-solving skills. Everyday care for children requires constant problem solving. Many times professionals give advice or recommendations without encouraging the parents to solve the problem independently or to try their own actions first. When others direct parents, they become more dependent. However, when parents successfully solve a problem, they become empowered to act independently in daily decision making. Problem solving can be taught and modeled. Espe-Sherwindt and Kerlin suggested that teaching problem-solving skills in daily caregiving could be critical to parents' development of caregiving competence.[36]

When occupational therapists work with parents with intellectual or mental health impairments, it becomes essential to know the parents' learning styles and abilities. Many times instructions need to be repeated and reinforced. Therapists must use good judgment in what techniques are taught to these parents, with emphasis on safe and simple methods.

The occupational therapist should also recognize the need for additional support to help parents with intellectual delays access those needed services. Regular visits in the home by aides, nurses, or teaching assistants can meet the level of support needed. If the occupational therapist communicates his or her goals and strategies to the visiting aide, therapy activities are more likely to be implemented by the parents and other professionals working with the family.

Working with parents with intellectual or mental health impairments can be frustrating when appointments are missed or requests are not followed. Therefore, an understanding of the parents' needs is essential. The development of simple, repetitive routines and systems that the parents can learn and follow enables them to become competent caregivers. With support, they can offer a child a positive and loving environment that fosters both health and development.

Professionals use a variety of strategies to deal with challenging families. When families have continual stress and problems, it is important for therapists to begin to build trust slowly, to share observations and concerns, and to accept parents' choices.[31] When parents do not seem to understand the intervention process, professionals can attempt to establish rapport by using concrete, simple terms; by providing both graphic and oral information; and by providing ideas that would immediately help the child. Professionals also report that parents can better articulate their concerns when services are home based, when lay terminology is used, and when services are presented in a slow, nonjudgmental way.[31] Focusing on the child's strengths and developing trust and responsiveness are also important when parents are coping with their own challenges.

SUMMARY

Working with families is one of the most challenging and rewarding aspects of pediatric occupational therapy. The family's participation in intervention is of critical importance in determining how much the child can benefit. Therapy goals and activities that reflect the family's priorities often result in meaningful outcomes.

This chapter described families as systems with unique structures and interactive patterns. The potential effects of a child with a disability on a family's occupations were related to implications for the occupational therapist's role. Issues that arise during different stages of the family's life cycle were described. In the final section, principles and strategies for working with families were discussed. The strategies included communication methods to inform and involve parents in the intervention program. It is critically important that the occupational therapist show sensitivity to and respect for the family's values and interests, maintain a positive attitude, continually update skills, obtain current information to give parents, and offer consistent, positive support of family members.

REFERENCES

1. Allen, K. R., Fine, M. A., & Demo, D. H. (2000). An overview of family diversity: Controversies, questions and values. In D. H. Demo, K. R. Allen, & M. A. Fine (Eds.), *Handbook of family diversity* (pp. 1-14). New York: Oxford University Press.

2. Alvarado, M. I. (2004). Mucho camino: The experiences of two undocumented Mexican mothers participating in their child's early intervention program. *American Journal of Occupational Therapy, 58*, 521-530.

3. Amato, P. R. (2000). Diversity within single-parent families. In D. H. Demo, K. R. Allen, & M. A. Fine (Eds.), *Handbook of family diversity* (pp. 149-172). New York: Oxford University Press.

4. Anderson, C. (2003). The diversity, strengths and challenges of single-parent households. In F. Walsh (Ed.), *Normal family processes: Growing diversity and complexity* (3rd ed., pp. 121-152). New York: Guilford Press.

5. Anderson, D. (1983). He's not "cute" anymore. In T. Dougan, L. Isbell, & P. Vyas (Eds.), *We have been there* (pp. 90-91). Nashville, TN: Abington Press.

6. Aran, A., Shalev, R. S., Biran, G., & Gross-Tsur, V. (2007). Parenting style impacts on quality of life in children with cerebral palsy. *Journal of Pediatrics, 151*, 56-60.

7. Bailey, D. B., Bruder, M. B., Hebbeler, K., Carta, J., Defosset, M., Greenwood, C., et al. (2006). Recommended outcomes for families of young children with disabilities. *Journal of Early Intervention, 28*, 227-251.

8. Baird, A., John, R., & Hayslip, B. (2000). Custodial grandparenting among African Americans: A focus group perspective. In B. Hayslip & R. G. Glen (Eds.), *Grandparents raising grandchildren: Theoretical, empirical, and clinical perspectives* (pp. 125-144). New York: Springer Publishing.

9. Barakat, L. P., Patterson, C. A., Tarazi, R. A., & Ely, E. (2007). Disease-related parenting stress in two sickle cell disease caregiver samples: Preschool and adolescent. *Families, Systems, & Health, 25*, 147-161.

10. Barnett, S., & Boyce, G. C. (1995). Effects of children with Down syndrome on parents' activities. *American Journal of Mental Retardation, 100*(2), 115-127.

11. Bedell, G. M., Cohn, E. S., & Dumas, H. M. (2005). Exploring parents' use of strategies to promote social participation of school-age children with acquired brain injuries. *American Journal of Occupational Therapy, 59*, 273-284.

12. Bernheimer, L. P., & Keogh, B. K. (1995). Weaving interventions into the fabric of everyday life: An approach to family assessment. *Topics in Early Childhood Special Education, 15*, 415-433.

13. Bernheimer, L. P., & Weisner, T. S. (2007). "Let me just tell you what I do all day…": The family story at the center of intervention research and practice. *Infants & Young Children, 20*(3), 192-201.

14. Betz, C. L. (2006). Parent-professional partnerships: Bridging the disparate worlds of children, families, and professionals [Editorial]. *Journal of Pediatric Nursing: Nursing Care of Children & Families, 21*(5), 333-335.

15. Blue-Banning, M., Summers, J. A., Frankland, H. C., Nelson, L. L., & Beegle, G. (2004). Dimensions of family and professional partnerships: Constructive guidelines for collaboration. *Exceptional Children, 70*(2), 167-184.

16. Boone, H. A., McBride, S. L., Swann, D., Moore, S., & Drew, B. S. (1998). IFSP practices in two states: Implications for practice. *Infants and Young Children, 10*(4), 36-45.

17. Booth, T., & Booth, W. (2004). Brief research report: Findings from a court study of care proceedings involving parents with intellectual disabilities. *Journal of Policy and Practice in Intellectual Disabilities, 1*, 179-181.

18. Bradley, R. H., Corwyn, R. F., McAdoo, H. P., & Coll, C. G. (2001). The home environments of children in the United States: Part 1. Variations by age, ethnicity, and poverty status. *Child Development, 72*, 1844-1867.

19. Brinker, R. P. (1992). Family involvement in early intervention: Accepting the unchangeable, changing the changeable, and knowing the difference. *Topics in Early Childhood Special Education, 12*(3), 307-332.

20. Britner, P. A., Morog, M. C., Pianta, R. C., & Marvin, R. S. (2003). Stress and coping: A comparison of self-report measures of functioning in families of young children with cerebral palsy or no medical diagnosis. *Journal of Child and Family Studies, 12*, 335-348.

21. Bronfenbrenner, U. (1990). Discovering what families do. In D. Blankenhorn, S. Bayme, & J. B. Elshtain (Eds.), *Rebuilding the nest* (pp. 27-38). Milwaukee: Family Service America.

22. Carlson & Harwood. (2003). Attachment, culture, and the caregiving system: The cultural patterning of everyday experiences among Anglo and Puerto Rican mother-infant pairs. *Infant Mental Health Journal, 24*, 53-73.

23. Case-Smith, J. (2004). Parenting a child with a chronic medical condition. *American Journal of Occupational Therapy, 58*, 551-560.

24. Case-Smith, J., & Nastro, M. (1993). The effect of occupational therapy intervention on mothers of children with cerebral palsy. *American Journal of Occupational Therapy, 46*, 811-817.

25. Case-Smith, J., Sainato, D., McQuaid, J., Deubler, D., Gottesman, M., & Taber, M. (2007). IMPACTS project: Preparing therapists to provide best practice early intervention services. *Physical & Occupational Therapy in Pediatrics, 27*(3), 73-90.

26. Christian, L. G. (2006). Understanding families: Applying family systems theory to early childhood practice. *Journal of the National Association for the Education of Young Children* (electronic), Retrieved April 28, 2008, from http://journal.naeyc.org/btj/200601/ChristianBTJ.asp.

27. Coll, C. G., & Pachter, L. M. (2002). Ethnic and minority parenting. In M. H. Bornstein (Ed.), *Handbook of parenting* (2nd ed., Vol. 4) (pp. 1-20). Mahwah, NJ: Lawrence Erlbaum.

28. Connard, C., & Novick, R. (1996). The ecology of the family: A background paper for a family-centered approach to education and social service delivery. Retrieved January 28, 2008, from http://www.nwrel.org/cfc/publications/ecology2.html.

29. Crowe, T. K. (1993). Time use of mothers with young children: The impact of a child's disability. *Developmental Medicine and Child Neurology, 35*, 612-630.

30. Crowe, T. K., & Florez, S. I. (2006). Time use of mothers with school-age children: A continuing impact of a child's disability. *American Journal of Occupational Therapy, 60*, 194-203.

31. DeGangi, G. A., Wietlesbach, S., Poisson, S., Stein, E., & Royeen, C. (1994). The impact of culture and socioeconomic status on family-professional collaboration: Challenges and solutions. *Topics in Early Childhood Special Education, 14*(4), 503-520.

32. DeGrace, B. W. (2004). The everyday occupation of families with children with autism. *American Journal of Occupational Therapy, 58*, 543-550.

33. Dolev, R., & Zeedyk, M. S. (2006). How to be a good parent in bad times: Constructing parenting advice about terrorism. *Child: Care, Health & Development, 32*(4), 467-476.

34. Dunst, C. J., Trivette, C. M., & Jodry, W. (1997). Influences of social support on children with disabilities and their families. In M. J. Guralnick (Ed.), *The effectiveness of early intervention* (pp. 499-522). Baltimore: Brookes.

35. Edin, K., & Lein, L. (1996). Work, welfare, and single mothers' economic survival strategies. *American Sociological Review, 61*, 253-266.

36. Espe-Sherwindt, M., & Kerlin, S. L. (1990). Early intervention with parents with mental retardation: Do we empower or impair? *Infants and Young Children, 2*(4), 21-28.

37. Falicov, C. J. (2003). Immigrant family processes. In F. Walsh (Ed.), *Normal family processes: Growing diversity and complexity* (3rd ed., pp. 280-300). New York: Guilford Press.

38. Fiese, B. H., & Tomcho, T. J. (2001). Finding meaning in religious practices: The relation between religious holiday ritual and marital satisfaction. *Journal of Family Psychology, 15,* 597-609.

39. Fine, M. A., Demo, D. H., & Allen, K. R. (2000). Family diversity in the 21st century: Implications for research, theory and practice. In D. H. Demo, K. R. Allen, & M. A. Fine (Eds.), *Handbook of family diversity* (pp. 440-448). New York: Oxford University Press.

40. Fox, L., Vaughn, B. J., Wyatte, M. I., & Dunlap, G. (2002). "We can't expect other people to understand": Family perspectives on problem behaviors. *Exceptional Children, 68,* 437-450.

41. Gallagher, P. A., Fialka, J., Rhodes, C., & Arceneaux, C. (2001). Working with families: Rethinking denial. *Young Exceptional Children, 5*(2), 11-17.

42. Gallagher, P. A., Rhodes, C. A., & Darling, S. M. (2004). Parents as professionals in early intervention: A parent educator model. *Topics in Early Childhood Special Education, 24*(1), 5-13.

43. Gallimore, R., & Lopez, E. M. (2002). Everyday routines, human agency and ecocultural context: Construction and maintenance of individual habits. *Occupational Therapy Journal of Research, 22,* 70-77.

44. Gavidia-Payne, S., & Stoneman, Z. (1997). Family predictors of maternal and paternal involvement in programs for young children with disabilities. *Child Development, 68,* 701-717.

45. Gordon, P. A., Tschopp, M. K., & Feldman, D. (2004). Addressing issues of sexuality with adolescents with disabilities. *Child and Adolescent Social Work Journal, 21*(5), 513-527.

46. Grant, G., Ramcharan, P., & Goward, P. (2003). Resilience, family care and people with intellectual disabilities. *International Review of Research in Mental Retardation, 26,* 135-173.

47. Grant, G., & Whittell, B. (2000). Differentiated coping strategies in families with children or adults with intellectual disabilities: The relevance of gender, family composition and the life span. *Journal of Applied Research in Intellectual Disabilities, 13,* 256-275.

48. Greene, M. (1999). A parent's perspective. *Topics in Early Childhood Special Education, 19,* 147.

49. Greene, S. M., Anderson, E. R., Hetherington, E. M., Forgatch, M. S., & DeGarmo, D. S. (2003). Risk and resilience after divorce. In F. Walsh (Ed.), *Normal family processes: Growing diversity and complexity* (3rd ed., pp. 96-120). New York: Guilford Press.

50. Haley, S. M., Coster, W. J., Ludlow, L. H., Haltiwanger, J. T., & Andrellos, P. J. (1992). *Pediatric Evaluation of Disability Inventory.* San Antonio: Psychological Corporation.

51. Hanft, B. E., Rush, D. D., & Shelden, M. L. (2004). *Coaching families and colleagues in early intervention.* Baltimore: Paul H. Brookes.

52. Harrison, C., Romer, T., Simon, M. C., & Schulze, C. (2007). Factors influencing mothers' learning from paediatric therapists: A qualitative study. *Physical & Occupational Therapy in Pediatrics, 27,* 77-96.

53. Harwood, R. L., Leyendecker, B., Carlson, J., Asencio, M., & Miller, A. M. (2002). Parenting among Latino families in the U.S. In M. H. Bornstein (Ed.), *Handbook of parenting: Social conditions and applied parenting* (2nd ed.). Mahwah, NJ: Lawrence Erlbaum Associates.

54. Hasselkus, B. R. (2002). *The meaning of everyday occupation.* Thorofare, NJ: Slack.

55. Hastings, R. P. (2003). Child behavior problems and partner mental health as correlates of stress in mothers and fathers of children with autism. *Journal of Intellectual Disability Research, 47,* 231-237.

56. Hayslip, B., Emick, M. A., Henderson, C. E., & Elias, K. (2002). Temporal variations in the experience of custodial grand parenting: A short-term longitudinal study. *Journal of Applied Gerontology, 21,* 139-156.

57. Helitzer, D. L., Cunningham-Sabo, L. D., VanLeit, B., & Crowe, T. K. (2002). Perceived changes in self-image and coping strategies of mothers of children with disabilities. *Occupational Therapy Journal of Research, 22*(1), 25-33.

58. Hibbard, R. A., Desch, L. W., & the Committee on Child Abuse and Neglect and Council on Children with Disabilities. (2007). Maltreatment of children with disabilities. *Pediatrics, 119*(5), 1018-1025.

59. Hinojosa, J. (1990). How mothers of preschool children with cerebral palsy perceive occupational and physical therapists and their influence on family life. *Occupational Therapy Journal of Research, 10*(3), 144-162.

60. Hinojosa, J., Sproat, C. T., Mankhetwit, S., & Anderson, J. (2002). Shifts in parent-therapist partnerships: Twelve years of change. *American Journal of Occupational Therapy, 56,* 556-563.

61. Hodapp, R. M. (2007). Families of persons with Down Syndrome: New perspectives, findings, and research and service needs. *Mental Retardation and Developmental Disabilities Research Reviews, 13,* 279-287.

62. Hoff, E., Laursen, B., & Tardif, T. (2002). Socioeconomic status and parenting. In M. H. Bornstein (Ed.), *Handbook of parenting* (2nd ed., Vol. 2, pp. 231-252). Mahwah, NJ: Lawrence Erlbaum Associates.

63. Holloway, R. L. (2007). Families and chronic illness: Introduction to the special section for. *Families, Systems, and Health. Families, Systems, & Health, 25,* 243-245.

64. Hombeck, G. N., Gorey-Ferguson, L., Hudson, T., Seefeldt, T., Shapera, W., Turner, T., et al. (1997). Maternal, paternal, and marital functioning in families of preadolescents with spina bifida. *Journal of Pediatric Psychology, 22,* 167-181.

65. Hummelinck, A., & Pollock, K. (2006). Parents' information needs about the treatment of their chronically ill child: A qualitative study. *Patient Education and Counseling, 62,* 228-234.

66. Humphry, R. (1995). Families living in poverty: Meeting the challenge of family-centered services. *American Journal of Occupational Therapy, 49,* 687-693.

67. Humphry, R. (2002). Young children's occupations: Explicating the dynamics of developmental processes. *American Journal of Occupational Therapy, 56,* 171-179.

68. Humphry, R., & Wakeford, L. (2008). Development of everyday activities: A model for occupation-centered therapy. *Infants & Young Children, 21*(3), 230-240.

69. Individuals with Disabilities Education Act of 2004 (IDEA). (P.L. 108-446.)

70. Jinnah, H. A., & Stoneman, Z. (2008). Parents' experiences in seeking child care for school age children with disabilities—where does the system break down? *Children and Youth Services Review, 30*(8), 967-977.

71. Johnson, C. P., Kastner, T. A., & the Committee/Section on Children With Disabilities. (2005). Clinical report: Helping families raise children with special health care needs at home. *Pediatrics, 115*(2), 507-511.

72. Joslin, D. (2000). Emotional well-being among grandparents raising children affected and orphaned by HIV disease. In B. Hayslip, & R. G. Glen (Eds.), *Grandparents raising grandchildren: theoretical, empirical, and clinical perspectives* (pp. 87-105). New York: Springer Publishing.

73. Kaiser, A. P., & Hancock, T. B. (2003). Teaching parents new skills to support their young children's development. *Infants and Young Children, 16,* 9-22.

74. Kellegrew, D. (2000). Constructing daily routines: A qualitative examination of mothers with young children with disabilities. *American Journal of Occupational Therapy, 54,* 252-259.

75. Kelley, S. J., Whitley, D., Sipe, T. A., & Yorker, B. C. (2000). Psychological distress in grandmother kinship care providers: The role of resources, social support and physical health. *Child Abuse and Neglect, 24,* 311-321.

76. King, G. A., King, S. M., & Rosenbaum, P. L. (1996). How mothers and fathers view professional caregiving for children with disabilities. *Developmental Medicine and Child Neurology, 38,* 397-407.

77. King, G., Law, M., Hanna, S., King, S., Hurley, P., Rosenbaum, R., et al. (2006). Predictors of the leisure and recreation participation

of children with physical disabilities: A structural equation modeling analysis. *Children's Health Care, 35*(3), 209-234.

78. King, G., Law, M., King, S., Rosenbaum, P., Kertoy, M. K., & Young, N. L. (2003). A conceptual model of factors affecting the recreation and leisure participation of children with disabilities. *Physical and Occupational Therapy in Pediatrics, 23,* 63-89.

79. King, G., Tucker, M. A., Baldwin, P., Lowry, K., LaPorta, J., Martens, L., et al. (2002). A life needs model of pediatric service delivery: Services to support community participation and quality of life for children and youth with disabilities. *Physical & Occupational Therapy in Pediatrics, 22*(2), 53-77.

80. Kirk, S. (1998). Families' experiences of caring at home for a technology-dependent child: A review of the literature. *Child: Care, Health and Development, 24*(2), 101-114.

81. Knott, F., Lewis, C., & Williams, T. (2007). Sibling interaction of children with autism: Development over 12 months. *Journal of Autism and Developmental Disorders, 37,* 1987-1995.

82. Knox, M., Parmenter, T. R., Atkinson, N., & Yezbeck, M. (2000). Family control: The views of families who have a child with an intellectual disability. *Journal of Applied Research in Intellectual Disabilities, 13,* 17-28.

83. Koramoa, J., Lynch, M. A., & Kinnair, D. (2002). A continuum of child-rearing: Responding to traditional practices. *Child Abuse Review, 11,* 415-421.

84. Kotchick, B. A., & Forehand, R. (2002). Putting parenting in perspective: A discussion of the contextual factors that shape parenting practices. *Journal of Child and Family Studies, 11,* 255-269.

85. Kroll, B. (2007). A family affair? Kinship care and parental substance misuse: Some dilemmas explored. *Child and Family Social Work, 12,* 84-93.

86. Laird, J. (2003). Lesbian and gay families. In F. Walsh (Ed.), *Normal family processes: growing diversity and complexity* (3rd ed.). New York: Guilford Press.

87. Larson, R. (2001). Mothers' time in two-parent and one-parent families: The daily organization of work, time for oneself, and parenting of adolescents. In *Minding the time in family experiences: emerging perspectives and issues* (Vol. 3, pp. 85-109). New York: Elsevier Science.

88. Larson, R. W., & Verma, S. (1999). How children and adolescents spend time across the world: Work, play, and developmental opportunities. *Psychological Bulletin, 125,* 701-736.

89. Law, M., Teplicky, R., King, S., King, G., Kertoy, M., Moning, T., et al. (2005). Family-centred service: Moving ideas into practice. *Child: Care, Health & Development, 31,* 633-642.

90. Lawlor, M. C., & Mattingly, C. F. (1998). The complexities embedded in family-centered care. *American Journal of Occupational Therapy, 52,* 2059-2067.

91. Lawlor, M. C., & Mattingly, C. F. (2001). Beyond the unobtrusive observer: Reflections on researcher-informant relationships in urban ethnography. *American Journal of Occupational Therapy, 55*(2), 147-154.

92. Lea, D. (2006). 'You don't know me like that': Patterns of disconnect between adolescent mothers of children with disabilities and their early interventionists. *Journal of Early Intervention, 28*(4), 264-282.

93. Leiter, V. (2004). Dilemmas in sharing care: Maternal provision of professionally driven therapy for children with disabilities. *Social Science & Medicine, 58,* 837-849.

94. LeRoy, B. W. (2004). Mothering children with disabilities in the context of welfare reform. In S. A. Escaile, & J. A. Olson (Eds.), *Mothering occupations: challenge, agency, and participation* (pp. 372-390). Philadelphia: F.A. Davis.

95. Lyon, J. (1989). I want to be Zak's mom, not his therapist. *Developmental Disabilities Special Interest Section Newsletter, 12*(1), 4.

96. MacKean, G. L., Thurston, W. E., & Scott, C. M. (2005). Bridging the divide between families and health professionals' perspectives on family-centred care. *Health Expectations, 8,* 74-85.

97. Magill-Evans, J., Wiart, L., Darrah, J., & Kratochvil, M. (2005). Beginning the transition to adulthood: The experiences of six families with youths with cerebral palsy. *Physical & Occupational Therapy in Pediatrics, 25*(3), 19-36.

98. Margetts, J. K., Le Couteur, A., & Croom, S. (2006). Families in a state of flux: The experiences of grandparents in autism spectrum disorder. *Child: Care, Health and Development, 32,* 565-574.

99. Markson, S., & Fiese, B. H. (2000). Family rituals as a protective factor for children with asthma. *Journal of Pediatric Psychology, 25,* 471-479.

100. McBride, S. L., Brotherson, M. J., Joanning, H., Whiddon, D., & Dermitt, A. (1993). Implementation of family-centered services: Perceptions of families and professionals. *Journal of Early Intervention, 17,* 414-430.

101. McCubbin, M., Balling, K., Possin, P., Frierdich, S., & Bryne, B. (2002). Family resilience in childhood cancer. *Family Relations. 51,* 103-111.

102. McGuire, B. K., Crowe, T. K., Law, M., & VanLeit, B. (2004). Mothers of children with disabilities: Occupational concerns and solutions. *OTJR: Occupation, Participation and Health, 24,* 54-63.

103. McIntosh, J., & Runciman, P. (2008). Exploring the role of partnership in the home care of children with special health needs: Qualitative findings from two service evaluations. *International Journal of Nursing Studies, 45,* 714-726.

104. McKay, E. A. (2004). Mothers with mental illness: an occupation interrupted. In S. A. Escaile & J. A. Olson (Eds.), *Mothering occupations: Challenge, agency, and participation* (pp. 238-258). Philadelphia: F.A. Davis.

105. McLanahan, S., Garfinkel, I., Reichman, N., Teitler, J., Carlson, M., & Audigier, C. N. (2003). *The fragile families and child wellbeing study: Baseline national report.* Retrieved March 18, 2008, from http://www.fragilefamilies.princeton.edu/publications.asp

106. McWilliam, R. A., Tocci, L., & Harbin, G. L. (1998). Family-centered services: Service providers' discourse and behavior. *Topics in Early Childhood and Special Education, 18*(4), 206-221.

107. Meadow-Orlans, K. P. (1995). Sources of stress for mothers and fathers of deaf and hard of hearing infants. *American Annals of the Deaf, 140*(4), 352-357.

108. Melamed, B. G. (2002). Parenting the ill child. In M. H. Bornstein (Ed.), *Handbook of parenting* (2nd ed., Vol. 5, pp. 329-348). Mahwah, NJ: Lawrence Erlbaum.

109. Merenstein, D., Diener-West, M., Krist, A., Pinneger, M., & Cooper, L. A. (2005). An assessment of the shared-decision model in parents of children with acute otitis media. *Pediatrics, 116,* 1267-1275.

110. Meyer, D. J., & Vadasy, P. F. (1994). *Sibshops: workshops for siblings of children with special needs.* Baltimore: Paul H. Brookes.

111. Missiuna, C., Moll, S., King, S., King, G., & Law, M. (2007). A trajectory of troubles: Parents' impressions of the impact of developmental coordination disorder. *Physical & Occupational Therapy in Pediatrics, 27*(1), 81-101.

112. Morton, K. (1985). Identifying the enemy: A parent's complaint. In H. R. Turnbull & A. Turnbull (Eds.), *Parents speak out: Now and then* (pp. 143-148). Columbus, OH: Merrill.

113. Murphy, K. E. (1997). Parenting a technology assisted infant: Coping with occupational stress. *Social Work in Health Care, 24*(3/4), 113-126.

114. Murray, M., Bynum, M. S., Brody, G. H., Willert, A., & Stephens, K. (2001). African American single mothers and children in context: A review of studies on risk and resilience. *Clinical Child and Family Psychology Review, 4,* 133-155.

115. Nagy, S., & Ungerer, J. (1990). The adaptation of mothers and fathers to children with cystic fibrosis: A comparison. *Children's Health Care, 19*(3), 147-154.

116. Nastro, M. (1992). *An ethnographic study of mothers of children with cerebral palsy and the effect of occupational therapy intervention on their lives.* Unpublished master's thesis, Ohio State University, Columbus.

117. National Center for Health Statistics. (2000). *Unmarried Childbearing.* Retrieved July 2003 from www.cdcgov/nchs/fastats/unmarry.htm

118. Ninio, A., & Rinott, N. (1988). Fathers' involvement in the care of their infants, and their attributions of cognitive competence to infants. *Child Development, 59,* 652-663.

119. O'Keefe, N., & O'Hara, J. (2008). Mental health needs of parents with intellectual disabilities. *Current Opinion in Psychiatry, 21*(5), 463-468.

120. Olsson, M. B., & Hwang, C. P. (2001). Depression in mothers and fathers of children with intellectual disability. *Journal of Intellectual Disability Research, 45,* 535-543.

121. Opacich, K., & Savage, T. A. (2004). Mothers with chronic illness: reconstructing occupation. In S. A. Escaile, & J. A. Olson (Eds.), *Mothering occupations: Challenge, agency, and participation* (pp. 217-237). Philadelphia: F.A. Davis.

122. Oswald, R. F., & Culton, L. S. (2003). Under the rainbow: Rural gay life and its relevance for family providers. *Family Relations, 52,* 72-81.

123. Parish, S. L., Cloud, J. M. (2006). Child care for low-income school-age children: Disability and family structure effects in a national sample. *Children and Youth Services Review, 28,* 927-940.

124. Parish, S. L., & Cloud, J. M. (2006). Financial well-being of young children with disabilities and their families. *Social Work, 51*(3), 223-232.

125. Park, C. A. (1998). Lesbian parenthood: A review of the literature. *American Journal of Orthopsychiatry, 68,* 376-389.

126. Parke, R. D. (2002). Fathers and families. In M. H. Bornstein (Ed.), *Handbook of parenting* (2nd ed., Vol. 3, pp. 27-74). Mahwah, NJ: Lawrence Erlbaum.

127. Patterson, C. J. (2002). Lesbian and gay parenthood. In M. H. Bornstein (Ed.), *Handbook of parenting* (2nd ed., pp. 317-338). Mahwah, NJ: Lawrence Erlbaum Associates.

128. Patterson, J. M. (2002). Integrating family resilience and family stress theory. *Journal of Marriage and Family, 64,* 349-360.

129. Patterson, J. M., & Blum, R. W. (1996). Risk and resilience among children and youth with disabilities. *Archives of Pediatric Adolescent Medicine, 1150,* 692-698.

130. Patterson, J. M., Garwick, A. W., Bennett, F. C., & Blum, R. W. (1997). Social support in families of children with chronic conditions: Supportive and nonsupportive behaviors. *Developmental and Behavioral Pediatrics, 18,* 383-391.

131. Piggot, J., Hocking, C., & Paterson, J. (2003). Parental adjustment to having a child with cerebral palsy and participation in home therapy programs. *Physical & Occupational Therapy in Pediatrics, 23*(4), 5-29.

132. Porterfield, S. L. (2002). Work choices of mothers in families with children with disabilities. *Journal of Marriage and Family, 64,* 972-981.

133. Powers, K., Hogansen, J., Geenen, S., Powers, L. E., & Gil-Kashiwabara, E. (2008). Gender matters in transition to adulthood: A survey study of adolescents with disabilities and their families. *Psychology in the Schools, 45*(4), 349-364.

134. Rivers, J. W., & Stoneman, Z. (2003). Sibling relationships when a child has autism: Marital stress and support coping. *Journal of Autism and Developmental Disorders, 33*(4), 383-394.

135. Rogoff, B. (2003). *The cultural nature of human development.* New York: Oxford University Press.

136. Sameroff, A. J., & Fiese, B. H. (2000). Transactional regulation: The developmental ecology of early intervention. In J. P. Shonkoff & S. J. Meisels (Eds.), *Handbook of early childhood intervention* (2nd ed. pp. 135-159). New York: Cambridge University Press.

137. Schimoeller, G. L., & Baranowski, M. D. (1998). Intergenerational support in families with disabilities: Grandparents' perspective. *Families in Society: The Journal of Contemporary Human Services, 79,* 465-476.

138. Schteingart, J. S., Molnar, J., Klein, T. P., Lowe, C. B., & Hartmann, A. H. (1995). Homelessness and child functioning in the context of risk and protective factors moderating child outcomes. *Journal of Clinical Child Psychology, 24,* 320-331.

139. Schultz-Krohn, W. (2004). Meaningful family routines in a homeless shelter. *American Journal of Occupational Therapy, 58*(5), 531-542.

140. Schulz, J. B. (1985). The parent-professional conflict. In H. R. Turnbull, & A. P. Turnbull (Eds.), *Parents speak out: Then and now* (2nd ed., pp. 3-22). Columbus, OH: Merrill.

141. Seccombe, K., James, D., & Walters, K. B. (1998). "They think you ain't much of nothing": The social construction of the welfare mother. *Journal of Marriage and the Family, 60,* 849-865.

142. Segal, R. (2000). Adaptive strategies of mothers with children with ADHD: Enfolding and unfolding occupations. *American Journal of Occupational Therapy, 54,* 300-306.

143. Segal, R. (2004). Family routines and rituals: A context for occupational therapy interventions. *American Journal of Occupational Therapy, 58*(5), 499-508.

144. Segal, R., & Beyer, C. (2006). Integration and application of a home treatment program: A study of parents and occupational therapists. *American Journal of Occupational Therapy, 60*(5), 500-510.

145. Segal, R., & Hinojosa, J. (2006). The activity setting of homework: An analysis of three cases and implications for occupational therapy. *American Journal of Occupational Therapy, 60*(1), 50-59.

146. Shonkoff, J. P., & Phillips, D. A. (2000). *From neurons to neighborhoods: The science of early childhood development.* Washington, DC: National Academy Press.

147. Skogrand, L. & Shirer, K. (2007). Working with low-resource and culturally diverse audiences. *The Forum for Family and Consumer Issues, 12*(1), Retrieved March 25, 2008, from http://ncsu.edu/ffci/publications/2007/v12-n1–2007-spring/skogrand-shirer/fa-9-skogrand-shirer.php.

148. Smith, L. K., Draper, E. S., Manktelow, B. N., Dorling, J. S., & Field, D. J. (2007). Socioeconomic inequalities in very preterm birth rates. *Archives of Disease in Childhood—Fetal and Neonatal Edition, 92,* F11-F14.

149. Spagnola, M., & Fiese, B. H. (2007). Family routines and rituals: A context for development in the lives of young children. *Infants & Young Children, 20*(4), 284-299.

150. Spratt, E. G., Saylor, C. F., & Macias, M. M. (2007). Assessing parenting stress in multiple samples of children with special needs (CSN). *Families, Systems, & Health, 25*(4), 435-449.

151. Stacey, J., & Biblarz, T. J. (2001). How does the sexual orientation of parents matter? *American Sociological Review, 66,* 159-183.

152. Steinberg, L., & Silk, J. S. (2002). Parenting adolescents. In M. H. Bornstein (Ed.), *Handbook of parenting* (2nd ed., Vol. 1, pp. 103-133). Mahwah, NJ: Lawrence Erlbaum.

153. Stewart, D., Law, M., Burke-Gaffney, J., Missiuma, C., Rosenbaum, P., King, G., et al. (2006). Keeping It Together™: An information KIT for parents of children and youth with special needs. *Child: Care, Health & Development, 32,* 493-500.

154. Stoneman, Z. (2001). Supporting positive sibling relationships during childhood. *Mental Retardation and Developmental Disabilities Research Reviews, 7,* 134-142.

155. Suarez-Orozco, C., Todorova, L. G., & Louie, J. (2002). Making up for lost time: The experiences of separation and reunification among immigrant families. *Family Process, 41,* 625-643.

156. Summers, J. A., Dell'Oliver, C., Turnbull, A. P., Benson, H., Santelli, E., Campbell, M., et al. (1990). Examining the individualized family service plan process: What are family and practitioner preferences? *Topics in Early Childhood Special Education, 10*(2), 78-99.

157. Tetreault, S., Parrot, A., & Trahan, J. (2003). Home activity programs in families with children presenting with global developmental delays: Evaluation and parental perceptions. *International Journal of Rehabilitation Research, 26,* 165-173.

158. Trent-Stainbrook, A., Kaiser, A. P., & Frey, J. R. (2007). Older siblings' use of responsive interaction strategies and effects on their younger siblings with Down syndrome. *Journal of Early Intervention, 29*(4), 273-286.

159. Trivette, C. M., & Dunst, C. J. (2005). DEC recommended practices: Family-based practices. In S. Sandall, M. L. Hemmeter, B. J. Smith, & M. E. McLean (Eds.), *DEC recommended practices: A comprehensive guide for practical application in early intervention/early childhood special education* (pp. 107-126). Missoula, MT: Division for Early Childhood.

160. Turnbull, A. P., Blue-Banning, M., Turbiville, V., & Park, J. (1999). From parent education to partnership education: A call for a transformed focus. *Topics in Early Childhood Education, 19,* 164-172.

161. Turnbull, A. P., & Ruef, M. (1997). Family perspectives on inclusive lifestyle issues for people with problem behavior. *Exceptional Children, 63,* 211-227.

162. Turnbull, A. P., Summers, J. A., Turnbull, R., Brotherson, M. J., Winton, P., Roberts, et al. (2007). Family supports and services in early intervention: A bold vision. *Journal of Early Intervention, 29*(3), 187-206.

163. Turnbull, A. P., Turbiville, V., & Turnbull, H. R. (2002). Evolution of family-professional partnerships: Collective empowerment as the model for the early twenty-first century. In J. P. Shonkoff & S. J. Meisels (Eds.), *Handbook of early childhood intervention* (2nd ed., pp. 630-650). New York: Cambridge University Press.

164. Turnbull, A. P., & Turnbull, H. R. (1990). *Families, professions and exceptionality: A special partnership* (pp. 156-157). Columbus, OH: Merrill.

165. Turnbull, A. P., & Turnbull, H. R. (1997). *Families, professionals, and exceptionality: A special partnership.* (3rd ed.). Columbus, OH: Merrill.

166. Turnbull, A., & Turnbull, R., Erwin, E. J., Soodak, L. C. (2006). *Families, professionals, and exceptionality: Positive outcomes through partnerships and trust* (5th ed.). Columbus, OH: Merrill.

167. Tymchuk, A. J., Andron, L., & Unger, O. (1987). Parents with mental handicaps and adequate child care: A review. *Mental Handicap, 15,* 49-54.

168. U.S. Bureau of the Census. (2002). 169. *America's families and living arrangements: Population characteristics.* Retrieved August 2003 from www.census.gov U.S. Department of Commerce Economics and Statistics Administration

169. Valencia, L. S., & Cromer, B. A. (2000). Sexual activity and other high-risk behaviors in adolescents with chronic illness: A review. *Journal of Pediatric and Adolescent Gynecology, 13,* 53-64.

170. VanLeit, B., & Crowe, T. K. (2002). Outcomes of an occupational therapy program for mothers of children with disabilities: Impact on satisfaction with time use and occupational performance. *American Journal of Occupational Therapy, 56,* 402-410.

171. Wacharasin, C., Barnard, K. E., & Spieker, S. J. (2003). Factors affecting toddler cognitive development in low-income families: Implications for practitioners. *Infants and Young Children, 16,* 175-187.

172. Walker, S. (2002). Culturally competent protection of children's mental health. *Child Abuse. Review, 11,* 380-393.

173. Wall, S., Kisker, E. E., Peterson, C. A., Carta, J. J., & Jeon, H. (2006). Child care for low-income children with disabilities: Access, quality, and parental satisfaction. *Journal of Early Intervention, 28*(4), 283-298.

174. Walsh, F. (2002). A family resilience framework: Innovative practice applications. *Family Relations, 51,* 130-137.

175. Walsh F. (Ed.). (2003). *Normal family processes: Growing diversity and complexity* (3rd ed.). New York: Guilford Press.

176. Weiss, K. L., Marvin, R. S., & Pianta, R. C. (1997). Ethnographic detection and description of family strategies for child care: Application to the study of cerebral palsy. *Journal of Pediatric Psychology, 22,* 263-278.

177. Williams, L. (2007). The many roles of families in family-centered care—Part III. *Pediatric Nursing, 33*(2), 144-146.

178. Williams, P. D., Williams, A. R., Graff, J. C., Hanson, S., Stanton, A., Hafeman, C., et al. (2002). Interrelationships among variables affecting well siblings and mothers in families of children with chronic illness or disability. *Journal of Behavioral Medicine, 25,* 411-424.

179. Young, D. M., & Roopnarine, J. L. (1994). Fathers' childcare involvement with children with and without disabilities. *Topics in Early Childhood Special Education, 14*(4), 488-502.

A Parent's Perspective

Beth Ball

When I was first asked to contribute to this chapter, I reflected on the myriad experiences and feelings that have emerged as a result of having children with disabilities. This seemed too vast a topic to be captured in a few typed pages. The following is a brief glimpse into my thoughts and feelings about life with my three children. There is much more than facts or history about our lives. There is, of course, emotion—deep and undeniable—and there is poetry. There is the first shed tear of realization that my child will have a life that is more difficult than most. There is the happy smile of childhood shared with supportive therapists and teachers. There is the frustrated panic of adolescence, when social situations are hard and troublesome and the phone does not ring on Saturday night.

INITIAL RESPONSE

Learning about the disabilities of each of my children came at different times in their lives. The impact varied because of the timing of the news and the disability of each child. Benjamin was born on a warm June day in 1971. On the delivery table, the nurse turned the mirror away, and I didn't understand why I couldn't see the baby. Everything seemed to happen in slow motion. The physician held him up and announced that he was a boy, but there was a small problem. His right arm tapered from the elbow to a thumb-like digit for a right hand, and his left arm ended in a modified claw hand, having a center cleft halfway into his palm and syndactyl webbing between the outside fingers.

The nurse placed him on my tummy, and he peed a fountain all over the sterile drapes. She said, "That works," which was comforting, but scary, because I considered that other things could be wrong. It was not until that night when I had him all to myself in the privacy of my own room that I felt the bifid femur of his right leg; the block at his knee that refused to let it extend; the very thin lower leg, which turned out to be missing the tibia; and the clubfoot. I discovered these problems one at a time. The sick feeling in my stomach was guilt. There must have been something that I had done wrong that had caused this. Even though I had followed all the doctor's instructions, I must have missed something. What would everyone think? I must not be good enough to have a child.

Mick, my husband, and I were lucky to have a wonderful pediatrician whose first advice was exactly what we needed to hear. He told us not to withdraw from our family and friends (alluding to the feelings of shame and guilt that we had not overtly expressed). He told us to allow them to give us support—they would only want to help. The unspoken message that they would not judge us was very important.

And so we started on our journey of new experiences with orthopedic surgeons, prosthetists, genetic counselors, neurologists, urologists, internists, and pediatricians. Later came more professionals, occupational therapists, physical therapists, ENT (ear, nose, and throat) specialists, vision therapists, special education teachers, and psychologists. We searched for answers to "Why?" We searched for options to deal with the issues of discrepancies in leg length and hand function. We searched for resolution to our own feelings. But we were fortunate because, as husband and wife, we never blamed each other.

Mick and I started the journey together, and we have always turned to each other for support. Sometimes it was an "us against the world" attitude and a fierce, protective response that got us through the hard times. When joyous times came, they did so with the realization that it had taken all our efforts to get there. The reason that we have been able to deal with the problems and come out on top is that we have a commitment to each other and a deep faith in God. This statement is much too simplistic for the deep feelings of need, grace, and oneness that we have. This oneness has allowed us to go forward to meet challenges as they have come.

Another reason we have been able to go forward is that we see each of our children as a gift. They are grace without gracefulness. They are charm without all the social skills. They are fun with a sometimes struggling sense of humor. They are individuals who have enriched our lives and given us humility, wonder, and awe at their commitment to living, loving, and succeeding.

ACCESSING SERVICES AND RESOURCES

Gaining services and resources for our children has not come without pain, questioning, depression, and anger. It has been a struggle that has required persistence and patience. We faced the first barrier when we attempted to find the money to cover the costs of prosthetics for our son. When we were told that it would be better to amputate Benjy's leg above the knee than to try to keep it and work through the lack of joints and musculature, we were also told about the costs of prosthetics. One of the first things our orthopedic surgeon told us was that we needed to find a source of funding, because prosthetics would cost more than a small house by the time Benjy was 16. I will not go into all the details, but parents have to be persistent if they do not know where to turn to find funds. The doctors have a few ideas, but they are not the best source of information in this area. Agencies and hospitals may have more information, but getting connected to the right person to gain the information is not an easy task.

In the search for money to cover the costs of prosthetics, we approached a well-known agency that worked with individuals who had physical disabilities. This agency had fund-raising campaigns that were earmarked for this purpose. After being told that providing prosthetics was not among its services, and because this was the third or fourth rejection that we had encountered, Mick broke down and joined me in some tears. We were then informed by the agency personnel that we had better pull ourselves together. This was our child and our responsibility, and we had better "face it." Shame turned to anger as we left. I felt judged, and included in the anger was the fear that we would not be able to provide for Benjy. How could this man judge us? Why didn't this administrator of an agency that provides services to children with disabilities and parents have more empathy for our situation? If he didn't help, then to whom could we turn?

This experience made us more leery of asking for assistance. Luckily, the Shriners accepted our application, and they provided most of the funds for Benjy's prosthetics until he turned 18. I do not want to think of what might have happened if we had not had their help. Dealing with financial issues created a new level of trauma that was added to our earlier pain. Because the Shriners helped with the finances for the prosthetics, we could focus our energy on education plans and homework and hope.

However, what we discovered from this process were the necessary and valuable aspects of networking. It was through work, friends, and family that we made contact with the Shriners. It was through people at school that we were put in touch with the local Special Education Regional Resource Center and became a part of the Parent Advisory Council. It was through many of the parents that we met in these places that we learned about the Ohio Coalition for the Education of Children with Disabilities. It has always been invaluable to us to be able to share with other parents who have similar feelings, frustrations, and breakthroughs. If it had not been for these people and these agencies, we would not have received the valuable personal, educational, and emotional support that we needed.

WHOSE DISTRESS, WHOSE STRUGGLE?

When my children were small, the feelings about their disabilities could be set aside for the new dream of having the brightest, cutest, most wonderful child with special needs. I dreamed of the well-spoken poster child. These dreams might have also been called denial and led others to believe that I was unaware of the true impact of my children's problems. In truth, that may have been, but I chose to live with faith.

The feelings do not come from the big picture of the disability. They come from all the little incidents. For example, when Benjy was 12 or 13 months old, I took him out of a nice, warm tub of sudsy water and stood his chubby, slippery little nude body next to the tub so that he could hold on while I toweled him dry. He stood straight and tall on his left leg, but as I watched, he tried to bear weight on his useless, dangling right leg. He bent his left leg so that his right toes touched the floor, and then he leaned forward to see why he could not reach the floor with his right foot. It was a moment of revelation for me. Until that moment, I think that all the focus had been on me: my inadequacy, my problem, my pain. This was harder; it was too deep even for tears. This was Benjy's life, *his* surgeries, *his* pain, and *his* inability to run swiftly through life. My role was and is to help and support him. Of course, every now and then, I have my own private pity party. However, it is not my pain that is the issue; it is theirs. Somehow, for me, there is a deeper pain in watching someone I love struggle than the pain I feel when struggling myself.

In our minds, Jessica, our second child, had no disabilities through her first 5 years of life. My dream was of a baby ballerina with grace and coordination. She did have four eye surgeries by age 5 (due to crossed eyes, muscle imbalance, and rotary nystagmus). During her preschool years, she attended a church-related preschool. At parent conference times, when the teacher would indicate problems or ask pointed questions about behaviors at home, I would justify Jessica's performance by telling myself, or Mick, that every surgery sets a child back about 3 months.

When Jessica was old enough to go to kindergarten, we were called into a special conference in which we were carefully told that she was not ready to do so. I did not hear anything else that day. The impact of that statement and the carefully worded explanation was like an icy shower. It was almost as if I had awakened from a dream with a clear vision of how disabled and delayed my daughter really was. I felt guilty and ashamed. I am an occupational therapist, and I know developmental milestones. I had let my doctor and others calm my fears about delays in walking, ataxia, and fine motor challenges because I did not want to believe that this second child of mine could have more than visual impairments. I was in denial for 5 years, helped by well-meaning people who did not want to hurt me.

The night after Jessica's conference, I received an answer to my prayer of "Where do I go from here?" I attended a presentation by Ken Moses, a psychologist and counselor who writes and speaks about parenting children with disabilities. I then experienced a new step on my journey. He spoke about the grief cycle and how we are grieving not for a lost child but for a lost dream. His discussion supported what I had been feeling and experiencing. The most important factor to me was the permission he gave me to feel the way I did. He emphasized how important denial is in helping us to deal with life-affecting decisions. He pointed out that denial buys us the time to gather our resources so that we can deal head on with problems.

Ken Moses also spoke about the importance of recognizing that anger gives us the energy to take action. Many times, my children's disabilities required so many appointments, surgeries, exercises, prescriptions, Individualized Education Program (IEP) meetings, and other details that I was left with only enough energy to put one foot in front of the other. I ignored, or put on hold, things or decisions that I should have taken care of immediately. Often it was anger that got me off my duff and sparked my determination to get things done. I learned that anger can actually help as long as it is not turned inward or unleashed on others. I came away from this talk with a sense of relief. To have these feelings was normal, and I was not a bad person, mom, or therapist.

Some parents believe that the word "denial" should not be used to describe parents' reactions to their children's disabilities. Instead they assert that parents' reactions are "hope." Denial has been a word that has allowed professionals to make judgments about parental actions. They have used the word denial when parents are not following through on something recommended or are having difficulty accepting decisions about educational programs or medical diagnoses. Having been on both sides of the table, I understand the issues. I have what I think is a realistic view that the word denial is not going to go away. Also, the spring of anticipation and hope for each of my children's futures cannot be erased by a word called denial. My hopes are real and if I choose to live with them, I don't mind if someone calls them denial. I embrace my whole journey and all aspects of my children. I can wallow with the best of them, dig in my heels, and go in the direction that I believe is right—no matter whether someone thinks I am denying reality. I believe that parents "in denial" need to hold onto their hope and/or don't yet have the resources they need to deal with their child's disability. So, dear OTs, give them some!

I have also recently come to believe that the stage, or being, or phase called denial by some comes from fear as well as hope. I have been afraid that I would not do the "right" things for my children. I wanted so much to allow them to be and do their best. I wanted for them to have the "right" experiences. I wanted them to experience the "right" education. I wanted them to be in the "right" situations. I wanted them to see the "right" doctors. In two recent meetings as an OT, as I explained about sensory processing and reflexive movement patterns affecting their child's ability to stay on task and to coordinate to perform motor tasks, both of the fathers cried. Each of them said that I was describing them, not their sons. They talked about their own experiences and how hard school had been for them. They explained how afraid they had been for their sons because of their own experiences. I told each of them how fortunate that his son had him for a father. Turning from being angry and defensive and letting go of the fears requires courage. Both of these fathers melted. What they heard was an explanation of their child's differences but explained with a belief in their potential. What I offered were resources and hope. Sometimes the fear in the room is palpable. It *is* within our ability to restore the link to the melody of hope that lies beneath.

Mick says that he believes, regardless of the words, parents' behaviors and attitudes are justified: "If the judgment word is denial, parents need that time to buy time to accumulate resources. If the word is hope, they need to be buoyed up out of some of the harsh realities. Empowerment of parents in impossible situations is a noble mission. As parents, we want to be powerful advocates and capable guardians. To do that, we need to be emotionally healthy and grounded in reality. We arrive at that point by working though the emotions associated with our disillusionment, our fear, our anger, and our denial to ultimately achieve acceptance and the feeling of victory at having arrived *each* time we encounter another in the endless series of emotion-filled transitions of life."

WHERE DO WE GO FROM HERE?

Decisions are forced on parents. There are medical decisions, therapy decisions, educational decisions, second opinion decisions, and decisions made in the middle of the night and in the emergency room. Some decisions are avoided until the last possible moment. Decision making starts immediately with a diagnosis or with the search for a diagnosis. What doctor should we use? What hospital? What about insurance? How much intervention do we need? How much do we want? What will *they* think if we say no to this thing that they think is important for our family? Is it important?

When Jessica was in elementary school, we would wait for the bus together. Each morning while sitting on our staircase landing, Jessica and I spent 20 minutes practicing eye exercises. Some days it was easy; other days Jessica would complain, resist, and attempt to divert my attention from the task. One day, when she was 7 or 8 years old, we were doing her exercises and discussing her braces, her eye surgery, and her occupational therapy session scheduled for that afternoon. She wanted to know for the thousandth time why we had to do these things. I explained that we were trying to fix things so she would have an easier time of it. She suddenly looked up at me and asked, "Is there anything about me that you don't have to fix?" I quickly named all of her gifts and attributes that I treasured. Later, as Jessica's bus turned the corner, I was left sitting on the steps with emptiness and guilt. I also had a new insight into the impact of countless therapy sessions, surgeries, and home programs.

This incident also made me face another aspect of denial. There is an unavoidable fact that there are some aspects of disabilities that cannot be fixed. I became an occupational therapist so that I could help people and make things better for them. I truly believed (and believe) that I could help eliminate some problems, that I could help heal hurts, and that I could provide training so that people could be more independent. Once I saw Jessica's problems, I was off and running. I wanted to make up for lost time. Fear drove me to leave no stone unturned if I thought that it would help Jessica get better. As a result of this revelation I stopped doing many of the recommended home programs. I found out that I needed to be "Mom" and others could be therapists. When professionals criticize parents for not following through on recommendations, I tell them that each family has its own story and now may be the time for regrouping and just being the Mom instead of the scheduler, therapist, taxi driver, MD, or counselor.

SCHOOL

Other than their child's medical issues, qualifying for special education is one of the greatest traumas parents of a special needs child will encounter. It was obvious that Benjy had an orthopedic handicap. However, to qualify for special education, we had to go through an intake process. Benjy had to be tested, and we waited with bated breath. He did qualify, and Benjy attended kindergarten through third grade in a school that had an orthopedic handicap program. He was in a self-contained classroom for disabled children until third grade.

When attention turned to education instead of surgeries and therapies, we found that physical disabilities are more apparent than learning disabilities (LDs). Soon our priorities switched to cognition and classroom skill building. During that time, Benjy was retained in first grade because the teachers had decided that he had a LD. This evaluation provided another chance for the ever-present grief cycle to jump up and bite us. Acceptance of the physical part of the disability was almost in place. However, this new evaluation crushed my new dream of having the brightest, most socially adept physically disabled child. I went through an equally bitter (if not more so) period of blame. Once again, I also feared for his success.

When Jessica was tested, *we* requested the testing because the preschool had prepared us for the possibility that she would have trouble learning. The school said that it was too early to find a discrepancy, but we pursued it, and one was found. She qualified for the learning-disabled program. For each of the next 5 years, Jessica's resource room moved from one school to another. This meant that each year, she had to adjust to a new building, new teachers, and new classmates. When Jessica was in fourth grade, we were told to take her to counseling because she was withdrawn and had no friends on the playground. Guess why? When she was in sixth grade, we moved to another district because it had neighborhood schools with special education resources in each building. There, too, the resource room for her particular grade level was not in the neighborhood school. She couldn't win! She still struggles with feelings of not belonging.

When Benjy was in the third grade, Mick and I decided that he would benefit from being in the regular classroom for most of his instruction. We were a little ahead of the curve regarding inclusion, and our request received quite a response! In 1980, Benjy was a pioneer. That year was difficult for us because we decided to change priorities to allow the learning-disabled program to meet his needs instead of the orthopedic handicapped program. One of the most intimidating places in the world is a room full of educators, including heads of programs, psychologists, teachers, occupational therapists, and physical therapists, and the only people who believe that you are doing the right thing for your child seem to be you and your spouse. Allowing the school's LD program to meet our son's needs turned out to be the right decision, but I still get stomach cramps when it is time for an IEP meeting (even an IEP meeting in which I am the occupational therapist).

Mick and I always helped our children with their homework and school projects. I rationalized that their success with their schoolwork would help them achieve in life. Their work ethic for school was high. Unfortunately, because we provided continual support in completing their homework, they never had the opportunity to fail. It is now very clear to me that children have to learn responsibility for themselves and that failure is a vital part of the learning process. I wanted to cushion my children's self-esteem by ensuring that they were successful in school. However, with the complex pattern of learning and growth, there is no clear path for children who have more challenges than most. Children with disabilities do need more help with schoolwork, but how much is too much? Lessons learned later are just as valuable, but they are more challenging because there is more at stake.

When we find ourselves making judgments about families, a red flag needs to go up. As was pointed out earlier in this chapter, each family has a different structure and different values. Decision making in each family is complicated and sacred. I know many people thought we were crazy when we decided to have a third child. Some were even brave enough to tell us so to our faces. Service providers held their breath, and educators looked for another Ball child in their classrooms. Having another child was a decision about which Mick and I prayed.

This time in our lives was like a pause in a heartbeat, filled with hope and fear but also with the knowledge that we were in it together.

Alexander was born on a cold day in February of 1981. He had no physical problems, but he was just as colicky as the other two children. He walked at 9 months and never stopped after that. He was very busy. In preschool meetings, I was the one to point out discrepancies in Alexander's progress. The teacher complimented me on being accepting, and I carefully informed her that I had been through this twice before and had not been as accepting then. I told her that that was okay, too. My children had not fallen off the face of the earth because it took time for me to face their delays. They were doing just fine, and parents need to be allowed to feel the way they do. However, that does not mean that professionals should not be honest with them!

Receiving sympathetic and respectful honesty from professionals is the only way to know I have all the facts before I make a decision. Honesty is a gift that you, as a therapist, give parents. It does not mean that parents will hear you, follow your suggestions, or even believe that you are always right. But your honest appraisal of the situation gives parents a piece of the picture and the truth that they need to help their child succeed. It helps if you take the time to listen to the parents' dreams or if you help them put words to those dreams. Many times I could not even express my dreams because they were caught under the lump of fear deep in my soul. There were, and still are, weeks that I cannot deal with the long term. I can only take it one crisis at a time. There are days when I do not even know that I have a dream for my children. But there are other days when I clearly see the life that my children may achieve, and that is where I like to be.

Alexander has turned out to be gifted and learning disabled, with attention deficit disorder and dyslexia. Auditory and visual processing problems and sensory defensiveness completed the picture. His disabilities were identified between kindergarten and first grade, again at our insistence. Alexander continues to reverse letters as he reads and writes. He often reads the end of words first. At age 9, he wrote out, in bold letters on a T-shirt, a commitment to avoid drugs: "Lust say on." Classic notes left for me on the kitchen counter often told me that his "homework is bone" or the "bog has ben out."

Alexander's disability has also been difficult for me and my husband. The feelings of loss and sadness that accompanied identification again resurfaced. Again I had to fight for services. I also had to watch him struggle through years of extra tutoring, vision therapy, and occupational therapy just to begin to decode words. Alexander has borne the burden of being the articulate, social child in the family. He has struggled with feelings of guilt that his disabilities are not as great as those of his siblings. He has received counseling to help him deal with these feelings as well as feelings of his own inadequacy.

However, part of Alexander's disability was a gift for me. He always needed books read to him for school. When he could not get a particular book on tape or he needed to complete one in a hurry, I spent time reading with him. We have shared insights on comparisons of religions, how Native Americans smoke peace pipes, and how to save yourself if you become lost in the middle of a forest. It has been cherished time that would not have occurred if he had the ability to read on his own.

GIFTS AND DREAMS

Recently I heard that old saying, "I'm playing the hand I've been dealt." I think that applies to all of us. It seems to me that everyone has many sources of distress in their lives. We, as the parents of children with disabilities, often focus on the delays and the fears. We should be allowed to feel the feelings that are associated with this situation. However, I think that you'll find that most of us are proud of our children's accomplishments: learning to put on a prosthesis independently, learning to turn a somersault, or hitting the right key on the keyboard to match the computer screen.

There are some things our children will never be able to do, activities they choose not to attempt. Jessica has chosen not to pursue bike riding. Benjy has chosen not to alternate his feet on the stairs. Alexander has chosen not to read piano music. All of these things would be next to impossible for them, but I never told them they couldn't do them. Parents are always in the position of encouraging the impossible. However, the reality is that it is the child who will ultimately determine what he or she can or cannot do. We have made and will make many mistakes parenting our children with disabilities, but we refuse to let their disabilities limit the possibilities.

I remember crying over *The Velveteen Rabbit* when I read it to the kids. It seemed that the problems of my children kept them from being "real" too. I knew that all the love I was showering on them could not change their physical makeup; however, I also knew that the love I was showering on them might help them cope with their "realness." Benjy has told me that he will run in heaven, and I believe that. I also know that all three of them run in their hearts every day here, and that others seeing them are challenged to be more themselves.

As part of my job, I was asked to evaluate a student who had hands similar to Benjy's "claw" hand. He had a hearing impairment, and the special education team met to determine how best to serve him in the school setting. When we sat down in the meeting, one of my colleagues made a comment about his hands. She said she couldn't understand why his parents didn't have his hands "fixed"—they looked so strange. I sucked in a breath and my heart pounded. I could not respond. I felt immobilized in my chair, without a voice. How did my colleague have the right to judge that the boy's hands needed fixing? My pounding heart was accompanied by the resounding thought, "He has a right to those hands, his hands. He has a right to be different." In part I had these feelings because I had evaluated his hand skills and knew that despite how different his hands appeared, he was able to use them skillfully. Only after the meeting was I able to express what I thought and felt. I realized that this person had made the comment because she thought that "fixing" his hands would take away the staring and teasing that always accompany looking different.

To express my feelings, I wrote my colleague a letter. In it I explained that my husband and I had made the decision to increase function in Benjy's left hand when he was 7 months old, wishing it would look more like everyone else's. It was hard to admit that I had those feelings. I told her that Benjy's right arm, which we affectionately call "Super Pinky," will never look like everyone else's. I told her about the scars on his hand and the scars on his wrist from the site where the graft skin was taken. I talked about Benjy's surgery allowing for a little stronger grasp but not full extension or flexion. I told her that the young man about whom she had commented had an adapted grasp for scissors and functional cutting skills.

My letter also explained that this is a bigger issue than hands; it is about attitudes. I see our roles as professionals who work with children who are different as teaching not only the children, but also everyone else. The message about our kids needs to be that *different is not worse, just different.* I know that people have the capacity to be open to difference. If we lived in a perfect world, all differences would be OK, and we would not feel that we have to fix them. However, we live in the ever-present face-lift, nose fix, and "Extreme Makeover" society. People are judged on their appearance. Part of our role as professionals is to learn to accept differences, particularly in appearance, and not to try to fix everything. Our job is to help others understand that different is not wrong. This is a very simplistic view of a complex problem.

When I told Benjy about the incident, he said, "That person is not cold. She just doesn't know all the facts. If God wanted everyone to look like everyone else, He wouldn't have made handicapped people. There have been times when I wanted to look like everyone else. True people are the ones who remember you for more than your physical side, and that's what really matters. True people are able to look at you and not think you are different, but that you are unique."

Benjy is now 31 and has married a young lady with spina bifida. He has a new diagnosis of spinal muscle atrophy. He is gradually losing function in his remaining leg. He and I are in denial about this, but we know that we have always taken one day at a time. He and his wife are working toward independence in all areas of their lives. Jessica is working in a grocery and has had several poems published. Alexander is a carpentry apprentice, married to a wonderful young lady, and has a beautiful daughter and a new son. As parents of children with disabilities, we continue to be very involved in our children's lives beyond the usual time. My dreams for them remain the same as when they were small: that they will be happy, that they will be as independent as they can be, and that they will always have someone who loves them. As the kids have grown into adults, we have had to practice involvement and support—without control. We also continue to deal with emotions, because the disabilities our children have are for life.

In all stages and at all ages, families of people with disabilities value support and resources. If you take the time to hear a parent's dream, you may hear the sound of laughter and tears. You may hear the strong heartbeat of anger or the resistance to a life that is less than it could be. As a therapist, you are a gift to the parents whose lives you touch. You have a solution to some of their frustrations. You can help uncover the hope. You have the opportunity to be as honest as you can be and provide them with the information they need to make decisions. You have the answer to some parent's question.

Thank you.

Beth Ball is the mother of three children with disabilities. She is also an occupational therapist and has worked in the public school system for a number of years.

Common Conditions That Influence Children's Participation

Sandra L. Rogers

Burn injury
Cardiopulmonary dysfunctions
Depression and suicide
Developmental disabilities
Infectious conditions
Musculoskeletal disorders
Neuromuscular disorders

Pediatric obesity
Pervasive developmental disorder (PDD)/autism spectrum disorder (ASD)
Toxic agents
Traumatic brain injury (TBI)

1. Describe the incidence, signs and symptoms, causes, and pathologic conditions of common medical diagnoses in children.
2. Describe the primary medical conditions associated with major developmental disabilities.
3. Explain how functional performance is affected by various medical, pathologic, and developmental conditions.
4. Explain precautions and special considerations for working with children who have specific medical conditions and/or developmental disabilities.

This chapter is intended to familiarize the occupational therapist with some of the major medical conditions, diseases, and disabilities of children who receive occupational therapy services. Pediatric conditions can be differentiated in several ways: congenital or acquired, acute or chronic, stable or aggressive, discrete or pervasive, occurring at different stages of development, or according to body systems affected. None of these alone is totally satisfactory; however, the body systems approach is the simplest and most useful for educational and reference purposes.

The chapter is therefore organized in a body systems format; it also includes sections on traumatic brain injury, neurodevelopmental disorders, burn injury, and pervasive developmental disorders. The chapter provides information on the incidence

and prevalence, signs and symptoms, causes, pathologic abnormalities, general medical treatment, and prognosis of the conditions described. Functional performance and treatment issues are also introduced. Pediatric psychiatric conditions are reviewed in Chapter 13, and neonatal medical conditions are described in Chapter 22. No single chapter can provide complete information about all conditions that may affect children. Many of the other chapters detail the appropriate occupational therapy evaluation, planning, treatment, and follow-up guidelines for specific conditions. A list of more comprehensive medical texts is provided at the end of the chapter.

CARDIOPULMONARY DYSFUNCTIONS

Cardiopulmonary dysfunctions are conditions that affect the cardiac and respiratory systems of the infant and child; they include congenital and acquired conditions that affect the child's health and ability to participate fully in life's occupations and roles.

Congenital Heart Disease

Most cardiac problems in children are congenital or occur secondary to other conditions. These disorders are serious, frightening, and sometimes life-threatening. This section discusses several of the major common anomalies found in the heart and major vessels.

Congenital heart disease is the major cause of death in the first year of life (other than prematurity) and occurs in approximately 9.6 children per 1000 births.[27] Heart defects are also common components of syndromes and have a higher prevalence in chromosomal disorders. The cause of most congenital heart defects is unknown, but numerous studies have linked congenital heart disease to specific chromosomal abnormalities, and several diseases have been linked to specific gene defects.

Three major cardiovascular changes must take place at birth. The foramen ovale, the hole between the right and the left atria, must close. In addition, the ductus arteriosus and the ductus venosus must close to allow blood to flow to the lungs and to the liver, respectively. Many complications can arise if these changes do not occur. Another cardiovascular complication that may occur during the perinatal period is *intracranial hemorrhage*. This condition may occur prenatally, during the birth process, or postnatally. The site and the extent of the bleeding affect the prognosis. For example, extracranial bleeding, resulting in *cephalohematoma*, is considered minor and usually does not cause permanent damage. Conversely, subdural, subarachnoid, and intraventricular hemorrhages are more serious and, depending on the extent of damage, may cause seizures, brain damage, cerebral palsy, or death.[18]

Heart defects are classified according to the hemodynamic characteristics of blood flow deficits—that is, deficits that result in (1) increased pulmonary blood flow, (2) decreased pulmonary blood flow, (3) obstructed blood flow, or (4) mixed blood flow.[50] Deficits that increase the amount of pulmonary blood flow include one of the most common conditions found in premature newborns, *patent ductus arteriosus (PDA)*. In this condition the ductus arteriosus does not constrict, which can lead to heart failure and inadequate oxygenation of the brain. Treatment includes administration of the drug indomethacin, which often triggers closure of the arterial wall. Surgery follows if the drug is not an effective treatment.[18] The other major congenital malformations that result in an increase in pulmonary blood flow are *atrial septal defects (ASDs)* and *ventricular septal defects (VSDs)*. An ASD is an opening in the septum between the right and left atrial chambers (Figure 6-1). It can be of any size and can occur anywhere along the septum. Because of the opening, when the left atrium contracts, blood is sent into the right atrium; this is called a *left-to-right shunt*. Left-to-right shunts cause more blood than normal to be sent to the lungs, resulting in *wet lungs*, a condition that makes the lungs more susceptible to upper respiratory infection. A left-to-right shunt also causes the right atrium, and especially the right ventricle, to work much harder and eventually can cause heart failure in the older child. Symptoms include poor exercise tolerance and small size for age. Information for diagnosis is gathered from the physical examination (i.e., detection of the characteristic heart murmur), evaluation of chest x-ray films and electrocardiograms, and the use of echocardiography or heart catheterization.[18]

Surgical procedures are implemented if the child is in distress. The surgery may be performed early, or it may be postponed until the child is 4 or 5 years of age. Until that time the child is watched closely for complications, especially for signs of heart failure.[18] VSDs are the most common type of congenital cardiac malformation and are often more serious than ASDs. A VSD consists of a hole or opening in the muscular or membranous portions of the ventricular septum (Figure 6-2).

In a VSD, the blood flows from the left ventricle to the right ventricle (a left-to-right shunt), and as in an ASD, an increased amount of blood is pumped to the lungs. The defect is considered less serious if the opening is in the membranous section of the septum and more serious if multiple muscular holes are present.[50]

Symptoms associated with VSDs include feeding problems, shortness of breath, increased perspiration, fatigue during physical activity, increased incidence of respiratory infections, and delayed growth. Causative factors are often idiopathic, but congenital infections, various teratogenic agents, and genetic predisposition may contribute.[92]

As with an ASD, the diagnosis of VSD is based on the murmur and on the findings of chest x-rays, electrocardiograms, echocardiograms, and heart catheterization. Improvement often occurs after 6 months of age, and more than 50% of cases correct themselves by 5 years of age.[92] However, if the extent of damage is great or if the hole does not repair itself, surgical procedures to close the defect may be needed early in the child's life.

Children with a VSD must be monitored carefully to avoid the life-threatening condition known as *Eisenmenger's complex*, in which pulmonary vascular obstruction can occur as a result of prolonged exposure to increased blood flow and high pressure. Eventually, the heart is no longer capable of pumping against the increased pulmonary pressure, the child goes into congestive heart failure, and blood pools in the right ventricle. This development is a medical emergency that requires immediate surgical intervention.

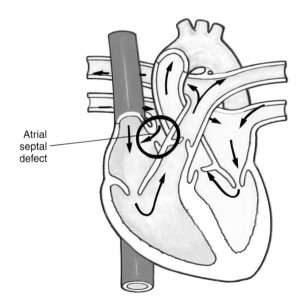

FIGURE 6-1 Atrial septal defect. (From Hockenberry, M. J. & Wilson, D. [2009]. *Wong's essentials of pediatric nursing* [8th ed.]. St. Louis: Mosby.)

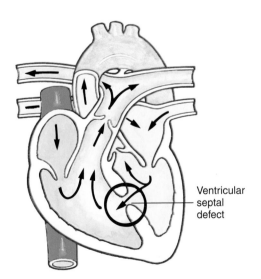

FIGURE 6-2 Ventricular septal defect. (From Hockenberry, M. J., & Wilson, D. [2009]. *Wong's essentials of pediatric nursing* [8th ed.]. St. Louis: Mosby.)

The prognosis for infants with VSDs continues to improve with advances in surgical techniques and the management of heart failure. These children are at risk for several serious complications, including cardiovascular accident (CVA), embolism, brain abscess, growth restriction, seizures, and death.[92]

Tetralogy of Fallot (TOF) is a defect of decreased pulmonary blood flow. As its name implies, TOF is associated with four different problems: (1) pulmonary valve or artery stenosis with (2) a VSD present prenatally, causing (3) right ventricular hypertrophy and (4) override of the ventricular septum by the aorta (Figure 6-3). Physiologically, the unoxygenated returning blood cannot exit easily to the lungs because of the pulmonary stenosis. Instead, it takes two paths of least resistance: the defect, creating a right-to-left shunt, and the aorta.[18]

Signs and symptoms of TOF include central cyanosis, coagulation defects, clubbing of the fingers and toes, feeding difficulties, failure to thrive, and dyspnea.[50] The cause of TOF is probably similar to that of VSD. The insult to the developing fetus is believed to occur in the early weeks of fetal development, when the right ventricle is at a critical stage.[92] The diagnosis of TOF is usually based on the presence of cyanosis; analysis of the heart murmur; electrocardiographic demonstration of right ventricular hypertrophy and right axis deviation; chest x-ray films that show the characteristic boot-shaped heart; and echocardiographic demonstration of the overriding aorta.[18,92]

TOF is managed initially with medication, and surgery is delayed as long as possible. In severe cases a temporary shunt may be inserted to bypass the stenosis. Usually the Blalock-Taussig surgical procedure is used until complete corrective surgery can be performed, in which the pulmonary outflow obstruction is removed, the VSD is closed, and the aorta may be enlarged. As with VSDs, the prognosis is improving as techniques and maintenance improve. The operative mortality rate

has been reduced from 10% to 5%, but the surgery is still a dangerous and complicated procedure.[50]

A common congenital heart defect that affects mixed pulmonary flow is *transposition of the great vessels (TGV),* also known as *transposition of the great arteries (TGA).* In this condition, the pulmonary artery leaves the left ventricle and the aorta exits the right ventricle, with no communication between the systemic and pulmonary circulations. The severity of the condition depends on the amount of circulatory mixing that occurs between the two sides. Circulatory mixing occurs as a result of coexisting congenital cardiac defects (e.g., a VSD or pulmonary stenosis) or congenital transposition of the ventricles, called *corrected transposition.*[92] The severity of the symptoms varies, but cyanosis, congestive heart failure, and respiratory distress are common.

The diagnosis of TGV is made through heart catheterization and through echocardiography; both procedures can identify the transposition. The condition is treated surgically. One technique involves enlargement of the foramen ovale. To accomplish this, a catheter with a balloon tip is inserted through the foramen ovale into the left atrium and then pulled back through the opening, enlarging it and thereby increasing the flow of oxygenated blood to the right atrium.[18] Another procedure involves excision of the atrial septum and insertion of a patch that redirects the blood flow. In a third, more recently developed technique, the great vessels are severed at their bases and reattached to the proper ventricles. The main pulmonary artery is anastomosed to the proximal aorta, and the ascending aorta is anastomosed to the proximal pulmonary artery.[92]

The operative mortality rate for TGV is 5% to 10%, regardless of the surgical procedure used. Later in life these children have been known to develop arrhythmias and ventricular dysfunctions.

A child with congenital cardiac defects that have not yet been repaired can be expected to have reduced endurance for exertion but may be normal in other ways. This child may want to participate in a range of self-care and play activities. Pacing and the selection of appropriate activities may be essential to the child's health and ability to participate in family and peer activities. After surgery and throughout life, general health maintenance is essential in these individuals, including a well-balanced diet, aerobic exercise, and avoidance of smoke inhalation.[18]

The occupational therapist may deal directly or indirectly with the consequences of congenital cardiac defects. For example, these defects are often secondary diagnoses in children with genetic syndromes. Children with Down syndrome or other types of cognitive impairment may have a history of congenital heart problems. In these cases, occupational therapists must be aware of associated signs and symptoms, treatment procedures, complications of medications, and the effect of the condition on the child's functioning.

Dysrhythmias

Irregular cardiac rhythms, or *dysrhythmias,* are not as common in children as in adults. However, the incidence of these problems is increasing, possibly because more children with congenital heart defects are surviving surgery, which may leave them with a residual dysrhythmia. The three classes of

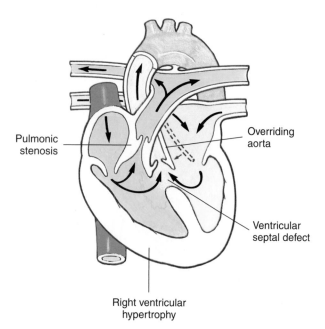

Pulmonic stenosis

Overriding aorta

Ventricular septal defect

Right ventricular hypertrophy

FIGURE 6-3   Tetralogy of Fallot.   (From Hockenberry, M. J., & Wilson, D. [2009]. *Wong's essentials of pediatric nursing* [8th ed.]. St. Louis: Mosby.)

dysrhythmia are bradydysrhythmia, tachydysrhythmia, and conduction disturbances. The diagnosis of dysrhythmia is based primarily on standard and 24-hour electrocardiographic monitoring.[92]

Bradydysrhythmia is an abnormally slow heart rate. The most common type is a complete heart block, or *atrioventricular (AV) block*. This condition is common after surgery or myocardial infarction and occasionally may require a pacemaker. Sinus bradycardia can be caused by anoxia or autonomic nervous system disorder. In this condition the child's heart rate may be reduced to less than 60 beats per minute (bpm), and extra beats and slow nodal rhythms also may be present.[92]

Tachydysrhythmia is an abnormally fast heart rate. Sinus tachycardia can be a sign of several other conditions, including fever, anxiety, anemia, and pain. *Supraventricular tachycardia (SVT)* is a heart rate of 200 to 300 bpm and is among the most common disturbances in children. SVT is a serious condition that can lead to congestive heart failure. The child with SVT is irritable, eats poorly, and is pale. In some cases a vagal maneuver, such as the Valsalva maneuver, can reverse the SVT, but in other cases the child may require hospitalization, esophageal overdrive pacing, or synchronized cardioversion.[50]

Conduction disturbances are common after surgery and may be temporary. Premature contractions may be atrial, ventricular, or junctional. These sometimes can be handled with interim or permanent pacing, depending on the nature and severity of the disturbance.[18]

Neonatal Respiratory Problems

Respiratory problems are common in newborns and can be dangerous. Some of these problems are acute, and others are considered chronic lung diseases. Respiratory distress problems may be caused by prematurity, aspiration of amniotic fluid or meconium, malformation or tumors of the respiratory organs, neurologic disease, central nervous system (CNS) damage, drugs, air trapped in the chest or pericardium (the sac surrounding the heart), and pulmonary hemorrhages.[44]

An acute respiratory problem often found in newborns, especially preterm infants, is *respiratory distress syndrome*. This disease is caused by a deficiency of *surfactant*, the chemical that prevents the alveoli from collapsing during expiration. Because surfactant is not produced until about the 34th to the 36th week of gestation, many premature infants are born with this deficiency. As the air sacs collapse, oxygen absorption and carbon dioxide elimination are hindered. Treatment includes administration of surfactant and supplemental oxygen, and ventilator support may be needed. Most infants begin to recover after 3 to 4 days of treatment, as the baby's body begins to produce surfactant. In some newborns, respiratory distress syndrome results in chronic lung problems.[103]

Chronic lung disease implies a long-term need for supplemental oxygen. A chronic lung disease often seen in neonatal centers is *bronchopulmonary dysplasia (BPD)*. These newborns have had some type of acute respiratory problem that required prolonged use of mechanical ventilation and other types of necessary but perhaps traumatic intervention. In BPD, the airways thicken, excess mucus forms, and alveolar growth is restricted. As a result, these children often are susceptible to respiratory infections and other respiratory problems. Problems such as BPD that are associated with the techniques used to save newborns' lives are called *iatrogenic disorders*.

The artificial respirators currently used are sophisticated machines that allow careful control of oxygen mixtures. They are designed to maintain a constant pressure on the alveoli, thus keeping them open in the absence of surfactant. This is known as *positive end-expiratory pressure (PEEP)*, which has significantly lowered the rate of fetal death and the overall risk of severe developmental delays.[103] Currently, many newborns with respiratory distress are given surfactant at birth, which allows them to breathe independently despite lung immaturity. Early administration of surfactant has greatly reduced the incidence of BPD and has reduced the mortality rate in very premature infants.

Asthma

Asthma is a chronic inflammatory disorder characterized by bronchial smooth muscle hyperreactivity that causes airway constriction in the lower respiratory tract, difficulty breathing, and bouts of wheezing. It is one of the most common long-term respiratory disorders of childhood. In most children with asthma, the first symptoms appear in early childhood, before 5 years of age.[83] Asthma appears to be an inherited trait and is often associated with familial patterns of allergy.

Exposure to an allergen, smoking, cold air, exercise, inhaled irritants, and viral infection may trigger asthma attacks.[50] The attacks are characterized by smooth muscle spasm of the bronchi and bronchioles and inflammation and edema of the mucous membranes, with accumulation of mucous secretions. The child has difficulty breathing, particularly in expiration; the forceful expiration through the narrowed bronchial lumen creates the characteristic wheezing. The child also has a hacking, nonproductive cough. This experience can be frightening for the child, and the symptoms may worsen in response to the panic. The effort of breathing may also result in sore ribs and exhaustion. *Status asthmaticus* is a serious asthmatic condition in which medications typically prescribed do not result in improvement and emergency medical intervention is needed.[44,83]

Treatment for asthma may include environmental control measures, skin testing, immunotherapy for allergies, emotional support, and a combination of pharmacologic agents, usually beta-adrenergic agonists and methylxanthine.[50,83] These drugs may be related to school performance problems and can cause dependency in some cases. Monitoring the child's schoolwork and teaching him or her about the use and abuse of the medications should minimize difficulties in this area. The goal of nonpharmacologic therapy is prevention, and occupational therapists can help prevent or reduce the child's exposure to airborne allergens and irritants in a therapy setting. The goal of pharmacologic therapy is to prevent or control asthma symptoms, reduce the frequency and severity of asthma exacerbations, and reverse airflow obstruction. Occupational therapists, therefore, should be knowledgeable about the use of asthma medications, including metered-dose inhalers.[83]

Children with asthma may be fearful of overexertion and may be concerned about contact with triggering allergens. This may result in a self-limiting lifestyle. Teaching the child to manage the condition, respond calmly to stress, and pace activities can be essential to maintaining a normal childhood pattern.

Structured peer group activities can also be useful in preventing social isolation. Breathing exercises, stretching, and controlled breathing can assist in management of the attacks.[83]

Cystic Fibrosis

The most common serious pulmonary and gastrointestinal problem of childhood is *cystic fibrosis (CF)*. This inherited autosomal recessive disorder is related to a gene located on chromosome 7. In the United States, the incidence of CF is 1 in 3500 births among white children and 1 in 17,000 births among African American children.[21] CF is a multisystem disease that appears to be related to an impermeability of epithelial cells to chloride; as a result, the exocrine (mucus-producing) glands malfunction, producing secretions that are thick, viscous, and lacking in water.[21] The thick secretions block the pancreatic ducts, bronchial tree, and digestive tract.

One of the earliest signs of CF, *meconium ileus,* occurs in the newborn. A thick, putty-like substance that cannot be eliminated blocks the small intestine.[50] The abdomen becomes distended, and the child is unable to pass stools; if the condition goes untreated, vomiting and dehydration occur.[21]

Chronic pulmonary disease is the most serious complication of CF. A chronic cough, wheezing, lower respiratory infections, abscesses and cysts, hemoptysis, and recurrent pneumothorax are examples of the serious pulmonary manifestations of CF. Other complications often include hypoxemia, nasal polyps, and enlargement of the right side of the heart (right ventricular hypertrophy), which eventually may cause heart failure.[50]

In addition, CF typically affects sodium absorption–inhibiting factor, and as a result, excessive amounts of sodium chloride are secreted from the sweat glands onto the skin. Mothers may detect a salty taste when they kiss their children. This may alert the physician, who can perform a simple diagnostic procedure known as the *sweat test.* For this test, an electrode is placed on the skin, causing the child to sweat at the contact site, and a sample of the sweat is taken. Detection of an excessive level of sodium chloride establishes the diagnosis.[50]

Pancreatic insufficiency causes characteristic foul-smelling, greasy stools. Associated problems include malabsorption; clinical diabetes; deficiencies of vitamins A, E, and K; and gastrointestinal obstruction. In the liver, bile ducts also become blocked, resulting in destruction of cells behind the blocked ducts. Although this is a serious problem, a positive point is that children's livers are often capable of regeneration.

Medical management of CF generally consists of vigorous pulmonary therapy, inhalation therapy, chest physical therapy, antibiotic therapy, bronchodilator therapy, anti-inflammatory treatment, endoscopy and lavage, and nutritional therapy.[21] Efforts are made to keep the lungs as free as possible of secretions; these may involve physical or respiratory therapy techniques such as mist tent therapy, intermittent positive-pressure breathing, aerosol therapy, and postural drainage techniques.[50]

A child with CF frequently spends time in and out of hospitals with various complications and for various treatments. These children may have a series of crises alternating with periods of comparative health, although a general degeneration occurs. Children whose primary symptoms are related to gastric inflammation have a better prognosis than those whose initial problems are related to respiratory functioning. All require a careful balance of nutrition, fluid intake, and exercise. Boys generally have a longer life span than girls, but degeneration of body functions and death occur for many in their teens and early twenties.[50] Early detection and treatment have been shown to prolong life. The child and family may need assistance in dealing with grief and impending death.

Medical, nursing, dietary, and respiratory therapy are central to the treatment of a child with CF. Respiratory therapists may play a key role by providing postural drainage, chest clapping, and chest expansion exercises. The occupational therapist may be concerned with energy conservation (activities that promote efficient breathing) and prevocational, recreational, and psychosocial support groups. Social, psychologic, and pastoral staff may provide essential family support.

MUSCULOSKELETAL DISORDERS

Bone tissue is one of the few body tissues that actively regenerate. The skeletal system is malleable; it deposits or reabsorbs bone based on the stresses it receives. Elements of the skeletal system include the bones, joints, cartilage, and ligaments. The muscular system includes the muscle fibers and their covering of fascia; it is activated by the nerves and moves the bones to create functional motion. Tendons connect the muscular and skeletal systems at the origins and insertions of the muscles.[109]

Bone is mesenchymal tissue. As the child develops, the bone is first laid down as either membranous or cartilaginous tissue and gradually becomes ossified through a calcium deposition process called *endochondral ossification.* The bones are initially formed early in fetal development. The growth and ossification processes in long bones occur at the epiphyseal plates; these structures, which are located at the ends of the bones and are covered in articular cartilage, form the associated joints. Growth and ossification continue until the age of 25 years, at which time the epiphyses fuse.[109] Bones without physeal plates (i.e., the pelvis, scapulae, carpals, and tarsals) grow by appositional bone growth from their surrounding perichondrium and periosteum. The bones of the spine, metacarpals, metatarsals, and phalanges grow by a combination of appositional and endochondral ossification.[113]

The musculoskeletal system can be affected by genetic and congenital disorders, trauma, infection, and metabolic, endocrine, circulatory, and neurologic disorders.[109] This section addresses some of the major musculoskeletal disorders.

Congenital Anomalies and Disorders

A relatively large number of the conditions that affect the musculoskeletal system have a genetic or congenital cause. These conditions often affect the child throughout life, causing disability, deformity, and sometimes death.

Osteogenesis imperfecta (OI), also called *brittle bones,* is a disorder characterized by decreased bone deposition caused by an inability to form type 1 collagen. In most cases, OI is transmitted by an autosomal dominant gene. However, the most severe fetal type has an autosomal recessive inheritance pattern.[73] This condition can run several different courses, from mild to severe, with most individuals having a milder form of the disease. OI has an incidence of 1 in 20,000 births.

TABLE 6-1 Age at Onset Effects of Osteogenesis Imperfecta

Type	Severity	Effect
Fetal	Most severe	Fractures occur in utero and during birth; mortality is high.
Infantile	Moderately severe	Many fractures occur in early childhood; severe limb deformities and growth disturbances also occur.
Juvenile	Least severe	Fractures begin in late childhood; by puberty, bones often begin to harden, and fewer fractures occur. Dental problems may be present.

In all cases, the bones are unusually fragile, and even minor trauma can cause a fracture. The severity of the disorder varies greatly, depending on the time of onset (Table 6-1). Multiple fractures or repeated fracture of the same bone may cause a limb to become misshapen and eventually muscularly underdeveloped because of the long periods of immobilization and disuse. Prevention must be attempted at least with padded arm and leg protectors and orthoses. Surgical insertion of metal rods and segmental osteotomies may be helpful for providing internal support and correcting deformities that may develop. As the child grows, the rods must be replaced to accommodate the growth.

Over time, children with OI can be expected to develop progressive deformities. In addition, their activity patterns are affected by caution and time spent in casts. With the fetal and infantile forms of the disorder, maternal education in handling and positioning is essential to prevent fractures during childcare activities. Children with OI need to be involved in monitored movement activity so that muscle strength and the postural effects of weight bearing and exercise can be achieved.[109] Children with less severe forms of OI may participate in many normal activities, including some sports. Novel treatments for OI are being tested. They include medications that stop bone resorption (and thereby increase bone density), bone marrow transplantation, and gene therapy to replace the incorrect message in collagen metabolism.[73]

Marfan's syndrome, or *arachnodactyly,* is an autosomal dominant trait marked by excessive growth at the epiphyseal plates (i.e., tall stature), arachnodactyly (the fingers are long, slender, and curved, resembling a spider's legs), skull asymmetry, and alterations in the joints, eyes, heart, and aorta. The incidence is 1 to 2 per 100,000 individuals. The joints are lax and hypermobile, and striated muscles are poorly developed. Visual problems are often present because of the dislocation of the lens.[109] Symptoms include increased height and decreased weight for age, excessively long extremities, scoliosis, coxa vara, depressed sternum, stooped shoulders, elastic skin, and fragility of the blood vessels. A child with Marfan's syndrome may begin walking later than usual because of decreased postural stability, but the child will not necessarily have developmental delays. Longevity is diminished because of cardiac complications. Treatment is symptomatic and addresses any skeletal deformities, such as scoliosis, that interfere with function.[88]

Achondroplasia, or *chondrodystrophia,* is the most common cause of dwarfism. Dwarfism is caused by stunting of epiphyseal plate growth and cartilage formation. Achondroplasia is an autosomal dominant trait, and frequent spontaneous mutations are known to occur. The limb bones continue to grow to appropriate widths but are abnormally short. Individuals with achondroplasia rarely grow to more than 4 feet in height. Although skull size is normal, face size may be small, with a prominent forehead and jaw and a small nose. Trunk growth is near normal. Skeletal abnormalities include lumbar lordosis, coxa vara, and cubitus varus. There is no cure for achondroplasia. Adults may experience back pain and occasionally paralysis caused by spinal stenosis. Surgical treatment occasionally may be necessary to relieve neurologic complications, improve functional movement, or correct extreme deformities.[109]

Arthrogryposis multiplex congenita is characterized by incomplete fibrous ankylosis, or contracture of many or all of the child's joints at birth. With amyoplasia, the primary form of arthrogryposis, both the upper and lower extremities are involved. The cause is unknown, but these children have few anterior horn cells in the spinal cord, which may indicate a neuropathic cause. The child has stiff, spindly, and deformed joints and may also have clubfoot, hip dislocation, or characteristic posturing. The knee and elbow joints may appear thickened, and muscles may be absent or incompletely formed. The anterior horn cells of the spinal cord may be absent, in which case the child may also experience paralysis. Treatment focuses on maintaining and increasing functional range of motion (ROM) and strength. Splints, serial casts, surgery, and daily stretching may be included in this regimen.[109] Adapted equipment and training for activities of daily living (ADLs), school, play, and work performance may assist the child in optimal functioning.

A common abnormality of the foot is *congenital clubfoot,* or *talipes equinovarus.* The incidence of congenital clubfoot is high (1 to 2 per 1000) and much higher when a sibling has clubfoot (1 in 35). Boys are affected twice as frequently as girls.[52,109] The pattern of presentation suggests inheritance through a single autosomal dominant gene. The condition may be unilateral or bilateral, and the major clinical features are forefoot adduction and supination, heel varus, equinus of the ankle, and medial deviation of the foot (Figure 6-4). Some of the bones involved may be malformed, and the muscles of the lower leg are often underdeveloped. In a small number of cases, paralysis and permanent deformity may be present.

In some cases, clubfoot is associated with other congenital problems and conditions, but the exact cause or causes of clubfoot are unclear. During fetal development, development of the muscles on the medial and posterior aspects of the legs is adversely affected, and as a result, these muscles are shorter than normal.[52] These contractions, in turn, lead to the bone and joint problems. The clubfoot deformity can be corrected with taping, the use of malleable splints, serial casting, or orthopedic surgery. The soft tissue surgeries may be combined with bony operations, such as arthrodesis of joints, osteotomies, and insertion of a bone wedge on the medial side of the calcaneus, to correct the line of weight bearing.[52] This treatment reduces foot mobility but increases function and stability. The prognosis is good for children who are treated early.

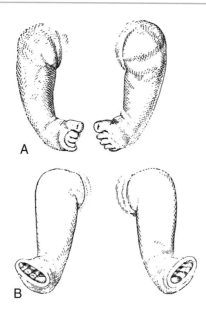

FIGURE 6-4 Bilateral congenital talipes equinovarus. **A**, Before correction. **B**, Undergoing correction in plaster casts. (From Brashear, H. R., & Raney, R. B. [1986]. *Handbook of orthopedic surgery* [10th ed., p. 39]. St. Louis: Mosby.)

The analogous condition in the upper extremity, *congenital clubhand,* is far less common and is associated with partial or full absence of the radius and bowing of the ulnar shaft. The radial musculature, nerves, and arteries may be absent or underdeveloped. Often the hand remains functional. Treatment includes progressive casting and ROM exercises, static or dynamic splinting, or surgery; however, these procedures provide more cosmetic than functional benefit. The child with congenital clubhand may occasionally require some training or adaptations for school or ADLs.[109]

Developmental dysplasia of the hip (congenital hip dislocation) is almost as common as clubfoot, having an incidence of 1.5 per 1000 live births.[53] The condition is often bilateral and occurs nine times more often in girls than in boys. The causes of congenital hip dislocation (head out of the socket) and subluxations (head partly out of the socket) are both genetic and environmental. Hip laxity may be genetically inherited or may be a result of a hormonal secretion of the uterus. Environmental factors related to hip dislocation include birth complications from uterine pressure and poor presenting positions. Dislocation or subluxation of the unstable hip also may be caused by sudden, passive extension or by positioning that keeps the legs extended and adducted.[50]

Early diagnosis of congenital dislocation of the hip is critical because delay can cause serious and permanent disabilities. Three clinical observations that may be used in diagnosing this condition in infants are Ortolani's sign, Galeazzi's sign, and Barlow's test. The result of the Barlow test (the most critical test for newborns) is considered positive if the unstable hip clicks out of the acetabulum when the leg is abducted and pressure is placed on the medial thigh.[109] Ortolani's sign is elicited by a maneuver to reduce a recently dislocated hip. For this maneuver, the infant's knees and hips are flexed, and the femur is alternately adducted and pressed downward and then abducted and lifted. If the hip is unstable, it dislocates when adducted but returns to the socket when abducted. The evaluator feels and often hears a click as this happens. With Galeazzi's sign, one knee is lower than the other when the child is placed in the supine position on a table with the knees flexed to 90 degrees. This results from the dislocated femur's lying posterior to the acetabulum.[53]

In the older child with congenital hip dislocation, Trendelenburg's sign is seen. With this sign, the hip drops to the opposite side of the dislocation and the trunk shifts toward the dislocated hip when the child is asked to stand on the foot of the affected side.[109]

If treatment is begun within the first few weeks of life, normal development of the hip nearly always can be ensured. The longer the dislocation goes unresolved, the poorer the prognosis. Specific treatment techniques vary according to the age of the client when treatment is initiated, but generally the techniques involve stabilizing the hip in an abducted and flexed position to facilitate femoral and acetabular development. This stabilization may be accomplished with splints, traction, the hip spica plaster cast, or the pillow splint.[53] If these methods do not correct the disorder, several surgical procedures may be performed to correct bony and soft tissue problems. In severe cases, arthrodesis or total replacement arthroplasty may be performed. Again, every infant should be examined for this deformity in the first weeks of life to prevent the complications this defect can cause.

Limb Deficiencies

Limb deficiencies in children are most commonly attributable to congenital malformations. A small number of cases are the result of accidents or of surgery to prevent the spread of cancer, such as Ewing's sarcoma. Congenital limb deficiencies occur more frequently in the upper extremities. Limb deficiencies and malformations may be familial or may result from early fetal insult or, rarely, from congenital constricting bands. With congenital constricting bands, the soft tissue and overlying skin on a small body part fail to grow in circumference. If the constriction is severe enough, the band stops distal limb circulation, causing gangrene and intrauterine amputation.[109] Traumatic amputations are becoming less common because of better emergency care and the improved ability of surgeons to reattach a traumatically removed body part. Congenital malformations of the hands or feet, usually in the fingers and toes, occur in 1 per 600 live births. According to the Centers for Disease Control and Prevention (CDC), more than 3200 infants are born with polydactyly, syndactyly, or adactyly each year.[85]

Polydactyly is an excess of fingers or toes. This is a relatively common condition that may involve one or more extra complete digits or duplication of only part of a digit. Bony changes may be present or just extra soft tissue. In most cases surgical amputation or reconstruction is performed early in childhood, particularly if the hand is involved. *Syndactyly,* or webbing between the fingers or toes, occurs frequently. It is most common in the upper extremity and in boys. It sometimes coexists with polydactyly, which makes repair more complicated. In simple cases, the fingers are surgically separated in early childhood (Skinner, 2006; Staheli, 2006).[108,109] Extensive hand therapy is usually unnecessary, although splinting and scar reduction may be helpful in some cases. *Bradydactyly* and *microdactyly* are overly large or small digits, respectively. Plastic surgery may be performed if the digits are unsightly or impair function.[109]

Congenital limb deficiencies include amelia, phocomelia, paraxial deficiency, and transverse hemimelia (Figure 6-5). *Amelia* is the absence of a limb or the distal segments of a limb. With *phocomelia*, the child may have a fully or partly formed distal extremity but is missing one or more proximal segments of the limb. With *paraxial deficiencies*, the proximal part of the limb is correctly developed, but either the medial or lateral side of the rest of the limb may be missing. *Transverse hemimelia* is the amputation of a limb segment across the central area. It is common for a child with malformation of one body part to have bilateral or hemilateral problems.[109]

Children with congenital limb deficiencies may require surgery for removal of skin flaps or "nuisance" parts if these interfere with function. It is common for children to have some shoulder, trunk, and rib asymmetries as well. These children are fitted with prostheses as early as 2 months but usually by 6 months of age. Hybrid and myoelectric prosthesis have developed significantly in the past 10 years, eliminating some of the prior limitations of prosthetic use (e.g., lack of combination of both force and manipulation in one device), making the use of a prosthesis more realistic and appropriate.[109] Early and appropriate matching of the child to the prosthetic device allows the child to incorporate the prosthesis into his or her body image; it promotes balance, prevents scoliosis, facilitates bilateral function, and reduces dependence on the residual limb for tactile input. A multidisciplinary prosthetic team often follows the child's development into adolescence.[109]

Prosthetic device use can be instituted between 15 and 24 months of age. Hybrid and myoelectric devices should be considered as the initial prostheses. When these devices are applied early in development, the child develops a more intuitive use of the available muscle groups to power the prosthesis. As the child grows and matures, new prostheses are fabricated that reflect the child's increased size and skills.[109]

Acquired limb deficiencies are treated much like those in adults, except that tasks must be developmentally structured and sequenced. Bimanual activities for play, school, and self-care are emphasized. Learning to independently apply, remove, and care for the prosthesis is also part of the treatment process for school-aged children. The child must be taught ADL skills, with and without the prosthesis, and may require assistance and adaptations for some school, work, and play tasks. Occasionally, children experience overgrowth of the long bones, resulting in pain and possibly skin penetration and infection. Conservative skin stretching and surgical revision may be necessary.[36] Psychosocial, self-concept, and social play experiences may assist these children, particularly as they approach puberty.

Juvenile Rheumatoid Arthritis

Juvenile rheumatoid arthritis (JRA) is a major cause of physical disability in children younger than 16 years of age. It has an overall prevalence of 10 to 20 per 100,000 children.[82] JRA usually begins between 2 and 4 years of age and is more common in girls.[82] It is the most common form of arthritis in children. There is no single test to diagnose the disease; the diagnosis is made on the basis of persistent arthritis in one or more joints for at least 6 weeks after other possible illnesses have been ruled out. Sometimes a variety of tests may be needed to arrive at a firm diagnosis.

Arthritis is best described by four major changes that may occur in the joints. The most common features of JRA are joint inflammation, joint contracture (stiff, bent joint), joint damage, and/or alteration or change in growth. Other symptoms include joint stiffness after rest or decreased activity (also referred to *morning stiffness* or *gelling*) and weakness in muscles and other soft tissues around involved joints. Children vary in the degree to which they are affected by any particular symptom.[50]

Rheumatoid arthritis is a systemic disease that affects every aspect of an individual's life. It is characterized primarily by inflammatory changes in and destruction of the synovial joints (Figure 6-6). The exact cause of JRA is unknown, but factors believed to play undefined roles in its cause include genetics, emotional trauma, histocompatibility antigens, viruses, and antigen-antibody immune complexes.[82]

JRA is usually described as having three different forms: (1) pauciarticular, (2) polyarticular, and (3) systemic. The pauciarticular form usually affects fewer than five joints.

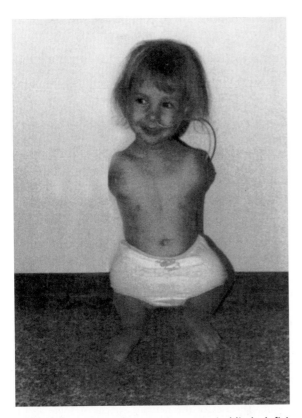

FIGURE 6-5 Child with multiple congenital limb deficiencies, including bilateral transverse upper arm deficiency and bilateral proximal femoral focal deficiency. (From Stanger, M. [2006]. Limb deficiencies and amputations. In S. Campbell, D. W. Vander Linden, & R. J. Palisano [Eds.], *Physical therapy for children* (3rd ed). Philadelphia: Saunders.)

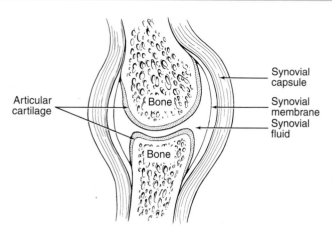

FIGURE 6-6 Components of a typical synovial joint.

Involvement is often asymmetric, and there are few or no systemic manifestations. The joints most often affected are the knees, hips, ankles, and elbows. Overgrowth of the long bones surrounding the inflamed joint often causes gait problems and flexion contractures. Many children who have pauciarticular JRA develop iridocyclitis, an inflamed condition of the iris and ciliary body of the eye that can lead to blindness if not treated.

With polyarticular JRA, the onset is often abrupt and painful, with symmetric involvement of the wrists, hands, feet, knees, ankles, and sometimes the cervical area of the spine. This resembles adult rheumatoid arthritis, and rheumatoid nodules on extensor surfaces indicate a more severe course. Five or more joints are affected, and as many as 20 to 40 separate joints may be involved; other symptoms include a low-grade fever, malaise, anorexia, listlessness, and irritability.[82]

Systemic JRA, or *Still's disease,* consists of polyarticular symptoms plus involvement of other organs, such as the spleen and lymph nodes.[109] Signs and symptoms include high fever, rash, anorexia, enlargement of the liver and spleen, and an elevated white blood cell count. Epiphyseal plates adjacent to an affected joint may initially show an acceleration of growth but later may be destroyed, causing local growth delay.

Medical management centers primarily on the use of therapeutic drugs, such as nonsteroidal anti-inflammatory analgesics. Corticosteroids are used to manage overwhelming inflammatory or systemic illness or as a bridge therapy in children who are not yet responsive to other medications. Surgical repair and reconstruction are seldom recommended for children. Other forms of treatment may include splinting, active and passive ROM exercises, and monitoring of joint motion to maintain maximal function and prevent deformity.

The prognosis for JRA varies depending on a number of factors, but it is important to remember that the largest percentage of children (with the pauciarticular type of JRA) recover completely within 1 to 2 years. Only about 15% of all children with JRA have permanent disabilities.[82]

Children with JRA may have pain at times, may show signs of fatigue, and may have reduced ROM in one or more joints. As a result, they may have difficulty performing ADLs and certain school tasks. Use of adaptive equipment such as pen and pencil grips, dressing aids, and built-up handles on utensils or other adaptations to feeding equipment often improves functioning and reduces fatigue and stress on joints. Seating needs must be monitored to help reduce fatigue and prevent harmful pressure on joints.[36,96]

Play and recreational activities may be adapted to allow full participation and to maintain strength and ROM. Children with severe deficits may require prevocational evaluation and treatment. Child and parent education in joint protection and energy conservation techniques is essential for children with JRA at all ages and stages.[96]

Curvature of the Spine

Lordosis, kyphosis, and scoliosis are the three major deformities of the spine. These conditions may occur functionally, posturally, and structurally; they may occur secondary to muscle imbalance, bony deformities, or other pathologic conditions such as cerebral palsy; or they may occur idiopathically. They may be congenital or acquired. In most cases, the cause of these disorders is unknown, although some familial patterns exist (Figure 6-7).[109] *Lordosis* is an anteroposterior curvature in which the concavity is directed posteriorly. Also called *hollow back,* this condition often occurs secondary to other spinal deformities or to an anterior pelvic tilt. Usually, it is predominantly in the lumbar area of the back and occasionally is painful. It can also occur secondary to extreme obesity, hip flexion contractures, or conditions such as muscular dystrophy. Lordosis may occur during the adolescent growth spurt experienced by many girls. Treatment focuses on correcting the underlying conditions, stretching tight hip flexors, and strengthening the abdominal musculature. Postural training and, occasionally in severe cases, back bracing are included.

The opposite anteroposterior curvature, with the convexity posterior, is called *kyphosis.* With this condition, also called *round back* and, in adolescents, *Scheuermann's disease,* the curvature is usually primarily in the upper back. The deformity is common in children and adolescents and usually is the result of faulty posture. This is particularly true as the teenage girl's skeletal growth outpaces her muscular growth. The deformity can occur in children with spina bifida cystica or arthritis. Treatment depends on the cause and severity of the problem. In mild cases postural training and strengthening activities such as weight training, swimming, and dance are often useful. Thoracic kyphosis requires the use of a Milwaukee brace. In severe cases, a combination of anterior spinal release and fusion and posterior spinal fusion and instrumentation may be used to guide and support the spine.[50]

Scoliosis is the most common and serious of the spinal curvature disorders, usually involving lateral curvature, spinal rotation, and thoracic hypokyphosis. Treatment is considered when a lateral curvature of more than 10 degrees is present. Lateral curvature of the spine is often accompanied by rotation of the vertebral bodies. Functional scoliosis is flexible and can be caused by poor posture, leg length discrepancy, poor postural tone, hip contractures, or pain. Congenital scoliosis is usually structural, caused by abnormal spinal or spinal cord structure. Diseases of the nervous system or spine also may result in scoliosis. However, most cases of scoliosis have no known cause.

Scoliosis is rarely painful. The diagnosis is based on careful examination and history taking. If preliminary evaluation and palpation suggest the condition, radiographic analysis is also used. Structural scoliosis often progresses over time; the

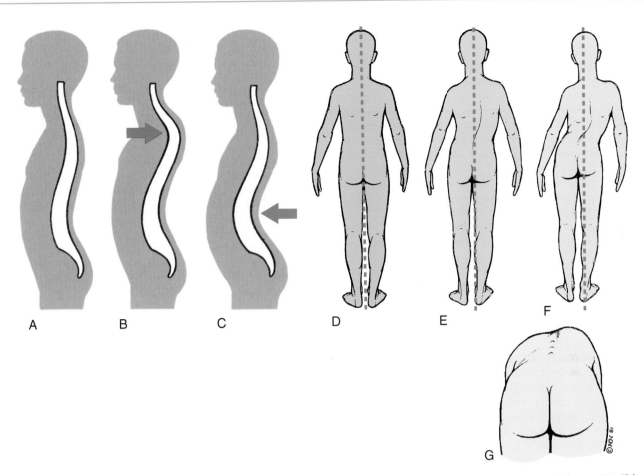

FIGURE 6-7   Defects of the spinal column. **A,** Normal spine. **B,** Kyphosis. **C,** Lordosis. **D,** Normal spine in balance. **E,** Mild scoliosis in balance. **F,** Severe scoliosis not in balance. **G,** Rib hump and flank asymmetry seen in flexion caused by rotary component.   (Redrawn from Hilt, N. E., & Schmitt, E. W. [1975]. From Hockenberry, M. J., & Wilson, D. [2009]. *Wong's essentials of pediatric nursing* [8th ed.]. St. Louis: Mosby.)

vertebral bodies may become wedge shaped and rotate toward the convex part of the curve, and the intervertebral disk may shift and deform.[109] Curves of less than 20 degrees are considered mild. Those of more than 40 degrees may result in permanent deformity, and those of 65 to 80 degrees may result in reduced cardiopulmonary function. Skin breakdown between the ribs and pelvis may also develop in some cases.

Treatment includes orthotic intervention and surgical spinal fusion. The two most common types of bracing are the Boston brace, created from prefabricated plastic shells, and a thoracolumbosacral orthotic (TLSO). Exercise alone is rarely effective for managing scoliosis but may be helpful in strengthening spinal and abdominal muscles during treatment. If surgery is indicated, postoperative therapy and ADL adaptions are sometimes needed; in general, children and adolescents progress well after surgery and maintain a normal lifestyle into adulthood.[108,109]

NEUROMUSCULAR DISORDERS

Children with neuromuscular disorders constitute a large percentage of the clients of occupational therapy practice. Several conditions involve impairment of the neurologic system,

resulting in interference with the child's ability to interact effectively with the environment. The site of damage may be the brain, spinal cord, peripheral nerves, neuromuscular junction, or the muscle itself. The disorder may interfere with the reception and processing of sensory input or the ability to act effectively on the environment, or a combination of these may result. Neuromuscular deficits may occur before, at, or after birth. This section addresses several of the major conditions in this category.[88,94]

Cerebral Palsy

Cerebral palsy (CP) is characterized by nonprogressive abnormalities in the developing brain that create a cascade of neurologic, motor, and postural deficits in the developing child. The incidence of CP is estimated to be 1.4 to 2.4 per 1000 live births, and although this rate has remained constant over a 30-year period, the causes have changed. Because of a rise in the survival rate of very premature infants in both the very-low-birth-weight and extremely-low-birth-weight categories, a rise in the incidence of CP with spastic diplegia, often associated with prematurity and low birth weight, has been noted. On the other hand, athetoid CP, often attributed to fetal asphyxia and hyperbilirubinemia, has decreased in developed countries.[94] It is estimated that 5000 infants and 1200 to 1500 preschool children are diagnosed with CP each year.

Although a pattern of motor and postural deficits is a defining feature of CP, many secondary disorders typically coexist with this diagnosis. Cognitive, sensory, and psychosocial deficits often compound motor impairments and subsequent functioning.[94] Although CP is usually the result of injury or disease at or before birth (congenital CP), children injured in early childhood display similar symptoms and are sometimes classified as having CP (acquired CP). CP is expressed through variable impairments in motor and postural control, coordination of muscle action, and sensation that typically are classified according to the type and distribution of motor impairment.[110]

The various causes of congenital CP can be grouped according to premature birth or term birth. Prematurity now accounts for the majority of known causes for CP. This increased rate may be associated with the central nervous system's vulnerability to insult (i.e., increased sensitivity to bleeding near the lateral ventricles, which has a cascading effect on further CNS development) during gestational weeks 26 to 32.

Cerebrovascular accident (CVA), developmental brain abnormalities, placental abruption, fetomaternal hemorrhage, placental infarction, and maternal exposure to environmental toxins have also been associated with CP. In addition, maternal infections such as cytomegalovirus, syphilis, varicella virus, and toxoplasmosis can be secondary causes of CP. Causes of acquired CP include trauma, intracranial hemorrhage, CNS infections, near-drowning, hypoxia, and metabolic disorders.

Early diagnosis of CP is important to elicit the services that the child and family may need to optimize the child's potential for development and to prevent secondary disabilities. To develop a definitive diagnosis, a team of developmental specialists conducts thorough physical and developmental evaluations. These evaluations usually take place over a period of months in early development. The team may include a pediatrician, an occupational and a physical therapist, a developmental nurse, and a speech-language pathologist. Retention of primitive reflexes and automatic reactions, variable tone, hyperresponsive tendon reflexes, asymmetry in the use of extremities, clonus, poor sucking or tongue control, and involuntary movements may indicate the presence of CP. Motor delays coupled with delays in other developmental areas or with a discrepancy in cognitive development are also strong indicators. Infants who weigh less than 1500 g at birth are particularly vulnerable and must be monitored closely.[102] Each child with CP has a unique set of problems. Comprehensive ongoing medical assessment is necessary in children diagnosed with CP to treat medical sequelae associated with the condition.

Characteristically, the child with CP shows impaired ability to maintain normal postures because of a lack of muscle coactivation and the development of abnormal movement compensations. These compensatory patterns develop in certain muscle groups to maintain upright postures and to effect movement against gravity. For example, the child's poor head control, resulting from poor coactivation of cervical flexors and extensors, causes the center of gravity to move anteriorly; this results in compensatory reactions in the thoracic and lumbar spine as the child attempts to stay upright. Likewise, hyperreactive responses to tactile, visual, or auditory stimuli may result in fluctuations of muscle tone that often adversely affect

postural control and further diminish coordinated responses in everyday activities.[88]

Classification of Cerebral Palsy

The locale of the lesion affects the development and quality of movement patterns present in the child with CP. For example, CP with spasticity indicates a lesion in the motor cortex. Lesions in the basal ganglia typically cause fluctuations in muscle tone that are described as *diakinesis, dystonia,* or *athetosis.* Cerebellar damage tends to produce the unstable movements characteristic of the ataxic child.[94]

The variability of the movement and postural disorder may be classified according to which limbs are affected. Involvement of the upper and lower extremities on one side is *hemiplegia;* involvement of all limbs is *tetraplegia* or *quadriplegia* and *diplegia* when the child demonstrates quadriplegia with mild upper-extremity involvement and significant impairment of function in lower extremities.[94] See Figure 6-8 for classifications of limb involvement.

Several classifications of CP have been developed according to the quality of tone, disorder distribution, and locale of brain lesions. These classifications are featured in Table 6-2. Characteristics are described according to quality and distribution of muscle tone, ROM, quality of movement, presence of reflexes and reactions, oral motor problems, associated problems, and personality characteristics.

Although CP is considered nonprogressive, abnormal movement patterns, muscle tone, and sensory function, combined with the effects of gravity and normal growth, may cause the child to develop contractures and deformities over time. Function may become more limited as the child grows to adulthood. Furthermore, the effects of normal aging may result in decreased function, physical discomfort, and arthritic responses over time.[88]

Language and intellectual deficits often coexist with CP. Delays in cognitive development and below-average intelligence have been seen in 50% to 75% of children with CP. This impairment may range from mild to profound.[94] Speech disturbances occur in approximately 30% of these children. Artic-

text continues on page 160

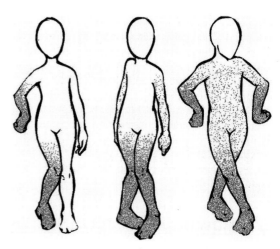

FIGURE 6-8 Limb involvement classification and severity in cerebral palsy: *Left,* Hemiplegia; *middle,* diplegia; *right,* tetraplegia or quadriplegia.

TABLE 6-2 Cerebral Palsy Classifications

Clinical Feature	Severe Spasticity	Moderate Spasticity	Mild Spasticity	Pure Athetosis	Athetosis with Spasticity	Athetosis with Tonic Spasms	Choreoathetosis	Flaccidity	Ataxia
Quality of tone	Severely increased tone; flexor and extensor co-contraction is constant; tone is high at rest, during sleep, or when awake; tone pattern is more proximal than distal	Moderately increased tone; near normal at rest but increases with excitement, movement attempts, effort, emotion, speech, sudden stretch; agonists and distal muscles more spastic	Mildly increased or normal tone at rest increases with effort or attempts to move or attempts at quicker movements	Fluctuation of tone from low to normal; no or little spasticity; no co-activation of flexors and extensors	Fluctuates from normal to high; some ability to stabilize proximally; moderate proximal spasticity and distal athetosis	Unpredictable tone changes from low to very high; either all flexion or extension of extremities	Constant fluctuations from low to high with no co-contraction; jerky involuntary movements more proximal than distal	Fluctuating, markedly low muscle tone; seen at birth, or toddler initially classified as flaccid, later classified as spastic, athetoid, or ataxic	Ranges from near normal to normal; increased tone, when present, usually involves lower extremity flexion
Distribution of tone	Quadriplegia, but may also manifest as diplegia or paraplegia	Same as in severe spasticity	Same as in severe spasticity, but diplegia and hemiplegia more common	Quadriplegia with occasional hemiplegia	Same as in athetosis	Quadriplegia, hemiplegia, or monoplegia	Quadriplegia	Quadriplegia	Quadriplegia
Range of motion	Abnormal patterns can lead to scoliosis, kyphosis, hip/knee/finger deformity; forearm pronation contracture, hip subluxation, heel cord subluxation with equinovarus or equinovalgus; decreased trunk, shoulder, and pelvic girdle mobility; limited midrange control where co-contraction is least balanced.	More available movement and more flexor/extensor imbalance can lead to kyphosis, lordosis, hip subluxations or dislocations, hip and knee flexion contractures; tight hip internal rotators and adductors; heel cord shortening; foot rotation	Limitations more distal than proximal; minimal deformities	Transient subluxation of joints such as shoulders and fingers; may have valgus on feet or knees; rarely any deformities	Incidence of scoliosis; some flexion deformities at hips, elbows, and knees; usually full range of motion proximally and hypermobile distally	More pronounced scoliosis; more dislocation of arm because of flailing spasm; possible kyphoscoliosis, hip dislocation, or skull dislocation, flexion contracture on hips/knees, subluxation of hips, fingers, or lower jaw	Many involuntary movements with extreme ranges but no control at midrange; deformities rare, but tendency for shoulder and finger subluxation	Hypermobile joints that tend to subluxate; flat chest; later, range limitations due to limited movement	Range usually not a problem; decreased range, when present, usually in flexion

Continued

TABLE 6-2 Cerebral Palsy Classifications—Cont'd

Clinical Feature	Severe Spasticity	Moderate Spasticity	Mild Spasticity	Pure Athetosis	Athetosis with Spasticity	Athetosis with Tonic Spasms	Choreoathetosis	Flaccidity	Ataxia
Quality of movement	Decreased midrange, voluntary, and involuntary movements; slow and labored stereotypical movements	May be able to walk; stereotypical, asymmetric, more associated reactions; total movement synergies	Often able to walk; seems driven to move; has increased variety of other movements, some stereotypical	Writhing involuntary movements, more distal than proximal; no change with intention to move; many fixation attempts caused by decreased ability to stabilize	Decreased ability to grade movements; decreased midline control and selective movement; proximal stability and distal choreoathetosis; varies with case	Extreme tonic spasm without voluntary control; some involuntary movement, distal more than proximal	Wide movement ranges with no gradation; jerky movements more proximal than distal; no selective movement or fixation of movement; weak hands and fingers	Ungraded movements; slow movements difficult; many static postures, as if hanging on to anatomic structures instead of active control	Lacks point of stability, therefore co-activation is difficult; uses primitive rather than abnormal patterns, hence gross, total patterns; incoordination, thus dysmetria disdiadochokinesia, tremors at rest, symmetric problems
Reflexes and reactions	Obligatory primitive reflexes (positive support, ATNR, STNR, neck righting); protective, righting, and equilibrium reactions are often absent	Strong primitive reflexes— Moro, startle, TNR, TLR, positive support prominent; decreased neck righting; associated reactions strong; righting may be present, but equilibrium reaction develops to sitting and kneeling	Primitive reflexes used for functional purposes and not obligatory; righting, protective, and equilibrium reactions delayed but established; may not develop higher level reactions	Primitive reflexes not usually obligatory or evoked; protective and equilibrium reactions usually present but involuntary movements affect grading	TNR/TLR strong but intermittent and modified by involuntary movements; equilibrium reactions, when present, unreliable and may or may not be used	Strong ATNR, STNR, TLR; protective and equilibrium reactions absent during spasm, otherwise present, unreliable, or absent	Intermittent TNR; righting and equilibrium reactions present to some extent, but abnormal coordination; abnormal upper extremity protective extension possible, but often absent	Usually less reactive because of decreased tone; righting is delayed; delayed protective extension more available than equilibrium reaction	May develop righting reactions, but these are uncoordinated, exaggerated, and poorly used; equilibrium reactions, when developed, are not coordinated; needs wide base of support because of poor weight shifting
Oral motor	Immobile, rigid chest; shallow respiration and forced expiration; lip retraction with decreased lip closure and tongue thrust; communication through forced expiration	Not as involved as in severe spasticity	Increased mobility, thus more respiratory function for phonation; shortness of breath limits sentence length; better ability to dissociate mouth parts, but poor lip closure causes drooling	Fluctuations adversely affect gross and fine motor performance; volume of speech may go up or down with breath; feeding may be decreased due to instability and tongue/jaw/swallow incoordination	Difficulty with head control, thus decreased oral motor, strained speech; decreased coordination of suck/swallow, resulting in decreased feeding and speech	Feeding may be difficult because aspiration is unpredictable; severe language and speech impairment caused by decreased control	Facial grimaces, dysarthria, irregular breathing, difficulty sustaining phonation, poor intraoral and extraoral surfaces	Quiet, soft voice because of decreased respiration; delayed speech; increased drooling; often expressionless face	Speech is monotone, very slow; uses teeth to stabilize tongue or hold cup to mouth when drinking; decreased articulation

Associated problems	Seizures, cortical blindness, deafness, ID, malnutrition, prone to URTI	Seizures, ID, perceptual motor problems, imbalance of eye musculature	Seizures, less ID, perceptual problems	Hearing loss, less ID	Same as in athetosis	Same as in athetosis	Obesity, sensory impairment, URTI	Nystagmus, MR, sensory problems; uses vision for righting and as reference point for movement
Personality characteristics	Passive, dependent; resistant and adapts poorly to change; anxious and fearful of being moved; generally less frustrated than athetoid individuals	Lesser degree of traits seen in severe spasticity	More frustrated and critical about self because of awareness of better performance; more patient than children of same age	Emotional lability; less fearful of movement; more outgoing, but tends to be frustrated	Same as in athetosis	Same as in athetosis	Visually attentive, cannot move, therefore is a "good" baby; decreased motivation	Does not like to move

ATNR, Asymmetric tonic neck reflex; *ID*, intellectual disabilities; *STNR*, symmetric tonic neck reflex; *TNR*, tonic neck reflex; *TLR*, tonic labyrinthine reflex; *URTI*, upper respiratory tract infection. *Classification of types of cerebral palsy based on the quality of postural tone.* London: The Bobath Centre.
Modified from Bobath, B. (1978).

ulation problems may be associated with impairment of tongue and lip movements. Speech and language problems may be receptive or expressive, relating to central processing impairment. Limitations in communication tend to isolate the child, may create stress and frustration for the child and parent, and can negatively affect the development of psychosocial skills. Use of augmentative communication equipment can prevent some of these consequences of speech impairment and is critical for increasing the communication abilities of children with severe CP.[88]

Seizure disorders occur in approximately 40% of children with CP, and the incidence appears to be higher among children with spastic disorders. In children with severe seizures, some degeneration may continue after birth. Partial epilepsy is the most common form of seizures in children with CP.[94] Anticonvulsant drugs are commonly used to control seizure activity. These drugs must be carefully monitored and may affect the state of the child's digestion and gums, requiring feeding adjustments and good dental care.[55]

Feeding problems are associated with the abnormal oral movements, tone, and sensation. The child may be hypersensitive or hyposensitive to touch around and in the mouth, and sucking, chewing, and swallowing may be difficult to initiate or control.[94] The child's diet may need to be adjusted, and special feeding techniques may be required. These children also may require medication to maintain regularity of elimination. Positioning helps improve postural stability for feeding and toileting.[88]

Several sensory deficits may be present. Problems with the visual system may include impaired vision, blindness, limitations in eye movements and eye tracking, squinting, strabismus, eye muscle weaknesses, and eye incoordination. In addition, children with CP may have visual perception problems that can interfere with school progress. It is estimated that 40% to 50% of children with CP have visual defects of some type and require glasses or low-vision and visual-perceptual training. Auditory disturbances include hearing problems (acuity), which can range from slight hearing loss to total deafness. Auditory-perceptual problems and agnosia are also common. An estimated 25% of children with CP have some type of auditory disturbance and may require hearing aids.[110]

Children with CP must be monitored for signs of behavioral problems and psychosocial delays that can become serious if not found and corrected early. Evaluation of these areas, emotional support, normalization of social experiences, and behavior management programs should be integral parts of the total assessment and treatment regimen for these special children.[94]

Antispasticity oral medications (e.g., diazepam, baclofen, dantrolene) have shown limited effectiveness in improving muscle tone in children with spasticity. The medications can reduce spasticity or rigidity and improve comfort in older children for short periods. These medications work on the neurotransmitter acetylcholine (ACh) and are fast acting. Significant side effects occur with many children, including drowsiness, excessive drooling, and physical dependency, all of which tend to outweigh the potential benefit of the medication.[94]

Several injectable agents are now available that can target localized areas of spasticity more effectively. Implanted medication pumps are being used with children who have severe spasticity. The pump is inserted into the skin of the abdomen, and the catheter is routed to the lumbar spine, where it is placed in the intrathecal space. This placement allows delivery of antispasticity medication (primarily baclofen) into the spinal cord, where it can directly inhibit motor nerve conduction. The major advantages of the pump include lower and more controlled doses of medication and decreased spasticity.[96,110] Mechanical failures, infection, and the need for intensive medical intervention may preclude use of this treatment in some children. When spasticity is severe, neural blocks may be used to disrupt the reflex arc.[94] Recently, injectable botulinum toxin has been used to effectively block the nerve-muscle junction. Botulinum toxin is deadly in the general circulation, but when injected intramuscularly in minute quantities, it blocks the neuromuscular junction effectively for 3 to 6 months. This allows the child to use the muscle without the interference of spasticity. The long-term benefits of treatment have yet to be well researched, but no serious side effects have been documented.

Orthopedic surgery traditionally has been used to correct joint deformities, to balance uneven muscular action, and to reduce contractures that have resulted from abnormal and asymmetric tone. The most frequently performed surgeries include tendon release (permanent lengthening of a muscle) and tendon transfer (moving the point of attachment of a tendon on bone). Both procedures require the use of a cast for 6 to 8 weeks after surgery, and because overall muscle tone is not changed, the procedures may need to be repeated.[79]

Other possible surgeries include correction of hip deformities or dislocations and scoliosis. Orthotic management in support of surgery or to reduce tone, prevent contractures, or stabilize or position often improves and increases functional activity. Tone-reducing or inhibitive casts made for the lower extremity can gently strengthen and lengthen spastic muscles. Often, a series of casts is applied to increase ROM gradually. When ROM within normal limits has been achieved, the cast is worn intermittently to maintain the increased muscle length. Active and passive ROM activities, positioning and handling to enhance postural tone, and orthotics may be used alone or in combination to improve the child's functional independence.[88]

Neurosurgical intervention for spasticity has been aimed at the brain, spinal cord, and peripheral nerves. For example, cerebellar or dorsal column stimulators have been implanted, but the results have been disappointing. Currently, selective posterior rhizotomy (SPR) is the most widely used neurosurgical procedure. In SPR, 50% of the dorsal rootlets at L2-S2 are severed to muscles determined to be spastic, as tested by electromyography (EMG) during surgery. Good candidates for SPR include children with a diagnosis of spastic diplegia, normal cognitive status, no fixed deformities, and good underlying muscle strength in the spastic muscles.[64,94,114] The initial studies for SPR provide encouraging data for functional changes, although others have indicated that long-term risks must be balanced with the potential for sustained functional improvements. Reported changes include improved motor control, gait, upper extremity functioning, sitting balance, and responsiveness to other treatment strategies.[64,114]

Although the prognosis varies for each type of CP, children with CP typically live to adulthood, but their life expectancy may be less than that of the normal population. The reason for the shorter life expectancy is not known. Some speculate that it is related to persistent alterations in physiologic and immunologic functioning, the implications of which are not fully understood.[100] The functional prognosis varies greatly from type to type, with hemiplegia and spastic diplegia having a better prognosis than the more severe, rigid types. Depending on their ability to attain independence or modified independence with assistive devices and technology, children with CP may experience the full range of life events,[94] although they may have limitations in all areas of human occupation to some degree. The most effective motor intervention to occur in the past decade is that of *constraint-induced intervention,* sometimes called *forced-used intervention,* which has now been contrasted with a less restrictive form of intervention, that of Hand-Arm Bimanual Intensive Training (HABIT) for children with hemiplegic-type cerebral palsy. Current evidence in the past 6 years has been very encouraging and may indicate that intensive motor training, using specific protocols, significantly improves use of the affected arm. The next decade may prove it to be the most effective method for improving hand function in those children with spastic hemiplegic-type cerebral palsy.

Functional performance in self-care and independent living, school and work performance, play, and recreation all may need to be addressed at some point in the child's life. Parents may require support and respite, as well as education, to care for the child with CP and to meet the needs of the family as a whole.[88]

Seizure Disorders and Epilepsy

Epilepsy is a chronic neurologic condition of recurrent seizures that occur with or without the presence of other brain abnormalities. A *seizure* may be defined as a temporary, involuntary change of consciousness, behavior, motor activity, sensation, or automatic functioning.[119] Provoked seizures occur frequently in children as a result of fever, acute illness, or CNS infection or after traumatic brain injury.[79]

A seizure starts with an excessive rate and hypersynchrony of discharges from a group of cerebral neurons that spreads to the adjoining cells, called the *epileptogenic focus.*[119] Some seizures may be directly attributed to the factor or factors that trigger the seizure. For example, acute factors often described are hypoglycemia, fever, trauma, hemorrhages, tumors, infections, and anoxia. Other seizures may be attributed to previous scarring and structural damage or to hormonal changes. Many seizures, especially in children, have no discernible underlying disease and are therefore idiopathic.[79]

Seizures are classified by their clinical signs or symptoms and electroencephalographic characteristics. The two major types of seizure according to this form of categorization are (1) *generalized seizures,* which involve the entire cerebral cortex, and (2) *partial seizures,* which begin in a single location and remain limited or spread to become more generalized. Generalized seizures can be further divided into tonic-clonic, absence, atypical absence, myoclonic, and atonic forms. Partial seizures can be either simple or complex and are the most common type of seizure disorder found in childhood; approximately 60% of cases are partial seizures. An individual may experience both generalized and partial seizures, which is called a *mixed seizure disorder.*[50]

Of the generalized seizures, the tonic-clonic type occurs most frequently. A child having a *tonic-clonic seizure* may have an aura, or sensation, that the seizure is about to begin. This nonspecific seizure can occur at any age and involves excessive neuronal firing from both hemispheres in a symmetric pattern. This is usually followed by a loss of consciousness, during which the body becomes rigid, or tonic, and then rhythmic clonic contractions of all the extremities occur. Incontinence is common. The seizure may last 5 minutes and is followed by a postictal period that may last 1 to 2 hours, during which the child is drowsy or in a deep sleep.[119]

A second type of generalized seizure, *absence seizure,* is characterized by a momentary loss of awareness and the absence of motor activity except eye blinking or rolling. There is no aura, the seizure usually lasts less than 30 seconds, and there is no postictal period. The onset of these seizures occurs in the first decade of life. Abrupt interruption of an activity, a glazed look, stares, and unawareness of surroundings characterize a child having an absence seizure. This may be mistaken for daydreaming. Absence seizures are uncommon in children and early adolescents, accounting for only 5% of all seizures.[119]

Two other mild forms of generalized seizure are (1) *myoclonic seizures,* which consist of contractions by single muscle or small groups of muscles, and (2) *akinetic seizures,* in which the primary problem is a loss of muscle tone. Children rarely have serious seizures for an extended period (30 minutes or longer). These extended seizures are called *status epilepticus* and require medical management to maintain body functions and hydration. Intravenous anticonvulsant medication is also indicated to treat this condition.

In *complex partial seizures,* which usually originate in the temporal lobe, children may show automatic reactions such as lip smacking, chewing, and buttoning and unbuttoning of clothing. These seizures are focal, and the characteristics are similar to those of absence seizures. In addition, the individual may appear to be confused and disorganized and may have sensory experiences, such as smelling and tasting items not in the environment and hearing sounds of various types.

Simple partial seizures usually involve the motor cortex and result in clonic activity of the face or extremities. Psychic symptoms include visual hallucinations, illusions, auditory hallucinations, or olfactory sensations. The typical seizure includes nighttime awakenings and twitching of facial muscles; this twitching interferes with speech and spreads to the hands.[119]

Infantile spasms pose a serious threat to development. They typically begin at 6 months and disappear by 24 months. During this time, development appears to stop and skills may be lost. Early treatment with adrenocorticotropic hormone can inhibit the seizure activity; however, the effects on development are almost inevitable. More than 90% of children with known causes for their seizures have intellectual impairments.[119]

The incidence and prevalence of seizures are difficult to estimate. The incidence of generalized seizures, including tonic-clonic, absence, and myoclonic seizures, has been reported to be approximately 2.5 per 1000 children. The incidence of partial seizures has been reported to be 1.7 to 3.6 per 1000 children, and unclassified and mixed seizures account for 2 per 1000.[79] Many of these unclassified and mixed seizures may occur infrequently and cease as the child matures.

A child who has a seizure must undergo a thorough evaluation to determine the factors that caused it. A family history, medical history, and developmental history must be completed, as well as an electroencephalogram (EEG) to help determine the type of seizure.

Anticonvulsive medications are administered in an attempt to control the seizures. In theory, these medications increase the intensity required to trigger the seizure or eliminate the recruitment of surrounding cells. Weinstein and Gaillard[119] have described some of the common side effects of these anticonvulsive medications, including cataracts, weight gain, high blood pressure, pathologic fractures, drowsiness, hair loss or gain, nausea, liver damage, vomiting, gum enlargement, hyperactivity, anorexia, and lymphoma-like syndrome. Commonly prescribed medications include valproic acid (Depakene), phenytoin (Dilantin), phenobarbital, ethosuximide (Zarontin), and carbamazepine (Tegretol).

Balancing the dosage of anticonvulsant medications can be a difficult process and is often repeated at various times as the child grows and matures. Antiepileptic medication is often withdrawn or reduced in dose if the child has been seizure-free with a normal EEG for at least 2 years. Withdrawal is done slowly and with caution, and health care workers are often asked to monitor the child closely during the withdrawal period.[79]

A number of antiepileptic therapies based on old treatments are regaining favor as a result of new research. One example is the ketogenic diet, which consists of a carefully monitored intake of fats, sugars, and carbohydrates that forces the body to use fat rather than carbohydrates for energy and alters neurotransmitters.[47] The urine must be monitored to ensure adequate spillage of ketones. Short-term side effects include metabolic acidosis and electrolyte disturbances, uric acid kidney stone formation, and diarrhea and vomiting. When the child has been seizure-free for a period of 9 months, the diet can be terminated. Currently, there are only large observational studies that suggest an effect on controlling seizures if medication is not effective; there are no reliable randomized controlled trials to support the use of ketogenic diets for people with epilepsy.[68]

Surgical intervention is used if adequate control of the seizures cannot be achieved with medication. Surgical interventions that seek to cure epilepsy have been shown to be effective by reducing the seizure focus of the brain, particularly in complex partial seizures arising from the mesial temporal lobe. *Hemispherectomy,* involving removal of most of one side of the brain, is used for seizures that arise from multiple foci in one side of the brain and for progressive unilateral disorders. Palliative surgical interventions include corpus callosotomy and electrical stimulation of the vagus nerve or the thalamus for intractable mixed seizures that have an onset that cannot be localized to one area or that arise from both hemispheres. The timing for surgery is determined by the effectiveness of medication, seizure severity, and the impact of epilepsy on the child's functioning.[79]

Even with optimal care, only about 50% to 75% of children can achieve complete seizure control with medication. Having a seizure can be frightening to the child and those around him or her. When a child has a seizure, staff members must remain calm, move spectators away, and protect the child. Box 6-1 presents an outline of the emergency treatment procedures for seizures. Most children with seizure disorders have normal intelligence scores, achieve seizure control with a single antiepilepsy drug, and lead typical lives. The prognosis depends primarily on the type of seizure and the underlying brain pathology.[50]

Muscular Dystrophies

The muscular dystrophies are the most common muscle diseases of childhood. They cause changes in the biochemistry and structure of the surface and internal membranes of the muscle cells and result in progressive degeneration and weakness of various muscle groups, disability, deformity, and sometimes death. For most of the neuromuscular disorders, which

---

BOX 6-1   Emergency Treatment of Seizures

1. Remain calm.
2. Time seizure episode.
3. Protect child during seizure:
   - Do not attempt to restrain child or use force.
   - If child is standing or sitting in wheelchair at beginning of attack, ease child down so that he or she will not fall; when possible, place cushion or blanket under child.
   - Do not put anything in child's mouth.
   - Loosen restrictive clothing.
   - Prevent child from hitting hard or sharp objects that might cause injury during uncontrolled movements.
   - Remove objects.
   - Pad objects.
   - Move furniture out of the way.
   - Allow seizure to end without interference.
4. When seizure stops:
   - Check for breathing; if not present, use mouth-to-mouth resuscitation.
   - Time postictal period.
   - Keep child on his/her side.
   - Check mouth, head, and body for possible injuries.
5. Check around mouth for evidence of burns or suspicious substances that might indicate poisoning.
6. Remain with child.
7. Seek help if the child is not breathing, there is evidence of injury or the child is diabetic, seizure lasts for more than 5 minutes, status epilepticus occurs, pupils are not equal after seizure, child vomits for more than 30 minutes after seizure, child cannot be awakened and is unresponsive to pain, seizure occurs in water, this is the child's first seizure.

Adapted from Hockenberry, M. J., & Wilson, D. (2009). *Wong's essentials of pediatric nursing* (8th ed.). St. Louis: Mosby.

---

all have a genetic basis, the chromosomal location is known and the causal gene has been identified.[30]

Types of muscular dystrophy include limb-girdle, facioscapulohumeral, congenital, and Duchenne's (pseudohypertrophic) muscular dystrophy.[50] Figure 6-9 shows the differential distribution of paralysis with these dystrophies.

In *limb-girdle muscular dystrophy,* the initial muscles affected are the proximal muscles of the pelvis and shoulder girdles. The onset may occur anywhere from the first to the third decade of life, with progression usually slow but sometimes moderately rapid. The hereditary pattern is autosomal recessive, as with the congenital form.[104]

Facioscapulohumeral muscular dystrophy is autosomal dominant, and the onset usually occurs in early adolescence. Although the severity varies greatly among clients, involvement is primarily in the face, upper arms, and scapular region, as the name implies. Clinical manifestations include a slope to the shoulders, decreased ability to raise the arms above shoulder height, and decreased mobility in the facial muscles, resulting in a masklike appearance.

The most common and most severe form of muscular dystrophy is *Duchenne's muscular dystrophy.* It is inherited as an X-linked recessive disorder. Because it is an X-linked disorder, the condition affects boys, and the incidence is 1 per 3500 live male births. This disorder is caused by a deficiency in the production of dystrophin, which is a component of the plasma

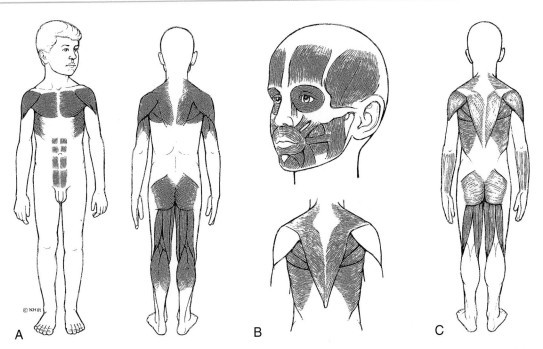

FIGURE 6-9 Initial muscle groups involved in muscular dystrophies. **A,** Pseudohypertrophic. **B,** Facioscapulohumeral. **C,** Limb-girdle. (From Hockenberry, M. J., & Wilson, D. [2009]. *Wong's essentials of pediatric nursing* [8th ed.]. St. Louis: Mosby.)

membrane of muscle fibers. Muscles cannot function and degenerate without dystrophin.[104]

Children show typical development at birth, and symptoms usually begin to appear between the second and sixth years of life. Parents describe their child as having increasing difficulty climbing stairs and rising from a sitting or lying position. The child stumbles and falls excessively and tires easily. A distinctive characteristic of this form is the enlargement of calf muscles and sometimes of forearm and thigh muscles, giving the appearance of strong, healthy muscles. However, this enlargement is caused by extensive fibrosis and proliferation of adipose tissue, which when combined with the other pathologic changes in the muscle tissue actually causes muscle weakness. This phenomenon is referred to as *pseudohypertrophy of muscles.*[38]

Involvement begins in the proximal musculature of the pelvic girdle, proceeds to the shoulder girdle, and finally affects all muscle groups. As leg and pelvic muscles weaken, the child often uses his or her arms to "crawl" up the thighs into a standing position from a kneeling position. This maneuver is known as *Gower's sign* and is diagnostically significant (Figure 6-10). Independent ambulation is one of the first functions to be lost, and dependence on a wheelchair is common by 9 years of age. Gradually, the simplest ADLs become difficult and then impossible. In the advanced stages of the disease, lordosis and kyphosis are common, as are contractures at various joints. Death, usually as a result of infection, respiratory problems, or cardiovascular complications, often occurs before the early twenties.[45]

Currently, no treatment is available that arrests or reverses the dystrophic process, but antibiotic therapy and other advances in dealing with pulmonary complications have helped

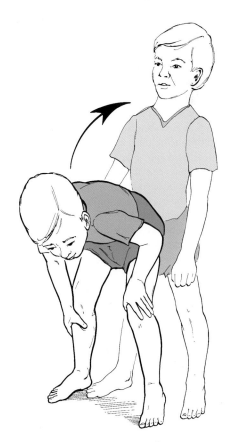

FIGURE 6-10 Child with Gower's sign.

extend life expectancy. Steroids can help, but their use remains controversial because of their side effects. Myoblast transfer has been used on a trial basis. Although gene therapy is still in the preclinical trial phase, it is a promising option for treatment of Duchenne's and Becker's muscular dystrophies. Two types of treatment are being explored: the use of adenovirus-mediated dystrophin gene transfer and upregulation of a natural dystrophin analog.[104]

The goals of rehabilitation in patients with neuromuscular disease are to maximize and prolong independent function and locomotion, inhibit physical deformity, and provide access to full integration into society. A multidisciplinary team consisting of physicians, nurses, therapists, social and vocational counselors, and psychologists, among others, is needed to manage the symptoms of these dystrophies. Stretching, ROM activities, timely surgical correction of spinal deformities and contractures, and bracing may improve or prolong ambulation and enhance functional use of the extremities. Moderate-resistance (submaximal) weight lifting and aerobic exercise may improve strength and cardiovascular performance in slowly progressive neuromuscular diseases. For patients with advanced restrictive lung disease, positive pressure ventilation may improve breathing and comfort. Cardiac complications in some neuromuscular diseases can be severe and may require monitoring. Nutritional, psychologic, and vocational considerations should also be part of the management of neuromuscular disease. Major advances in biomedical and computer engineering continue to provide more functional equipment, enabling better strategies for improvement of quality of life.[45]

Congenital muscular dystrophies (CMDs) make up a heterogeneous group of muscle disorders with onset in utero or during the first year of life. Several forms of CMD show brain involvement in addition to the neuromuscular disorder.[102] CMD is marked by hypotonia, generalized muscle weakness, and multiple contractures. Four categories have been identified: classic CMD I without severe impairment of intellectual functioning; CMD II, involving muscle and brain abnormalities; and the less severe types CMD III and IV, involving muscle, eye, and brain abnormalities.[104] Associated problems include clubfoot, torticollis, diaphragmatic involvement, and congenital heart and spinal defects. Often little or no progression of the disease is seen after childhood, and some functional improvement may be seen around this time.[104] The diagnosis is established by the presence of high serum levels of the muscle enzyme creatine kinase, by EMG analysis, and by examination of muscle tissue taken during biopsy.[104] Clinical examination often reveals a "floppy" child with muscle weakness in the face, neck, trunk, and limbs; decreased muscle mass; and absent deep tendon reflexes.

The use of orthopedic devices and adaptive equipment and activity can increase mobility, minimize contractures, delay or prevent spinal curvatures, and increase participation in physical activities. Maintaining the child's independent mobility for as long as possible is a major goal. Children with CMDs appear to degenerate more rapidly once in a wheelchair. Because these children are generally aware of their situation, the therapist working with this child should also be prepared to work with the issues of death and dying. Genetic counseling for parents and female siblings and family support programs are also of value.[45]

Myopathies are muscle disorders with symptoms that are similar to those of the dystrophies. The child may exhibit proximal muscle weakness of the face, neck, and limbs. Congenital myopathies are rare in infants; when they occur, they are usually caused by autosomal dominant patterns of inheritance but may also be caused by prolonged treatment with certain drugs, such as steroids. The congenital dislocation of the hip, scoliosis, seizures, and reduced cognitive skills may also be present. The diagnosis is made by muscle biopsy. Unlike the dystrophies, congenital myopathies progress slowly or not at all, which improves the prognosis.[102]

Neural Tube Defects and Spina Bifida

Neural tube defects (NTDs) are malformations that occur early in uterine development of the CNS, likely because of genetic and environmental factors. The prevalence of NTDs is falling, primarily caused by the ability to conduct prenatal screenings for NTD and improvement in nutritional status, principally that of folic acid. Because the incidence of NTDs varies so widely, it is assumed that both genetic and environmental factors play a part in vulnerability.[69] Recently, the research suggests that a combination of heredity and a folic acid deficiency may account for up to 50% of cases.[69] Studies have indicated that supplemental daily doses of folic acid can reduce the risk of NTDs by more than 50%. Even more convincing evidence for the role of folic acid is the ability of women to reduce their risk by 70% by taking the supplement when they are susceptible to the recurrence of an NTD. The prevalence of NTDs is falling worldwide as a result of screening, use of folic acid, and incidence of spina bifida cystica, which is believed to be 0.2 to 4.2 per 1000 live births.[27] The CDC reported an annual rate of 900 babies born with spina bifida or meningocele in the United States.[27] In Wales and Ireland, the prevalence is 3 to 4 times higher, and in Africa it is much lower, reflective of the genetic and environmental influences. The degree of impairment in NTDs depends on the level and degree of spinal cord involvement. This continuum of impairment can include no functional impairment, mild muscle imbalances and sensory losses, paraplegia, or even death in severe cases.

The three major forms of neural tube deficits are encephalocele, anencephaly, and spina bifida. *Encephalocele* is a result of protrusion in the occipital region of the brain. The overall incidence is approximately 2 per 1000 births.[27] These children typically have severe deficits, including cognitive impairment, hydrocephalus, motor impairments, and seizures. *Anencephaly* indicates a lack of neural development above the level of the brainstem; anencephalic children do not survive infancy. Females are three to seven times more likely to be affected than their male counterparts.[79]

Spina bifida is the term most commonly used to describe a congenital defect of the vertebral arches and spinal column. This condition occurs in the fourth week of prenatal development and can be identified by amniocentesis.[63] This defect may be mild, with the laminae of only one or two vertebrae affected (spina bifida occulta) and no malformation of the spinal cord, or it may involve an extensive spinal opening with an exposed pouch made up of cerebrospinal fluid (CSF) and the meninges (*meningocele*) or CSF, meninges, and nerve roots (*myelomeningocele*).

Spina bifida occulta is the most common and the most benign form; there is a separation of the vertebrae but no abnormalities are visible, no pouch is evident, and no symptoms are present (Figure 6-11).[63] In *occult spinal dysraphism (OSD)* (not to be confused with occulta) the infant is born with a visible abnormality on the lower back in the form of skin overlying the defect that may be dimpled, pigmented, or covered with hair.

Myelomeningocele is more serious and complex. A sac, or meningocele, visible above the bony defect characterizes this form of spina bifida. This sac is covered with skin and subcutaneous tissue and contains CSF, and although the meninges extend into the sac, the spinal cord remains confined to the spinal canal. In the neonatal period, great care must be taken

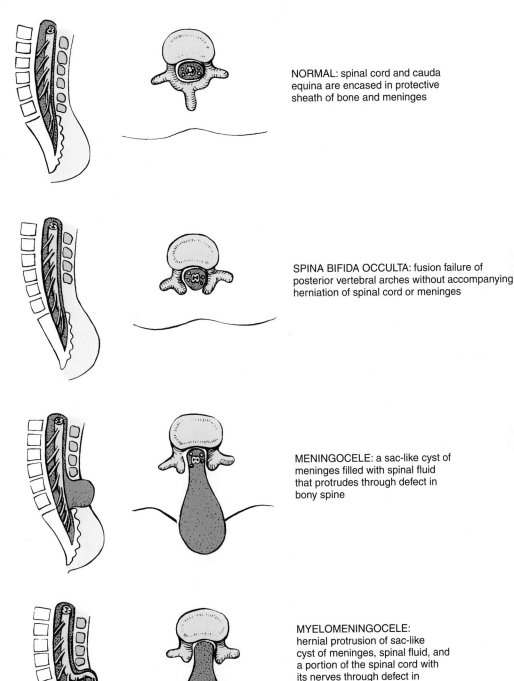

NORMAL: spinal cord and cauda equina are encased in protective sheath of bone and meninges

SPINA BIFIDA OCCULTA: fusion failure of posterior vertebral arches without accompanying herniation of spinal cord or meninges

MENINGOCELE: a sac-like cyst of meninges filled with spinal fluid that protrudes through defect in bony spine

MYELOMENINGOCELE: hernial protrusion of sac-like cyst of meninges, spinal fluid, and a portion of the spinal cord with its nerves through defect in vertebral column

FIGURE 6-11 Three forms of spina bifida. (From Hockenberry, M. J., & Wilson, D. [2009]. *Wong's essentials of pediatric nursing* [8th ed.]. St. Louis: Mosby.)

not to rupture the sac and to prevent infection. Surgical skin closure is usually performed soon after birth to protect the cyst. In some cases part or all of the sac is removed.[79]

Children with myelomeningocele usually display sensory and motor disturbances below the level of the lesion. Most lesions are in the thoracic or lumbar spine, resulting in lower-extremity paralysis and loss of sensation. Some children also demonstrate hip, spinal, or foot deformities. Orthotic interventions include lightweight bracing, casting, orthopedic shoes, and assistive devices for ambulation. Bowel and bladder incontinence is often a problem. Cognitive impairments and learning issues are also common with this form of spina bifida. Family education in skin care, urology, and diet enhances the child's independence. Medication, bowel training, and intermittent catheterization may assist significantly in this area.[63,69] Case Study 6-1 illustrates specific medical issues and outcomes in a child with spina bifida.

Complications with these forms of spina bifida include meningitis and hydrocephalus. Infection is contracted easily because of environmental exposure of the meninges and spinal cord. Hydrocephalus is a common secondary complication that may be caused either by a developmental defect in the brain (e.g., aqueduct stenosis) or by slippage of the lower portion of the brain (and part of the cerebellum) through the foramen magnum, a condition known as *Arnold-Chiari syndrome*.[69]

Hydrocephalus

Hydrocephalus is the result of a buildup of CSF in the ventricles of the brain. This occurs when an imbalance exists in the amount of CSF produced and the amount absorbed. Noncommunicating ventricles that obstruct the outflow of CSF from the ventricles can produce this phenomenon, as can an *Arnold-Chiari malformation* or occasionally a tumor.

An early sign of the condition in infants is an enlarged head. In an older child, whose head cannot grow, intracranial pressure increases. Definitive diagnosis may be made by sonography, computed tomography (CT), or magnetic resonance imaging (MRI) scans.[119]

Clinical signs of hydrocephalus in infants include abnormal head growth, with bulging fontanels, dilated scalp veins, and separated sutures; eyes that appear to deviate downward, producing a "sunset" appearance of the iris and visible sclera; and, after time, lethargy, irritability, and problems with reflexes, feeding, and tone. In older children, headache, irritability, development of strabismus or nystagmus, and cognitive changes may occur.[61]

The pressure produced by the hydrocephalus can result in visual and perceptual deficits, cognitive impairment, and seizures and in extreme cases, death. Children with hydrocephalus may demonstrate sensory processing and perceptual problems. Often they exhibit fine motor delays in association

---

CASE STUDY 6-1 Angela

Angela is a 6-year-old child who was born at term to a 23-year-old mother and did not receive consistent prenatal care. At the time of birth, a thoracic-level spina bifida with meningomyelocele (also called myelomeningocele) was evident. It was surgically closed at 2 days of age, and a ventriculoperitoneal shunt was inserted at 8 days of age to correct the hydrocephalus associated with her Chiari II malformation (common in children with meningomyelocele; the brainstem and cerebellum are displaced downward). At age 4, she needed to have her shunt surgically corrected for a blockage. She required a vesicostomy to treat the recurrent urinary tract infection, allowing urine to drain into her diaper continuously at 1 year of age. It is anticipated that she will continue to require use of a catheter. Angela is currently on a bowel and bladder program. Scoliosis is common at this level of lesion and it is anticipated that Angela will require orthotics and surgical intervention to prevent scoliosis and the development of further impairments.

During her first year, Angela received early intervention services, including physical and occupational therapy, speech language pathology, and an early childhood development program. She made good progress and at 12 months she was speaking several single words, sitting independently, and crawling by propelling herself with her arms. She was able to stand using a parapodium (an external flexible skeleton). By 3 years of age, Angela was independently using the parapodium for mobility and is still using this for mobility, but it is anticipated that as she grows she will require a wheelchair.

Fine motor impairments include difficulty with handwriting and in-hand manipulation skills. She is able to use a tripod grasp but is unable to maintain her grasp and frequently drops her pencil and quickly moves to other tasks. She forms all of her letters, but her handwriting quickly becomes illegible. She is age appropriate and is able to independently feed herself, with assistance for cutting foods. She demonstrates age-appropriate development and is independent in dressing her upper body, brushing her teeth and hair, and bathing with adaptive equipment. She requires maximum assistance with lower extremities and management of her bowel and bladder functions and for transfers. She enjoys watching sports with her father, watching movies, and making art projects. Her artwork adorns many rooms in the house.

She had psychoeducational testing before school entry at 5 years of age, which indicated that she had low-average intelligence (an IQ score of 90) and learning impairments. Her learning impairments include a short attention span, lack of frustration tolerance, difficulty with spatial relationships, and poor organizational skills. Executive functions including the ability to plan, initiate, sequence, sustain, and pace work are impairing her school participation more than her cognitive level. Her medical concerns and impairments have challenged her socially, although she is outgoing and has a positive affect. She has few friends and interacts with peers as a younger child. She will be placed in an inclusive class with a teacher's aide and resource help in reading and arithmetic. She receives direct occupational therapy services to improve in self-care skills and school occupations using both compensatory and skill-building approaches.

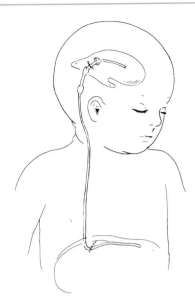

FIGURE 6-12   Ventriculoperitoneal shunt. Catheter is threaded subcutaneously from small incisions at the sites of ventricular and peritoneal insertions. (From Hockenberry, M. J., & Wilson, D. [2009]. *Wong's essentials of pediatric nursing* [8th ed.]. St. Louis: Mosby.)

with visual-perceptual impairment or dyspraxia. With problems in sensory, neuromotor, and perceptual performance areas, therapists often emphasize self-care, instrumental ADLs, and functional mobility skills.[63] If the hydrocephalus is caused by an obstruction, removal of the obstruction may alleviate the condition. The usual medical treatment for idiopathic hydrocephalus is placement of a ventriculoperitoneal (VP) shunt. This procedure (Figure 6-12) reduces the CSF pressure by means of a catheter that runs under the skin from one of the ventricles to the abdominal cavity, where the fluid can be absorbed safely. These shunts are usually effective but must be monitored regularly for signs of infection, clogging, kinking, or migration of the tube. Even with shunting, however, many of these children have cognitive, perceptual, visual, or other functional problems.[61]

Peripheral Nerve Injuries

Birth Injuries

Infants and children occasionally have traumatic injuries, perinatally and postnatally, that temporarily or permanently cause peripheral nerve impairment. For example, breech deliveries with after-coming arms can cause *brachial plexus lesions*. These infants may demonstrate weakness or wasting of the small muscles of the hands and sensory diminution in the area of the hand and arm served by this plexus.[118] This condition, called *Erb-Duchenne palsy*, is typically unilateral and related to the upper brachial plexus only. It is usually a result of extreme shoulder flexion (with the hand over the head). The condition is a common problem, and the incidence is 0.38 to 1.56 per 1000 live births. Paralysis of the arm results and is often more pronounced in the shoulder musculature than in the hand. The child often holds his or her arm in a characteristic posture,

with the shoulder adducted and internally rotated, elbow extended, forearm pronated, and wrist flexed. The prognosis depends on the extent of the damage to the nerves but can be good with early intervention.[118] In *Klumpke's palsy*, or lower brachial plexus paralysis, the stretching injury generally is more severe. Klumpke's palsy results in paralysis of the hand and wrist muscles. A severe brachial palsy injury results in paralysis of the entire arm, and a true Klumpke paralysis is very rare.

Partial immobilization and appropriate positioning to prevent contractures are required. Occupational therapy often involves fabrication of a sling that fits proximally around the humerus and passive and active assistive exercises. Later in infancy, resistive exercises may be recommended for development of optimal strength in the affected arm. If paralysis persists without improvement between 3 and 6 months of age, neuroplasty, neurolysis, end-to-end anastomosis, and nerve grafting are likely to be recommended.[3]

Traumatic Injury of Peripheral Nerves

In older children, injury to a peripheral nerve is usually caused by an accident, either through severing of the nerve or secondary to fractures, dislocations, excessive exercise, or occasionally medical treatments such as injections. Injuries of this type commonly occur to the radial, ulnar, and median nerves and the brachial plexus, lumbar plexus, peroneal nerves, or sciatic nerves.[48]

The diagnosis is made using a combination of measures, including nerve conduction studies, observations of sensory and motor involvement, muscle biopsies, electromyographs (EMGs), and, with serious accidents, surgical exploration.

Nerve injuries are categorized as class I, class II, or class III. A class III injury, the most severe type, is a *neurotmesis*, which means the axon and endoneurium have been severed. A class II injury is referred to as an *axonotmesis*, meaning that the endoneurium is intact but the axon degenerates distal to the lesion. A class I injury is a *neurapraxia*, in which there is some degree of paralysis but no peripheral degeneration. Depending on the severity of the injury, impairments range from diminished strength, absence of deep tendon reflexes (DTRs), and impairment of sensation with spontaneous recovery to complete disruption of connective tissues, in which regeneration of the damaged nerves may not occur without surgical intervention.

Specific treatment depends on the extent, progression, location, and especially the cause of the nerve damage. In general, treatment includes rest, splinting, nerve and local anesthetic injections (medication injected into the injured nerve), and surgical intervention to relieve nerve compression or to repair the damaged nerve.[48]

TRAUMATIC BRAIN INJURIES

Traumatic brain injuries (TBIs) or *head injuries (HIs)* during childhood constitute a major medical and public health problem. Among children ages 0 to 14 years, TBI results in an estimated 2,685 deaths, 37,000 hospitalizations, and 435,000 emergency department visits annually. If adolescents 14 to 18 years of age are included, the number of deaths and injuries rises dramatically and doubles for those years. Approximately 1 in 500 children are seriously injured and must endure prolonged hospitalizations and lifelong complications to some degree.[65,81] Trauma is the leading cause of both morbidity and mortality in the pediatric population, and traumatic injury causes 50% of all childhood deaths.[34] Significant mortality rates have been reported for children with TBI. Although children have better survival rates than adults with TBI, the long-term sequelae and consequences are often more devastating in children because of their age and developmental potential.[77] The costs involved in the care of a child with severe TBI, extended over the individual's lifetime, are significant.

Medical practitioners also have begun to recognize the importance of diagnosing minor head injuries, which may result in more subtle but persistent cognitive and functional impairments. According to the CDC, the most common causes of head injuries in young children, in order of frequency, are falls, motor vehicle accidents, assault or child abuse, and sports and recreation injuries. In older children, most head injuries are caused, in order of frequency, by motor vehicle accidents, sports-related injuries, and falls. As children reach adolescence, motor vehicle accidents remain the major cause of TBIs, followed by assault (primarily abuse and gunshot wounds), sports and recreation injuries, and falls.[65]

Head traumas are classified by the nature of the force that causes the injury and the severity of the injury. Forces that cause head trauma are referred to as either *impact* or *inertial forces*. Impact forces result from the head striking a surface or a moving object striking the head; these forces most often cause skull fractures, focal brain lesions, and epidural hematomas. Inertial forces are typically the result of rapid acceleration and deceleration of the brain inside the skull, resulting in a shearing or tearing of brain tissue and nerve fibers. Most TBIs are the result of both types of forces. The severity of HIs is rated as a range, from relatively mild concussion to more serious injury.[81] Damage to nervous system tissue occurs both at the time of impact or penetration and through secondary damage caused by brain swelling, intracranial pressure, hematomas, emboli, and hypoxic brain conditions. Early medical intervention can prevent or at least minimize these secondary causes of nervous system damage.[4]

Loss of consciousness is a prime indicator of a significant head injury. TBI also is implicated if the child does not lose consciousness or loses it only momentarily at the time of injury but later develops symptoms of lethargy, confusion, severe headache, irritability, vomiting, or speech or motor impairment. If consciousness is lost longer than momentarily, immediate medical attention is indicated.[81]

Once the child's medical condition has been stabilized, the severity of brain injury is determined. An assessment tool often used for this purpose is the Glasgow Coma Scale (GCS).[112] The GCS rates several parameters, including eye opening (4 [spontaneous] to 1 [no response]), best motor response (6 [obeys] to 1 [no response]), and verbal response (5 [oriented] to 1 [no response]). The score range, therefore, is 3 to 15, and a score of 8 or lower is considered an indicator of severe TBI. Initial diagnostic procedures typically include MRI or CT scanning, EEG, angiography, and radiography to determine the extent and location of fractures.[81] Medical treatment for moderate and severe TBIs includes close monitoring and control of cerebral circulation and intracranial pressure through the use of sophisticated devices and control systems. If the intracranial pressure cannot be controlled by traditional means, a large dose of barbiturate (e.g., phenobarbital) may be administered. If this fails to control the pressure, lowering the body temperature may help. Withdrawal from the barbiturate and body temperature treatments is difficult and may cause sleep disturbances, behavioral problems, apnea, and diminished intellectual functioning.[121]

Fortunately, most children who sustain a head injury have only a minor TBI (score of 13 to 15 on the GCS). Children with residual minor head injury deficits may require educational support, environmental modifications, and psychologic support. In most cases, the prognosis for these children is very good.[65]

Children who have sustained moderate or severe brain injuries typically follow a behavioral pattern of gradual and full return to consciousness. Depending on the severity of damage, the individual initially does not respond to any external stimuli or responds in a stereotypic manner. Only a small number of children remain in comas. At the first stage of recovery, children exhibit eye opening to external stimuli and generalized responses to noxious stimuli. The next stage of recovery can be the most difficult for family members because the individual is often agitated and combative; however, the child is rarely aware of his or her actions. As the agitation resolves, the child demonstrates increasingly appropriate responses to commands, ability to attend and concentrate, and recognition of family members. As the child progresses, intervention becomes more functional and goal oriented.[81]

An unfortunate perception of many health professionals is that children have better outcomes from severe TBI than adults; however, this belief is not substantiated by fact. The mortality rate for children with severe TBI (36% with a GCS score over 8) is similar to that for adults and, as do adults, these children make a guarded recovery.[4] Persistent deficits can vary widely; individuals who sustain moderate brain damage generally have fewer residual deficits. Performance skills deficits may include impairments in motor skills, process skills, and communication/interaction skills. Specific client factors likely to be involved are mental functions, sensory functions, and neuromusculoskeletal and movement-related functions. Typically, academic achievement is hindered, and the child requires modifications to the educational setting, including assistive technology and related services.[46,59,111]

DEVELOPMENTAL DISABILITIES

This section addresses disorders found in childhood that are not specifically associated with one body system and that delay the child's developmental progress. In general, developmental disabilities are characterized by prenatal, perinatal, or early childhood onset. Some of the factors that negatively affect developmental outcomes are maternal in origin, and others are caused by infant complications. Chapter 22 discusses medical factors during and immediately after birth that place the infant at risk for long-term disability. Each of the developmental disabilities described in this section has the potential to affect several areas of the child's development and to impair the child's performance and roles.

Intellectual Disabilities

Intellectual disability is the most common developmental disability, affecting 0.8% to 3% of the population, depending on the definition used.[15] Definitions of intellectual disabilities

(IDs) have three key factors: significantly impaired intellectual ability, usually measured on standardized psychoeducational tests; onset before 18 years of age; and impairment of the adaptive abilities necessary for independent living (i.e., communication, ADLs, instrumental activities of daily living (IADLs), work, play/leisure, education, and social participation).

Formal testing and the history are used to make a diagnosis of intellectual impairment. Assessment usually includes intelligence quotient (IQ) testing and tests of adaptive behavior (basic reasoning, environmental knowledge, and developmentally appropriate daily living and self-maintenance skills). Although the use of IQ scores is controversial, significantly below-average scores remain a good predictor of future cognitive functioning. Fortunately, intelligence is composed of a wider range of skills than is demonstrated on IQ tests. In addition, as in typically developing children, the developmental outcomes of children with IDs are significantly influenced by socioeconomic conditions, environmental events, having at least one parent who is highly committed to the child, and the individual's unique resilience.[14] A child is usually considered to have an ID if he or she scores more than two standard deviations below the normative range for age. In the fourth edition of the *Diagnostic and Statistical Manual of Mental Disorders* (DSM-IV-TR), ID is classified into four levels: mild, moderate, severe, and profound.[7] Although this classification has changed over the years and is somewhat artificial (i.e., it does not always directly equate with function), it is commonly used to describe children with ID (Figure 6-13).

Intensive debate persists in the literature regarding the rate of development in individuals with intellectual impairment and the ultimate potential of these individuals. These issues have significant implications for the identification and education of individuals with MR and their integration into society. The modes and strategies by which individuals with ID learn and the ways they differ in development are critical issues that must be resolved to facilitate education and the most appropriate therapeutic intervention.[51] Children with mild ID have an IQ range of approximately 55 to 70. Characteristics include the ability to learn academic skills at the third- to seventh-grade level and the usual achievement of social and vocational skills adequate for living in the community with intermittent support. The employment rate for adults with mild intellectual impairment is 80%, and 80% are married.

Children with moderate ID have an IQ range of approximately 40 to 55. These individuals require support to function in society. They are unlikely to progress past the second grade level in academics, but they can usually handle routine daily functions and do unskilled or semiskilled work in sheltered workshop conditions. A group home or supervised housing situation is usually the placement that families choose for these individuals as adults.

Children with severe ID have an IQ range of approximately 25 to 40. These individuals can usually learn to communicate, and they can be trained in basic health habits; however, they require extensive support and supervision to accomplish most tasks.

Children with profound ID have IQs below 25. These children need caregiver assistance for basic survival skills, and they usually have minimal capacity for sensorimotor or self-care functioning. Individuals with profound ID also often have interrelated neuromuscular, orthopedic, or behavioral deficits.

Intellectual impairment can occur secondary to another condition or without apparent cause.[15] These causes are usually categorized as (1) problems acquired in childhood (e.g., through toxins, trauma, or infection); (2) problems of fetal development and birth; (3) chromosomal problems; (4) CNS malformations; (5) congenital anomalies; and (6) neurocutaneous, metabolic, and endocrine disorders.

Approximately 80% of children with ID have additional problems. For example, it is estimated that approximately 50% have speech problems, 50% have ambulation problems, 20% have seizures, 25% have visual problems, and 40% have chronic conditions such as heart disease, diabetes, anemia, obesity, and dental problems.[14]

Parents, physicians, and allied health professionals involved in well-baby care and screening often express concerns about children later diagnosed with ID. Early signs of cognitive impairment include delays in meeting motor and speech milestones, unresponsiveness to handling and physical contact, reduced alertness or spontaneous play, feeding difficulties, and neurologic "soft" signs (i.e., balance, motor symmetry, perceptual motor skills, and fine motor skills). A formal diagnosis

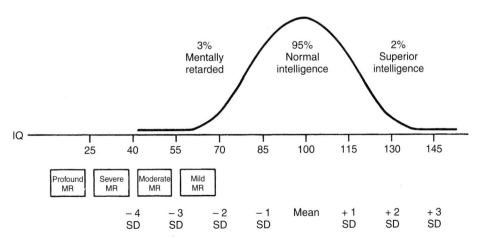

FIGURE 6-13 Criteria for determining the four degrees of severity in intellectual disabilities.

of ID generally is made when the child reaches school age because intellectual testing in preschool is limited by test sensitivity. Referrals for psychologic, educational, developmental, and speech and hearing evaluation may be made and the findings then interpreted for the parents. Services must be determined, and parents, siblings, and other family members must be given support and advice.[90]

Today, health care professionals, educators, and the general public practice a philosophy of inclusion of individuals with intellectual impairment. Beginning with early intervention, services and programs provide opportunities that enable these individuals to reach their maximum level of functioning in the least restrictive environment.[90]

Early programs for children with intellectual impairment usually focus on facilitating the attainment of developmental milestones; enriching the environment; developing self-help, language, and motor skills; and educating and supporting the parents. As the child grows, specific deficits may be addressed in special education programs. For the adolescent with ID, the development of vocational interests and skills, social skills and sex education, and community mobility skills are essential.[51]

Autism Spectrum Disorders or Pervasive Developmental Disorders

Autism spectrum disorder (ASD) or pervasive developmental disorders (PDDs) constitute a broad class of conditions that reflect a range of deficits, of which autism is the most well-documented form. ASDs are characterized by severe and complex impairments in reciprocal social interaction and communication skills and by the presence of stereotypical behavior, interests, and activities.[7] Onset typically is before 3 years of age, and the deficits persist throughout life. The most current prevalence rates indicate that ASD is seen at an aggregate rate of 16.8 per 10,000 persons.[40,116] Some surveys have suggested that the rate for all forms of ASD is about 3 per 1000 people, but more recent surveys suggest that the estimate may be as high as 6 per 1000.[40] These rates are almost twice as high as for early epidemiologic reports of autism and may partly be the result of an increase in recognition and of the clarification of diagnostic criteria. In 2002, the CDC estimated that approximately four times as many boys as girls have autism. Children with ASD are found in families of all racial, ethnic, intellectual, and socioeconomic backgrounds.[40] ASD includes autism, Asperger's syndrome, pervasive developmental disorder–unspecified, Rett syndrome, and other childhood disintegrative disorders.[7]

The unusual combinations of sensory, communication, and behavioral characteristics seen with ASDs have significant negative effects on a child's ability to participate in home, school, and community activities. Particularly associated with autism are severe limitations in relating to others and the display of ritualistic, stereotypical behaviors. Since Kanner's original description of 11 children who had "extreme autistic aloneness," many theories on the cause of autism have been proposed.[58]

Currently, autism is considered a neurobiologic disorder. Although none of the mechanisms is definitively known, many reliable studies suggest that the impairment occurs during the sculpting or wiring of the brain in utero. Neuroimaging studies have suggested that differences in cell density (e.g., brains are heavier) and reduced neuron size in areas critical to the trilogy of social-behavioral-communication disorders may be responsible for the impairments seen in PDDs.[99] Individuals with autism also exhibit abnormal cortical convolutions. Specifically, some of their sulci appear to be deeper and slightly out of place compared with those of healthy control subjects.[22]

In typical development, connections in the brain are shaped by experience and learning; with PDDs, it appears that synaptic and dendritic growth occur without guidance in areas related to communication and interaction skills; therefore, the correct migration and synaptic connections are not made.[29] Furthermore, studies show that when input is received in those with autism, communication between nearby cortical areas increases, whereas communication with more distant areas decreases. As a result, these persons have difficulty filtering or ignoring irrelevant stimuli and shifting attention when it is appropriate to do so.[116]

Some theories hold that abnormal action of the genes that control myelination and the creation of synapses and dendritic connections may be responsible for incorrect selective molding and elimination of synaptic connections.[19,22,60] Despite the compelling evidence for a strong genetic contribution to the etiology of autism (from twin and family studies), the unequivocal detection of a gene or susceptibility genes remains elusive.[70] The areas primarily affected include the amygdala, cerebellum, right somatosensory cortex, and orbitofrontale cortex, as well as the cingulated gyri. Initial pathologic anomalies seem to occur at higher-level cognitive processing pathways and involve the cerebral cortex as well.[54]

Neurochemical alterations also play a major role in autism. Studies consistently show elevated serotonin levels, hypothalamic-pituitary-adrenal axis (HPA) dysfunctions, and abnormalities in neuroendocrine functioning.[116] Although popular claims about the origins of autism abound, no evidence indicates that the disorder is correlated with diet or vaccinations (e.g., mumps, measles, and rubella vaccine) or that these affect the development or prevention of autistic disorders.[23]

Autism

Autism often coexists with neuropsychiatric disorders, including seizures, attention deficit–hyperactivity disorder, affective disorders, anxiety disorders, obsessive-compulsive disorders, and Tourette's syndrome.[72] The behavioral characteristics of autism are critical to the diagnosis of the disorder. These characteristics can be categorized into the following four subclusters of disturbances[7]:

1. Disturbances in social interactions
2. Disturbances in communication
3. Disturbances in behaviors
4. Disturbances of sensory and perceptual processing and associated impairments

Disturbances in social interactions affect the child's ability to establish meaningful relationships with people and inanimate objects. Although abnormalities in this area vary with age and in severity, they directly involve interactions that require initiative or reciprocal behavior from the child. Specific behaviors observed are poor or deviant eye contact, failure to develop peer relationships, delayed or inappropriate facial expression, apparent aversion to physical contact, lack of social reciprocity, delayed or absent anticipatory response to being picked up, and lack of spontaneous seeking of another to share enjoyment, an apparent preference for being alone.

Disturbances in communication may be thought of as a continuum from mild to severe. At the mild end of the continuum, normal language accompanied only by slight articulation or tonal deficits may be observed. At the severe end is a complete lack of speech (mute). Many other communication problems have been described at points along the continuum. For instance, much of the speech of children with autism is repetitive, or *echolalic*. Classic echolalia consists of parrot-like repetitions of phrases immediately after the child has been exposed to them; delayed or deferred echolalia consists of the repetition of phrases at a later time. Echolalic speech occurs out of social context and appears to have little or no communicative value. Other types of speech and language problems include syntax problems, atonal and arrhythmic speech, pronoun reversals, and lack of inflection and emotion during communication.

Disturbances in behaviors are seen in the intolerance of deviation from routine, resistance to any type of change, and patterns of behaviors that are best categorized as stereotypical, perseverative, and lacking in representational or pretend play. In addition, bizarre attachments to unusual objects develop (e.g., intense interest in a vacuum cleaner or a sheet of paper versus stuffed animals or dolls). These patterns of behavior are obsessive rituals, from which any deviation is not tolerated.[54] Deviations from the routine, however slight, often elicit intense temper tantrums.

Deviant motor patterns may involve the arms, hands, trunk, lower extremities, or entire body. Motor patterns in the upper extremities are common and include wiggling and flicking of the fingers, alternating flexion and extension of the fingers, and alternating pronation and supination of the forearm. Other motility patterns often seen include head rolling and banging, body rocking and swaying, lunging and darting movements, toe walking, involuntary synergies of the head and proximal segments of the limbs, and inability to perform two motor acts at the same time.[8]

For almost 40 years, *disturbances of sensory and perceptual processing* have been reported in children with autism. These include abnormal responses to various visual, vestibular, and auditory stimuli. In particular, children with autism appear to be overly sensitive to sound and may have difficulty coping with everyday environmental noises.[35] Some studies have reported auditory under-responsivity.[10] Over-responsivity to tactile input has also been reported in the literature.[11] Children with tactile hypersensitivity are more likely to exhibit inflexible behaviors, such as stereotypies and repetitive actions.

Associated impairments in autism include intellectual impairment, seizure disorders, and discontinuities in developmental rates. The fact that a large percentage of children with autism also suffer from cognitive deficiencies has been a controversial but relatively accepted issue. The cognitive deficiencies exhibited by children with autism significantly affect potential outcomes and may result in significant, long-term disability. The incidence of seizure disorders in children with autism is high, and both tonic-clonic and complex partial seizures have been reported in this population.[54]

Although most children with autism have normal life expectancies, the functional prognosis is diverse. Some individuals with high-functioning autism or other types of PDD live and work independently in the community; some are fairly independent, needing only minimal support to work, whereas others continue to depend on support from family and friends. In general, the prognosis for children in the autism spectrum is closely related to communication skills and intelligence.

Higher-functioning children may become high-functioning adults with deficits in social interactions. The prognosis for independent functioning through behavioral and sensory interventions is encouraging.[116]

Comprehensive intervention, including parental counseling, behavioral treatment, special education in highly structured environments, sensory integrative therapy, social skills training, speech-language therapy, medications, and family support, constitutes the best management for children with autism and other types of PDD.[116] Various types of therapies have been advocated, including auditory integration training, dietary interventions, discrete trial training, medications, music therapy, and vision therapy. Despite wide use of these programs and the claims of benefits derived from them, most of these approaches lack rigorous scientific support.[24] In general, studies to date indicate that individuals with autism respond best to a highly structured, specialized educational program that includes elements of communication therapy, social skills training, and sensory integration therapy.[116] The medications used for these children include sedatives, stimulants, major and minor tranquilizers, antihistamines, antidepressants, and psychotropic medications. It is believed that these medications work best when used in conjunction with an interdisciplinary special education program.[54] However, significant progress has been made in the efficacy and safety of pharmacotherapeutic agents, primarily the selective serotonin reuptake inhibitors.

Asperger's Syndrome

Asperger's syndrome can be distinguished from autism by the fact that these children do not exhibit clinically significant delays in language skills. The essential features of Asperger's syndrome are severe and sustained impairments in social interaction and the development of restricted, repetitive patterns of behavior, interests, and activities. The interference with functional daily living skills must be significant.[7] Children with Asperger's syndrome show typical cognitive development and age-appropriate self-help skills or adaptive behavior aside from social interaction impairments.[116] Although language skills are age appropriate, individuals with Asperger's syndrome display idiosyncrasies in verbal communication, characterized by highly circumstantial utterances, long-winded and tangential accounts of events, failure to convey a clear thought, and one-sidedness. Often an obsessive interest in letters and numbers absorbs most of the person's attention and energy. In addition, these individuals display a lack of nonverbal communication and of empathy; they tend to intellectualize feelings and show a poor understanding of others' affect.[116]

Epidemiologic studies suggest an overall incidence of 8.4 per 10,000 births, and the syndrome is five times more prevalent in boys. Treatment currently consists of supportive and symptomatic intervention. These services include special education programs, assistance with generalizing adaptive functioning to a wider variety of settings, problem-solving strategies, social skills training, speech and language skills training, and vocational training.[116]

Rett Syndrome

Rett syndrome is an X-linked, dominant progressive neurologic disorder (i.e., it occurs exclusively in girls). It is caused by mutations in the gene *MeCP2*, which is responsible for coding the methyl-CpG–binding protein 2, a protein critical to early brain development. This disorder is extremely rare, having a pooled estimated incidence across studies of 0.2 per 10,000 births. The presence of the abnormal gene on the X chromosome of the male embryo results in miscarriage.[54] The condition is diagnosed by genetic analysis, and although its early symptoms are indistinguishable from those of autism, its progressive nature makes it unlike the other PDDs.[56]

Development appears normal in children with Rett syndrome until about 6 months of age; thereafter, the child demonstrates rapid degeneration in head growth, loss of hand skills, and poorly coordinated gait or trunk movements. Difficulties with social interaction are similar to those seen with autism, but are transient in nature. Initially there is a loss of social engagement, but then social skills re-emerge later in the disorder. Microcephaly, spasticity, and seizures occur, and the child develops autistic-like behaviors such as hand mouthing, flapping, or wringing. Functional hand use disappears, and waking hyperventilation is characteristic. Children with Rett syndrome can survive for some time but are usually nonambulatory and nonverbal by late childhood. This is an incurable condition, but carbamazepine may be helpful in reducing symptoms and improving alertness.[56]

Attention Deficit–Hyperactivity Disorder

Regarded as the most common childhood neurobehavioral disorder, *attention deficit–hyperactivity disorder* (ADHD) is a heterogeneous behavioral disorder of uncertain cause that always is evident in childhood but that typically persists through adolescence and, for some, into adulthood.[37] Because of past and recurring difficulties with strict definitions of ADHD, accurate prevalence data are difficult to determine.[12] Using DSM-IV-TR criteria as a standard, prevalence estimates for ADHD vary between 3% and 5% of the school-age population, or approximately 2 million children.[7] The disorder occurs approximately three times more often in boys than in girls.

The prevalence of ADHD subtypes may differ according to the source of referral, with hospital-based clinics, pediatric neurologists, and child psychiatrists treating predominantly a combined subtype and primary care practitioners treating a higher number of the inattentive subtype. The CDC estimates 4.4 million youth ages 4 to 17 have been diagnosed with ADHD by a health care professional, and as of 2003, 2.5 million youth ages 4 to 17 are currently receiving medication treatment for the disorder. In 2003, 7.8% of school-aged children were reported to have an ADHD diagnosis by their parent.[115]

Children with ADHD exhibit inattention, hyperactivity, and impulsivity, which cause impairment in ADLs before 7 years of age. Inattention is demonstrated by failure to attend to details, difficulty sustaining attention during play, inability to listen actively to instructions or conversation, difficulty organizing tasks, and avoidance of tasks that require sustained attention. This child is easily distracted and is often forgetful in daily activities. Examples of hyperactivity are frequent fidgeting, inability to sit when remaining seated is expected (e.g., in a classroom), difficulty playing quietly, excessive talking, and being "constantly on the go." Impulsivity can be seen in the inability to wait one's turn, frequent and incessant interruptions, and blurting out of answers before a question is

asked. Other related features include low frustration tolerance, sleep disorders, bossiness, excessive and frequent demands for attention, mood lability, demoralization, dysphoria, peer rejection, and poor self-esteem.[13] Children with ADHD are also at high risk for injuries associated with increased risk-taking behavior and impulsivity.[13]

The symptoms vary in degree of impairment, frequency of occurrence, and pervasiveness across settings. They must occur "often" (to distinguish single symptoms from typical behavior observed in 48% to 52% of children) and across multiple settings (e.g., school, play, home, daycare). The symptoms must persist for at least 6 months to a degree that is maladaptive and that subsequently interferes with all occupational activities, including self-care, academic performance, and peer relationships.

Over the past few decades, researchers have sought to develop and test theories about the etiology of ADHD. One theory that persists in popular literature is that ADHD is related to food allergies or food additives and the amount of sugar in a child's diet. The National Institutes of Health (NIH) concluded that there is no evidence that diet is responsible for the onset of ADHD and that only in a fraction of children with ADHD is a restricted diet efficacious in reducing symptoms associated with this disorder.[41] The current etiologic theories, widely supported but still under investigation, include genetic factors, neurologic factors, and neurochemical imbalances.

In neural imaging studies, a significant decrease in brain activity in the frontal parietal lobes, which inhibit impulsiveness and control attention, has been demonstrated in adults with ADHD; however, the primary cause of this decreased activity is still unknown.[43] Studies of the heritability of this disorder are perhaps the best support that researchers have for linking ADHD with a neurobiologic etiology.[9,39] It is clear that ADHD runs in families, and this may be one mechanism underlying ADHD symptoms. Siblings of children diagnosed with ADHD are five to seven times more likely to be diagnosed with ADHD as are children from unaffected families.[43]

Three genes are hypothesized to be related to the onset of ADHD. Although these genes do not account for a majority of ADHD symptoms, the specific alleles of these genes may impart an increased susceptibility to ADHD.[43] Neurochemical research into potential causes has failed to identify a single neurotransmitter that is responsible for the clinical deficits in ADHD.[13] However, medications that influence neurotransmitter functioning are effective in treating some aspects of ADHD, leading researchers to believe that a neurochemical cause remains a viable theory. The selective availability of dopamine and norepinephrine are both candidates for a significant role in this disorder.[13]

Two theories have been proposed for the cognitive impairments seen in ADHD. Barkley suggests that the symptoms seen in ADHD are a result of response inhibition, which prevents accurate self-regulation to environmental stimuli.[13] He suggests that the response inhibition stems from underfunctioning of the orbital frontal cortex and its subsequent connections to the limbic system.

Two primary medical intervention strategies include stimulant pharmacotherapy (e.g., amphetamines, methylphenidate) and behavioral interventions. Pharmacotherapy allows 9 of 10 affected children to focus and to be more successful at school, home, and play.[13] There is no evidence that prolonged use of stimulant drugs is addictive, promotes addictive behavior in adolescence, makes children "high" or jittery, or sedates the child. The realistic side effects of these drugs include weight loss, loss of appetite, interrupted sleep patterns and, in some children, slowed growth. Pharmacologic treatment seems to improve overactivity, attention span, impulsivity and self-control, compliance, physical and oral aggression, social interactions with peers, and academic productivity and accuracy.[13] Rarely, however, are medications alone sufficient to allow a child to function in most settings.[43] Deficits that seem to persist are those in reading skills, social skills, learning, academic achievement, and antisocial behavior.

Consequently, one or more behavioral interventions are typically needed. The most frequently recommended therapies include cognitive-behavioral therapy, behavior modification, educational interventions, social skills training, and psychotherapy.[93] Although the definitive efficacy of any one strategy has not yet been determined, it is clear that a consistency in responses in all of the child's settings, the environmental adaptations, and counseling to alleviate low self-esteem contribute to improvement in learning and attainment of social skills.[42] School-based occupational therapists often receive referral for children with ADHD and provide a variety of strategies to the classroom to improve attention and focus. Examples include modifying the classroom environment, social skills training, self-management techniques, and interventions to enhance sensory modulation.

Learning Disabilities

The term *learning disabilities* describes a group of problems that affect a child's ability to master school tasks, process information, and communicate effectively. These disabilities are often not associated with a specific neurologic insult.[105] Learning disabilities (LDs) are often associated with a variety of other neurologic problems (e.g., ADHD). Specific LDs include auditory processing, language disabilities, and perceptual impairments.

Most children with a learning disability have average or above-average intelligence and adequate sensory acuity (are not blind or deaf) and have been provided with appropriate learning opportunities. Despite all of these positive features, a significant discrepancy exists between the child's academic potential and his or her educational performance. LDs include a variety of conditions such as perceptual disabilities, dyslexia, and developmental aphasia. Not included in this category are learning problems that stem from primary sensory deficits, MR, socioeconomic conditions, or psychosocial impairments. The National Joint Committee on Learning Disabilities defines *learning disability* as a generic term that refers to a heterogeneous group of disorders manifested by significant difficulties in the acquisition and use of listening, speaking, reading, writing, reasoning, or mathematic abilities.[7]

Although different studies and agencies report varying incidence figures, the figure most often given is approximately 4% to 5% of the school population, or about 2 million children. More boys than girls are affected in this instance at a ratio of 4:1. In this case, however, some researchers suggest that the gender difference is related to the tendency of girls not to exhibit oppositional defiant behavior and girls therefore are infrequently diagnosed.[105]

A child with LD may display any number of the behaviors in the following nine categories:

1. *Disorders of motor function:* These include disorders both of motor skills and of motor activity level. Motor skills dysfunction may range from clumsiness, to poor performance in gross or fine motor skills, to problems planning new tasks (dyspraxia), to equilibrium deficits, to sensorimotor problems in a number of areas. Sometimes tics, grimaces, and choreoathetoid movements in the hands may be observed. The child may be described as always being in motion (hyperactive) or as being slow and lethargic (hypoactive).

2. *Educational disorders:* Educational disorders can occur in one or more academic subjects. Related educational skills that are often limited or delayed are copying from the blackboard, printing and cursive writing, organizing time and materials, understanding written and oral directions, symbolic confusion (reversing letters), cutting, coloring, drawing, and keeping place on the page.

3. *Disorders of attention and concentration:* Examples of these disorders include short attention span and other attention deficits, restlessness, impulsivity, and motor and verbal perseveration.

4. *Disorders of thinking and memory:* These types of disorders are characterized by difficulty with abstract reasoning and concept formation and by poor short- and long-term memory capabilities.

5. *Problems with speech and communication:* In these cases, the child may show difficulty shifting topics of conversation; difficulty with "small talk"; difficulty with the sequencing of words, sentences, or sounds; slurred words; and articulation problems.

6. *Auditory difficulties:* Auditory difficulties associated with LD often stem from auditory perceptual and auditory memory problems and not from acuity (hearing) problems. Children with these types of problems are often the ones who cannot remember the oral directions just given to them (auditory memory), cannot sound out words or blend sounds into words (phonemic synthesis), cannot block out background noise (speech-in-noise), and cannot remember the sequencing of sounds, words, or numbers (auditory sequencing). These types of problems often affect school performance and should be explored by an audiologist who is familiar with the specific instruments and programs available to assess and treat auditory-perceptual (central auditory processing) problems. The high incidence of allergies and ear infections in children with LD puts them at risk for auditory-perceptual problems.

7. *Sensory integrative and perceptual disorders:* Children with LD often have various sensory integrative and perceptual disorders. Many of these children have difficulty with laterality and directionality concepts and tasks that require visual perception skills.

8. *Psychosocial problems:* These disorders may be manifested as temper tantrums or antisocial behavior, and the child's social competencies may be delayed compared with his or her chronologic age and mental age. Many of these children are sensitive and decidedly at risk for poor self-esteem and for self-concept problems because they have the intelligence to know when they are being teased

and to know the frustration of being good at some things and not at others.

9. *Specific learning difficulties that accompany the learning disability:* This is most frequently a specific reading disability.[105]

Most children with LD retain some degree of disability as adults; however, most are contributing members of society. As with all disorders, the prognosis is affected by the severity of the disability. Therefore, individuals with limited impairment should not be limited in their life and career skills, but those with severe LD may need vocational planning, counseling, and adaptations to ensure as high a level of social, emotional, and vocational functioning as possible.

The occupational therapist's role in an intervention program for the child with LD may change as the child develops, depending on the nature and extent of the child's specific disability. With young children, sensory integration, play, and basic socialization and self-help skills may be the focus of early intervention and parent education. As the child progresses into school, sensory integration intervention may continue, but additional programs to promote social play, perceptual motor integration, and writing skills are indicated. By early adolescence, the focus of evaluation and intervention shifts to independent living skills, social skills, and the development of compensatory and adaptive techniques, as well as vocational skills and interests.

Developmental Coordination Disorder

Developmental coordination disorder has been known by many names, some of which are still used today. It has been called clumsy child syndrome, clumsiness, developmental disorder of motor function, and congenital maladroitness. Developmental coordination disorder is usually first recognized when a child fails to reach such normal developmental milestones as walking or beginning to dress him or herself. The essential feature of developmental coordination disorder is impairment in the development of motor coordination. The diagnosis is made if the coordination difficulties are not the result of a general medical condition or pervasive developmental disorder.[7]

Children with developmental coordination disorder often have difficulty performing tasks that involve both fine and gross motor skills, including forming letters when they write, throwing or catching balls, and buttoning buttons. Children who have developmental coordination disorder may exhibit typical development in all other ways. The disorder can, however, lead to social or academic problems for children. Because of their underdeveloped coordination, they may choose not to participate in activities on the playground. This avoidance can lead to conflicts with or rejection by their peers. Also, children who have problems forming letters when they write by hand, or drawing pictures, may become discouraged and give up academic or artistic pursuits.[28]

The manifestations of developmental coordination disorder vary greatly from child to child. The general characteristic is that the child has delayed or deficit development of one or more types of motor skills when the child's age and IQ are taken into account. In some children these coordination deficiencies manifest as an inability to tie shoes or catch a ball, whereas in other children they appear as an inability to draw objects or properly form printed letters.[7]

It is estimated that as many as 6% of children between the ages of 5 and 11 have developmental coordination disorder.[7] Males and females are thought to be equally likely to have this disorder, although males may be more likely to be diagnosed. Developmental coordination disorder and speech-language disorders seem to be closely linked, and children with one disorder are more likely to have the other.

No interventions are known to work for all cases of developmental coordination disorder. Experts recommend that a specialized course of treatment, possibly involving work with an occupational therapist, be designed to improve the child's performance. Many children can be effectively helped in special education settings to improve handwriting, keyboarding, and manipulation of materials. For other children, physical education classes designed to improve general motor coordination, with emphasis on skills the child can use in playing with peers, can be very successful. Any kind of physical training that allows the child to safely practice motor skills and motor control may be helpful.[49]

It is important for children who have developmental coordination disorder to receive individualized therapy, because for many children the secondary problems that result from extreme clumsiness can be very distressing. Self-esteem may be lower because they lack the skills needed to participate with peers in many games and sports. Exclusion from these activities can lead to poor self-image. Children may go to great lengths to avoid physical education classes and similar situations in which their motor coordination deficiencies might be noticeable. Treatments that focus on skills that are useful on the playground or in the gymnasium can help to alleviate or prevent these problems.[49]

Children with developmental coordination disorder also frequently have problems writing letters and numbers, or performing other motor activities required in the classroom—including coloring pictures, tracing designs, or making figures from modeling clay. These children may become frustrated by their inability to master tasks that their classmates find easy and, therefore, may stop trying or become disruptive. Individualized programs designed to help children master writing or skills related to arts and crafts may help them regain confidence and interest in classroom activities. For many people, developmental coordination disorder lasts into adulthood. Through specialized attention and teaching techniques, many children develop the motor skills that they lack. Some children, however, never fully develop the skills required in sports and other physical tasks. Although many children improve their motor skills significantly, in most cases their motor skills will never match those of their peers.[7]

Genetic and Chromosomal Abnormalities

Human beings normally have 23 pairs of chromosomes in each cell of the body, and each chromosome contains 250 to 2000 genes. Genetic anomalies involve one gene, whereas chromosomal abnormalities can involve thousands of genes. Smaller or larger numbers of chromosomes can cause significant developmental disabilities. These syndromes may present characteristic symptom patterns and can often be identified by chromosomal analysis of the child's body tissues. Genetic disorders range from addition or loss of an entire chromosome in each cell, to loss of part of a chromosome, to microdeletion of a number of contiguous genes within a chromosome. As a general rule, the larger the defect, the more severe the ensuing disorder.[14] Analysis of the amniotic fluid may identify these children before they are born.[50]

Chromosomal Disorders

During cell division, chromosomes pass their identical genetic information to daughter cells. The two types of cell division are mitosis and meiosis. *Mitosis* creates two daughter cells from one parent cell. In *meiosis,* four daughter cells are created from one parent cell, with only 23 chromosomes passed on. Mitosis occurs in all cells, meiosis only in germ cells (i.e., it creates sperm and eggs). A number of events can occur during cell division that will adversely affect development.

One such event, *nondisjunction of autosomes* (i.e., unequal division of chromosomes during cell division) yields an excess or loss of chromosomal material. The most common condition is evidenced in the trisomy syndromes. The most common trisomy syndrome is *trisomy 21,* or *Down syndrome,* which is characterized by one additional chromosome 21. The egg that is fertilized has 23 chromosomes, and the resulting embryo has three copies of chromosome 21. This syndrome, found in approximately 1 in 660 newborns, causes specific mental and physical problems. Although a range of physical characteristics may be associated with Down syndrome, a few are common to most children, such as a short, stocky stature and a protruding abdomen. The head is often small and flattened at the back, and the eyes have an upward slant and abnormal epicanthal folds. Other common facial features include low-set ears, a flat nose, and often a mouth held slightly open with the tip of the tongue protruding. The extremities are shorter than normal, and the fingers and toes are usually broad and short. The palms of the hands typically have a single crease, known as the *simian crease.*[101]

Related health problems often include cardiovascular abnormalities, obesity, a higher incidence of respiratory infections and other infections caused by immune system inefficiency, thyroid deficiencies, gastrointestinal problems, and an apparent increase in the risk of leukemia.[101] Often, visual acuity is poor and requires correction. One problem that is potentially dangerous to the child is atlantoaxial dislocation, which results in a tendency for dislocation between the first and second cervical vertebrae. A severe dislocation can result in spinal cord damage. If this dislocation is found through radiographic films, surgery may be performed, and the family may be given precautions about roughhouse play or participation in activities that put stress on this joint.

The life expectancy for children with Down syndrome has improved greatly over the past several years. Those without cardiac anomalies can be expected to live into late adulthood. However, it is common for these older individuals to develop a syndrome similar to Alzheimer's disease.[101]

Children with Down syndrome are usually recognized at birth by their facial characteristics. They frequently also have low muscle tone, hypermobile joints, and problems with sucking. A medical examination is performed to detect any related congenital cardiac and medical problems, which could extend the child's hospital stay. As the child grows, developmental delays in all areas of function are noted, although the degree can vary greatly from case to case. Motor planning skills, language, and cognitive skills develop slowly. Early intervention

and special education, as well as support and education of the parents, help these children achieve their optimal function.

Other trisomies occur, but most of these are uncommon, and many of them result in abortion of the fetus, or stillbirth. *Trisomy 18,* or *Edwards' syndrome,* occurs in approximately 1 in 3000 births.[14] These children have a long, narrow skull; low-set, malformed ears; a prominent occiput; small mouths and a weak cry; syndactyly and webbed neck; congenital heart and kidney malformations; severe MR; failure to thrive; and early death.[79] The survival rate beyond infancy is only about 10%.

Trisomy 13, or *Patau's syndrome,* occurs in 1 in 5000 births.[79] Children with Patau's syndrome have multiple anomalies, including eye, ear, and nasal anomalies; cleft lip and palate; polydactyly and syndactyly; and microcephaly and neural tube defects. About 20% of these children survive, and most of these are severely retarded and have seizure disorders.

A decrease in the number of chromosomes (45 or fewer) also causes problems. Fetuses with this genetic abnormality often die early in gestation. One exception is children born with *Turner's syndrome,* which is found in approximately 1 in 5000 girls and is caused by one missing sex chromosome. These babies may be born with webbing of the neck or congenital edema of the extremities and may have cardiac problems. Small stature, obesity, and underdeveloped ovaries, resulting in infertility and absence of secondary sexual characteristics, are clinical features that must be dealt with in the school-aged child and adolescent with Turner's syndrome. Although visual perception problems are common, most of these children do not have intellectual impairment; therefore, their functional prognosis is good.[14]

Other chromosomal abnormalities are caused by a missing portion of an individual chromosome (deletion) or by a portion of a chromosome breaking off and reattaching to another chromosome (translocation). The incidence of these events is lower than that of the chromosomal problems described, and because the amount of chromosomal material that is missing or duplicated varies, the resulting conditions are expressed differently. Problems common in these types of conditions are MR, abnormal brain development, and facial abnormalities.

Cri du chat syndrome is rare (1 in 50,000 live births) and is caused by deletion of part of chromosome 5. This condition is so named because the affected baby has a weak, mewing cry. These children have a small head and widely spaced, downslanting eyes, cardiac abnormalities, failure to thrive, and microcephaly. They also have MR, hypotonia, and feeding and respiratory problems.[14]

Nondisjunction of sex chromosomes, the most common type of which is *Klinefelter's syndrome,* is caused by an XXY sex chromosomal pattern. In this condition, the male is born with an extra X chromosome, derived primarily from the mother. This gives the child a total of 47 chromosomes instead of the usual 46. The syndrome occurs in approximately 1 in 500 live male births and results in a mild disorder that may not be recognized until adulthood. LDs and emotional and behavioral problems are characteristic of Klinefelter's syndrome. Males with this syndrome are tall and slim, have small genitalia, and are infertile. An XYY chromosomal pattern occurs in 4 in 1000 male births, and those with this pattern also are tall. These individuals may be expected to have mildly depressed IQ scores, tremors, reduced coordination, radioulnar synostosis, and an increased incidence of temper tantrums, impulsiveness, and inability to plan or handle frustration and aggression.[50]

Genetic Disorders

The foregoing syndromes represent the presence or absence of genes resulting from extra or deleted chromosomal material. Genetic disorders that stem from an abnormality in a single gene, of which there are an estimated 100,000 in the human genome (the set of all genes), can also occur. Genes are responsible for producing specific protein products and for regulating development and functions in the body.

Single-gene, or *Mendelian trait*, genetic disorders are inherited abnormalities caused by abnormal genes that have had a negative effect on development.[14] Four different patterns of single-gene inheritance are recognized:

1. *Autosomal dominant inheritance*, in which an abnormal gene is present on one of the non-sex chromosomes. Usually this gene is passed directly from one of the parents to the child. On rare occasions, the gene is not present in either the mother or the father, in which case it is known as a new, or "fresh," mutation. There is no carrier state; if the gene is present, the baby will have the abnormal characteristics. An example of an autosomal dominant illness is von Recklinghausen's disease (neurofibromatosis).

2. *Autosomal recessive inheritance*, in which an abnormal gene must be in a paired condition because it is less potent. This also exists on non-sex chromosomes. Commonly, both parents are carriers but have no symptoms of the illness. Examples of conditions with autosomal recessive patterns are cystic fibrosis, phenylketonuria, and diabetes. Many of the inherited diseases and illnesses have this pattern of inheritance, and in many instances the carrier states can be detected with various diagnostic procedures.

3. *X-linked inheritance*, in which the abnormal gene sits on the female sex chromosome, the X chromosome. Because this gene is recessive, in girls the normal gene on the second sex chromosome prevents expression of the disease. However, a boy who inherits the abnormal gene on his mother's X chromosome will be affected. Duchenne's muscular dystrophy and hemophilia (factor VIII deficiency) are examples of diseases inherited through this pattern.

4. *Polygenic*, or *multifactorial, inheritance*, which is a result of the interaction of heredity and the environment. Some congenital heart problems, cleft lip and palate, and meningomyelocele are examples of polygenic inheritance problems.

Fragile X syndrome accounts for one third of all X-linked causes of MR. This condition is most evident in boys, who have only one X chromosome. The prevalence is estimated at 0.4 to 0.8 per 1000 boys and 0.2 to 0.6 per 1000 girls. Genetic transmission of this disorder is complex, and outcomes can vary when the mother passes on the defective gene. The clinical manifestations become progressively more severe in subsequent generations of expression of fragile X syndrome. The underlying gene defect is the result of an abnormality of the X chromosome that causes a portion of the chromosome to become constricted; this defect has been named the *FMR1 gene*. The FMR1 gene affects body functions, primarily brain development. It is responsible for a protein that is important in brain development, and production of this protein is decreased. The progression in this disorder is caused by the expanded section of DNA on the X chromosome; the sequence that is repeated is a series of three nucleotide bases or a triplicate repeat of cytosine-guanine-guanine (CGG) at four fragile X locations. These mutations lead to a host of characteristics.[80]

In addition to intellectual impairment, children with fragile X syndrome have craniofacial deformities, including elongated face; prominent jaw and forehead; large, protruding ears; a high-arched palate; hyperextensible joints; and flat feet. Other features, including prolapse of the mitral valve and enlarged testicles, become more pronounced with age. Some cognitive features seem to be preserved in males (e.g., simultaneous processing) even while they are identified as having MR with poor auditory memory and reception. In addition, participation in daily living skills is preserved, whereas communication and social skills are impaired.[80] Speech tends to be echolalic, cluttered, and perseverative. Furthermore, these children may be identified as having ASD because of the presence of stereotypical behavior, poor eye contact, unusual sensory stimuli responses, and lack of social skills.[50]

Neurofibromatosis, or *von Recklinghausen's disease*, manifests in two forms, which have different genetic patterns. *Peripheral neurofibromatosis* (type 1) is the more common form; the other is *central neurofibromatosis* (type 2). The incidence is estimated at 1 in 3000 to 5000 live births, and the condition occurs more often in boys.[79] Neurofibromatosis causes multiple tumors, usually neurofibromas, on the central and peripheral nerves, café-au-lait spots on the skin, and vascular and visceral lesions. If these tumors occur in critical areas, they may cause death. Mild MR and LD are associated with the condition, as are speech disorders. Hypertension, optic nerve gliomas (type 1), auditory nerve tumors (type 2), skeletal anomalies, and short stature are also associated with the disease. Intervention for the condition may include surgical removal of dangerous or disfiguring lesions, reduction of symptoms, special education, and monitoring for cerebral tumors.

Prader-Willi syndrome is a genetic disorder associated with a defect in chromosome 15. This condition causes severe obesity, short stature, decreased muscle tone, a long face and slanted eyes, poor thermal regulation, and underdeveloped sex organs. Moderate MR and extreme food-seeking behaviors are classic signs. This condition occurs in 1 in 15,000 live births.[79]

Williams syndrome has been traced to a microdeletion on chromosome 7 in the region of the gene that codes for elastin. Although the condition is rare (1 per 20,000 live births), its clinical features are dramatic. The syndrome yields a unique combination of cerebral maldevelopment and cardiovascular abnormalities. This inherited syndrome is characterized by mild mental retardation, yet striking preservation of musical aptitude, social skills, and writing, and an inability to draw even simple objects. The facial characteristics include a wide mouth, almond-shaped eyes, upturned nose, and small, pointed ears.[102] Sensitivity to auditory stimuli is paired with a delay in the acquisition of speech and deficits in visual, spatial, and motor skills. These individuals are virtually the converse of autism in their sociability and empathy.

Inborn Errors of Metabolism

Several genetic problems produce errors in the metabolism of environmental and internal substances. Left untreated, these conditions may cause serious disability and sometimes death. For some, early diagnosis allows treatment or prevention of these consequences, but for others, no known treatment has yet been found. For individuals with errors of metabolism, prenatal diagnosis and genetic counseling may be the only options.

Phenylketonuria (PKU) is an inborn error in the metabolism of phenylalanine, an amino acid commonly found in some proteins. This silent (i.e., produces acute toxicity) condition affects 1 in 15,000 children but is rare in individuals of Jewish origin and in African American children. These children predominantly have blond hair and blue eyes. If the condition is untreated, severe cognitive and behavioral disabilities will develop and will, at times, mimic autism. The diagnosis can be made at birth with the Guthrie test. Treatment, which is effective, is with dietary modification involving withholding foods that have the precursors of phenylalanine to prevent toxic accumulation. It is believed that the restrictive diet must be maintained until the age of 10 years.[16]

A similar condition, *galactosemia*, is the inability to convert galactose, a milk sugar, into glucose. Galactose builds up in the blood and causes hepatic and splenic dysfunction. If the condition goes untreated, the consequences include jaundice, vomiting and diarrhea, drowsiness and lethargy, cataracts, systemic infections, and death. Urine testing can detect the condition and is required for newborns in many states. Treatment involves a diet without galactose (no milk, milk products, or breast milk) and is usually effective in compliant children. In poorly controlled cases, some intellectual dulling, perceptual problems, tremors, choreoathetosis, and ataxia may be present.[50]

Lesch-Nyhan syndrome is a rare (1 in 380,000) progressive neuromuscular disease that is limited to boys and is characterized by an inability to metabolize purines. Affected children appear normal for the first year but then experience significant MR, neuromotor degeneration, and spasticity, as well as a compulsive need to bite their lips and fingers and rub their faces. This behavior is involuntary and becomes self-mutilating if it goes unchecked. Vocal tics may also be a feature. Arthritis, anemia, and renal calculi are also common. Treatment usually includes protecting the child from self-mutilation, developmentally focused therapies, and medication to prevent secondary problems and reduce mutilation. Naltrexone, an opioid antagonist, improves some of the clinical signs of this syndrome.[102]

DIABETES

Diabetes mellitus is a metabolic disorder of the pancreas in which the hormone insulin is secreted in insufficient amounts. Increased concentrations of glucose are found in the blood, and several systemic problems occur. The causes of diabetes are unknown, but the disease has a familial pattern and is now thought to be an autoimmune response to a viral infection in some cases.[50]

There are two major types of diabetes. Type 1 results in the destruction of pancreatic beta cells, usually leading to absolute insulin deficiency. The onset usually is around age 10 but may be earlier or later. This form of the disease tends to be more acute and requires the administration of insulin, carefully balanced with food intake and exercise, to provide adequate metabolic balance. Type 2 diabetes occurs more frequently in adults over 40 years of age. Type 2 is characterized by a resistance to insulin action, and it sometimes can be controlled by diet, exercise, or oral medications. Insulin may also be required in some stages of this form of diabetes. Maturity-onset diabetes of the young is transmitted as an autosomal dominant disorder; it is characterized by the formation of structurally abnormal insulin that has decreased biologic activity. The onset typically is before 25 years of age, and the condition often can be controlled with dietary modifications and oral hypoglycemic agents.[50]

Early symptoms of type 1 diabetes include polyuria, increased thirst, weight loss, and dehydration. Later symptoms may include acidosis, vomiting, hyperventilation, and coma.[5] Overdose of insulin may cause insulin shock or hypoglycemia. Over many years, even with good care, microvascular lesions may occur in multiple organs and result in retinopathy that leads to blindness, nephropathy, and peripheral nerve damage. Sensory loss and increased infection, especially in the extremities, may occur. Individuals with diabetes are at increased risk for heart disease, and diabetic women are at increased risk for complications in pregnancy.[5] Because this is a lifelong condition, the child and parents must be taught to administer insulin medications and adjust and monitor blood glucose levels and life and dietary patterns. These children must also adjust to being drug-dependent. This adjustment often is particularly difficult in adolescence.

The general goals of treatment are to ensure satisfactory growth and emotional development, help the child acquire some degree of normal life, resolve the symptoms, and prevent ketoacidosis and long-term sequelae, such as renal and cardiac damage and eye disease.[5] Achievement of these goals is difficult, because a delicate balance must be maintained among so many factors, specifically exercise, nutritional intake, hormones, emotions, and many other internal and external influences on blood sugar levels.

TOXIC AGENTS

Prenatal Toxins

Several birth defects may be caused by adverse changes in the fetal environment. Substances and factors that negatively affect the developing fetus are called toxic agents, or *teratogens*. Drugs, radiation, and chemicals are the most common teratogens known to affect fetal development. Table 6-3 lists some common teratogens and their possible effects on the developing fetus. Several factors determine whether a teratogen will affect the fetus. The dosage, the gestational stage of the infant, and the specific sensitivity of the developing organs at the time of exposure to the teratogen are all factors that contribute to the outcome.

Fetal Alcohol Syndrome Disorders

Prenatal exposure to alcohol can cause a range of disorders in the child that are known as *fetal alcohol syndrome disorders (FASDs)*. This umbrella term refers to *fetal alcohol syndrome*

TABLE 6-3 Effects of Common Teratogens on the Developing Fetus and Child

Substance	Effect on Fetus or Child
DRUGS	
Alcohol	Intrauterine growth retardation, mental deficiency, stillbirth. Infants may have complete fetal alcohol syndrome (including facial feature anomalies) or more mild fetal alcohol effects. They may experience withdrawal symptoms, mental retardation, hyperactivity, behavioral disorders, and learning disabilities.
Aspirin	In large amounts may be fatal or cause hemorrhagic manifestations
Cortisone	Possible factor in cleft palate
Caffeine	At extremely high levels, increased incidence of miscarriage and limb and skeletal malformations; mild intake shows no effect on the fetus
Dilantin	Fetal hydantoin syndrome (growth and mental deficiency, abnormalities of the face, anomalies of the hands)
Heroin, codeine, morphine	Hyperirritability, shrill cry, vomiting and withdrawal symptoms, decreased alertness and responsiveness to visual and auditory stimuli; can be fatal. Narcotic exposure has been associated with learning disabilities later in life.
Lysergic acid diethylamide (LSD)	Spontaneous abortion, chromosomal changes, suspected anomalies
Tetracycline	Staining of teeth, inhibition of bone growth
Thalidomide	Phocomelia, hearing loss, cardiac anomalies; can be fatal
Tobacco	Intrauterine growth retardation
Tranquilizers	All may cause withdrawal symptoms during neonatal period
Radiation therapy	Congenital anomalies, growth retardation, chromosomal damage, mental deficiency, stillbirth
CHEMICALS	
Methylmercury	Congenital abnormalities, growth retardation; can cause abortions
Pesticides (some types)	Congenital anomalies
Lead	Spontaneous abortion, intrauterine growth retardation, congenital anomalies, anemia; can be fatal

Modified from Schuster, C. S., & Ashburn, S. S. (1986). *The process of human development: A holistic approach* (2nd ed.). Boston: Little, Brown; and Healthline. (2006). *Pregnancy and teratogens.* Retrieved on March 29, 2009, at http://www.healthline.com/yodocontent/pregnancy/teratogens.html.

(FAS), which is the most serious example of a fetal syndrome caused by maternal exposure to a teratogen, and other conditions in which individuals have some, but not all, of the clinical signs of FAS. FAS includes a specific pattern of altered growth structure and function seen in infants of women who ingest high amounts of alcohol during pregnancy.[102] Infants with alcohol-related birth defects (ARBDs) or alcohol-related neurodevelopmental disorder (ARND) have milder forms of FASD may lack the distinct facial morphology and growth deficiencies, but share many of the neurobehavioral deficits found in infants with FAS.[1,84] The mechanism of injury includes a reduction in brain size, with the basal ganglia and cerebellum most impaired.[75]

Conservative estimates indicate that alcohol is the third leading cause of birth defects and the leading cause of cognitive impairments. The incidence of FAS has been reported as 0.2 to 1.5 per 1000 live births worldwide. The estimate for children born with other FASDs is even higher, 3 to 5 per 1000 live births worldwide.[84,76] The risk of FASD in children born to mild-to-moderate drinkers currently is the subject of controversy; some investigators show a high incidence of effects with even small amounts of alcohol, whereas others show few, if any, effects.[97] Investigators have demonstrated that the nature and extent of fetal injuries produced by alcohol depend on several factors, including (1) the amount of alcohol consumed per day, (2) the time during the pregnancy when the alcohol was taken, (3) other stressors experienced by the mother, (4) whether food was eaten near the time of alcohol consumption, (5) whether other substance abuse occurred during the pregnancy, and (6) the mother's general health.[33]

Like other teratogens, alcohol causes a spectrum of defects that vary from severe physical and mental problems that are readily detectable at birth to more subtle learning problems that may not be detected until school age.[97] The principle features of FAS include prenatal and postnatal growth deficiencies, a pattern of craniofacial malformations, and CNS dysfunction. Newborns typically are small for gestational age (SGA) and continue to show height, weight, and head circumference differences. The pattern of craniofacial malformations seen with FAS includes microcephaly, epicanthal folds, a long philtrum, short palpebral fissures, a flat midface, and a thin vermilion of the upper lip (Figure 6-14).[102] Musculoskeletal problems include congenital dislocations, foot positional defects, cervical spine abnormalities, specific joint alterations, flexion contractures at the elbows, and tapering of the terminal phalanges. Many of these craniofacial and skeletal defects occur secondary to the effect of alcohol on brain development, and although craniofacial deficits may even recede with growth, microcephaly does not.[123]

Although CNS dysfunction can vary, intellectual impairment is the disability most frequently noted with FASD. This impairment ranges from moderate ID to average intellectual function, with an average IQ of 70 being most recently cited.[75] Other characteristics include hyperactivity, attention deficits, vestibular problems, impulsivity, poor social skills, learning disabilities, memory deficits, and deficits in visuospatial-perceptual skills, as well as sensory problems affecting ocular, auditory, and possibly vestibular functioning.[31]

The prognosis for children with FASD varies with the extent and severity of the various malformations and growth deficiencies. Two important factors are the severity of the

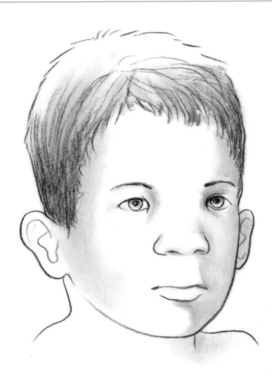

FIGURE 6-14   Typical facial features of a child with fetal alcohol syndrome (FAS).

maternal alcoholism and the quality and stability of the home environment.[1] Studies of the long-term effects of FASD are beginning to provide information about the influence of alcohol on the growth and development of the affected child. Size delays appear to continue for some time, with head circumference remaining smaller into middle childhood. Children with FASD show persistent delays in self-care, school activities, and play. Performance areas typically evaluated include mental function, interactions, sensory functions, and neuromusculoskeletal functions.

Families of children with FASD have multiple psychosocial issues, and the clinician must involve the entire family in the child's therapy program. Many health care professionals believe that with intensive family intervention (e.g., alcohol recovery programs for the mother, early intervention for the child) and with social, medical, and financial support, a better prognosis is possible. Preventive measures can have a significant effect on the prevalence of FASD, and the prevalence of the disorder can be substantially reduced by educating the public about the deleterious effects of alcohol on unborn infants.[123]

Cocaine and Opiates

The effects of cocaine, crack, and opiates on infants are of increasing concern to developmental specialists. Use of these drugs increased noticeably in the 1990s and continues to be a social concern, particularly the use of cocaine and "crack," a relatively cheap cocaine derivative. Also, maternal drug use is complicated by the tendency of these individuals to abuse other substances, such as alcohol and tobacco, and many mothers using these drugs are poorly nourished and receive less than adequate prenatal care. It is estimated that more than 100,000 infants each year are born to mothers who use drugs during pregnancy, although accurate counts are difficult because of the social and legal implications of reporting drug use.[123]

Cocaine is extremely addictive; it causes ecstatic "highs" and significant and prolonged "lows." Addiction to crack is said to be possible after one or two uses.[123] Cocaine increases the levels of norepinephrine, serotonin, and dopamine and has strong vasoconstrictive effects. It crosses the placenta and has similar effects in the fetus, and this vasoconstriction is believed to be damaging to the fetus. Use of opiates, heroin, or methadone by the mother results in an addicted infant who experiences drug withdrawal after birth.

Longitudinal studies that have followed mothers from early in their pregnancies and their children from birth into early childhood, studies that take into account many confounding factors that are associated with cocaine use, show a pattern of subtle neurobehavioral effects associated with prenatal cocaine exposure. These include effects on the child's attention and alertness, IQ, and motor skills. The effects are not as profound as some early reports suggested, but they are very damaging to later academic success. Research in the area continues, but controlled studies are difficult to complete. Several general patterns are emerging. Babies born of addicted mothers are often SGA, with reduced head size and irritability and hypersensitivity to stimuli.[117]

Cocaine has been associated with congenital anomalies, limb deficiencies, cerebral hemorrhage, increased muscle tone, necrotizing enterocolitis, and rapid shifts of arousal state.[50] Newborns who had been exposed to narcotics in utero go through active withdrawal, during which they are irritable, hypertonic, and poor feeders. Often, they frantically suck on their hands. Motor coordination is reduced, and the activity level may be high. Respiratory distress has also been noted.[117] These infants tend to require quiet, low-stimulus environments and may respond positively to swaddling. Parenting of these children can be difficult for several months.

The long-term effects are becoming evident. Longitudinal studies, like those conducted by Accornero,[2] examined the influence of prenatal cocaine exposure on attention and response inhibition measured by continuous performance tests (CPTs) at ages 5 and 7 years. The sample included 415 children from the Miami Prenatal Cocaine Study (219 cocaine-exposed, 196 non–cocaine-exposed as determined by maternal self-report and infant bioassays). Children were enrolled prospectively at birth and assessed comprehensively through age 7 years. Deficits in attention and response inhibition were correlated with prenatal cocaine exposure using generalized estimating equations within the general linear model. Results indicate cocaine-associated increases in omission errors at ages 5 and 7, as well as increases in response times for target tasks (i.e., slower reaction times) and decreased consistency in performance at age 7.[2] Studies have found that by school age, these children perform at lower than age-level expectations. Most studies have reported performance problems, including hyperactivity and organizational problems, subtle learning and cognitive deficits, and play deficits. Furthermore, the mothers of these children often have few social supports and may be young or homeless or may remain addicted, and the children may be placed in foster care. Early intervention and school intervention programs may be necessary to identify, prevent, or minimize the long-term effects of the maternal substance abuse.[123]

Heavy Metals

Heavy metal poisoning is a serious health concern. Because small children often put things in their mouths, they are at particular risk for poisoning by these substances.[102] Mercury can enter the body by means of ingestion or inhalation, resulting in *mercury poisoning*, which can cause tremors, memory loss, anorexia, weight loss, diarrhea, and acrodynia (painful extremities). Liquid mercury evaporates quickly and should be cleaned up immediately to prevent this problem.

Lead poisoning is usually caused by ingestion of environmental lead, such as the lead paint used in buildings before World War II. Lead paint has caused a significant problem in some inner-city communities and in older houses that have been renovated.[71] Lead water pipes and some ceramic glazes have also been associated with lead poisoning.

A child may be acutely or chronically affected. Lead affects three body systems in particular: the renal, circulatory, and nervous systems. Renal damage occurs in the proximal tubules of the kidneys, resulting in abnormal excretion of important nutrients and impairment of vitamin D synthesis. Lead severely limits the body's ability to synthesize heme, leading to accumulation of alternate metabolites in the body and, ultimately, anemia.[50] The most significant and irreversible effects of lead poisoning on the body occur in the nervous system. Fluid builds up in the brain, and intracranial pressure can reach life-threatening levels.[79] Cortical atrophy and lead encephalitis are usually associated with high blood levels of lead. This can lead to intellectual impairments, paralysis, blindness, and convulsions. Low-level exposure has been associated with LDs, ADHD, hearing impairment, and milder intellectual deficits. Other lead poisoning symptoms include cramping, digestive difficulty, lethargy, headache, and fever.[79]

INFECTIOUS CONDITIONS

Maternal Infections

The fetus may be infected by a variety of organisms. Some of these infectious conditions are passed from the mother to the fetus during pregnancy (transplacental infections), and others are present in the vagina and are passed to the infant at birth (ascending infections). These infections invade the fetus at a time when it has a limited capacity to ward off disease and, in the case of transplacental infections, at a time when the infection may have a profound effect on the formation or growth and development of tissues and organs.[50]

The most common maternal infections are the *STORCH infections* (i.e., syphilis, toxoplasmosis, rubella, cytomegalovirus, and herpesvirus), which are also called *TORCH* or *TORCHS*. Each of these conditions is caused by a specific virus or bacterium and has a different set of characteristics. A summary of these five infections and their effects on the fetus can be found in Table 6-4. *Congenital syphilis* can be transmitted in the late stages of pregnancy or during delivery. It is the most virulent form of syphilis and requires isolation of the infected infant. The usual treatment for congenital syphilis is penicillin. Early-stage congenital syphilis is characterized by hepatitis, failure to thrive, neurologic involvement, fever, anemia, restlessness, irritability, and syphilitic rhinitis. Characteristic lesions may be present, and the hair and nails may be damaged. Osteochondritis at the joints and other bone abnormalities are relatively common. Because of residual damage from the infection, late-stage congenital syphilis is marked by bony and dental anomalies and visual and auditory deficits.[50]

Toxoplasmosis can be contracted by the mother through ingestion of raw meat or contact with the feces of newly infected cats and can be transmitted to the fetus at any point during the pregnancy. Toxoplasmosis is also an increasingly common opportunistic infection in acquired immunodeficiency syndrome (AIDS).[78] In the United States, the incidence of toxoplasmosis is about 1.3 in 1000 live births.[78] Stillbirth and death are common, but some newborns are asymptomatic. Children born with this condition are often severely mentally disabled. Hydrocephalus, cerebral calcification, and chorioretinitis are classic symptoms. CP, seizures, cardiac and liver damage, and gastrointestinal problems are also found. Treatment with sulfonamides and pyrimethamine is usually initiated in infected mothers and children. Once acquired, the neurologic deficits related to the disease in the fetus can be reduced but not eliminated by maternal treatment.[78]

Rubella, a common and fairly mild disease in children, can be devastating when contracted by a pregnant woman, particularly in the first trimester. With the advent of a preventive vaccine, the frequency of congenital rubella syndrome has declined 99% in the past 25 years; however, the dangers to unvaccinated mothers are significant. Congenital defects, spontaneous abortion, and stillbirth may occur. Central processing and hearing loss, intellectual impairment, microcephaly, and seizures are possible outcomes. Congenital heart defects, including patent ductus arteriosus, are characteristic,

TABLE 6-4 Intrauterine Infections (STORCH)

Infection	Cause	Type	Effects on Fetus
Syphilis	Parabacterial infection	A, T	Enlarged liver and spleen, jaundice, anemia, rash, rhinorrhea
Toxoplasmosis	Parasitic infection	T	Deafness, blindness, ID, seizures, pneumonia, enlarged liver and spleen
Rubella	Viral infection	T	Meningitis, hearing loss, cataracts, cardiac problems, ID, retinal defects
Cytomegalovirus	Viral infection	T	Hearing loss; in severe form, problems are similar to those seen with rubella
Herpes	Viral infection	A	Localized form: lethargy, rash, respiratory distress, jaundice, enlarged liver and spleen. Generalized form: virus attacks CNS, causing ID, seizures, and other problems.

STORCH, Syphilis, toxoplasmosis, rubella, cytomegalovirus, and herpes; *A*, ascending; *T*, transplacental; *ID*, intellectual disability; *CNS*, central nervous system.

as are visual deficits, hepatomegaly, and splenomegaly.[74] These children may be SGA and may suffer from numerous respiratory infections in infancy. Late-occurring symptoms include diabetes, encephalitis, hearing loss, and thyroid problems. Functionally, children with congenital rubella symptoms may be expected to have mixed developmental delays and hearing and vestibular deficits. The child's therapy program may need to be adjusted to accommodate cardiorespiratory problems.[74]

Transmission of *cytomegalovirus* (i.e., cytomegalic inclusion disease) is similar to that for rubella, and the effects also are similar. This herpes-type viral infection may be transmitted before, during, or after birth. The infection may be active or latent in the newborn; therefore, infection control precautions are appropriate for therapists working with these children. Clinical manifestations include low birth weight, sensorineural hearing loss, microcephaly, hepatomegaly, splenomegaly, and purpuric rash. Jaundice and hepatitis may also be present. Children with cytomegalovirus infection may be asymptomatic at birth. Symptomatic newborns have a poor prognosis with regard to neurologic deficits. These children often have learning disabilities and diminished cognitive skills.[50]

The newborn most often contracts *congenital herpes* infection during or after delivery by a mother with herpes simplex infection, often genital herpes.[50] Infected children frequently develop skin, mouth, or eye lesions within 6 to 10 days of contact, although some children do not develop overt symptoms. In the disseminated form, a sepsis-like picture presents itself, and the child may develop internal organ lesions and encephalitis with CNS involvement. Early signs are fever, lethargy, poor feeding, irritability, and vomiting. Infusion of antiviral agents may reduce the severity of this condition noticeably and has been known to prevent serious brain damage. Cesarean sections are sometimes used as a preventive measure for mothers with active lesions.[50]

The sexually transmitted diseases *gonorrhea* and *chlamydia* are passed to the infant late in fetal development or during delivery. Both may result in eye infections, and gonococcal arthritis, septicemia, and meningitis may also occur. Fortunately, both infections respond well to antibiotic therapy if discovered early. Other maternal infections known to affect neonatal health are listeriosis, Lyme disease, hepatitis B, and AIDS, as well as infections caused by parvovirus, coxsackievirus, and varicella virus (the agent of chickenpox).[50]

Acquired Immunodeficiency Syndrome

Acquired immunodeficiency syndrome (AIDS) is caused by the human immunodeficiency virus (HIV), which is a retrovirus transmitted by lymphocytes and monocytes, in blood, semen, vaginal secretions, and breast milk. It has changed from a rapidly fatal disease, when originally identified in 1981, to a chronic, but terminal, disease. In the United States, since the beginning of the HIV/AIDS epidemic, an estimated 8460 children who contracted HIV from their mothers have been diagnosed with AIDS. Nearly 5000 of these children have died.[85] The transmission of HIV to children is primarily the result of perinatal contact with the mother (96% of the cases); however, perinatally acquired AIDS peaked in 1992 and has been significantly declining since then. This trend can be attributed primarily to implementation of recommended HIV counseling and voluntary testing practices and the use of

highly active antiretroviral therapy (HAART).[50] Regularly testing pregnant women for HIV and providing antiretroviral drugs if they are infected has dramatically reduced the number of children born with HIV. In 1992, 855 children in the United States developed AIDS, but in 2005 only 57 children developed AIDS—a decline of 93%. Currently, it is estimated that 6015 children and young adults who got HIV from their mothers were living with HIV/AIDS at the end of 2005.[85] Most perinatal transmission occurs in utero by transplacental passage of the virus, intrapartum through contact with infected maternal blood and cervical secretions, or postpartum through breast-feeding. HIV infection can be diagnosed between 1 and 6 months of age. Children with AIDS represent the most serious disease manifestations of HIV.[17]

HIV infects and damages cells of the immune system, rendering the child vulnerable to life-threatening illnesses that do not affect children with normal immunity. HIV-positive newborns are often asymptomatic at birth. The interval from birth to the development of AIDS among perinatally affected infants varies widely. Evaluation of the most current data indicates that there is a subset of perinatally infected children who do not have significant disease for years after infection and a subset of children who develop the most serious manifestations of infection by 2 years of age (rapid progressors). The onset, which often occurs before 6 months of age, of serious clinical disease is a prognostic indicator of survival. Cases of rapid progression of the disease are currently under intensive study. Although investigators can identify the factors involved in rapid progression, they cannot yet offer reasons for this subset of pathogenesis.[66]

Clinical management of HIV-infected children remains intensive, with recommendations for clinical evaluations and laboratory assessment to be completed every 3 months. Any viral or bacterial infection is considered a serious breach of immune system integrity and is carefully monitored. Most HIV specialists believe that early and aggressive treatment for children with HIV should include antiretroviral drug therapy and administration of intravenous (IV) gamma globulin. These treatments decrease the viral load, preserve the immune system, extend the interval preceding the development of AIDS, and prolong survival. As indicated by the diagnostic features, infections are a common occurrence after HIV infection. Children tend to have a greater number of minor bacterial infections, including otitis media, urinary tract infections, and pneumonia. Fungal infections include oral candidiasis and candidal dermatitis. Children with recurrent infections may benefit from IV administration of gamma globulin. *Pneumocystis carinii pneumonia* (PCP), caused by *Pneumocystis jiroveci*, is the most common opportunistic infection seen in children. PCP prevention has become an important focus of care in both HIV and AIDS.

Although no cure currently exists for HIV infection or AIDS, antiretroviral drugs are successfully prolonging survival.[66] The antiretroviral drugs commonly used in children fall into three categories: nucleoside transcriptase inhibitors, nonnucleoside reverse transcriptase inhibitors, and protease inhibitors. These drugs result in a significant slowing of progression of the disease and are associated with prolonged survival times. Therapy is started immediately after birth, and medical visits include monitoring of the HIV infection as well as routine care and immunizations. The goal of each class of drug is to prevent the virus from producing progeny. Other drugs are in development to prevent HIV from infecting the CD4 cells in the first place.[17]

If the disease progresses to a severe level, suppression of the immune system, chronic respiratory illness, skin and other types of infection, and diarrhea often noticeably weaken infected children. These conditions often respond slowly to treatment.[50] Developmental delays and degeneration may result in delayed or lost motor, speech, and independent living skills. Neurologic deficits, including ataxia, spasticity, rigidity, tremor, and seizures, may be expected as the disease progresses. Early intervention and rehabilitative and educational services are often indicated.[50]

Interdisciplinary care is essential for the assessment and treatment of pediatric HIV infection. The team guides the family through well-child visits, immunizations, nutritional support, antiretroviral therapy, adherence to medication regimens, monitoring of antiretroviral treatment, and coping with adverse drug reactions. Developmental assessment and educational programs may aid the child with multiple environmental influences, including socioeconomic factors, family environment, and failure to thrive. Other services that may need to be considered are social support, infection control at home and school, and possibly the need for placement outside the home.[17,50]

Encephalitis and Meningitis

Encephalitis and meningitis, which are infections of the brain and its coverings, can be life-threatening and can result in permanent disability. *Encephalitis,* or inflammation of the brain, may be caused by bacteria, spirochetes, or other organisms, but is usually caused by a viral infection. The specific cause is often not identified clinically. The condition may be localized or may include the spinal cord or meninges. Infection of the brain may occur directly or secondary to another infection. Because mosquitoes spread several viral forms, a summer onset is common. Herpes simplex has also been associated disproportionately with encephalitis in young children.[50]

The severity of these conditions varies with the cause. The onset may be sudden or gradual, and the condition often is difficult to distinguish from other infections. Signs and symptoms include fever, headache, dizziness, stiff neck, nausea and vomiting, tremors, and ataxia. In severe cases, stupor, seizures, disorientation, coma, and death may occur. The diagnosis is based on environmental patterns of infection, clinical findings, EEG and MRI results, and laboratory examination of blood, brain tissue, or CSF. Treatment may include antibiotics if bacterial infection is suggested but is primarily supportive while the acute disease runs its course.[50]

Unfortunately, encephalitis can result in mild to severe residual brain damage. The degree of damage depends on the child's age, the type of infection, and the care provided. Young children are at increased risk for neurologic complications. The health care staff must monitor the child's progress and neurologic status after the infection resolves. MR, LDs, behavior disorders, seizures, and neuromotor deficits are common. Neurorehabilitation techniques are applied to limit the disability, and compensatory interventions, including assistive technology, may help the child in school, play, and, later, prevocational activities.

Meningitis is an infection of the meninges, the tissue covering the brain and spinal cord. Like encephalitis, meningitis may have a tubercular, fungal, protozoal, viral, or (most commonly) bacterial cause. Clinical manifestations of meningitis vary slightly in newborns, infants, older children, and adolescents, but the clinical picture is not unlike that for encephalitis. Headache, fever, and rigidity in the neck are classic signs. These may be accompanied by seizures, vomiting, spasticity, behavioral and arousal state changes, and, in young children, bulging fontanels. In newborns, jaundice, cyanosis, hypothermia, and respiratory distress may also be present.[95]

Diagnostic evaluation may include lumbar puncture, analysis of the CSF, and blood, throat, and nasal cultures. Interventions include management of the underlying infection with antibiotics, hydration, maintenance of intracranial pressure, and treatment of symptoms and complications. Because many forms of the disease are highly contagious, the acutely ill client may be isolated. The child may be monitored for apnea and cardiac function. As with encephalitis, neuromotor, visual, auditory, seizure, and learning disorders may remain after the acute infection abates. Anticonvulsant and rehabilitative therapy is necessary to manage and remediate these sequelae.[95]

BURNS

Major burn injury accounts for a large number of children who must undergo prolonged, painful, and restrictive hospitalizations. Countless other children suffer from minor burns. Thermal, electrical, chemical, and radioactive sources can cause burns, but thermal burns are by far the most common. Most burns can be attributed to accidents; however, 10% to 20% of hospital admissions for burns may be attributed to child abuse. Children under 3 years of age account for a majority of thermal burns, and of these, hot water and hot beverage scalds account for 50% to 60% of injuries. About 30% of burns in older children are related to flame (e.g., match, gasoline, firecracker) or chemical burns. Short periods of high heat or long periods of low heat can both cause significant burns. Chemical burns can cause serious injury, but their effect often can be stopped with prompt emergency treatment. Electrical burns may damage not only the skin but also underlying bone, muscle, and nerve tissue along the conduction path. Further damage can be caused by smoke inhalation, respiratory failure, shock, and posttraumatic infection.[50]

The criteria that determine the prognosis for survival of a child with a burn injury include the percentage of body area burned, the depth and location of the burn, the child's age, the causative agent, whether respiratory involvement is a factor, the length of the hospital stay, and whether other injuries are present.[67]

The percentage of area injured in children is assessed according to the total body surface area (TBSA) affected, either by the rule of nines in children older than 10 years or by charts specifically designed to accurately estimate the body proportions involved in children of different ages.[50] The *rule of nines* ascribes 9% of the TBSA to the head and neck, 9% to each upper extremity, 18% to each lower extremity, 36% to the trunk (18% anterior and 18% posterior), and 1% to the perineum and genitals. In children under 10 years of age, the accuracy of TBSA estimations are improved through use of various charts to estimate the modified rule of nines (Figure 6-15). The mortality rate for children under 4 years of age with burns covering more than 30% of the TBSA is significantly higher than that for older

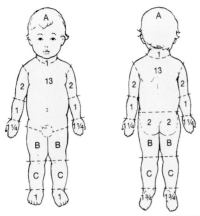

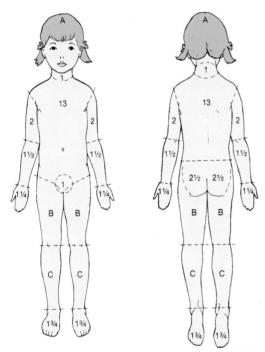

RELATIVE PERCENTAGES OF AREAS AFFECTED BY GROWTH

AREA	BIRTH	AGE 1 YR	AGE 5 YR
A = ½ of head	9½	8½	6½
B = ½ of one thigh	2¾	3¼	4
C = ½ of one leg	2½	2½	2¾

A

RELATIVE PERCENTAGES OF AREAS AFFECTED BY GROWTH

AREA	AGE 10 YR	AGE 15 YR	ADULT
A = ½ of head	5½	4½	3½
B = ½ of one thigh	4½	4½	4¾
C = ½ of one leg	3	3¼	3½

B

FIGURE 6-15 Estimation of distribution of burns in children. **A,** Children from birth to 5 years of age. **B,** Older children. (From Hockenberry, M. J., & Wilson, D. [2009]. *Wong's essentials of pediatric nursing* [8th ed.]. St. Louis: Mosby.)

The American Burn Association also classifies burns as minor, moderate, or severe.[6] In minor burns, less than 10% of the TBSA is covered by a partial-thickness burn; these burns can be adequately treated on an outpatient basis. In a moderate burn, 10% to 20% of the TBSA is covered by a partial-thickness burn, and the child requires hospitalization. A major burn is considered to be any full-thickness burn or any burn injury in which more than 20% of the TBSA is covered by a partial-thickness burn.[6]

The depth of the burn is assessed according to the number of layers of tissue involved in the injury (Figure 6-16). *Superficial burns*, or first-degree burns, demonstrate minimal tissue damage, although they can be painful. In these burns, the skin is red and dry, and healing typically occurs without scarring. *Partial-thickness burns*, or second-degree burns, involve the epidermis and dermis in varying degrees and can be further classified as deep or superficial burns. Superficial partial-thickness burns involve the epidermis and a portion of the dermis, but many of the dermal elements are left intact. Partial-thickness burns appear slightly raised, blistered, reddened, and moist, and they blanch to the touch. These are the most painful of burns and may result in some scarring, although superficial partial-thickness burns may heal spontaneously. In deep partial-thickness burns, both the epidermis and dermis are damaged, but the sweat glands and hair follicles of the dermis are left intact. In many cases, a deep partial-thickness burn resembles a full-thickness burn. The appearance of these injuries is dry, soft, and waxy, with no edema or raised appearance. In *full-thickness burns*, or third- or fourth-degree burns, all layers of the skin are destroyed, as may be some of the underlying subcutaneous tissue (see Figure 6-16). Full-thickness burns are hard, insensate, and leathery, with inflexible eschar. Some systems include a fourth-degree burn classification when the damage extends to underlying muscle, bone, and fascia. These burns may be charred, brown, or red; nerve endings and blood vessels may be damaged; and pain may not be present in the central area. Most third- and fourth-degree burns also have borders of second-degree burns that are painful.[6]

With a moderate or major burn, critical care focuses on maintenance of breathing if there is evidence of respiratory involvement, as well as immediate replacement of fluids, nutrition, and pain management. The intensive pathophysiologic response to a major burn creates a need to balance the amount of fluid replacement and nutrition carefully to compensate for the loss of blood, the presence of edema, and critical sodium or potassium changes. Sedation is needed to allow tolerance of treatment and for comfort. Pain management continues throughout treatment. Morphine combined with methadone, ketamine, propofol, and nitrous oxide have all demonstrated usefulness in pain management for victims of major burns.[50]

In addition to emergency care, prevention of secondary infection, wound débridement, and wound closure are critical. Application of antimicrobial agents to prevent secondary infection is an ongoing process until the wound is closed. A variety of topical antimicrobial agents are used to help prevent infection. Silver nitrate, silver sulfadiazine, mafenide acetate, nystatin, neomycin, povidone-iodine, and bacitracin are the most common.[50] However, after a deep partial- or full-thickness burn, primary excision is often required before treatment with topical agents is effective. Physicians also are beginning to use

children with a burn of the same size (46.9% versus 12.5%, respectively).[6] Inhalation injuries are significantly correlated with death. In addition, major burns of less than 30% TBSA in children under 4 years of age may result in death despite excellent emergency and burn care.

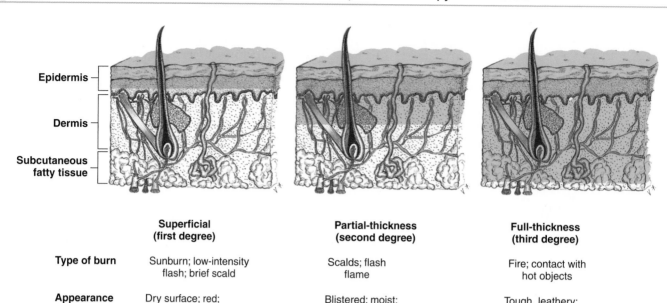

	Superficial (first degree)	Partial-thickness (second degree)	Full-thickness (third degree)
Type of burn	Sunburn; low-intensity flash; brief scald	Scalds; flash flame	Fire; contact with hot objects
Appearance	Dry surface; red; blanches on pressure and refills	Blistered; moist; mottled pink or red, reddened; blanches on pressure and refills	Tough, leathery; brown, tan, black, or red; does not blanch on pressure; dull, dry
Sensation	Painful	Very painful	Variable pain, often severe

FIGURE 6-16   Classification of burn depth.   (From Hockenberry, M. J., & Wilson, D. [2009]. *Wong's essentials of pediatric nursing* [8th ed.]. St. Louis: Mosby.)

growth hormone, which has been shown to enhance wound healing and decrease nutritional requirements.[6]

Débridement of necrotic tissue is essential to recovery. Hydrotherapy is used to remove debris, cleanse the wound, and allow increased ROM in all body parts. This is an extremely painful process that must be done twice a day, and typically the child must be sedated. Tissue is redressed with topical antimicrobial agents and gauze.[50] Full-thickness, partial-thickness, or meshed skin grafts may be used to cover large burned areas. Wound healing procedures may need to be repeated if the grafts do not take. Skin grafting procedures using synthetic and animal skins have significantly improved the prognosis for skin healing. In severe burns, reconstructive surgeries often are needed to limit the long-term effects of burn injuries.

The team approach is essentially universal in burn care units in the United States. The American Burn Association has established guidelines for the personnel that make up a burn unit team.[6] The team consists of physicians with specialized training in burn care, nurses, occupational therapists, physical therapists, speech therapists, psychologists, and social workers. Occupational therapists are typically involved very early after the burn injury, often within 24 hours.[20]

The major goals of burn rehabilitation are early skin coverage, correction of cosmetic damage, restoration of function, and integration back into the environment. During the acute period, positioning, hydrotherapy, splinting, active and passive ROM, and ADL modalities are used to prevent contractures and ensure optimal functional and physical outcomes. Many of these procedures are painful, and infection is a continued threat until all burned areas have been closed. During this period, the child also experiences malaise and may be heavily sedated. Ongoing treatment goals include minimizing problems with

scarring, optimizing active ROM, decreasing hypersensitivity, preventing contractures, ensuring good use of the hands, and optimizing skills for self-care and for home and school activities.[20] These goals include the use of various techniques, including fitting and maintenance of pressure garments, splinting, active and passive ROM, client and family education about scar formation, emotional support, massage to prevent hypertrophied scarring, and adaptation of ADLs.

Outcome measures used to determine successful burn rehabilitation include resumption of typical daily living skills (e.g., return to school), scar rating, and sensorimotor skills (e.g., ROM, gross and fine motor skills). Numerous rating scales have been developed to characterize or assess a scar. Reliable assessment of the scar surface (e.g., to evaluate healing) includes border height, thickness, and color of a scar.[124] Each of these four characteristics is rated from 1 to 4, with pictorial definitions used for each characterization; a composite score is then generated for the overall scar appearance.

Scar appearance and location typically are believed to influence psychosocial adaptation. A scar on the face or neck has been correlated with lower self-esteem, less engagement in typical activities, and fewer interpersonal interactions; however, the accuracy of these beliefs is controversial.[50] Ongoing scar massage techniques have been shown to be effective if initiated before the development of invasive hypertrophied scarring. Splinting continues to be used, primarily after limitations in ROM are noted, except for full-thickness or deep partial-thickness burns. in which loss of ROM and the likelihood of scar contractures are greatest.[106] The process of scar remodeling, plastic surgery, and revision of skin grafts may be required for up to 2 years after a major injury.

Possibly more important measures are developmental and return-to-school outcomes. Developmental outcomes, especially language development and social skills, are delayed after burn injury in children, even if physical and functional skills are within normal limits.[89] Adjustment to school after a burn injury generally is successful regardless of the severity of the burn, provided the return to school reentry program is comprehensive (i.e., includes peer counseling, encouragement to return to school promptly, early contacts with the school, a comprehensive school plan, engagement of parents in reentry efforts, and social skills training).[50] Therapists can be involved in each step of the rehabilitation and return-to-school process, providing ongoing direct services, consultation, and monitoring.

GENERAL DEVELOPMENTAL CONCERNS

Pediatric Obesity

According to the National Health and Nutrition Examination Survey (NHANES) IV, 16.3% of children aged 6 to 19 years are obese, and obesity rates have increased from earlier decades.[86,91] Nearly 31% of children are at risk for becoming overweight or they are already overweight, representing a nearly 300% increase since the 1960s and a 45% increase since the last complete NHANES survey for 1988-1994. In addition, there is health disparity between ethnic groups, with African American girls (24%) and Hispanic boys (22%) and girls having the highest rates of obesity or overweight status.[86,91] Poverty has also been associated with higher prevalence rates of obesity and being overweight.[86]

Pediatric obesity has been associated with significant health consequences including high blood pressure, high cholesterol, type 2 diabetes, and it potentially predisposes a child/adolescent to cardiovascular disease, sleep disorders, and musculoskeletal disorders and associated limitations in physical activity later in life.[120]

Development of overweight or obesity status results from a complex interplay between genetic risk, behavioral risk factors, and environment that causes a dysregulation of caloric intake and energy expenditure. Obesity results from an individual's genetic predispositions and the environment. The combination of which affects an intricate system that controls appetite and energy expenditure. The best predictor of being overweight is high birth weight, probably linked to maternal obesity or maternal diabetes. Paradoxically, lower birth weight appears to place people at risk for later central obesity. Children who are overweight are more likely to be overweight as adults, with the likelihood increasing as the age of the overweight child increases. The strongest predictor of childhood overweight, as well as later adult obesity, is parental obesity. Parental obesity doubles the risk of adult obesity among children younger than 10 years of age, regardless of current weight.[107]

Obesity and overweight status are classified by age- and gender-specific body mass index (BMI). Obesity is considered to be present in children at or above the 95th percentile of the 2000 BMI-for-age growth charts, and overweight status is at the 85th percentile.[91] (See Figure 6-17 for BMI-for-age growth charts.[25]) Online calculators are available for determination of BMI, calculated as weight in pounds divided by height in inches squared and multiplied by 703 (BMI = [lbs ÷ inches^2] × 703).[87] Alternative diagnostic assessment measures include skinfold thickness and waist circumference.[62]

Fortunately, although obesity is a condition with medical consequences, it is also a modifiable risk factor, and treatment involves primarily behavioral and lifestyle changes. Consequently, physicians engage the assistance of other members of the health care team to provide the needed education and facilitation of behavioral changes. Frequently, the team includes nurses, nurse practitioners, physician assistants, and physical and occupational therapists. Because treatment involves behavioral and lifestyle changes, it also proves exceptionally difficult to successfully treat. Of equal challenge is that health care providers must actively engage both the child and his or her family in behavioral and lifestyle changes.[57] Evidence clearly suggests that merely educating and treating a child for obesity has little long-term effect unless parents are also involved in changing their lifestyle and habits. One example of the most effective and studied programs is The Traffic Light Childhood Weight Control and Prevention Program at the University of Buffalo.[122]

The general recommendations for obesity prevention include limiting consumption of sugar-sweetened beverages, increasing the amount of fruits and vegetables consumed, limiting television and other screen time to less than 2 hours per day and removing computer screens from children's sleeping areas, eating daily breakfast, limiting fast food, encouraging family meals, and limiting portion sizes. Other suggestions include eating a diet rich in calcium and fiber, breast-feeding infants, and participating in 60 minutes of moderate to vigorous physical activity daily. Occupational therapy interventions include a focus on reinforcement of healthy diets, habits, routines, and physical activity patterns. This may include working at a range of levels including population (schools and communities to educate and institute programs that promote healthy lifestyles and physical activity) and with the person (developing healthy habits, roles, and routines that include regular physical activity).[32]

Suicide and Depression

Suicide is the third leading cause of death in adolescents and young adults ages 10 to 24 years,[26] making suicide prevention one of the most critical health objectives for adolescents and young adults. Teen suicide statistics draw a correlation between gender and suicide. Males are four times more likely to die from suicide than females. However, teen girls are more likely than teen boys to attempt suicide. So, although teenage girls make more attempts on their own lives than teenage boys, the boys are more likely to actually succeed at a suicide attempt. Males do not allow for intervention, and are less likely to "call for help" through a suicide attempt, because there is often little opportunity to get males into treatment because their suicide completion rate is higher than that of females.

Several different factors may lead a teenager to take his or her life, but the most common is depression. Feelings of hopelessness and anxiety, along with feelings of being trapped in a life that one can't handle, are very real contributors to teen suicide. In some cases, teenagers believe that suicide is the only way to solve their problems. The pressures of life seem too much to cope with, and some teenagers view suicide as a welcome escape. Depression plays on the often tumultuous feelings experienced by teenagers. Intense feelings can contribute to a teen's sense of helplessness and to a general feeling that life is not worth living. Taking these feelings seriously is an important part of preventing teen suicide.

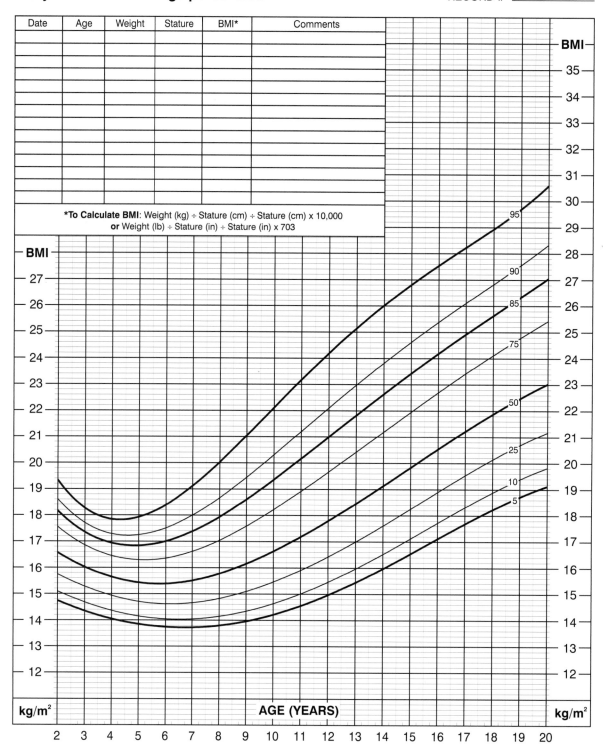

2 to 20 years: Boys
Body mass index-for-age percentiles

NAME _____

RECORD # _____

*To Calculate BMI: Weight (kg) ÷ Stature (cm) ÷ Stature (cm) x 10,000
or Weight (lb) ÷ Stature (in) ÷ Stature (in) x 703

Published May 30, 2000 (modified 10/16/00).
SOURCE: Developed by the National Center for Health Statistics in collaboration with
the National Center for Chronic Disease Prevention and Health Promotion (2000).
http://www.cdc.gov/growthcharts

SAFER·HEALTHIER·PEOPLE™

FIGURE 6-17 Body weight indexes. **A,** Boys. **B,** Girls. (From Centers for Disease Control and Prevention, 2000.)

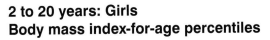

2 to 20 years: Girls
Body mass index-for-age percentiles

NAME _____

RECORD # _____

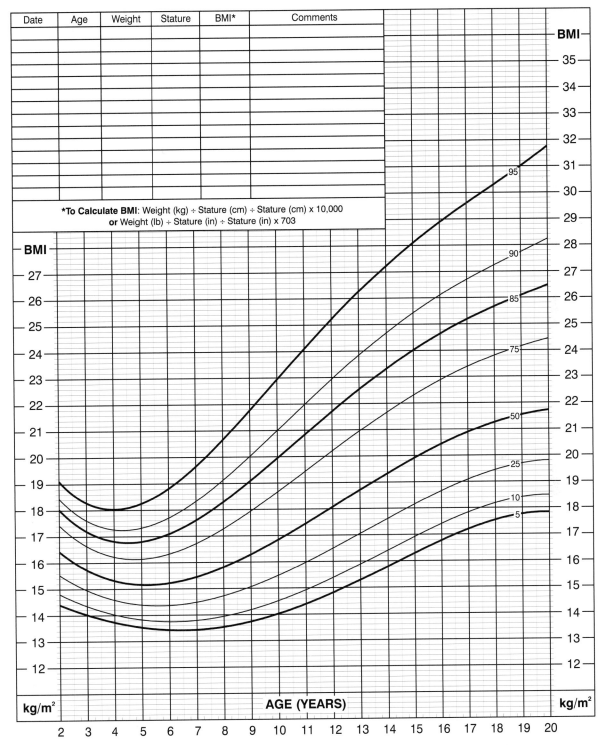

*To Calculate BMI: Weight (kg) ÷ Stature (cm) ÷ Stature (cm) x 10,000
or Weight (lb) ÷ Stature (in) ÷ Stature (in) x 703

AGE (YEARS)

Published May 30, 2000 (modified 10/16/00).
SOURCE: Developed by the National Center for Health Statistics in collaboration with
the National Center for Chronic Disease Prevention and Health Promotion (2000).
http://www.cdc.gov/growthcharts

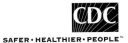

SAFER·HEALTHIER·PEOPLE™

FIGURE 6-17 cont'd

Other factors that may contribute to teen suicide include (1) divorce of the parents, (2) violence in the home, (3) inability to find success at school, (4) feelings of worthlessness, (5) rejection by friends or peers, (6) substance abuse, (7) death of someone close to the adolescent, and (8) suicide of a friend, or someone he or she "knows" online.

Another factor to consider is the presence of firearms. Because firearms are used in more than half of teen suicides, it is important to realize that easy access to a firearm and ammunition can contribute to a teenage death by suicide. Teenagers who express suicidal thoughts and feelings should not have ready access to firearms.

Prevention is the obvious solution for suicide. For any suicide attempt, it is most critical to realize that an attempted suicide is a cry for help. The most effective treatment is to recognize the pattern of behaviors—warning signs—that might indicate suicidal thoughts and feelings. These include the following: (1) expression of thoughts of death, dying, and a desire to leave this life; (2) changes in normal habits, such as eating and sleeping, and spending time with friends and family; (3) dramatic weight fluctuations, in any direction; (4) evidence of substance abuse (alcohol and drugs, both legal and illegal); (5) dramatic mood swings (becomes very happy after feeling very depressed); and (6) loss of interest in schoolwork and extracurricular activities (including declining grades). Although not all of these factors are necessarily indications of suicidal thoughts and feelings when taken separately, or happening rarely, a pattern can exhibit a serious problem, as can a combination of factors. Taking note of how often the foregoing behaviors appear is an essential monitoring of depression. Troubled teenagers who make suicide attempts are signaling that they feel overwhelmed with life and the stresses that come with it. An attempted suicide is usually an indication of depression as well. This can mean that a teenager has feelings, thoughts, and stressors that he or she cannot handle any more. Because of their underdeveloped coping skills, they see suicide as a solution to intense problems.

Teens are helped by concerned adults (i.e., parents, teachers, spiritual leaders, and counselors) showing support and guiding them to obtain the assistance needed to learn to deal with issues. Medical, physical, and cognitive/emotional evaluations are needed after a teenage suicide attempt. The primary recommendations for treatment for suicidal thoughts or a suicide attempt may typically include one or more of the following:

- *Individual therapy.* This is suicide treatment that involves therapy just for the teenager to help him or her work through feelings and suicidal thoughts.
- *Family therapy.* Sometimes family therapy works best in instances of teen suicide treatment. This can provide a supportive environment for the teenager, as well as help the family learn how to cope with the problem and work together.
- *Hospitalization.* In some cases, it is necessary to provide a teenager with a secure, safe, and constantly supervised environment. Most in-patient treatment protocols for the suicidal teenager include therapeutic aspects and offers the kind of supervision that might be necessary in extreme cases.

Entering therapy can be a good idea for many teenagers. In some cases, family therapy may be a good idea. This can help the family members of the suicidal teen receive the support they need, and it can show the teenager that the family cares about him or her and is willing to receive counseling as well.

Showing support and unconditional love is a necessary part of helping a suicidal adolescent.

Depression and other mood disorders are described in detail in Chapter 13. Occupational therapy intervention models of practice that have been used with these conditions include cognitive behavioral, occupational adaptation, and social skills groups. These models of practice ideally include a focus on occupation-based intervention in a naturally occurring context, primarily home and school. Performance skills addressed are emotional regulation, cognitive skills, communication, and social skills. In addition, therapists may help to foster development of healthy habits, roles, and routines to support engagement in a balance of activities.

SUMMARY

This chapter provides an overview of medical diagnoses in children who often receive occupational therapy services. Knowledge about the child's medical condition is important for developing appropriate intervention plans and for communicating with family and team members. Application of this information should consider that each child's presentation of the diagnosis is unique and that the effect of the disease or disability on the child's function is highly influenced by environmental and developmental variables. The field of medicine continually expands, and the occupational therapist must stay abreast of new developments and current information. Best practice requires thorough research of each diagnosis incurred. To assist the student in researching the implication of the medical diagnoses discussed in this chapter, key references have been cited and should be consulted for additional information.

REFERENCES

1. Abel, E. L. (1998). *Fetal alcohol abuse syndrome.* New York: Plenum Press.
2. Accornero, H., Amado, A. J., Morrow, C. E., Xue, L., Anthony, J. C., & Bandstra, E. S. (2007). Impact of prenatal cocaine exposure on attention and response inhibition as assessed by Continuous Performance Tests. *Journal of Developmental Behavioral Pediatrics, 28*(3), 195-205.
3. Adams-Chapman, I., & Stoll, B. J. (2007). Fetal and neonatal infant: Nervous system disorders. In R. M. Kliegman, R. E. Behrman, H. B. Jenson, & B. F. Stanton (Eds.), *Nelson textbook of pediatrics* (18th ed., pp. 713-721). Philadelphia: Saunders.
4. Adelson, P. D., & Kochanek, P. M. (1998). Head injury in children. *Journal of Child Neurology, 13*(1), 2-15.
5. Alemzadeh, R., & Wyatt, D. T. (2007). Diabetes mellitus in children. In R. M. Kliegman, R. E. Behrman, H. B. Jenson, & B. F. Stanton (Eds.), *Nelson textbook of pediatrics* (18th ed., pp. 2404-2429). Philadelphia: Saunders.
6. American Burn Association. (2009). Educational Resource Center. Retrieved August 2009 from http://www.ameriburn.org/. Chicago: American Burn Association.
7. American Psychiatric Association. (2000). *Diagnostic and statistical manual of mental disorders IV-TR.* (4th-TR ed.). Washington, DC: APA.
8. Baird, G., Cass, H., & Slonims, V. (2003). Diagnosis of autism. *British Medical Journal, 327*(7413), 488-493.
9. Ballard, S., Bolan, M., Burton, M., Snyder, S., Pasterczyk-Seabolt, C., & Martin, D. (1997). The neurological basis of attention deficit hyperactivity disorder. *Adolescence, 32*, 855-862.

10. Baranek, G. T. (1999). Autism during infancy: a retrospective video analysis of sensory-motor and social behaviors at 9-12 months of age. *Journal of Autism and Developmental Disorders, 29,* 213-224.

11. Baranek, G. T., Foster, L. G., & Berkson, G. (1997). Tactile defensiveness and stereotypic behaviors. *American Journal of Occupational Therapy, 51,* 91-95.

12. Barkley, R. A. (2003). Issues in the diagnosis of attention-deficit/hyperactivity disorder in children. *Brain & Development, 25*(2), 77-83.

13. Barkley, R. A. (2005). *Attention-deficit hyperactivity disorder* (3rd ed.). New York: Guilford Press.

14. Batshaw, M. L. (2007). Genetics and Developmental Disabilities. In M. L. Batshaw, L. Pellegrino, & N. J. Roizen (Eds.), *Children with disabilities* (6th ed., pp. 3-22). Baltimore: Brookes.

15. Batshaw, M. L., Shapiro, B., & Farber, M. L. Z. (2007). Developmental delay and intellectual disability. In M. L. Batshaw, L. Pellegrino, & N. J. Roizen (Eds.), *Children with disabilities* (6th ed., pp. 245-262). Baltimore: Brookes.

16. Batshaw, M. L., & Tuchman, M. (2007). Inborn errors of metabolism. In M. L. Batshaw, L. Pellegrino, & N. J. Roizen (Eds.), *Children with disabilities* (6th ed.). Baltimore: Brookes.

17. Bell, M. J. (2007). Infections and the Fetus. In M. L. Batshaw, L. Pellegrino, & N. J. Roizen (Eds.), *Children with disabilities* (6th ed., pp. 71-82). Baltimore: Brookes.

18. Bernstein, D. (2007). Congenital heart disease. In R. M. Kliegman, R. E. Behrman, H. B. Jenson, & B. F. Stanton (Eds.), *Nelson textbook of pediatrics* (18th ed., pp. 1878-1941). Philadelphia, PA: Saunders.

19. Bespalova, N., & Buxbaum, J. D. (2003). Disease susceptibility genes for autism. *Annals of Medicine, 35*(4), 274-281.

20. Biggs, K. S., de Linde, L., Banaszewski, M., & Heinrich, J. J. (1998). Determining the current roles of physical and occupational therapists in burn care. *Journal of Burn Care And Rehabilitation, 19*(5), 442-449.

21. Boat, T. F., & Acton, J. D. (2007). Cystic fibrosis. In R. M. Kliegman, R. E. Behrman, H. B. Jenson & B. F. Stanton (Eds.), *Nelson textbook of pediatrics* (18th ed., pp. 1803-1816). Philadelphia: Saunders.

22. Boddaert, N., Chabane, N., Gervais, H., Good, C. D., Bourgeois, M., Plumet, M. H., et al. (2004). Superior temporal sulcus anatomical abnormalities in childhood autism: A voxel-based morphometry MRI study. *Neuroimage, 23*(1), 364-369.

23. Brown, N. J., Berkovicand, S. F., & Scheffer, E. (2007). Vaccination, seizures and 'vaccine damage.' *Current Opinions in Neurology, 20,* 181-187.

24. Case-Smith, J., & Arbesman, M. (2008). Evidence-based review of interventions for autism used in or of relevance to occupational therapy. *American Journal of Occupational Therapy, 62,* 416-429.

25. Centers for Disease Control and Prevention. (2000). *Body Mass Index Charts for Boys and Girls 2-20.* Retrieved November 1, 2008, from http://www.cdc.gov/nchs/about/major/nhanes/growthcharts/clinical_charts.htm

26. Centers for Disease Control and Prevention. (2006). *Leading Causes of Death by Age Group.* Retrieved November 3, 2008, from http://www.cdc.gov/nchs/fastats/lcod.htm

27. Centers for Disease Control and Prevention. (2008). *Metropolitan Atlanta Congenital Defects Program.* Atlanta: CDC.

28. Cermak, S. A., & Larkin, D. (2002). *Developmental coordination disorders.* Albany, NY: Delmar.

29. Chakrabarti, S., & Fombonne, E. (2001). Pervasive developmental disorders in preschool children. *Journal of the American Medical Association, 285,* 3093-3099.

30. Chance, P. F., Ashizawa, T., Hoffman, E. P., & Crawford, T. O. (1998). Molecular basis of neuromuscular diseases. *Physical Medicine & Rehabilitation Clinics of North America, 9,* 49-81.

31. Church, M. W., & Abel, E. L. (1998). Fetal alcohol syndrome. Hearing, speech, language, and vestibular disorders. *Obstetrics and Gynecology Clinics of North America, 25,* 85-97.

32. Clark, F., Reingold, F. S., Salles-Jordan, K., & Commission on Practice. (2007). Obesity and occupational therapy. *American Journal of Occupational Therapy, 61*(6), 701-703.

33. Coles, C. (1994). Critical periods for prenatal alcohol exposure. *National Institutes of Health: Alcohol Health and Research World, 18*(1), 112-115.

34. Coronado, G., Thomas, K. E., & Kegler, S. R. (2007). Rates of hospitalization related to traumatic brain injury. *Morbidity and Mortality Weekly Report, 56*(8), 167-170.

35. Dahlgren, S. O., & Gillberg, C. (1989). Symptoms in the first two years of life: A preliminary population study of infantile autism. *European Archives of Psychology and Neurological Sciences, 238,* 169-174.

36. DeLisa, J. A., Gans, B. M., Walsh, N. E., Bockenek, W., & Frontera, W. R. (Eds.). (2004). *Physical medicine and rehabilitation: Principles and practice* (4th ed.). Philadelphia: Lippincott Williams & Wilkins.

37. Elia, J., Ambrosini, P., & Rapoport, J. (1999). Treatment of attention-deficit-hyperactivity disorder. *New England Journal of Medicine, 340,* 780-788.

38. Escolar, D. M., Tosi, L. L., Rocha, A. C. T., & Kennedy, A. (2007). Muscles, bones, and nerves. In M. L. Batshaw, L. Pellegrine, & N. J. Roizen (Eds.), *Children with disabilities* (6th ed., pp. 203-216). Baltimore: Brookes.

39. Faraone, S. V., & Biederman, J. (1998). Neurobiology of attention-deficit hyperactivity disorder. *Biological Psychiatry, 44,* 951-958.

40. Fombonne, E. (2003). Epidemiological surveys of autism and other pervasive developmental disorders: An update. *Journal of Autism and Developmental Disorders, 33*(4), 365-382.

41. Gadoth, N. (2008). On fish oil and omega-3 supplementation in children: The role of such supplementation on attention and cognitive dysfunction. *Brain & Development, 30*(5), 309-312.

42. Gillberg, C. (2003). Deficits in attention, motor control, and perception: A brief review. *Archives of Disease in Childhood, 88,* 904-910.

43. Glanzman, M. M., & Blum, N. J. (2007). Attention deficits and hyperactivity. In M. L. Batshaw, L. Pellegrino, & N. J. Roizen (Eds.), *Children with disabilities* (6th ed., pp. 345-366). Baltimore: Brookes.

44. Haddad, J. (2007). Disorders of the respiratory tract. In R. M. Kliegman, R. E. Behrman, H. B. Jenson, & B. F. Stanton (Eds.), *Nelson textbook of pediatrics* (18th ed., pp. 1742-1848). Philadelphia: Saunders.

45. Hallum, A. (2007). Neuromuscular disease. In D. A. Umphred (Ed.), *Neurological rehabilitation* (5th ed., pp. 475-531). St. Louis: Mosby.

46. Haydel, M. J. (2003). Prediction of intracranial injury in children aged five years and older with loss of consciousness after minor head injury due to nontrivial mechanisms. *Annals of Emergency Medicine, 42*(4), 507-514.

47. Hemingway, C., Freeman, J. M., Pillas, D. J., & Pyzik, P. L. (2001). The ketogenic diet: A 3- to 6-year follow-up of 150 children enrolled prospectively. *Pediatrics, 108*(4), 898-905.

48. Hentz, R., & Koi, K. (2005). Traumatic brachial plexus injury. In D. P. Green, R. N. Hotchkiss, W. C. Pederson, & S. W. Wolfe (Eds.), *Green's operative hand surgery* (Vol. 2, pp. 1319-1371). Philadelphia: Saunders.

49. Hillier, S. (2007). Intervention with children with developmental coordination disorder: A systematic review [Electronic version]. *Internet Journal of Allied Health Sciences and Practice, 5,* Retrieved Feb. 28, 2009, from http://ijahsp.nova.edu

50. Hockenberry, M. J., & Wilson, D. (2009). *Wong's essentials of pediatric nursing.* (8th ed.). St. Louis, MO: Mosby.

51. Hodapp, R. M., & Dykens, E. M. (2007). Behavioral effects of genetic mental retardation disorders. In J. W. Jacobson, J. A. Mulick, & J. Rojahn (Eds.), *Handbook of intellectual and developmental disabilities* (pp. 115-130). New York: Springer.

52. Hosalkar, H. S., Spiegel, D. A., & Davidson, R. S. (2007). The foot and toes. In R. M. Kliegman, R. E. Behrman, H. B. Jenson, & B. F. Stanton (Eds.), *Nelson textbook of pediatrics* (18th ed., pp. 2778-2779). Philadelphia: Saunders.

53. Hosalkar, H. S., & Wells, L. (2007). Bone and joint disorders. In R. M. Kliegman, R. E. Behrman, H. B. Jenson, & B. F. Stanton (Eds.), *Nelson textbook of pediatrics* (18th ed., pp. 2771-2847). Philadelphia: Saunders.

54. Hyman, S. L., & Towbin, K. E. (2007). Autism spectrum disorders. In M. L. Batshaw, L. Pellegrino, & N. J. Roizen (Eds.), *Children with disabilities* (6th ed., pp. 325-344). Baltimore: Brookes.

55. Johnston, M. V. (2007). Encephalopathies. In R. M. Kliegman, R. E. Behrman, H. B. Jenson & B. F. Stanton (Eds.), *Nelson textbook of pediatrics* (pp. 2494-2495). Philadelphia: Saunders.

56. Johnston, M. V. (2007). Neurodegenerative disorders of childhood. In R. M. Kliegman, R. E. Behrman, H. B. Jenson, & B. F. Stanton (Eds.), *Nelson textbook of pediatrics* (18th ed., pp. 2499-2505). Philadelphia: Saunders.

57. Johnston, C. A., & Steele, R. C. (2007). Treatment of pediatric overweight: An examination of feasibility and effectiveness in an applied clinical setting. *Journal of Pediatric Psychology, 32*(1), 106-110.

58. Kanner, L. (1943). Autistic disturbances of affective contact. *Nervous Child, 2,* 217-250.

59. Keenan, H. T., Runyan, D. K., Marshall, S. W., Nocera, M. A., Merten, D. F., & Sinal, S. H. (2003). A population-based study of inflicted traumatic brain injury in young children. *Journal of the American Medical Association, 290*(5), 621-626.

60. Kinnear, K. J. (2003). Purkinje cell vulnerability and autism: A possible etiological connection. *Brain & Development, 25*(6), 377-382.

61. Kinsman, S. L., & Johnston, M. V. (2007). Congenital anomalies of the central nervous system. In R. M. Kliegman, R. E. Behrman, H. B. Jenson & B. F. Stanton (Eds.), *Nelson textbook of pediatrics* (pp. 2443-2455). Philadelphia: Saunders.

62. Krebs, N. F., Himes, J. H., Jacobson, D., Nicklas, T. A., Guilday, P., & Styne, D. (2007). Assessment of child and adolescent overweight and obesity [Electronic Version]. *Pediatrics, 120,* S193-S228. Retrieved on November 5, 2008, from http://www.pediatrics.org/cgi/content/full/120/Supplement_4/S193

63. Krosschell, K. J., & Pesavento, M. J. (2007). Congenital spinal cord injury. In D. Umphred (Ed.), *Neurological rehabilitation* (5th ed., pp. 567-604). St. Louis: Mosby.

64. Langerak, N. G., Lamberts, R. P., Fieggen, A. G., Peter, J. C., van der Merwe, L., Peacock, W. J., et al. (2008). A prospective gait analysis study in patients with diplegic cerebral palsy 20 years after selective dorsal rhizotomy. *Journal of Neurosurgery, Pediatrics, 1*(3), 180-186.

65. Langlois, J. A., Rutland-Brown, W., & Thomas, K. E. (2006). *Traumatic brain injury in the United States: Emergency department visits, hospitalizations, and deaths.* Atlanta: Centers for Disease Control and Prevention, National Center for Injury Prevention and Control.

66. Langston, C., Cooper, E. R., Goldfarb, J., Easley, K. A., Husak, S., Sunkle, S., et al. (2001). Human immunodeficiency virus–related mortality in infants and children: Data from the pediatric pulmonary and cardiovascular complications of vertically transmitted HIV (P(2)C(2)) study. *Pediatrics, 107*(2), 328-338.

67. Latenser, B. A. (2008). Burn treatment guidelines. In R. E. Rakel & E. T. Bope (Eds.), *Conn's current therapy* (60th ed., pp. 1121-1126). Philadelphia: Saunders.

68. Levy, R. G., & Cooper, P. P. (2003). Ketogenic diet for epilepsy. *Cochrane Database of Systematic Reviews, 3.*

69. Liptak, G. S. (2007). Neural tube defects. In M. L. Batshaw, L. Pellegrino, & N. J. Roizen (Eds.), *Children with disabilities* (6th ed., pp. 419-438). Baltimore: Brookes.

70. Losh, M., Sullivan, P. F., Trembath, D., & Piven, M. D. (2008). Current developments in the genetics of autism: from phenome to genome. *Journal of Neuropathology and Experimental Neurology, 67*(9), 829-837.

71. Mahaffey, K. R. (1992). Exposure to lead in childhood. *New England Journal of Medicine, 327,* 1308-1309.

72. Mahoney, W. J., Szatmari, P., MacLean, J. E., Bryson, S. E., Bartolucci, G., Walter, S. D., et al. (1998). Reliability and accuracy of differentiating pervasive developmental disorder subtypes. *Journal of the American Academy of Child & Adolescent Psychiatry, 37,* 278-285.

73. Marini, J. C. (2007). Osteogenesis imperfecta. In R. M. Kliegman, R. E. Behrman, H. B. Jenson, & B. F. Stanton (Eds.), *Nelson textbook of pediatrics* (18th ed., pp. 2887-2890). Philadelphia: Saunders.

74. Mason, W. H. (2007). Rubella. In R. M. Kliegman, R. E. Behrman, H. B. Jenson, & B. F. Stanton (Eds.), *Nelson textbook of pediatrics* (18th ed., pp. 1337-1341). Philadelphia: Saunders.

75. Mattson, S. N., & Riley, E. P. (1998). A review of neurobehavioral deficits in children with fetal alcohol syndrome or prenatal exposure to alcohol. *Alcoholism, Clinical & Experimental Research, 22*(2), 279-294.

76. May, P. A., & Gossage, J. P. (2001). Estimating the prevalence of fetal alcohol syndrome: A summary. *Alcohol Research & Health, 25*(3), 159-167.

77. Mazzola, C. A., & Adelson, P. D. (2002). Critical care management of head trauma in children. *Critical Care Medicine, 30,* S393-S401.

78. McLeod, R., & Remington, J. S. (2007). Toxoplasmosis. In R. M. Kliegman, R. E. Behrman, H. B. Jenson, & B. F. Stanton (Eds.), *Nelson textbook of pediatrics* (18th ed., pp. 1486-1494). Philadelphia: Saunders.

79. Menkes, J. H., Sarnat, H. B., & Maria, B. L. (Eds.). (2005). *Childhood neurology* (7th ed.). Baltimore: Lippincott Williams & Wilkins.

80. Meyer, G. A. (2007). X-linked syndromes causing intellectual disability. In M. L. Batshaw, L. Pellegrino, & N. J. Roizen (Eds.), *Children with disabilities* (6th ed.). Baltimore: Brookes.

81. Michaud, L. J., Duhaime, A. C., Wade, S. L., Rabin, J. P., Jones, D. O., & Lazar, M. F. (2007). Traumatic brain injury. In M. L. Batshaw, L. Pellegrino, & N. J. Roizen (Eds.), *Children with disabilities* (pp. 461-478). Baltimore: Brookes.

82. Miller, M. L., & Cassidy, J. T. (2007). Juvenile rheumatoid arthritis. In R. M. Kliegman, R. E. Behrman, H. B. Jenson, & B. F. Stanton (Eds.), *Nelson textbook of pediatrics* (18th ed., pp. 1001-1010). Philadelphia: Saunders.

83. National Asthma Education and Prevention Program. (2007). Expert panel report: guidelines for the diagnosis and management of asthma. Retrieved November 23, 2008, from http://www.nhlbi.nih.gov/guidelines/asthma/asthmafullrpt.pdf

84. National Center for Birth Defects and Developmental Disabilities. (2006). Fetal alcohol syndrome disorders. Retrieved March 19, 2009, from http://www.cdc.gov/ncbdd/fas/fasask.htm

85. National Center for Health Statistics. (2007). Health, United States. Retrieved December 2, 2008, from http://www.cdc.gov/nchs/

86. National Health and Nutrition Examination Survey (NHANES). (2000). Retrieved October 22, 2008, from http://www.cdc.gov/nchs/about/major/nhanes/survey_results_and_products.htm

87. National Institute of Health. (2008). Calculate your body mass index [Electronic Version]. Retrieved July 21, 2008, from http://www.nhlbisupport.com/bmi/

88. Nelson, C. A., & Senesac, C. (2007). Management of clinical problems of children with cerebral palsy. In D. A. Umphred (Ed.), *Neurological rehabilitation* (5th ed., pp. 357-385). St. Louis: Mosby.

89. Neugebauer, C. T., Serghiou, M. S., Herndon, D. N., & Suman, O. E. (2008). Effects of a 12-week rehabilitation program with music and exercise groups on range of motion in young children with severe burns. *Journal of Burn Care Research, 29,* 939-948.

90. Odom, S. L., Horner, R. H., Snell, M. E., & Blacher, J. (Eds.). (2007). *Handbook of developmental disabilities*. New York: Guilford Press.

91. Ogden, C. L., Carroll, M. D., Curtin, L. R., McDowell, M. A., Tabak, C. J., & Flegal, K. M. (2006). Prevalence of overweight and obesity in the United States, 1999-2004. *Journal of the American Medical Association, 295*, 1549-1555.

92. Park, M. K. (2008). *Pediatric cardiology for practitioners* (5th ed.). St. Louis: Mosby.

93. Pelham, W. E., & Fabiano, G. A. (2008). Evidence-based psychosocial treatments for attention-deficit/hyperactivity disorder. *Journal of Clinical Child & Adolescent Psychology, 37*(1), 184-214.

94. Pellegrino, L. (2007). Cerebral palsy. In M. L. Batshaw, L. Pellegrino, & N. J. Roizen (Eds.), *Children with disabilities* (6th ed., pp. 387-408). Baltimore: Brookes.

95. Prober, C. G. (2007). Central nervous system infections. In R. M. Kliegman, R. E. Behrman, H. B. Jenson, & B. F. Stanton (Eds.), *Nelson textbook of pediatrics* (18th ed., pp. 2512-2523). Philadelphia: Saunders.

96. Radomski, M. V., & Latham, C. A. T. (Eds.). (2008). *Occupational therapy for physical dysfunction* (6th ed.). Baltimore: Lippincott Williams & Wilkins.

97. Riley, E. P., & McGee, C. L. (2005). Fetal alcohol spectrum disorders: an overview with emphasis on changes in brain and behavior. *Experimental Biology and Medicine, 230*, 357-365.

98. Robinson, L. K., & Fitzpatrick, E. (2007). Marfan syndrome. In R. M. Kliegman, R. E. Behrman, H. B. Jenson, & B. F. Stanton (Eds.), *Nelson textbook of pediatrics* (18th ed., pp. 2890-2893). Philadelphia: Saunders.

99. Rodier, P. M. (2000). The early origins of autism. *Scientific American, 282*(2), 56-63.

100. Rogers, S. L., Coe, C. L., & Karaszewski, J. W. (1998). Immune consequences of stroke and cerebral palsy in adults. *Journal of Neuroimmunology, 2*, 113-120.

101. Roizen, N. J. (2007). Down syndrome. In M. L. Batshaw, L. Pellegrino, & N. J. Roizen (Eds.), *Children with disabilities* (6th ed., pp. 263-274). Baltimore: Brookes.

102. Ropper, A. H., & Samuels, M. A. (2009). *Principles of neurology* (8th ed.). New York: McGraw-Hill Medical.

103. Sarnaik, A. P., & Heidemann, S. M. (2007). Respiratory system. In R. M. Kliegman, R. E. Behrman, H. B. Jenson, & B. F. Stanton (Eds.), *Nelson textbook of pediatrics* (pp. 1719-1730). Philadelphia: Saunders.

104. Sarnat, H. B. (2007). Neuromuscular disorders. In R. M. Kliegman, R. E. Behrman, H. B. Jenson, & B. F. Stanton (Eds.), *Nelson textbook of pediatrics* (18th ed., pp. 2531-2567). Philadelphia: Saunders.

105. Shapiro, B., Church, R. P., & Lewis, M. E. B. (2007). Specific learning disabilities. In M. L. Batshaw, L. Pellegrino, & N. J. Roizen (Eds.), *Children with disabilities* (6th ed., pp. 367-386). Baltimore: Brookes.

106. Sharp, P., & Kagan, R. (2007). The effect of positioning devices and pressure therapy on outcome after full-thickness burns of the neck. *Journal of Burn Care Rehabilitation, 28*, 451-459.

107. Skelton, J. A., & Rudolph, C. D. (2007). Overweight and obesity. In R. M. Kliegman, R. E. Behrman, H. B. Jenson, & B. F. Stanton (Eds.), *Nelson textbook of pediatrics* (18th ed.). Philadelphia: Saunders.

108. Skinner, H. B. (2006). *Current diagnosis and treatment in orthopedics* (4th ed.). New York: McGraw-Hill Medical.

109. Staheli, L. T. (2006). *Practice of pediatric orthopedics* (2nd ed.). Philadelphia: Lippincott Williams & Wilkins.

110. Stanley, F. J., Blair, E., & Alberman, E. (2000). Cerebral palsies: Epidemiology and causal pathways. *Clinics in Developmental Medicine, 151*.

111. Teasdale, T. W., & Engberg, T. W. (2003). Cognitive dysfunction in young men following head injury in childhood and adolescence: A population study. *Journal of Neurology, Neurosurgery, and Psychiatry, 74*, 933-936.

112. Teasdale, T., & Jennett, B. (1974). Assessment of coma and impaired consciousness. *Lancet, 2*, 81-84.

113. Canale, S. T., & Beaty, J. H. (2008). *Campbell's operative orthopedics* (11th ed., Vol. II). Philadelphia: Mosby.

114. Trost, J. P., Schwartz, M. H., Krach, L. E., Dunn, M. E., & Novacheck, T. F. (2008). Comprehensive short-term outcome assessment of selective dorsal rhizotomy. *Developmental Medicine & Child Neurology, 50*, 765-771.

115. Visser, S. V., & Lesesne, C. A. (2005). Mental health in the United States: Prevalence of diagnosis and medication treatment for attention-deficit/hyperactivity disorder—United States, 2003. *Morbidity and Mortality Weekly Report, 54*(34), 842-847.

116. Volkmar, F. R., Paul, R., Klin, A., & Cohen, D. J. (Eds.). (2005). *Handbook of autism and pervasive developmental disorders* (3rd ed.). New York: Wiley.

117. Wagner, C. L., Katikaneni, L. D., Cox, T. H., & ryan, R. M. (1998). The impact of prenatal drug exposure on the neonate. *Obstetrics & Gynecology Clinics of North America, 25*(1), 169-194.

118. Waters, P. M. (2005). Pediatric brachial plexus palsy. In D. P. Green, R. N. Hotchkiss, W. C. Pederson, & S. W. Wolfe (Eds.), *Green's operative hand surgery* (5th ed., Vol. 2, pp. 1297-1318). Philadelphia: Saunders.

119. Weinstein, S. L., & Gaillard, W. D. (2007). Epilepsy. In M. L. Batshaw, L. Pellegrino, & N. J. Roizen (Eds.), *Children with disabilities* (6th ed., pp. 439-460). Baltimore: Brookes.

120. Whitaker, R. C., Wright, J. A., Pepe, M. S., Seidel, K. D., & Dietz, W. H. (1997). Predicting obesity in young adulthood from childhood and parental obesity. *New England Journal of Medicine, 37*(13), 869-873.

121. Whyte, J., Hart, T., Laborde, A., & Rosenthal, M. (2004). Rehabilitation issues in traumatic brain injury. In J. A. DeLisa, B. M. Gans, N. E. Walsh, W. L. Bockenek, & W. R. Frontera (Eds.), *Physical medicine & rehabilitation: Principles and practice* (5th ed., Vol. 2, pp. 1677-1713). Philadelphia: Lippincott Williams & Wilkins.

122. Wrotniak, B. H., Epstein, L. H., Paluch, R. A., & Roemmich, J. N. (2004). Parent weight change as a predictor of child weight change in family-based behavioral obesity treatment. *Archives of Pediatric and Adolescent Medicine, 158*, 342-347.

123. Wunsch, M. J., Conlon, C. J., & Scheidt, P. C. (2007). Newborn screening: opportunities for prevention of developmental disabilities. In M. L. Batshaw, L. Pellegrino, & N. J. Roizen (Eds.), *Children with disabilities* (6th ed., pp. 97-106). Baltimore: Brookes.

124. Yeong, E. K. (1997). Improved burn scar assessment with use of a new scar-rating scale. *Journal of Burn Care and Rehabilitation, 18*(4), 353-364.

SUGGESTED READINGS

Batshaw, M. L., Pellegrino, L., & Roizen, N. J. (2007). *Children with disabilities* (6th ed.). Baltimore, MD: Brookes.

Bowyer, P., & Cahill, S. M. (2009). *Pediatric occupational therapy handbook: A guide to diagnoses and evidence-based interventions*. St. Louis: Mosby.

Bruni, M. (2006). Fine motor skills in children with Down syndrome (2nd ed.). Bethesda, MD: Woodbine House.

Carey, W. B., Crocker, A. C., Elias, E. R., Feldman, H. M., & Coleman, W. L. (2009). *Developmental-behavioral pediatrics* (4th ed.). Philadelphia: Saunders.

Cermak, S. A., & Larkin, D. (2002). *Developmental coordination disorders*. Albany, NY: Delmar.

Dewey, D., & Wilson, B. (2001). Developmental coordination disorder: what is it? *Physical & Occupational Therapy in Pediatrics, 20*, 5.

Eliasson, A.-C., & Burtner, P. (2008). Improving hand function in children with cerebral palsy. London: MacKeith Press.

Gross, M. A. (1997). *The ADD brain: Diagnosis, treatment and science of attention deficit disorder (ADD/ADHD) in adults, teenagers and children.* Hauppauge, NY: Nova Science Publishers.

Hockenberry, M. J., & Wilson, D. (2009). *Wong's essentials of pediatric nursing* (8th ed.). St. Louis: Mosby.

Jacobson, J. W., Mulick, J. A., & Rojahn, J. (2008). *Handbook of intellectual and developmental disabilities.* New York: Springer.

Kliegman, R. M., Behrman, R. E., Jenson, H. B., & Stanton, B. F. (2007). *Nelson textbook of pediatrics* (18th ed.). Philadelphia: Saunders.

National Research Council. (2001). *Educating children with autism.* Washington, DC: National Academy Press.

Neistein, L. S. (2007). *Adolescent health care: A practical guide* (5th ed.). Philadelphia: Lippincott Williams & Wilkins.

Puttkammer, C. H. (1998). *Working with substance exposed children.* San Antonio, TX: Therapy Skill Builders.

Volkmar, F. R., Paul, R., Klin, A., & Cohen, D. J. (Eds.). (2005). *Handbook of autism and pervasive developmental disorders* (3rd ed.). New York: Wiley.

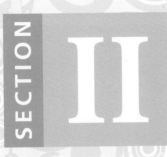

Occupational Therapy Evaluation in Pediatrics

7

Purposes, Processes, and Methods of Evaluation

Katherine B. Stewart

KEY TERMS

Evaluation
Occupational profile
Analysis of
   occupational
   performance
Screening
Comprehensive
   evaluation
Standardized tests
Norm-referenced
   measures

Skilled observations
Criterion-referenced
   measures
Reevaluation
Clinical research
Evaluation plan
Ecologic assessments
Interview
Arena assessment

OBJECTIVES

1. Apply the Occupational Therapy Practice Framework to the evaluation process for children and their families.
2. List five primary reasons to conduct evaluations.
3. Discuss the variety of decisions pediatric occupational therapists make throughout the evaluation process.
4. Describe the specific steps pediatric occupational therapists follow in the process of evaluating children
5. Describe the primary evaluation methods commonly used in pediatric occupational therapy.
6. Discuss the major factors therapists should consider when selecting evaluation methods and measures.
7. Apply the knowledge gained in this chapter to specific case studies of children who have or are at risk for disabilities.

Those who observe human behavior must be vigilant when examining the details of the behavior and when relating those details to each other in the context of that behavior. Occupational therapists involved in the evaluation of children face this challenge daily. To examine fully a child's occupational performance, the occupational therapist first analyzes how the physical demands and social expectations of the home, school, and community environments influence the child's participation. After identifying the areas of occupation most important to the child and the caregivers, the occupational therapist assesses the child's performance skills and performance patterns essential to his or her participation in everyday activities.

The evaluation process is one of the most fundamental, yet complex, aspects of occupational therapy services. According to the Standards of Practice for Occupational Therapy, evaluation is "the process of obtaining and interpreting data necessary for intervention. This includes planning for and documenting the evaluation process and results" (p. 663).[2] On the basis of the evaluation results, the occupational therapist makes important decisions regarding the type and intensity of occupational therapy intervention. The following factors influence these decisions: how the occupational therapist views the evaluation process; whether the therapist is open to new ways of understanding the child and family; which methods and measures the therapist selects to evaluate the child; and how the therapist interprets and documents the evaluation data.

This chapter describes the occupational therapy evaluation for children and adolescents. The first section explains the purposes of evaluating children based on the Occupational Therapy Practice Framework (OTPF).[1] A case study illustrates the application of the OTPF to the evaluation of a child. The second section describes the evaluation process, including sequential steps used by pediatric occupational therapists. The third section describes the general methods, measures, and principles used in selecting and administering pediatric occupational therapy assessments.

Four primary concepts are reinforced throughout this chapter:

1. The evaluation of a child or adolescent is an ongoing, dynamic process that begins with the initial referral for therapy and continues throughout the intervention and discharge phases of occupational therapy services.
2. The views and priorities of the child's primary caregiver and of the child are central throughout the evaluation process.
3. Evaluations should be ecologically and culturally valid.
4. The outcome of the evaluation is an in-depth understanding of the child's participation in occupations meaningful to him or her and to the caregivers.

EVALUATION PURPOSES

Occupational therapists evaluate children and their environments to gather information needed to make decisions about intervention services. This section discusses the decisions that therapists make during the various steps of careful screening and comprehensive evaluation of children who have or are at risk for disabilities.

The five primary purposes of occupational therapy evaluation are as follows:

1. Comprehensive evaluation to develop an intervention plan
2. Screening to decide if further evaluation of the child is warranted
3. Eligibility or diagnostic testing to decide if the child is eligible for occupational therapy services or to assist in the diagnostic process
4. Reevaluation to determine the child's progress in therapy and determine whether further therapy is warranted
5. Research or outcomes testing to evaluate the efficacy of intervention services and therapy outcomes

Comprehensive Evaluation for Intervention Planning

Comprehensive evaluation allows the occupational therapist to establish goals and plan intervention. The occupational therapist uses a top-down approach, assessing what the child wants and needs to do and then identifying those factors that act as supports or barriers to the child's participation in those childhood occupations. Consistent with the International Classification of Functioning, Disability and Health (ICF),[56] the OTPF supports the notion that an individual's performance and participation are inextricably linked to context, activity demands, and client factors. Occupation-centered assessment of children "acknowledges the importance of individual activities that are part of a particular occupation, as well as the context, but is most concerned with the overall process of participation."[15] Initially the therapist develops an *occupational profile* of the child based on referral concerns, interviews with caregivers and the child (if possible), and direct observations of the child performing

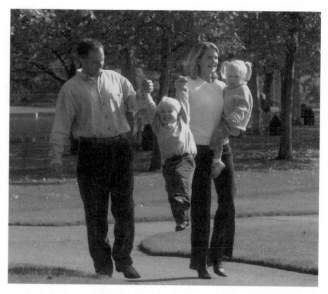

FIGURE 7-1 Family environment: parents playing with their two children at the park. (Courtesy Susan Phillips.)

self-care, play, and school-related activities. This profile describes the child's past occupational history and experiences, his or her current performance in occupational areas (e.g., self-help, play, and school activities), and the caregiver's (and child's) priorities regarding the child's participation in everyday activities. After identifying the limitations on the child's participation, the therapist develops a working hypothesis regarding possible reasons for identified problems and concerns. The occupational profile is the foundation for the next step in the evaluation process, which is the analysis of the child's occupational performance.

The analysis of occupational performance includes an evaluation of the child's physical, cognitive, and psychosocial performance and of important environmental factors that influence the child's participation in everyday occupations. Evaluation of the child's occupations consists of the child's performance skills (e.g., motor skills, process skills), performance patterns (e.g., habits, routines, roles), contexts (e.g., cultural, physical, social, personal, spiritual, temporal), activity demands (e.g., objects, space demands, social demands, sequencing and timing, required actions, required body functions and structures), and child factors (e.g., body functions and body structures).

To gain an in-depth understanding of the child's performance abilities and limitations, the occupational therapist evaluates the features of the environment in which the child performs the activities. Children and their families (Figure 7-1) are embedded in a network of social systems, including extended family, friends, neighbors, day care, schools, medical and religious institutions, and cultural groups. An ecologic model of development delineates the important dynamic process by which children and their environments interact.[10,52] Occupational therapists view the child in the context of his or her social environments. With an increased focus on participation in everyday occupations, occupational therapists are incorporating evaluation measures that allow them to move beyond impairment-based measures to ecologic assessments that facilitate a better understanding of the child's social and community participation.

Coster, Deeney, Haltiwanger, and Haley, the authors of the School Function Assessment (SFA), provide an exemplary model of pediatric assessment.[16] Coster and her colleagues recognized the need to develop an assessment tool that measures children's ability to participate in the academic and social aspects of the school environment. The SFA fills an important gap for therapists and educators interested in using a top-down, problem-solving approach by first considering the student's current level of participation in the educational programs and activities expected of his or her peers and then identifying the activity settings in which the student's participation is less than expected. This instrument is based on key concepts of the ICF and is consistent with the OTFP.

Other measures of participation in childhood occupations are used by pediatric occupational therapists. The Activities Scale for Kids is a measure of a child's self-report of activities done every day.[58] The child describes what he "did do" and what he "could do" during the past week, to help determine the effect of the child's physical disability on engagement in everyday occupations. The Children's Assessment of Participation and Enjoyment (CAPE) and the Preferences for Activities of Children (PAC) measure a child's day-to-day participation in activities and the child's preference for those activities.[34] The CAPE is a 55-item questionnaire designed to examine how children and youth participate in everyday activities. The questionnaire provides information about the diversity, intensity, and enjoyment in five types of activities (recreational, active physical, social, skill-based, and self-improvement activities). The PAC contains the 55 activities also included in the CAPE. The PAC scores are average preference ratings for each of the five activity categories. The Miller Function & Participation Scales measure the child's participation at school with an emphasis on fine motor, gross motor, and visual motor performance.[45]

An understanding of the child's participation in everyday activities is gained by using multiple measures, over multiple times, in multiple settings. In addition to the measures described earlier, evaluation data are obtained through direct observation of the child and through interviews with the child, the child's parents, and others who know the child.

Interviews with parents and other adults working with the child are another primary source of data regarding the child's performance and level of participation. For intervention planning, norm-referenced instruments may have limited value. Norm-referenced developmental assessments measure skills commonly seen in children who are typically developing, but they do not necessarily measure what is critical for functional performance in children with disabilities. For example, several of the items on the Peabody Developmental Motor Scales-2 (PDMS-2) (Figure 7-2) require the stacking of 1-inch cubes.[23] Is this specific skill critical for the child's success on everyday tasks? A common mistake of therapists is to design intervention goals directly from norm-referenced test items. This approach not only misses the mark with regard to writing functional outcomes, but may invalidate the use of these test items during reevaluation because of the practice effect on the child.

Therapists use criterion-referenced and curriculum-based assessments when the primary evaluation purpose is treatment planning. These measures provide information about specific skills important to the child's functional performance in activities of daily living, play, or school-related tasks. The Hawaii Early Learning Profile (HELP) is a curriculum-based assessment tool used to identify developmental needs and track progress in children from birth to 3 years of age.[25] The Assessment, Evaluation and Programming Systems for Infants and Young Children (AEPS) (2nd ed.) is an activity-based system that links assessment, intervention, and evaluation for children from birth to 6 years.[8] The Carolina Curriculum for Infants and Toddlers with Special Needs (3rd ed.) is an assessment and intervention program designed for use with young children from birth to 5 years who have mild to severe disabilities.[32] The Transdisciplinary Play-Based Assessment (TPBA) (2nd ed.) measures the child's cognitive, social-emotional, communication, and sensorimotor skills during a play session in a natural environment.[40] The School Assessment of Motor and Process Skills (School AMPS) is an innovative observational assessment tool used by occupational therapists to measure the quality of a student's performance on goal-directed tasks.[22] The School AMPS addresses functional performance issues in the classroom and provides information for effective programs and consultation in the school setting. An observational tool that measures an important dimension of children's play is the Test of Playfulness.[53] This criterion-based tool examines the key elements of playfulness: intrinsic motivation, suspension of reality, and internal locus of control.

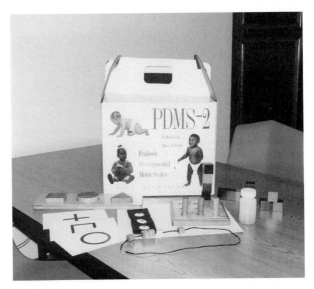

FIGURE 7-2 Fine motor materials from the Peabody Developmental Motor Scales-2 (PDMS-2) assessment tool.

Application

Case Study 7-1 illustrates the application of the OTPF to the evaluation of a child with developmental delays and environmental risk factors.

Screening

The primary reason for screening children is to determine whether they warrant a more comprehensive evaluation. Occupational therapists may participate in two levels of screening. The first level is a basic screening of developmental skills (e.g., motor, social, language, personal and adaptive skills). In

CASE STUDY 7-1   Kobe

Kobe is a second-grade boy with a diagnosis of spastic quadriplegia cerebral palsy who is 8 years 5 months of age. When he entered public school 2 years ago, Kobe qualified for special education based on the results of a multidisciplinary evaluation. He currently attends a special education classroom that consists of 12 children ranging from 7 to 11 years of age who exhibit mild to severe developmental delays in cognitive, speech and language, or motor skills. Kobe is being reevaluated in occupational therapy to determine his functional performance at school and identify the most appropriate goals to address in his individual education plan (IEP). The teacher reports that he becomes easily frustrated with fine motor tasks such as printing and cutting. In addition to his fine motor difficulties, she wonders if Kobe has visual perceptual difficulties that affect his school performance.

Kobe lives with his mother, father, and younger brothers, ages 2 and 4 years. The mother, who works full-time outside the home, reports that she is interested in how Kobe does at school, but has little time to help him with his schoolwork at home. When asked what she hopes Kobe can accomplish at school in the next year, she says she wants him to drive his power wheelchair safely, print his first name (Figure 7-3), and make friends with other children at school.

and family-centered approaches, the therapist gains an understanding of Kobe's perspective and his parents' concerns and priorities for his development and function. Kobe's occupational profile reveals that he has difficulty engaging in childhood occupations of play, self-help, and school-related tasks. The therapist hypothesizes that his occupational performance difficulties stem from his neurologic deficits and his need for adaptations to support his participation at school and home. The school-based occupational therapist selects a variety of methods and measures to further analyze Kobe's occupational performance in the context of his school environments.

TABLE 7-1   Methods and Measures for Kobe's Evaluation

Occupational Therapy Practice Framework	Methods and Measures
Occupational profile	Initial teacher interview Initial interview with parent Direct observation of Kobe at school
ANALYSIS OF OCCUPATIONAL PERFORMANCE	
School-related performance Performance skills (motor and process)	School Function Assessment Skilled Observations of Neuromotor Status Developmental Test of Visual Perception (DTVP-2) (Figure 7-4)
Activity demand	In-depth observation and analysis of Kobe performing a classroom activity

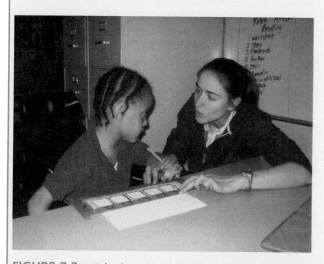

FIGURE 7-3   Kobe learning to print his letters at school.

Given the performance concerns noted by the teacher and parents, the evaluation methods and measures listed in Table 7-1 are appropriate options for the school-based occupational therapist to consider. Data for Kobe's occupational profile are collected during the initial contact with him, but his evaluation occurs over time. In this case, the therapist develops Kobe's occupational profile based on information gathered during interviews with him, his teacher, and parents regarding his performance in his environments (e.g., classroom, playground, lunchroom, home). Using client-centered

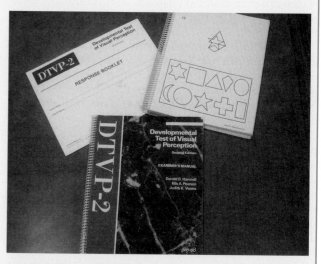

FIGURE 7-4   Materials for the Developmental Test of Visual Perception (2nd ed.) (DTVP-2).

some settings, such as public school programs, occupational therapists may participate in the screening of large numbers of children to determine which children should receive further testing. Public policies and regulations, including the Individuals with Disabilities Education Act (IDEA),[30,31] Head Start, and Medicaid programs for children, mandate early developmental screening to identify children at risk for disabilities. Some examples of this first level of screening include the Ages & Stages Questionnaires,[9] the Bayley Scales of Infant and Toddler Development-Screening Test,[7] the Denver Developmental Screening Test-II (Denver-II),[24] and the FirstSTEP.[43]

More frequently, pediatric occupational therapists participate in the second level of child screening. This type of screening usually occurs after a health care professional or teacher identifies the child as being at risk for developmental delays or functional limitations. At this point in the screening process, the occupational therapist administers more comprehensive screening tools specific to a particular functional area of concern.

For example, second-level screening of a child might proceed as follows: A first grade teacher observes her student's unusual responses to sensory experiences during art projects and his motor clumsiness on the playground at recess. The teacher refers the child to the occupational therapist for screening to determine if he needs a more comprehensive evaluation. In this case, the therapist might choose the Short Sensory Profile[17] and the Bruininks-Oseretsky Test of Motor Proficiency (BOT-2) (Short Form)[11] (Figure 7-5) to screen the child and determine the need for further evaluation.

In addition to administering standardized screening tests, the occupational therapist gathers pertinent information from parents and teachers and observes informally the child's performance in his or her natural environments (e.g., classroom, playground, and home). Regardless of the setting and the level of screening, the therapist considers the following points when screening children to determine whether further evaluation is warranted:

1. Standardized screening tools are implemented whenever possible to ensure that the results of the screening are reliable and valid. Standardized tests require uniform procedures for administration and scoring. Chapter 8 provides more information on the use of standardized instruments.

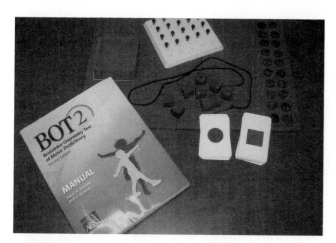

FIGURE 7-5 Materials for the Bruininks-Oseretsky Test of Motor Proficiency (BOT-2).

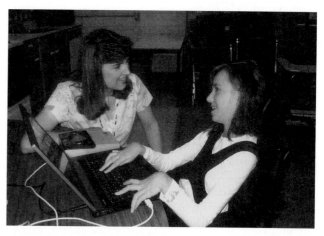

FIGURE 7-6 Therapist interviewing an adolescent about her preference for assistive technology.

2. In addition to standardized screening tools, the therapist gathers relevant information from the child and the child's teachers, parents, or other caregivers (Figure 7-6).
3. Information gathered during the screening process includes the child's performance across various developmental domains (e.g., motor, social, self-help) and in different environments to substantiate the need for further evaluation.
4. Screening tools are evaluated carefully for their cultural validity, and the results are interpreted cautiously when administered to children from diverse cultural backgrounds. A few instruments have established norms for children of different ethnic groups. For example, the Miller FirstSTEP[43] is published in Spanish (Primer PASO),[44] with norms established on 500 Spanish-speaking children.

Eligibility and Diagnostic Purposes

To determine children's eligibility for services, standardized measures are used to ensure that the test results are reliable and valid. Common assessment tools that occupational therapists use with children and adolescents are listed in Appendix 7-A.

Many public school systems mandate the use of norm-referenced tests by school personnel when qualifying students for special services. For example, to qualify in the developmentally delayed category, children between 3 and 6 years of age in Washington State must perform at least two standard deviations below the mean on a standardized, norm-referenced test in one developmental area or 1.5 standard deviations below the mean in two developmental areas.[55]

Standardized, norm-referenced measures determine how the individual child's performance compares with that of children in the normative sample. Because most norm-referenced instruments do not include children with disabilities in their standardization sample,[21] the therapist must use caution when interpreting the performance of a child with a disability. For example, a child with Down syndrome may score more than two standard deviations below the mean for his or her chronologic age, but this standard score does not reveal how he or she performs relative to other children with Down syndrome.

The IDEA mandates that "any assessment and evaluation procedures and materials that are used are selected and administered so as not to be racially or culturally discriminatory" (§ 300.304).[32] Unfortunately, many measures standardized on the U.S. population have limited cultural validity for children from ethnic groups not fully represented in the U.S. norms.

In summary, standardized, norm-referenced tools have an important, but limited, function in the occupational therapy evaluation process. Some service systems may require their use for determining a child's eligibility. However, standard scores, when used alone, do not provide a complete picture of a child and may be misleading, particularly for children with established disabilities or those from diverse cultural or ethnic backgrounds.

The occupational therapist also participates in multidisciplinary evaluations to determine a child's diagnosis. To assist in the diagnostic process, the therapist considers a combination of standardized norm-referenced tools, caregiver interviews, and skilled observations. Skilled observations (Figure 7-7) are nonstandardized methods developed by therapists to gather objective data on the quality, frequency, and duration of the child's performance. The "Evaluation Methods" section in this chapter presents specific information about the use of skilled observation. Box 7-1 provides a sample form for skilled observations of a child's neuromotor status. Scores from a norm-referenced measure provide the basis for the child's developmental status relative to other children the same age. In addition, the therapist's skilled observations of a child's performance provide important information on the quality of performance and possible reasons for the child's delayed or poor performance on the norm-referenced test. Case Study 7-2 describes how norm-referenced measures are used in combination with nonstandardized, skilled observations.

Reevaluation Purposes

In the reevaluation of a child's performance, progress is measured and the need for continued therapy is determined. The content and format of the reevaluation vary according to the specific purpose of the reevaluation. If the purpose is to determine whether the child continues to qualify for early intervention or special education services, the reevaluation may include a norm-referenced measure to ensure valid and reliable results. However, if the primary purpose of the reevaluation is to determine whether the child is making progress in therapy, criterion-referenced measures or the specific therapy goals and objectives are generally more appropriate and sensitive to the functional changes in the child.

For example, an infant with Down syndrome may show a drop in scores on a norm-referenced test over the course of the intervention year. However, these standard scores indicate only that the infant is developing at a slower rate compared with the test's norms. Measures of progress more sensitive to the developmental changes seen in this infant may be the long-term goals and short-term objectives written by the early intervention therapist. Short-term objectives are developed by therapists through careful task analysis and lead sequentially to more advanced behaviors stated in the long-term, functional goals. When written as criterion-referenced, measurable behaviors, short-term objectives can be used to evaluate the child's progress toward the long-term goal.

The process of reevaluation of children is ongoing and dynamic. Each time a therapist works with a child, the therapist evaluates the child's response to the therapeutic activities and assesses the child's performance on functional tasks. The therapist analyzes and interprets the data gathered during each therapy session to determine whether the intervention plan needs adjustment. In summary, although a formal reevaluation of the child is conducted at specific times during the course of therapy services, the occupational therapist embeds evaluation probes within each therapy session.

Clinical Research

Occupational therapy researchers carefully select standardized measures to evaluate the child's performance and participation in everyday activities. A more complete discussion of standardized tests used for clinical research is presented in Chapter 8, but a few major points are offered here:

1. Whether the research design includes a large group of children or a single subject, the instruments used must be reliable and valid measures of the dependent variable.

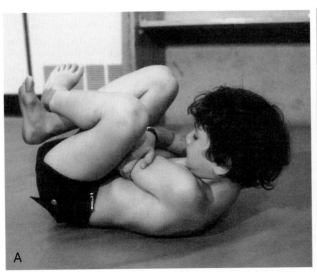
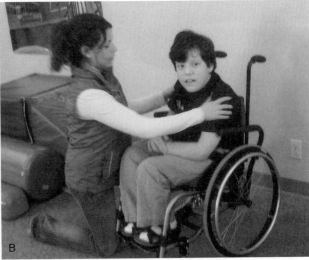

FIGURE 7-7 **A,** Skilled observation of a child in supine flexion. **B,** Skilled observation of a child's posture in a wheelchair.

BOX 7-1 Checklist for Skilled Observations of Neuromotor Status

As the child participates in everyday activities, note the quality of the child's posture, coordination, and transitional movement patterns. If a question or concern arises regarding the quality of motor performance during functional tasks, examine the child's muscle tone, range of motion, primitive postural reflexes, automatic reactions, oculomotor skills, strength and endurance, and response to handling and movement.

Use the following ratings:

1 = within normal limits
2 = mild to moderate abnormalities, but completes task
3 = severe abnormalities that limit completion of task

POSTURE (note asymmetries and alignment)

___ Supine
___ Prone
___ Sit
___ Quadruped
___ Stand

COORDINATION (GROSS MOTOR) (note asymmetries)

___ Rolling
___ Pivot in prone
___ Getting in/out of sitting
___ Crawling in quadruped
___ Pulling to stand
___ Cruising
___ Walking
___ Moving from stand to sit/sit to stand
___ Climbing up and down stairs
___ Jumping
___ Galloping
___ Skipping

COORDINATION (FINE MOTOR) (note asymmetries)

___ Reaching
___ Grasping
___ Releasing
___ Transferring objects
___ Crossing midline of body
___ Bilateral hand use
___ Using eating utensils
___ Using writing utensils
___ Manipulating objects within the hand
___ Cutting with scissors
___ Buttoning clothing

MUSCLE TONE (note asymmetries)

___ Left upper extremity ___ Right upper extremity
___ Left lower extremity ___ Right lower extremity
___ Trunk muscles
___ Neck muscles

RANGE OF MOTION

___ Left upper extremity ___ Right upper extremity
___ Left lower extremity ___ Right lower extremity
___ Trunk (flexion, extension, rotation of spine)
___ Neck (flexion, extension, rotation)

PRESENCE OF PRIMITIVE POSTURAL REFLEXES

___ Asymmetric tonic neck reflex
___ Symmetric tonic neck reflex
___ Tonic labyrinthine reflex (prone, supine)
___ Walking reflex
___ Grasp reflex
___ Plantar reflex

DELAYED AUTOMATIC REACTIONS (note asymmetries)

___ Head righting (flexion, extension, lateral)
___ Equilibrium (sitting, standing)
___ Protective arm extension (forward, sideward, backward)

OCULOMOTOR ABILITIES (note asymmetries)

___ Focuses on object
___ Shifts gaze
___ Tracks slow-moving object (horizontal, vertical, circular)
___ Eyes converge
___ Esotropia (eyes turn inward)
___ Exotropia (eyes turn outward)
___ Depth perception
___ Visual neglect (left, right)
___ Nystagmus

STRENGTH

___ Left upper extremity ___ Right upper extremity
___ Left lower extremity ___ Right lower extremity
___ Trunk muscles
___ Neck muscles
___ GENERAL ENDURANCE
___ RESPONSE TO PHYSICAL HANDLING
___ RESPONSE TO BEING MOVED

2. The measures selected depend on the research design. Standardized, norm-referenced, or criterion-referenced instruments are used in large-group designs. Occupational therapists working in rehabilitation settings use the Functional Independence Measure for Children (WeeFIM) to document clinical outcomes related to children's self-care, mobility, communication, and social problem solving.[27] Criterion-referenced instruments or operationally defined therapy objectives are used for single-subject research.

3. An important area of research in pediatric occupational therapy is the measurement of outcomes to document treatment effectiveness. Goal attainment scaling (GAS) is a technique used to evaluate the functional goal attainment of children receiving therapy.[35] GAS is an individualized, criterion-referenced measure of change that has been used to assess occupational therapy outcomes for children with learning disabilities,[57] children with traumatic brain injury,[47] and children with sensory integration disorders.[41]

Examples of research instruments include the tools that have been developed by Kielhofner and his colleagues to measure occupation based on the Model of Human Occupation. These instruments assess a child's volition, providing specific information about the child's interests and values. The Pediatric Volitional Questionnaire obtains information about the child's motivation, values, and interests.[6] The Child Occupational Self Assessment (COSA) is a self-report in which the child rates his performance competency and the importance of the skill.[33] By objectively quantifying information that occupational therapists typically obtain through informal interview, interest and motivation can be used as variables in research studies.

Law used an earlier version of the ICF[56] as a framework to develop a computerized, self-directed software program designed to help pediatric therapists select relevant and appropriate outcome measures for client, service, or program evaluation.[38] With a large database of pediatric measures, this

---

CASE STUDY 7-2   Jason

Jason is an 8-year-old boy with mild motor coordination deficits and hypersensitivities to touch and movement. The therapist administers a norm-referenced tool, the Sensory Integration and Praxis Tests,[5] to obtain standard scores on his sensory and motor performance (Figure 7-8). In addition, through skilled observations, the therapist obtains qualitative data regarding Jason's muscle tone, righting and equilibrium reactions, posture, and bilateral hand use. Combining this information enables the examiner to understand how Jason's sensory processing and motor planning abilities affect his everyday performance.

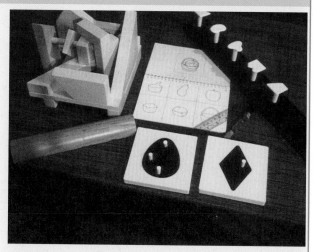

FIGURE 7-8   Materials for the Sensory Integration and Praxis Tests.

---

software program is an excellent resource for practitioners and researchers in occupational therapy who are conducting clinical outcome studies on children with disabilities.

EVALUATION PROCESS

This section provides a logical sequence of steps that pediatric occupational therapists follow in the process of evaluating children. Kobe's case, discussed previously, is a good illustration of the evaluation process. Based on Kobe's occupational profile, the therapist identifies several methods and measures to evaluate Kobe's occupational performance. Not all the methods and measures listed in Table 7-1 need to be completed before occupational therapy can commence for Kobe. The process of evaluation in occupational therapy starts with the referral and continues for the duration of therapy services. Key areas of the child's performance are evaluated before the intervention plan is developed and therapy is initiated. Other areas of evaluation are completed as the therapist learns more about the child and family. The therapist, therefore, continually considers the new challenges the child faces and other priorities that emerge for the family.

According to the Standards of Practice for Occupational Therapy,[2] the occupational therapist and the occupational therapy assistant have important but different roles in the evaluation of clients. The occupational therapist is responsible for selecting evaluation methods and measures and interpreting and analyzing assessment data. The occupational therapy assistant, under the supervision of the occupational therapist, may contribute to the child's evaluation by administering some of the assessments and documenting some of the results (Figure 7-9).

To conduct thorough evaluations and provide accurate interpretation and documentation of evaluation results, occupational therapists follow logical steps in the evaluation process. Figure 7-10 shows a flowchart for the evaluation sequence.

Referral

Children who have or are at risk for disabilities are referred to occupational therapists by health care providers, educators, and other professionals for evaluation of and intervention for occupational performance deficits. The referral form often lists the child's diagnosis or deficits in specific developmental areas. To ensure that the referrals to occupational therapy are appropriate, the occupational therapist should be involved in the development of the referral form used in his or her work setting.

Development of the Child's Occupational Profile

Once the therapist receives the referral, he or she consults with the child's parents and professionals from other disciplines to determine which measures to use, the evaluation setting, and the schedule for the occupational therapy evaluation activities. Most therapists find it helpful to formulate an evaluation plan based on the child's chronologic age, presenting problems, theoretical frames of reference, parents' priorities regarding reasons for referral, availability of evaluation tools, type of service delivery model, and amount of time and resources available for initial evaluation activities. The therapist lists the major concerns and the evaluation methods and measures that specifically assess those concerns (Table 7-2). Box 7-2 provides a checklist of the important steps therapists take in the process of selecting appropriate methods and measures when evaluating children.

Kramer and Hinojosa described how philosophical foundations and theoretical frames of reference guide the occupational therapist in the selection, use, and interpretation of assessment measures.[37] Kobe's case (Case Study 7-3) illustrates the application of theory to the evaluation process. As mentioned previously, the therapist hypothesized, on the basis of Kobe's occupational profile, that his performance deficits are likely a result of his significant motor challenges, possible visual processing deficits, and some environmental barriers. In this case, the therapist draws on specific models of practice

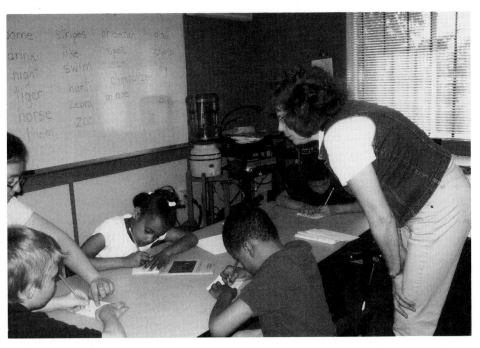

FIGURE 7-9 Occupational therapy assistant evaluating children's performance during a handwriting activity school.

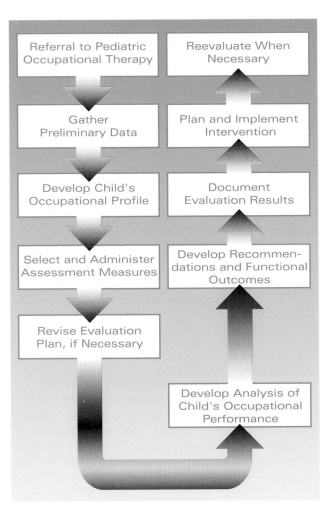

FIGURE 7-10 Flowchart for the evaluation process using the Occupational Therapy Practice Framework.

(e.g., client-centered approach, person-environment-occupation model, compensatory approach, motor learning theory) to select methods and measures for Kobe's evaluation.

As mentioned previously, the evaluation process occurs over time. In view of the complexity of problems in children referred to pediatric occupational therapists, it may be difficult to formulate a comprehensive evaluation plan based on the limited referral information. Therefore, the therapist usually revises the evaluation plan when more information is obtained regarding the family's priorities and the child's functional status. In Kobe's example, the therapist learned from a phone interview with the mother that she is most concerned about his safety while driving his powered wheelchair.

Administration of Evaluation

Using key information from the child's occupational profile, the therapist decides which methods and measures to administer to evaluate more fully the child's performance skills and the contexts that may be limiting his or her participation in everyday occupations. In Kobe's case, the therapist selects a series of methods and measures to evaluate his performance at school, his neuromotor status, and his visual processing skills. Although data from these methods and measures provide an initial picture of Kobe, the therapist recommends further assessment of his computer skills and his preferences related to school and home activities.

For most entry-level therapists in pediatrics, one of the most challenging aspects of the evaluation process is managing the child's behavior during administration of the evaluation measures, particularly when the measures are more formal, structured, and standardized. The evaluation of infants and young children in a structured situation is demanding for the children, the parents, and the therapist. Box 7-3 outlines several strategies therapists can use to manage young children's behavior during structured, standardized assessments.

TABLE 7-2 Selection of Appropriate Evaluation Methods

Purpose of Assessment	Evaluation Methods				
	Norm Referenced	Criterion Referenced	Skilled Observation	Interview	Checklists
Comprehensive evaluation to determine intervention plan		X	X	X	X
Screening	X	X	X	X	
Evaluation to determine eligibility	X				
Evaluation to assist in diagnosis	X	X		X	
Reevaluation to monitor child's progress	X	X	X	X	X
Research to investigate treatment outcomes	X				

The administration of nonstandardized tools, skilled observations, environmental assessments, and interviews with the child's caregivers should receive the same careful attention and preparation by the occupational therapist as the standardized measures require. For some children, a combination of standardized tests and nonstandardized measures is appropriate, but for many children with severe disabilities, norm-referenced tests are neither valid nor meaningful. In these cases, data gathered from criterion-referenced and nonstandardized measures provide the essential information for planning intervention.

Analysis of the Child's Occupational Performance

After most of the evaluation information on a child's performance and participation is gathered, the therapist analyzes the quantitative and qualitative data from the various methods and measures used. When a standardized test is used, the therapist carefully follows procedures outlined in the test manual to interpret accurately the test results. When nonstandardized measures are used, the therapist skillfully identifies any patterns of strength and areas of concern across all measures. Often data obtained from nonstandardized measures are instrumental in identifying the possible underlying reasons for a child's specific performance on standardized tests. To illustrate this point, consider Kobe's case. His teacher wondered if he had visual perceptual deficits that affected his performance on school-related tasks. Although Kobe scored significantly better on the visual-perceptual test items than on the visual-motor test items, other observations of his performance across school settings (e.g., classroom, lunchroom, and playground) revealed his difficulties with figure-ground perception. For example, he had a difficult time finding letters on a busy worksheet, locating his spoon on a crowded tray, and finding his way through a maze of children in the hallway (see Case Study 7-3).

Accurate and complete interpretation of all accumulated data is an important and demanding task in the evaluation process. The occupational therapist must be thorough in examining the details of a child's performance and viewing the child's behaviors in the context of environmental demands and supports. Accurate and complete interpretation of evaluation data allows therapists to make sound clinical decisions, including whether the child would benefit from occupational therapy services and, if so, the appropriate frequency, duration, and type of therapeutic intervention. Once the evaluation data are analyzed, the therapist turns to the task of developing recommendations for the child.

Development of Recommendations Based on Evaluation Results

One of the first factors the therapist considers when developing recommendations is the functionality of the recommendations. The term *functionality* refers to the relevance of the recommendation to the child's daily life.[49] When developing recommendations for a child, the occupational therapist asks the following two questions:

1. Does this recommendation relate to the child's occupational performance?
2. Is this recommendation relevant to the child's participation in everyday activities?

Writing therapy goals and objectives gives therapists the opportunity to think about and determine the most important skills a child needs to meet the demands of his or her environment(s). Bundy suggests that functional outcomes for children be viewed as an expression of possibilities of what children can do with support from their families and therapists.[12] The following examples illustrate how therapists can translate evaluation findings into functional, measurable

CASE STUDY 7-3   Occupational Therapy Evaluation Report for Kobe

BACKGROUND INFORMATION

Kobe is an African American boy with a diagnosis of spastic quadriplegia cerebral palsy who is 8 years 5 months of age. He attends a second grade special education class that includes 10 other children with moderate to severe developmental disabilities. He lives with his parents and two younger brothers in a small suburban home. Kobe uses a powered wheelchair for his mobility at home and at school.

REFERRAL INFORMATION

Kobe's special education teacher referred him to occupational therapy for a comprehensive reevaluation to determine his current functional performance at school and to identify appropriate goals and objectives to address in his individual education plan. He has participated in special education since he started public school 2 years ago.

OCCUPATIONAL PROFILE

A brief interview with Kobe's teacher reveals he has difficulty learning to print, maneuvering his power wheelchair around the school, and managing utensils at lunchtime. In an interview with Kobe's mother, she reports that she is worried that he is going to hurt himself or others while driving his power wheelchair. Kobe says he wants to learn to play games on the computer and he enjoys racing his wheelchair around the playground. He says he does not like "getting in trouble" at school or home.

Kobe's occupational profile suggests that he is having difficulty engaging in some childhood occupations of play, self-help, and school-related tasks. It appears that his occupational performance limitations stem from underlying neurologic deficits, possible visual processing deficits, and physical barriers in his home and school environments.

ASSESSMENTS USED

School Function Assessment (SFA) was used to measure Kobe's performance on school-related tasks that are important for successful participation at school.

Skilled observations of Kobe's neuromotor status were done to assess his muscle tone, posture in sitting, range of motion, oculomotor abilities, and functional gross and fine motor skills.

The Developmental Test of Visual Perception (2nd ed.) (DVPT-2) was administered to compare his performance on items that require a visual response with his performance on items that require a motor response.

ASSESSMENT SITUATION

The assessments were conducted over a 2-week period at the beginning of the school year. The occupational therapist, the certified occupational therapy assistant, and the teacher each completed portions of the SFA. The occupational therapist directly observed Kobe's neuromotor status and administered the DTVP-2. Kobe was a friendly child who easily engaged in conversation with the evaluators. He had significant difficulty on the motor items, but with encouragement from the evaluators, he tried hard to complete the tasks.

The scores obtained appear to be an accurate reflection of his actual abilities.

ASSESSMENT RESULTS

School Function Assessment

Participation—Kobe spends most of his time in the special education classroom. He meaningfully participates in some aspect or portion of the classroom tasks, but requires significant assistance while he is moving around the classroom and when he is completing a fine motor activity. His participation in other school settings varies widely. For example, he is extremely limited in the lunchroom and the bathroom because of his significant motor impairments. However, with the use of his powered wheelchair, he has access to other parts of the school, where he can engage in some activities on the playground and can get on and off the bus with a lift.

Needs for Supports and Activity Performance—Kobe uses his powered wheelchair at school throughout the day. He moves around most settings at school, but needs extra verbal cues and physical assistance when getting through congested areas, doorways, and around obstacles. He frequently bumps into people and objects. Kobe participates in all field trips and uses the adapted bus for transportation to and from school. He requires moderate assistance when changing his position into or out of his wheelchair. Kobe bears some of his weight when transferring on and off the toilet, but needs extensive assistance for dressing. He needs frequent cues to sit upright in his wheelchair while doing most activities. Kobe goes out on the playground at recess, but does not engage in any activities except to drive his powered wheelchair to "chase" the other children. At lunchtime, he needs extensive assistance to carry his tray and use utensils for eating. He usually needs support in finding his spoon on a crowded tray. In the classroom, he needs extensive assistance with fine motor tasks such as printing with an adapted pencil and cutting with adapted scissors. Kobe can use his left index finger to press the keys on the computer, but cannot use a mouse to select items on the screen. He reaches for, grasps, and places objects such as pencils, paper, lightweight books, and larger math manipulatives. He needs extensive assistance with complex fine motor tasks such as managing his seat belt, turning doorknobs, or carrying things that spill. Kobe independently communicates most information, but he needs some assistance to express complex ideas compared with his peers. He requires frequent reminders to stay on task when in groups or in noisy environments. He also needs extra cues to discriminate his letters or numbers from a busy background on his worksheets. Kobe engages positively in adult and peer interaction. He follows most routines at school, but does not always follow the rules about restricted areas or materials. He needs moderate assistance in avoiding dangerous situations when maneuvering his powered chair on the playground and in the hallways.

Summary of Strengths and Concerns—Kobe is a socially engaging child who communicates most of his needs and ideas. He follows the school routines with only occasional reminders. Kobe enjoys being at school and frequently

Continued

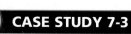

CASE STUDY 7-3 | **Occupational Therapy Evaluation Report for Kobe—cont'd**

initiates learning activities in the classroom. He needs extensive support in following safety rules, particularly when maneuvering his powered wheelchair. He also needs extensive support and adaptations for completion of fine motor activities such as printing, cutting, and eating with utensils.

Observations of Neuromotor Status

Skilled observations revealed increased muscle tone in extremities and low muscle tone in trunk and neck muscles. Active range of motion is limited in shoulder flexion, elbow extension, forearm supination, and finger extension. Posture is affected by abnormal tone, and Kobe sits with a rounded back and reduced head control. Equilibrium and protective extension reactions are delayed. He has difficulty visually tracking moving objects. These neuromotor deficits underlie most of Kobe's performance difficulties.

Visual Perception

On the DTVP-2, Kobe obtained a percentile rank of 1 (-2.33 SD) on the visual-motor subtests and a percentile rank of 15 (-1.04 SD) on the visual-perceptual subtests. He scored in the low-average range on some of the motor-reduced (visual perception) items, including the Figure Ground and Form Constancy subtests. The items on the motor-enhanced (visual-motor integration) subtests, including the Eye-Hand Coordination and Copying subtests, were particularly difficult for Kobe.

SUMMARY AND ANALYSIS OF OCCUPATIONAL PERFORMANCE

Kobe is an 8-year, 5-month-old boy with spastic quadriplegia cerebral palsy who is currently enrolled in a second-grade classroom. This evaluation reveals that he participates in most school activities, but he requires extensive support and modifications for fine and gross motor functions. His significant neuromotor deficits, including abnormal muscle tone, limited active range of motion in extremities, delayed equilibrium reactions, and ocular pursuits, underlie most of his performance difficulties. Kobe's overall performance on the DTVP-2 fell significantly below the mean compared with other children his age. His scores were low on some of the visual-perceptual subtests, but he had substantially more difficulty on items that required visual-motor integration. Kobe is a friendly, engaging boy who wants to do well at school, but his severe motor deficits and mild cognitive and communication deficits limit his performance on most tasks at school.

RECOMMENDATIONS

Kobe would benefit from occupational therapy services in which intervention activities are carefully designed to improve his function in school activities. Adaptations to his school environment and materials should be made to lessen the support he needs from adults and increase his participation. Further assessment of his computer skills is necessary to determine the type of assistive technology he needs to complete his written schoolwork. Administration of the Preferences for Activities of Children (PAC) may reveal more information about Kobe's interests related to school and home activities. Kobe needs a specific training program to improve the wheelchair skills he needs to maneuver safely in his school and home environments. His parents may benefit from suggestions for low-cost materials and simple adaptations for Kobe at home to enhance his functional performance. If there are any questions regarding this report, please contact this therapist at 123-4567.

BOX 7-3 | Behavior Strategies for Testing Young Children

1. Be prepared. Know your testing procedures so well that you can focus on the child's behavior and performance, not on the test manual or your paperwork.
2. Be sensitive to the child's and the parents' physical and emotional needs. Whenever possible, adjust the pace of the examination to match the child's style and acknowledge any concerns the parents may express.
3. Be purposeful in carrying out the examination. Keep the situation friendly, interesting for the child, and informative for the parent.
4. Be sure that the testing room supports the child's optimal performance. The chair and table should be of the appropriate size, and lighting should be sufficient. Remove all auditory and visual distractions. Use test materials attractive to children.
5. Build a rapport with the child before physically interacting with or handling him or her. Some children may do better starting with tabletop tasks in which the child sits across from the examiner and observes the situation before being handled physically for motor testing. Other children may do better if allowed to engage in a spontaneous play situation while the examiner focuses on the parent interview before directly testing the child. Be flexible and follow the child's lead whenever possible.
6. Use positive reinforcement that is meaningful to the child (e.g., praise, stickers, or a fun activity). Be sure to reinforce the child's effort rather than his or her success.
7. Begin and end with some easy items for the child. This helps the child feel more comfortable at the beginning and provides a positive ending to the test session for both the child and the parents.
8. Watch the complexity of your language. Be clear and concise in your instructions to the child.
9. Be organized. Keep the test materials arranged neatly in an area that is easily accessible to you but not to the child. Place an attractive toy (not from the test kit) on the table or nearby for the child to play with while you are not directly testing him or her.
10. Try to develop reciprocal interactions with the child. When you first show a test object, allow the child to explore it briefly in his or her own way before you give the test instructions. This extra time provides an excellent opportunity for informal observations. Then give the test instructions and allow the child to demonstrate his or her skill. If the child continues to be actively engaged with the object when you want to present the next test item, present the new test object as you remove the old one.

treatment goals that are relevant to the everyday activities of children.

1. *Evaluation finding.* Because of imprecise release of objects, Jill does not stack 1-inch cubes on the PDMS-2. Given a 6-month time frame:
   a. *Inadequate treatment goal.* Jill will stack two 1-inch cubes, three out of four trials.
   b. *Functional goal.* When playing with small toys, Jill will independently pick up and place small toys in a container, three out of four trials.
2. *Evaluation finding.* Because of increased muscle tone and poor reciprocal movements in the lower extremities, Ryan does not assume the half-kneel position on either leg when coming to stand, an item on the Gross Motor Function Measure (2nd ed.) (GMFM-II).[51] Given a 6-month time frame:
   a. *Inadequate treatment goal.* Ryan will maintain the half-kneel position for 30 seconds, three times over two consecutive therapy sessions.
   b. *Functional goal.* Ryan will step up with either leg on a 6-inch stool to use the classroom toilet without losing his balance, three out of four times.

A second factor to consider when making recommendations is the parents' or teachers' priorities for the child. Hanft suggests that every recommendation from an occupational therapist to a parent of a child with special needs should be followed by a question to the caregiver[29]: "How will this suggestion work for you and your child?" For example, during a feeding evaluation in a child's home, a therapist observes a mother and her child who has cerebral palsy and failure to thrive. The therapist notes that the mother placed the child in an infant walker at mealtime. Because infant walkers are unsafe and because this particular child would benefit from a more stable seating device that provides trunk and head support for optimal oral-motor performance, the therapist recommends the use of the infant walker be discontinued and a special feeding seat be ordered. However, unless the therapist asks the mother what the implications of this recommendation are for her child and family, the mother may not implement this important recommendation. In this case, additional information from the mother revealed that the child refused to eat in any other position than in the walker. She was more concerned about her child's adequate nutrition for growth than his feeding position. Based on the mother's input, the therapist provided the parents with information on the safety of infant walkers and the importance of proper positioning when swallowing to prevent aspiration.

A third factor for therapists to consider when developing recommendations from evaluation findings is the service delivery model. Dunn defined service delivery models as direct services, integrated or supervised therapy, and consultation.[19] The therapist's recommendations should be consistent with the program's service delivery model. For example, if the therapist's primary role with the child is consultation, recommendations from the initial evaluation center on how to teach the parents and other adults working with the child to adapt the child's environment.

The therapist must be able to reconcile these three, sometimes conflicting factors when developing meaningful recommendations for children. Years of experience can teach a therapist to negotiate through the maze of issues regarding the child, family, team, environments, and service delivery systems. Entry-level therapists, however, can use several basic strategies to help them become more competent in evaluating children:

1. Find a mentor who is experienced in working with children with various diagnoses and families from diverse backgrounds.
2. Be willing to search continually for new knowledge and resources that are relevant in working with children with special needs.
3. Be open to new ways of viewing children and families.
4. Learn to build effective communication and collaboration skills with team members, including the child's parent.

Documentation of Evaluation Results and Recommendations

The next step in the evaluation process is to provide written and oral reports on the evaluation findings and recommendations. The primary purpose of documenting the results of the pediatric occupational therapy evaluation is to describe to individuals working with the child the child's current abilities and limitations on various functional tasks. McClain suggested: "Effective documentation is telling a true story with a particular style. It calls for the ordinary tasks of day-to-day experience to be succinctly stated in writing. The true story about any child who has a disability is not a simple tale" (p. 213).[42]

When providing written documentation, the therapist must first consider for whom the reports are intended, then carefully construct reports that are understandable and useful to those individuals. The format and content of evaluation reports may vary significantly, depending on the referral concern, the complexity of the child's problem, and the regulations of the service delivery system in which the child is served (e.g., public school setting, hospital, or outpatient clinic). For eligibility purposes, written evaluation reports usually include specific standard scores documenting developmental delay. In all pediatric occupational therapy settings, documentation creates a chronological record of the child's status, the occupational therapy services provided to the child, and the child's outcomes.[3]

Experienced therapists recognize that their words have significant impact on the child's family. Hanft cautioned pediatric therapists that "words convey powerful personal images that can be positive and supportive or negative and destructive" (p. 5).[28] Pediatric occupational therapists should use words that reflect positive attitudes toward children with disabilities. Unfortunately, some therapy reports include jargon or technical terms that may not convey the intended message and often confuse or alienate parents. Therapists should use "person first" language in their documentation (e.g., a child with cerebral palsy; not a cerebral-palsied child).

Case Study 7-3 provides a written example of how the therapist documents Kobe's evaluation findings and recommendations. An important point is that the therapist words the report so that the information is helpful to Kobe's parents and teacher. The format and terminology of the evaluation report are consistent with the OTPF.[1]

In summary, to ensure the evaluation process provides a family-centered, occupation-based approach using valid and reliable measures, occupational therapists should ask the following questions:

1. Are the caregiver's concerns about the child addressed?
2. Does the evaluation measure the child's engagement in occupations and activities and identify the factors that support and hinder the child's participation?
3. Are multiple methods of evaluation used, including interviews, direct observations of the child in the natural environment, and standardized tools?
4. Is the child's cultural background considered in selecting evaluation methods and measures and in developing recommendations for intervention?
5. Are administration procedures correctly applied in using standardized tests?
6. Are the child's strengths and interests documented?
7. Does the evaluation report contribute meaningful, user-friendly information about the child's functional skills?

This section described the evaluation process, including important sequential steps for conducting accurate, thorough evaluations of children and documenting the evaluation findings to parents and other professionals working with the child.

EVALUATION METHODS

Several evaluation methods are available to occupational therapists. The challenge for therapists is to determine which evaluation methods to select for a particular child or group of children. This section describes the primary evaluation methods commonly used in pediatric occupational therapy practice and discusses the major factors that therapists consider when selecting a particular method.

The starting point in the selection process is to identify clearly the purpose of the evaluation and to match appropriate evaluation methods with the identified purpose. For example, if the only purpose of the evaluation is to determine a child's eligibility for special education services in a public school setting, the primary evaluation method is a norm-referenced, standardized test. If the primary purpose of the evaluation is to gain information useful for planning an intervention program for the child, the evaluation measures include skilled observations of the child's functional performance and interviews with the child's caregivers. Often the initial evaluation of a child serves more than one purpose; therefore, therapists frequently use multiple measures and methods when conducting child evaluations.

Standardized Assessments

Norm-referenced measures are tests based on norms of a sample that represent the population to be tested. The child's score on a norm-referenced test is compared with the scores of the normative sample. To evaluate the usefulness of a norm-referenced measure, the pediatric occupational therapist reads the test manual carefully to learn about the characteristics of the normative sample, how the norms were derived, and how to interpret accurately an individual child's scores.

Criterion-referenced measures are standardized tests that consist of a series of skills on functional or developmental tasks, usually grouped by age level or performance area. These tests compare the child's performance on each test item with a criterion that must be met if the child is to receive credit for that item. The items on a criterion-referenced test are selected because of their importance to the child's function on everyday tasks. Therefore, the items often become intervention targets when the child exhibits difficulty in successfully completing them.

Some examples of criterion-referenced measures used by occupational therapists are the Hawaii Early Learning Profile Checklist,[25] the revised Erhardt Developmental Prehension Assessment,[20] the Assessment and Programming System for Infants and Young Children (2nd ed.),[8] and the Evaluation of Children's Handwriting (ETCH) (Figure 7-11).[4] Information

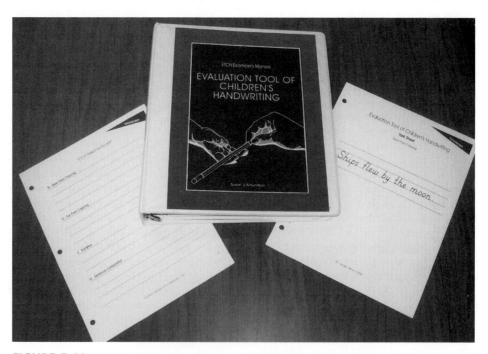

FIGURE 7-11   Materials for the evaluation of children's handwriting.

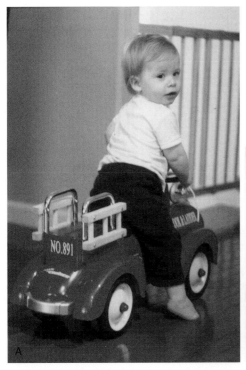
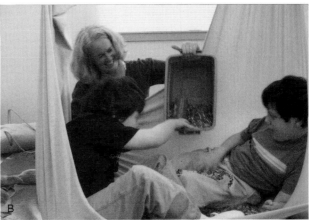

FIGURE 7-12 *A,* Observation of child in his natural environment. *B,* Observation of peer interaction during play.

gained from criterion-referenced tests is particularly helpful for evaluation of the child's functional skills and for planning appropriate intervention activities to enhance those skills (see Appendix 7-A).

Ecologic Assessments

Neisworth and Bagnato defined ecologic assessments as "the examination and recording of the physical, social, and psychological features of a child's developmental context."[48] Consistent with the transactional approach,[52] ecologic assessments are also concerned with the interaction between the child and his or her physical and social environments (Figure 7-12).

Occupational therapists are particularly interested in ecologic measures because these tools are a primary mechanism for obtaining data relevant to the child's performance context. An ecologic assessment of a child uses techniques that consider the cultural influences, socioeconomic status, and value system of the family. These assessments also consider the physical demands and social expectations of the child's environment. Some of these methods include naturalistic observations, interviews, and rating scales. Ecologic measures that are often administered by occupational therapists include the Knox Preschool Play Scale,[36] the revised HOME Inventory,[13] and the TPBA[40] The SFA is another example of an ecologic assessment.[16] The Sensory Processing Measure provides a comprehensive measure of children's sensory functioning in the context of their occupational performance and roles in the home, school, and community.[46,50]

Skilled Observation

An essential skill of the pediatric occupational therapist is the ability to observe keenly and to record accurately children's behavior in an objective manner. Although formal,

standardized assessments are highly valued in pediatric practice, skilled observation of a child performing a functional task offers different but equally important information about the child's performance (Figure 7-13).

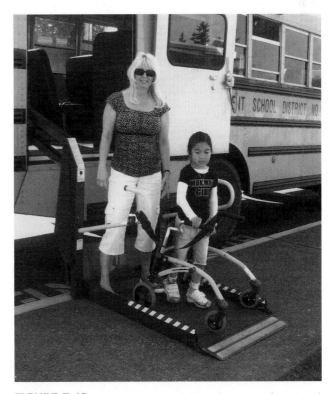

FIGURE 7-13 Observation of child performing a functional task at school.

Dunn proposed that skilled observation is one of the essential tools available to occupational therapists.[18] Dunn described the following key competencies required to conduct skilled observations: (1) do not interfere with the natural course of events, (2) pay attention to the physical and social features of the environment that support or limit a child's performance, and (3) record the child's behavior in observable and neutral terms. When skilled observations are used in the evaluation process, therapists must select a systematic, objective recording procedure so that data collected are accurate and reliable. Clark and Miller proposed a problem-solving approach to functional assessments and data-based decision making for occupational therapists working with children in school settings.[14] Based on direct observations of the child's performance at school, the occupational therapist and other team members define the outcome behaviors and design a useful data collection system to monitor the child's progress.

A word of caution is due, however, about the use of skilled observations of the child in his or her natural environments. If the examiner is not experienced in observing children, he or she may not recognize key behaviors or patterns of behavior in the child and the meaning of those behaviors within the demands of the task and the environment. Therapists entering the field of pediatric occupational therapy should seek out master clinicians and mentors who are willing to help new therapists hone their observation skills.

Interviews

Another primary method used in pediatric occupational therapy evaluation is the interview with the child, the child's parent, the teacher, and other adults working with the child.

Interviews used in conjunction with other evaluation methods provide a more comprehensive view of the child. An important outcome of the interview is an accurate, meaningful exchange of information between the professional and the client (e.g., parent, older child, or adolescent). When done well, interviews can provide an opportunity for building rapport between the therapist and the client. They provide a unique opportunity for parents, children, and adolescents to identify and discuss issues that are important to them. Interviews, therefore, are particularly useful when the therapist is interested in individuals' perceptions of their own abilities, the influence of specific events on them, and their priorities for intervention. When interviews are conducted in a flexible, sensitive manner, therapists and clients are able to explore areas of concern as they arise.

The Canadian Occupational Performance Measure (COPM) is a well-researched tool that uses a structured interview format to obtain information on the client's performance and satisfaction in the areas of self-care, leisure, and productivity.[39] This tool was designed to help occupational therapists identify the targets for intervention based on the individual's most important concerns. The COPM manual discusses some cautions and considerations when interviewing children. The authors suggest "that even as young as 5 or 6 years, children can tell us what they are having trouble with and what they are willing to work on" (p. 39).[39] When the child is very young or not capable of expressing his or her thoughts, parents are interviewed to gain their perspectives and concerns related to raising their child.

BOX 7-4 Basic Strategies for Interviewing Parents, Older Children, and Adolescents

1. Begin the session by clarifying the purpose of the interview with the individual in terms that are meaningful to him or her.
2. Be sensitive to the individual's physical and emotional needs throughout the interview.
3. Promote interaction by asking open-ended questions and guide the individual to where he or she may sit to participate fully in the conversation.
4. Through careful questioning, attempt to understand the individual regarding his or her values and cultural beliefs.
5. Carefully plan when to take notes, preferably after the interview or when the individual is involved in another task (e.g., parent tending to the child's needs).
6. Remain positive in your approach and realistic in the information you provide the individual.
7. Be flexible throughout the interview, responding sensitively to the individual's questions and need for information. If you cannot answer a question, let him or her know and develop a plan to find the needed information.
8. Use effective verbal and nonverbal communication skills. Often, nonverbal communication can override verbal information.
9. Avoid the use of therapy and medical jargon. If technical terms are used, be sure they are explained adequately.

Interviews may include closed- or open-ended questions or a combination of these. Specific questions, which are often closed-ended, allow the therapist to gather a predetermined set of information from the individual in a relatively short time. Unstructured interviews using open-ended questions allow the child or parent to take the lead and set the priorities in the discussion. Open-ended questions invite the individual to elaborate on a topic and provide critical information (Box 7-4). An important decision the therapist makes when conducting interviews with parents is whether the interview is done in the presence of the child. Most parents are uncomfortable describing their child's deficits in front of the child, particularly if the child is older than 3 years of age and possibly aware of his or her difficulties. Therapists and parents should carefully plan when, how, and where to conduct the interview(s).

In summary, a skilled therapist interviews children (older than 5 or 6 years) and caregivers by carefully selecting questions and sensitively listening to the responses. Interviews offer a unique opportunity for an exchange of information between the child or adolescent, the parents or teacher, and the therapist. During the interview, the therapist should reciprocate by providing accurate, relevant information about the functional abilities of the child or adolescent, the intervention services, and community resources.

Inventories and Scales

A variety of inventories and scales are used to gather data on a child's development, on caregiver–child interactions, or on the child's environments.

The Pediatric Evaluation of Disability Inventory (PEDI) is an evaluation of functional capabilities and performance in children 6 months to 7.5 years of age.[26] The PEDI is judgment-based inventory completed by the parent and professionals who are familiar with the child. It measures both capability and performance of the child during functional activities (e.g., self-care, mobility, and social function). The inventory consists of 197 functional skills items; the child is scored either 1 (has capability) or 0 (has not yet demonstrated capability, unable) on each item. Twenty additional items rate the amount of caregiver assistance required to complete key functional tasks. The PEDI was designed for use with young children who have a variety of disabling conditions, particularly physical disabilities. The authors completed a series of reliability and validity studies and developed criterion scores using Rasch analysis techniques. As a result, the PEDI stands as a well-developed instrument for evaluating the functional performance and capabilities of children.

A rating scale may rate the quality, degree, or frequency of a behavior. (For example, the Caregiver/Parent–Child Interaction Feeding and Teaching Scales are designed to assess parent–child interactions in the context of feeding and teaching events).[54] Figure 7-14 shows the type of data obtained using the feeding scale's rating system.

A parent, teacher, or other caregiver can complete some inventories and rating scales. For example, the Ages & Stages Questionnaires rely exclusively on parent report.[9] On this scale, the items are clearly described, and many are illustrated so that parents can record specific behaviors of their children. After each item, parents check the appropriate box—"yes," "sometimes," or "not yet." The Sensory Profile[17] and the Infant/Toddler Sensory Profile[19] are caregiver questionnaires that may be completed through a parent interview.

Arena Assessments

In many settings serving children with disabilities, a team of professionals evaluates the child. The form and scope of team evaluations vary widely, depending on the philosophy of the intervention program and the expertise of the professionals. For example, in some settings, each professional provides an individual evaluation of the child, then the team members meet to discuss their evaluation findings and recommendations. Sometimes little or no communication occurs among team members before or during the evaluation. In contrast, a team in another setting may use the transdisciplinary approach, in which one primary team member conducts the evaluation while other key team members contribute their expertise to the evaluation process through consultation.

The arena assessment uses a transdisciplinary approach that allows the child and primary caregiver to interact with one professional throughout the evaluation session while other professionals observe and, on occasion, directly test the child or interview the caregiver. An example of an arena assessment is the TPBA.[40] This assessment places major emphasis on a team approach to the evaluation of young children. The purpose of the TPBA is to obtain developmental information on the child using multidimensional, functional observations of the child during a play session. Parents and professionals together plan, observe, and analyze the child's play session.

Arena assessment of feeding difficulties in children is an effective way to gather relevant information without over-testing the child or requiring the caregiver to participate in repeated interviews with different professionals. For example, an arena feeding assessment for a child with cerebral palsy and failure to thrive may include an occupational therapist, a nurse, a psychologist, and a nutritionist. One professional is

IV. COGNITIVE GROWTH FOSTERING	YES	NO
42. Caregiver provides child with objects, finger foods, toys, and/or utensils.		
43. Caregiver encourages and/or allows the child to explore the breast, bottle, food, cup, bowl, or the caregiver during feeding.		
44. Caregiver talks to the child using two words at least three times during the feeding.		
45. Caregiver verbally describes food or feeding situation to child during feeding.		
46. Caregiver talks to child about things other than food, eating, or things related to feeding.		
47. Caregiver uses statements that describe, ask questions, or explain consequences of behavior, more than commands, in talking to child.		
48. Caregiver verbally responds to child's sound within 5 seconds after child has vocalized.		
49. Caregiver verbally responds to child's movement within 5 seconds of child's movement of arms, legs, hands, head, trunk.		
50. Caregiver avoids using baby talk.		

FIGURE 7-14 Examples of items from the Caregiver/Parent–Child Interaction Feeding Scale.

designated the lead evaluator, depending on the primary referral concern. The occupational therapist may take the lead if the child has oral-motor deficits, such as chewing or swallowing difficulties, postural difficulties that create the need for external support of posture at mealtime, or fine motor difficulties that limit self-feeding skills. The nurse or the psychologist may take the lead in the evaluation process if the child exhibits behavioral difficulties, if the parent's caregiving skills appear limited, or if parent–child interactions are at risk. The nutritionist may take the lead if the child's diet needs careful analysis and if the family would benefit from specific information on types and amounts of food the child should eat. The benefit of an arena feeding assessment is that the child and the caregiver are subjected to the mealtime evaluation only once, rather than several times. The arena assessment provides an opportunity for collaboration among parents and professionals to observe, discuss, and solve problems in critical areas together.

SUMMARY

Accurate, reliable evaluation of a child is one of the most challenging and rewarding services an occupational therapist offers. This chapter described the purposes, processes, and methods of evaluation in pediatric occupational therapy. Having an awareness of the many purposes of evaluation and the ability to match carefully appropriate methods and measures with those purposes are critical skills of the pediatric occupational therapist. Careful observation of the details of a child's performance on tasks and recognition of the importance of the context in which the child performs those tasks are also essential to skillful evaluation. Equally important in the evaluation process is the therapist's collaborative skills when working with the child's caregiver and other team members to gain an in-depth understanding of the child and his or her environments. A comprehensive view of the child's participation in settings and activities important to the child and family leads to the development of relevant, appropriate occupational therapy interventions.

REFERENCES

1. American Occupational Therapy Association (AOTA). (2008). Occupational therapy practice framework: Domain and process. *American Journal of Occupational Therapy, 62(6)*, 625–683.
2. American Occupational Therapy Association (AOTA). (2005). Standards of practice for occupational therapy. *American Journal of Occupational Therapy, 59*, 663–665.
3. American Occupational Therapy Association (AOTA). (2008). *Guidelines for documentation of occupational therapy. American Journal of Occupational Therapy, 62(6)*, 684–690.
4. Amundson, S. (1995). Evaluation of children's handwriting. In A. K. Homer (Ed.), OT kids. http://psychtest.com/
5. Ayres, A. J. (1989). *Sensory Integration and Praxis Tests*. Los Angeles: Western Psychological Services.
6. Basu, S., Kafkes, A., Geist, R., & Kielhofner, G. (2002). *The Pediatric Volitional Questionnaire (PVQ) (2.0)*. Chicago: Model of Human Occupation Clearinghouse, Department of Occupational Therapy, College of Applied Health Sciences, University of Illinois.
7. Bayley, N. (2005). *Bayley Scales of Infant and Toddler Development* (3rd ed.). San Antonio, TX: The Psychological Corporation.
8. Bricker, D. (Ed.). (2002). *Assessment, evaluation, and programming system* (2nd ed.). Baltimore: Brookes.
9. Bricker, D., & Squires, J. (1999). *Ages & stages questionnaires: A parent-completed, child-monitoring system* (2nd ed.). Baltimore: Brookes.
10. Bronfenbrenner, U. (1977). Toward an experimental ecology of human development. *American Psychologist, 32*, 513–531.
11. Bruininks, R., & Bruininks, B. (2005). *Bruininks-Oseretsky Test of Motor Proficiency (BOT-2)*. Circle Pines, MN: American Guidance Service.
12. Bundy, A. (1991). Writing functional goals for evaluation. In C. B. Royeen (Ed.), *AOTA self-study series: School-based practice for related services* (pp. 7–30). Bethesda, MD: American Occupational Therapy Association.
13. Caldwell, B. M., & Bradley, R. H. (1984). *Home observation for measurement of the environment* (rev. ed.). Little Rock, AR: University of Arkansas.
14. Clark, G. F., & Miller, L. E. (1996). Providing effective occupational therapy services: Data-based decision making in school-based practice. *American Journal of Occupational Therapy, 50(9)*, 701–708.
15. Coster, W. (1998). Occupational-centered assessment of children. *American Journal of Occupational Therapy, 52(5)*, 337–344.
16. Coster, W., Deeney, T., Haltiwanger, J., & Haley, S. (1998). *School Function Assessment*. San Antonio: Psychological Corporation.
17. Dunn, W. (1999). *Sensory Profile: User's manual*. San Antonio, TX: Psychological Corporation.
18. Dunn, W. (Ed.). (2000). *Best practice occupational therapy in community service with children and families*. Thorofare, NJ: Slack.
19. Dunn, W. (2002). *Infant/Toddler Sensory Profile: User's manual*. San Antonio, TX: Psychological Corporation.
20. Erhardt, R. P. (1994). *Erhardt Developmental Prehension Assessment* (revised). Maplewood, MN: Erhardt Developmental Publications.
21. Farran, D. C. (2000). Another decade of intervention for children who are low income or disabled: What do we know now? In J. P. Shonkoff & S. J. Meisels (Eds.), *Handbook of early childhood intervention* (2nd ed., pp. 510–548). Cambridge, UK: Cambridge University Press.
22. Fisher, A. G., Bryze, K., Hume, V., & Griswold, L. A. (2005). *School AMPS: School version of the assessment of motor and process skills* (2nd ed.). Fort Collins, CO: Three Star Press.
23. Folio, M. R., & Fewell, R. R. (2000). *Peabody Developmental Motor Scales* (2nd ed.). Austin, TX: Pro-Ed.
24. Frankenburg, W., & Dodds, J. (1992). *Denver Developmental Screening Test-II*. Denver: Denver Developmental Materials.
25. Furuno, S., O'Reilly, K., Hosaka, C. M., Zeisloft, B., & Allman, T. (2004). *The Hawaii Early Learning Profile*. Palo Alto, CA: VORT.
26. Haley, S. M., Coster, W. J., Ludlow, L. H., Haltiwanger, M. A., & Andrellos, P. J. (1992). *Pediatric Evaluation of Disability Inventory*. San Antonio, TX: Psychological Corporation.
27. Hamilton, B. B., & Granger, C. U. (1991). *Functional Independence Measure for Children (WeeFIM)*. Buffalo, NY: Research Foundation of the State University of New York.
28. Hanft, B. (1989). How words create images. In B. Hanft (Ed.), *Family-centered care: An early intervention resource manual* (Unit 2, pp. 77–78). Bethesda, MD: American Occupational Therapy Association.
29. Hanft, B. (1994). The good parent: A label by any other name would not smell as sweet. *AOTA's Developmental Disabilities Special Interest Section Newsletter, 17(2)*, 5.
30. Individuals with Disabilities Education Act of 1997. (1997). (Public Law 105-17) 20 USC 1400 et seq.
31. Individuals with Disabilities Education Improvement Act of 2004. (2004). (Public Law 108-446). 20 USC 1400 et seq.

32. Johnson-Martin, N. M., Jens, K. G., Attermeier, S. M., & Hacker, B. J. (2004). *The Carolina Curriculum for Infants and Toddlers with Special Needs* (2nd ed.). Baltimore: Brookes.

33. Keller, J., Kafkas, A., Basu, S., Federico, J., & Kielhofner, G. (2005). *Child Occupational Self-Assessment (COSA), Version 2.1.* Chicago: Model of Human Occupation Clearinghouse, Department of Occupational Therapy, College of Applied Health Sciences, University of Illinois.

34. King, G., Law, M., King, S. Hurley, P., Rosenbaum, P., Hanna, S., et al (2005). *Children's Assessment of Participation and Enjoyment (CAPE) and Preferences for Activities of Children (PAC).* San Antonio, TX: Harcourt Assessment.

35. King, G. A., McDougall, J., Palisano, R. J., Gritzan, J., & Tucker, M. (1999). Goal attainment scaling: Its use in evaluating pediatric therapy programs. *Physical and Occupational Therapy in Pediatrics, 19*(2), 31–52.

36. Knox, S. (2008). Development and current use of the Knox Preschool Play Scale. In L. D. Parham & L. S. Fazio (Eds.). *Play in occupational therapy for children* (pp. 55–70). St. Louis: Mosby.

37. Kramer, P., & Hinojosa, J. (1998). Theoretical basis of evaluation. In J. Hinojosa & P. Kramer (Eds.), *Occupational therapy evaluation: Obtaining and interpreting data* (pp. 17–28). Bethesda, MD: American Occupational Therapy Association, Inc.

38. Law, M. C. (1999). *All about outcomes: An educational program to help you understand, evaluate, and choose pediatric outcome measures* (CD-ROM). Thorofare, NJ: Slack.

39. Law, M. C., Baptiste, S., McColl, M., Carswell, A., Polatajko, H., & Pollock, N. (2005). *Canadian Occupational Performance Measure* (4th ed.). Ottawa, ON: Canadian Association of Occupational Therapy Publications.

40. Linder, T. W. (2008). *Transdisciplinary play-based assessment: a functional approach to working with young children.* Baltimore: Brookes.

41. Mailloux, A., May-Benson, T. A., Summers, C. A., Miller, L. J., Brett-Green, B., Burke, J. P., et al. (2007). Goal attainment scaling as a measure of meaningful outcomes for children with sensory integration disorder. *American Journal of Occupational Therapy, 61*(2), 254–259.

42. McClain, L. H. (1991). Documentation. In W. Dunn (Ed.), *Pediatric occupational therapy: Facilitating effective service provision* (pp. 213–244). Thorofare, NJ: Slack.

43. Miller, L. J. (1993). *First STEp Screening Tool.* San Antonio, TX: Psychological Corporation.

44. Miller, L. J. (2003). *Primer PASO Screening Tool.* San Antonio, TX: Psychological Corporation.

45. Miller, L. J. (2006). *Miller Function & Participation Scales.* San Antonio, TX: Psychological Corporation.

46. Miller-Kuhaneck, H., Henry, D. A., & Glennon, T. J. (2007). *Sensory Processing Measure (Main Classroom and School Environments Forms).* Los Angeles: Western Psychological Services.

47. Mitchell, T., & Cusik, A. (1998). Evaluation of a client-centred paediatric rehabilitation programme using goal attainment scaling. *Australian Journal of Occupational Therapy, 45*(1), 7–17.

48. Neisworth, J. T., & Bagnato, S. J. (1988). Assessment in early childhood special education: A typology of dependent measures. In S. L. Odom & M. B. Karnes (Eds.), *Early intervention for infants and children with handicaps: An empirical base* (pp. 23–49). Baltimore: Brookes.

49. Notari, A., & Bricker, D. (1990). The utility of a curriculum-based assessment instrument in the development of individualized education plans for infants and young children. *Journal of Early Intervention, 14*, 117–132.

50. Parham, D., & Ecker, C. (2007). *Sensory processing measure (Home Form).* Los Angeles: Western Psychological Services.

51. Russell, D. J., Rosenbaum, P. L., Avery, L. & Lane, M. (2002). *Gross motor function measure. User's manual.* Malden, MA: Blackwell Publishing.

52. Sameroff, A. J., & Fiese, B. H. (2000). Transactional regulation: The developmental ecology of early intervention. In J. P. Shonkoff & S. J. Meisels (Eds.), *Handbook of early childhood intervention* (2nd ed., pp. 135–159). Cambridge, UK: Cambridge University Press.

53. Skard, G., & Bundy, A. (2008). Test of playfulness. In L. D. Parham & L. S. Fazio (Eds.), *Play in occupational therapy for children* (2nd ed., pp. 71–94). St. Louis: Mosby.

54. Sumner, G., & Spietz, A. (1994). *NCAST caregiver/parent-child interaction scales.* Seattle: NCAST Publications, University of Washington, School of Nursing.

55. Washington [State] Administrative Code. (1998). *Rules for the provision of special education: Eligibility criteria for students with disabilities (WAC 392–172–114).* Olympia, WA: Office of Superintendent of Public Instruction.

56. World Health Organization. (2001). *ICF: International classification of functioning, disability and health.* Geneva: WHO.

57. Young, A., & Chesson, R. (1997). Goal attainment scaling as a method of measuring clinical outcomes for children with learning disabilities. *British Journal of Occupational Therapy, 60*(3), 111–114.

58. Young, N. L. (1997). *Activities Scale for Kids.* Toronto, ON: Pediatric Outcomes Research Team, Hospital for Sick Children.

Common Measures Used in Pediatric Occupational Therapy

The following list represents a selection of measures used in occupational therapy. Occupational therapists working with infants, children, and adolescents should stay current with the research literature on pediatric measures and should carefully evaluate the reliability and validity of new instruments as they become available to practitioners.

Adolescent/Adult Sensory Profile

Brown, C., & Dunn, W. (2002)

This self-questionnaire, for individuals 11 years of age or older, measures possible contributions of sensory processing to the person's daily performance patterns. The classification system is based on normative information. (www.sensoryprofile.com)

Ages & Stages Questionnaires

Bricker, D., & Squires, J. (2009)

These parent questionnaires are designed to screen children from birth to 5 years of age in communication, gross motor, fine motor, problem-solving, and personal–social development. (www.brookespublishing.com/store/books/bricker-asq/index.htm)

Alberta Infant Motor Scale (AIMS)

Piper, M. C., & Darrah, J. (1994)

A norm-referenced measure designed to identify and monitor infants with gross motor delays from birth to 18 months of age.

Bayley Scales of Infant and Toddler Development (3rd Edition)

Bayley, N. (2005)

A norm-referenced assessment tool that measures the cognitive, language, motor, social–emotional, and adaptive behavior in infants and toddlers from 1 to 42 months of age. A screening test, caregiver report, and growth scores/charts are also available. (www.psychcorp.com)

Bayley Scales of Infant and Toddler Development—Third Edition Motor Scale

Bayley, N. (2005)

A norm-referenced measure used to identify young children with developmental delay of motor function and assist the practitioner in intervention planning. Includes growth charts for plotting motor growth over time. (www.psychcorp.com)

Beery-Buktenica Developmental Test of Visual–Motor Integration, 5th Edition (BEERY VMI)

Beery, K. E., Buktenica, N. A., & Beery, N. A. (2006)

This standardized tool is used to screen for visual–motor integration deficits. The short format is used with children ages 2 to 8 years. The full format is used with individuals up to 100 years old. Supplemental visual perception and motor coordination tests can be used if further testing is indicated. These supplemental tests help compare an individual's test results with relatively pure visual and motor performances. (www.pearsonassessments.com/tests/vmi.htm)

Bruininks-Oseretsky Test of Motor Proficiency (BOT-2)

Bruininks, R. & Bruininks, B. (2005)

A norm-referenced assessment of the motor proficiency of children 4 to 21 years of age, ranging from those who are typically developing to those with moderate motor-skill deficits. A short form is available for brief screening. (www.agsnet.com)

Canadian Occupational Performance Measure (4th edition)

Law, M., Baptiste, S., McColl, M., Carswell, A., Polatajko, H., & Pollock, N. (2005)

This interview tool helps identify the family's priorities for their child with special needs and assists in developing therapy goals with the child's primary caregivers. Distributed by the Canadian Association of Occupational Therapy. (www.caot.ca)

Child Occupational Self-Assessment (COSA)

Keller, J., Kafkas, A., Basu, S., Federico, J., & Kielhofner, G. (2005)

A self-report that asks children to rate their performance competency and the importance of that activity.

Available through the Model of Human Occupational Clearinghouse. (www.moho.uic.edu)

Childhood Autism Rating Scale (CARS)

Schopler, E., Reichler, R. J., & Renner, B. R. (2002)

The CARS is an observational tool designed to identify children older than 2 years of age who have mild, moderate, or severe autism and to distinguish those children from children with developmental delay without autism. (www.wpspublish.com)

Children's Assessment of Participation and Enjoyment (CAPE)

King, G., Law, M., King, S., Hurley, P., Rosenbaum, P., Hanna, S., Kertoy, M., & Young, N. (2004)

The CAPE is designed to explore an individual's day-to-day participation to plan intervention or measure outcomes. The CAPE may be used independently or with the Preferences for Activities for Children (PAC). (www.psychcorp.com)

Denver Developmental Screening Test (Revised) (Denver-II)

Frankenburg, W. K., Dodds, J., & Archer, P. et al. (1996)

The Denver-II is a standardized screening tool for children from birth to 6 years of age who are at risk for developmental problems in the areas of personal-social, fine motor adaptive, language, and gross motor skills. (www.denverii.com)

Developmental Test of Visual Perception (Second Edition) (DTVP-2)

Hammill, D. D., Pearson, N. A., & Voress, J. K. (1993)

A norm-referenced tool that measures the visual perception and visual-motor integration skills in children 4 to 10 years of age. (www.proedinc.com/store)

Developmental Test of Visual Perception—Adolescent and Adult

Reynolds, C. R., Pearson, N. A., & Voress, J. K. (2002)

A battery of six subtests that measures different but interrelated visual-perceptual and visual-motor abilities in individuals 11 to 75 years of age. (www.proedinc.com/store)

Early Coping Inventory

Zeitlin, S., Williamson, G. G., & Szczepanski, M. (1988)

This observation instrument is used to assess coping-related behavior, including sensorimotor organization, reactive behaviors, and self-initiated behaviors, in children functioning at the 4-month to 36-month developmental level. (www.ststesting.com/early.html#EAR)

Evaluation Tool of Children's Handwriting (ETCH)

Amundson, S. J. (1995)

A criterion-referenced tool designed to evaluate the manuscript and cursive handwriting skills of children in grades 1 through 6. (www.theraproducts.com/index)

FirstSTEP: Screening Test for Evaluating Preschoolers

Miller, L. J. (1993)

This standardized screening tool is used to identify children 2 years 9 months to 6 years 2 months of age who need in-depth diagnostic testing in the areas of cognition, communication, and motor development. (http://marketplace.psychcorp.com)

Functional Independence Measure for Children (WeeFIM)

Hamilton, B. B., & Granger, C. U. (1991)

This measure assesses the functional outcomes in children and adolescents with acquired or congenital disabilities. The WeeFIM was designed to document the need for assistance and the severity of disability in children functioning within the developmental level of 6 months to 7 years in the areas of self-care, mobility, and cognition. (www.udsmr.org/wee_index.php)

Gross Motor Function Measure (Revised) (GMFM)

Russell, D., Rosenbaum, P., Avery, L. & Lane, M. (2002)

A clinical measure designed to evaluate change in gross motor function in children with cerebral palsy. The GMFM is appropriate for use in children whose motor skills are at or below those of a 5-year-old child without any motor disability. (www.fhs.mcmaster.ca/canchild)

Hawaii Early Learning Profile (HELP)

Furuno, S., O'Reilly, K. A., Hosaka, C. M., Zeisloft, B., & Allman, T. A. (2004)

A curriculum-based assessment of children from birth to 6 years of age and their families. The HELP is a family-centered, interdisciplinary approach to identify developmental needs, determine intervention goals, and track children's progress. (www.vort.com)

Home Observation for Measurement of the Environment (HOME)

Caldwell, B., & Bradley, R. H. (1984)

The initial version of this inventory, the Infant/Toddler HOME, was designed to measure the quality and quantity of stimulation and support available to a child from birth to 3 years of age in his or her home environment. More recent versions include the Early Childhood HOME (ages 3 to 6 years), the Middle Childhood HOME (ages 6 to 10 years), and the Early Adolescent HOME (ages 10 to 15 years). (http://.ualr.edu/case/)

Infant/Toddler Sensory Profile

Dunn, W. (2002)

This standardized, norm-referenced tool is a judgment-based caregiver questionnaire designed to describe behavioral responses to various everyday sensory experiences in children from birth to 3 years of age. (www.sensoryprofile.com)

Knox Preschool Play Scale (Revised)

Knox, S. (2008)

This scale is a naturalistic observation tool used to assess play behaviors in children from birth to 6 years of age. The four parameters measured include space management, material management, pretense-symbolic, and participation. Available in Parham & Fazio (2008), *Play in occupational therapy for children*. (2nd ed.) St. Louis: Mosby.

Miller Function & Participation Scales

Miller, L. J. (2006)

This norm-referenced measure assesses a child's performance in functional tasks needed to successfully participate in classroom and school activities with an emphasis on motor skill performance. Uses the ICF as a framework and addresses participation, activity, and body function. Video clips on writing and cutting exercises are available on the publisher's website. (http://harcourtassessment.com)

Motor-Free Visual Perception Test (MVPT-3)

Colarusso, R. R., & Hammill, D. D. (2002)

The MVPT-3 is a norm-referenced test used for individuals 4 to 70 years of age to assess visual-perceptual abilities that do not require motor involvement to make a response. (www.academictherapy.com)

NCAST Caregiver/Parent–Child Interaction Scales

Sumner, G., & Spietz, A. (1994)

These scales measure caregiver–child interactions during a feeding situation (with infants from birth to 12 months) and a teaching situation (with children from birth to 3 years). (www.ncast.org/)

Occupational Therapy Psychosocial Assessment of Learning (OT PAL)

Townsend, S. C., Carey, P. D., Hollins, N. L., Helfrich, C., Blondis, M., Hoffman, A., Collins, L., Knudson, J., & Blackwell, A. (2001)

The OT PAL measures psychosocial factors that influence a child's learning. The tool uses observation and interview to assess volition, habituation, and environmental fit within the classroom in children ages 6 to 12 years.

Peabody Developmental Motor Scales (2nd edition) (PDMS-2)

Folio, M. R., & Fewell, R. R. (2000)

The PDMS-2 is a norm-referenced and criterion-referenced measure of gross and fine motor skills used for children from birth through 5 years of age. (www.proedinc.com)

Pediatric Evaluation of Disability Inventory (PEDI)

Haley S. M., Coster W. J., Ludlow, L. H., Haltiwanger, J. T., & Andrellos, P. J. (1992)

The PEDI is a standardized, criterion-referenced assessment of key functional capabilities and performance by observing self-care, mobility, and social function in children from birth to 7 years of age. Standard and scaled performance scores are calculated. (http://harcourtassessment.com)

Pediatric Volitional Questionnaire (PVQ) (2.1)

Basu, S., Kaflas, A., Schatz, R., Kiraly, A., & Kielfhofner, G. (2008)

This observational assessment is designed to evaluate a young child's volition, including motivation, values, and interests, and the impact of environment. For children ages 2 to 7 years.

Available through the Model of Human Occupational Clearinghouse. (http://www.moho.uic.edu)

Preferences for Activities of Children (PAC)

King, G., Law, M., King, S., Hurley, P., Rosenbaum, P., Hanna, S., Kertoy, M., & Young, N. (2004)

The PAC is used to assess an individual's preference for activities. The PAC may be used independently or together with the CAPE. (http://harcourtassessment.com)

Quality of Upper Extremity Skills Test (QUEST)

DeMatteo, C., Law, M., Russell, D., Pollock, N., Rosenbaum, P., & Walter, S. (1992)

This outcome measure was designed to evaluate movement patterns and hand function in children with cerebral palsy from 8 months to 8 years of age. The four domains measured are dissociated movements, grasp patterns, protective extension reactions, and weight-bearing ability. (http://www.canchild.ca/)

School Function Assessment (SFA)

Coster, W., Deeney, T., Haltiwanger, J., & Haley, S. (1998)

The SFA is a judgment-based questionnaire designed to measure a student's performance of functional tasks that support his or her participation in the academic and social aspects of an elementary school program (grades K-6). Three scales evaluate the student's level of participation, the type and amount of task supports needed, and his or her activity performance on specific school tasks. The SFA was designed to facilitate collaborative program planning for students with a variety of disabling conditions. (http://harcourtassessment.com)

School Assessment of Motor and Process Skills (School AMPS)

Fisher, A. G., Bryze, K., Hume, V., & Griswold, L. A. (2005)

The School AMPS is a standardized, criterion-referenced assessment for students 3 to 12 years. This naturalistic observation tool is used to measure the student's schoolwork task performance in his or her classroom setting during the typical school routines. The School AMPS is a sensitive measure that can document change in schoolwork performance and outcomes of intervention. (www.schoolamps.com)

Sensory Integration and Praxis Tests (SIPT)

Ayres, A. J. (1989)

The SIPT is a battery of standardized, norm-referenced tests designed to measure the sensory integration processes that underlie learning and behavior in children 4 to 9 years of age. The 17 tests assess visual perception, somatosensory and vestibular processing, and various types of praxis. Extensive training is required to administer and interpret the SIPT. (www.wpspublish.com)

Sensory Processing Measure (SPM)

Parham, D., & Ecker, C. (Home Form) and Miller-Kuhaneck, H., Henry, D. A., & Glennon, T. J. (School Form) (2007)

The SPM was developed to allow assessment of sensory processing, praxis, and social participation in the home, classroom, and other school environments and to compare an individual child's performance with normative samples of other school-aged children.

Sensory Profile

Dunn, W. (1999)

This caregiver questionnaire was designed to measure the frequency of behaviors related to sensory processing, modulation, and emotional responsivity to sensory input in children 3 to 12 years of age. (www.sensoryprofile.com)

The Short Child Occupational Profile (SCOPE) (2.2)

Bowyer, P., Ross, M., Schwartz, O., Kielhofner, G., & Kramer, J. (2008)

This measure determines how volition, habituation, skills, and the environment facilitate or restrict a child's participation.

Available through the Model of Human Occupational Clearinghouse. (http://www.moho.uic.edu)

Test of Playfulness (ToP)

Bundy, A. (1997); Skard, G., & Bundy, A. (2008)

This naturalistic observational tool measures three elements of playfulness in children of all ages: perception of control, source of motivation, and suspension of reality.

Available in Parham & Fazio (2008) *Play in occupational therapy for children.* (2nd ed.) St. Louis: Mosby.

Test of Environmental Supportiveness (TOES)

Bundy, A. C. (1999)

TOES assesses the extent to which environment supports a child's play. This measure investigates caregiver's actions, rules, and boundaries during the child's play; identifies peer, younger, and older playmates' use of cues and domination of interaction; describes natural and fabricated objects used during play; and

describes the amount and configuration of space, the sensory environment, and the safety and accessibility of space.

Available at Colorado State University, Department of Occupational Therapy, Fort Collins, CO 80523.

Test of Visual-Motor Skills (Revised) (TVMS-R)

Gardner, M. F. (1995)

The TVMS-R measures eye-hand coordination skills needed to copy geometric designs in children 3 to 13 years of age. (www.academictherapy.com)

Test of Visual-Motor Skills—Upper Level (TVMS-UL)

Gardner, M. F. (1992)

The TVMS-UL measures eye-hand skills needed to copy geometric designs in individuals 12 to 40 years of age. (www.academictherapy.com)

Test of Visual–Perceptual Skills (Non-Motor) (TVPS-3)

Martin, N. (2006)

The TVPS-R assesses visual-perceptual skills (e.g., discrimination, memory, spatial relations, form constancy, sequential memory, figure-ground, and closure) in children 4 to 18 years of age. (www.academictherapy.com)

Toddler and Infant Motor Evaluation (TIME)

Miller, L. J., & Roid, G. H. (1994)

This standardized, norm-referenced assessment measures the motor abilities of children ages 4 months to 3.5 years. Test items assess mobility, stability, motor organization, functional performance, and social-emotional abilities. The TIME tool was designed to measure neuromotor changes in children who have atypical development. (http://harcourtassessment.com)

Transdisciplinary Play-Based Assessment (TPBA)

Linder, T. W. (2008)

The TPBA tool is a naturalistic observation tool that uses an arena assessment approach in which early childhood professionals evaluate a child's development in cognitive, social-emotional, communication and language, and sensorimotor domains during play sessions. The TPBA can be used with children from infancy to 6 years of age in home- and center-based environments. (www.pbrookes.com)

8

Use of Standardized Tests in Pediatric Practice

Pamela K. Richardson

Standardized test
Performance-based test
Context-based test
Reliability
Norm-referenced test
Criterion-referenced test
Normative sample

Measures of central tendency
Measures of variability
Standard score
Correlation coefficient
Validity
Ethics in testing

1. List the characteristics of commonly used standardized pediatric tests.
2. Describe the differences between norm- and criterion-referenced tests and give the purpose of each type of test.
3. Describe the differences between performance- and observation-based tests.
4. Explain the descriptive statistics used in standardized pediatric tests.
5. Discuss the types of standard scores used in standardized pediatric tests.
6. Explain the concepts of reliability and validity.
7. Discuss the importance of test validity.
8. Describe the procedures necessary to become a competent user of standardized tests.
9. Understand the ethical considerations involved in the use of standardized tests.
10. Demonstrate knowledge of standardized test applications to information found in a case study.

What are standardized tests, and why are they important to occupational therapists? A test that has been standardized has uniform procedures for administration and scoring.[63] This means that examiners must use the same instructions, materials, and procedures each time they administer the test, and they must score the test using criteria specified in the test manual. A number of standardized tests are in common use. Most schoolchildren have taken standardized achievement tests that assess how well they have learned the required grade-level material. College students are familiar with the Scholastic Aptitude Test (SAT), the results of which can affect decisions on admission at many colleges and universities. Intelligence tests, interest tests, and aptitude tests are other examples of standardized tests frequently used with the general public.

Pediatric occupational therapists use standardized tests to help determine the eligibility of children for therapy services, to monitor their progress in therapy, and to make decisions on the type of intervention that would be most appropriate and effective for them. Standardized tests provide precise measurements of a child's performance in specific areas, and this performance is described as a standard score. The standard score can be used and understood by other occupational therapists and child development professionals familiar with standardized testing procedures.

Using anthropometric measurements and psychophysical testing to measure intelligence, Galton and Cattell developed the initial concept of standardized assessments of human performance late in the 19th century. The first widespread use of human performance testing was initiated in 1904, when the minister of public education in Paris formed a commission to create tests that would help to identify "mentally defective children," with the goal of providing them with an appropriate education. Binet and Simon developed the first intelligence test for this purpose. Terman and Merrill incorporated many of Binet and Simon's ideas into the construction of the Stanford-Binet Intelligence Scale,[60] which remains widely used today.[58] Although intelligence was the first human attribute to be tested in a standardized manner, tests have been developed over the past several decades that assess children's developmental status, cognition, gross and fine motor skills, language and communication skills, school readiness, school achievement, visual-motor skills, visual-perceptual skills, social skills, and other behavioral domains. Although the number and types of tests have changed radically since the time of Simon and Binet, the basic reason for using standardized tests remains the same: to identify children who may need special intervention or programs because their performance in a given area is outside the norm, or average, for their particular age.

The use of standardized tests requires a high level of responsibility on the part of the tester. The occupational therapist who uses a standardized test must be knowledgeable about scoring and interpreting the test, must know for whom the test is and is not appropriate, and must understand how to report and discuss a child's scores on the test. The tester must also be aware of the limitations of standardized tests in providing information about a child's performance deficits. This, in turn, requires a working knowledge of standardized testing concepts and procedures, familiarity with the factors that can affect performance on standardized tests, and awareness of the ethics and responsibilities of testers when using standardized tests.

This chapter introduces pediatric standardized testing used by occupational therapists. The purposes and characteristics of standardized tests are discussed, technical information about standardized tests is presented, practical tips to help the student become a competent user of standardized assessments are given, and ethical considerations are explained. The chapter concludes with a summary of the advantages and disadvantages of standardized tests and a case study that incorporates the concepts presented in the chapter into a "real life" testing scenario. Throughout the chapter, several standardized assessments commonly used by pediatric occupational therapists are highlighted to illustrate the concepts of test administration, scoring, and interpretation.

INFLUENCES ON STANDARDIZED TESTING IN PEDIATRIC OCCUPATIONAL THERAPY

When standardized tests became widely used in pediatric practice in the 1970s and 1980s, the tests available for occupational therapists focused primarily on the developmental domains of gross motor skills, fine motor skills, and visual-motor/visual-perceptual skills. These early tests were developed by educators and psychologists. The first pediatric standardized test developed by an occupational therapist was the Southern California Sensory Integration Tests (SCSIT), published by A. Jean Ayres in 1972.[3] The SCSIT assessed sensory integration and praxis, domains that were of specific interest to occupational therapists, and was instrumental in defining the measurement standards in these areas.

In the ensuing years, the number of standardized tests created by and for pediatric occupational therapists has increased dramatically, and the number of behavioral and performance domains assessed has expanded. This evolution in standardized testing in occupational therapy has been influenced by developments both inside and outside the profession. Some key developments are briefly summarized next:

- Individuals with Disabilities Education Act (IDEA) Part B defined the role of occupational therapy as a related service in school-based settings for children age 3 to 21 years. In this setting, standardized tests provide information that is used to determine children's eligibility for services, measure progress, and develop individualized education programs (IEPs).
- IDEA Part C created federal support for family-centered services for children age 0 to 3 and their families. Occupational therapy is a supportive service that participates in multidisciplinary evaluations to determine eligibility for services, assessment of family needs, resources, and priorities to support development of an individualized family service plan (IFSP), and periodic review of progress. Standardized tests of children's developmental status, caregiver–child interactions, and the home environment are an important part of this process.

- The development of occupational therapy frameworks that consider environmental characteristics and the performance of activities within daily contexts expanded evaluation to include information about how individuals engage with their environment and how environments may support or inhibit participation in daily life. This new focus required the development of evaluation procedures that assessed characteristics of the environment and the quality of children's interactions within the environment. Key frameworks that define this person-environment interaction include the model of human occupation,[40] the ecology of human performance,[20] and the person-environment-occupation model.[43]
- The development of client-centered models of practice that advocated involvement of the client and family in the evaluation and intervention planning process required the development of evaluation methods that collected information from clients about their needs, priorities, and satisfaction with their performance. The Canadian Occupational Performance Measure (COPM) is frequently used for this purpose.[42] In pediatric practice this information is generally collected from parents/caregivers and teachers. Increasingly, however, the importance of obtaining information directly from children is being acknowledged, and evaluation methods to obtain this information are being developed.[38,41]
- Recognition of the limitations of collecting evaluation data focused on sensorimotor skills and the need to address multiple aspects of children's occupational performance created a call for a "top down" evaluation process,[13] whereby initial focus of the evaluation shifted to the quality and quantity of children's engagement in daily occupations. Assessments such as the School Function Assessment (SFA)[14] and the Pediatric Evaluation of Disability Inventory (PEDI)[34] incorporate this approach to assessment.
- The International Classification of Functioning, Disability, and Health (ICF) identified three levels of focus for interventions: body structure or function (impairment), whole body movements or activities (activity limitations), and involvement in life situations (participation restrictions).[66] Incorporation of participation restrictions as an area of intervention created a new focus on the effect of impairments or activity limitations on children's ability to participate in all aspects of daily life. As a result, methods to assess children's participation needed to be developed. Participation measures are incorporated into some standardized pediatric assessments such as the SFA[14] and the Miller Function & Participation Scales (M-FUN).[48] In addition, children's participation is evaluated in the Children's Assessment of Participation and Enjoyment (CAPE) and Preferences for Activities of Children (PAC).[41]

The preceding discussion illustrates how evolution of the occupational therapy profession has contributed to the ongoing development of standardized testing practices. One of the most significant changes in standardized testing over the past 30 years involves the inclusion of multiple information sources in the standardized testing process. Pediatric occupational therapists no longer draw conclusions about a child's abilities and needs based only on the child's performance on test items administered in a highly structured setting. Context-based assessments allow therapists to obtain information about children's performance and participation in a variety of daily contexts based on information provided by adults who are familiar with the child and in some cases from the children themselves. These multiple sources of information provide a well-rounded picture of how personal and environmental factors interact to influence children's ability to engage productively in age-appropriate occupations. Table 8-1 lists some of the most commonly used pediatric standardized assessments.

PURPOSES OF STANDARDIZED TESTS

Standardized tests are used for several reasons. For example, a standardized test can be used as a screening tool to assess large numbers of children quickly and briefly and identify those who may have delays and are in need of more in-depth testing. Examples of screening tests frequently used by occupational therapists include the Miller Assessment for Preschoolers (MAP),[46] the revised Denver Developmental Screening Test (Denver-II),[28] and the FirstSTEP (Screening Test for Evaluating Preschoolers).[47]

Screening tests typically assess several developmental domains, and each domain is represented by a small number of items (Table 8-2). Screening tests generally take 20 to 30 minutes and can be administered by professionals or by paraprofessionals such as classroom aides, nurse's aides, or teaching assistants. Therapists who work in settings that primarily serve typically developing children (e.g., a public school system or Head Start program) may become involved in developmental screening activities. In addition, occupational therapists frequently use assessment tools to evaluate children with specific developmental problems. Therefore it is important for all therapists to be aware of the strengths and weaknesses of specific tests used in their settings. Although the screening tools mentioned are not discussed in greater depth, the concepts of developing, administering, scoring, and interpreting standardized tests (discussed later in this chapter) should also be considered when using screening tools.

Occupational therapists most frequently use standardized tests as in-depth assessments of various areas of occupation and performance skills. Standardized tests are used for four main purposes:

1. to assist in the determination of a medical or educational diagnosis
2. to document a child's developmental and functional status
3. to aid the planning of an intervention program
4. to measure variables in research studies

Assistance with Medical or Educational Diagnoses

A primary purpose of standardized tests is to assist in the determination of a diagnosis through use of normative scores that compare the child's performance with that of an age-matched sample of children. Standardized tests are frequently used to determine if a child has developmental delays or functional deficits significant enough to qualify the child for remedial services such as occupational therapy. Many funding agencies and insurance providers use the results of standardized testing as one criterion in deciding whether a child will receive occupational therapy intervention. In school-based practice, standard scores are helpful for identifying specific student problems that may indicate that the involvement of an occupational therapist is appropriate. Funding approval for special services generally depends on documentation of a predetermined degree of delay or deficit in one or more developmental or academic domains, and standardized test results are an important component of this documentation. The results of standardized testing performed by occupational therapists, when used in conjunction with testing done by other professionals, can help physicians or psychologists arrive at a medical or educational diagnosis.

Documentation of Developmental and Functional Status

Another purpose of standardized testing is to document a child's status. Many funding and service agencies require periodic reassessment to provide a record of a child's progress and to determine if the child continues to qualify for services. Standardized testing is often a preferred way of documenting progress because the results of the most current assessment can be compared with those of earlier ones. Periodic formal reassessment can also provide valuable information to the therapist working with the child. Careful scrutiny of a child's test results can help identify areas of greatest and least progress. This can assist the therapist in prioritizing intervention goals. Many parents are also interested in seeing the results of their child's periodic assessments. Standardized tests used in periodic assessments must be chosen carefully so that areas of occupation or performance skills addressed in the intervention plan are also the focus of the standardized testing.

A discussion about the child's progress in areas that may not be measured by standardized testing should accompany the discussion of test performance. Structured or unstructured observations of the child's play, academic, social, and/or self-care performance; interviews with the caretaker or teacher about the child's home or school routine; the developmental, educational, and medical histories; and a review of pertinent medical or educational records are equally important components of the assessment process (see Chapter 7 for more information about the assessment process).

Planning of Intervention Programs

A third purpose of standardized testing is program planning. Standardized tests provide information about a child's level of function, and they help therapists determine the appropriate starting point for therapy intervention. Most commonly, criterion-referenced standardized tests are used as the basis for developing goals and objectives for individual children and for measuring progress and change over time. Criterion-referenced tests are used extensively in educational settings and include such tools as the Hawaii Early Learning Profile (HELP)[51]; the Assessment, Evaluation, and Programming System for Infants and Children[9]; and the SFA.[14] Criterion-referenced tests are described in more detail in the following section.

TABLE 8-1　Summary of Selected Pediatric Standardized Tests

Test	Age Range	Domains Tested	Sources of Information	Standard Scores Used	Time to Administer
Bayley Scales of Infant & Toddler Development Motor Scale (3rd ed.) (BSID-III)	1–42 mo	*Fine Motor Subtest:* Prehension, perceptual-motor integration, motor planning, motor speed *Gross Motor Subtest:* Static positioning, locomotion and coordination, balance, motor planning	Performance-based	Scaled scores Composite scores Percentile ranks Confidence intervals Growth scores Developmental age equivalent	15–20 min
Peabody Developmental Motor Scales (2nd ed.) (PDMS-2)	1–84 mo	*Fine Motor Scale:* Grasping, hand use, eye-hand coordination, manual dexterity *Gross Motor Scale:* Reflexes, balance, locomotor, nonlocomotor, receipt and propulsion	Performance-based	Z-scores T-scores Scaled scores Age-equivalent scores Developmental motor quotient scores	45–60 min for total test, 20–30 min for each scale
Miller Function & Participation Scale (M-FUN)	2 yr 6 mo–7 yr 11 mo	*Fine Motor, Visual Motor, and Gross Motor* subtests each assess aspects of four neurologic foundations: hand function, postural abilities, executive function and participation, nonmotor visual perception *Test Observations:* Examiner rating of child's behavior during testing session *Home Observations:* Caregiver rating of child's participation in activities of daily living (ADLs) and leisure activities at home *Classroom Observations:* Teacher or examiner rating of participation in classroom activities	Performance-based Context-based: examiner, caregiver, and teacher ratings	Scaled scores Confidence intervals Percentile scores Age equivalents Progress scores Criterion-referenced participation scores	40–60 min for performance activities 5–10 min for participation checklists
Bruininks-Oseretsky Test of Motor Proficiency (2nd ed.) (BOT-2)	4 yr 0 mo–21 yr 11 mo	*Fine Manual Control:* Motor skills for drawing and writing *Manual Coordination:* Motor skills for reaching, grasping, and manipulating objects; emphasis on speed, dexterity, and coordination *Body Coordination:* Motor skills involved in balance and coordination of upper and lower extremities *Strength and Agility:* Large muscle strength, motor speed, motor skills for maintaining body position for walking and running	Performance-based	Scale scores Composite standard scores Percentile ranks Total motor composite Age-equivalent scores Descriptive categories Confidence intervals	40–60 min for complete form; individual subtests can also be administered
Pediatric Evaluation of Disability Inventory (PEDI)	6 mo–7 yr	*Social Function, Self Care,* and *Mobility* scales: Each scale is scored according to functional skills, amount of caregiver assistance, and modifications	Context-based: caregiver and/or therapist/professional ratings; can be completed by one or more respondents	Normative standard score Scaled score	40–60 min when scoring by caregiver report

Continued

TABLE 8-1 Summary of Selected Pediatric Standardized Tests—Cont'd

Test	Age Range	Domains Tested	Sources of Information	Standard Scores Used	Time to Administer
School Function Assessment (SFA)	Grades K–6	*Participation* in nonacademic school tasks *Task Supports:* Five assistance and five adaptation scales *Activity Performance:* Physical tasks and cognitive/behavioral tasks	Context-based: teachers and other school staff ratings. Can be completed by one or more respondents	Criterion scores for each scale Cutoff scores for each scale for grades K–3 and grades 4–6	Total time 1.5–2 hr; 5–10 min per scale
Sensory Profile (SP)	3–10 yr	*Sensory Processing:* Auditory, visual, vestibular, touch, multisensory, and oral sensory processing *Modulation:* Sensory Processing Related to Endurance/Tone, Modulation Related to Body Position and Movement, Modulation of Movement Affecting Activity Level Modulation of Sensory Input Affecting Emotional Responses *Behavioral and Emotional Responses:* Emotional/Social Responses, Behavioral Outcomes of Sensory Processing, Thresholds for Response	Context-based: completed by caregiver	Cut score and classification system based on normative information: typical performance, probable difference, definite difference	20–30 min
Adolescent/Adult Sensory Profile (AASP)	11 yr and up	Sensory processing categories—Taste/Smell, Movement (vestibular/proprioceptive), Visual, Touch, Activity Level, and Auditory—are evaluated for each quadrant: *Low Registration, Sensation Seeking, Sensory Sensitivity,* and *Sensation Avoiding,* on a neurologic threshold continuum and behavioral response/self-regulation continuum	Context-based self report	Cut score and classification system based on normative information: Quadrant grid Quadrant summary Quadrant profile	10–15 min
Sensory Processing Measure (SPM)	5–12 yr (Grades K–6)	Social participation Vision Hearing Touch Body awareness Balance and motion Planning and ideas Total sensory systems	Context-based: completed by caregiver (Home Form), teacher (Main Classroom Form), teacher and other school staff (School Environments Form)	Standard scores, T-score, percentile score (Home and Main Classroom Forms) Cutoff scores (School Environments form)	15–20 min for Home and Main Classroom forms 5 min for each of six rating sheets for School Environments Form
Assessment of Motor and Process Skills (AMPS)	3 yr and up	Quality of motor and process skills in performance of basic and instrumental activities of daily living (IADLs)	Performance-based	ADL ability measure Logit scores for motor and process scales	30–40 min
School Assessment of Motor and Process Skills (School AMPS)	3–11 yr	Quality of occupational performance in school motor and process skills in five classroom tasks: *Pen/pencil writing, drawing and coloring, cutting and pasting, computer writing, manipulatives*	Performance-based	Logit scores for motor and process scales	30–40 min

TABLE 8-2 Developmental Domains Assessed in Four Screening Tools

Screening Tool	Age Range	Domains Assessed
Denver Developmental Screening Test (Revised)	1 mo–6 yr	Personal-social, fine motor adaptive, language, gross motor
Developmental Indicators for Assessment of Learning (Revised)	2.5–6 yr	Motor, language, concepts
FirstSTEP: Screening Test for Evaluating Preschoolers	2 yr, 9 mo–6 yr, 2 mo	Cognition, communication, physical, social and emotional, adaptive functioning
Miller Assessment for Preschoolers	2 yr, 7 mo–5 yr, 8 mo	Foundations, coordination, verbal, nonverbal, complex tasks

Measurement Instruments for Research Studies

Due to the psychometric properties of standardized tests, standard scores obtained from these tests can be statistically manipulated and analyzed. This allows test scores to be used for both descriptive and experimental research. Standardized tests can be used to obtain descriptive data about particular populations or groups. Experimental studies compare scores obtained before and after interventions, or compare two different interventions for efficacy. Data obtained through descriptive and experimental studies enhance our knowledge about client groups, and provide evidence regarding the efficacy of occupational therapy interventions.

CHARACTERISTICS

As stated earlier, standardized tests have uniform procedures for administration and scoring. These standard procedures permit the results of a child's tests to be compared either with his or her performance on a previous administration of the test or with the test norms developed by administration of the test to a large number of children.

Standardized tests characteristically include a test manual that describes the purpose of the test (i.e., what the test is intended to measure). The manual should also describe the intended population for the test. For pediatric assessments, this generally refers to the age range of children for whom the test was intended, but it may also refer to specific diagnoses or types of functional impairments. Test manuals also contain technical information about the test, such as a description of the test development and standardization process, characteristics of the normative sample, and studies done during the test development process to establish reliability and validity data. Finally, test manuals contain detailed information about the administration, scoring, and interpretation of the test scores.

Another characteristic of standardized tests is that they are composed of a fixed number of items. Items may not be added or subtracted without affecting the standard procedure for test administration. Most tests have specific rules about the number of items that should be administered to ensure a standardized test administration. These rules may differ significantly from test to test. For instance, the Bruininks-Oseretsky Test of Motor Proficiency (2nd ed.) (BOT-2) specifies that within each subtest the entire item set be administered regardless of the child's age.[10] In contrast, the Bayley Scales of Infant and Toddler Development (3rd ed.) (BSID-III) has 17 start points for the test.[7]

Examiners are instructed to begin testing at the start point corresponding to the child's chronologic age (or corrected age, if the child was born prematurely) and to move to easier or more difficult items, depending on the child's performance. Box 8-1 explains how to compute ages corrected for prematurity.

A third characteristic of standardized tests is fixed protocol for administration. The term *fixed protocol for administration* refers to the way each item is administered and the number of items administered. Generally, the protocol for administration specifies the verbal instruction or demonstration to be provided, the number of times the instructions can be repeated, and the number of attempts the child is allowed on the item. For some tests, instructions for each item are printed in the manual, and the tester is expected to read the instructions verbatim to the child without deviating from the text. However, other tests allow for more freedom of instruction, especially when the test involves a physical activity (Figure 8-1).

Standardized tests also have a fixed guideline for scoring. Scoring guidelines usually accompany the administration guidelines and specify what the child's performance must look like to receive a passing score on the item. Depending on the nature of the item, passing performance may be described using text, a picture, or a diagram. The administration and scoring guidelines for a test item from the BOT-2 are shown in Figure 8-2. In this example, the instructions to be given to the child are printed in bold type. Also included are the criteria for a passing score on the item, examples of incorrect responses, the number of trials and the time allowed for completion of the item. This example (Figure 8-2) describes how to present the item and what constitutes a passing score and includes a diagram of what a passing performance looks like.

TYPES OF STANDARDIZED TESTS

The two main types of standardized tests are norm-referenced tests and criterion-referenced tests. Many pediatric occupational therapists use both types in their practices. Each type has a specific purpose, and it is important for testers to be aware of the purpose of the test they are using.

A norm-referenced test is developed by giving the test in question to a large number of children, usually several hundred or more. This group is called the normative sample, and *norms,* or average scores, are derived from this sample. When a norm-referenced test is administered, the performance of the child being tested is compared with that of the normative sample. The purpose of norm-referenced testing, then, is to determine how a child performs in relation to the average performance of the normative sample.

BOX 8-1 Calculating the Chronologic Age and Corrected Age

Many standardized tests require that the examiner calculate the child's exact age on the date of testing. The method for calculating both the chronologic and the corrected age is presented below.

CALCULATING THE CHRONOLOGIC AGE

First, the date of testing and the child's birth date are recorded in the following order:

	YEAR	MONTH	DAY
Date of testing	99	6	15
Birth date	95	3	10
Chronologic age	4	3	5

Beginning on the right (the Day category), the day, month, and year of the child's birth date are subtracted from the date of testing. In the above example, the child's chronologic age is 4 years, 3 months, 5 days at the time of testing.

The convention in calculating age is, if the number of days in the chronologic age is 15 or less, the month is *rounded down*. Therefore in the above example, the child's age would be stated as 4 years, 3 months, or 4-3. If the number of days in the chronologic age is between 16 and 30, the month is *rounded up*. If the above child's chronologic age had been 4 years, 3 months, 16 days, the chronologic age would be expressed as 4 years, 4 months, or 4-4.

Sometimes, "borrowing" is necessary to subtract the birth date from the date of testing correctly:

	YEAR	MONTH	DAY
Date of testing	99	6	15
Birth date	95	10	22
Chronologic age	3	7	23

Begin with the Day category. Twenty-two cannot be subtracted from 15 without borrowing from the Month category. One month must be borrowed and placed in the Day category. One month equals 30 days; 30 is added to the 15 days in the Date of testing, giving a total of 45. Twenty-two is subtracted from 45, leaving 23 days. Moving to the Month category, 1 month has been borrowed by the Day category, leaving 5 months. Because 10 cannot be subtracted from 5, 1 year must be borrowed from the Year

category. One year equals 12 months; therefore, 12 will be added to the 5 in the Month category for Date of testing, totaling 17. Ten is subtracted from 17, leaving 7 months. Moving to the Year category, 1 year has been borrowed by the Month category, leaving 98. Ninety-five can be subtracted from 98, leaving 3 years. Therefore this child's chronologic age is 3 years, 7 months, 23 days. Using the rounding convention as discussed, the month is rounded up, giving a chronologic age of 3 years, 8 months.

CALCULATING THE CORRECTED AGE

Corrected age is used for children who were born prematurely to "correct" for the number of weeks they were born prior to the due date. Generally, the age is corrected until the child turns 2 years of age, although this convention can vary. Given 40 weeks' gestation as full term, the amount of correction is the difference between the actual gestational age at birth and the 40 weeks' full-term gestational age. Therefore a child born at 30 weeks' gestation is 10 weeks, premature. Many practitioners consider 36 or 37 weeks or above to be full-term gestation; therefore, children with a gestational age of 36 weeks or above do not receive a corrected age. Because there is some variation in how and when corrected age is used, it is wise for the therapist to learn the procedures of his or her facility and to adhere to them when calculating corrected age.

If the expected due date and birth date are both known, subtracting the birth date from the due date yields an exact measurement of prematurity.

	YEAR	MONTH	DAY
Due date	98	9	20
Birth date	98	6	12
	—	3	8

This child is 3 months, 8 days premature. To calculate corrected age, subtract the prematurity value from the chronologic age:

	YEAR	MONTH	DAY
Chronologic age	1	1	25
Prematurity	—	3	8
	—	10	17

The child's corrected age is 10 months, 17 days or, when rounded, 11 months.

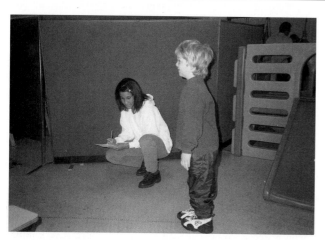

FIGURE 8-1 A therapist prepares to test a child on the broad jump item from the Bruininks-Oseretsky Test of Motor Proficiency 2.

Test developers generally attempt to include children from a variety of geographic locations, ethnic and racial backgrounds, and socioeconomic levels so that the normative sample is representative of the population of the United States, based on the most recent U.S. Census data. Generally, the normative sample is composed of children who have no developmental delays or conditions, although some tests include smaller subsamples of clinical populations as a means of determining whether the test discriminates between children whose development is proceeding normally and those who have known developmental delays.

Norm-referenced tests address one or more areas of behavior. If the test evaluates more than one area, each area typically has one or more subtests. For instance the BOT-2 assesses performance in four motor-area composites: fine manual control, manual coordination, body coordination, and strength and agility. Items are chosen to represent a broad range of skills within these composite areas. Additionally, items are chosen to incorporate materials and activities that are reasonably

Item 8: Standing Heel-to-Toe on a Balance Beam

Number of Trials	Maximum Raw Score
2	10 seconds

Procedure

- The examinee stands with preferred foot on the balance beam and non-preferred foot on the floor.
- The examinee places hands on hips.
- The examinee takes one step forward, placing non-preferred foot on the balance beam and touching heel of front foot to toe of back foot, and looks at the target.
- Conduct the second trial *only if* the examinee does not earn the maximum score of 10 seconds on the first trial.

Scoring

- Record the number of seconds, to the nearest tenth of a second, that the examinee maintains proper form, up to 10 seconds.
- Stop the trial after 10 seconds or if the examinee fails to keep feet heel-to-toe, fails to keep hands on hips, or steps or falls off the beam.

Equipment

Balance Beam
Target
stopwatch

Administration

Teach the task to the examinee. Then, say,

Stand heel-to-toe on the beam until I tell you to stop. Ready? Begin.

Begin timing *when the examinee attains proper form*. After 10 seconds or when the examinee breaks proper form, say,

Stop.

If the examinee does not earn the maximum score of 10 seconds, conduct the second trial. If necessary, reteach the task after you say,

Let's try it again.

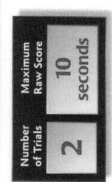

FIGURE 8-2 Administration and scoring protocol for Bruininks-Oseretsky Test of Motor Proficiency 2, subtest 5, item 8. (From Bruininks, R. H., & Bruininks, B. [2005]. *Bruininks-Oseretsky Test of Motor Proficiency 2.* Circle Pines, MN: American Guidance Service.)

familiar and typical for children of the age group being tested. A child's performance on an individual test item is not as important as the overall subtest or area score. However, it is important for the therapist to observe the quality and characteristics of a child's performance on each item, as these qualitative observations provide important information to complement the obtained standard scores.

Norm-referenced tests have standardized protocols for administration and scoring. The tester must adhere to these protocols so that each test administration is as similar as possible to that of the normative sample. This is necessary to compare any child's performance fairly with that of the normative sample.

Sometimes the examiner must deviate from the standard protocol because of special needs of the child being tested. For instance, a child with visual impairments may need manual guidance to cut with scissors, or a child with cerebral palsy may need assistance stabilizing the shoulder and upper arm to reach and grasp a crayon. If changes are made in the standardized procedures, the examiner must indicate this in the summary of assessment, and standard scores cannot be used to describe that child's performance in comparison with the normative sample.

Norm-referenced tests have specific psychometric properties. They have been analyzed by statisticians to obtain score distributions, mean or average scores, and standard scores. This is done to achieve the primary objective of norm-referenced tests: comparability of scores with the normative sample. A test under development initially has a much larger number of items than the final version of the test. Through pilot testing, items are chosen or rejected based partly on how well they statistically discriminate between children of different ages and/or abilities. Items are not chosen primarily for their relevance to functional skills. Consequently, some norm-referenced tests are not intended to link test performance with specific objectives or goals for intervention. Other norm-referenced tests, such as the Sensory Profile, are designed to specifically evaluate the effect of sensory processes on functional performance in daily life and, when combined with other evaluation and observation data, to allow therapists to develop intervention goals. A portion of the Sensory Profile questionnaire is presented in Figure 8-3.

A criterion-referenced test, by contrast, is designed to provide information on how children perform on specific tasks. The term *criterion-referenced* refers to the fact that a child's performance is compared with a particular *criterion*, or level of performance of a particular skill. The goal of a criterion-referenced test is to determine which skills a child can and cannot accomplish, thereby providing a focus for intervention. In general the content of a criterion-referenced test is detailed and in some cases may relate to specific behavioral or functional objectives. The intent of a criterion-referenced test is to measure a child's performance on specific tasks rather than to compare the child's performance with that of his or her peers.

Many developmental checklists have been field tested and then published as criterion-referenced tests. The HELP is a good example of a developmental checklist designed to be used with children from birth to 3 years of age. It contains a large number of items in each of the domains of gross motor, fine motor, language, cognitive, social-emotional, and self-help skills. Each item correlates with specific intervention objectives. For instance, if a child is not able to pass Fine Motor item 4.81, Snips with Scissors, a list of intervention ideas are presented in the HELP activity guide.[30] The activity guide is meant to accompany the test and is designed to help the therapist or educator by providing ideas for developmentally appropriate activities to address areas of weakness identified

Sensory Processing				ALWAYS	FREQUENTLY	OCCASIONALLY	SELDOM	NEVER
Item			A. Auditory Processing					
🔊	L	1	Responds negatively to unexpected or loud noises (for example, cries or hides at noise from vacuum cleaner, dog barking, hair dryer)					
🔊	L	2	Holds hands over ears to protect ears from sound					
🔊	L	3	Has trouble completing tasks when the radio is on					
🔊	L	4	Is distracted or has trouble functioning if there is a lot of noise around					
🔊	L	5	Can't work with background noise (for example, fan, refrigerator)					
🔊	H	6	Appears to not hear what you say (for example, does not "tune-in" to what you say, appears to ignore you)					
🔊	H	7	Doesn't respond when name is called but you know the child's hearing is OK					
🔊	H	8	Enjoys strange noises/seeks to make noise for noise's sake					
			Section Raw Score Total					

Comments

FIGURE 8-3   A portion of the caregiver questionnaire for the Sensory Profile.   (From Dunn, W. [1999]. *Sensory Profile user's manual*. San Antonio, TX: Psychological Corporation.)

BOX 8-2   Administration and Assessment Procedures and Processes for Hawaii Early Learning Profile: Item 4.81—Snips with Scissors (23 to 25 Months)

Definition: The child cuts a paper edge randomly, one snip at a time, rather than using a continuous cutting motion.
Example observation opportunities: *Incidental*—May observe while the child is preparing for a tea party with stuffed animals or dolls. Demonstrate making fringe on paper placemats and invite the child to help. *Structured*—Using a half piece of sturdy paper and blunt scissors, make three snips in separate places along the edge of the paper while the child is watching.

Exaggerate the opening and closing motions of your hand. Offer the child the scissors and invite him or her to make a cut. Let the child explore the scissors (if interested), helping him or her position the scissors in his or her hand as needed.
Credit: Snips paper in one place, holding the paper in one hand and scissors in the other (see also Credit Notes in this strand's preface).

From Parks, S. (2006). Inside HELP: Administration and reference manual for the Hawaii Early Learning Profile. Palo Alto, CA: VORT.

BOX 8-3   Administration and Assessment Procedures and Processes for Hawaii Early Learning Profile Item 4.81—Snips with Scissors: Activity Guide Suggestions

The child cuts with the scissors, taking one snip at a time rather than doing continuous cutting.
1. Let the child use small kitchen tongs to pick up objects and to practice opening and closing motions.
2. Let the child use child-sized scissors with rounded tips.
3. Demonstrate by placing your finger and thumb through the handles.
4. Position the scissors with the finger holes one above the other. Position the child's forearm in midsupination (i.e., thumb up). Let the child place his or her thumb through the top hole and the middle finger through the bottom hole. If the child's fingers are small, place the index and middle

fingers in the bottom hole. The child will adjust his or her fingers as experience is gained.
5. Let the child open and close the scissors. Assist as necessary by placing your hand over the child's hand.
6. Let the child snip narrow strips of paper and use it for fringe in art work.
7. The different types of scissors available for children are a scissors with reinforced rubber coating on the handle grips; a scissors with double handle grips for your hand and the child's hand; a left-handed scissors; and a scissors for a prosthetic hook. Use the different types of child's scissors appropriately as required.

From Furuno, S., O'Reilly, K. A., Hosaka, C. M., Zeisloft, B., & Allman, T. (2005). *HELP activity guide.* Palo Alto, CA: VORT.

---

in the criterion-based assessment. The administration protocol for this item and the associated intervention activities are presented in Boxes 8-2 and 8-3.

Administration and scoring procedures may or may not be standardized on a criterion-referenced test. The HELP has standard procedures for administering and scoring each item. In contrast, the SFA is a judgment-based questionnaire completed by one or more school professionals familiar with the child's performance at school.[14] Criteria for rating the child's performance on each item are provided. School professionals are encouraged to collaborate in determining ratings and to use these ratings as a basis for designing an intervention plan. Figure 8-4 shows a category of activity performance with the associated rating scale. Many other criterion-referenced tests take the form of checklists, in which the specific performance needed to receive credit on an item is not indicated. Many therapist-designed tests for use in a particular facility or setting are nonstandardized, criterion-referenced tests.

Criterion-referenced tests are not subjected to the statistical analyses performed on norm-referenced tests. No mean score or normal distribution is calculated; a child may pass all items or fail all items on a particular test without adversely affecting the validity of the test results. The purpose of the test is to learn exactly what a child can accomplish, not to compare the child's performance with that of the peer group. This goal is also reflected in the test development process for criterion-referenced tests. Items are generally chosen based on a process of task analysis or identification of important developmental milestones rather than for their statistical validity. Therefore the specific items on a criterion-referenced test have a direct

relationship with functional skills and can be used as a starting point for generating appropriate goals and objectives for therapy intervention. To be useful for intervention planning, the summary scores from criterion-referenced tests should relate closely to the child's current pattern of performance.[26]

The characteristics of norm- and criterion-referenced tests are compared in Table 8-3. As is shown in the table, some tests are both norm-referenced and criterion-referenced. This means that although the items have been analyzed for their ability to perform statistically, they also reflect functional or developmental skills that are appropriate for intervention. These tests permit the therapist to compare a child's performance with that of peers in the normative sample, and they also provide information about specific skills that may be appropriate for remediation.

The Peabody Developmental Motor Scales (2nd ed.) (PDMS-2) is an example of both a norm- and criterion-referenced test. Although the PDMS-2 has been subjected to the statistical analyses used in norm-referenced tests, many individual items on the test also represent developmental milestones that can be addressed as part of the intervention plan. The SFA, although primarily a criterion-referenced test, provides a criterion score and standard error for each raw score based on a national standardization sample.

TECHNICAL ASPECTS

The following discussion of the technical aspects of standardized tests focuses on the statistics and test development procedures used for norm-referenced tests. Information on how

Behavior Regulation

1. Displays appropriate restraint regarding self-stimulation (e.g., refrains from head banging, hand flapping).................	1 2 3 4
2. Accepts unexpected changes in routine...........	1 2 3 4
3. Refrains from provoking others..................	1 2 3 4
4. Uses nonaggressive words and actions...........	1 2 3 4
5. Maintains behavioral control in large groups of students (e.g., cafeteria, assemblies).............	1 2 3 4
6. Hears constructive criticism without losing temper..	1 2 3 4
7. Uses words rather than physical actions to respond when provoked or angry at others........	1 2 3 4
8. Seeks adult assistance, if necessary, when experiencing peer conflict, especially conflicts involving violence............................	1 2 3 4
9. Responds to/handles teasing in a constructive way..	1 2 3 4
10. Handles frustration when experiencing difficulties with school tasks/activities.....................	1 2 3 4
11. Shows common sense in words and actions around bullies, gangs, or strangers....................	1 2 3 4
12. Resolves ordinary peer conflicts or problems adequately on his/her own without requesting teacher assistance...........................	1 2 3 4

Respondent's Initials	Behavior Regulation Raw Score	

Ratings Key for Activity Performance

1: Does not perform **2:** Partial performance **3:** Inconsistent performance **4:** Consistent performance

FIGURE 8-4 One category of activity performance and corresponding rating scale for the School Function Assessment (SFA). (From Coster, W., Deeney, T., Haltiwanger, J., & Haley, S. [1998]. *School Function Assessment.* San Antonio, TX: Psychological Corporation.)

TABLE 8-3 Comparison of Norm-Referenced and Criterion-Referenced Tests

Characteristic	Norm-Referenced Test	Criterion-Referenced Test
Purpose	Comparison of child's performance with normative sample	Comparison of child's performance with a defined list of skills
Content	General; usually covers a wide variety of skills	Detailed; may cover specific objectives or developmental milestones
Administration and scoring	Always standardized	May be standardized or nonstandardized
Psychometric properties	Normal distribution of scores; means, standard deviations, and standard scores computed	No score distribution needed; a child may pass or fail all items
Item selection	Items chosen for statistical performance; may not relate to functional skills or therapy objectives	Items chosen for functional and developmental importance; provides necessary information for developing therapy objectives
Examples	BSID-III; PDMS-2; BOT-2; PEDI	PDMS-2, PEDI, HELP, Gross-Motor Function Measure, SFA

BOT-2, Bruininks-Oseretsky Test of Motor Proficiency (2nd ed.); *BSID-III,* Bayley Scales of Infant and Toddler Development (3rd ed.); *HELP,* Hawaii Early Learning Profile; *PDMS,* Peabody Developmental Motor Scales; *PEDI,* Pediatric Evaluation of Disability Inventory; *SFA,* School Function Assessment.

standard scores are obtained and reported is included, as well as on how the reliability and validity of a test are evaluated. It is the responsibility of the test author to provide initial data on test reliability and validity. However, these test characteristics are never definitively determined, and ongoing evaluation of validity and reliability is necessary. A knowledge of technical aspects of standardized tests is important to occupational therapists for the following reasons:

1. Therapists must be able to analyze and select standardized tests appropriately, according to the child's age and functional level and the purpose of testing.
2. Therapists must be able to interpret and report scores from standardized tests accurately.
3. Therapists must be able to explain test results to caregivers and other professionals working with the child in a clear, understandable manner.

Presented next is information on (1) descriptive statistics, (2) standard scores, (3) correlation coefficients, (4) reliability, and (5) validity.

Descriptive Statistics

Descriptive statistics provide information about the characteristics of a particular group. Many human characteristics, such as height, weight, head size, and intelligence, are represented by a distribution called the *normal curve* (or *bell-shaped curve*) (Figure 8-5). The pattern of performance on most norm-referenced tests also follows this curve. The greatest number of people receive a score in the middle part of the distribution, with progressively smaller numbers receiving scores at either the high or the low end. Descriptive statistics also provide information about where members of a group are located on the normal curve. The two types of descriptive statistics are the measure of central tendency and the measure of variability.

The measure of central tendency indicates the middle point of the distribution for a particular group, or sample, of children. The most frequently used measure of central tendency is the *mean*, which is the sum of all the scores for a particular sample divided by the number of scores. It is computed mathematically using a simple formula

$$\bar{X} = \frac{\Sigma X}{n}$$

where Σ means to sum, X is each individual score, and n is the number of scores in the sample (the mean is also often called the average score).

Another measure of central tendency is the *median*, which is simply the middle score of a distribution. Half the scores lie below the median and half above it. The median is the preferred measure of central tendency when outlying or extreme scores are present in the distribution. The following distribution of scores is an example:

2   3   13   14   17   17   18

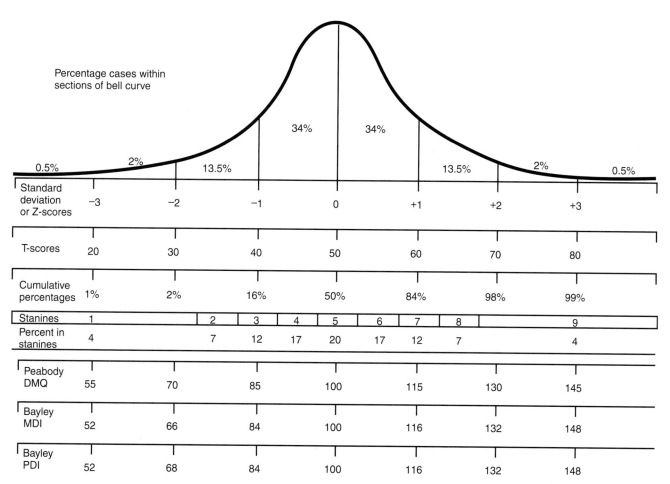

FIGURE 8-5   The normal curve and associated standard scores.

The mean score is 12 [i.e., $(2 + 3 + 13 + 14 + 17 + 17 + 18) \div 7$]. The median, or middle score, is 14. In this case the score of 14 is a more accurate representation of the middle point of these scores than is the score of 12 because the two low scores, or *outliers,* in the distribution pulled down the value of the mean.

The measure of variability determines how much the performance of the group as a whole deviates from the mean. Measures of variability are used to compute the standard scores used in standardized tests. As with measures of central tendency, measures of variability are derived from the normal curve. The two measures of variability discussed are the variance and the standard deviation.

The *variance* is the average of the squared deviations of the scores from the mean. In other words, it is a measure of how far the score of an average individual in a sample deviates from the group mean. The variance is computed using the following formula:

$$S^2 = \frac{\Sigma(X - \overline{X})^2}{n}$$

where S^2 is the variance, $\Sigma(X - X)^2$ is the sum of each individual score minus the mean score, and n is the total number of scores in the group. The standard deviation is simply the square root of the variance. To illustrate, calculations are provided for the mean, the variance, and the standard deviation for the following set of scores from a hypothetical test:

$$17 \quad 19 \quad 21 \quad 25 \quad 28$$

To calculate the mean, the following equation is used:

$$\frac{(17 + 19 + 21 + 25 + 28)}{5} = 22$$

To calculate the variance, the mean must be subtracted from each score, and that value then must be squared:

$$17 - 22 = (-5)^2 = 25$$
$$19 - 22 = (-3)^2 = 9$$
$$21 - 22 = (-1)^2 = 1$$
$$25 - 22 = (3)^2 = 9$$
$$28 - 22 = (6)^2 = 36$$

The squared values are summed and then divided by the total number of scores:

$$25 + 9 + 1 + 9 + 36 = 80$$
$$80 \div 5 = 16$$

The variance of this score distribution is 16. The standard deviation is simply the square root of the variance, or 4.

The *standard deviation (SD)* is an important number because it is the basis for computing many standard scores. In a normal distribution (see Figure 8-5), 68% of the people in the distribution score within 1 SD of the mean (± 1 SD); 95% score within 2 SD of the mean (± 2 SD); and 99.7% score within 3 SD of the mean (± 3 SD). In the score distribution with a mean of 22 and a standard deviation of 4, three of the five scores were within 1 SD of the mean (22 ± 4; a score range of 18 to 26), and all five scores were within 2 SD of the mean (22 ± 8; a score range of 14 to 30). The standard deviation, then, determines the placement of scores on the normal curve. By showing the degree of variability in the sample, the standard deviation reveals how far the scores can be expected to range from the mean value.

Standard Scores

Standardized tests are scored in several different ways. Scoring methods include Z-scores, T-scores, deviation intelligence quotient (IQ) scores, developmental index scores, percentile scores, and age-equivalent scores.

The *Z-score* is computed by subtracting the mean for the test from the individual's score and dividing it by the standard deviation, using the following equation:

$$z = \frac{X - \overline{X}}{SD}$$

For the score distribution above (i.e., 17 19 21 25 28), the person receiving the score of 17 would have a Z-score of $(17 - 22) \div 4 = -1.25$. The person receiving the score of 28 would have a Z-score of $(28 - 22) \div 4 = 1.5$. The negative value of the first score indicates that the Z-score value is below the mean for the test, and the positive value of the second score indicates that the Z-score value is above the mean. Generally, a Z-score value of -1.5 or less is considered indicative of delay or deficit in the area measured, although this can vary, depending on the particular test.

The *T-score* is derived from the Z-score. In a T-score distribution, the mean is 50 and the standard deviation is 10. The T-score is computed using the following equation:

$$T = 10(Z) + 50$$

For the two Z-scores computed above, the T-score values are as follows: for the first Z-score of -1.25, the T-score is $10(-1.25) + 50 = 37.50$. For the second Z-score of 1.5, the T-score is $10(1.5) + 50 = 65$. Note that all T-scores have positive values, but because the mean of a T-score distribution is 50, any number below 50 indicates a score below the mean. Because the standard deviation of the T distribution is 10, the first score of 37.50 is slightly more than 1 SD below the mean. The second score of 65 is 15 points, or 1.5 SD, above the mean.

Two other standard scores that are frequently seen in standardized tests are the *deviation IQ score* and the *developmental index score*. Deviation IQ scores have a mean of 100 and a standard deviation of either 15 or 16. These are the IQ scores obtained from such tests as the Stanford-Binet[61] or the Wechsler Intelligence Scale for Children (WISC).[65] On these tests, individuals with IQ scores 2 SD below the mean (IQs of 70 and 68, respectively) are considered to have an intellectual disability. Individuals with IQ scores 2 SD above the mean (IQs of 130 and 132, respectively) are considered gifted. Developmental index scores are used in developmental tests such as the PDMS-2 and the BSID-III. Like the deviation IQ scores, they have a mean of 100 and a standard deviation of 15 or 16. Children who receive a developmental index score of 2 SD below the mean (index score of 68 or 70) in one or more skill areas are considered to be in need of remedial services. In many cases children who receive developmental index scores lower than -1.5 SD (index score of 85) may also be recommended for occupational therapy services.

Two other types of scores (i.e., percentile scores and age-equivalent scores) are frequently used in standardized tests. These are not standard scores in the strictest sense, because they are computed directly from raw scores rather than through the statistically derived measures of central tendency and variability. However, they give an indication of a child's performance relative to that of the normative sample.

The *percentile score* is the percentage of people in a standardization sample whose score is at or below a particular raw score. A percentile score of 60, for instance, indicates that 60% of the people in the standardization sample received a score that was at or below the raw score corresponding to the 60th percentile. Tests that use percentile scores generally include a table in the manual by which raw scores can be converted to percentile scores. These tables usually indicate at what percentile rank performance is considered deficient. Raw scores can be converted to percentile rank (PR) scores by a simple formula:

$$PR = \frac{\left(\begin{array}{c} \text{Number of people} \\ \text{below score} \end{array} + \begin{array}{c} \text{One half of} \\ \text{people at score} \end{array}\right) \times 100}{\text{Total number of scores}}$$

Using the previous sample data (i.e., 17 19 21 25 28), percentile ranks for the highest and lowest scores can be computed. The raw score of 17 is the lowest score in the distribution and is the only score of 17. Therefore the equation is as follows:

$$\frac{(0 + 0.5)}{5} \times 100 = \frac{0.5}{5} \times 100 = 10$$

The highest score in the distribution is 28; therefore four people have lower scores and one person received a score of 28. The equation is as follows:

$$\frac{(4 + 0.5)}{5} \times 100 = \frac{4.5}{5} \times 100 = 90$$

In this distribution, then, the lowest score is at the 10th percentile and the highest score is at the 90th percentile.

Although PR scores can be easily calculated and understood, they have a significant disadvantage: the percentile ranks are not equal in size across the score distribution. Distances between percentile ranks are much smaller in the middle of the distribution than at the ends; consequently, improving a score from the 50th to the 55th percentile requires much less effort than improving a score from the 5th to the 10th percentile (see Figure 8-5). As a result, an improvement in performance by a child functioning at the lower end of the score range may not be reflected in the PR score the child achieves. Other standard scores are more sensitive at measuring changes in the performance of children who fall at the extreme ends of the score distribution.

The *age-equivalent score* is the age at which the raw score is at the 50th percentile. The age-equivalent score generally is expressed in years and months, e.g., 4-3 (i.e., 4 years, 3 months). It is a score that is easily understood by parents and caregivers who may not be familiar with testing concepts or terminology. However, age-equivalent scores have significant disadvantages. Although they may provide a general idea of a child's overall developmental level, it may be misleading to say, for example, that a 4-year-old is functioning at the 2.5-year level. The age-equivalent score may be more or less an average of several developmental domains, some of which may be at the 4.5-year level and some at the 1.5-year level. Therefore the child's performance may be highly variable and may not reflect that of a typical 2.5-year-old. In addition, because the age-equivalent score represents only the score that a child of a particular age who is performing at the 50th percentile would receive, a child who is performing within normal limits for his or her age but whose score is below the 50th percentile would receive an age-equivalent score below his or her

chronologic age. This can cause parents or caregivers to conclude incorrectly that the child has delays. Age equivalents, then, are a type of standard score that can contribute to an understanding of a child's performance, but they are the least psychometrically sound, can be misleading, and should be used only with the greatest caution.

Correlation Coefficients

Test manuals often report correlation coefficients when describing the test's reliability and validity. A correlation coefficient tells the degree or strength of the relationship between two scores or variables. Although the standard scores are used to compute individual scores, correlation coefficients are used to determine the relationship between scores from one measurement and those from another. Correlation coefficients range from −1.00 to +1.00. A correlation coefficient of 0.00 indicates that no relationship exists between the two variables measured. Any relationship that occurs is strictly by chance. The closer the correlation coefficient is either to −1.00 to +1.00, the stronger is the relationship between the two variables. A negative correlation means that a high score on one variable is accompanied by a low score on the other variable. A positive correlation means that a high score on one variable is accompanied by a high score on the other variable and that a low score on one variable is accompanied by a low score on the other variable.

Examples of two variables that generally have a fairly high positive correlation are height and weight. Taller individuals are also generally heavier than shorter individuals. However, this is not always true. Some tall individuals are light, and some short individuals are heavy. Consequently, the correlation between height and weight for a given population is a positive value, but it is not a perfect 1.00. Examples of two variables that are unrelated are eye color and height. The correlation coefficient for these two variables for any population is close to zero, because a person's eye color cannot be predicted by the individual's height.

An example of two variables that have a negative correlation might be hours spent studying and hours spent watching television. A student who spends many hours studying probably watches fewer hours of television, and a student who watches many hours of television probably spends fewer hours studying. Hence, a negative relationship exists between these two variables. As one variable increases, the other decreases. Several different correlation coefficients may be calculated, depending on the type of data used. Some correlation coefficients commonly used in test manuals include the Pearson Product-Moment Correlation Coefficient or Pearson r, the Spearman Rank-Order Correlation Coefficient, and the Intraclass Correlation Coefficient (ICC).

Why are correlation coefficients important? As the following sections on reliability and validity illustrate, correlation coefficients are important tools for evaluating the properties of a test. Knowledge of test characteristics helps testers know how best to use a test and makes them aware of the strengths and limitations of individual tests.

Reliability

The reliability of a test describes the consistency or stability of scores obtained by one individual when tested on two different occasions with different sets of items or under other variable examining conditions.[63] For instance, if a child is given a test and receives a score of 50 and 2 days later is given the same test and receives a score of 75, the reliability of the test is questionable. The difference between the two scores is called the *error variance* of the test, which is a result of random fluctuations in performance between the two testing sessions. Some amount of random error variance is expected in any test situation because of variations in such things as mood, fatigue, or motivation. Error variance can also be caused by environmental characteristics such as light, temperature, or noise. However, it is important that error variance caused by variations in examiners or by the characteristics of the test itself be minimal. Confidence in the scores obtained requires that the test have adequate reliability over a number of administrations and low error variance.

Most standardized tests evaluate two or three forms of reliability. The three forms of reliability most commonly used in pediatric standardized tests are (1) test–retest reliability, (2) inter-rater reliability, and (3) standard error of measurement (SEM).

Test–Retest Reliability

Test–retest reliability is a measurement of the stability of a test over time. It is obtained by giving the test to the same individual on two different occasions. In the evaluation of test–retest reliability for a pediatric test, the time span between test administrations must be short to minimize the possibility of developmental changes occurring between the two test sessions. However, the time span between tests should not be so short that the child may recall items administered during the first test session, thereby improving his or her performance on the second test session (this is called the *learning,* or *practice, effect*).

Generally, the time span between testing sessions is no more than 1 week for infants and very young children and no more than 2 weeks for older children. During the process of test development, test–retest reliability is evaluated on a subgroup of the normative sample. The size and composition of the subgroup should be specified in the manual. The correlation coefficient between the scores of the two test sessions is calculated. This coefficient is the measure of the test–retest reliability. A test that has a high test–retest reliability coefficient is more likely to yield relatively stable scores over time. That is, it is affected less by random error variance than is a test with a low test–retest reliability coefficient. When administering a test with a low test–retest reliability coefficient, the examiner has less confidence that the score obtained is a true reflection of the child's abilities. If the child were tested at a different time of day or in a different setting entirely, different results might be obtained.

A sample of 197 children was evaluated twice within 2 weeks (mean retest interval of 6 days) to assess the test–retest reliability (stability) of the BSID-III Motor Scale.[7] Overall stability coefficients were 0.80 for the Fine Motor Scale, 0.82 for the Gross Motor Scale, and 0.83 for the Motor Composite. Test–retest stability was slightly higher for the older age groups. The performance of a young child often varies within short periods because it is highly influenced by variables such as mood, hunger, sleepiness, and irritability. The test–retest reliability coefficients for 50 children tested twice within 1 week with the PDMS-2 ranged from 0.73 for the Fine

Motor Quotient and 0.84 for the Gross Motor Quotient for 2- to 11-month-old children to 0.94 for the Fine Motor Quotient and 0.93 for the Gross Motor Quotient for 12- to 17-month-old children.[27]

To evaluate test–retest reliability of the Sensory Processing Measure (SPM),[50] a rating scale of sensory processing, praxis, and social participation in home and school environments for children age 5 to 12, caregivers and teachers of 77 typically developing children completed the rating scale two times within a 2-week interval. Correlation coefficients for the scales ranged from .94 to .98. These three examples of good to excellent test–retest reliability are typical examples of scales that measure children's sensory processing and motor performance. The rapid and variable development of young children and the practice effect are two factors that negatively influence the tests' stability over time. The test–retest reliability of a test is critical to its use as a measure of the child's progress or of intervention efficacy.

Inter-rater Reliability

Inter-rater reliability refers to the ability of two independent raters to obtain the same scores when scoring the same child simultaneously. Inter-rater reliability is generally measured on a subset of the normative sample during the test development process. This is often accomplished by having one rater administer and score the test while another rater observes and scores at the same time. The correlation coefficient calculated from the two raters' scores is the inter-rater reliability coefficient of the test. It is particularly important to measure inter-rater reliability on tests for which the scoring may require some judgment on the part of the examiner.

Although the scoring criteria for many test items are specific on most tests, scoring depends to a certain extent on individual judgment, and scoring differences can arise between different examiners. A test that has a low inter-rater reliability coefficient is especially susceptible to differences in scoring by different raters. This may mean that the administration and scoring criteria are not stated explicitly enough, requiring examiners to make judgment calls on a number of items. Alternatively, it can mean that the items on the test call for responses that are too broad or vague to permit precise scoring.

No universal agreement has been reached regarding the minimum acceptable coefficient for test–retest and inter-rater reliability. The context of the reliability measurement, the type of test, and the distribution of scores are some of the variables that can be taken into account when determining an acceptable reliability coefficient. One standard suggested by Urbina and used by a number of examiners is 0.80.[63]

Not all tests have test–retest or inter-rater reliability coefficients that reach the 0.80 level. Lower coefficients indicate greater variability in scores. When examiners use a test that has a reliability coefficient below 0.80, scores must be interpreted with great caution. For example, if one subtest of a test of motor development has test–retest reliability of 0.60, the examiner who uses it to measure change over time must acknowledge that a portion of the apparent change between the first and second test administration is a result of the error variance of the test.

The inter-rater reliability of the M-FUN[48] was evaluated by having pairs of examiners score the performance of

29 children on the M-FUN using the scoring rubrics developed for the standardization edition of the test. One examiner administered and scored while the second examiner observed and scored independently. Correlation coefficients were 0.91 for Visual Motor, 0.93 for Fine Motor, and 0.91 for Gross Motor. A second aspect of inter-rater reliability, decision agreement, was also evaluated. Decision agreement is the degree to which examiner's scores agree in the identification of a child as performing in the average range or as having an impairment. Since standardized tests are used frequently to qualify children for services, it is important to know whether different examiners can consistently identify whether or not a child has impairments. On the M-FUN, decision agreement was 96% for Visual Motor, 97% for Fine Motor, and 93% for Gross Motor. The results of the inter-rater reliability studies on the M-FUN suggest that examiners can reliably score children's performance and based on the obtained scores can make reliable determinations about the presence of impairment.

Inter-rater reliability for the PDMS-2 was evaluated using a slightly different method. Sixty completed test protocols were randomly selected from the normative sample and were independently scored by two examiners. The resulting correlation coefficients were 0.97 for the Gross Motor Composite and 0.98 for the Fine Motor Composite.[27] It should be noted that this method of determining reliability is not based on two independent observations of the child's performance but on review of completed scoring protocols. Hence, potential error related to the way examiners interpreted and applied the scoring criteria to determine scores on individual items was not addressed. This could result in spuriously high inter-rater reliability coefficients. In a test such as the DTVP-II, in which scores are based on a written record of the child's response, inter-rater reliability is excellent. When two individuals scored 88 completed DTVP-II protocols, the interscorer reliability was 0.98.[35]

When individual subtests of a comprehensive test have a low reliability coefficient, it is generally not recommended that the standard scores from the subtests be reported. Often the reliability coefficient of the entire test is much higher than that of the individual subtests. One reason for this is that reliability increases with the number of items on a test. Because subtests have fewer items than the entire test, they are more sensitive to fluctuations in the performance or scoring of individual items. When this occurs, it is best to describe subtest performance qualitatively, without reporting standard scores.

Standard scores can be reported for the total, or comprehensive, test score. Examiners should consult the reliability information in the test manual before deciding how to report test scores for individual subtests and for the test as a whole. The inter-rater reliability coefficients reported in the manual are estimates based on the context and conditions under which they were studied by the test developers. This reliability coefficient is an estimate; inter-rater reliability may vary when children are tested in different contexts or when examiners have differing levels of training and experience.

Examiners can exert some control over the inter-rater reliability of tests they use frequently. It is good practice for examiners to check inter-rater reliability with more experienced colleagues when learning a new standardized test before beginning to administer the test to children in the clinical setting.

Also, periodic checking of inter-rater reliability with colleagues who are administering the same standardized tests is a good practice. Some simple methods for assessing inter-rater reliability are discussed in more detail later in the chapter.

For context-based tests, inter-rater reliability is generally not a meaningful indicator of the psychometric integrity of the test, since each individual who contributes information to the test does so based on knowledge of the child in a specific environment with unique demands. However, since different raters may be evaluating the child on similar constructs, some agreement between ratings should be expected. This is known as cross-rater concordance, and is a measure of the validity of the instrument rather than reliability. For instance, on the SPM, concordance between caregiver (home) and teacher (school) ratings ranged from a coefficient of 0.31 for balance and motion to 0.55 for planning and ideas. These represent moderate to high correlations, but are lower than minimum inter-rater reliability standards for performance-based tests. These results are acceptable for a context-based instrument, and reflect the importance of gathering data on children's ability to engage in daily life tasks, activities, and occupations based on observations of the child over time in daily environments.

Standard Error of Measurement

The *standard error of measurement (SEM)* is a statistic used to calculate the expected range of error for the test score of an individual. It is based on the range of scores an individual might obtain if the same test were administered a number of times simultaneously, with no practice or fatigue effects. Obviously, this is impossible; the SEM, therefore, is a theoretical construct. However, it is an indicator of the possible error variance in individual scores.

The SEM creates a normal curve for the individual's test scores, with the obtained score in the middle of the distribution. The child has a higher probability of receiving scores in the middle of the distribution than at the extreme ends. The SEM is based on the standard deviation of the test and the test's reliability (usually the test–retest reliability). The SEM can be calculated using the following formula:

$$SEM = SD\sqrt{(1 - r)}$$

where SEM is the standard error of measurement, SD is the standard deviation, and r is the reliability coefficient for the test (test–test reliability coefficients are the ones most commonly used). Once the SEM has been calculated for a test, that value is added to and subtracted from the child's obtained score. This gives the range of expected scores for that child, a range known as the *confidence interval*. The SEM corresponds to the standard deviation for the normal curve: 68% of the scores in a normal distribution fall within 1 SD on either side of the mean, 95% of the scores fall within 2 SD on either side of the mean, and 99.7% of the scores fall within 3 SD on either side of the mean. Similarly, a child receives a score within 1 SEM on either side of his or her obtained score 68% of the time; a score within 2 SEM of the obtained score 95% of the time; and a score within 3 SEM of the obtained score 99.7% of the time.

Generally, test manuals report the 95% confidence interval. As can be seen by the equation above, when the SD of the test is high or the reliability is low, the SEM increases. A larger SEM means that the range of possible scores for an individual child is much greater (i.e., a larger confidence interval) and consequently that there is a greater degree of possible error variance for the child's score. This means that the examiner is less confident that any score obtained for a child on that test represents the child's true score.

An example may help to illustrate this point. Two tests are given, both consisting of 50 items and both testing the same skill area. One test has an SD of 1.0 and a test–retest reliability coefficient of 0.90. The SEM for that test is calculated as follows:

$$SEM = \sqrt{(1 - 0.90)}$$
$$SEM = 0.32$$

The second test has an SD of 5.0 and a test–retest reliability coefficient of 0.75. The SEM for that test would be calculated as follows:

$$SEM = 5\sqrt{(1 - 0.75)}$$
$$SEM = 2.5$$

Using the SEM, a 95% confidence interval can be calculated for each test. A 95% confidence interval is 2 SEM; therefore, test 1 has a confidence interval of ±0.64 points from the obtained score, or a total of 1.28 points. Test 2 has a confidence interval of ±5 points, or a total of 10 points. If both tests were available for a particular client, an examiner could use test 1 with much more confidence that the obtained score is truly representative of that individual's abilities and is not caused by random error variance of the test.

Occupational therapists who use standardized tests should be aware of how much measurement error a test contains so that the potential range of performance can be estimated for each individual. Currently, the trend is to report standardized test results as confidence intervals rather than as individual scores.[17,32] Several tests, such as the BSID-III, the M-FUN, and the BOT-2, include confidence intervals for subtest or scaled scores so that examiners can determine the potential score range for each child. According to Bayley, "Confidence intervals also serve as a reminder that measurement error is inherent in all test scores and that the observed test score is only an estimate of true ability" (p. 104).[7]

Consideration of the SEM is especially important when the differences between two scores are evaluated (e.g., when the progress a child has made with therapy over time is evaluated).[63] If the confidence intervals of the two test scores overlap, it may be incorrect to conclude that any change has occurred. For instance, a child is tested in September and receives a raw score of 60. The child is tested again in June with the same test and receives a raw score of 75. Comparison of the two raw scores would seem to indicate that the child has made substantial progress. However, the scores should be considered in light of an SEM of 5.0. Using a 95% confidence interval (the 95% confidence interval is 2 SEM on either side of the obtained score), the confidence interval for the first score is 50 to 70, and the confidence interval of the second score is 65 to 85.

Based on the two test scores, it cannot be conclusively stated that the child has made progress because the confidence intervals overlap. It is conceivable that a substantial amount of the difference between the first and second scores is a result of error variance rather than actual change in the child's abilities. (See the article by Cunningham-Amundson and Crowe for a more in-depth discussion of the use of the SEM in pediatric assessment, particularly the effect of the SEM in the interpretation of test scores and the qualification of children for remedial services.[16])

Validity

Validity is the extent to which a test measures what it says it measures.[63] For example, it is important for testers to know that a test of fine motor development actually measures fine motor skills and not gross motor or perceptual skills. The validity of a test must be established with reference to the particular use for which the test is being considered.[63] For instance, a test of fine motor development is probably highly valid as a measure of fine motor skills. It is less valid as a measure of visual motor skills and has low validity as a measure of gross motor skills.

The information on validity reported in test manuals has been obtained during the test development process. In addition, after a test becomes available commercially, clinicians and researchers continue to evaluate validity and to publish the results of their validation studies. This information about test validity can help examiners make decisions about appropriate uses of standardized tests. The four categories of validity are construct-related validity, content-related validity, criterion-related validity, and Rasch analysis.

Construct-Related Validity

Construct-related validity is the extent to which a test measures a particular theoretic construct. Some constructs frequently measured by pediatric occupational therapists include fine motor skills, visual-perceptual skills, self-care skills, gross motor skills, and functional performance at home or school. There are many ways to determine construct validity, a few of which are discussed in this chapter.

One method of establishing construct validity involves investigating how well a test discriminates among different groups of individuals. For instance, a developmental test (e.g., BSID-III, PDMS-2, BOT-2) is expected to differentiate between the performance of older and younger children. Older children should receive higher scores than younger children, providing clear evidence of developmental progression with advancing age. Because these tests are also intended to discriminate typically developing children from children with developmental delays, children in specific diagnostic categories should receive lower scores than children with no documented deficits. This type of construct validity analysis is termed the "known groups" method.[54]

For example, during the development process for the Sensory Profile,[18] the sensory processing patterns of children in the following clinical groups were evaluated: attention deficit hyperactivity disorder, autism/pervasive developmental disorder, fragile X disorder, sensory modulation disorder, and other disabilities. The scores for children in each of these groups differed from that of the standardization sample, with the score ranges for all factors generally lower than those for the standardization sample. This indicates that the Sensory Profile is able to differentiate children with typical sensory processing from those who have sensory processing differences. In addition, score patterns for various clinical groups were identified, allowing therapists to compare client scores with those of the corresponding clinical group. Subsequent research using the

Sensory Profile has identified specific differences in sensory processing scores and sensory processing profiles for children with Asperger's syndrome, autism, fragile X disorder, and fetal alcohol syndrome.[21,29,55,62,64]

Factor analysis can be used as another method of establishing construct-related validity. *Factor analysis* is a statistical procedure for determining relationships between test items. In a test of motor skills that includes gross motor items and fine motor items, factor analysis is expected to identify two factors on which items showed the strongest correlation, one composed mostly of gross motor items and one composed mostly of fine motor items. Factor analysis of the Sensory Integration and Praxis Tests (SIPT)[4] resulted in identification of four primary factors. The constructs that emerged from the analysis demonstrated that the test primarily measures praxis (motor planning). The constructs measured were visual-perceptual skills (related to praxis); somatosensory-praxis skills; bilateral integration and sequencing of movements; and praxis on verbal command.[5] Factor analysis helped establish the functions that are measured by the SIPT and that can be used to interpret the results of testing individual children.

The third method of establishing construct-related validity requires repeated administration of a test before and after a period of intervention. For example, a group of children are given a test of visual-perceptual skills and subsequently receive intervention focused on improving those skills. They are then retested with the same test and the difference in scores is analyzed. A rise in test scores supports the assertion that the test measured visual-perceptual skills and provides evidence of construct-related validity.

Content-Related Validity

Content-related validity is the extent to which the items on a test accurately sample a particular behavior domain. For instance, to test self-care skills, it is impractical to ask a child to perform every conceivable self-care activity. A sample of self-care activities must be chosen for inclusion on the test, and conclusions can be drawn about the child's abilities on the basis of the selected items. Examiners must have confidence that self-care skills are adequately represented so that accurate conclusions regarding the child's self-care skills can be made. Test manuals should show evidence that the authors have systematically analyzed the domain being tested. Content validity is established by review of the test content by experts in the field, who reach some agreement that the content is, in fact, representative of the behavioral domain to be measured.

Criterion-Related Validity

Criterion-related validity is the ability of a test to predict how an individual performs on other measurements or activities. To establish criterion-related validity, the test score is checked against a criterion, an independent measure of what the test is designed to predict. The two forms of criterion-related validity are concurrent validity and predictive validity.

Concurrent validity describes how well test scores reflect current performance. The degree of relationship between the test and the criterion is described with a correlation coefficient. Most validity correlation coefficients range from 0.40 to 0.80; a coefficient of 0.70 or above indicates that performance on one test can predict performance on a second test.

Concurrent validity is examined in the test development process to determine the relationship between a new test and existing tests that measure a similar construct. For instance, during the development of the Sensory Profile, children were scored with both the Sensory Profile and the SFA. The SFA was chosen because some aspects of children's performance at school depend on sensory processing and modulation.[18] High correlations between SFA performance items and the Fine Motor/Perceptual factor on the Sensory Profile were expected, because both tests address hand use. In addition, the SFA socialization and behavior interaction sections were expected to correlate highly with the modulation sections and factors on the Sensory Profile, because problems with regulating sensory input could result in problems with generating appropriate responses. The scores on the two tests were compared for a random sample of 16 children enrolled in special education programs. Portions of the correlational data are presented in Table 8-4. The correlations are negative because of the different scoring systems on the two tests; lower scores are desirable on the SFA but undesirable on the Sensory Profile.

TABLE 8-4 Correlations between the Sensory Profile and the School Function Assessment

	School Function Assessment			
	Behavioral Regulation		Positive Interaction	
Sensory Profile				
FACTOR	ADAPTATIONS	ASSISTANCE	ADAPTATIONS	ASSISTANCE
1 Sensory Seeking	−0.434	−0.436	−0.095	−0.328
2 Emotionally Reactive	−0.372	−0.360	−0.245	−0.282
3 Low Endurance/Tone	−0.584*	−0.721*	−0.584*	−0.716*
4 Oral Sensory Sensitivity	−0.199	−0.320	.007	−0.300
5 Inattention/Distractibility	−0.582*	−0.584*	−0.495	−0.373
6 Poor Registration	−0.615*	−0.340	−0.348	−0.388
7 Sensory Sensitivity	−0.452	−0.478	−0.546*	−0.388
8 Sedentary	−0.551*	−0.554*	−0.545*	−0.368
9 Fine Motor/Perceptual	−0.502	−0.720†	−0.703†	−0.681†

Modified from Dunn, W. (1999). *Sensory Profile user's manual* (p. 54). San Antonio, TX: Psychological Corporation.
*Correlation is significant at the 0.05 level (2-tailed).
†Correlation is significant at the 0.01 level (2-tailed).

As Table 8-4 shows, there are areas of moderate to high correlation and areas of low correlation between the two tests. Factor 9, which consists of items describing product-oriented behaviors, correlated strongly with three sections of the SFA. Factors 3, 6, and 8 on the Sensory Profile contain items that indicate low responsiveness, whereas Factor 5 contains items indicating overresponsiveness. These four factors correlated moderately with the Behavioral Regulation and Positive Interaction sections of the SFA, suggesting relationships between sensory processing and modulation, and children's social/behavioral repertoires.[18] This pattern of correlation coefficients supports the research hypotheses about relationships between the constructs measured by the two tests and also supports the validity of the Sensory Profile as a measure of sensory processing and modulation.

In contrast with concurrent validity, *predictive validity* identifies the relationship between a test given in the present and some measure of performance in the future. Establishing predictive validity is a much lengthier process than establishing other forms of validity because often several years must elapse between the first and second testing sessions. The predictive validity of a test often is not well documented until it has been in use for several years. Barbosa, Campbell, and Berbaum studied the predictive validity of the Test of Infant Motor Performance (TIMP).[6] These researchers examined how well the TIMP, when administered shortly after birth, predicted the infant's outcome at 12 months. Using a sample of 96 at-risk infants recruited from special care nurseries, the infants were categorized as developmentally delayed, cerebral palsy, or typical at 12 months on the basis of their scores on the Alberta Infant Motor Scale and physician's clinical judgment. The TIMP scores at 13 weeks correctly classified all of the infants at 12 months. Two items, hand-to-mouth and fingering objects, were identified as highly accurate predictors of cerebral palsy (i.e., children with cerebral palsy did not exhibit fingering or hand-to-mouth movements).

One final point about criterion-related validity: the meaningfulness of the comparison between a test and its criterion measure depends on both the quality of the test and the quality of the criterion. Because no single measure of criterion-related validity provides conclusive evidence of the test's validity, multiple investigations should be undertaken. Important standardized assessments undergo extensive evaluation of validity after publication. The resulting information helps the test user decide when and with whom the test results are most valid.

In summary, validity is an important but sometimes elusive concept that rests on a number of judgments by authors of the tests, users of the tests, and experts in the field of occupational therapy. It is important to remember that validity is not an absolute and that a test that is valid in one setting or with one group of children may not be valid for other uses. Test users must not assume that because a test has been developed and published for commercial distribution, it is universally useful and appropriate. An examiner must apply his or her clinical knowledge and experience, knowledge of normal and abnormal development, and understanding of an individual child's situation when deciding whether a test is a valid measure of the child's abilities.

Rasch Model of Measurement

The Rasch models of measurement[1] have been used to develop item scaling for several tests in the field of occupational therapy. The SFA, the PEDI,[34] and the Assessment of Motor and Process Skills (AMPS)[23,24] have used Rasch methodology in the test development process. Rasch methodology has also been used to develop a school version of the AMPS (School AMPS).[2,25]

A test instrument developed using Rasch methodology must meet several assumptions.[14] The construct being measured (e.g., activities of daily living) can be represented as a continuous function with measurement covering the full range of possible performance from dependent to independent. The instrument (or individual scale of the instrument) measures one characteristic (or construct) of performance, and each item represents a sample of the characteristics measured. The scale provides estimates of item difficulty that are independent of the sample of persons tested, and an individual's ability estimate is independent of the specific items tested.

The Rasch model generates a hierarchical ranking of items on the test from easiest to most difficult, creating a linear scale of items from ordinal observations. With the items ranked along the continuum within each skill area, an individual's performance can be assessed in light of an item's difficulty rather than against a normative sample. The ranking of items creates an expected pattern of mastery of items; the model predicts that more difficult items on the continuum are mastered only after easier items have been. Therefore therapists who administer an assessment tool developed using Rasch methodology generally can assume that the most appropriate goals for intervention will be the items and/or skills immediately above the items successfully passed by the client.

Occupational therapy tests developed using Rasch methodology emerge from a different philosophical base than traditional standardized tests. The two main methods of data collection are naturalistic observation and parent/teacher/caregiver report. The tasks observed are the ones the child engages in daily (e.g., schoolwork, self-care, social participation, mobility) rather than items administered in a controlled testing situation. Intervention recommendations can be generated directly from the child's observed and/or reported performance and participation.

Tests developed using the Rasch model are not considered norm-referenced tests because individual performance is not compared against that of a normative sample. However, the Rasch model provides an objective measure of performance that can be linked directly to desired occupational performance outcomes. The Rasch model has been applied to a variety of rating scales and traditional measurement instruments to assess disablement and functional status.[33,56] It is a model that can be used alone or in conjunction with traditional test development and measurement theory to produce measurement tools that provide a clearer connection between the assessment process and intervention planning.

BECOMING A COMPETENT TEST USER

The amount of technical information presented here might make the prospect of learning to administer a standardized test seem daunting. However, potential examiners can take a number of specific steps to ensure that they administer and score a test reliably. These steps also help examiners interpret test results accurately so that they provide a valid representation of each child's abilities. This section discusses the process of learning to administer and interpret any standardized test, be it a screening tool or a comprehensive assessment.

Choosing the Appropriate Test

The therapist's first step is to decide which test, or tests, to learn. A number of standardized tests used by pediatric occupational therapists address a wide age span and a number of different performance skills and areas of occupation. The examiner must decide which tests are most likely to meet the assessment needs of his or her particular work setting and of the children served in that setting. For instance, an occupational therapist working in an early intervention setting might use the BSID-III or the PEDI.[34] A therapist working in preschools might use the M-FUN or the PDMS-2. A therapist working in a school-based setting might use the SFA, the School AMPS, or BOT-2. Instruments such as the PEDI or the AMPS can be used in a variety of settings.

A number of other standardized tests are available that assess more specialized areas of function, such as the SIPT, the Developmental Test of Visual-Motor Integration,[8] the Sensory Profile, or the DTVP-II. Examiners should consult with other therapists working in their practice settings to determine which tests are most commonly used. In addition, they should examine the characteristics of the children referred to them for assessment to determine which tests are most appropriate. Some children may not be able to comply with standardized testing procedures. In particular, children who are diagnosed with an autism spectrum disorder often do not cooperate with a structured testing environment. Occupational therapists evaluating these children often make adjustments in the standardized testing procedures or use nonstandardized assessments.[59] Observation-based standardized tests that obtain information from adult ratings or observation of the child in typical daily contexts are a useful alternative. See Table 8-1 for a list of selected standardized tests arranged by information source.

Learning the Test

Once a decision has been made about which test to learn, the therapist should read the test manual carefully. In addition to administration and scoring techniques, the technical attributes of the test should be studied. Particular attention should be paid to the size and composition of the normative sample, the reliability coefficients, the validation data, and the intended population for the test. The examiner should determine the standardized administration procedures and whether they can be altered for children with special needs. He or she should also understand how the scores should be reported and interpreted if the standardized procedure is changed.

It may also be appropriate to consult other sources for information about a test. The *Seventeenth Mental Measurements Yearbook*[31] and *Tests in Print VII*[49] publish descriptions and critical reviews of commercially available standardized tests written by testing experts. These resources can also be accessed online through most university library systems. In addition, published studies of the validity or reliability of tests relevant to pediatric occupational therapists appear throughout the occupational therapy literature.

The next step in learning a test is to observe it being administered by an experienced examiner. If possible, the therapist should also discuss administration, scoring, and interpretation of the test results. One observation may suffice; however, it may be helpful to watch several administrations of the test to children of different ages and abilities. Observation is an excellent way to learn how other examiners deal with the practical aspects of testing (e.g., arranging test materials, sequencing test items, handling unexpected occurrences, managing behavior). A discussion with the examiner about the interpretation of a child's performance can also be extremely helpful for acquiring an understanding of how observed behaviors are translated into conclusions and recommendations.

Once these preparatory activities have been completed, the learner should practice administering the test. Neighborhood children, friends, or relatives can be recruited to be "pilot subjects." It is a good idea to test several children whose ages are similar to those for whom the test is intended. Testing children, rather than adults, provides the realism of the mechanical, behavioral, and management issues that arise with a clinical population (Figure 8-6).

Checking Inter-rater Reliability

When possible, an experienced examiner should observe the testing and simultaneously score the items as a check of inter-rater reliability (Research Note 8-1). A simple way to assess inter-rater agreement is to use *point-by-point agreement*.[37] With this technique, one examiner administers and scores the test while the other observes and scores (Figure 8-7). The two examiners then compare their scores on each item. The number of items on which the examiners assigned the same score is then added.

Inter-rater agreement then is computed using this formula:

$$\text{Point-by-point agreement} = \frac{A}{A+D} \times 100$$

where *A* equals the number of items on which there was agreement and *D* equals the number of items on which there was disagreement.

The following example illustrates point-by-point agreement.

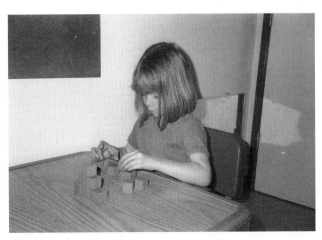

FIGURE 8-6 A child performs a fine motor item from the PDMS-2.

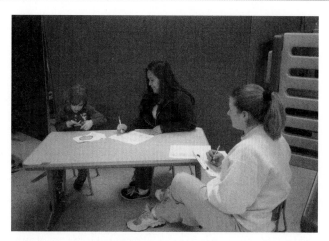

FIGURE 8-7 Two therapists check their inter-rater reliability by scoring the same testing session.

Two examiners score a test of 10 items. The child receives either a pass (+) or fail (−) for each item. The scores for each examiner are shown in Table 8-5. According to the data, the raters agreed on 7 of the 10 items. They disagreed on items 2, 7, and 9.

Their point-by-point agreement would be calculated as follows:

$$\frac{7}{7+3} = 0.70 \times 100 = 70\% \text{ Point-by-point agreement}$$

This means that the examiners agreed on the scores for 70% of the items. To benefit from this exercise, the two examiners should discuss the items on which they disagreed and their reasons for giving the scores they did. A new examiner may not understand the scoring criteria and may be making scoring errors as a result. The experienced examiner can help clarify scoring criteria. This procedure helps bring the new examiner's administration and scoring techniques in line with the standardized procedures.

The point-by-point agreement technique can also be used for periodic reliability checks by experienced examiners, and it is particularly important if the examiners may be testing the same children at different times. No universally agreed-on standard exists for a minimum acceptable level for point-by-point agreement. However, 80% is probably a good guideline. Examiners would be well advised to aim for agreement in the range of 90% if possible. Organization of the testing environment and materials can improve reliability by creating a standard structured environment.

Selecting and Preparing the Optimal Testing Environment

The testing environment should meet the specifications stated in the test manual. Generally, the manual specifies a well-lighted room free of visual or auditory distractions. If a separate room is not available, a screen or room divider can be used to partition off a corner of the room. An example of an appropriate test setup is shown in Figure 8-8.

Testing should be scheduled at a time when the child is able to perform optimally. For young children, caregivers should be consulted about the best time of day for testing so that the test session does not interfere with naps or feedings. Older children's school or other activities should be considered in the scheduling of assessments. For instance, a child who has just come from recess or a vigorous physical education session may have decreased endurance for gross motor activities.

The test environment should be ready before the child arrives. Furniture should be appropriately sized so that children sitting at a table can rest their feet flat on the floor and can comfortably reach items on the table. If a child uses a wheelchair or other adaptive seating, he or she should be allowed to sit in the equipment during testing. Infants or young children generally are best seated on the caregiver's lap unless particular items on the test specify otherwise. The examiner should place the test kit where he or she can easily access the items but not where the child can see or reach the kit. Often a low chair placed next to the examiner's chair is a good place to put a test kit.

Each examiner should consider what adaptations are necessary to administer the test efficiently. In many cases a test manual is too large and unwieldy to have at hand during testing, and the score sheet does not provide enough information about administration and scoring criteria. Examiners have developed many ways to meet this need. A common method

TABLE 8-5 Raters' Scores for Point-by-Point Agreement

Item	Rater 1	Rater 2
1	+	+
2	+	−
3	+	+
4	−	−
5	−	−
6	+	+
7	−	+
8	−	−
9	−	+
10	+	+

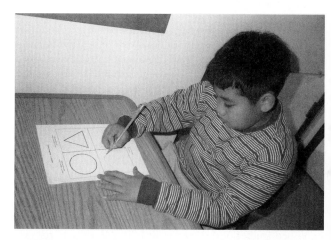

FIGURE 8-8 A child completes a portion of the visual-motor subtest of the Bruininks-Oseretsky Test of Motor Proficiency 2.

is preparation of a cue card on which the examiner records specific criteria for administration and scoring, including the instructions to be read to the child. This can be accomplished by making a series of note cards, putting color codes on a score sheet, or developing a score sheet with administration information.

Administering Test Items

Most important, the examiner must be so familiar with the test that his or her attention can be focused on the child's behavior and not on the mechanics of administering the test. This is a critical part of preparation, because much valuable information can be lost if the examiner is unable to observe carefully the quality of the child's responses because he or she instead must devote energy to finding test materials or looking through the test manual. In addition, young children's attention spans can be short, and the examiner must be able to take full advantage of the limited time the child is able to attend to the activities.

Familiarity with the test also allows the examiner to change the pace of activities if necessary. The child can be given a brief break to play, have a snack, or use the bathroom while the examiner interviews the caregiver or jots down notes. Most standardized tests have some flexibility about the order or arrangement of item sets, and an examiner who knows the test can use this to his or her advantage. Sometimes, because of the child's fatigue or behavior or because of time constraints, a test cannot be administered completely in one session. Most tests provide guidelines for administering the test in two sessions, and examiners should be familiar with these guidelines before starting to test.

Interpreting the Test

Before administering the test, the examiner should read the test interpretation section of the examiner's manual and discussion interpretation of the test with experienced examiners. It is essential for examiners to understand what conclusions can and cannot be drawn about a child's performance based on the items administered and standard scores obtained. In addition to the guidelines and interpretation standards specified in the test manual, the examiner must take into account a number of other factors when interpreting an individual child's test score. The following questions should be asked when interpreting test results:

- How representative or typical was the child's response to the testing situation? If the child did not appear to perform optimally during testing, what influenced the child's performance? When the parent observes the testing, the examiner should ask the parent if the child's performance was typical. The parent's judgment of the child's performance during testing can be included in the report of findings.
- How closely does the information obtained by the occupational therapist concur with standardized or nonstandardized test results, observations or reports by caregivers, teachers, or other professionals? Possible reasons for discrepancies can include different performance demands or expectations in various environments, differences in characteristics and

environmental supports provided to the child, differing levels of tolerance for children's behavior, or discrepant ability in different developmental or performance domains (may be identified when several disciplines are evaluating a child).
- Were there any strategies used during the testing that were either particularly effective or ineffective in organizing, motivating, or facilitating the child's best performance? Evaluating and discussing the efficacy of management strategies can provide important information to augment test results and recommendations.
- Did the tests administered provide a complete picture of the child's occupational performance and participation, or is additional testing, observation, or interview required?

Evaluating the Clinical Usefulness of the Test

The final area of preparation is to evaluate the clinical usefulness of the test. The learner should discuss the test with colleagues: What are its strengths and weaknesses? What important information does it give? What information needs to be collected through other techniques? For which children does it seem to work especially well and for which is it an especially poor choice? Can it be adapted for children with special needs? Does it measure what it says it measures? Do other tests do a better job of measuring the same behavioral domain? Is it helpful for program planning or program evaluation? An ongoing dialog is an important way to ensure that the process of standardized testing meets the needs of the children, families, therapists, and service agencies that use the tests. The steps to becoming a competent user of standardized tests are summarized in Box 8-4.

ETHICAL CONSIDERATIONS IN TESTING

All pediatric occupational therapists who use standardized tests in their practice must be aware of their responsibilities to the children they evaluate and their families. Urbina has discussed several ethical issues relevant to standardized testing, including (1) examiner competency, (2) client privacy, (3) communication of test results, and (4) cultural bias.[63]

BOX 8-4 Steps to Becoming a Competent Test User

1. Study the test manual.
2. Observe experienced examiners; discuss your observations.
3. Practice using the test.
4. Check inter-rater agreement with an experienced examiner.
5. Prepare administration and scoring cue sheets.
6. Prepare the testing environment.
7. Consult with experienced examiners about test interpretation.
8. Periodically recheck inter-rater agreement.

Examiner Competency

Examiner competency was discussed in detail in the previous section. However, it is important to reemphasize here that examiners must achieve a minimal level of competency with a test before using it in practice. Along with knowing how to administer and score a test, a competent examiner should know for whom the test is intended and for what purpose. This also means knowing when it is *not* appropriate to use a particular standardized instrument. The examiner should be able to evaluate the technical merits of the test and should know how these characteristics may affect its administration and interpretation. The examiner also should be aware of the many things that can affect a child's performance on a test, such as hunger, fatigue, illness, or distractions, as well as sources of test or examiner error.

The competent examiner draws conclusions about a child's performance on a standardized test only after considering all available information about the child. Such information can include the results of nonstandardized tests, informal observations, caregiver interviews, and reviews of documentation from other professionals. It is extremely important to put a child's observed performance on standardized testing in the context of all sources of information about the child; this ensures a more accurate and meaningful interpretation of standard scores.

Client Privacy

The Privacy Rule of the Health Insurance Portability and Accountability Act (HIPAA) mandates that all recipients of health care services be notified of their privacy rights; that they have access to their medical information, including provision of copies at their request; and that they be notified of any disclosure of medical information for purposes other than treatment or billing. For minor children, the parent or legal guardian must provide consent prior to initiation of any evaluation or intervention procedures. Agencies have different forms and processes for obtaining consent, and examiners must be aware of the procedures for their particular institution. Informed consent generally is obtained in writing and consists of an explanation of the reasons for testing, the types of tests to be used, the intended use of the tests and their consequences (i.e., program placement or qualification for remedial services), and the testing information that will be released and to whom it will be released. Parents/guardians should be given a copy of the summary report and should be informed about who will receive the additional copies. If test scores or other information will be used for research purposes, additional consent procedures must be followed.

Verbal exchanges about the child should be limited. Although it is often necessary to discuss a case with a colleague for the purposes of information sharing and consultation, it is not acceptable to have a casual conversation about a particular child in the elevator, lunchroom, or hallway. If others overhear the conversation, a violation of confidentiality could result.

Communication of Test Results

Reports should be written in language that is understandable to a nonprofessional, with a minimum of jargon. Each report should be objective in tone, and the conclusions and recommendations should be clearly stated. When the results of tests are discussed, the characteristics of the person receiving the information should be taken into account.

Speaking with other professionals and speaking with family members require different communication techniques. When sharing assessment results with family members, the examiner should be aware of the general level of education and, in the case of bilingual families, the level of proficiency with English. Even if family members have a reasonable capability in the English language, it may be a good idea to have an interpreter available. Often the family members most skilled in English act as interpreters. However, this may not be the optimal arrangement for sessions in which test results are discussed because of the technical nature of some of the information. The ideal interpreter is one who is familiar with the agency and the kinds of testing and services it offers and who has developed techniques for helping examiners offer information in an understandable and culturally meaningful way.

When presenting information to family members, examiners must also consider the anticipated emotional response. A parent who hears that his young child has developmental delays may be emotionally devastated. Therefore the information should be communicated sensitively. Every child has strengths and attributes that can be highlighted in the discussion of his or her overall performance. The examiner should also avoid any appearance of placing blame on the parent for the child's difficulties, because many parents are quick to blame themselves for their child's problems. The tone of any discussion should be objective, yet positive, with the emphasis placed on sharing information and making joint decisions about a plan of action.

Cultural Bias

A number of authors have discussed the cultural bias inherent in standardized tests.[44,45,53,63] Tests developed primarily on a white, middle-class population may not be valid when used with children from diverse cultural backgrounds. It is important for examiners to be aware of the factors that may influence how children from diverse cultures perform on standardized tests.

Children who have not had any experience with testing may not understand the unspoken rules about test taking. They may not understand the importance of doing a task within a time limit or of following the examiner's instructions. They may not be motivated to perform well on tasks because the task itself has no intrinsic meaning to them. The materials or activities may be seen as irrelevant, or the child, having had no experience with the kinds of materials used in the tests, may not know how to interact with them. Establishing a rapport may be difficult either because of language barriers or because of a cultural mismatch between the child's social interaction patterns and those of the examiner. If the examiner is aware of these potential problems, steps can be taken to minimize possible difficulties.

The caregiver or an interpreter can be present to help put the child more at ease. The caregiver can be questioned about the child's familiarity with the various test materials; this information can help the examiner determine whether the child's failure to perform individual items is the result of unfamiliarity with the materials or of inability to complete the task. The caregiver can also be shown how to administer some items, particularly those involving physical contact or proximity to the child. This may make the situation less threatening for the child. However, if these adjustments are made, standard procedure has been violated, and it may be inappropriate to compute a standard score. Even so, the test can provide a wealth of descriptive information about the child's abilities.

Standardized tests should be used cautiously with children from diverse cultures. Occupational therapists who find themselves frequently evaluating children from cultural or ethnic groups that are underrepresented in the normative samples of most standardized tests may want to consider developing "local norms" on frequently used instruments that reflect the typical patterns of performance among children of that culture. This information can help provide a more realistic appraisal of children's strengths and needs. Several studies have evaluated the performance of children from different countries and/or different cultural groups on pediatric standardized tests developed in the United States and identified differences in test outcomes.[11,12,15,22,36,39] In addition, observation of the child in a variety of contexts and communication with the family, caregivers, and others familiar with the child are essential to the assessment process.

Clearly, when using standardized tests, occupational therapists must have a number of skills beyond the ability simply to administer test items. Professional communication skills are essential when administering tests and reporting information. Awareness of family and cultural values helps put the child's performance in a contextual framework. An understanding of the professional and ethical responsibilities involved in dealing with sensitive and confidential information is also extremely important. A competent examiner brings all of these skills into play when administering, scoring, interpreting, and reporting the results of standardized tests.

ADVANTAGES AND DISADVANTAGES OF STANDARDIZED TESTING

Standardized tests have allowed occupational therapists and other professionals to develop a more scientific approach to assessment, and the use of tests that give statistically valid numeric scores has helped give the assessment process more credibility. However, standardized tests are not without their drawbacks. This section discusses the advantages and disadvantages of using standardized tests, and presents suggestions on how to make test results more accurate and meaningful.

Advantages

Standardized tests have several characteristics that make them a unique part of the assessment inventory of pediatric occupational therapists. For example, they are tests that in general are well known and commercially available. This means that a child's scores on a particular test can be interpreted and understood by therapists in other practice settings or geographic locations.

Standard scores generated by standardized tests allow testers from a variety of professional disciplines to "speak the same language" when it comes to discussing test scores. For example, a child may be tested by an occupational therapist for fine motor skills, by a physical therapist for gross motor

skills, and by a speech pathologist for language skills. All three tests express scores as T-scores. An average T-score is 50. The child receives a fine motor T-score of 30, a gross motor T-score of 25, and a language T-score of 60. It is apparent that although this child is below average in both gross and fine motor skills, language skills are an area of strength; in fact, they are above average. These scores can be compared and discussed by the assessment team, and they can be used to identify areas requiring intervention and areas in which the child has particular strengths.

Standardized tests can be used to monitor developmental progress. Because they are norm-referenced according to age, the progress of a child with developmental delays can be measured against expected developmental progress compared with the normative sample. In this way, occupational therapists can determine if children receiving therapy are accelerating their rate of development because of intervention. Similarly, children who are monitored after discharge from therapy can be assessed periodically to determine whether they are maintaining the expected rate of developmental progress or are beginning to fall behind their peers without the assistance of intervention.

Standardized tests can be used for program evaluation to determine response to intervention across a large number of clients. Standard test scores can be subjected to statistical analysis to evaluate efficacy of interventions. These data can contribute to evidence-based practice and provide information about areas of strength and weakness in the intervention program that can be addressed through quality improvement processes.

Disadvantages

The importance of assessing standardized testing results within the child's performance context is discussed in Chapter 7. A standardized test cannot stand alone as a measure of a child's abilities. Clinical judgment, informal or unstructured observation, caregiver interviews, and data gathering from other informants are all essential parts of the assessment process. These less structured evaluation procedures are needed to provide meaning and interpretation for the numeric scores obtained by standardized testing.

Several other considerations must be taken into account when standardized tests are used. For example, a test session provides only a brief "snapshot" of a child's behavior and abilities. The performance a therapist sees in a 1-hour assessment in a clinic setting may be different from that seen daily at home or at school. Illness, fatigue, or anxiety, or lack of familiarity with the test materials, the room, or the tester can adversely affect a child's performance. The tester must be sensitive to the possible impact of these factors on the child's performance.

A competent tester can do a great deal to alleviate a child's anxiety about testing and to ensure that the experience is not an unpleasant one. However, any test situation is artificial and usually does not provide an accurate indication of how the child performs on a daily basis. Therefore it is important for the therapist to speak to the child's parent, caregiver, or teacher at the time of testing to determine whether the observed behavior is truly representative of the child's typical performance, and the representativeness of the behavior must be taken into account when the child's test scores are interpreted and reported.

Another concern about standardized tests is the rigidity of the testing procedures themselves. Standardized tests specify both particular ways of administering test items and, in many cases, exactly what instructions the tester must give. In view of these administration requirements, children who have difficulty understanding verbal instruction (e.g. with autism, hearing impairment, or attention deficit) or lack control of movement (e.g., with muscle weakness or lack of coordination) may be disadvantaged on performance-based tests. Although this issue is not addressed by all standardized tests, some provide guidelines for administering the test under nonstandard conditions, and some are specifically designed to evaluate functional performance and participation of children with disabilities using performance-based and observation-based formats. For example, the PDMS-2 provides case illustrations of how the test can be adapted for children with vision impairment and cerebral palsy. The BSID-III and the Sensory Profile provide normative data for several clinical groups. Piper and Darrah, in developing the AIMS, used infants who were preterm or born with congenital anomalies, as well as those who were full term and those who did not have an unusual diagnosis.[52] The PEDI, the Gross Motor Function Measure (GMFM),[57] and the SFA are examples of tests that evaluate function and participation of children with identified disabilities. The PEDI measures the level of caregiver assistance and environmental modifications required for children to perform specific functional tasks. The PEDI assesses the level of independence and the quality of performance of children whose disabilities may prevent them from executing a particular task in a typical way. The GMFM is a criterion-referenced test that measures the components of a gross motor activity accomplished by children with cerebral palsy. It provides information necessary for designing intervention programs and measuring small increments of change. The SFA evaluates the child's performance of functional tasks that support participation in the academic and social aspects of an elementary school program.

It is important to reiterate that although it is permissible to alter the administration procedures of most performance-based tests to accommodate children's individual needs, the child's performance cannot be expressed as a standard score. Rather, the purpose of the testing is to provide a structured format for describing the child's performance (Case Study 8-1). The test manual should always be consulted for guidelines on alterations in test procedures.

CASE STUDY 8-1 Caitlin

Caitlin is a 5.5-year-old kindergarten student referred for occupational therapy assessment by her teacher, Mrs. Clark, who notes that Caitlin is having difficulty learning to write; she holds her pencil awkwardly and exerts too much pressure on the paper. On the playground she has difficulty keeping up with her peers, falls frequently, appears uncoordinated, and has difficulty learning new motor skills. Her energy level is low. She is easily overwhelmed by typical classroom activity and often has emotional outbursts, which affect her ability to complete her work and interact with classmates.

The occupational therapist, Debra, spoke to Caitlin's parents and discovered that Caitlin received physical therapy as an infant because of low muscle tone and slow achievement of developmental milestones. Her parents were worried about her ability to cope with the increase in writing assignments in first grade and her social acceptance by other children.

Debra considered Caitlin's age (5.5 years) and the areas of concern (gross and fine motor skills and social adjustment) in choosing which standardized tests to use. She decided to administer the PDMS-2, along with clinical observations of Caitlin's posture, muscle tone, strength, balance, motor planning, hand use and hand preference, attention, problem-solving skills, and visual skills. She asked Caitlin's teacher to complete the SFA to provide information on Caitlin's performance of functional school-related behaviors. In addition, she had the teacher complete the Sensory Profile School Companion (SPSC) (Dunn, 2006) to determine whether sensory processing problems were contributing to Caitlin's motor delays.

TEST RESULTS

Caitlin's testing session was scheduled at midmorning to avoid possible effects of fatigue or hunger. She attended well, although she needed encouragement for the more challenging items. By the end of the session she complained of fatigue, but Debra believed she was able to get a representative sample of Caitlin's motor skills and that the scores obtained were reliable.

On the PDMS-2 Caitlin received a gross motor quotient of 81, placing her at the 10th percentile for her age. Her fine motor quotient was 76, placing her at the 5th percentile. In the gross motor area, ball skills were an area of relative strength, but she had difficulty with balance activities and activities involving hopping, skipping, and jumping. In the fine motor area, Caitlin used a static tripod grasp on the pencil, frequently shifting into a fisted grasp if the writing task was challenging. Based on the small number of visual-motor items on this test, visual-perceptual skills appeared to be an area of strength, whereas tasks involving speed and dexterity were difficult.

Debra found that Caitlin had low muscle tone overall, particularly in the shoulder girdle and hands, and strength was somewhat decreased overall. Caitlin's endurance was poor. Motor planning difficulties were evident in the way she handled test materials and moved about the environment. She had difficulty devising alternate ways to accomplish tasks that were challenging for her and required manual guidance to complete some tasks.

Debra obtained a functional profile on the SFA based on Mrs. Clark's responses to the items on the test. On the scales of recreational movement, using materials, clothing management, written work, and task behavior and/or completion, Caitlin received scores below the cutoff for her grade level. Other scales were within grade-level expectations, with strengths in the scales of memory and understanding, following social conventions, and personal care awareness.

On the SPSC, scores indicated that Caitlin had definite differences in Environmental Sensations–Auditory and Body Sensations–Movement. She also received definite difference scores in School Factors 1, indicating a need for external

CASE STUDY 8-1 Caitlin—cont'd

support for sensory input, and School Factor 3, a low tolerance for sensory input. The scale confirmed that she could easily become overloaded by environmental stimuli.

OBSERVATIONS AND RECOMMENDATIONS

According to her scores on the PDMS-2, Caitlin had mild delays in her gross motor skills and mild to moderate delays in her fine motor skills. Although Debra believed that the PDMS-2 gave a good indication of what Caitlin could do under optimal circumstances (i.e., a nondistracting environment, individual attention and encouragement, and structuring of tasks to maximize success and minimize frustration), she also thought it did not represent the level of performance that would be seen over the course of a typical day.

In the classroom Debra observed that Caitlin avoided motor activities and completed writing and drawing activities rapidly, resulting in poor quality of the endproduct. Her materials were disorganized, she required multiple reminders to complete tasks, and she became upset when unable to finish on time. SFA results indicated that her performance of tasks involving fine and gross motor coordination and task organization was below grade-level expectations.

Debra met with the teacher, psychologist, principal, and Caitlin's parents to determine a plan of action. The SFA was used to facilitate collaborative problem solving by helping to identify which specific areas of school function could be targeted in the classroom and which skills should be identified as functional outcomes.

The team determined that Debra would provide recommendations to Mrs. Clark about classroom modifications and activities that would increase Caitlin's success and build her motor skills. The team members also collaborated to design strategies and routines that could be used at school and at home to improve Caitlin's on-task behavior, sensory responsiveness, organization, and ability to manage daily tasks at school.

Debra provided a chair that fit Caitlin better and allowed better positioning for writing. She provided Mrs. Clark with ideas for appropriate activities and ways of teaching Caitlin new motor skills and addressing her sensory needs. Debra provided Caitlin's parents with suggestions for family activities that would improve general strength and endurance (e.g., bicycle riding and swimming) and provided specific ideas for ways they could build Caitlin's fine motor skills at home. She also agreed to be available to Mrs. Clark for periodic informal consultation. It was agreed that a reassessment would be scheduled at the end of the school year so that the team could make a decision about further intervention and program planning for the next school year.

SUMMARY

Standardized testing, specifically the PDMS-2, SFA, and SPSC, provided a helpful framework for Debra's assessment of Caitlin and gave specific information about areas of strength and difficulty. Debra made use of her clinical observations and information gathering from a variety of sources to recommend interventions she felt would be beneficial, efficient, and relatively easy to implement. The standardized scores helped her identify Caitlin's problems in fine and gross motor skills, and the test items provided activities that revealed the challenges Caitlin faced when performing motor tasks. However, if Debra had simply relied on the standardized test scores, she would not have acquired the breadth of knowledge that led to her decision-making process for developing intervention options. This example illustrates the important roles of both standardized testing and other methods of data collection in arriving at meaningful and realistic conclusions about children's intervention needs and modes of service delivery.

RESEARCH NOTE 8-1

Jankovich M., Mullen J., Rinear E., Tanta K., & Deitz, J. (2008). Revised Knox Preschool Play Scale: Interrater agreement and construct validity. American Journal of Occupational Therapy, 62, 221–227.

ABSTRACT

The purpose of this study was to evaluate inter-rater agreement and construct validity of the Revised Knox Preschool Play Scale. Two raters who were trained separately evaluated 38 typically developing children, ages 36 to 72 months. For each child, the raters observed two 15-minute free-play sessions. For the overall play age, the scores of the two raters were within 8 months of each other 86.8% of the time; for the 4 dimension scores, they were within 12 months of each other 91.7% to 100% of the time; and for the 12 category scores, they were within one age level of each other 81.8% to 100% of the time. Construct validity results showed a general match between the children's chronological ages and their overall play age scores. The authors made three recommendations for future instrument development: (1) provide more detail on how to interpret and score play behaviors, (2) provide guidelines for using open-ended questions to children to clarify play scenarios, and (3) consider allowing use of a prompt by the examiner so that a greater variety of play behaviors can be observed.

IMPLICATIONS FOR PRACTICE

- Two raters can achieve acceptable consistency in scoring this instrument.
- The scores on the test reflect a developmental progression in play skills, supporting the construct validity of the instrument.
- If a child's score is within 8 months of chronological age, play skills should be considered age-appropriate. If scores are more than 8 months below chronological age, additional assessment should be considered.
- Information obtained in this study provides occupational therapists with psychometric data to support the use of this instrument for evaluating play skills of preschool children.
- Recommendations made by the authors could improve the validity and reliability of the instrument.

REFERENCES

1. Andrich, D. (1988). *Rasch models for measurement.* Beverly Hills, CA: Sage Publications.
2. Atchison, B. T., Fisher, A. B., & Bryze, K. (1998). Rater reliability and internal scale and person response validity of the School Assessment of Motor and Process Skills. *American Journal of Occupational Therapy, 52,* 843–850.
3. Ayres, A. J. (1972). *Southern California Sensory Integration Tests.* Los Angeles: Western Psychological Corporation.
4. Ayres, A. J. (1989). *Sensory Integration and Praxis Test manual.* Los Angeles: Western Psychological Corporation.
5. Ayres, A. J., & Marr, D. (1991). Sensory Integration and Praxis Tests. In A. Fisher, E. Murray, & A. Bundy (Eds.), *Sensory integration: Theory and practice* (pp. 201–233). Philadelphia: F.A. Davis.
6. Barbosa, V. M., Campbell, S., Berbaum, M. (2007). Discriminating infants from different developmental outcome groups using the Test of Infant Motor Performance (TIMP) Item Responses. *Pediatric Physical Therapy, 19,* 28–39.
7. Bayley, N. (2006). *Bayley Scales of Infant and Toddler Development, Motor Scale* (3rd ed.). San Antonio, TX: PsychCorp.
8. Beery, K. E., Buktenica, N. A., & Beery, N. A. (2004). *Developmental Test of Visual-Motor Integration* (5th ed.). Los Angeles: Western Psychological Services.
9. Bricker, D. (Ed.). (2002). *Assessment, evaluation, and programming system for infants and children* (2nd ed.). Baltimore: Brookes.
10. Bruininks, R. H., & Bruininks, B. D. (2005). *Bruininks-Oseretsky Test of Motor Proficiency* (2nd ed.) Manual. Circle Pines, MN: AGS Publishing.
11. Chow, S. M. K. (2005). The suitability of the Sensory Profile for diagnosing sensory modulation dysfunctions in Chinese children. *International Journal of Rehabilitation Research, 28,* 153–158.
12. Chow, S. M. K., Henderson, S. E., & Barnett, A. L. (2001). The Movement Assessment Battery for Children: A comparison of 4-year-old to 6-year-old children from Hong Kong and the United States. *American Journal of Occupational Therapy, 55,* 55–61.
13. Coster, W. (1998). Occupation-centered assessment of children. *American Journal of Occupational Therapy, 52,* 337–344.
14. Coster, W., Deeney, T., Haltiwanger, J., & Haley, S. (1998). *School Function Assessment.* San Antonio, TX: Psychological Corporation.
15. Crowe, T. K., McClain, C., & Provost, B. (1999). Motor development of Native American children on the Peabody Developmental Motor Scales. *American Journal of Occupational Therapy, 53,* 514–518.
16. Cunningham-Amundson, S. J., & Crowe, T. K. (1993). Clinical applications of the standard error of measurement for occupational and physical therapists. *Physical and Occupational Therapy in Pediatrics, 12*(4), 57–71.
17. Deitz, J. C. (1989). Reliability. *Physical and Occupational Therapy in Pediatrics, 9*(1), 125–147.
18. Dunn, W. (1999). *Sensory Profile User's Manual.* San Antonio: Psychological Corporation.
19. Dunn, W. (2006). *Sensory Profile School Companion.* San Antonio, TX: Psychological Corporation.
20. Dunn, W., Brown, C., & McGuigan, A. (1994). The ecology of human performance: A framework for considering the effect of context. *American Journal of Occupational Therapy, 48,* 595–607.
21. Dunn, W., Myles, B. S., & Orr, S. (2002). Sensory processing issues associated with Asperger syndrome: A preliminary investigation. *American Journal of Occupational Therapy, 56,* 97–102.
22. Egilson, S. T., & Coster, W. J. (2004). School Function Assessment: Performance of Icelandic students with special needs. *Scandinavian Journal of Occupational Therapy, 11,* 163–170.
23. Fisher, A. G. (2003). *Assessment of Motor and Process Skills. Vol. 1: Development, standardization, and administration manual* (5th ed.). Fort Collins, CO: Three Star Press.
24. Fisher, A. G. (2003). *Assessment of Motor and Process Skills. Vol. 2: User manual* (5th ed.). Fort Collins, CO: Three Star Press.
25. Fisher, A. G., Bryze, K., & Atchison, B. T. (2000). Naturalistic assessment of functional performance in school settings: Reliability and validity of the School AMPS scales. *Journal of Outcome Measurement, 4,* 504–522.
26. Fisher, W. P. (1993). Measurement-related problems in functional assessment. *American Journal of Occupational Therapy, 47,* 331–338.
27. Folio, M. R., & Fewell, R. R. (2000). *Peabody Developmental Motor Scales* (2nd ed.). Austin, TX: Pro-Ed.
28. Frankenburg, W. K., & Dodds, J. B. (1990). *Denver II Developmental Screening Test.* Denver, CO: Denver Developmental Materials.
29. Franklin, L., Deitz, J., Jirikowic, T., & Astley, S. (2008). Children with Fetal Alcohol Spectrum Disorders: Problem behaviors and sensory processing. *American Journal of Occupational Therapy, 62,* 265–273.
30. Furuno, S., O'Reilly, K. A., Hosaka, C. M., Inatsuka, T. T., Allman, T. L., & Zeisloft, B. (2005). *HELP activity guide (0–3).* Palo Alto, CA: Vort.
31. Geiger, K. F., Spies, R. A., Carlson, J. F., & Plake, B. S. (2007). *Seventeenth mental measurements yearbook.* Lincoln, NE: Buros Institute of Mental Measurements.
32. Gregory, R. J. (2000). *Psychological testing: History, principles and applications* (3rd ed.). Needham Heights, MA: Allyn & Bacon.
33. Grimby, G., Andren, E., Holmgren, E., Wright, B., Linacre, J. M., & Sundh, V. (1996). Structure of a combination of functional independence measure and instrumental activity measure items in community-living persons: A study of individuals with cerebral palsy and spina bifida. *Archives of Physical Medicine and Rehabilitation, 77,* 1109–1114.
34. Haley, S. M., Coster, W. J., Ludlow, L. H., Haltiwanger, J. T., & Andrellos, P. J. (1992). *Pediatric Evaluation of Disability Inventory: Development, standardization and administration manual.* San Antonio, TX: Psychological Corporation.
35. Hammill, D. D., Pearson, N. A., & Voress, J. K. (1993). *Developmental Test of Visual Perception* (2nd ed.). Austin, TX: Pro-Ed.
36. Katz, N., Kizony, R., & Parush, S. (2002). Visuomotor organization and thinking operations of school-age Ethiopian, Bedouin, and mainstream Israeli children. *Occupational Therapy Journal of Research, 22,* 34–43.
37. Kazdin, A. E. (1982). *Single-case research designs.* New York: Oxford University Press.
38. Keller, J., Kafkes, A., & Kielhofner, G. (2005). Psychometric characteristics of the Child Occupational Self Assessment (COSA), Part One: An initial examination of psychometric properties. *Scandinavian Journal of Occupational Therapy, 12,* 118–127.
39. Kerfeld, C. I., Guthrie, M. R., & Stewart, K. B. (1997). Evaluation of the Denver-II as applied to Alaska Native children. *Pediatric Physical Therapy, 9,* 23–31.
40. Kielhofner, G. (2007). *Model of human occupation: Theory and application* (4th ed.). Philadelphia: Lippincott Williams & Wilkins.
41. King, G., Law, M., King, S., Hurley, P., Hanna, S., Kertoy, M., et al. (2004). *Children's Assessment of Participation and Enjoyment (CAPE) and Preferences for Activities of Children (PAC).* San Antonio, TX: Harcourt Assessment, Inc.
42. Law, M., Baptiste, S., Carswell, A., McColl, M., Polatajko, H., & Pollock, N. (1998). *Canadian Occupational Performance Measure* (3rd ed.). Ottawa: CAOT Publications.
43. Law, M., Cooper, B., Strong, S., Stewart, D., Rigby, P., & Letts, L. (1996). Person-environment-occupation model: A transactive approach to occupational performance. *Canadian Journal of Occupational Therapy, 63,* 9–23.
44. Leavitt, R. L. (1999). *Cross-cultural rehabilitation: An international perspective.* London: W.B. Saunders.
45. Lynch, E. W., & Hanson, M. J. (Eds.). (1998). *Developing cross-cultural competence: A guide for working with young children and their families.* Baltimore: Brookes.

46. Miller, L. J. (1988). *Miller Assessment for Preschoolers: MAP manual* (rev. ed.). San Antonio, TX: Psychological Corporation.

47. Miller, L. J. (1990). *First STEp screening tool.* San Antonio, TX: Psychological Corporation.

48. Miller, L. J. (2006). *Miller Function and Participation Scales Examiner's Manual.* San Antonio, TX: The Psychological Corporation.

49. Murphy, L. L., Spies, R. A., & Plake, B. S. (Eds.). (2006). *Tests in print VII.* Lincoln, NE: Buros Institute of Mental Measurements.

50. Parham, L. D., Ecker, C., Kuhaneck, H. M., Henry, D. A., & Glennon, T. J. (2007). *Sensory Processing Measure Manual.* Los Angeles: Western Psychological Services.

51. Parks, S. (2006). *Inside HELP: Administration manual (0–3).* Palo Alto, CA: Vort.

52. Piper, M. C., & Darrah, J. (1994). *Motor assessment of the developing infant.* London: W.B. Saunders.

53. Polgar, J. M. (2003). Critiquing assessments. In B. Crepeau, E. S. Cohn, & B. A. Boyt Schell (Eds.), *Willard and Spackman's occupational therapy* (10th ed., pp. 299–313). Philadelphia: Lippincott Williams & Wilkins.

54. Portney, L. G., & Watkins, M. P. (2006). *Foundations of clinical research: Applications to practice.* Upper Saddle River, NJ: Prentice Hall Health.

55. Rogers, S. J., Hepburn, S., & Wehner, E. (2003). Parent reports of sensory symptoms in toddlers with autism and those with other developmental disorders. *Journal of Autism and Developmental Disorders, 25,* 61–70.

56. Roth, E. J., Heinemann, A. W., Lovell, L. L., Harvey, R. L., McGuire, J. R., & Diaz, S. (1998). Impairment and disability: Their relation during stroke rehabilitation. *Archives of Physical Medicine and Rehabilitation, 79,* 329–335.

57. Russell, D., Rosenbaum, P., Avery, L. M., & Lane, M. (2002). *Gross Motor Function Measure.* (GMFM-66 and GMFM-88). User's manual. Cambridge, UK: Cambridge University Press.

58. Sternberg, R. J. (1990). *Metaphors of mind: Conceptions of the nature of intelligence.* Cambridge, UK: Cambridge University Press.

59. Stuhec, V., & Gisel, E. G. (2003). Compliance with administration procedures of tests for children with pervasive developmental disorder: Does it exist? *Canadian Journal of Occupational Therapy, 70,* 33–41.

60. Terman, L. M., & Merrill, M. A. (1937). *Measuring intelligence.* Boston: Houghton Mifflin.

61. Thorndike, R. L., Hagen, E. P., & Sattler, J. M. (1986). *Technical manual, Stanford-Binet Intelligence Scale* (4th ed.). Chicago: Riverside.

62. Tomchek, S. D., & Dunn, W. (2007). Sensory processing in children with and without autism: A comparative study using the Short Sensory Profile. *American Journal of Occupational Therapy, 61,* 190–200.

63. Urbina, S. (2004). *Essentials of psychological testing.* Hoboken, NJ: Wiley.

64. Watling, R. L., Deitz, J., & White, O. (2001). Comparison of Sensory Profile scores of young children with and without autism spectrum disorders. *American Journal of Occupational Therapy, 55,* 416–423.

65. Wechsler, D. (1991). *Wechsler Intelligence Scale for Children.* San Antonio, TX: Harcourt.

66. World Health Organization. (2001). *The International Classification of Functioning, Disability, and Health.* Geneva, Switzerland: World Health Organization.

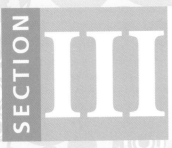

Occupational Therapy Intervention: Performance Areas

CHAPTER 9

Application of Motor Control/Motor Learning to Practice

Jane O'Brien   •   Harriet Williams

KEY TERMS

Dynamical systems
Postural control
Motor control
Motor learning
Vestibular

Balance
Visual perception
Feedback
Transfer of learning

OBJECTIVES

1. Understand the concepts of motor control and motor learning theories.
2. Develop interventions for children with motor control deficits based on current motor control/motor learning research.
3. Compare and contrast intervention using motor control/motor learning approaches.
4. Describe components of motor control that influence movement, including postural control, balance, visual perception, and body awareness.
5. Define concepts of motor learning including transfer of learning, feedback, practice, sequencing and adapting tasks, modeling or demonstration, and mental rehearsal.

Typically-developing children move into and out of positions fluidly and with ease, exploring their worlds, learning about their bodies, and developing motor, cognitive, sensory, and social skills. They use their hands for feeding, dressing, bathing, play, and academics (Figure 9-1). They practice sitting, walking, jumping, and crawling. They play in a variety of positions and show variability in their movements. Conversely, children with motor control deficits have difficulty in such activities and may not have the same opportunities to explore their surroundings; they may take longer and often do not master movements. Because motor control is central to participation, occupational therapists are concerned with how to help children control movements so that they may engage in their occupations.

This chapter presents case examples to illustrate the principles of motor control and motor learning related to occupational therapy practice, beginning with a definition of motor control and an overview of past motor approaches. Next, dynamical systems theory and the components of movement, including postural control, balance, visual perception, and body awareness are explained to help readers understand the complexity of movement. A definition of related motor learning and a review of related key concepts, including practice, feedback, modeling or demonstration, and mental rehearsal, also are provided.

Case Studies 9-1 through 9-3 illustrate the diversity of motor control deficits found in children. Motor control deficits interfere with activities of daily living, self-care, social participation,

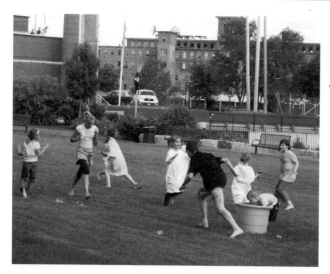

FIGURE 9-1 Children playing involves a variety of motor skills.

CASE STUDY 9-2 Georgia

Georgia is a 2-year-old girl who has difficulty playing on the playground. She is diagnosed with cerebral palsy, right hemiplegia. She walks but her movements are awkward and slow. She leans to the left and drags her right toe on the ground. Her right leg is positioned in the "typical" hemiplegic pattern (internally rotated, foot pronated, ankle extended). She does not use her right hand when playing with her toys and has difficulty manipulating objects. The other children run quickly past her. Georgia falls frequently. She looks frustrated at times that her body will not cooperate with her intentions.

CASE STUDY 9-3 Devin

Devin is a 10-year-old boy who has difficulty with fine-motor tasks, such as tying his shoes, buttoning, and, especially, writing. He takes longer than his peers to get ready for recess. Devin is awkward in his movements, falls frequently, and experiences difficulty with balance and coordination skills. He cannot skip, hop, or ride a bicycle. Eye-hand coordination is poor as shown in his inability to catch a ball or play games such as baseball or Frisbee. Devin has been diagnosed with developmental coordination disorder (DCD) (Box 9-1). He has above average intelligence and enjoys playing with other children, although he tends to stay on the "fringes" of the activity.

BOX 9-1 Description of Developmental Coordination Disorder

Developmental coordination disorder (DCD) refers to children who exhibit motor coordination markedly less effective than expected for their chronological age and intellectual ability. The motor coordination impairments must significantly interfere with activities of daily living and cannot be a result of physical, sensory, or neurological impairments.

From the American Psychiatric Association. (1994). *The diagnostic and statistical manual of mental disorders: DSM-IV* (4th ed.). Washington, DC: American Psychiatric Association.

CASE STUDY 9-1 Teagan

Teagan is a 4-year-old boy who loves to play tee-ball and especially run the bases. He loves getting ready (like the pros) for the swing. Teagan has Down syndrome. His gross motor skills are awkward and he must take breaks when running around the bases. However, he is able to play tee-ball for long periods of time and enjoys pushing his tricycle, sliding down the slide, and swinging (see the Evolve website for accompanying video). Closer analysis of Teagan's gross motor skills shows that he has low muscle tone throughout, as is characteristic of Down syndrome. He runs with a wide-based gait, and holds his arms close to his body for balance. His posture is asymmetrical (he elevates his shoulders and leans) when he runs. He holds objects in a palmar grasp and exhibits delayed visual-perceptual skills, interfering with his fine-motor performance. Teagan's speech is delayed, he mumbles words, he attempts to communicate, and is able to express simple needs through signs (e.g., I want). Teagan engages in parallel play with other children at his day care center, not really interacting with them. When he does interact with his peers, he engages at a much younger level and frequently interferes in their play.

---

play, and academics (Figure 9-2). The following section presents an overview of motor control and a review of the motor control approaches that led to the development of dynamical systems theory.

MOTOR CONTROL: OVERVIEW AND DEFINITION

Motor control is defined as the "ability to regulate or direct the mechanisms essential to movement" (p. 4).[108] Motor control refers to how the central nervous system organizes movement, how we quantify movement, and the nature of

movement. Researchers interested in motor control examine the mechanisms, strategies, and development of movement, as well as causes of motor dysfunction. Occupational therapy practitioners use this knowledge to design effective intervention so that children with motor control deficits may participate in their desired occupations.

Movement deficits occur in numerous conditions including cerebral palsy, developmental coordination disorder (DCD), pervasive developmental disorder, Down syndrome, sensory integration disorders, and acquired brain injury. Historically, intervention strategies used by practitioners varied according to the etiology and nature of motor impairments.[71,108] Traditionally, therapists have used bottom-up approaches, hypothesizing that if they treat the underlying causes of motor dysfunction, the child's function will improve. Therefore, the

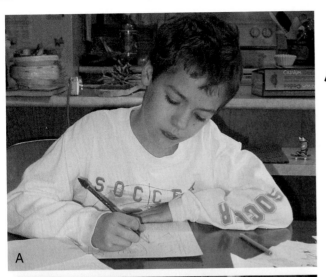

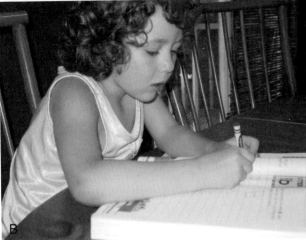

FIGURE 9-2 A and **B,** Children working on academics. (Courtesy Tracy Whitten.)

goals of intervention included improving abnormal muscle tone, sensory dysfunction, weakness, and poor endurance. Bottom-up approaches include sensory integration intervention, neurodevelopmental treatment, strength training, and perceptual motor training.[5,11,25] These interventions focus on decreasing the underlying deficit and improving performance.[11,73] These motor control approaches support a hierarchical model of control—that is, the brain (central nervous system) controls movements. Case Study 9-4 illustrates a bottom-up approach.

Overall, bottom-up approaches have not been found to be effective in improving the occupations of children.[60,66,71,77,78,92,111,112] Bottom-up approaches do not take into consideration the dynamical nature of movement or the multiple systems that interact with one another to produce movement. In contrast, dynamical systems theory was developed to describe how systems interact and how these interactions are responsible for motor performance.[108,117]

CASE STUDY 9-4 Rachel

Rachel, an occupational therapist, works with Gavin, a 2-year-old boy with Down syndrome who exhibits low muscle tone and consequent motor deficits. Gavin has difficulty achieving and participating in feeding, dressing, bathing, and play. Using techniques based on Margaret Rood's sensory approach to motor control intervention (see Box 9-2 for a description of Rood's approach), Rachel focuses on activating muscle fibers, resulting in improved motor performance. Sensory techniques, such as those proposed by Margaret Rood,[101] including bouncing, tapping the muscle belly and fast movement, are included regularly in intervention sessions. By working to increase Gavin's muscle tone, Rachel hopes to increase motor performance.

BOX 9-2 Rood's Sensory Techniques

Margaret Rood proposed the use of sensory stimulation (such as icing, brushing, stroking, manual joint compression, quick stretching, tapping, and proprioceptive pressure) to facilitate muscles for movement. She proposed such activities as neutral warmth, slow rocking, and sustained pressure to inhibit muscle tone. She also used other senses (e.g., olfactory or gustatory) to stimulate responses in clients.[101]

DYNAMICAL SYSTEMS THEORY

Dynamical systems theorists propose that movement derives from a variety of sources and takes place within a variety of contexts.[108,117] This contemporary motor control theory assists therapists in framing evaluation and subsequent intervention to promote movement in children and youth with motor dysfunction. Dynamical systems theory suggests that movement is dependent on task characteristics and an interaction among cognitive, neuromusculoskeletal, sensory, perceptual, socio-emotional, and environmental systems (Figure 9-3). The interaction among systems is essential to predictive and adaptive control of movement; motor performance results from an interaction between adaptable and flexible systems. Dysfunction occurs when there is a lack of flexibility or adaptability of movements to accommodate task demands and environmental constraints.

This lack of adaptability or flexibility is observed in children with motor impairments, who frequently move in limited or stereotypical ways—that is, they have a small repertoire of movements. For example, 3-year-old Sakina, who experienced motor planning deficits, had only one motor pattern for climbing onto a tricycle and could not get on the tricycle when it was turned at a different angle. Case Study 9-5 illustrates the complexity and dynamical nature of movement.

As depicted in this case, Teagan's movement arises from interactions and organization among many systems and is not simply a matter of muscle tone and central nervous system functioning (as bottom-up approaches suggest). The occupational therapy practitioner simplified the task by using a tee-stand, instead of requesting that Teagan hit a moving target.

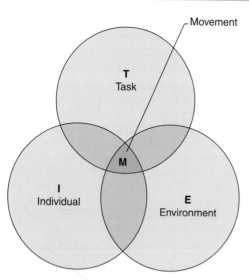

FIGURE 9-3 Dynamical systems theory. (From Shumway-Cook, A., & Woollacott, M. H. [2007]. *Motor control: translating research into clinical practice* [3rd ed.]. Philadelphia: Lippincott Williams & Wilkins.)

CASE STUDY 9-5 · Teagan (cont'd)

Teagan can hit the ball in tee-ball, but not on the playground at day care. A simple explanation for the difference in performance may be that the ball is stationary in tee-ball and someone throws the ball toward Teagan at day care (e.g., different task demands/environments). This explanation shows the importance of looking at the task itself. However, dynamical systems theory suggests that many factors may interact with motor performance (such as limited endurance, delayed visual perception, inadequate timing, and difficulty sequencing). Teagan's low muscle tone may result in poor postural control and subsequent difficulty with gross and fine motor activities. Furthermore, if Teagan is "nervous" or "anxious" with new people tossing the ball at him, this emotional factor may interfere with his performance. Teagan may not be motivated to run at day care on a hot day. He may feel this is not part of his routine; instead he wants to wait until the tee-ball game later that evening. Teagan's mother also reports that he loves "showing off" when he is at the tee-ball games. He may need the contextual cues (e.g., uniforms, ball field, peers and parents watching) to perform.

Stationary tasks (e.g., ball placed on tee-stand) are more easily accomplished than dynamic tasks (e.g., hitting a moving target).

The difficulty of planning and executing movement may also be changed by altering the degrees of freedom required to accomplish a movement. Degrees of freedom are defined as possible planes of motion in the joints controlled by the musculoskeletal and central nervous system.[9,108] Decreasing the degrees of freedom required for movement may result in more functional movement. Holding the bat close to the ball and hitting it while it is on the tee-stand require that Teagan control fewer planes of motion, thereby limiting the degrees

of freedom for the movement when compared with hitting a moving ball.

Teagan may also learn to contract movements together (i.e., synergistically) to decrease the degrees of freedom. For example, synergistic movements (or coupling) occur when children reach for objects, because the elbow, wrist, and fingers tend to extend toward the object.[109,113,121] Other synergistic patterns have been found with walking, tapping tasks, and throwing.[18,142]

Teagan may adopt movement tendencies or patterns in which he is comfortable, such as running with his arms close to his body. Dynamical systems theorists use the term *attractor state* to describe the tendency to stay in the patterns of the status quo.[18] For example, a child may have the tendency to sit in a posterior pelvic tilt. This pattern may not be most efficient and may even prevent the child from achieving other milestones (e.g., such as reaching with ease). The therapist's role is to identify the attractor state and help facilitate movement away from this state (i.e., perturbation), if it is not functional for the client. W-sitting (Figure 9-4) is a common attractor state children use to maintain stable sitting but is not recommended because it may dislocate hips and limit trunk strengthening. Facilitating a child away from an attractor state is often referred to as a perturbation—a force that alters the movement pattern. Perturbations can be used to help children move in different ways.

Dynamical systems theory integrates well with occupational therapy principles and can be used to facilitate intervention. Specifically, a child learns movement more easily and effectively if (1) the movement is taught as a whole (versus part); (2) the movement is performed in variable situations; (3) the child is allowed to actively problem-solve the actions required; and (4) the activity is meaningful to the child. Summarized next are findings from motor control literature on the non-linear dynamical systems concepts of whole learning, variability, problem-solving, and meaning, and their influence on occupational therapy practice.

Whole Learning

According to dynamical systems theory, many systems are involved and interact with each other to plan and execute movement.[108] Therefore, engaging in the whole activity

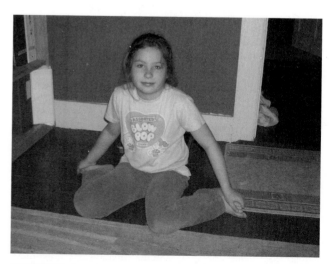

FIGURE 9-4 W-sitting.

(occupation) targets and facilitates multiple systems and the interactions required for effective movement. Overall, learning the whole motor task is more effective and motivating than learning only a part of the movement.[74,110]

Children perform whole tasks more efficiently and with better coordination than when they are asked to perform only a part or component of the movement.[35] Van der Weel and colleagues found that children with cerebral palsy used more supination when banging a drum than when simply exercising.[124] Not only did children perform the task more efficiently, but they also engaged in the task for longer periods of time and activated more areas of the brain during the activity. In addition, functional magnetic resonance imaging (fMRI) studies indicate that more areas of the brain are activated when subjects engage in meaningful whole tasks versus parts of the tasks.[62]

Engaging in the whole activity or occupation requires children to use multiple systems and to respond to changes within and between systems. The ability to respond to this variability within systems is a hallmark of functional movement. Typically developing children, for example, use multiple strategies when moving, as opposed to children with DCD who have been found to exhibit limited variability and adaptability in their movement.[71,104] Therefore, one goal of occupational therapy intervention is to promote variability and flexibility in movements.

Variability

Dynamical systems theorists propose that movement requires an ability to adapt to changes within and between systems; in other words, variability is central to functional movement. Variability is inherent in activity (e.g., reaching for different objects, environmental stimuli) as well as within and between systems (e.g., interactions between visual and sensory systems).

Movement occurs in a variety of settings and requires that children adapt to environmental changes (using visual and auditory systems) or internal changes (perceived through vestibular and proprioceptive systems) changes. For example, children may need to adjust movements in response to interpretations of visual input (e.g., the ball is coming fast versus slow); children may experience physiological changes (e.g., low energy) affecting movement patterns. The environment may pose changes (e.g., weather, terrain, other children). Functional movement, the goal of motor control intervention, requires that children possess a variety of motor skills.

Because variability is essential to functional movement, occupational therapists teach children to move in variable ways while engaging in occupations. Thus, the expectation of intervention is that the child perform movements in a variety of ways versus repeating and learning one pattern of movement. For example, requesting a child sit in a corner seat to repeatedly pick up a block and drop it into a stationary container requires no adaptability on the child's part. The child is repeating the same motion. A better intervention session would include placing the blocks scattered on the floor and requiring the child reach in different directions (for different sized blocks) (Figure 9-5).

Performing movements in multiple ways requires that children problem-solve and self-correct. For example, to learn to build a sand castle, the child problem-solves his or her position in the sand and how to scoop and place the sand. Learning a

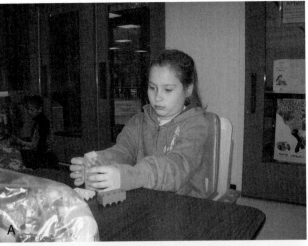

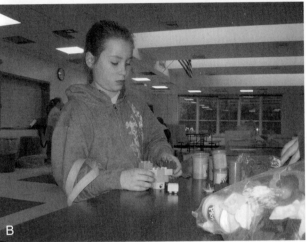

FIGURE 9-5   A and **B**, Playing with blocks in varied positions promotes motor control.

new motor task is more likely to occur if this is a meaningful, socially engaging activity for the child. The child must position his or her body away from the structure and use adequate timing and force to make the castle of his choice. All children use problem-solving to develop and refine movement; therefore, problem-solving is an important part of motor control.

Problem-solving

Improved retention of motor skills occurs when children problem-solve and self-correct for motor errors.[12,50,76,79,93] Children learn and retain motor skills more from intrinsically problem-solving a motor action than from receiving external feedback during an action (such as hand-over-hand assistance). Self-correcting enables children to rely on internal cues that indicate the effectiveness of movement and thereby help them adapt and modify movements in a variety of contexts.[40,48]

Therefore, therapists working to improve a child's motor performance provide many opportunities for the child to actively solve motor problems by doing, rather than repetitive practicing of a part of the movement. Setting up the environment to facilitate physical, social, and cognitive tasks encourages the child to discover how to move, explore options, and self-correct movement errors beneficial to motor learning.

Not only do children benefit from problem-solving how to move, they also benefit from engaging in activities that they find meaningful. Participation in meaningful activities is central to occupational therapy practice and also improves the child's motor control.

Meaning

Dynamical systems theory proposes that the interactions between systems (including the emotional system) influence movements. Occupational therapists have historically viewed the meaningfulness of activities as essential to practice and acknowledge the benefits of purposeful activity in motivating clients to perform.[33,61,85,119] Kielhofner uses the term *volition* to describe one's motivations, goals, desires, and belief in skill.[61] A child's participation in motor tasks is influenced by the extent to which he can identify his own interests and goals and believes he will be effective in those motor tasks. Illustrative of these concepts is that children are more motivated to engage in difficult motor skills if they find the activity important and fun and if they believe they can be successful.[64]

In addition, subjects participate for longer periods of time and perform more repetitions when activities are meaningful.[110,141] Not only do subjects perform longer, but, in addition, the quality of movement improves when the activity has meaning to the child.[41] Meaning may be determined by asking children directly using semi-structured interviews. Cohn, Miller, and Tickle-Degnen[22] and O'Brien et al.[86] found that children with motor deficits wanted to participate in "regular" activities with friends. These expressed interests suggest that practitioners promote meaningful physical activity (such as skiing, swimming, cycling, running, and skating) for children who have motor impairments.

To design effective motor control intervention, occupational therapists must acknowledge the meaning a child attaches to the activity by learning the child's goals and desires.[3,61,71] Meaning is derived from an individual's experience and viewpoint; thus therapists involve the child in selecting and designing the activity.

DEVELOPMENT OF MOTOR CONTROL

The development of motor skills occurs in three stages—cognitive, associative, and autonomous—and involves an interaction among three processes (i.e., cognition, perception, and action).[108] These stages and processes are considered dynamic in that they are constantly changing and interacting with each other in relation to the motor skill or performance requirements.

The cognitive stage refers to the skill acquisition stage. In this stage, the learner practices new movements, errors are common, and movements are inefficient and inconsistent. During this stage, learners need frequent repetition and feedback. Children learning to hold a spoon, for example, may need reminders to take little scoops of food, and to move the spoon to the mouth slowly.

The associative stage involves skill refinement, increased performance, decreased errors, and increased consistency and efficiency. During this stage the learner relates past experiences to the present, thereby "associating" movements (e.g., the child may realize that the last time he moved his hand too

quickly, the food dropped off the spoon, so he reminds himself to slow down).

During the autonomous stage, the learner retains the skills and can perform the movement functionally. During this stage, skills are transferred easily to different settings and refined. For example, during this stage a child can feed himself or herself a variety of foods using a spoon and simultaneously carry on a conversation at the table.

Each stage of movement involves interactions among the processes of cognition, perception, and action.[108] Cognition refers to intent or the child's motivation to move, and also to the ability to plan the movement. Cognitive processes are used in decisions about how to use an object (e.g., throw versus catch).

Perception refers to how the individual receives and makes sense of a stimulus (visual, auditory, tactile, kinesthetic, vestibular, olfactory). Perception involves attributing meaning to sensory input. Perception refers to both peripheral sensory mechanisms and higher level processing that add interpretation and meaning to stimuli.[108] For example, the child must be able to identify the object coming toward him or her or "feel" balance.

The process of action includes muscle contractions, patterns, and precision and nature of the movement (dynamic versus static). Research devoted to the action stage explores factors such as strength, ability to co-activate muscles groups, reaction time, and timing and sequencing, all contributors to movement.[87,91,97]

Each stage and process of movement involves a variety of factors that contribute to the motor performance. The following section provides an overview of factors that contribute to motor performance.

FACTORS AFFECTING MOTOR PERFORMANCE

A variety of factors are involved in producing motor skills and participation in occupations. After identifying the child's desires and occupational goals, occupational therapists examine factors within a variety of systems (e.g., social-emotional, physical, sensory) to determine what may be interfering with or facilitating optimal movement.

Social-Emotional Factors

Emotion is a psychological state that may affect motor performance. Individuals are able to achieve motor challenges in which they attribute positive feelings.[88,96,103] For example, athletes use the "power of positive thinking" to visualize achievement and subsequently exhibit improved motor performance as a result.[81] Conversely, children may experience difficulty performing at their best when they are experiencing negative emotions (such as anxiety or fear). Children may perform less effectively if they are feeling pushed or judged; they may be afraid of failure. Children may want to perform an activity or skill and feel frustrated when they cannot. Watching the child's expressions during therapy can provide cues to therapists about the degree of difficulty (Figure 9-6).

The practitioner's therapeutic use of self can facilitate the child's motor control. Pushing children too hard (e.g., to the point of tears) produces chaos versus self-organization and is not conducive to motor learning. A child who is crying is

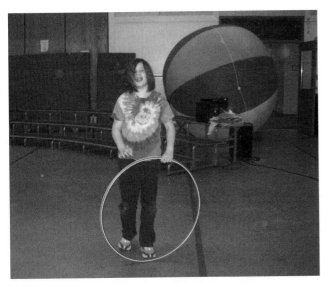

FIGURE 9-6 Children can become frustrated when learning new motor skills or tasks.

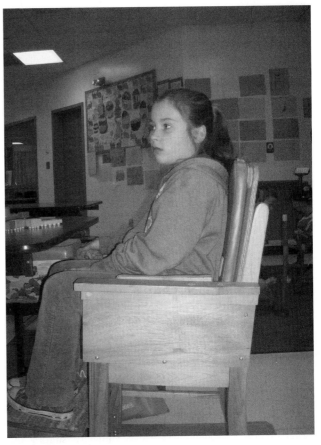

FIGURE 9-7 Sitting in an adapted seat with tabletop helps postural control.

not actively problem-solving or ready to learn a new motor skill. Children learn movement best when they are challenged at a level at which success is achievable and they are emotionally ready to engage in problem-solving.

Physical Factors

While social-emotional factors are important for movement, physical limitations (and/or strengths) must be equally considered. Occupational therapy practitioners examine physical client factors using knowledge of biomechanics and kinesiology. The following section provides a brief overview of these client factors.

Range of motion is necessary for movement to occur. Impairments in range of motion may require children learn how to move differently (to compensate) or make adaptations in how activities are performed. Interventions are developed to help children increase range of motion to improve function. When examining range of motion, therapists also observe the physical appearance of the structures such as symmetry, physical anomalies, scar tissue, and stature. Not only is it important to evaluate these things, but also to consider how these areas affect movement. Occupational therapy intervention for physical anomalies often includes teaching children to compensate by performing activities in a different manner or providing adaptive equipment to help children perform occupations.

Muscle tone affects movement patterns and is considered in evaluation of motor performance. Muscle tone is defined as the resting state of the muscle. Typical muscle tone allows movement into and out of positions with ease. Children with hypertonicity exhibit increased muscle tone, resulting in limited movements; those with hypotonicity exhibit low muscle tone, which results in excessive range of movement but limited control over movement.

The goal of occupational therapy intervention is not to change the muscle tone, but rather to improve the child's ability to perform occupations. This may be accomplished by providing children with assistive support, such as a supportive seat or an alternative tabletop (Figure 9-7). Case Study 9-6

CASE STUDY 9-6   Kiera

Kiera is a 4-year-old girl with spastic quadriplegia who has difficulty sitting independently and playing. Kiera is unable to reach accurately for objects. Rather than working to decrease Kiera's muscle tone, the occupational therapist provided Kiera with an adaptive seat, which supported her trunk and allowed her to sit upright. Kiera was able to sit upright and interact with others, play, and work her trunk muscles in this seated position. As a consequence of engaging in play in supported sitting, her muscle tone improved and she was able to play with improved physical coordination.

illustrates how engaging the child in play and supporting an upright posture may improve muscle tone or, conversely, how despite abnormal muscle tone, a child can learn to move.

Strength limitations may interfere with motor performance. Strength is defined as the voluntary recruitment of muscle fibers. In strength training, the child repeats movements, often with added resistance or weight. Although it is possible to increase a child's strength through exercise routines, engaging the child in play is more suitable to occupational therapy. Kaufman and Schilling reported changes in muscle strength, motor function and proprioceptive position in space in a young child with DCD after a strength training program.[59] However, the authors did not examine how the program affected the child's occupational performance.

RELATING DYNAMICAL SYSTEMS THEORY TO BALANCE

Because balance is an integral part of movement, occupational therapy practitioners frequently address balance issues in children. For example, children must possess adequate standing balance to dress and play. Children require adequate sitting balance for handwriting, feeding, and academic tasks. Balance involves the interaction of multiple systems (e.g., sensory, neuromuscular, skeletal, cognition, and environmental). How dynamical systems theory relates to balance is discussed next.

Balance: An Overview

For children to carry out skillful, coordinated, and effective movements, whether they are fine motor or gross motor actions, they must have an adequate foundation of balance and postural control. Children with poor posture and/or balance often exhibit limited motor skills, in part because the foundation for carrying out skillful movements is not well developed (e.g., posture is inappropriate and/or control of balance is poor or inconsistent).[133,136] Frequently, it is the core muscles of the trunk and muscles of the lower extremity, along with the timing of activity in the muscles of the trunk and lower extremities, that contribute to the motor control issues observed in children who have difficulty carrying out both fine and gross motor tasks.[13,94] Thus, it is important to have a rich understanding of the nature of the processes and developmental milestones associated with developing and maintaining balance.

To understand posture and balance and their intricate interrelationships, it is important to define and describe these terms. *Posture* is defined as the alignment of body parts and involves the relationships among various segments of the body. The optimal alignment of body parts (e.g., posture) for standing is close to a straight line from the ankles through the hips, shoulders, and ears. In contrast with posture, *balance* has to do with overall body equilibrium or stability. Biomechanically, it is described as the maintenance of the center of mass over the base of support. Maintaining the center of mass over the base of support requires that the child equalize differences between two opposing forces: gravity, which is constantly pulling on the body and moving it out of alignment, and the internal force of muscular activity, which acts against gravity to maintain the body in its appropriate or desired alignment.[133]

Stability is required for movement and functional activities such as hand skills, feeding, dressing, bathing, and play. Stability and balance change as children modify their posture (e.g., the alignment of body parts). For example, if a child raises the arms over the head (as when reaching for a toy), the center of mass increases and stability diminishes, whereas if a child bends the knees, the center of mass decreases and stability increases. Generally, the higher the center of mass, the less stable balance is, and the lower the center of mass, the more stable the balance. Assuming different foot positions add to the effect by changing the child's posture on the base of support. Standing with the feet in a tandem position narrows the base of support and thus decreases stability whereas standing with the feet shoulder width apart provides a wider base of support and increases stability in relation to standing with feet in tandem. Thus, when planning intervention, occupational therapy practitioners should keep in mind that it is more difficult for children to perform activities standing with one foot forward than with feet shoulder width apart. If a child then stands on the balls of the feet, this both raises the center of mass and reduces the base of support and decreases stability. These examples illustrate the subtle and intricate relationship between posture and balance. Both are controlled by the part of the sensory-motor systems referred to as the *postural control system*.[133]

The postural system maintains the body's stability by maintaining (1) the body in a stationary position when necessary (e.g., static balance); (2) balance when changing from one discrete position to another (e.g., moving from supine to sitting or from sitting to standing); and (3) equilibrium while the body is in continuous motion (e.g., walking, running). Multiple physiological systems are involved in carrying out these highly interrelated functions and include the musculoskeletal, neuromuscular, and sensory systems (i.e., visual, vestibular, and proprioceptive or somatosensory).

To carry out these functions, the child must first detect the presence of instability—that is, any perturbation or disturbance to balance, must be detected and evaluated with regard to its potential for leading to a loss of balance (Figure 9-8) (Case Study 9-7). This is the job of the visual, vestibular, and proprioceptive systems. Generally, input from these systems is transmitted to the brain and a motor plan for correcting or adapting to the changes is developed. This motor plan is transmitted through the primary motor systems to the periphery to appropriate musculature. These muscle groups contract, moving the skeleton as dictated by the muscular activity, and balance is maintained or recovered.[136]

Sensory Organization and Control of Balance/Posture

To maintain balance, the child must be able to detect when balance has been challenged and equilibrium or stability is changing. The vestibular, proprioceptive, and visual systems work together to provide information to detect changes in postural stability, as discussed next.

Vestibular System

The vestibular system is a powerful source of information about orientation of the body, position of the head, and movement of the head. Children use vestibular information to understand where their head and body are in space.[52,53] One set of sensory receptors in the inner ear signals the position of the head in relation to gravity (otoliths); another set helps to detect the speed and direction of body movement based in part on what is happening to the head (semicircular canals). The vestibular system provides critical input regarding head position, body orientation, balance, and equilibrium.[2] It helps to detect and interpret the following:

- Is the head in upright, midline alignment?
- If not, is it forward, backward, to the side?
- Is the head moving?
- How fast is the head moving and in what direction?

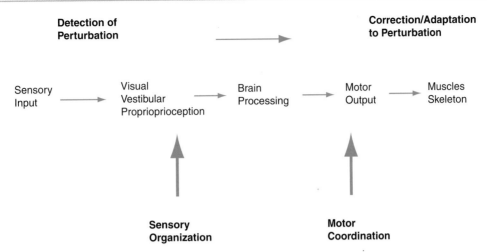

FIGURE 9-8   What is involved in posture/balance control?   (From Neumann, D. A. [2002]. *Kinesiology of the musculoskeletal system: Foundations for physical rehabilitation.* St. Louis: Mosby.)

| CASE STUDY 9-7 | Margi |

Margi is a 3-year-old girl who has awkward movements, labeled as generalized ataxia. She is unable to control her arms and hands. She over-reaches and under-reaches for toys. She lacks controlled release of objects (e.g., into a container) and often drops them. Margi has difficulty using both hands together. She stumbles frequently as she walks, falls in sitting, and prefers to sit with both hands touching the ground. Along with poor visual perception, all of the foregoing are examples of Margi's poor balance and posture, which affects her ability to sit, stand, walk, and use her arms and hands effectively. The occupational therapist begins the intervention to improve Margi's ability to use her hands for feeding and playing by targeting Margi's posture and balance.

Margi must first detect the instability—that is, she must "feel" and be aware that she is unstable or about to lose balance. This may be difficult for a child with ataxia and thus requires that the therapist focus on activities to help her feel the changes. Consequently the therapist may begin with large perturbations, using verbal cues to prepare the child for the perturbation. This can be accomplished during a play session on a swing, where the therapist moves the swing in extreme directions and says "to the left and to the right" so Margi has a verbal cue to relate to the change. Therapists also consider the sensory systems requirements for Margi to control balance and posture as they play an important role in developing these foundational behaviors.

Proprioceptive/Somatosensory Systems

The proprioceptive system contributes information critical to maintaining posture and balance. It provides information from the sensory receptors in the muscles (muscle spindle), tendons (Golgi tendon organs), and joints (joint receptors) throughout the body to the brain. Children use this proprioceptive information to detect body position, determine stability, and maintain posture and balance. The proprioceptive system conveys critical information about the position of the joints of the body and their relationship or alignment with each other, and gives children a sense of overall position of the body. The proprioceptive system also provides information about joint movement (e.g., changes in joint position), along with speed and direction of those changes/movements.[23,56,107,133] Thus, the proprioceptive system helps children detect:

- What is the position of the body?
- How are body parts aligned?
- Which joints are stationary/which are moving?
- If joint positions are changing, how fast and in what direction (e.g., flexion, extension, rotation) are they moving?

Visual System

The visual system also contributes to posture and balance control. Briefly, the visual system may be thought of as a monitoring system that tracks a variety of aspects of information integral to maintaining balance and postural control.[29,47,90,107,115,133] For example, the visual system:

- Monitors the environment and provides information that addresses:
  - What are the primary features of the environment?
  - What is present in the environment (objects, people)?
  - Are these objects/people moving or stationary?
  - Where are the objects/people in the environment in relation to each other?
  - Where are the objects in relation to the child?
- Monitors the body and its movement in the environment and transmits information about:
  - Self-motion: is the body stationary or moving?
  - Speed and direction of body movement
  - Verticality of the body: where is the head/body in relation to gravity?
  - Is this changing or constant?
- Monitors vestibular and proprioceptive input and indicates:
  - Is this information consistent with the current and continuing visual input?

Intersensory Function

Many of the foregoing functions are intersensory functions because they involve synthesizing and integrating visual, proprioceptive and/or vestibular information in making decisions related to the stability of the body. It is well known that the sensory systems do not work in isolation of each other; rather they work in tandem and share information that is needed to detect instability and help correct that instability. Three conditions reveal how intersensory functions contribute to balance control: (1) redundancy of information, a condition in which all three sources of sensory information (visual, proprioceptive, and vestibular) are present and accurate; (2) removal or substitution of sensory information, a condition in which one or more of the three inputs is missing or degraded; and (3) sensory conflict, a condition in which input from any one of the three sensory systems is in conflict with other inputs (e.g., visual input may indicate that balance is unstable, whereas proprioceptive or vestibular information indicates that balance is stable).[42,107,133,138]

The redundancy condition is the most common condition in which children maintain balance; balance is generally well controlled in conditions where all three sources of sensory information are present and accurate. In many instances, one or more of these primary sensory inputs is not available or is inadequate, and in this case (removal or substitution of sensory information) the child must rely on other inputs to determine the nature or status of the equilibrium of the body. For example, children with visual impairments maintain balance based solely on inputs from the vestibular and proprioceptive systems. The third condition, sensory conflict, creates the greatest challenge to balance because the brain must determine which input is conflicting or erroneous and which is accurate, and then ignore or suppress the conflicting information. In this case, the child uses the remaining sources to judge the nature and degree of instability.[133]

Intersensory function and the effect of different sensory inputs on balance control can be measured by the amount of postural sway a child exhibits under different sensory conditions. To examine this, a child stands upright on a force platform and attempts to maintain balance under different combinations of sensory conditions (Figure 9-9):
1. Redundant information
2. No vision (proprioceptive/vestibular information present)
3. Conflicting visual information (proprioceptive/vestibular information present)
4. Conflicting/degraded proprioceptive information (visual/vestibular information present and accurate)
5. No vision and conflicting/degraded proprioceptive information (vestibular information accurate)
6. Conflicting visual information and conflicting/degraded proprioceptive information (vestibular information present and accurate)

In each of these conditions, changes in the amount of sway and/or in sway patterns can indicate deficits in a particular sensory system.[107,133,139]

When all three sensory inputs are available (Condition 1), sway is minimal; when visual input is removed (Condition 2), sway increases slightly suggesting that visual input is important in maintaining balance. It is interesting that in any condition when ankle proprioception is conflicting or degraded (e.g., Conditions 4, 5, 6) sway increases dramatically compared with when it is not degraded (e.g., Conditions 1, 2, 3). Sway is greatest when only vestibular information is present and "accurate"

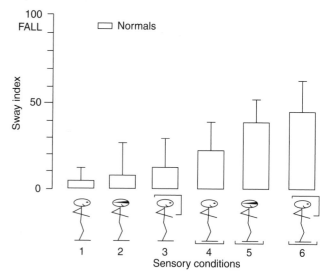

FIGURE 9-9 Sway and sensory conditions. 1 = visual, proprioceptive, and vestibular inputs all present and accurate; 2 = visual input is not available; 3 = conflicting visual information is present; 4 = ankle proprioception information is degraded; 5 = visual is not available and proprioceptive information is degraded; 6 = conflicting visual information is present, proprioceptive information is degraded. (From Horak, F., Diener, H., & Nasher, L. [1990]. Postural strategies associated with somatosensory and vestibular loss, *Experimental Brain Research, 82,* 167–177.)

(Conditions 5, 6). The most difficult condition for maintaining balance is when ankle proprioception is degraded and visual input is conflicting and has to be suppressed. This type of condition may occur in children with hemiplegia who have limited sensation in the affected extremity (e.g., decreased ankle proprioception) and poor visual perceptual skills.

Motor Coordination Aspects of Posture/Balance Control

Once a child becomes posturally unstable, some correction for the disturbance to balance must take place quickly to avoid loss of balance. The response to instability and recovery of balance is a function of the motor control system and is referred to as the Motor Coordination component of balance control.

Corrective responses to disturbances of stability involve different levels of the motor control system. Some responses are "wired-in," that is, they are reflexive or automatic and may involve lower levels of the nervous system (e.g., the stretch reflex, postural reflexes). Other responses may require higher-order analysis of visual, proprioceptive, and vestibular information and have been shown to involve supraspinal mechanisms, including the cortical regions. These latter responses include the postural synergies and integrative responses, both of which are adaptable or modifiable and are affected by practice and experience. These supraspinal responses or types of postural control include reactive responses (responses that occur after an instability or disturbance to balance have occurred) and anticipatory responses (responses planned before the occurrence of instability and designed to avoid instability). Presented next is a brief review of the postural reflexes, postural synergies, and integrative responses.[16,17,82,83,122,136,140]

Postural Reflexes

Children tend to develop postural reflexes in a predictable sequence: prone and supine positions to quadruped to standing. Postural reflexes act primarily to align the head with the body, keep the head in an upright position, and maintain equilibrium. There are three major categories of postural reflexes: attitudinal (also known as primitive), righting, and equilibrium and protective reflexes (Table 9-1). Attitudinal reflexes appear within the first year and are designed to align the head with the body (limbs) and the upper body with lower body. For example, when an infant changes his head position, the position of his limbs automatically shift (e.g., the symmetrical tonic neck and asymmetrical tonic neck reflexes). Most attitudinal reflexes are suppressed early in infancy but may reappear after injury or trauma to the brain.[8,43,44,51,107,133]

Righting reflexes are typically observed at about 3 months of age and persist to 6 months of age. When rotation is imposed on the body, the righting reflexes realign the segments of the body and bring the body into appropriate alignment. They are designed to align the head with gravity (keep the child's head upright) and include, among others, the optical righting and labyrinthine righting reflexes. These two reflexes realign the head vertically when the body is displaced and are mediated, respectively, by the visual and vestibular systems.

The third category, equilibrium and protective reflexes, are present at about 6 months of age and persist throughout life to help the child remain upright. Equilibrium and protective reflexes are whole-body responses to instability. Shoves or pushes to the body or tilting of surfaces on which the child is standing or sitting will elicit these responses. These reflexes help children protect the body from injury during loss of balance; if some instability occurs that could lead to a fall, the child extends the appropriate set of limbs to protect the body. Children develop equilibrium reactions in supine and prone positions between 5 and 8 months of age and continue to develop equilibrium in more upright positions throughout early childhood.

Occupational therapy practitioners evaluate reflexes and reactions as an indication of the child's neuromotor status, and the intervention emphasis is on improving postural stability and equilibrium to enhance the child's occupational performance. Thus, therapists help children improve balance and equilibrium reactions for play, mobility, feeding, dressing, self-care, and school functions.

TABLE 9-1 Age of Postural Reactions Acquisition

Balance Reactions	Age (mos.)
RIGHTING REACTIONS	
Neck on body	
Immature	Birth
Mature	4–5
Body on body	
Immature	Birth
Mature	4–5
Body on head	
Prone (partial)	1–2
Mature	4–5
Supine	5–6
Landau	
Immature	3
Mature	6–10
Flexion	
Partial (head in line)	3–4
Mature (head forward)	6–7
Vertical	
Partial (head in line)	2
Mature (head to vertical)	6
PROTECTIVE REACTIONS	
Forward	6–7
Lateral	6–11
Backward	9–12
EQUILIBRIUM REACTIONS	
Prone	5–6
Supine	7–8
Sitting	7–10
Quadruped	9–12
Standing	12–21

Postural Synergies

Postural synergies are an important part of posture and balance development. A synergy consists of a group of muscles acting as a single unit; it involves the "coupling" of muscle activation in a particular set of muscles. Postural synergies act to help correct for disturbances to balance or equilibrium, and although they are believed to be an inherent part of the motor system, they appear to be regulated at supraspinal levels. For this reason, postural synergies are often referred to as "long-loop" reflexes, indicating that they can be modified through practice and experience. Three major postural synergies—ankle, hip, and step—react to disturbances to equilibrium when the individual is in an upright stance. These are present as early as 2 years but continue to develop and undergo refinement until 7 to 10 years of age.

The ankle strategy involves the sequential contraction of the lower extremities in a disto-proximal direction (i.e., from the ankles up).[83,84,107,133] The ankle strategy is usually activated when/if the child is standing on a firm surface that is wider than a foot (e.g., a large platform or a beam 6" or wider). Typically it is elicited when the child's center of mass is displaced by a small amount (see Figure 9-9).

The hip strategy involves the sequential contraction of the muscles of the lower body in a proximo-distal direction (from the hips downward).[82,83,107,133,140] The hip strategy is typically activated when/if the child is standing on a narrow or unstable/compliant surface. The strategy is elicited primarily with a fast, large perturbation to body stability (a quick but substantial jerk). This often occurs in young children when they attempt to walk a narrow (2") beam or stand on a balance board. When standing balance is perturbed in a backward direction, muscles on the anterior of the body contract in a consistent sequence (see Figure 9-9).

The third postural synergy is the step strategy; although this is elicited easily, the muscle activity involved is not well documented because this is a more complex strategy for regaining equilibrium.[107] The step strategy typically occurs when or if the perturbation to balance is great enough to cause the center of mass to fall outside the base of support. This can be elicited under a variety of conditions, depending on the level of control of the child. In these instances, the response is a step/hop that serves to restore equilibrium. Children may use a variety of different combinations of strategies, depending on the task, individual, or circumstance.

Integrative Responses

Another set of responses often involved in responding to perturbations to balance are those referred to as integrative responses. These fall into the category of higher-order, conscious or voluntary responses that are thought to be anticipatory in nature. Integrative responses are preplanned and are designed to accommodate known or anticipated disturbances to balance. Integrative responses by definition involve intersensory functions, where the brain must either substitute one source of sensory information for another (e.g., when visual input is not available) or if there is a need to suppress erroneous incoming sensory information. Postural synergies can and do occur under such conditions as well.[70,106,107,133] A common example of the use of integrative, anticipatory responses may be seen in the form of preplanning for possible changes in equilibrium when a child is asked to move through an obstacle course. In this case, the system must plan for maintaining balance control as the child moves through a series of obstacles that require the body move in a variety of positions and on, over, and/or around a number of stable and unstable objects.

Balance Control Issues in Children with Developmental Coordination Disorder

Children with DCD exhibit a variety of motor control disorders that include deficits in balance and postural control and other gross motor and fine motor eye-hand coordination skills that interfere with activities of daily living, school, feeding, and social participation.[38,75,130,135] Examining the differences in balance and sensory processing between children with and without DCD may provide some insight into the motor coordination difficulties of children with DCD.

Vision and Proprioception

Children integrate and use information from visual, proprioceptive, and vestibular systems to control balance. Several studies indicate that children with DCD rely more heavily on visual input in controlling balance than typical children.[128] It is possible that children with DCD who rely on vision to regulate balance may do so in part because of the inability to process and use proprioceptive input effectively.

Proprioceptive feedback is believed to play an important role in correcting for externally or internally induced errors in balance, as well as in modifying the speed and force of corrective actions. Effective processing of proprioceptive input is especially important in recognizing when one is becoming or close to becoming unstable. Children with DCD have more difficulty with this than typical children and thus lose control

of balance more often. They also have difficulty in recovering balance after onset of instability. That is, when balance is lost or they become unstable, they cannot easily regain a stable state. Recovery of stability is also thought to be in large part a proprioceptive-related function.[20]

The brain may place greater weight on proprioceptive, visual, or vestibular inputs in regulating static balance. Inder and Sullivan reported that visual and vestibular functions in older children with DCD lagged behind those of their age-related peers.[55] Based on performances on the Test of Visual-Perceptual Skills, it is clear that many children with DCD have less well-developed visual perception skills than typical children.[120] Young children with DCD (4 to 6 years of age) have more difficulty regulating balance (e.g., they exhibit more sway) when proprioceptive input is degraded than when it is not.[20] Children with DCD may rely more on proprioceptive input for balance control than typical children because of visual perception deficits. However, such deficits are not present in all of these children.[37,95] They often have difficulty effectively integrating visual and proprioceptive information, a process important to maintaining and recovering control of balance.[57,128]

Overall evidence suggests that many children, including those with DCD, have deficits not in any one sensory system but in sensory organization (i.e., integration of visual, proprioceptive and/or vestibular inputs). For that reason, many young children, in particular children with DCD, tend to rely more on vision than proprioception for balance control. The child's age certainly plays an important role in this integrative process because younger children do appear to have less well-developed integrative capacities than older children (10 years and older).[87,135]

Improving Balance: Intervention

Planning for and organizing a program of intervention activities to promote balance control is of critical importance to occupational therapists. Such planning and organization requires that therapists use as much information as possible about various aspects of balance so that tasks can be designed to provide a gradual, orderly, and sequential program of activities to promote and enrich the child's ability to maintain stability. Therapists design tasks that are both varied and interesting to the child for whom the program is intended.

Occupational therapy practitioners help children perform a variety of daily living activities, play, and academic activities, all of which require balance. One perspective on how to approach analyzing and developing tasks to challenge balance in a systematic way is to consider the major ways in which the body and the environment can be structured to challenge different aspects of balance.[134] These can be thought of as components of balance, which can be varied or combined in different ways to encourage adaptive balance control. By analyzing and facilitating components in an occupation-based intervention, the child can easily generalize new skills to his or her everyday natural environment. Components of balance may be grouped as primary or secondary, as described next.

Primary Components

Primary components involve aspects of balance that are integral to developing efficient balance control and consist of the following: body movement, use of vision, and external base of support. Therapists address these first in planning balance interventions.

Body Movement

An important component in any balance activity or task is whether the child is maintaining balance in a stationary position (static) or maintaining balance while the body is moving (dynamic). Because static and dynamic balance skills are important for effective stability in a wide variety of situations, and because they tend to be somewhat independent of each other, it is important to provide opportunities to develop control under conditions where the body remains stationary and where the body is moving or changing positions. Therefore, occupational therapy intervention to improve sitting balance may include sitting in one position and coloring (static) and sitting on an unstable surface (e.g., therapy ball) and playing catch (dynamic).

Use of Vision

Balance is almost always better when visual information is available than when it is not. Most experts agree that it is important to provide opportunities to practice balance under a variety of visual conditions; such practice also has the indirect benefit of providing opportunities to enhance the capacity to use vestibular and proprioceptive input regulating balance. Efforts to improve balance should include tasks where the child balances with vision, with vision occluded, as well as with varying kinds of distortion of visual information (e.g., blocking peripheral vision, wearing goggles, moving in lower levels of illumination). Occupational therapists can incorporate games with children, such as wearing various "funny" glasses.

External Base of Support

The nature of the external surface on which the child is asked to balance is an important part of developing effective balance control. Therapists structure the environment to challenge balance in a variety of ways. For example, the external base of support may be selected to include surfaces that range from:

- Wide to narrow
- Rigid to compliant
- Stable to unstable
- Flat to tilted or inclined

Occupational therapy practitioners can use a wide range of combinations of different types of surfaces to provide interesting and relevant challenges that encourage improved balance control.

Secondary Components

Secondary components of balance are aspects of balance that can be used to add new and different challenges to balance control and include position of the body, internal base of support, and elevation.

Position of the Body

Examining the position of the body and/or the alignment of different parts or segments of the body provides another set of possibilities for challenging balance. Some common positions that challenge balance include upright position, trunk flexed forward, arms extended in front, hands on hips, arms overhead, and/or any combination of the foregoing. All of these have the effect of modifying the location of the center of mass (even though only slightly in many cases). Thus, occupational therapy practitioners modify the position in which the child balances to challenge stability and improve balance control whether the child is stationary or moving through space.

Internal Base of Support

The internal base of support is a component of balance that involves varying the nature and number of body parts used to maintain balance. Modifications in the internal base of support are an integral ingredient in challenging balance. Some examples of varying the internal base of support are activities requiring the child to balance on two feet or a single foot, knee and a hand, or one foot and a knee. Changing the internal base of support creates different demands on the balance system and in that way adds to the range of adaptations that the child must make. Occupational therapists can make this fun by incorporating different positions into play sessions or relay races (e.g., walk with right hand on left knee).

Elevation

A third and final secondary component important in challenging balance is that of elevation. This has to do with structuring the environment so that the element of height is added. Children tend to perceive a greater risk or challenge to balance with elevation than when they balance on the ground (e.g., non-elevated surface). Typical uses of elevation include balancing on large, very stable boxes of different heights (4″, 8″, 12″ high). Overall, the potential combinations of the foregoing components are almost endless and thus provide a guideline for developing interventions to promote improved balance as well as the child's confidence in his or her ability to adapt to everyday balance challenges.

Occupational therapists may play climbing games with stacked heights on soft surfaces to promote balance. For example, encouraging children to walk on the blocks without falling into the "water" is a fun game that works on balance.

Examining Balance: Process Characteristics

When the goal is to improve balance for occupational performance, it is important to assess the nature and extent of the control exhibited in carrying out various balance tasks. Box 9-3 provides an assessment of balance. Figure 9-10 is a checklist that includes a series of process characteristics occupational therapists can observe as the child balances in various positions.[134]

VISION, VISUAL PERCEPTION, AND MOTOR CONTROL

Visual perception refers to making sense and attributing meaning to what is seen. Depth perception, for example, refers to the ability to determine distance visually. This section defines the importance of visual perception on controlled movement and balance and explains the theoretical and practical aspects of visual perception related to balance and movement.

Perception and action are coupled in the sense that rapid and accurate perception of the visual components of the environment is intricately linked to the effective planning and execution of associated actions/movements. In general, children rely on vision and the processing of visual information for almost all interactions with the environment. For example the simple acts of reaching for an object on a table, walking down the street, using a computer, and writing a sentence within the boundaries of a defined space all require the ability to perceive and use visual information from the environment. To illustrate, the way a child prepares to reach for and grasp

---

BOX 9-3   Assessment of Balance

NON-STANDING BALANCE

The ease with which the child moves through and assumes the sequence of positions provides another window for gauging the nature of this foundational base for balance control. Typically, the individual is asked to balance in or assume five different positions:

- *Pivot prone*: a position in which the child lies face down with the hands/arms at the sides and the head and shoulders raised. This position provides a broad base of support (nearly the whole body) and requires appropriate head control and back extensor strength.
- *Prone on elbows*: in this position, the head, shoulders, and upper trunk are lifted and the body weight is borne on the forearms and the lower body; this position also involves a broad base of support and requires improved head and upper trunk control.
- *All fours (quadruped)*: the body is positioned on the forearms and lower legs (dog position); the base of support is considerably smaller in this position and the demand for efficient head, shoulders, and trunk (horizontal position) strength is increased.
- *Full kneel*: in this position, the body weight is centered on an even smaller base of support, that of the lower legs. Greater control of the head and vertical position trunk is integral to stability in this position; strength of the core muscles also plays an important role.
- *Half kneel*: body weight is centered on the foot (with the leg up and the knee flexed) on one side and on the whole of the

lower leg on the other side; the base of support is still smaller than in the full kneel, and appropriate head control and adequate trunk and leg strength are integral to stability in this position.

STATIONARY AND MOVING UPRIGHT BALANCE

The suggested sequence of acquisition and/or practice of these skills is as follows:

- *Two-foot stance* with feet in the following sequence of positions: shoulder width apart, standing with feet together, standing with feet in semi-tandem, and, finally, standing with feet in tandem (heel-toe) position; varying arm/hand positions adds an important element here.
- *One-foot stance* (dominant and non-dominant) superimposing a sequence of positions of the hands/arms, (a) standing with the hands/arms free, (b) with hands/arms in other positions (arms overhead, one arm extended in front and one raised over head, etc.), and finally (c) with hands on hips.
- *Walking a single line or between two lines* (wide to narrow) (a) with one foot on/one foot off the line; (b) using a non-alternating forward pattern (inching the feet forward on the line); (c) using a side-stepping (non-alternating sideways gait) in forward and backward directions; (d) using an alternating foot pattern forward and backward; and (e) using a tandem or heel-toe walk forward and backward;
- *Walking on a beam* (wide to narrow raised surface) using the sequence of foot patterns described for walking a line.

---

an object clearly differs for blind versus sighted children; a child with vision tends to reach directly toward the target object and automatically shapes the hand as it approaches the object to be grasped. This is accomplished by processing visual information that indicates the distance and direction of the object to be grasped (the transport phase) as well as the processing of the size, shape, and orientation of the object (the grasp phase). In contrast, a child without vision reaches less accurately toward the object to be grasped, and only when the object is touched is the hand shaped in an appropriate way for grasping.[21,58,107,125,137,143]

It is also clear that it is not by chance that children with motor dysfunctions frequently have perceptual difficulties or limitations.[125] For example, the incidence of visual perception difficulties is significantly greater in children with DCD (poor motor coordination) than is the case for children without motor skill problems. In comparison with children with age-appropriate motor skill development, children with DCD also perform more poorly on visual perception tasks that involve judgments about form and space and exhibit deficits in the ability to retain visual information in short-term memory.[105] In addition, children with DCD also have great difficulty coordinating eye movements needed to stabilize the focus on moving objects; in other words, they have difficulty synchronizing eye movements with the speed and direction of the path of a moving object.[65]

A Theoretical Perspective

Visual perception may be thought of as a process that involves the pick-up, processing, analysis/interpretation, and/or

retrieval of visual information stored in the brain. Visual perception involves the capacity to discriminate among various visual stimuli and interpret or give meaning to those stimuli. In many ways, visual perception is a learned phenomenon; children learn to use the eyes, to attend to and fixate on visual stimuli, and to search these stimuli for information about the nature and meaning of what is being viewed.[72,98,123,126,127] It also involves the capacity to track objects moving in the environment and move the eyes effectively in that process.

Children use information from the visual system, including visual structures and visual perception to understand the nature of the environment so they can respond to what they perceive and act on it.[4,31,63,105,131] These components are described in Chapter 12.

Eye Movement Control

Eye movements may be helpful in identifying subgroups of children with movement or motor skill problems, particularly those with eye-hand coordination issues. Eye movements may act as a "window" to understanding general motor control processes; more specifically, they may serve as an early biological marker of motor control problems in children born prematurely and especially those with DCDs.

Tracking/Pursuit Movements

In typical development, von Hofsten and Rosander found that smooth pursuit or tracking of predictable targets (0.1-0.3 Hz sinusoidal motion) develops rapidly in the first 3 months of postnatal life.[127] The tracking action was carried out predominantly by movement of the eyes, with some head motion.

Overall Balance Control
1. What are the general characteristics of the balance performance?

_____easy stability throughout
_____stable but with effort throughout
_____often unstable but recovers easily
_____often unstable often; has difficulty recovering
_____unstable more than 50% of time
_____other

Specific Aspects of Balance Control
1. How are the arms used?

_____appropriate action (based on task/developmental level)
_____out for balance
_____at sides
_____hands on hips
_____other
_____inappropriate action
_____flail
_____held in a contorted position
_____other (Please describe)

2. How are the feet/legs used?

_____appropriate action (based on task/developmental level)
_____heel toe pattern
_____alternating pattern
_____non-alternating pattern (inching forward)
_____feet placed toes pointing straight ahead (on line/beam)
_____knees are soft (slightly flexed)
_____walks or moves with ease
_____other
_____inappropriate action
_____knees are stiff (extended)
_____feet are placed crosswise on line/beam
_____steps on toe of trail foot
_____executes foot patterns inconsistently/with difficulty/hesitation
_____alternating/ side stepping
_____heel tie (frequently leaves space between heel/toe
of front foot and toe of trail foot)
_____other

3. What is the status of the trunk?

_____relaxed and upright
_____stiff and upright
_____flexed forward
_____leans to right or left
_____slumped
_____other

4. What is the status of the hands/fingers?

_____relaxed
_____extended/tense (fingers)
_____spread/tense (fingers)
_____contorted (hands/fingers)
_____other

5. What is the status of the face?

_____relaxed
_____tense
_____grimace/contorted
_____tongue protruding
_____other

Comments:

FIGURE 9-10 Williams' checklist of process characteristics of balance performance.[134]

Other data indicate that tracking (pursuit)[63] of slowly moving targets matures by age 7 but continues to improve into adolescence,[102] whereas horizontal tracking of faster moving targets (12°/sec) takes longer to develop.[1,102] Overall tracking skill appears early in development and continues to improve into adolescence.[45] The long time course in acquiring skillful tracking movements may be due partly to incomplete maturation of the tracking/pursuit system and higher-level cognitive factors. For example, the ability to track a ball through space and judge its speed and direction is not fully developed until after 12 years of age.[129] Early in development, the head and eyes tend to move together as a single unit in tracking moving objects; the separation of eye and head movement continues to be refined throughout early childhood.[129]

Langaas et al. studied differences between the tracking movements in children (5-7 years) with and without DCD.[65] These workers examined (1) how closely the speed of eye movements matched the speed of target movement and (2) whether eye movements lag behind or ahead of target movement. Typical children tracked moving targets well and needed just a few quick saccades to get back on the target. Children with DCD consistently failed to match target velocity with eye movement speed and thus fell behind the target, suggesting that messages to the brain for making sensory decisions were slower or were incomplete. In addition, children with DCD had difficulty catching up to the target and had significantly more shifts away from the target than those noted in typical children. Thus children with DCD received less sensory input to the brain about the moving object and the surrounding environment. Visual acuity was within normal limits for all of the children and therefore did not account for the differences between children with and without DCD.

It is important to consider the effect that reduced ocular-motor control has on children's perceptual development. For example, in children with DCD, the lack of effective tracking movements makes anticipatory judgments about speed and direction of moving targets difficult (i.e., they have difficulty judging when and where to go to catch an object). Many young children and those with DCD in particular have problems with catching or intercepting moving objects. The association between ocular-motor control and more general motor impairment has not been verified by research.[34]

Fixation/Search Movements

Infants develop the capacity to fixate on stationary objects with some degree of control within 4-5 days after birth and during the first two postnatal years. In terms of search processes (e.g., finding information in a picture) and determining the nature of the object or figure being viewed, refinement of this process undergoes important changes between 3 and 6 or 7 years. Whereas young children tend to be unsystematic and spend as much time fixating off target as they do on target (the time and number of fixations also varies widely), older children are more systematic and tend to use more rapid fixations of short duration that are directed to the salient parts of the stimulus being viewed (e.g., they follow the object's contours). The important difference is that the patterns of fixation of the older child are adapted to fit the characteristics of the object/figure of interest, whereas the young child's are not.[127,129]

Body Awareness and Motor Control

Several different terms are used in defining and discussing body awareness. Generally the development of the concept of the physical self involves at least three major components: body schema, body image, and body awareness. Figure 9-11 shows a schematic of the components of the concept of the physical self and the behavioral components specific to body awareness.

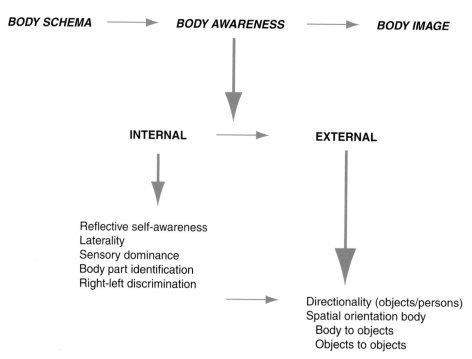

FIGURE 9-11 Schematic: components of body awareness.

Body Schema

The body schema is the neural substrate for body awareness. It is present at birth, and as children grow and develop, this so-called diagram of the body (homunculus) in the sensory and motor areas of the brain is modified, in part, through the sensory-motor experiences (active movement, interaction with the environment, and the feedback derived from those interactions) the child undergoes. The child's own body representations are processed in distinct regions of the intact brain. An example of the manifestation of the body schema may be seen in the phantom limb phenomenon. Children who have had a limb amputated often report that they "feel" both pain and sensation from the missing limb just as if it were physically present. Children who have cerebral palsy (hemiplegia) tend to ignore the affected limbs.

These clinical observations suggest that sensations received when the limb was intact are stored in the brain and when stimulated cause the child to experience feelings and sensations of the missing limbs. The general consensus is that the body schema becomes defined through sensory input from receptors in the skin, muscles, tendons, joints, and the vestibular system, which act to define the boundaries of the limb(s) in the body schema. These receptors are stimulated through body movement and through the actions of the child that are involved in interacting with persons and objects in the environment. The importance of body schema in motor control lies in its relation to motor planning (e.g., the planning of actions). Children develop body schema through active use of the body. Adequate planning of action is based, in part, on the fullness of the body schema. Theoretically, it is proposed that if information children receive and store in the brain in the form of the body schema is incomplete, imprecise, or simply unavailable, children will have difficulty planning or adequately preparing specific plans for action or movement.

Body Image

Body image refers to the image one has of oneself as a physical entity; it includes the perception that one has of the body's physical or structural characteristics (e.g., am I short, tall, heavy, lean?) and of one's physical performance abilities. By its nature, body image has an important emotional component that evolves as the child compares himself or herself to others in the environment in terms of both physical and motor performance characteristics. Integral to the development of an adequate body image is the input from significant others who interact with the child and provide feedback (verbal and nonverbal) about the importance and uniqueness of the child. Clearly, the nature of the interactions between the child and the family, teachers, peers, and others is an important element in the development of a positive self-image.[6,15,36,67-69,94,99,118]

An interesting aspect of the development of body image is seen in attempts by very young children (e.g., 30 months) to do things that the body size/shape simply will not allow; for example, they often try to fit themselves onto or into miniature toys that are clearly too small for them.[27] This suggests that they are still developing body image in terms of the ability to accurately judge the physical characteristics of the body in relation to objects in the environment. Development of body image continues to evolve and be refined throughout early and later childhood, and into adolescence.

Body Awareness

A second component of the physical self-concept is body awareness; it is closely related to body schema in that it involves the conscious awareness of the location, position, and movement of the body and its parts, as well as the relationship between the body and the external environment. The importance of body awareness to motor control is seen in the many challenges that the young child, typical or atypical, faces in judging the characteristics of the body and of objects, people, and events in the surrounding environment. Children use the capacity to hold information about their own body in relation to other objects in the world as the foundation for developing effective plans for execution of movements necessary to achieve specific end goals. For example, the child uses body awareness when moving through obstacle courses, whether they be of natural origin or structured for specific purposes in a clinical setting or when manipulating objects of different sizes and shapes to learn about concepts such as spatial orientation; relationships among shape, size, and weight; and functional uses of objects.[27,100,129]

Body awareness is defined as the ability to visually discriminate, recognize, and identify labels for various aspects of the body's physical and motor dimensions. Body awareness can be divided into internal (body-related) and external (environmental) aspects. Internal aspects involve the development and refined awareness of the body itself; external aspects are associated with development and awareness of the relationship of the body to the environment (external space), as well as the extension of select internal aspects of body awareness to external space. Internal aspects of body awareness tend to develop slightly in advance of external components.[10,14,80,129] The internal and external aspects of body awareness and the relationships between the two are discussed next (see Figure 9-11).

Internal Aspects

As shown in Figure 9-11, there are five important behavioral indicators of the development of the internal aspects of body awareness.

Reflective self-awareness is manifested, in part, in young children's ability to recognize themselves in the mirror, to refer to themselves by name, and to point to themselves referentially.[15,68,80] Visual self-recognition exemplifies the emergence of the objective self and of body awareness. The development of this aspect of body awareness begins with the toddler's discrimination of his own real-time limb movements as different from those of other toddlers when viewing paired videos or watching himself and another child in a mirror. Recognition of the movements of the limbs is an early form of the differentiation of the body (self) from the external environment (space). This recognition also serves as the perceptual/perceptual-motor foundation for later development of refined self-awareness and in particular the acquisition of conceptual knowledge about the body.[6,99] This reflective self and body awareness typically are present in 2-year-olds. The significance of the awareness of the body's movements is that it involves a kind of visual-kinesthetic-motor matching that is integral to effective planning and execution of actions.[67] For example, children develop self-awareness as they begin to feed themselves and understand where their mouth is in relation to their body.

Laterality refers to the awareness that the body has two sides, that the body is separate from space, and that the limbs on each side of the body can move independently of each other. Initially the infant has only a crude awareness of the distinctness of the body as separate from space.[129] Early in development, the infant does not distinguish between the two sides and often moves the two arms/hands and two legs together as a single unit. Gradually, the child begins to be "aware" that the limbs on either side of the body can be used independently of one another. Although at this early stage, the infant does not have "verbal labels" for any aspect of the body, he or she "knows" what is and what is not the body. Much of the defining of the body's dimensions is derived from feedback from the movement of the body itself. Awareness that the body has two sides is an important part of the development of the perception of other internal aspects of the body and provides the foundation for the acquisition of directionality.

Therapists assess laterality clinically, using a series of both individual and coupled arm and leg movements (child lies in supine and moves various individual and combinations of arm and leg movements as requested by the clinician). The coupled arm/leg movements include both ipsilateral and contralateral (e.g., right arm/right leg versus right arm/left leg). Laterality is established when the child can discriminate and coordinate various individual and combinations of movements of the ipsilateral and contralateral sides of the body. Clearly, then laterality involves both sensory (awareness of limbs) and motor (coordination/control of movements) systems. Children need to develop a sense of laterality (i.e., understand the body has two sides) to move in a coordinated fashion. Awareness of both sides of the body is observed in movements required for feeding, dressing, bathing, play, and academics. Therefore, occupational therapy practitioners facilitate mastery of laterality to help children function in a variety of daily life skills (Figure 9-12).

Sensory dominance develops as the child becomes aware of his or her body and its parts and its separateness from space. Sensory dominance helps to further define the body, especially the two sides of the body. It manifests in the development of the preferential use of one side of the body. Most children have a well-defined preferred hand and foot by the age of 6 years.[130] Occasionally, children as young as 4 years of age have established a hand preference; however most do not. The two categories of sensory dominance are mixed and pure. Pure dominance refers to the preferential use of the eye, hand, and foot on the same side of the body; mixed dominance involves the situation in which the preferred limbs and eye are on opposite sides of the body—that is the child may be right-handed, right-eyed, and left-footed. A large percentage of the adult population has mixed dominance (about 95%).

Hand dominance appears to be associated with cerebral dominance; approximately 90% of the population is right-handed and left cerebral dominant. The left cerebral hemisphere houses the major motor and speech control centers and regulates the actions of the right side of the body. The remaining 10% of the population has been reported to be either right cerebral dominant or have dual dominance. Interestingly, some of these individuals are right-handed, whereas others are left-handed. Handedness also appears to have a familial component. Clearly, mechanisms underlying sensory dominance, in particular handedness, are complex and not well understood.

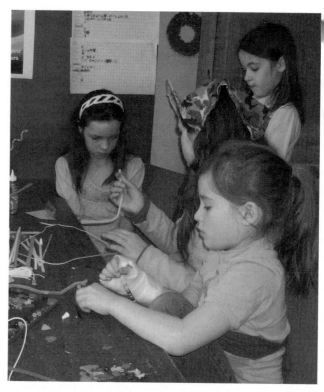

FIGURE 9-12   Laterality refers to developing an understanding of both sides of the body and having a preferred side for tasks. Craft activities can be used to help children develop a sense of laterality.

The period from 4 to 8 years is an important period in the development of hand, eye, and foot preference. By 6 years of age, 81% of children have established a preferred hand, 73% have a preferred eye, and 94% have a preferred foot. Eye preference appears, in general, to be more variable than hand or foot preference. Foot preference is interesting in that there may be two types of foot preference: a preferred balance/strength foot and a preferred skill foot (Figure 9-13). This is most evident in comparing balance times on the right and left feet and examining the skill in kicking a ball. For example, balance is typically better on the side of the preferred foot. Although many children kick using the right foot, these children often have better balance on the left foot. In this case the left foot is considered the "balance foot" and the right foot, the "skill foot." This makes sense in terms of differentiating the role of each foot in skills such as kicking.[129]

Body part identification develops at different rates in children and depends, in part, on the experiences of the child and the emphasis placed on language and the learning of the names of body parts. Knowing verbal labels for different body parts further solidifies the distinctness of the body and its parts.[129] At 2 years, children can often identify some major body parts (e.g., nose, eyes, ears); by 3 years, they are aware of such parts as head, hand, and foot. By 5 years, a majority of children (55%) know more remote body parts (e.g., thumb, eyebrows) and at 6 to 7 years, 70% to 88% of children can name both major and minor parts of the body consistently (e.g., elbows, wrists, heels, shoulders, hips). At 8 or 9 years, it is rare that a

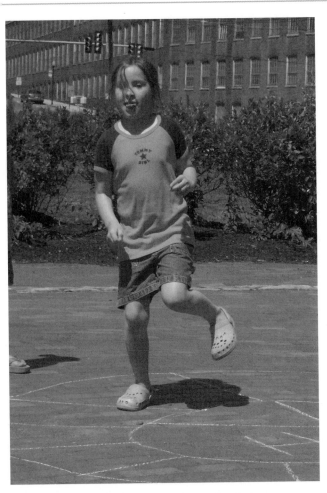

FIGURE 9-13 Playing hopscotch requires balance.

child fails to verbally label all body parts, major or remote (95%). Children recognize verbal labels of body parts (e.g., show me your hand; point to your ankles) slightly earlier than that of attaching verbal labels to those same body parts.

Identifying right and left body parts is the next step in defining the body. This step in the development of body awareness adds to the distinction of the two sides of the body and to the body parts on those distinct sides. Language and spatial awareness are important elements in acquiring the capacity to identify right and left on the body. Developmentally, consistency in naming right and left sides of the body has a linear relationship with age.[129] Young children (up to 5 years of age) typically have little concept of right and left; thus, 5-year-olds typically guess right and left on the body. A majority of 6-year-olds (70+%) are consistent in accurately and spontaneously identifying right and left on the body. This capacity continues to evolve so that by the age of 8 to 9 years, 90% to 94% of children have mastered this aspect of body awareness and readily label right and left parts of the body.

Children tend to master body awareness in the following order: (1) hand dominance, (2) body part identification, and (3) right-left discrimination. Overall, the internal aspects of body awareness tend to overlap in development and are loosely sequenced. Children need to develop internal body awareness, including reflective self-awareness, laterality, sensory dominance, body part identification, and right-left discrimination to be aware of their body to effectively move throughout the environment. For example, children with DCD frequently have difficulty "sensing" or "feeling" where their limbs are without looking at them. They may not possess an internal awareness of their body. This interferes with smooth and coordinated movement.

External Aspects

Children must also develop external awareness, including directionality and spatial awareness, to move their body through the environment. External aspects of body awareness are an extension or outgrowth of internal aspects and involve relating the body to space and to objects and other people in space.

Directionality refers to the child's ability to identify right/left and other dimensions (e.g., top/bottom, front/back, beside) on objects or other persons. Some hypothesize that children project or extend the concepts of right/left and other spatial dimensions of the body onto objects in space. Because the environment has variant spatial references, children appear to use their reflection in the mirror, to refer to themselves by name, and to point to themselves or their own bodies to reference directionality. Thus, knowledge about the body is expanded to objects and persons in space. Most work has focused on directionality defined as identifying right/left on objects and other people.[129] Mastery of directionality, in this case, is described as the ability to consistently and accurately identify right and left on another person and to understand the tenuousness of right and left on objects and how this varies with regard to their position (in relation to the object). Identification of other dimensions of objects is thought to be based on knowledge gained via experiences the child has had using language to describe dimensions of the body. Developmentally, with regard to right-left identification, approximately half of 6-to 7-year-olds have mastered directionality (50-52%); not until 9 years of age do a majority of children consistently and spontaneously identify right and left on another person.

Spatial awareness is the other major component of the external aspects of body awareness. This discussion focuses on two aspects of spatial awareness: awareness of the body in relation to objects in space and awareness of relationships between or among objects.[99,129] These aspects of body awareness rely heavily on language and the conceptual meaning of the so-called "spatial" words. The former involves relating objects to the body and the body to objects using language. A sample activity might involve the child holding an object (e.g., a doll) and the clinician asking the child to "put the doll behind you," and "put the doll in front of you," "put the doll on your right side," "place the doll on your right foot." Object-to-child relationships involve the child's identifying where the object is in relation to himself or herself. By placing a red ball to the right of the child and a blue balloon to the left of the child, and asking the child "where is the red ball/where is the blue balloon," one can examine the child's understanding of this relationship.

Object-to-object relationships are more complex and involve identifying where one object is in relation to (an)other object(s). Children 9 to 10 years of age are able to spontaneously identify relationships among objects. For example, place two objects (e.g., a key and a coin) on a table, one in front of the other and one to the right of the other and ask the child the following: "Which object is in front?" "Which object is to the right?" Development of body-object and object-object relationships overlap. Children typically develop these two aspects of spatial awareness as follows: placement of objects in front or back of self; identification of front and back of objects; placement of a standard object in front and back of an object with distinct features (e.g., a doll); placement of an object to one's own side and to the side of an object with distinct features (e.g., a doll). Development of optimal spatial awareness (including awareness of relationships between or among objects, as well as the relationship between the body and objects in the environment) is integral to adequate planning and carrying out skillful movements. If spatial awareness is lacking or underdeveloped, the child often has difficulty moving and interacting skillfully with the surrounding environment because the child cannot accurately judge these subtle but important relationships between the body and the environment. Spatial awareness is a critical aspect of the movement planning and execution process.

INFLUENCE OF NON-MOTOR FACTORS

Dynamical systems theory suggests that motor control is the result of interactions between many systems, including the environment. These factors include the physical, social, psychological, institutional, and societal influences that may affect occupational performance.[3]

The physical environment consists of the surroundings, surface (e.g., flat, inclined, smooth, rough, hilly), and setting (inside, outside, city, country) and influences motor demands. Playing tee-ball on a competitive team differs from playing at home with parents. Playing on a rocky surface versus soft grass changes movement and balance requirements. Therapists examine the physical environment to determine the movement required.

The social system is part of the environment and influences movement requirements as well. For example, different motor skill requirements exist for a 10-year-old boy who is eating at home with one parent on a quiet afternoon and for another boy who must feed himself in the busy cafeteria at school with three friends. While the child is in the cafeteria, he wants to interact with his peers, increasing the motor demands for self-feeding. Now the child must try to socialize and feed himself (quickly so he can get to recess), realizing his friends will notice if he spills. Social participation is important to children, and, consequently, the influence of this system must be considered. For example, some children may not want adaptive equipment or special considerations in the classroom that make them "look different" than their peers.

The effect of psychological factors on movement must also be considered.[19,88] Attention, concentration, and motivation to perform movements are necessary for motor learning.[26,32] The ability to imagine or think through movement (e.g., mental practice) increases motor performance. Children who are motivated to perform or succeed in motor challenges are able to achieve skills more quickly and with better quality than those who do not.[41,54,124]

Institutional factors include those aspects of the institution or setting that hinder or facilitate movement. For example, institutions may have policies requiring children participate in physical activity. These institutional policies make it possible for children to participate. Requiring children to go outside for recess, for example, is an institutional policy that promotes activity.

Finally, societal influences may influence movement. For example, in the United States, active children are viewed as healthy and thus activities in which children move are expected. For this society, movement (e.g., on the playground, in the backyard) is valued and viewed as important for the child's development. The environment plays a major role in children's learning of motor skills and thus must be considered in designing intervention strategies to teach children movement.

MOTOR LEARNING

Motor learning refers to the acquisition or modification of motor skills. Motor learning literature explores transfer of learning, sequencing, and adapting tasks, type and amount of practice, error-based learning, timing, and type of feedback and mental rehearsal. These concepts provide useful information on techniques involved in the teaching-learning process of movement. Being knowledgeable and aware of the teaching-learning process enables therapists to incorporate motor learning principles into practice so that children learn and retain motor function for their daily lives (Box 9-4).

Transfer of Learning

Transfer of learning, or generalization, refers to applying learning to new situations. The goal of occupational therapy intervention is that the child transfer learning performed in the clinic or intervention setting to the natural context. For example, after working on maneuvering a new wheelchair through an obstacle course at the clinic with ease, the therapist hopes the child will be able to maneuver the wheelchair through the school hallway.

Children are best able to transfer motor skills when they have practiced the motor skill within the natural context or in the "real world" situation. Therefore, the best way to help the child be successful in maneuvering the wheelchair through the school hallway is to practice in that setting. The occupational therapist may need to start by teaching some basic wheelchair skills to the child, practice in the hallway after school hours (to decrease obstacles) and work up to maneuvering the wheelchair during class change. Research suggests that children transfer the task more quickly with this intervention strategy than with practicing in a clinic setting only.[24,114]

Transfer of learning occurs more easily when the motor task is performed during a functional activity or actual occupation, scheduled at its natural time and place, and in the real context.[24,32,41,89] In addition, motor skills with similar components are more likely to transfer. For example, a child who has just successfully learned to throw a ball would more easily learn to throw a bean bag at a target.

Sequencing and Adapting Tasks

Grading and adapting motor tasks so that children are successful constitute part of the occupational therapy process

BOX 9-4 Williams' Motor Learning Principles

TRANSFER OF LEARNING
- Skill experiences need to be presented in logical progression.
- Simple, foundational skills should be practiced before more complex skills.
- Skill practice should include "real life" and simulated settings.
- Skills with similar components are more likely to show transfer effect.

FEEDBACK

Modeling or Demonstration
- Demonstration is best if it is given to the individual before practicing the skill and in the early stages of skill acquisition.
- Demonstration should be given throughout practice and as frequently as deemed helpful.
- Demonstrations should not be accompanied by verbal commentary because this can reduce attention paid to important aspects of the skill being demonstrated.
- It is important to direct the individual's attention to the critical cues immediately before the skill is demonstrated.

Verbal Instructions
- Verbal cues should be brief, to the point, and use 1 to 3 words.
- Verbal cues should be limited in terms of numbers of cues given during or after performance.
- Only the major aspect of the skill that is being concentrated on should be cued.
- Verbal cues should be carefully timed so they do not interfere with performance.
- Verbal cues can and should be initially repeated by the performer.

Knowledge of Results (KR) and Knowledge of Performance (KP)
- A variety of different combinations of both KR and KP typically helps to facilitate learning.
- KP error information may help performer change important performance characteristics and thus may help facilitate skill acquisition.
- Information about "appropriate" or "correct" aspects of performance helps to motivate the child to continue practicing.
- It is important to balance between feedback that is error based and that which is based on "appropriate" or "correct" characteristics of the performance.
- KP feedback can also be descriptive or prescriptive; prescriptive KP is more helpful than just descriptive KP in the early or beginning stages of learning.
- KP and KR should be given close in time to but after completion of the task.
- KP and KR typically should not necessarily be given 100% of the time.
- Learning is enhanced if KR/KP is given at least 50% of the time.
- A frequently used procedure for given KR/KP is to practice a skill several times and then provide the appropriate feedback.

DISTRIBUTION AND VARIABILITY OF SKILL PRACTICE
- Shorter, more frequent practice sessions are preferable to longer, less frequent practice.
- If a skill or task is complex and/or requires a relatively long time to perform or if it requires repetitive movements, relatively short practice trials/sessions with frequent rest periods are preferable.
- If the skill is relatively simple and takes only a brief time to complete, longer practice trials/sessions with less frequent rest periods are preferable.
- It can enhance skill acquisition to practice several tasks in the same session.
- If several tasks are to be practiced, divide the time spent on each and either randomly repeat practice on each or use a sequence that aids the overall practice.
- Providing a number of different environmental contexts in which the skill is practiced appears to facilitate learning.
- With regard to the "amount" of practice, more is not necessarily always better.
- Clinical judgment should be used to recognize when practice is no longer producing changes; at this time, a new or different task could and probably should be introduced.

WHOLE VERSUS PART PRACTICE
- Whole practice is better when the skill or task to be performed is simple.
- Part practice may be preferable when the skill is more complex.
- If part practice is used, be sure that the parts practiced are "natural units"—that they go together.
- To simplify a task, reduce the nature and/or complexity of the objects to be manipulated, e.g., use a balloon for catching instead of a ball.
- To simplify a task, provide assistance to the learner that helps to reduce attention demands—for example, provide trunk support during practice of different eye-hand coordination tasks.
- To simplify a task, provide auditory or rhythmic accompaniment; this may help to facilitate learning through assisting the learner in getting the appropriate "rhythm" of the movement.

MENTAL PRACTICE
- Mental practice can help to facilitate acquisition of new skills as well as the relearning of old skills.
- Mental practice can help the child to prepare to perform a task.
- Mental practice combined with physical practice works best.
- For mental practice to be effective, the individual should have some basic imagery ability.
- Mental practice should be relatively short, not prolonged.

Adapted from Williams, H. (2006). Motor control. In J. Solomon & J. O'Brien (Eds.), *Pediatric skills for occupational therapy assistants* (2nd ed., pp. 474-480). St. Louis: Mosby.

(Table 9-2). Generally, discrete tasks are easier to accomplish than continuous tasks. Tasks involving uni-manual movements are often learned or mastered before bi-manual movements.[133] Skills manipulating stationary objects develop before skills with moving objects.

"Closed tasks are those in which the environment is stationary during task performance" (p. 407),[108] whereas open tasks are ones in which the environment is changing or in motion and involve some inter-trial variability. Closed tasks are generally simpler for most children to accomplish.

Therapists also consider the cognitive demands of activities; children complete simple motor tasks that have fewer cognitive requirements more easily. Tasks with fewer steps are accomplished more readily than those with multiple steps (e.g., throwing at a target is easier than picking up a ball from the container, moving to the starting line, and then throwing

TABLE 9-2 Grading and Adapting Activity

Simple	Example	More Difficult	Example
Discrete	Jump over rope × 1	Continuous	Keep jumping rope
Uni-manual	Grasp toy in one hand	Bimanual	Grasp toy with two hands
Stationary	Hold toy	Dynamic	Catch a moving ball
Closed	Scribble on paper	Open	Follow with pen moving target on computer
One-step	Write name	Multi-step	Write name and draw picture
Simple	Place ball in container	Complex	Pick up the red ball and place in blue container (multiple choices)

at a target). Children acquire tasks that require less precision (e.g., scribbling will be easier than coloring within the lines) more easily than those that require more precision. When sequencing and adapting activities for children, therapists consider the amount of direction required; movement requiring less direction is easier to learn than those requiring multiple directions.

The structure of the environment plays an important role in the nature and complexity of the demands of the activity. For example, environments with variability and extraneous stimuli (e.g., other children) are more challenging and thus more difficult for children because they must continually adapt and adjust.

Practice Levels and Types

Practice is an essential feature of occupational therapy intervention. A considerable amount of research has been conducted on the use of practice to improve or develop motor skills.[49,89,114]

Massed practice (also known as blocked) is defined as practice in which the period performing the movement is greater than the rest period. This type of practice works best during the cognitive stage, as the subject is just beginning to learn the movements. An example of blocked practice may include working on grasp pattern and release by asking a child to pick up 10 blocks and put them all in a container before taking a break and then repeating the game again.

Distributed practice is defined as practice in which rest between trials is greater than the time of the trial and is most useful during the associative stage (Figure 9-14). A clinical example of distributed practice includes asking the child to pick up bean bags placed on the floor while engaged in a game of swinging. In this scenario, the child is still practicing grasp and release, but the child is also working on postural control and processing vestibular input. Therefore, the child grasps and releases a few bean bags, has a rest while swinging in which he must work on other aspects of skill, and then returns to grasp and release.

Variable or random practice is most effective during the autonomous stage. Variable practice requires that learners repeat the same patterns but make small changes as necessary (Figure 9-15). This type of practice increases the ability to adapt and generalize learning. In general, short frequent practice is better than longer, less frequent practice because it decreases fatigue and increases reinforcement.[132] For example, a child is doing random practice when working on grasp and release as he or she engages in a variety of play activities during the intervention. This type of practice is most closely related to the actual occupation. The child must pick up and release toys as the play requires. The child must pick up a variety of objects: small blocks, large swings, light toys, and heavy scooter boards.

Mental practice includes performing the skill in the imagination, without any action involved. It may consist of role playing, watching a video, or imagining. Mental practice is effective in teaching motor skills and re-training the timing and coordination of muscle group activity.[26,28,30,46,88,96,116] Much of the research on mental practice is conducted on athletes trying to maximize their performance.[81,88,103] However, the techniques used may be beneficial to children with motor difficulties. See Research Note 9-1 for a description of a study on mental practice in children. Taktek and colleagues found performance (in throwing a ball) obtained with mental imagery combined with physical practice was equal during the retention phase, but superior during the transfer of learning phase.[116] The researchers examined visual and kinesthetic imagery in young children and found that they were both effective in children as young as 8 years. Imagery techniques are relatively simple and have been shown to work with children as young as 6 years of age. Many theorists suggest it is effective because it requires cognitive processes and helps children problem-solve motor solutions.[30,46]

Driskell and colleagues provide some specific feedback that may assist therapists using mental practice in clinical settings.[30] They suggest that practitioners using mental practice consider the type of task, duration of mental practice, and time between practice and performance for retention. Tasks in which the child may have had some experience may be easier to imagine. However, the child may be able to imagine movements after observing them on a video or seeing someone else perform them. Therapists should be cautious not to incorporate a too-long mental practice because this may be difficult for children and result in a lack of motivation. Finally, therapists should incorporate actual performance shortly after the mental practice for the best retention. Techniques of watching a video, pointing out components of the movement, or simply reviewing mentally how the movement will look in combination with physical practice may provide improved motor learning.

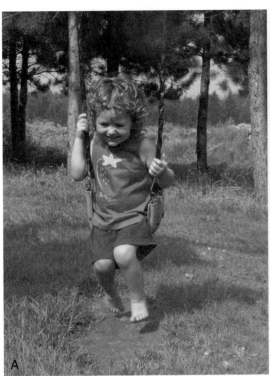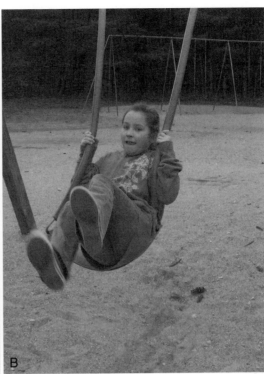

FIGURE 9-14   Distributed practice. **A,** Child begins to learn to swing with feet close to the ground and with frequent rests. **B,** As the child develops, she is able to swing with her feet off the ground, with few rests.

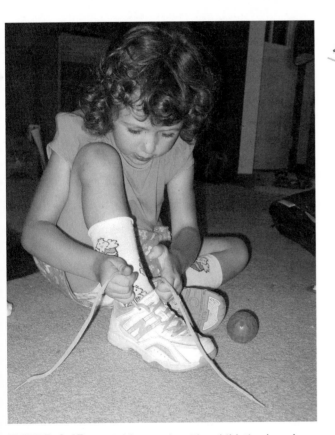

FIGURE 9-15   Variable practice. The child ties her shoes right before she goes outside to play. She is able to tie different sneakers and often she sits on the floor to complete the task.

RESEARCH NOTE 9-1

Jarus, T, & Ratzon, N. (2000). Can you imagine? The effect of mental practice on the acquisition and retention of motor skills as a function of age. The Occupational Therapy Journal of Research, 20, *163–181.*

The authors examined the effect of mental practice compared with physical practice for a bimanual coordination task on children, adults, and older adults. Subjects in each group were randomly assigned into a mental practice or a physical practice group. Thirty children (ages 9-10 years), 30 adults (21-40 years), and 29 older adults (65-70 years) participated in the study. Participants in the physical practice groups practiced 5 trials and rested for 15 seconds between each. The task involved holding a device with both hands and tracing a star (Lafayette Instrument Co., Model 32532). Participants in the mental practice group performed the physical practice and then were asked to image the performance for 10 seconds. Mental practice improved the performance for children and older adults in the acquisition phase. In the retention phase, older adults benefited.

This study suggests that children may benefit from mental practice when learning novel skills.

Error-Based Learning

Children learn movement by making errors or mistakes and self-correcting.[7,39,114] Therefore, clinicians must sometimes allow the challenge to exceed the capacity of the child so that he or she is given the opportunity to make errors, correct them (if possible), and learn from the experience. Children with disabilities must learn to adapt to new, different, or unexpected situations. In the past, therapists typically have been hesitant to allow children to learn through making errors. However, making errors in controlled settings allows children to resolve problems and is important for facilitating their motor skill learning. Encouraging children to explore, adjust movements, and evaluate their responses and reactions helps them learn and refine motor skills.

Feedback

Intrinsic feedback, which allows the child to self-correct, is most effective for sustaining motor performance and should be the goal of intervention sessions. Intrinsic feedback may be elicited through discovery, a situation in which the therapist sets up the environment and the child is allowed to explore and discover, make errors, and consequently learn new ways of moving.

Children may require extrinsic feedback in the early stages of motor skill development. Extrinsic feedback consists of providing verbal cueing or physical guidance. Demonstrative feedback refers to modeling or imitating movements. Demonstrative feedback is best if it is provided before the child actually practices the movement, as well as throughout early stages of skill acquisition. It should not be given with verbal commentary, because that decreases the child's attention to the movement.[24,114]

Knowledge of Performance

Feedback to improve movement is most helpful when it is specific and clear. Knowledge of performance helps children understand how they performed the desired movement. Knowledge of performance is helpful in refining and adjusting motor skills and therefore is useful after the child has established basic skills. Therapists may provide descriptive feedback to the child about performance of a specific task such as writing, such as "you held the pencil between thumb and fingers and pressed lightly" or therapists may provide prescriptive feedback, such as "next time, press a little more."

Knowledge of Results

Feedback related to the desired outcome helps children understand movement. Providing this knowledge is most effective when specific information on the movement's goal is stated. Thus, "each button is lined up with its buttonhole" is preferred over "good job." Knowledge of results is motivating and encourages children to continue; it is most helpful when learning new motor tasks.

Verbal Feedback

Verbal praise and reinforcement are useful in motivating clients and changing behaviors but may be overused in clinical settings. Allowing children to make their own assessments of their performance is beneficial and will increase their sense of efficacy.[114] Verbal feedback is best if provided immediately after completion of the task. Using one to three brief cue words that can be repeated easily by the performer is best. Knowledge of correct performance motivates a child to continue practicing, so such reinforcement may be used frequently. Positive feedback with specific cues improves performance such as "you pressed firmly with the pencil!"

APPLICATION OF MOTOR CONTROL/ LEARNING THEORY IN OCCUPATIONAL THERAPY PRACTICE

Case Study 9-8 illustrates how therapists may apply current motor control/motor learning principles to practice. Specifically, this example applies dynamical systems theory from an occupational therapy perspective to intervention of a child's motor deficits.

CASE STUDY 9-8 Paul

Paul is a 7-year-old boy referred to occupational therapy after his mother expressed concern that he has difficulty using his hands, completing school work, playing on the playground, and often falls on the playground. Paul's mother states "he has trouble coloring, doing anything with his hands, and can't climb up the slide or get on the swing."

OCCUPATIONAL PROFILE

Paul enjoys playing with trucks and being outside. He shows an interest in the swings, but does not get on them. Rather, Paul sits close by and watches others on the swings. His mother notes that Paul enjoys playing on the floor in the living room with his trucks. Paul's mother is concerned that he is not active on the playground and falls frequently. She is worried that his difficulty with coloring and writing will interfere with his school tasks and he will not like school. She has already noticed Paul seems to get stomachaches frequently and dislikes mornings.

Paul lives with his parents and 2-year-old sister in a quiet suburb. There are plenty of children in the neighborhood and they frequently play together outside. Paul states he has "one good friend" and he spends afternoons playing with that child. Paul participates in recreational soccer (although he says, "I'm not very good").

He is currently in the first grade and having trouble with handwriting and reading. The teacher is concerned that Paul is not "picking up things" as quickly as his peers, although verbally he has plenty to say and contributes to the class.

OCCUPATIONAL PERFORMANCE

Paul presented as a thin, small 7-year-old boy, who stood with his shoulders depressed. Range of motion was within normal limits. His muscle tone throughout was slightly low, especially in the trunk. He sat with a rounded back and could not maintain balance with eyes closed. Paul ran with his feet apart and his arms did not swing consistently or in rhythm. He had

CASE STUDY 9-8   Paul—cont'd

difficulty changing positions as observed by stopping and reorienting himself as his friend ran around him. Paul showed poor sequencing and timing of movements—he could not jump with both feet together and was unable to catch a ball.

Fine motor skills were delayed as well. Paul held a pencil in a tight pronated grasp and made dark marks on the paper. He was unable to draw a straight line (3 inches) within the ¼″ markings—his line went over in more than 5 places. He sat independently with his feet on the floor, his back was rounded, and his face was close to the paper. He showed some associated reactions (e.g., facial movements) when writing. He was unable to do alternating hand movements or imitate tasks.

Paul was able to put on his coat and hat. He had difficulty with the buttons, but was able to do it with adequate time. He could not tie his shoes, but made multiple knots instead. Paul was the last child to go outside for recess. He played with his friend and watched others. His friend waited for him and frequently repeated, "Hurry up, Paul."

SYSTEMS CONTRIBUTING TO PERFORMANCE
Environment
Paul lives in the country in a 3-bedroom home. He has access to toys inside and outside. His home is child-friendly. The backyard is fenced in and includes a swing set, slide, and sandbox. Paul plays with his best friend daily and sometimes will "hang out" with his sister. He likes being outdoors and looking for things in the woods. He does not ride a bike, swing, or go down the slide.

School
Paul attends a local elementary school; there are 15 students in his class. The teacher provides structure and is consistent. She expressed concern that Paul is falling behind his classmates and states he has great difficulty with handwriting, paying attention, and getting things done in a timely manner. She notices Paul is always the last one out the door, forgets things in the classroom, and seems frustrated at times. However, she also notes that Paul is verbal and answers questions readily. She states he is well liked by his peers and teachers and is always polite and well behaved.

Neuromuscular
Paul's low muscle tone, poor postural control, and difficulty with timing and sequencing are interfering with his ability to move in a coordinated fashion. Paul shows some soft neurological signs, such as associated reactions. He is unable to balance with his eyes closed.

Sensory
Paul's poor balance and motor planning may be a result of difficulty processing vestibular information. There is also some indication that he has some visual perceptual deficits interfering with motor control. Paul's body awareness is somewhat affected because he is unable to identify right-left, which would be expected at his age. His internal body awareness is not quite developed.

INTERVENTION PLANNING
The occupational therapist, Cora, a school-based practitioner, developed an intervention plan based on a top-down approach focusing on helping Paul play with his peers and perform in the classroom. This plan addresses the parents' concern that Paul's motor skills are interfering with his motivation to attend school and thus, the therapist felt this was the place to start. Secondly, working on Paul's handwriting ability will help him be successful in school.

Keeping in mind that children learn best when they are presented with the whole versus a part of the activity, Cora designed a variety of gross motor games. The intent of intervention was to help Paul play with peers by developing postural control, motor planning abilities, and body awareness while completing fun games and helping him feel better about his abilities. Furthermore, helping Paul develop postural control, motor planning, and body awareness may also help him with his handwriting abilities.

During the first session, the therapist targeted postural control and balance for play by setting up a detailed obstacle course, Cora demonstrated the moves and stood back, asking Paul to perform. Paul made many mistakes but started to problem-solve toward the end of the course. Upon completion, he said, "Let me try it again and see if I can go faster." Cora provided some key points about one particular part of the course with which he had trouble. Providing verbal feedback after the child has performed on only a few key aspects is recommended for motor learning. Furthermore, allowing Paul to make and learn from his own motor mistakes allowed him to internalize the motor learning. This technique has been found to improve generalization. The therapist periodically changed the format, allowing Paul to make some revisions in the course, to ensure that the course was meaningful. At the end of the session, Cora suggested that next week they go out on the playground and see what was there. She wanted to conduct the session in the actual context of the activity because she knew this provided the most variability and meaning for Paul and consequently was the best for motor control and motor learning. She did not invite peers yet to participate because she wanted Paul to feel comfortable in the setting first and meet some motor challenges on his own before increasing the emotional factors.

Cora ended the session by talking to Paul about his writing and discussing strategies that might help make it easier for him in terms of motor functioning. Paul decided he would do better if he held the paper down with his left thumb; he liked the idea of using a mechanical pencil with a new pencil grip. Research suggest that discussing handwriting performance may help children improve motor performance.[7] For example, Banks, Rodger, and Polatajko found that discussing strategies (so the children come up with the solutions) helped four children with developmental coordination disorder to improve handwriting performance more than physical practice alone.[7] This may not work with all groups of children and requires and adequate level of cognition. More research needs to be

Continued

done to show this is effective. Since mental practice has been found to be effective in motor learning, Cora also talked to Paul about visualizing how he would complete his writing tasks in school. The therapist asked Paul to sit and visualize this for a moment before beginning the writing task.

Cora provided Paul with a variety of activities to promote his postural control that were meaningful and fun for him. Periodically, she found she had to stop the activity and review a certain skill (e.g., catch the ball with two hands, like this). When she reviewed specific skills, she provided only a few key phrases and paid close attention to the non-verbal and verbal cues Paul gave her. She considered how to facilitate his learning through the therapeutic use of self. She used a block practice schedule to teach the new skills. As Paul becomes more able, she will move to a distributed practice schedule and later a random or variable schedule. Understanding how he views the challenge is important in motor learning. If the skill appeared to be too difficult, she quickly and almost effortlessly graded the activity to make it easier. Conversely, she could make the activity more difficult so Paul is adequately challenged.

Cora also considered the social-emotional aspects of the motor challenges. Paul stated "everyone else can tie their shoes, but I can't." This told her a great deal and Cora decided now is the time to work on this skill. She also considered how body schema interfered with his ability to tie his shoes—he did not seem to have a sense of his body in space. Thus, Cora decided to integrate body awareness and body image activities in sessions. She incorporated such games as "Where is the shoe? Is it close to you?" and "hide and seek" of objects. They also played Simon Says in the mirror (reflective self-awareness) and games involving laterality and directionality.

Throughout the sessions, the therapist examined how Paul's sensory functioning, specifically his poor visual and vestibular processing, interfered with his movement. Consequently, she decided to design activities to challenge these systems in movement. Key to her intervention is keeping the intervention client-focused and working with Paul to develop strategies.

The therapist designed intervention to improve Paul's ability to play with other children and handwriting. Further analysis of Paul's motor difficulties included an evaluation of balance and posture, sensory processing, and timing and sequencing. Using the natural environment to facilitate movement, Cora arranged occupational therapy sessions at times when the child was outside playing, initially. Because Paul enjoyed outside activities, Cora decided to work with him there until Paul felt comfortable and had some success. After therapy progressed, the therapist worked with Paul inside with smaller trucks to encourage Paul to manipulate smaller objects. By targeting activities that were meaningful, Cora used Paul's volition as a way to increase motor skills. Cora carefully chose activities in which Paul could be successful. Cora also included other children in therapy sessions as Paul developed skills. This increased the environmental stimulation and required Paul adapt to the unpredictability of the other children. Because variability is key to movements and motor control, intervention sessions were full of many activities promoting gross and fine motor functioning.

This example shows how therapists acknowledge the multiple systems involved in movement to evaluate and design intervention. Furthermore, the therapist used principles of variability, meaning, occupation, and natural context when designing intervention. The therapist also incorporated motor learning principles of feedback, demonstration, practice, and sequencing and adapting tasks.

By capturing the child's goals of playing outside and the parent's goal of helping him play with his peers and school, the therapist targeted intervention to help the child improve occupational performance in a meaningful way. This approach promotes practice and learning by empowering children to meet their own occupational goals.

SUMMARY

This chapter defined motor control and motor learning and presented case examples to illustrate how to apply current research to occupational therapy practice with children and youth. Also defined was dynamical systems theory, and the components of movement, including postural control, balance, visual perception, and body awareness were described. An overview of motor learning concepts of practice, feedback, modeling or demonstration, and mental practice was provided. A final case example illustrated the application of motor control/motor learning principles to occupational therapy practice.

REFERENCES

1. Accardo, P., Pensiero, S., Da Pozzo, S., & Perissutti, P. (1995). Characteristics of horizontal smooth pursuit eye movements to sinusoidal stimulation in children of primary school age. *Vision Research, 35,* 539–548.

2. Allum, J., Honegger, F., & Schicks, H. (1994). The influence of a bilateral vestibular deficit on postural synergies. *Journal of Vestibular Research, 4,* 49–70.

3. American Occupational Therapy Association. (2008). *Occupational therapy practice framework: Domain & process.* Bethesda, MD: AOTA, Inc.

4. Aslin, R., & Ciuffreda, K. (1983). Eye movements in preschool children. *Science, 222,* 75–78.

5. Ayres, A. J. (1972). *Sensory integration and learning disorders.* Los Angeles: Western Psychological Services.

6. Bahrick, L. (1995). Intermodal origins of self-perception. In P. Rochat (Ed.), *The self in infancy: Theory & research* (pp. 349–374). Amsterdam: Elsevier.

7. Banks, R., Rodger, S., & Polatajko, H. (2008). Mastering handwriting: How children with developmental coordination disorder succeed with CO-OP. *OTJR: Occupation, Participation and Health, 28*(3), 100–109.

8. Barnes, M., & Crutchfield, C. (1990). *Reflex and vestibular aspects of motor control, motor development and motor learning.* Atlanta: Stokesville.

9. Bernstein, N. (1967). *The coordination and regulation of movements.* London: Pergamon.

10. Bertoldi, A. L. S., Ladewig, E., & Israel, V. L. (2007). Influence of selectivity of attention on the development of body awareness in children with motor deficiencies. *Revista Brasileira de Fisioterapia, 11*, 319–324.

11. Bobath, B. (1971). Motor development, its effect on general development and application to the treatment of cerebral palsy. *Physiotherapy, 57*, 526–532.

12. Bouffard, M., & Wall, A. E. (1990). A problem-solving approach to movement skill acquisition: Implications for special populations. In G. Reid (Ed.), *Problems in movement control* (pp. 107–131). Amsterdam: Elsevier Science.

13. Brenière, Y., & Bril, B. (1998). Development of postural control of gravity forces in children during the first 5 years of walking. *Experimental Brain Research, 121*, 255–262.

14. Brownwell, C., & Zerwas, S. (2007). "So Big": The development of body self awareness in toddlers. *Child Development, 78*, 1426–1440.

15. Bullock, M., & Lutkenhaus, P. (1990). Who am I? Self-understanding in toddlers. *Merrill Palmer Quarterly, 36*, 217–238.

16. Burtner, P., Qualls, C., & Woollacott, M. (1998). Muscle activation characteristics of stance balance control in children with spastic cerebral palsy. *Gait & Posture, 8*, 163–174.

17. Burtner, P., Woollacott, M., & Qualls, C. (1999). Stance balance control with orthoses in a select group of children with and without spasticity. *Developmental Medicine and Child Neurology, 41*, 748–757.

18. Carson, R. G., Goodman, D., Kelso, J. A. S., & Elliott, D. (1995). Phase transitions and critical fluctuations in rhythmic coordination of ipsilateral hand and foot. *Journal of Motor Behavior, 27*, 211–224.

19. Chen, Y., & Yang, T. (2007). Effect of task goals on the reaching patterns of children with cerebral palsy. *Journal of Motor Behavior, 39*, 317–324.

20. Cherng, R. J., Hsu, Y. W., Chen, Y. J., & Chen, J. Y. (2007). Standing balance of children with developmental coordination disorder under altered sensory conditions. *Human Movement Science, 26*, 913–926.

21. Clarke, J., & Whitall, J. (2003). Perception-action coupling in children with developmental coordination disorder. *Journal of Sport and Exercise Psychology, 25*, 9.

22. Cohn, E., Miller, L. J., & Tickle-Degnen, L. (2000). Parental hopes for therapy outcomes: Children with sensory modulation disorders. *American Journal of Occupational Therapy, 54*, 36–43.

23. Coleman, R., Piek, J., & Livesey, D. (2001). A longitudinal study of motor ability and kinaesthetic acuity in young children at risk of developmental coordination disorder. *Human Movement Science, 20*, 95–110.

24. Correa, V., Poulson, C., & Salzberg, C. (1984). Training and generalization of reach-grasp behavior in blind, retarded young children. *Journal of Applied Behavior Analysis, 17*, 57–69.

25. Davidson, T., & Williams, B. (2000). Occupational therapy for children with developmental coordination disorder: A study of the effectiveness of a combined sensory integration and perceptual-motor intervention. *British Journal of Occupational Therapy, 63*, 495–499.

26. Deecke, L. (1996). Planning, preparation, execution, and imagery of volitional action. *Cognitive Brain Research, 3*, 59–64.

27. DeLoache, J., Uttal, D., & Rosengren, K. (2004). Scale errors offer evidence for a perception-action dissociation early in life. *Science, 304*, 1027–1029.

28. Denis, M. (1985). Visual imagery and the use of mental practice in the development of motor skills. *Canadian Journal of Applied Sport Sciences, 10*, 4S–16S.

29. Diener, H., Dichgans, J., Guschlbauer, B., & Bacher, M. (1986). Role of visual and static vestibular influences on dynamic posture control. *Human Neurobiology, 5*, 105–113.

30. Driskell, J. E., Cooper, C., & Moran, A. (1994). Does imagery practice enhance performance? *Journal of Applied Psychology, 79*, 481–492.

31. Dutton, G., Saaed, A., Fahad, B., Fraser, R., McDaid, G., McDade, J., et al. (2004). Association of binocular lower visual field impairment, impaired simultaneous perception, disordered visually guided motion and inaccurate saccades in children with cerebral visual dysfunction—a retrospective observational study. *Eye, 18*, 27–34.

32. Emanuel, M., Jarus, T., & Bart, O. (2008). Effect of focus of attention and age on motor acquisition, retention, and transfer: A randomized trial. *Physical Therapy, 88*, 251–260.

33. Fisher, A. G. (1998). Uniting practice and theory in an occupational framework. *American Journal of Occupational Therapy, 52*, 509–521.

34. Freedman, E. G., & Sparks, D. L. (2000). Coordination of the eyes and head: Movement kinematics. *Experimental Brain Research, 131*, 22–32.

35. French, K. E., & Thomas, J. R. (1987). The relation of knowledge development to children's basketball performance. *Journal of Sport Psychology, 9*, 15–32.

36. Gardner, R., Sorter, R., & Friedman, B. (1997). Developmental changes in children's body images. *Journal of Social Behavior and Personality, 12*, 1019–1036.

37. Geuze, R. H. (2003). Static balance and developmental coordination disorder. *Human Movement Science, 22*, 527–548.

38. Geuze, R. H., Jongmans, M. J., Schoemaker, M. M., & Smits-Engelsman, B. C. (2001). Clinical and research diagnostic criteria for developmental coordination disorder: A review and discussion. *Human Movement Science, 20*, 7–47.

39. Gilner, J. A. (1985). Purposeful activity in motor learning theory: An event approach to motor skill acquisition. *American Journal of Occupational Therapy, 39*, 28–34.

40. Goodgold-Edwards, S. A., & Cermak, S. A. (1990). Integrating motor control and motor leaning concepts with neuropsychological perspectives on apraxia and developmental dyspraxia. *American Journal of Occupational Therapy, 44*, 431–439.

41. Gordon, A., Schneider, J., Chinnan, A., & Charles, J. (2007). Efficacy of a hand-arm bimanual intensive therapy (HABIT) in children with hemiplegic cerebral palsy: A randomized control trial. *Developmental Medicine and Child Neurology, 49*, 830–839.

42. Grove, C. R., & Lazarus, J. A. (2007). Impaired re-weighting of sensory feedback for maintenance of postural control in children with developmental coordination disorder. *Human Movement Science, 26*, 457–476.

43. Hadders-Algra, M., Brogren, E., & Forssberg, H. (1996). Ontogeny of postural adjustments during sitting in infancy: Variation, selection, and modulation. *Journal of Physiology, 493*, 273–288.

44. Hadders-Algra, M., Brogren, E., & Forssberg, H. (1998). Development of postural control-differences between ventral and dorsal muscles. *Neuroscience and Biobehavioral Reviews, 22*, 501–506.

45. Haishi, K., & Kokubun, M. (1995). Developmental trends in pursuit eye movements among preschool children. *Perceptual and Motor Skills, 81*, 1131–1137.

46. Hall, C. R. (1985). Individual differences in mental practice and imagery of motor skill performance. *Canadian Journal of Applied Science, 10*, 17S–21S.

47. Hatziki, V., Zisi, V., Kollias, I., & Kioumourtzoglou, E. (2002). Perceptual-motor contributions to static and dynamic balance control in children. *Journal of Motor Behavior, 34*, 161–170.

48. Hay, J., & Missiuna, C. (1998). Motor proficiency in children reporting low levels of participation in physical activity. *Canadian Journal of Occupational Therapy, 65*, 64–71.

49. Hebert, E., Landin, D., & Solmon, M. (1996). Practice schedule effects on the performance and learning of low and high skilled students: an applied study. *Research Quarterly for Exercise and Sport, 67*, 52–58.

50. Henderson, S., & Sugden, D. (1992). *Movement Assessment Battery for Children*. Kent, England: Psychological Corporation.

51. Hirshfeld, H., & Forssberg, H. (1994). Epigenetic development of postural responses for sitting during infancy. *Experimental Brain Research, 97,* 528–540.

52. Horak, F., Diener, H., & Nashner, L. (1990). Postural strategies associated with somatosensory and vestibular loss. *Experimental Brain Research, 82,* 167–177.

53. Horak, F., Jones-Rycewicz, C., Black, F., & Shumway-Cook, A. (1992). Effects of vestibular rehabilitation on dizziness and imbalance. *Otolaryngology Head and Neck Surgery, 106,* 175–180.

54. Hsieh, C. L., Nelson, D. L., Smith, D. A., & Petersen, C. Q. (1996). A comparison of performance in added-purpose occupations and rote exercise for dynamic standing balance in persons with hemiplegia. *American Journal of Occupational Therapy, 50,* 10–16.

55. Inder, J. M., & Sullivan, S. M. (2005). Motor and postural response profiles of four children with developmental coordination disorder. *Pediatric Physical Therapy, 17,* 18–29.

56. Ingles, J., Horak, F., Shupert, C., & Rycewicz, C. (1994). The importance of somatosensory information in triggering and scaling automatic postural responses in humans. *Experimental Brain Research, 101,* 159–164.

57. Jung-Potter, J. O., Kim, S. J., Metcalfe, J. S., Horn, C., Wilms-Floet, A., McMenamin, S., et al. (2002). *Somatosensory-motor coupling in children with Developmental Coordination Disorder.* Banff, Alberta: Paper presented at the Fifth Biennial Workshop on Children with DCD.

58. Kagerer, F., Bo, J., & Contreras-Vidal, J. (2004). Visuomotor adaptation in children with developmental coordination disorder. *Motor Control, 8,* 450–560.

59. Kaufman, L. B., & Schilling, D. L. (2007). Implementation of a strength training program for a 5 year-old child with poor body awareness and developmental coordination disorder. *Physical Therapy, 87,* 455–467.

60. Kielhofner, G. (2004). *Conceptual foundations of occupational therapy* (3rd ed.). Philadelphia: FA Davis.

61. Kielhofner, G. (2008). *Model of human occupation: Theory and application* (4th ed.). Philadelphia: FA Davis.

62. Klingberg, T., Forssberg, H., & Westerberg, H. (2002). Increased brain activity in frontal and parietal cortex underlies the development of visuospatial working memory capacity during childhood. *Journal of Cognitive Neuroscience, 14,* 1–10.

63. Kowler, A., & Martins, J. (1982). Eye movements in preschool children. *Science, 215,* 997–999.

64. Kramer, J. M. (2007). Using a participatory action approach to identify habits and routines to support self-advocacy. *OTJR: Occupation, Participation and Health, 27,* 84S–85S.

65. Langaas, T., Mon-Williams, M., Wann, J., Pascal, E., & Thompson, C. (1998). Eye movements, prematurity and developmental coordination disorder. *Vision Research, 38,* 1817–1826.

66. Law, M., Russell, D., Pollock, N., Rosenbaum, P., Walter, S., & King, G. (1997). A comparison of intensive neurodevelopmental therapy plus casting and a regular occupational therapy program for children with cerebral palsy. *Developmental Medicine & Child Neurology, 39,* 664–670.

67. Lewis, M., & Brooks-Gunn, J. (1979). *Social cognition and the acquisition of self.* New York: Plenum.

68. Lewis, M., & Ramsay, D. (2004). Development of self recognition, personal pronoun use, and pretend play during the 2nd year. *Child Development, 75,* 1821–1831.

69. Lowes, J., & Tiggemann, M. (2003). Body dissatisfaction, dieting awareness and the impact of parental influence in young children. *British Journal of Health Psychology, 8,* 135–147.

70. Malouin, F., & Richards, C. (2000). Preparatory adjustments during gait initiation in 4–6-year-old children. *Gait & Posture, 11,* 239–253.

71. Mandich, A. D., Polatajko, H. J., Macnab, J. J., & Miller, L. T. (2001). Treatment of children with developmental coordination disorder: What is the evidence? *Physical and Occupational Therapy in Pediatrics, 20,* 51–58.

72. Martineau, J., & Cochin, S. (2007). Visual perception in children: Human, animal and virtual movement activates different cortical areas. *International Journal of Psychophysiology, 51,* 37–44.

73. Mathiowetz, V., & Bass-Haugen, J. (1994). Motor behavior research: Implications for therapeutic approaches to central nervous system dysfunction. *American Journal of Occupational Therapy, 48,* 733–745.

74. Miller, L., & Nelson, D. L. (1987). Dual-purpose activity versus single-purpose activity in terms of duration on task, exertion level, and affect. *Occupational Therapy in Mental Health, 7,* 55–67.

75. Missiuna, C. (1994). Motor skill acquisition in children with developmental coordination disorder. *Adapted Physical Activity Quarterly, 11,* 214–235.

76. Missiuna, C., & Mandich, A. (2002). Integrating motor learning theories into practice. In S. Cermak & D. Larkin (Eds.), *Developmental coordination disorder* (pp. 221–233). Delmar.

77. Missiuna, C., Rivard, L., & Bartlett, D. (2006). Exploring assessment tools and the target of intervention for children with developmental coordination disorder. *Physical and Occupational Therapy in Pediatrics, 26,* 71–89.

78. Miyahara, M. (1996). A meta-analysis of intervention studies on children with developmental coordination disorder. *Corpus, Psyche & Societas, 3,* 11–18.

79. Miyahara, M., & Wafer, A. (2004). Clinical intervention for children with developmental coordination disorder: A multiple case study. *Adapted Physical Activity Quarterly, 21,* 281–300.

80. Moore, C., Mealiea, J., Garon, N., & Povinelli, D. (2007). The development of body self-awareness. *Infancy, 11,* 157–174.

81. Murphy, S. M. (1994). Imagery interventions in sport. *Medicine and Science in Sports and Exercise, 26,* 486–494.

82. Nararro, A., Fukujima, M., Fontes, S., Matas, S., & Prado, G. (2004). Balance and motor coordination are not fully developed in 7 year old blind children. *Auquivos de Neuro-Psiquiatria, 62,* 654–657.

83. Nashner, L. (1990). Sensory, neuromuscular, and biomechanical contributions to human balance. In P. Duncan, (Ed.), *Balance proceedings of the APTA forum.* Alexandria, VA: American Physical Therapy Association.

84. Nashner, L., Shumway-Cook, A., & Marin, O. (1983). Stance posture control in select groups of children with cerebral palsy: Deficits in sensory organization and muscular coordination. *Experimental Brain Research, 49,* 393–409.

85. Nelson, D. L. (1988). Occupation: Form and performance. *American Journal of Occupational Therapy, 42,* 633–641.

86. O'Brien, J., Bergeron, A., Duprey, H., Olver, C., & St. Onge, H. (2009). Children with disabilities and their parents' views of occupational participation needs. *Occupational Therapy in Health Care, 25,* 1–17.

87. O'Brien, J., Williams, H., Bundy, A., Lyons, J., & Mittal, A. (2008). Mechanisms that underlie coordination in children with developmental coordination disorder. *Journal of Motor Behavior, 40,* 43–61.

88. Page, S., Sime, W., & Nordell, K. (1999). The effects of imagery on female college swimmers' perceptions of anxiety. *The Sport Psychologist, 13,* 458–469.

89. Painter, M., Inman, K., & Vincent, W. (1994). Contextual interference effects: I. the acquisition and retention of motor tasks by individuals with mild mental handicaps. *Adapted Physical Activity Quarterly, 11,* 383–395.

90. Patla, A. (1997). Understanding the roles of vision in the control of human locomotion. *Gait & Posture, 5,* 54–69.

91. Piek, J., & Skinner, R. (1999). Timing and force control during a sequential tapping task in children with and without motor coordination problems. *Journal of International Neuropsychological Society, 5,* 320–329.

92. Polatajko, H. J., Kaplan, B. J., & Wilson, B. N. (1992). Sensory integration treatment for children with learning disabilities: Its status 20 years later. *Occupational Therapy Journal of Research, 12,* 323–341.

93. Polatajko, H., Mandich, A., Miller, L., & Macnab, J. (2001). Cognitive orientation to daily occupational performance (CO-OP): Part II—the evidence. *Physical & Occupational Therapy in Pediatrics, 20,* 83–106.

94. Polivy, J., & Herman, C. P. (1993). Etiology of binge eating: Psychological mechanisms. In C. G. Fairburn & G. T. Wilson (Eds.), *Binge eating: Nature, assessment and treatment* (pp. 50–76). New York: Guilford Press.

95. Przysucha, E. P., & Taylor, M. J. (2004). Control of stance and developmental coordination disorder: The role of visual information. *Adapted Physical Activity Quarterly, 21,* 19–33.

96. Rathunde, K. (2001). Toward a psychology of optimal human functioning: What positive psychology can learn from the 'experiential turns' of James, Dewey, and Maslow. *The Journal of Humanistic Psychology, 41,* 135–153.

97. Raynor, A. (2001). Strength, power, and coactivation in children with developmental coordination disorder. *Developmental Medicine and Child Neurology, 43,* 676–684.

98. Rizzolatti, G., Fadiga, L., Gallese, V., & Fogassi, L. (1996). Premotor cortex and the recognition of motor actions. *Cognition and Brain, 3,* 131–141.

99. Rochat, P. (1995). Early objectification of the self. In P. Rochat (Ed.), *The self in infancy: Theory and research* (pp. 53–71). Amsterdam: Elsevier.

100. Rochat, P. (1998). Self perception and action in infancy. *Experimental Brain Research, 123,* 102–109.

101. Rood, M. (1956). Neurophysiological mechanisms utilized in the treatment of neuromuscular dysfunction. *American Journal of Occupational Therapy, 10,* 220–224.

102. Ross, R., Radant, A., & Hommer, D. (1993). A development study of smooth pursuit eye movements in normal children from 7 to 15 years of age. *Journal of American Academy of Child and Adolescent, 32,* 783–791.

103. Ryan, E. D., & Simons, J. (1982). Efficacy of mental imagery in enhancing mental rehearsal of motor skills. *Journal of Sports Psychology, 4,* 41–51.

104. Schoemaker, M. M., Niemeijer, A. S., Reynders, K., & Smits-Engelsman, B. C. (2003). Effectiveness of neuromotor task training for children with developmental coordination disorder: A pilot study. *Neural Plasticity, 10,* 153–163.

105. Schoemaker, M. M., van der Wees, M., Flapper, B., Verheij-Jansen, N., Scholten-Jaegers, S., & Geuze, R. H. (2001). Perceptual skills of children with developmental coordination disorder. *Human Movement Science, 20,* 111–133.

106. Shaefer, S., Krampe, R., Lindenberger, U., & Baltes, P. (2008). Age differences between children and young adults in the dynamics of dual-task prioritization: Body (balance) versus mind (mind). *Developmental Psychology, 44,* 747–757.

107. Shumway-Cook, A., & Woollacott, M. (2001). *Motor control: Theory and practical applications* (2nd ed.). Philadelphia: Lippincott Williams & Wilkins.

108. Shumway-Cook, A., & Woollacott, M. (2007). *Motor control: Theory and practical applications* (3rd ed). Philadelphia: Lippincott Williams & Wilkins.

109. Steenbergen, B., & Gordon, A. M. (2006). Activity limitation in hemiplegic cerebral palsy: Evidence for disorders in motor planning. *Developmental Medicine and Child Neurology, 48,* 780–783.

110. Steinbeck, T. (1986). Purposeful activity and performance. *American Journal of Occupational Therapy, 40,* 529–534.

111. Steultjens, E. M. J., Dekker, J., Bouter, L. M., Leemrijse, C. J., & van den Ende, C. H. M. (2005). Evidence of the efficacy of occupation therapy in different conditions: An overview of systematic reviews. *Clinical Rehabilitation, 19,* 247–254.

112. Sugden, D., & Dunford, C. (2007). Intervention and the role of theory, empiricism and experience in children with motor impairment. *Disability & Rehabilitation, 29,* 3–11.

113. Sugden, D., & Utley, A. (1995). Interlimb coupling in children with hemiplegic cerebral palsy. *Developmental Medicine and Child Neurology, 37,* 293–309.

114. Sullivan, K., Kantuk, S., & Burtner, P. (2008). Motor learning in children: Feedback effects on skill acquisition. *Physical Therapy, 88,* 720–732.

115. Sundermier, L., Woollacott, M., Jensen, J., & Moore, S. (1996). Postural sensitivity to visual flow in aging adults with and without balance problems. *Journal of Gerontology, 51,* M45–M52.

116. Taktek, K., Zinsser, N., & St.-John, B. (2008). Visual versus kinesthetic mental imagery: Efficacy for the retention and transfer of a closed motor skill in young children. *Canadian Journal of Experimental Psychology, 62,* 174–187.

117. Thelen, E., Kelso, J., Kelso, J. S., & Fogel, A. (1987). Self-organizing systems and infant motor development. *Developmental Review, 7,* 39–65.

118. Truby, H., & Paxton, S. (2002). Development of the children's body image scale. *British Journal of Clinical Psychology, 41,* 185–204.

129. Trombly, C. A. (1995). Occupation: Purposefulness and meaningfulness as therapeutic mechanisms. 1995 Eleanor Clarke Slagle Lecture. *American Journal of Occupational Therapy, 49,* 960–972.

120. Tsai, C. L., Wu, S. K., & Huan, C. H. (2008). Static balance in children with developmental coordination disorder. *Journal of Human Movement, 27,* 142–153.

121. Utley, A., & Sugden, D. (1998). Interlimb coupling in children with hemiplegic cerebral palsy during reaching and grasping at speed. *Developmental Medicine and Child Neurology, 40,* 396–404.

122. Vaillant, J., Vuillerme, N., Janvery, A., Louis, F., Braujou, R., Juvin, R., et al. (2008). Effect of manipulation of the feet and ankles on postural control in elderly adults. *Brain Research Bulletin, 75,* 18–22.

123. Vandenbussche, E. (2000). Deficits of visual perception in children with cerebral visual impairment due to early brain damage. *Perception, 29,* 6.

124. Van der Weel, F. R., Van der Meer, A. L., & Lee, D. N. (1991). Effect of task on movement control in cerebral palsy: Implications for assessment and therapy. *Developmental Medicine & Child Neurology, 33,* 419–426.

125. Van Waelvelde, H., De Weerdt, W., De Cock, P., Janssens, L., Feys, H., & Smits Engelsman, B. C. M. (2006). Parameterization of movement execution in children with developmental coordination disorder. *Brain and Cognition, 60,* 20–31.

126. Visser, T., Boden, C., & Giaschi, D. (2004). Children with dyslexia: Evidence for visual attention deficits in perception of rapid sequences of objects. *Vision Research, 44,* 2521–2535.

127. von Hofsten, C., & Rosander, K. (1996). The development of gaze control and predictive tracking in young infants. *Vision Research, 36,* 81–96.

128. Wann, J. P., Mon-Williams, M., & Rushton, K. (1998). Postural control and co-ordination disorders: The swinging room revisited. *Human Movement Science, 17,* 491–513.

129. Williams, H. (1983). *Perceptual and motor development.* Englewood Cliffs, NJ: Prentice-Hall.

130. Williams, H. (2002). Motor control in children with developmental coordination disorder. In S. A. Cermak, & D. Larkin (Eds.), *Developmental coordination disorder* (pp. 117–137). Delmar.

131. Williams, H. (2005). *A working model of visual perception: A manual for developing visual perception behaviors in children.* Columbia, SC: University of South Carolina Press.

132. Williams, H. (2006). Motor control. In J. Solomon, & J. O'Brien. (Eds.), *Pediatric skills for occupational therapy assistants* (2nd ed., pp. 461–480). St. Louis: Mosby.

133. Williams, H. (2007). *Balance control: A smart text.* Columbia, SC: University of South Carolina Press.

134. Williams, H. (2007). *Perceptual-motor development evaluation protocols: Process characteristics of balance.* Columbia, SC: University of South Carolina Press.

135. Williams, H., Fisher, J., & Tritschler, K. (1983). Descriptive analysis of static postural control in 4, 6, and 8 year old normal and motorically awkward children. *American Journal of Physical Medicine, 62,* 12–26.

136. Williams, H., & Ho, L. (2004). Balance and postural control across the lifespan. In D. Dewey & D. Tupper (Eds.), *Developmental motor disorders: A neurological perspective* (pp. 211–236). New York: Guilford Press.

137. Wilmut, K., Wann, J. P., & Brown, J. H. (2006). Problems in the coupling of eye and hand in the sequential movements of children with Developmental Coordination Disorder. *Child Care, Health & Development, 32,* 665–678.

138. Woollacott, M., Burtner, P., Jensen, J., Jasiewicz, J., Roncesvalles, N., & Sveistrup, H. (1998). Development of postural responses during standing in healthy children and in children with spastic diplegia. *Neuroscience Biobehavioral Review, 22,* 583–589.

139. Woollacott, M., & Shumway-Cooke, A. (1990). Changes in posture control across the life span: A systems approach. *Physical Therapy, 70,* 799–807.

140. Woollacott, M., & Sveistrup, H. (1992). Changes in the sequencing and timing of muscle response coordination associated with developmental transitions in balance abilities. *Human Movement Science, 11,* 23–36.

141. Yoder, R., Nelson, D., & Smith, D. (1989). Added purpose versus rote exercise in female nursing home residents. *American Journal of Occupational Therapy, 43,* 581–586.

142. Zanone, P. G., & Kelso, J. A. S. (1994). The coordination dynamics of learning: Theoretical structure and experimental agenda. In S. P. Swinnen, H. Heuer, J. Massion, & P. Casaer (Eds.), *Interlimb coordination: Neural, dynamical, and cognitive constraints* (pp. 461–490). San Diego, CA: Academic Press.

143. Zoia, S., Castiello, U., Blason, L., & Scabar, A. (2005). Reaching in children with and without developmental coordination disorder under normal and perturbed vision. *Developmental Neuropsychology, 27,* 257–273.

10 Evaluation and Interventions to Develop Hand Skills

Charlotte E. Exner

Visual-motor
  integration
Fine motor
  coordination
Fine motor skills
Dexterity

Hand skills
Reach and carry
Grasp
Voluntary release
In-hand manipulation
Bilateral hand use

OBJECTIVES

1. Describe the typical development of hand skills in children.
2. Identify factors that contribute to typical or atypical development of hand skills.
3. Explain the implications of hand skill problems for children's occupational performance, particularly in the areas of play, activities of daily living, and school performance.
4. Describe typical problems with children's development of hand skills.
5. Identify evaluation tools and methods useful in assessing hand skills in children.
6. Describe intervention approaches and strategies to assist children in improving or compensating for problems with hand skills.

Hand skills are critical to interaction with the environment. The hands allow action through human contact and contact with objects. Hands are the "tools" most often used to accomplish work and play and to perform activities of daily living. The child who has a disability affecting hand skills has less opportunity to take in sensory information from the environment and to experience the effect of his or her actions on the world.

COMPONENTS OF HAND SKILLS

Effective use of the hands to engage in a variety of occupations depends on a complex interaction of hand skills, postural mechanisms, cognition, and visual perception.

The term *visual-motor integration* refers to the interaction of visual skills, visual-perceptual skills, and motor skills. The term *hand skills* is used interchangeably with the terms *fine motor coordination, fine motor skills,* and *dexterity.* Because this chapter refers only to skills of the hands that are needed to attain and manipulate objects, the more specific term *hand skills* is used.

Although most therapists assume that the development of hand skills depends on adequate postural functions and sufficient visual-perceptual and cognitive development, these areas are not discussed in detail in this chapter. Hand skills are patterns that normally rely on both tactile-proprioceptive and visual information for accuracy. However, the child can accomplish these skills without visual feedback if somatosensory functions provide adequate information. The patterns include reach, grasp, carry, and voluntary release, as well as the more complex skills of in-hand manipulation and bilateral hand use. These patterns can be defined briefly as follows:

- Reach: extension and movement of the arm for grasping or placing objects
- Grasp: attainment of an object with the hand
- Carry: transportation of a hand-held object from one place to another
- Voluntary release: intentional letting go of a hand-held object at a specific time and place
- In-hand manipulation: adjustment of an object in the hand after grasp
- Bilateral hand use: use of two hands together to accomplish an activity

In the following discussion, the term *hand-arm* refers to the interactive movement and stabilization of different parts of the hand and arm to accomplish a fine motor task.

Visual skills constitute the use of extra-ocular muscles to direct eye movements. These skills include the ability to visually fix on a stationary object and the smooth, accurate tracking of a moving target. *Visual-perceptual skills* involve the recognition, discrimination, and processing of sensory information through the eyes and related central nervous system (CNS) structures. Visual-perceptual skills include the identification of shapes, colors, and other qualities; the orientation of objects or shapes in space; and the relationship of objects or shapes to one another and to the environment (see Chapter 12).

CONTRIBUTIONS OF CONTEXTUAL FACTORS TO HAND SKILLS

For occupational therapists, knowledge of context factors is critical for understanding, evaluating, and providing intervention for hand skill problems. Social and cultural factors, in particular, are likely to play important roles in the acquisition and use of various hand skills. Social factors that can affect the development of hand skills include socioeconomic status and gender and role expectations. Both cultural social factors are less likely to affect the development of more basic hand skills but may have a greater influence on skills needed for complex manipulation of objects and tool use. For example, children who live in conditions of poverty may not have the exposure to writing utensils, scissors, and other materials common to children from middle-class environments.

The objects that are important to the child's cultural group influence the development of object manipulation. Because tools that are important in one culture may not be available in another, children may not have the opportunity to develop some tool-specific skills. For example, eating utensils vary from chopsticks to forks and spoons. Scissors use may be important for school performance in some cultures but not in others.

In addition, the age at which children are expected to achieve skill in object manipulation can vary. Safety concerns influence parents in some cultural groups to delay introduction of a knife to their child, whereas parents in other cultural groups encourage independence in knife use. Some cultures introduce children to the use of writing materials before 1 year of age. Other cultures do not provide children with these materials until they can be expected to adhere to requirements such as using them only on paper (rather than on the wall or on clothing).

Culture also influences the perception of children's need for manipulative materials. Linked to this is the cultural group's view of the importance of play. Play materials that provide opportunities for the development of manipulative skills (e.g., building sets, beads, puzzles, table games) are highly valued in some cultural groups, whereas in other groups, play with gross motor objects (e.g., balls, riding toys) or play with animals is more valued. Some cultural groups do not view children's play as important; therefore, few play materials of any type are available.

Although the types of activities encouraged can promote the development of specific skills, acquisition of the basic hand skills of reach, grasp, release, and manipulation does not rely on the availability of any particular materials; rather, it relies on reasonable exposure to a variety of materials with the opportunity to handle them. Verdonck and Henneberg studied differences in performance on the Box and Block Test of Manual Dexterity in two groups of South African children between 6 and 17 years of age.[140] They found that children from the middle-class urban area performed significantly better than those from the poor rural area. Yim, Cho, and Lee found that school-aged Korean children had somewhat less strength in palmar and lateral pinch than that measured in Western children.[153]

CONTRIBUTIONS OF BODY FUNCTIONS TO HAND SKILLS

Body functions related to performance play a critical role in the development of hand skills. Although therapists usually give motor issues the most attention, many dimensions of development significantly influence effective hand use, including the child's visual skills, somatosensory functions, sensory integration, visual perception, cognition and, as discussed above, social factors and culture. As children mature, they begin to coordinate visual skills with hand skills effectively, and later they combine hand-eye coordination with visual-perceptual skills.[3]

Visual Skills

Visual skills play a major role in the development of hand function.[10,77,142] Vision is particularly important for learning new motor skills. At about 4 months of age, infants begin to move their hands under visual control as they reach for an object and make differentiated finger movements. The visuomotor development required for accurate reach matures by approximately 6 months of age. The infant's visual-motor coordination continues to refine, and by 9 months of age, the infant guides his or her hand movements using visual-somatosensory integration (i.e., these sensory inputs are combined and compared as the infant anticipates and plans movement). Vision is also important as the infant learns new fine motor skills or when an activity requires highly precise and accurate movements (e.g., stringing small beads or putting together a puzzle).

Somatosensory Functions

The relationship between somatosensory functions of the hands and hand skills is strong. Good hand skills are associated with intact somatosensory functioning; however, intact somatosensory functioning does not necessarily yield good hand skills. Huang, Gillespie, and Kuo found that adults with normal hand function had significant benefit from feedback that included both visual and haptic information to ensure consistency and rhythm while manipulating an object.[74]

The role of somatosensory information and feedback is critical to development in many areas of children's hand skills, particularly those involving isolated movements of the fingers and thumb. Typical infants develop the ability to match *haptic perception* (knowledge of objects gathered by means of active touch) of some three-dimensional objects with visual perception within the first 6 months of life. Bushnell and Boudreau reported that children as young as 2.5 years of age can identify common objects by touch alone and that children 5 years of age demonstrate good haptic recognition of unfamiliar objects.[16] Many aspects of haptic perception, such as identification of three-dimensional common objects and perception of spatial orientation, are well developed by 6 years of age. The adolescent has fully developed the refinement of haptic perception and the ability to discriminate all aspects of object characteristics through touch.[132]

The fingertips gather precise information about many types of object qualities. Children with impaired control of finger movement have limited access to somatosensory information, and/or the impaired control of finger movement may reflect their difficulties in perceiving and using sensory information. Initiating and sustaining grasp force requires tactile and proprioceptive input and integration.[60,64,78] The ability to hold objects in the hand (i.e., without dropping them) is related primarily to intact somatosensory functioning.[62] Gordon and Duff also noted that tactile information is critical for anticipating the amount of force needed to grasp and lift an object.[64] Apparently a minimum amount of tactile awareness, as measured by two-point discrimination, is needed for functional development of these fine motor skills.

Somatosensory functioning is difficult to study in children, particularly in young children and those with disabilities. In testing, the performance of these children varies from one session to another, which further complicates the assessment process. Given that the link between somatosensory functioning and hand skills is a strong one, further investigation of the relationship between tactile functioning and various hand skills will support the development of new intervention approaches for these children.

Sensory Integration

The types of sensory integration problems most likely to influence hand use are sensory registration problems, tactile hypersensitivity, poor tactile discrimination, and dyspraxia. Children with poor sensory registration engage in few activities involving hand skills. The child with tactile hypersensitivity is likely to avoid contact with certain materials, thus limiting exposure to various objects. Motor-planning deficits and clumsiness are associated with poor tactile and proprioceptive functioning. Praxis problems based on poor tactile and proprioceptive processing are referred to as *somatodyspraxia*.[4] Children with cerebral palsy can have sensory integration problems in addition to motor problems. Evidence of motor planning problems has been identified in children with cerebral palsy[130] as well as in children with other motor problems.

Visual Perception and Cognition

Perceptual development and cognitive development are difficult to isolate from each other, particularly as they relate to object-handling skills in children; for this reason, these areas are addressed together here. The development of hand skills allows for more complex interaction with objects, and perceptual and cognitive development allows the child to know the possibilities available for object use and interactions. Hand use and cognitive development seem to be particularly linked in infancy and very early childhood.[35]

The child's perception of object characteristics, movement speed required, and power needed affects his or her ability to effectively control objects.[44] The child acquires knowledge about objects through object manipulation. Early manual exploratory behavior plays an important role in the development of visual-spatial skills and learning about the environment.[34]

During the first 6 months, the infant uses visual and tactile perception to guide fine motor development and begins to develop an awareness of object placement in space. In the second half of the first year, the infant adjusts the actions of the hand in response to object characteristics, such as size, shape, and surface qualities.[28] Ruff, McCarton, Kurtzber, and Vaughan emphasized the importance of object manipulation in infants between 6 and 12 months of age for learning object characteristics, because this learning was believed to be important for concept and language development.[119] Infants demonstrate their perceptual and cognitive skills when reaching for objects. By 9 to 10 months of age, infants adapt their arm positions to horizontal versus vertical object presentations and shape their hands appropriately for convex and concave objects.

During the second year, infants learn to relate objects to one another with more accuracy and purpose. Before 18 months of age, infants modify their movement approach in anticipation of the weight of the object.[16,28]

Rao discussed the interaction of cognition and hand skill development.[114] Like perceptual development, cognitive development influences and is supported by the development of hand skills. For example, changes in attentional control and the development of problem-solving strategies are seen in the gradual improvement in infants' ability to handle two objects simultaneously. Without this development in cognition, bilateral skills would not be possible. The infant must be able to attend to two objects simultaneously to be able to bang objects together, stabilize an object with one hand while manipulating with the other, and manipulate two or more objects simultaneously. Because attention and planning demands are greater for two-handed activities than for one-handed activities, bilateral skill development lags behind unilateral skill development.[16,28]

Skeletal Integrity

The integrity of the hand's joint and bone structures is an important consideration in hand function. Children with congenital hand anomalies may be missing one or more digits, a condition that significantly affects the variety of possible prehension patterns. Refined finger movements and in-hand manipulation skills may also be limited or absent. Severe congenital anomalies can affect bilateral hand use. Involvement of the thumb has a more significant effect on acquisition and use of hand skills than impairment of any other digit.

Joint range of motion (ROM) has a significant effect on the positioning of the arm for hand use and on reaching and carrying skills. Effective hand function also depends on adequate mobilization of distal muscle groups that control palmar arches. Limitations in range can occur as a result of abnormal joint structure, muscle weakness, or joint inflammation. Any of the problems that reduce range of motion are likely to affect a child's ability to grasp larger objects or to flatten the hand to stabilize materials.

Muscle Function

Aspects of muscle functions include muscle power (strength), muscle tone, and muscle endurance. Sufficient strength is necessary to initiate all types of grasp patterns and to maintain these patterns during lifting and carrying. Children's grasp strength gradually increases through the preschool years,[88,89] the elementary school years,[153] and adolescence.[93,126] This increase allows them to engage in activities with objects of increasing weight and to use greater resistance. Children with poor strength may be unable to initiate the finger extension or the thumb opposition pattern necessary before grasp. They also may not have the flexor control to hold a grasp pattern. Many children with diminished strength are unable to use patterns that rely on the intrinsic muscles for control and therefore are unable to use thumb opposition or metacarpophalangeal (MCP) joint flexion with interphalangeal (IP) joint extension. Children with fair strength may be able to initiate a grasp pattern but may be unable to lift an object against gravity while maintaining the grasp. Endurance during an activity can be a problem for children with mildly diminished strength, particularly in situations in which they must use a sustained grasp pattern or hold an object against resistance (e.g., during eating with utensils, coloring, handwriting, and scissors activities).

Tone in muscle groups affects the stability of parts of the arms and hands during activities and the types of movements possible. Damage to the CNS may cause tonal abnormalities, which can affect joint ROM and, in general, decrease speed of movement.

Increased tone results in loss of ROM, whereas decreased tone results in exaggerated joint ROM and decreased stability. Children with fluctuating tone typically have full ROM but can maintain joint stability only at the extreme end of a joint position (full flexion or full extension). In addition, movements are less controlled and often are random or unrelated to the task.

GENERAL DEVELOPMENTAL CONSIDERATIONS

Developmental principles are further described in Chapter 3. Overall, hand skill development has a very long course, continuing through adolescence for many skills.[33,65] This long course of development mirrors other aspects of development and reflects the complexity of hand skills in expressing an understanding of objects and what they can be used to accomplish.

Two principles with particular application to hand skill development are the development of movement patterns from mass to specific and of motor control from proximal to distal. Two additional principles are discussed in this section: specifically, that mature movement patterns are characterized by integrated stability and mobility and that involuntary movement patterns precede associated movements that develop into isolated, voluntary movement and coordinated action.

The mass-to-specific principle of development means that less-differentiated movement patterns precede discrete, highly specialized skills. For example, the infant uses all fingers in early grasping and later uses only the specific number of fingers needed for object contact.

The proximal-to-distal principle means that development initially occurs proximally (in the head and trunk) and gradually progresses toward the distal parts of the body (hands and feet). Clinicians have interpreted this relationship to mean that improvement in postural control results in improvement in hand skills and/or that intervention should be sequential, proceeding from proximal to distal control. However, several clinical research studies[24,146] and some authors[105,106] have questioned this principle. The clinical studies have yielded weak correlations between postural or proximal control and hand function (approximately $r = 0.20$ to 0.35). Case-Smith and colleagues stated that "the correlations between the proximal and distal motor functions would be markedly higher if proximal motor control was necessary for the development of distal motor skill" (p. 661).[24] The relationship between proximal and distal control is a functional or biomechanical one in which postural control is necessary for placement of the hand in space and support of the hand during its execution of skills. These workers emphasized that "therapists should not assume that proximal control is a necessary precursor to fine motor skill; they should, however, assume that treating proximal weakness may affect distal function" (p. 661).[24] However, the degree of proximal control does not necessarily determine the child's degree of distal control.

Pehoski[106] used work by Lawrence and Kuypers[87] to explain why distal control is not directly linked to proximal control. Two motor systems are used in upper extremity control. One system is responsible for postural control and proximal control, including integrated body-limb and body-head movements. This system comprises primarily the ventromedial brainstem pathways that synapse primarily with interneurons to trunk and proximal muscles. In contrast, the corticospinal track system originates in the primary motor cortex, and its fibers directly synapse with the motoneurons for hand muscles. The latter system allows for isolated finger movements, which are needed for a precise pincer grasp and fine manipulation.[106] Thus development of upper extremity skills and hand skills occurs as a result of proximal *and* distal control mechanisms, rather than proximal *to* distal mechanism.

Refined movements also depend on the ability to combine patterns of stability and mobility effectively. The child must develop the ability to stabilize the trunk effectively and maintain it in an upright position without relying on the frequent use of one or both arms to maintain balance. In addition, the child sequentially develops patterns of stability and mobility in the scapulohumeral, elbow, and wrist joints; this permits arm use independent of, but effectively used with, trunk movement. Eventually the ability to use stability and mobility in the hand emerges.

For normal functioning, joints must be able to stabilize at any point in the normal range of movement and to move within small, medium-sized, or large segments of range. During most arm-hand activities (e.g., grasp and manipulation of objects), the proximal joints are stable while the fingers are moving. However, in carrying, the distal joints are stable while the arm is moving. In mature handwriting, the elbow, forearm, and wrist joints are relatively stable and the shoulder and finger joints are mobile.

An important sequence in the development of motor control is the use of straight movement patterns before the emergence of controlled rotation patterns. For example, the infant first develops controlled stability and mobility in basic flexion and extension of the shoulder, elbow, and wrist. This is followed by control of internal and external rotation of the shoulder and pronation and supination of the forearm.

In typical development the infant gradually learns to use both sides of the body together in effective ways and to use each side of the body independently of the other. Initially the infant uses his or her arms in asymmetrical patterns that are not coordinated. Movements of one arm often elicit reflexive, nonpurposeful reactions in the other arm. Gradually the infant develops the ability to move the two arms together in the same pattern. As skilled use of symmetrical hand and arm patterns is refined, the infant begins to use the two arms independently of one another for different parts of an activity. For example, one hand stabilizes an object while the other hand manipulates it. Overflow and associated movements gradually decrease to allow separate but coordinated action of the two hands.

DEVELOPMENT OF HAND SKILLS

As in all areas of occupational therapy, the therapist must supplement academic study of hand skill development and treatment with observations of typical infants and children and of children with differences in development. Imitating each of the normal and abnormal movements and patterns described in the following text also helps clarify the descriptions provided.

Reach and Carry

Rosblad stated that "in a reaching movement, the goal is to transport the hand to the target, with precision in both time and space" (p. 81).[117] Thus the development of reaching is described in terms of the changes that take place in the control and speed of the hand's movement toward the object and the preparation of the hand for grasp.

Within the first several days of life, the neonate shows visual regard of objects close to him or her and activation of the arms in response to objects.[141] Over the next few months the arms become more active and the infant swipes or bats at objects with the arm abducted at the shoulder. Reach with an extended arm is likely to occur between approximately 12 and 22 weeks of age.[136] Objects are rarely grasped and then only by accident. If grasped, they are released at random, generally in association with arm movements.

Gradually a midline orientation of the hands develops. Initially the hands are held close to the body. Soon, with an increased desire for visual regard of the hands and greater proximal arm stability, the child holds the hands further away to view them. This pattern precedes the onset of symmetric bilateral reaching, which usually occurs first in the supine and then in the sitting position. At this stage, the child initiates reach with humeral abduction, partial shoulder internal rotation, forearm pronation, and full finger extension.

As the infant shows increasing dissociation of the two body sides during movement, unilateral reaching begins. Abduction and internal rotation of the shoulder are less prominent in reach. The hand opens in preparation for grasping the object and is usually more open than necessary for the size of the object.

As scapular control and trunk stability mature, the infant begins to use shoulder flexion, slight external rotation, full elbow extension, forearm supination, and slight wrist extension during reaching. Active supination of the forearm is not seen until some external rotation is used to stabilize the humerus. In addition, well-controlled elbow extension evolves as the rotation elements are developing. Mature reach is usually seen with sustained trunk extension and a slight rotation of the trunk toward the object of interest. Over the next few years, the child refines this unilateral reaching pattern, increasing the accuracy of arm placement and the grading of finger extension as appropriate to the size of the object (Figure 10-1), as well as the timing of the various movement elements. To study the evolution of reaching behaviors after its primary development, Schneiberg, Sveistrup, McFadyen, McKinley, and Levin compared reaching behavior in typical 4- to 11-year-olds with that of adults.[121] Developmental changes during this period include decreased trunk movement when objects are within arm's length, enhanced smoothness, and decreased variability. With increasing age, arm movements were straighter and reaching patterns were more consistent.[121] The quality of reach with grasp continues to mature until approximately 12 years of age, at which time the child prepares the hand with the optimal hand opening for the object size at the initiation of reach.[84] Before this age the child needs to use visual monitoring for accuracy in hand opening during reach.

Carrying ("moving" and "lifting") involves a smooth combination of body movements accompanied by stabilization of an object in the hand. When carrying involves objects used in most occupational activities, small ranges of movements are used and adjusted in accordance with the demands of the activity. Co-contraction in the more distal joints of the wrist and hand often is present. The child must be able to hold the forearm stable while in any degree of rotation, and he or she must be able to modify the forearm and wrist positions during the carry so that the object remains in an optimal position. Similarly, the child must be able to use shoulder rotation movements simultaneously with shoulder flexion and abduction so that appropriate object orientation is maintained.

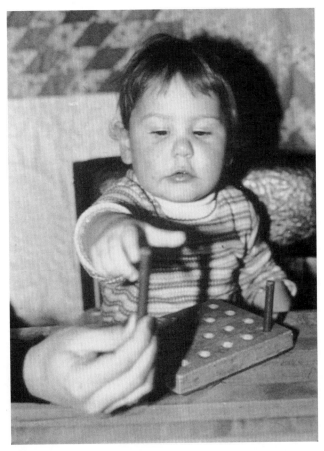

FIGURE 10-1 This typically developing child demonstrates reach with trunk rotation, full elbow extension, slight forearm rotation, and wrist stability, yet some degree of excess finger extension before grasp. (Courtesy Ed Exner, Greensburg, PA.)

Grasp Patterns

Classification

Napier proposed two basic terms to describe hand movements: prehensile and nonprehensile.[103] *Nonprehensile movements* involve pushing or lifting an object with the fingers or the entire hand. In contrast, *prehensile movements* involve grasp of an object and may be subdivided according to the purpose of the grasp: precision or power. *Precision grasps* involve opposition of the thumb to fingertips. *Power grasps* involve the use of the entire hand. In a power grasp, the thumb is held flexed or abducted to other fingers, depending on control requirements.

In most cases the activity and the object's characteristics determine the grasp pattern used. Small objects are generally held in a precision grasp, primarily because of the large amount of sensory feedback available through the fingertips and the control used to move them. Medium objects can be held with either pattern, and large objects are held with a power grasp. Napier noted a frequent interplay between precision and power handling of different objects based on the activity demands.[103]

Weiss and Flatt described a slightly different method of classification.[144] Grasps with no thumb opposition include hook grasp, power grasp, and lateral pinch. Patterns that use thumb opposition include tip and palmar pinches. The palmar pinch category is divided into standard, spherical, cylindrical, and disk grasps.

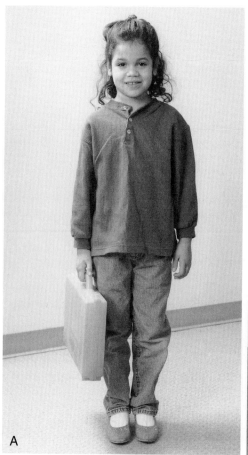

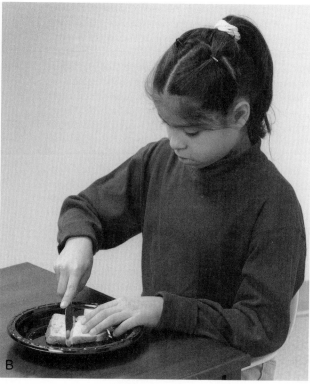

FIGURE 10-2 **A,** Hook grasp used to carry a child's art case. **B,** Power grasp with the right hand, used in cutting bread. (Courtesy Kanji Takeno, Towson University, Towson, MD.)

The *hook grasp* is used when strength of grasp must be maintained to carry objects. For this grasp, the transverse metacarpal arch is essentially flat, the fingers are adducted with flexion at the IP joints, and flexion or extension occurs at the MCP joints (Figure 10-2, *A*).[144] The thumb can be flexed over the fingers if additional power is needed. Observation of this pattern provides an indication of the child's ability to sustain wrist extension during finger flexion.

In contrast, the *power grasp* often is used to control tools or other objects. Oblique object placement in the hand, flexion of the ulnar fingers, less flexion with the radial fingers, and thumb extension and adduction facilitate precision handling with this grasp (e.g., for brushing the hair). Thus the child stabilizes the object with the ulnar side of the hand and controls the object for position and use with the radial side of the hand (Figure 10-2, *B*).[144] Observation of this pattern allows for assessment of the degree of radial-ulnar dissociation in the hand that the child can use and his or her control of thumb adduction with extension.

Lateral pinch is used to exert power on or with a small object. Partial thumb adduction, MCP flexion, and slight IP flexion are characteristics of this pattern. Although the index finger is slightly flexed, it is more extended than the other fingers. The pad of the thumb is placed against the radial side of the index finger at or near the distal interphalangeal (DIP) joint (Figure 10-3). This pattern involves controlling the index finger while adducting and flexing the thumb.

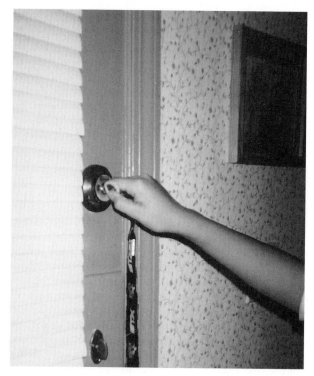

FIGURE 10-3 Lateral pinch with the right hand, used to open a lock on a door.

There are two types of standard pinches. Opposition of the thumb to the index finger pad describes only the *pad-to-pad, two-point pinch*[124] or *pincer grasp* (Figure 10-4, *A*).[57] Opposition of the thumb simultaneously to the index and middle finger pads, which provides increased stability of prehension, describes the *three-point pinch*[124] or *three-jaw chuck grasp* (Figure 10-4, *B*). In both cases, the thumb forms an oval or a modified oval shape with the fingers. In addition, the forearm is slightly supinated, which frees the thumb and radial fingers from contact with the surface and allows for an optimal view of the object. Observation of this pattern allows for assessment of the child's ability to control objects with the radial finger pads while controlling thumb opposition.

Opposition of the thumb tip and the tip of the index finger, forming a circle, describes a *tip pinch* (Figure 10-5). All joints of the index finger and thumb are partly flexed. This pinch pattern is used to obtain small objects. Observation of this grasp provides information about the child's ability to dissociate the two sides of the hand and to use the tips of the index finger and thumb. Edwards, Buckland, and McCoy-Powlen further explain and illustrate the development of grasping patterns.[38]

Differences in hand posture characterize the other palmar grasps. Significant wrist extension, finger abduction, and some degree of flexion at the MCP and IP joints describe the *spherical grasp* (Figure 10-6). Stability of the longitudinal arch is necessary to use this pattern to grasp large objects. The hypothenar eminence lifts to assist the cupping of the hand for control of the object.[144] Observation of this grasp pattern suggests the child's ability to balance control of the intrinsic and extrinsic hand muscles.

In the *cylindrical grasp*, the transverse arch is flattened to allow the fingers to hold against the object. The fingers are only slightly abducted, and IP and MCP joint flexion is graded according to the size of the object. When additional force is required, more of the palmar surface of the hand contacts the object (Figure 10-7).[144] Observation of this pattern allows

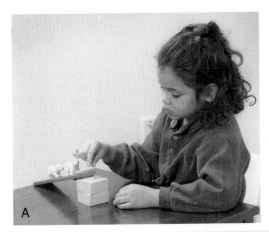

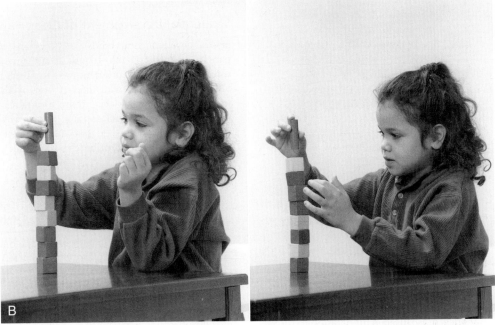

FIGURE 10-4 **A,** Pincer grasp, used to place "food" for the "climbing polar bears." **B,** This child uses variations of a three-jaw chuck grasp with her right hand, depending on task demands. (Courtesy Kanji Takeno, Towson University, Towson, MD.)

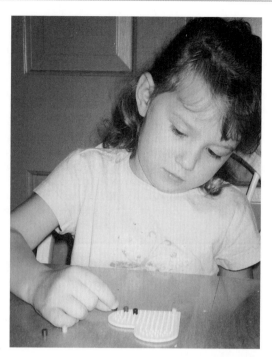

FIGURE 10-5 Tip pinch with the right hand, used to complete a bead craft project. Normal radial grasps, such as the tip pinch, are accompanied by slight forearm supination.

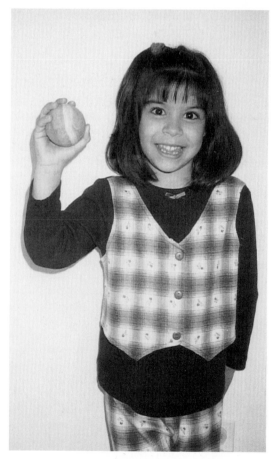

FIGURE 10-6 Spherical grasp, used in preparation to throw a ball.

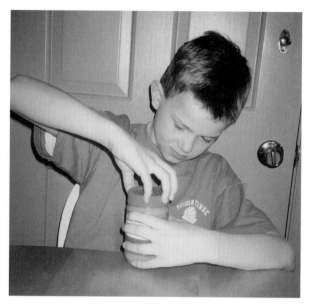

FIGURE 10-7 This child uses a cylindrical grasp with his left hand and a disk grasp with his right hand to open a jar. Note the grading of finger abduction with the left hand to provide adequate stability to the jar.

for assessment of palmar arch control during handling of a relatively large object.

A *disk grasp* incorporates finger abduction that is graded according to the size of the object held, hyperextension of the MCP joints, and flexion of the IP joints (see Figure 10-7).[144] The wrist is more flexed when objects are larger, and only the pads of the fingers contact the object. The amount of thumb extension also increases with object size. The transverse metacarpal arch is flattened in this prehension pattern. This pattern involves dissociation of flexion and extension movements and use of a combination of wrist flexion with MCP extension and IP flexion.

Sequential Development of Grasp Patterns

Several developmental trends affect the particular type of grasp pattern an infant is able to use at any time. The sequences listed in Box 10-1 are different ways to reflect the progressions in grasp; these sequences interact and overlap. The infant's growing interest in objects, desire to attain them, and desire to explore them and relate them to other objects influence these motor sequences. Haptic development and visual-perceptual development contribute to the infant's ability to shape

---

BOX 10-1 Approaches to Describing the Progression of Grasp Development

1. The part of the hand/fingers used in the grasping pattern: ulnar grasp to palmar grasp to radial grasp
2. The location of the object on the hand surface: palmar contact to finger surface contact to finger pad contact[76]
3. The muscle activity used in grasp: use of long finger flexors to increasing control of intrinsic muscles with extrinsic muscles

the hand appropriately for the object and to approach the object with optimal orientation of the arm and hand.

Another aspect of motor development that contributes to the infant's use of increasingly mature and more varied patterns is the ability to effect internal stability throughout upper extremity movement, forearm supination, and thumb opposition. Thumb activity and control are necessary to allow for patterns other than palmar grasp. The ability to stabilize the wrist in a slightly extended position is important for grasp patterns that use distal (fingertip) control. Slight forearm supination is important because it positions the hand so that the thumb and radial fingers are free for active object exploration, and it allows the infant to view fingers and thumb during grasp.[73]

A typical sequence can be seen during the infant's first 6 months. Initially the infant appears to have no voluntary hand use. The hands alternately open and close in response to various sensory stimuli. Gradually the traction response and grasp reflex decrease, and a voluntary palmar grasp begins to emerge (Figure 10-8). By approximately 6 months the infant progresses to being able to use a radial palmar grasp. Case-Smith, Bigsby, and Clutter found a marked increase in grasp skill between 4 and 5 months of age.[23] They noted less change between 5 and 6 months of age.

The second 6 months is a key period for the development of hand skills. The ability to grasp a variety of objects increases significantly between 6 and 9 months of age. During this time, grasp patterns with active thumb use emerge. Crude raking of a tiny object is present by about 7 months of age, and by 9 months of age the infant is able to hold a tiny object between the finger surface and the thumb. By 8 to 9 months of age, the infant holds a larger object between the thumb and the radial fingers (Figure 10-9) and readily varies the grasping pattern according to the shape of the object. Case-Smith et al. noted a particularly dramatic increase in skill between 8 and 9 months of age.[23] However, at this time intrinsic muscle control is not effective because the infant does not use grasp with MCP

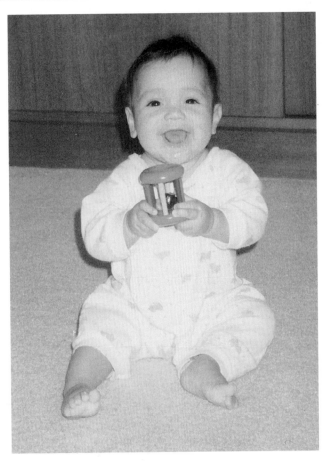

FIGURE 10-9 This baby uses a radial-digital grasp with both hands to hold a toy for shaking and mouthing.

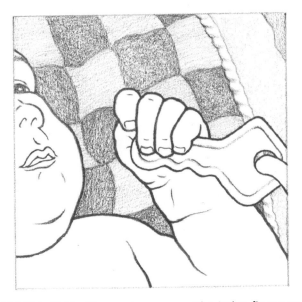

FIGURE 10-8 Ulnar-palmar grasp. The index finger and thumb are not used in this pattern.

flexion and IP extension. Between 9 and 12 months of age, refinement occurs in the ability to use thumb and finger pad control for tiny and small objects. More precise preparation of the fingers before initiation of grasp, more inhibition of the ulnar fingers, and slight wrist extension and forearm supination are characteristics of this refinement.

After 1 year of age, further refinement occurs in grasp patterns that were seen earlier, and more sophisticated patterns emerge. Between 12 and 15 months of age, the infant's ability to hold crackers, cookies, and other flat objects identifies an increasing control of the intrinsic muscles. Although studies are limited in terms of grasp development for patterns other than the pincer grasp, between 18 months and 3 years of age, most children with typical development acquire the ability to use a disk grasp, a cylindrical grasp, and a spherical grasp with control. Control of a power grasp continues to develop through the preschool years. The pattern for a lateral pinch may be present by 3 years of age, but children generally do not use this pattern with power until later in the preschool years. Overall grasp patterns for a variety of objects are well developed by 5 years of age, but those involving tools may continue to mature into the early school years.

In addition to quality of grasp, strength of grasp continues to increase throughout childhood. Lee-Valkow et al. reported on the development of grip and pinch strength in typical preschool-age children.[88] These workers noted significant increases in strength for palmar grip, key (lateral) pinch, and tripod (three-point) pinch for children between 3 and 4 years of age and 4 and 5 years of age. The increase in strength was greater between 4 and 5 years than between 3 and 4 years in both preferred and nonpreferred hands. Yim et al. found increases in grip, lateral pinch, palmar pinch, and tip pinch across the age range in 7- to 12-year-old Korean children; they also reported significant differences in grip strength between boys and girls in each age group for both right and left hands.[153] They noted that right-handed girls were stronger than left-handed girls in grip and lateral pinch with both hands. In a study of isometric strength of the index finger, Smits-Engelsman, Wilson, Westenberg, and Duysens found that isometric force increased gradually during the 5- to 10-year-old age span, reflecting corticospinal system maturation.[127] Compared with 10- to 12-year-olds, adults exhibited greater use of alternative strategies for selecting and monitoring force needed in an activity.

In-Hand Manipulation Skills

Classification

In-hand manipulation includes five basic types of patterns: finger-to-palm translation, palm-to-finger translation, shift, simple rotation, and complex rotation.[47] All skills require the ability to control the arches of the palm (Figure 10-10).

Long, Conrad, Hall, and Furler described translation as a linear movement of the object from the palm to the fingers or from the fingers to the palm; the object stays in constant contact with the thumb and fingers during this pattern.[90] The fingers and thumb maintain grasp but move into and out of MCP and IP flexion and extension. In contrast, Exner described the pattern of finger-to-palm translation as grasping the object with the pads of the fingers and thumb and moving it into the palm.[47] The finger pad grasp is released so that the object rests in the palm of the open hand or is held in a palmar grasp at the conclusion of the pattern. The object moves in a linear direction in the hand, and the fingers move from an extended position to a more flexed position during the translation. An example of this skill is picking up a coin with the fingers and thumb and moving it into the palm of the hand.

Palm-to-finger translation is the reverse of finger-to-palm translation.[47] However, palm-to-finger translation requires isolated control of the thumb and use of a pattern beginning with finger flexion and moving toward finger extension (see Figure 10-10). This pattern is more difficult for the child to execute than finger-to-palm translation. An example of this skill is moving a coin from the palm of the hand to the finger pads before placing the coin in a vending machine.

Shift involves linear movement of the object on the finger surface to allow for repositioning of the object on the pads of the fingers.[47] In this pattern the fingers move just slightly at the MCP and IP joints, and the thumb typically remains

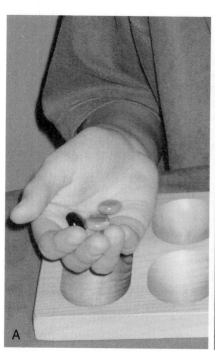
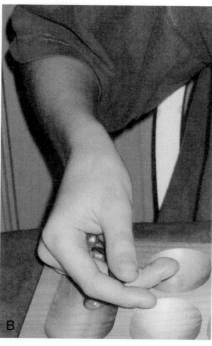
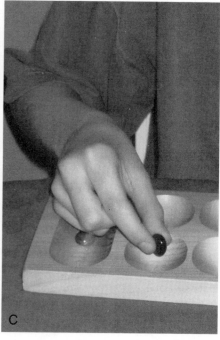

FIGURE 10-10 **A,** The child shows the ability to keep the palm in a cupped position to hold several stones for a game. The forearm is in almost full supination. **B,** Palm-to-finger translation with stabilization is initiated for one of the stones while the other stones are retained in the palm. The translation movement produced by the fingers is accompanied by forearm rotation into midposition. **C,** Palm-to-finger translation with stabilization is completed for one stone. The other stones are retained in the hand by flexion of the ulnar fingers. The forearm moves toward pronation to assist with placement of the stone on the game board.

opposed or adducted with MCP and IP extension throughout the shift. The object usually is held solely on the radial side of the hand. Examples of this skill are separating two pieces of paper, moving a coin from a position against the volar aspect of the DIP joints to a position closer to the fingertips (e.g., so that the coin can be easily inserted into the slot of a vending machine), and adjusting a pen or pencil after grasp so that the fingers are positioned close to the writing end of the tool. This skill is used frequently in dressing tasks such as buttoning, fastening snaps, lacing shoes, and putting a belt through belt loops.

The two patterns of rotation are simple rotation and complex rotation. Simple rotation involves the turning or rolling of an object held at the finger pads approximately 90° or less.[47] The fingers act as a unit (little or no differentiation of action is shown among them), and the thumb is in an opposed position. Examples of simple rotation are unscrewing a small bottle cap, reorienting a puzzle piece in the hand by turning it slightly before placing it in the puzzle, and picking up a small peg and rotating it from a horizontal to a vertical position for insertion into a pegboard.

Complex rotation involves the rotation of an object 180 to 360° once or repetitively.[47] During complex rotation the fingers and thumb alternate in producing the movement, and the fingers typically move independently of one another. An object may be moved end over end, such as in turning a coin or a peg over or in turning a pencil over to use the eraser.

In-hand manipulation skills can occur with only one object in the hand or with two or more objects in the hand. For example, a child typically unscrews a bottle lid with no other objects in his or her hand. In-hand manipulation skills also are used when the child is holding other objects in the hand. For example, a child may have two or more pieces of cereal in his or her hand but brings only one piece out to the finger pads before placing it in the mouth (see Figure 10-10). The term *with stabilization* refers to the use of an in-hand manipulation skill while other objects are stabilized in the hand. Therefore picking up multiple pieces of cereal involves palm-to-finger translation with stabilization, whereas unscrewing the bottle lid is simple rotation. In-hand manipulation skills with stabilization are generally more difficult to perform than the same skill without the simultaneous stabilization of other objects in the hand.

Developmental Considerations

Motor skill prerequisites for in-hand manipulation include the following[43]:

- Movement into and stability in various degrees of supination
- Wrist stability
- Opposed grasp with thumb opposition and object contact with the finger surface (not in the palm)
- Isolated thumb and radial finger movement
- Control of the transverse metacarpal arch
- Dissociation of the radial and ulnar sides of the hand
- Successive increases and decreases in fingertip forces

Children who are unable to use in-hand manipulation skills are likely to substitute other patterns. Substitution patterns are part of the typical strategies used in acquiring in-hand manipulation skills; however, their use does not necessarily represent abnormal fine motor control. Typical patterns a child uses when he or she shows very limited in-hand manipulation are (1) changing of hands (putting the object in the other hand for use) and (2) transferring from hand to hand (moving the object from one hand to the other and back to the hand that held it first). The child uses these patterns after the initial grasp when he or she realizes that the object in the hand needs to be repositioned for use but that the object cannot readily be adjusted in that hand. For example, a child picks up a crayon or marker with the right hand but is unable to shift it to place the fingers near the writing end; therefore, he or she grasps the object with the left hand and then transfers it back to the right hand with the fingers appropriately positioned. Some children preplan for this by picking up the crayon with the nonpreferred hand and changing it to the preferred hand.

Therapists observe several skills in children who are beginning to use in-hand manipulation skills or are preparing for the use of these skills. Infants typically engage in bilateral manipulation of objects by moving an object between the two hands. As the child moves the object between the hands, he or she turns and repositions it within the hands. Children use this strategy, called a *hand assist,* to substitute for palm-to-finger translation or rotation. In this case the object does not leave the hand that grasped it initially, but the other hand helps with repositioning of the object. Sometimes children use other surfaces or other parts of the body to provide support for the manipulation. Children commonly use assist strategies for shift and complex rotation.

Ongoing research is directed toward determining a sequence for the development of in-hand manipulation skills.[45,107,108] Based on these research studies, the following developmental sequence has emerged. By approximately 12 to 15 months of age, infants use finger-to-palm translation to pick up and "hide" small pieces of food in their hands. By 2 to 2.5 years of age, children use palm-to-finger translation and simple rotation with some objects. Complex rotation skills are observed in children at 2.5 to 3 years of age, although this age group often has difficulty with them. By 4 years of age, children consistently use complex rotation without using an external support.[107] Children between 3.5 and 5.5 years of age develop skills in rotating a marker (regardless of its initial orientation) and shifting it into optimal position for coloring and writing.[45,75] Shift typically is evident but inconsistent in children 3 and 3.5 years old.[45]

After 3 years of age the child uses in-hand manipulation skills with greater proficiency and consistency. Dropping of objects during in-hand manipulation tasks decreases through the preschool years.[108] Lee-Valkov et al. reported data on preschool-age children's object manipulation speed, as gathered with the Functional Dexterity test (using a pegboard with short pegs approximately 1 inch in diameter).[88] The test was administered to both hands, and scoring was based on the amount of time needed to rotate and place 16 pegs, accounting for use of substitution patterns or for dropping. Speed in performing the test improved yearly, with improvement in time to completion of approximately 7 to 8 seconds each year.

By 6 years of age, children develop the ability to use a variety of in-hand manipulation skills with stabilization.[45,108] Between 6 and 7 years of age, children more consistently use combinations of in-hand manipulation skills that must be used in an activity (e.g., palm-to-finger translation with stabilization followed by complex rotation with stabilization). A recent study by Pont, Wallen, Bundy, and Case-Smith illustrates the challenges of measuring in-hand manipulation skills in children between the ages of 5 and 6 years, including the variability in performance that still seems to be present at that age.[111]

Ongoing research by Exner and colleagues suggests that children continue to refine in-hand manipulation skills up to approximately 9 to 10 years of age and continue to develop speed of skill use through 12 years of age. Yim et al. used the Nine-Hole Pegboard test to evaluate dexterity skills (complex rotation skills) in Korean children without disabilities between the ages of 7 and 12 years.[153] In comparing their data for 12-year-olds with data for adults obtained by Kellor, Rost, Silberberg, Iversen, and Cummings,[79] they found that the girls' mean time scores were approximately the same as those for the youngest adults, but that the 12-year-old boys' mean time scores were slightly lower. The difference may reflect a cultural difference or possibly the continuing development of object manipulation speed during adolescence.

The ability to use a skill with one type of object is not always associated with an ability to use the skill with another size or shape of object. For example, the child may be able to use simple rotation to turn a small peg but may not be able to use simple rotation to orient a crayon for coloring. In general, small objects (e.g., smaller-diameter crayons) are easier for children to manipulate than slightly larger objects (e.g., larger-diameter crayons) or tiny objects. Tiny objects require precise fingertip control, whereas medium-sized and larger objects require control with more fingers.

In addition to object characteristics, other factors can contribute to a child's use of in-hand manipulation skills; such factors include the cognitive-perceptual demands of the activity, the child's interest in the manipulative materials or the activity, processing tactile-proprioceptive information, visual acuity, and the child's motor-planning skills. Problems in any of these areas can affect development of in-hand manipulation skills. Data collected by Lee-Valkov et al. suggest that dexterity in typical preschool children is not significantly correlated with grip or pinch strength.[88] However, it should be noted that typical children were likely to have grip and pinch strength generally within normal limits. Markedly diminished strength could have a negative effect on in-hand manipulation skills.

Voluntary Release

Voluntary release, like grasp, depends on control of arm and finger movements. To place an object for release, the arm must move into position accurately and then stabilize as the fingers and thumb extend. Gordon, Lewis, Eliasson, and Duff refer to the two components of voluntary release as *replacement* and *release*.[63]

Initially the infant does not voluntarily release an object; objects either drop involuntarily from the hand or must be forcibly removed from the hand. As the infant's nondiscriminative responses to tactile and proprioceptive stimuli decrease and visual control and cognitive development increase, volitional control of release emerges. With increases in the mouthing of objects and bringing of both hands to midline and playing

with them there, the infant begins to transfer objects from one hand to another. Initially the child stabilizes the object in the mouth during transfers or pulls it out of one hand with the other. Soon the infant begins to freely transfer the object from one hand to another. The receiving hand stabilizes the object, and the releasing hand is fully opened.

By 9 months of age, the infant begins to release objects without stabilizing then with the other hand. The arm is fairly extended during release. The infant exhibits increasing humeral control as he or she moves the arm to drop objects in different locations. The next step is the development of elbow stability in various positions, and the infant begins to release with the elbow in some degree of flexion. The child may stabilize the arm or hand on the surface during release. At about 1 year of age, the child can release objects with shoulder, elbow, and wrist stability; however, the MCP joints remain unstable during this pattern, therefore the infant continues to show excess finger extension (Figure 10-11, *A*). Gradually the child develops the ability to release objects into smaller containers (Figure 10-11, *B*) and to stack blocks (Figure 10-11, *C*). The release pattern is refined over the next few years until the child can release small objects with graded extension of the fingers, indicating control over the intrinsic hand muscles. These skills also illustrate the integration of perceptual, cognitive, and sensory skills with motor skills. For example, Eliasson and Gordon reported that typical children between 7 and 13 years of age demonstrate the ability to effectively modulate a decrease in force used to grasp a lighter object and a heavier object to allow for appropriate timing in voluntary release.[43]

Bilateral Hand Use

As discussed previously, the normal infant progresses from asymmetry to symmetry to differentiated asymmetrical movements, which are used in bilateral hand activities. Asymmetry is a characteristic of movement patterns until almost 3 months of age. Symmetric patterns predominate between 3 and 10 months of age, when bilateral reach, grasp, and mouthing of the hands and objects are primary activities. Control of these movements originates proximally at the shoulders, allowing the hands to engage at midline. By 9 to 10 months of age, the infant can hold one object in each hand and bang them together (see Figure 10-9). This ability to hold an object in each hand at the same time is critical for further bilateral skill development. By 10 months of age, bimanual action is well differentiated, with one hand grasping the object and the other manipulating parts of it.[50] More complex bilateral skills depend on this ability.

Bimanual activity emerges first as reciprocal or alternating hand movements, then as simultaneous hand movements. By 17 to 18 months of age, infants frequently use role-differentiated strategies (i.e., one hand stabilizes or holds the materials and the other manipulates or activates them).[113] For these skills to emerge, the infant must be able to dissociate the two sides of the body and begin to use the two hands simultaneously for different functions. Effective stabilization of materials also depends on adequate shoulder, elbow, and wrist stability.

Between 18 and 24 months of age, the child begins to develop skills that are precursors to simultaneous manipulation.

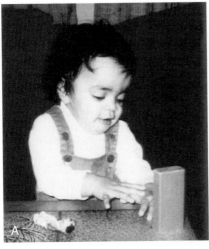
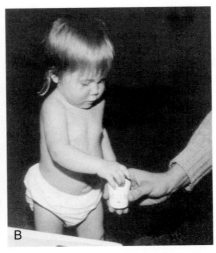
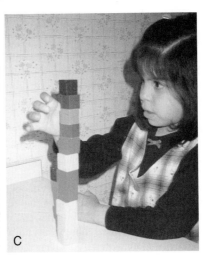

FIGURE 10-11 **A,** Full finger extension and some wrist movement occur with voluntary release. Note the visual regard of the object being released. **B,** The child's shoulder, elbow, and wrist are stable, and less finger extension occurs with release. The child visually monitors release of the object into a small container. **C,** Stability of the shoulder, elbow, forearm, wrist, and fingers combines with perceptual development to promote accurate placement of objects. This 5-year-old is able to use forearm supination to midposition with controlled finger extension. In this challenging task, only slight overextension of the fingers occurs. **(B,** Courtesy Kennedy Krieger Institute, Baltimore.)

Bilateral skill refinement depends heavily on continuing development of reach, grasp, release, and in-hand manipulation skills. Skills in visual-perceptual, cognitive, and motor areas become more integrated, leading to the child's effective use of motor planning for task performance. The child demonstrates simultaneous manipulation at 2 to 3 years of age. The mature stage of bilateral hand use, which is the ability to use opposing hand and arm movements for highly differentiated activities (e.g., cutting with scissors), begins to emerge at about 2.5 years of age. The child applies and refines the patterns from each stage of bilateral hand use in a variety of activities throughout childhood.

Once a child is able to differentially use the two hands, the task becomes more significant in eliciting the particular strategy to be used to accomplish a task than the particular motor action. For example, Kunde and Weigelt explored the challenge presented by different types of bilateral manipulative tasks.[85] They found that when the goal of a manipulative task was to orient two objects similarly, speed and efficiency were better even if arm-hand movements needed to differ to accomplish the task than when objects were to be oriented differently but the movement of the two hands was the same. This supports the concept that the goal of a motor action is more important in selecting a movement strategy than is the ease of the motor action itself.

Ball-Throwing Skills

Ball-throwing skills reflect the child's ability to use voluntary release skills. In throwing a small ball, the child must sequence and time movements throughout the entire upper extremity. The child must bring the arm into a starting position, then prepare for projection of the ball into space by moving the trunk with the scapulohumeral joint, stabilizing the shoulder while beginning to extend the elbow, stabilizing the

elbow while moving the wrist from extension to a neutral position, and simultaneously forcefully extending the fingers and thumb.

Children progress through a series of skill levels before they can smoothly sequence these movements and project the ball to the desired location. By 2 years of age, the child should be able to throw a ball forward and maintain balance so that his or her body does not also move forward.[123] At this age the child uses extensor movements to fling the ball but is unable to sustain shoulder flexion during the toss.[55] The child can dissociate trunk and arm movement but cannot dissociate humeral and forearm movements. By 2.5 to 3 years of age, the child can aim the ball toward a target and project the ball approximately 3 feet forward. This ability to control the direction of the ball to some degree implies that the child can control the humerus so that the elbow is in front of the shoulder when the ball is released. Thus the shoulder has sufficient stability to support controlled elbow and finger movement. By 3.5 years of age, the child is able to throw the ball 5 to 7 feet toward a target with little deviation from a straight line.[55] To accomplish this accuracy, the child positions his or her elbow in front of the shoulder before the ball is released.

Further refinement of ball-throwing skills continues over the next few years. Distance and accuracy improve as the child gains scapulohumeral control, the ability to sustain the humerus above the shoulder, and the ability to control the timing of elbow, wrist, and finger extension. Thus at approximately 5 years of age, the child is able to use an overhand throw to hit a target 5 feet away fairly consistently. Children between 6 and 7 years of age are able to hit a target 12 feet away by using an overhand throw.[55] Underhand throws to contact a target are also possible in children 5 years of age or older. This skill requires the ability to move the humerus into flexion while sustaining full external rotation.

Tool Use

Connolly and Dalgleish defined a *tool* as "a device for working on something ... tools serve as extensions of the limbs and enhance the efficiency with which skills are performed" (p. 895).[26] They defined *tool use* as "a purposeful, goal-directed form of complex object manipulation that involves the manipulation of the tool to change the position, condition or action of another object" (p. 895).[26] Tool-use skills are more complex than other hand skills, because the child must use a tool, rather than the hand, to act on objects.

The development of skill in using tools is critical to a variety of self-care, play and leisure, and school and work tasks. Skills in tool use for eating and play typically begin to emerge during the second year, after the child has mastered the basic skills of reach, grasp, and release. The skills emerge concurrently with in-hand manipulation skills, which are necessary for the progression of tool use skills beyond grasp and release proficiency. In-hand manipulation skills allow the tool to be adjusted in the hand after it has been grasped.

A key factor in the acquisition of tool-use skills is the high degree of interaction of these skills and cognitive development. Connolly and Dalgleish emphasized that an individual needs to know both what he or she wants to do (the intentional aspect of the task) and how he or she can accomplish it (the operational aspect of the task).[26] Both of these elements require development of the child's cognitive skills and operational aspects of the child's motor skills.

As with any new skill, when the child is developing tool use, the therapist sees inconsistencies in the child (even in the same session). The therapist is likely to record multiple strategies for children who are beginning to use a particular skill. Thus "inconsistency" in the strategy used to perform a skill should be considered an important stage in the skill-acquisition process. As skill acquisition progresses, practice allows the skill to progress from being performed with a high level of attention to being performed at a more automatic level. With such practice, performance becomes faster, more accurate, and smoother. Practice typically is necessary for a skill to become functional for execution in daily life tasks.

Researchers have studied the acquisition of children's skills in the use of three tools: drawing and writing, scissoring, and eating. Of these, most of the research has focused on drawing and writing tool use (see Chapter 19 for a description of this type of tool use).

Schneck and Battaglia described the development of scissors skills in young children.[120] This skill emerges when the child first learns to place his or her fingers in the holes and to open and close the scissors. Early cutting is actually snipping, a process of closing the scissors on the paper with no movement of the paper and with no ability to repetitively open and close the scissors while flexing the shoulder and extending the elbow to move across the paper. Three-year-old children may use a pronated forearm position or a forearm-in-midposition placement,[120] or they may alternate between the two forearm positions. By 4 years of age, children typically hold both forearms in midposition for the cutting activity.

The Peabody Developmental Motor Scales has established the following typical sequence for scissors skills[55]:

- By 2 years of age, children can snip with scissors.

- By 2.5 years of age, most children can cut across a 6-inch piece of paper.
- By 3 to 3.5 years of age, they can cut on a line that is 6 inches long.
- By 3.5 to 4 years of age, they can cut a circle.
- By 4.5 to 5 years of age, they can cut a square.

More complex cutting skills develop between 6 and 7 years of age. Other factors the therapist should consider when assessing a child's skill in cutting include the width of the line to cut on, the size of the paper, the size of the design to be cut, and the complexity of the design.

The child's grasp on the scissors changes over time. The thumb position in one hole remains consistent, but the finger positions change according to the child's level of maturation and the type of scissors used.[120] In a mature grasp, which may not be achieved until after 6 years of age, the child has the middle finger in the lower hole of the handle, the ulnar two fingers flexed (inside or outside the lower hole, depending on its size), and the index finger positioned to stabilize the lower part of the scissors.[102,120]

The general ages at which a child learns to use various utensils in eating are as follows: a spoon by 18 months of age, a fork by 2.5 years of age, and a knife by 6 years of age.[70] However, documentation regarding how these skills are acquired and how various components of movement interact to produce skill is limited. Connolly and Dalgleish conducted a longitudinal study on development of spoon use skills in infants between 11 and 23 months of age.[26] They analyzed videotapes of the infants' grasp patterns on the spoon; the placement of the spoon in the hand; movements used in filling the spoon, bringing it to the mouth, clearing the spoon, and taking it out of the mouth; and visual monitoring of the pattern, timing, and use of the nonpreferred hand in the eating process. They found that the mean number of grasp patterns decreased between 11 and 17 months of age and that most infants 17 months of age or older showed a clear hand preference for eating. The infants used 10 different grasp patterns, but none of them used an adult pattern. The most commonly used pattern was a transverse palmar grasp with all four fingers flexed around the handle of the spoon. In the next two most commonly used patterns, the spoon handle was held within the fingers rather than in the palm. The 17- to 23-month-old infants used some degree of index finger extension to hold and orient the spoon. The infants became increasingly efficient in spoon use during this period, and exhibited improved visual monitoring of the process.

Another component in the development of tool use in children is the role of the assisting hand. In handwriting and coloring, the assisting hand plays an important role in stabilizing the paper. However, in using scissors and eating, the assisting hand is likely to be much more active. In cutting, this hand must hold the paper and orient it through rotation by moving in the same or the opposite direction as the hand with the scissors. In eating, the child's assisting hand may be involved in a variety of activities, depending on the child's age and the utensils used. Connolly and Dalgleish found that infants between 18 and 23 months of age showed significantly more involvement of the assisting hand in stabilizing a dish during spoon feeding than did infants between 12 and 17 months of age.[26] Learning to use a knife entails the child learning to stabilize food with a fork in one hand while using a knife for spreading or cutting.

Hand Preference

Hand preference, previously referred to more frequently as *hand dominance,* is a complex concept. In typical children hand preference evolves over a long period of time and gradually becomes more consistent, as do other expressions of motor functioning. Fagard and Lochman studied young children between the ages of 6 months and 48 months with a variety of tasks involving hand use.[51] Greater variability was actually noted for less complex grasp activities. Activities and objects that elicited manipulative strategies were more likely to result in more consistent use of one hand for manipulation and the other for stabilization. Inconsistent use of one hand in a precision grasp task was noted in almost 20% of the infants under 12 months, but in none of the 2.5- to 3-year-old children, whereas about 60% of the children in this age group (and in the infants 6 to 24 months of age) were inconsistent in hand used for a simple grasp task. When one hand needed to be used as a stabilizer and one as a manipulator, 65% or more of the children over 18 months used the right hand as the manipulator. Inconsistency was noted in some children in the 2.5- to 3-year-old group but not in the 4-year-old group. Overall, Fagard and Lochman noted that the right hand was used more frequently than the left hand by infants and young children in every age group, even when it was not used consistently (on 80% or more of the trials).[51]

Hand preference continues to develop until at least 8 years of age, as illustrated in a study of a reaching activity that involved crossing the midline of the body. Carlier, Doyen, and Lamard found that with increasing age, children used the preferred hand with greater frequency to pick up cards in various locations, including crossing the midline with the preferred hand.[18] As with other areas of hand skill development, some degree of variability and inconsistency is the typical pattern for infants and young children. It is worrisome and atypical when infants (less than 7 months) consistently use one hand, and these infants should be further evaluated for possible neurologic impairment.

RELATIONSHIP OF HAND SKILLS TO CHILDREN'S OCCUPATIONS

Hand skills are vital to the child's interaction with the environment. Engagement in most occupations requires object handling, almost all of which is accomplished with the hands.

Play

Although infants engage with people and objects through their visual and auditory senses, these are distant senses and do not readily bring the infant key information, which can be gained only through touch. Ruff described object handling with visual exploration as essential for an infant to learn object properties.[118] The interaction of touching and looking helps enhance the infant's ability to integrate sensory information and to learn that objects remain the same regardless of visual orientation. Typically this object handling in infants is called *play* because it is purposeful and done with pleasure.

With increasing age, until at least the early school years, a great deal of play depends on competence in fine motor skills. These skills are reflected in the child's interest in activities such as cutting with scissors, dressing and undressing dolls, putting puzzles together, constructing with various types of building materials and model sets, participating in sand play, completing craft projects, and engaging in imaginary play with objects. Playing video games and using computers also require fine motor control. Some children may pursue play and leisure activities through organized groups such as the Girl Scouts or Boy Scouts and 4-H clubs, which tend to have projects requiring manual skills as a key component of their programs.

Activities of Daily Living

Activities of daily living also depend on the child's ability to use all types of hand skills. According to Henderson, the specific skills needed for skill development in this area are "(1) finger manipulation and grip ability, (2) the use of two hands in a complementary fashion, (3) the ability to use the hands in varied positions with and without vision, (4) the execution of increasingly complex action sequences, and (5) the development of automaticity" (p. 213).[70] Case-Smith found that in-hand manipulation speed, grasp strength, motor accuracy, and tool handling were each significantly positively correlated with self-care skills in preschool-age children receiving occupational therapy services.[21]

Dressing skills involve complex grasp patterns and in-hand manipulation skills in the use of fasteners, but the ability to use all types of bilateral skills and a variety of grasp patterns is useful for putting on and removing shirts, shoes, socks, and pants. The ability to put on jewelry relies on the ability to use delicate grasp patterns and in-hand manipulation.

Bathing, showering, and other personal hygiene skills depend on the child's increasing fine motor skills in handling slippery objects (e.g., soap). In addition, these skills are likely to be needed when an individual is in a standing position, such as when putting toothpaste on a toothbrush (Figure 10-12), brushing the teeth, shaving, or applying makeup. A high level of skill in tool use is needed for complex hygiene activities such as shaving, applying makeup, using tweezers, cutting nails, and styling hair (applying barrettes or rubber bands and using a curling iron, a brush, and a hair dryer).

Eating skills rely on refinement of the ability to use forearm control with a variety of grasp patterns and tools. The ability to use both hands together effectively is necessary for spreading and cutting with a knife, opening all types of containers, pouring liquids, and preparing food. In-hand manipulation skills are used to adjust eating utensils within the hand (Figure 10-13) and finger foods in the hand, to handle a napkin, and to manipulate the opening of packaged food and utensils.

In their studies of school-age children with developmental coordination disorder (DCD), Summers, Dawne, and Dewey[133] and Missiuna, Moll, King, King, and Law[99] illustrate the impact of hand skills on activities of daily living. Typically developing children 8 years of age and older are highly independent in an array of skills that rely on hand skill as well as postural control. In contrast, children with DCD demonstrated delayed development in dressing, personal hygiene, toileting, and independent eating skills. Older children who had

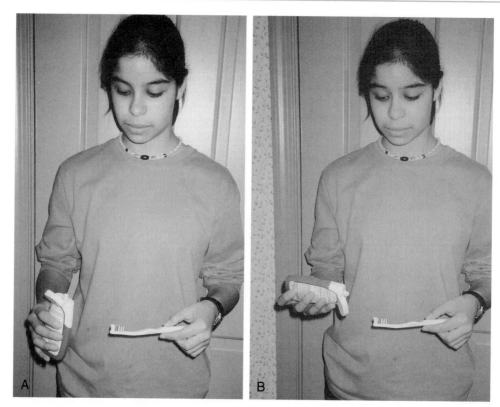

FIGURE 10-12 **A,** Different grasp patterns are used in preparation for putting toothpaste on a toothbrush. The child uses just-right force to stabilize the toothbrush with a modified power grasp (with supination to midposition) while using a cylindrical grasp on the toothpaste container. **B,** The child has used forearm supination and the in-hand manipulation skill of simple rotation to position the toothpaste container for application of the toothpaste to the toothbrush.

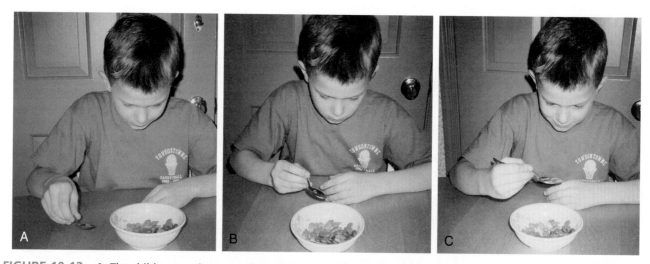

FIGURE 10-13 **A,** The child grasps the spoon from the table surface with a radial-digital grasp. The forearm is slightly supinated. **B,** He uses the in-hand manipulation skill of complex rotation to move the handle of the spoon from the palmar surface of his hand toward the web space between the index finger and thumb. Isolation and differentiation of the index finger and thumb are needed to produce this rotation. Forearm movement toward midposition assists. **C,** The child completes spoon positioning in his hand by moving the spoon so that the end of the handle is stabilized in the web space. Additional flexion of the metacarpophalangeal (MCP) joints of the fingers while extension of the interphalangeal (IP) joints is sustained assists with optimal positioning for eating.

DCD performed similarly to younger typical children. Parents provided cues, assistance, and substitutions for many of the needed skills far longer for their children with DCD than did parents of typically developing children.[99,133]

School Functions

Independent functioning in the school environment requires effective fine motor skills. The preschool classroom provides children with a variety of manipulative activities, including the use of crayons, scissors, small building materials, and puzzles, as well as simple cooking and art projects. During kindergarten and the early elementary school years, children use fine motor skills most of the school day. McHale and Cermak found that 45 to 55% of the school day for first and second grade children is spent in fine motor activities. Fourth grade children spend approximately 30% of their school day participating in fine motor tasks.[94] The primary fine motor activities in all of these grades are paper-pencil tasks. Any writing activity includes preparing one's paper, using an eraser, and getting writing tools in and out of a box. Other typical fine motor activities in children's classrooms include cutting with scissors, folding paper, using paste and tape, carrying out simple science projects, assuming responsibility for managing one's own snack and lunch items, and organizing and maintaining one's desk. Children also need computer skills in most elementary classrooms.

Older children and adolescents need fine motor skills for science projects, vocational courses (e.g., woodworking, metal shop, and home economics), art classes, music classes (other than vocal music), managing a high volume of written work and notebooks, keyboarding, and maintaining a locker. Greater speed (e.g., in writing and keyboarding) and greater strength (e.g., for physical education and vocational courses) are required. Adolescents should be able to demonstrate consistent hand skills that they can execute quickly in a variety of situations.

GENERAL MOTOR PROBLEMS THAT AFFECT HAND SKILLS

Children with a wide variety of types of disabilities are likely to have difficulty with hand function. These disabilities include cerebral palsy,[52,66] DCD,[92] attention deficit–hyperactivity disorder (ADHD),[112] and mental retardation and epilepsy.[9] As Mandich et al. noted, "Incompetence in everyday activities [has] serious negative effects for the children" (p. 583).[92]

Regardless of the nature of a specific disability, the affected child is likely to have impaired hand skills. Impairment of basic hand function (reach, grasp, carry, and release) in early childhood precludes emergence of more advanced hand skill and bilateral hand use. This section presents problems that may be observed as major or minor in any child with hand skill difficulties.

One of the more common problems is *inadequate isolation of movements*. Children who demonstrate significant problems in this area tend to use total patterns of flexion or extension throughout the upper extremities, and they are unable to combine wrist extension with finger flexion or elbow flexion with finger extension. Similarly, the child may be unable to perform differentiated motions with each arm and hand. More subtle problems may be seen in children who have difficulty isolating wrist and finger movements.

Another common problem is *poorly graded movement,* which may refer to movements not effectively graded in terms of range or strength. Eliasson and Gordon use the term *poor force scaling* to refer to difficulties in appropriately adjusting the force needed for grasp or release.[43] When joint stability in the hand or proximal to the hand is not effective, the child may be unable to hold the elbow in approximately 90° of flexion and the wrist in neutral position during a grasp activity. Thus, when initiating the grasp, the child may overflex the fingers in an attempt to obtain the object before the arm posture is lost. Another common pattern is difficulty shaping the hand in accordance with the object's properties prior to grasp.[83]

Children with poorly graded movements lack the ability to use the middle ranges of movement effectively; instead, during attempts at hand use they hold one or more joints in a locked position of full flexion or full extension (Figure 10-14, *A*). Typical patterns that children use to increase their stability include internal rotation of the shoulder, elbow extension, and hyperextension and/or abduction of the MCP joints (Figure 10-14, *B*). Problems with grading of movement are typically associated with tactile sensory problems, abnormal tone, and/or muscle weakness. The child with sensory problems has difficulty perceiving and evaluating feedback and therefore cannot accurately plan the extent of movements or force needed for a task. Gordon and Duff found that "spasticity may limit the ability to finely grade the fingertip force to the object's properties" (p. 590).[64]

Insufficient force may interfere with grasp control. Problems with force have been noted in children with developmental coordination disorder[148] and in children with cerebral palsy.[64] Difficulties with regulation of force may be due to poor tactile discrimination and/or spasticity.[64] Muscle weakness has also been suggested as a problem for individuals with cerebral palsy[31]; weakness could contribute significantly to insufficient force.

Poor timing of movements can also be a problem. Improper timing of muscle contractions leads to the use of movements that are too fast or too slow for the intended purpose. Movements that are too fast also tend to be poorly graded. Eliasson and Gordon describe difficulties in children with spastic hemiplegic cerebral palsy relative to the timing of "transitions between phases [and] sequential generation of forces" (p. 228) as needed for grasp and release of objects.[43] During voluntary release, children with increased tone are likely to place an object very quickly and then have slowed movement of the fingers away from the object.[43] Similarly, Kuhtz-Buschbeck et al. documented that children with traumatic brain injury also had impaired reaction times and slower movements when performing a task involving the combination of reach and grasp.[83] Wilson et al. similarly reported difficulties with timing of movements in children with DCD.[148] Tone problems or muscle weakness are often the underlying factors in movement that is too slow. Poor coordination of agonistic and antagonistic muscles and poor tactile discrimination are likely to be key factors in impaired timing of actions.[43] Speed and accuracy demands, particularly when these skills are required to place an object on an unstable

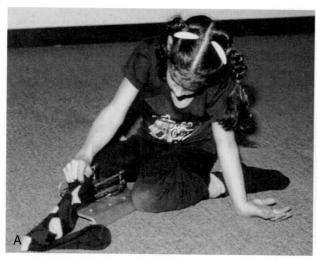
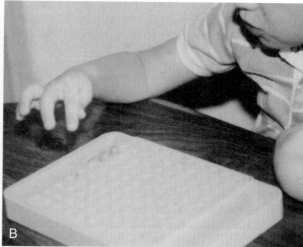

FIGURE 10-14 **A,** This child, who has involuntary movement, demonstrates the attempt to find stability by locking her left elbow with the arm in extension and by elevating her right shoulder during hand use. She also has difficulty isolating upper extremity movements and using the two hands together at midline. **B,** During voluntary release this child shows overextension and increased abduction of the fingers, with hyperextension at the MCP joints of the ulnar fingers. He also shows adduction of the thumb rather than slight abduction.   (**A,** Courtesy Kennedy Krieger Institute, Baltimore, MD.)

surface, lead to increased difficulty with motor timing and regulation of force.[63] Instability at joints can contribute to disordered sequences of hand and arm movements. For example, wrist extension may not be combined with the reach for an object but instead may occur after the grasp.

Another common motor problem is *limited variety of movement patterns*—a restricted repertoire often associated with biomechanical or neurologic issues affecting movement range and/or coordination. Other children may have marked variability in movement patterns[83] that result in substantial inefficiency of movement.

A fifth type of problem that affects hand function is a *disorder in bilateral integration of movements*. Some children are unable to bring both hands to midline effectively or to maintain the use of both hands at midline long enough to accomplish a task. Other children can hold objects symmetrically at midline but are unable to dissociate arm movements; they therefore have difficulty with activities that require reciprocal or simultaneous bilateral hand use.

Many children have difficulty with hand use because of *limitations in trunk movement and control*. CNS dysfunction or generalized muscle weakness can impair development or effective use of equilibrium reactions. Therefore the child may use one or both arms for support in maintaining sitting or standing positions. This significantly limits bilateral hand use and may limit the development of fine motor skills in the hand that the child most often uses for support.

Children with trunk instability or abnormal posture have difficulty with smooth, accurate placement of the hand and arm being used for a fine motor task. When the trunk is postured in flexion, functional ROM in the arm is limited (Figure 10-15). Conversely, arching of the trunk is accompanied by hyperextension of the humerus. The latter pattern typically causes one of three patterns of shoulder and elbow positioning: external rotation with elbow flexion, neutral rotation with elbow flexion, or internal rotation with elbow

extension. Posturing in any of these arm patterns affects the development of hand skills. Similarly, lateral trunk flexion causes the child to lean to one side and thus affects the child's ability to use the arm on the flexed side.

The problems discussed in this section can contribute to the child's use of *compensatory patterns of movement*. In an effort to increase function, the child seeks another pattern to substitute for movements impaired by the primary problem. For example, the child with weakness or instability may learn to use lateral trunk flexion to increase the height

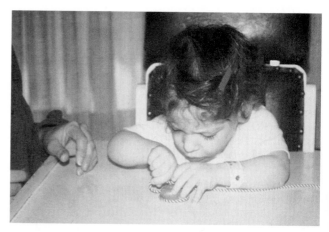

FIGURE 10-15 Poor trunk stability affects the upper extremity range of motion that this child can use. Note the right forearm pronation and wrist flexion. The child is unable to use a three-jaw chuck, or pincer, grasp effectively on the materials. However, she demonstrates awareness of the need to use both hands in this manipulative activity and good visual monitoring of the materials. (Courtesy Kennedy Krieger Institute, Baltimore, MD.)

of the opposite arm during reach, or a child with increased tone may compensate for limited finger extension by using a wrist tenodesis (flexion) action. Although these patterns are functional for certain tasks, continued use of compensatory movements may hinder the development of higher level skills.

OTHER FACTORS THAT AFFECT HAND SKILLS IN CHILDREN WITH DISABILITIES

Somatosensory Problems

Somatosensory problems can produce significant problems with hand function, even when motor control is good,[106] and poor hand skills can contribute to the child obtaining a limited amount of somatosensory information. Children with poor tactile discrimination receive less feedback about how their fingers move together and independently of one another. In addition, poor tactile discrimination has been found to be associated with difficulty anticipating the force needed in grasp, modulating the force needed for grasp, and transitioning from grasp to lift.[64]

Children with cerebral palsy are very likely to have tactile discrimination problems as well as motor control problems. Several studies of tactile dysfunction in children with cerebral palsy were conducted in the 1950s and 1960s. These studies verified the presence of a variety of tactile discrimination problems in the hands of a high percentage of children with this disorder.[80,101,139] Recent studies of children with spastic hemiplegia have resulted in similar findings. Cooper, Majnemer, Rosenblatt, and Birnbaum found that eight of the nine children with spastic hemiplegia whom they tested had bilateral sensory deficits.[27] Yekutiel, Jariwala, and Stretch found that 51% of the 55 children with cerebral palsy whom they tested had sensory deficits on two-point discrimination and/or stereognosis.[152] In a study of 25 children with spastic hemiplegia, Krumlinde-Sundholm and Eliasson found that 18 had impairment of the hemiplegic hand in two-point discrimination at 3 mm and more than half had difficulty with two-point discrimination at 7 mm.[82] For approximately one third of these children, tactile problems were noted in all five tests of tactile discrimination in the hemiplegic hand. A marked difference in stereognosis was seen between testing with common objects (11 children showed impairment) and testing with flat shapes (24 showed impairment). Arnould, Penta, and Thonnard also found deficits in stereognosis, proprioception, and perception of touch pressure in a large sample (approximately 100) of school-age and young adolescent children with cerebral palsy.[2] Some researchers have found that children with hemiplegia have deficits in the less (or non) involved upper extremity as well as the hemiplegic hand.[27]

Although some researchers note that the degree of tactile problems is not always associated with the degree of motor impairment,[2,27] Krumlinde-Sundholm and Eliasson found strong relationships between impairment in sensation and dexterity in the more impaired hand of children with spastic hemiplegia (i.e., r = 0.60 to 0.71).[82] They noted that bilateral hand skills were less associated with the level of tactile discrimination. Differences in these study findings may be associated with differences in tactile testing methodologies and sample sizes. Children with cerebral palsy tend to need more trials than nondisabled children to match tactile and proprioceptive information with force for grasp and lift of objects.[39]

The use of sensory information about objects to plan movements also appears to be impaired in children with cerebral palsy, thus affecting their skill in object handling. In their study of children with cerebral palsy, Gordon et al. found that when children used their hand with motor impairment they did not effectively plan initiation of grasp with well-controlled finger spacing for the object ("anticipatory control") relative to object weight, despite experience with the objects in the task.[61] Of interest, however, is that when grasping objects with the other hand, they appeared to reflect knowledge of object weight that was learned by grasping with the involved hand. Thus, Gordon et al. stated that "the findings suggest that the impaired anticipatory control may be due to an inability to integrate the sensory information with the motor command in the involved hand... and that intact sensory information alone is not enough for anticipatory control, but instead it must be integrated with motor-related information" (p. 590).[61]

Children with milder problems also are at risk for somatosensory problems that affect hand skills. Case-Smith studied the relationship between both tactile hypersensitivity and tactile discrimination and in-hand manipulation skills in 50 children between 4 and 6 years of age.[19] In this sample, which included 80% typical children, those having problems with either tactile defensiveness or decreased tactile discrimination showed no significant problems with performing the in-hand manipulation tasks presented. However, those who had both tactile discrimination problems and hypersensitivity had difficulty performing the in-hand manipulation tasks that were timed. Their performances were significantly less efficient than those of the children in the other groups.

Strategies and plans of action rely on knowledge of object properties that probably is gained through tactile and proprioceptive information. Children with DCD appear to have tactile problems, because they have difficulty with feed-forward strategies[127] and with planning for intentional actions that depend on the anticipation of force and timing.[148] Similarly Smyth and Mason found proprioception problems in a variety of tasks in children with DCD.[128]

Learned Nonuse Phenomenon in Children with Hemiplegia

Sterr, Freivogel, and Schmalohr conducted a study to assess available use in the more involved arm-hand of a sample of 21 children, adolescents, and young adults with hemiplegia.[131] Their research was based on several other studies with adults with learned nonuse as a result of strokes. They found that "the learned nonuse model predicts that even if the residual movement capacities of the hemiparetic arm should allow the person to carry out activities of daily living ... that arm is not, in fact, used in the real-life situation" (p. 1727).[131] The difference between these individuals' available movement skills and the use of them in spontaneous situations was significant. The authors concluded that the limited use of the hemiplegic arm appeared to be due to learned nonuse.

Hand Skill Problems in Children and Adolescents with Various Developmental Difficulties

Children with a wide variety of developmental problems show significant difficulties in hand skills. Common developmental conditions that are reported to result in hand skill or fine motor problems include visual impairment/blindness, ADHD, autism spectrum disorders (ASD), and DCD.

Hand skill problems that reflect motor coordination difficulties have been identified in children with ASD[58,116,146] and with ADHD.[54,58,116] In a number of studies, the problems with motor coordination have been particularly linked to either the inattentive type of ADHD[54] or the combined type (both inattention and hyperactivity)[115]; less correlation has been documented with children who have ADHD-hyperactive type alone. Overall, problems with hand skills have been documented in these diagnostic categories in both large- and small-scale studies across a variety of ages of children, with a variety of test instruments. These problems have been corroborated by parent and teacher reports and reflect evidence for persistent coordination difficulties beyond childhood.[54]

A study by Meyer and Sagvolden clarified the types of hand skill problems that may be noted in children with ADHD.[97] They compared typical South African children with a similar sample of children with ADHD relative to their skills in performing three fine motor tasks involving tool use, object manipulation, and finger tapping. Although the two groups did not differ on the repetitive tapping item, the children with ADHD were significantly slower and less accurate in performance on the more complex items involving object control. Children at the younger ages (6 to 9 years versus 10 to 13 years) appeared to have greater differences in the object manipulation task relative to their typical age-peers, but this may have been due to a ceiling effect on the measure used. The authors concluded that the combination of speed with demand for eye-hand coordination is very difficult for children with both hyperactivity and inattentiveness.

In clinical practice children with autism may be assumed to either not have specific hand skills problems[112] or have hand skill problems due to sensory avoidance of certain textures or materials or due to a limited repertoire of interests, which may interfere with the range and type of object manipulation activities. Some toddlers with autism have poorer fine motor skills than gross motor skills, but others may have similar performance in the two areas or poorer gross motor skills; all had at least some delay in motor skills.[112] Within the area of fine motor skills, the most common pattern identified was a delay in visual-motor integration and handling of objects.

In recent years, significant attention has been given to documenting the characteristics of children with developmental coordination disorder and to attempting to determine similarities and differences in the fine motor difficulties these children have relative to children with ASD[150] and ADHD.[115] Flapper, Houwen, and Schoemaker found that approximately 60% of a sample of children with DCD had attention deficit disorders.[53] In a subset of 12 of the children they studied, the children differed significantly from typical children on the manual dexterity section of the Movement Assessment for Children, with 9 of the children having notable fine motor problems and 2 others having borderline performance. Their problems were reflected in increased errors and slower speed of performance. Piek et al. noted that attention difficulties may cause motor performance to be more variable, whereas difficulties with motor skill interfered with performance speed.[110] One of the difficulties with motor skill may be related to poor control of force and torque using the finger tips.[104] The component of rotation/movement was more impaired in 7-, 9-, and 11-year-old children than was the component of pressure alone. Overall the typical 7-year-old children and the 9-year-olds with DCD had similar scores on the torque measure, while the force measure showed about a 1-year delay. The authors note that "impairments of torque control in children with DCD may result in a greater challenge in daily manipulative tasks" (p. 45)[104] because of the number of different digits that need to be controlled with relative force.

Differences in Developmental Trends between Children with and without Disabilities

Although information about normal development of hand skills can be useful to therapists in understanding difficulties with functioning and/or in guiding intervention planning, therapists also need to recognize that normal developmental sequences may not apply to children with some types of disabilities. For example, in a longitudinal study by Hanna et al., hand function in children with cerebral palsy generally improved in early childhood and then began to decline.[66] They found somewhat different patterns of development with children who had mild, moderate, and severe impairments and for children with hemiplegic cerebral palsy and with quadriplegic cerebral palsy. Hand skills increased more slowly in children with greater degrees of motor impairment. In general, the children with quadriplegic cerebral palsy showed more decrease in quality of functioning over time than did the children with hemiplegia. Overall the highest quality of functioning was found at the average age of 46 months, and the highest scores on the PDMS Fine Motor Scale were achieved at approximately 5 years of age.

Eliasson et al. also found a longer course of development of hand skills, but did not identify deterioration in the skills they tested over time.[42] The children with cerebral palsy in their study were initially tested when they were between 6 and 8 years of age and retested 13 years later, assessing their hand skill dexterity and their ability to time finger movements for grasp and use a direct approach for grasp of objects. Overall they became faster in object manipulation both as measured on a standardized test and on a task involving grasp and lift. Thus, the children demonstrated increases in motor skill, including greater speed and increased consistency in movement, but appeared to have a longer course of development than in typical children (Research Note 10-1). The differences in findings between Hanna et al.[66] and Eliasson et al.[42] may be related to use of different measures of hand function as well as different samples of children and may be influenced by intervention.

Similarly, it should be noted that individuals with DCD and other hand skill problems may continue to improve in performance over time, but problems with coordination persist that

RESEARCH NOTE 10-1

Eliasson, A., Forssberg, H., Hung, Y., & Gordon, A. M. (2006). Development of hand function and precision grip control in individuals with cerebral palsy: A 13-year follow-up study. Pediatrics, 118, e1226-e1236.

ABSTRACT

The purpose of this study was to add to the very limited knowledge regarding how hand skills develop in children with cerebral palsy, as a basis for being able to interpret outcomes and maintain improvements from intervention to improve hand skills in this population. Children with various degrees of cerebral palsy (spastic diplegia or hemiplegia) were tested at 6 to 8 years of age and again at 19 to 21 years of age. The Jebsen-Taylor Test of Hand Function and measures of grasp and lift of a small object were used on both occasions. By using these measures, information regarding basic hand functions and speed of use as well as functional performance in daily occupations was captured. In addition, the force and timing in coordinating actions for use of a fingertip grasp and lifting an object were measured. The findings show that across this group of individuals, improvements were noted on the Jebsen-Taylor test in speed of performance, with those with the slowest times initially showing the greatest improvements. They also were faster in completing a task involving precision grasp and lift of an object and increased in consistency of performance. Pressure on the object in the grasp-lift task decreased and the ability to modulate the grasp relative to object weight improved as well. Thus, although these individuals with cerebral palsy continued to have difficulty with coordination of movements and timing, continued improvement over time occurred. They also showed improved consistency in performance across the various tasks and the elements of the tasks.

IMPLICATIONS FOR PRACTICE

- Studies of intervention effects and retention of skills developed through intervention need to consider the ongoing development of hand skills in children and adolescents with cerebral palsy. Thus, use of a comparison group is very important in helping to differentiate change due to development versus change due to intervention.
- Individuals with cerebral palsy show evidence of changes in motor performance in congruence with motor learning theory (i.e., with practice and experience, they demonstrate enhanced consistency in skills and increased speed).
- The ability to use sensory information effectively to support motor performance appears to improve over the time period of ages 6 to 21 years in individuals with cerebral palsy. The course of development of these skills may be longer than it is in individuals without a disability.
- Evidence for ongoing development of hand skills in this population supports the premise that therapy is likely to positively influence skill development.

affect interactions with peers and have a negative impact on the children's emotional well-being.[99] The time demands associated with slower performance or inability to accomplish tasks can make it extremely difficult or impossible to effectively engage in academic work.[99] Such problems with hand skill use for complex tasks are reported to persist at least through adolescence.[54]

EVALUATION OF HAND SKILLS IN CHILDREN

The occupational therapist evaluates a child's hand skills when the evidence is sufficient to suggest that problems with performance of occupational skills are at least partly attributable to the child's problems with hand skills. A hand skill evaluation should not be performed simply to obtain information about the child's fine motor skills. The therapist first must have evidence suggesting that the child has a problem in at least one area of occupational performance. Parents, teachers, and the child often are the best sources of information about difficulties with participation in the family and the community, and this information can be obtained through the development of an occupational profile. See Chapter 7 for additional information on how to obtain an occupational profile.

Screening for Hand Skill Problems

When a problem with occupational performance has been identified, the therapist needs to continue gathering information on the child's performance of specific daily life activities. As part of this process, the therapist determines whether it is reasonable to carry out a full evaluation of fine motor and hand skill performance. This information must include data about the child's age and general information about motor skills, cognitive and perceptual skills, sensory processing, social situation and skills, and emotional functioning, as well as contexts that affect the child. The therapist can obtain screening information from parents, teachers, the child, and other professionals or from reports of other professionals.

Observation of the skills noted in Table 10-1 can help determine what standardized test and further analysis should be pursued. These observations about the child's quality of hand skills can supplement a standardized test. Some skills are inappropriate for younger children; an "X" designates the age group for which any activity may be used. When a skill emerges within a particular age group, ages are listed rather than an "X." For block stacking, the number represents the number of blocks a child in that age group should be able to stack. The therapist can vary the materials used for some of the items so that he or she can assess many of these skills during mealtime, dressing, hygiene, or play activity. For all categories, except Bilateral Skills and Tool Use, the therapist should ask the child to perform the activities with both the right hand and with the left hand. Evaluation of both hands is important, because subtle difficulties may not be readily apparent. For example, Gordon, Lewis, Eliasson, and Duff found mild problems in the timing of voluntary release components in the noninvolved hand of children with hemiplegia.[63]

Evaluation

A child with occupational performance problems who shows difficulties on screening for hand skills should be further

TABLE 10-1 Screening Activities for Hand Skills

Activities	Age Groups			
	6–12 mo	**1–2 yr**	**3–5 yr**	**6+ yr**
REACH				
Move both arms in full range of motion	X	X	X	X
Reach to midline, extended elbow	X	X	X	X
Reach across midline		X	X	X
GRASP				
Use full palmar grasp	X	X	X	X
Use radial-digital grasp	9 mo	X	X	X
Use standard pincer grasp	10 mo	X	X	X
Use spherical grasp		X	X	X
Use intrinsic-plus grasp		X	X	X
Use power grasp on tool			X	X
RELEASE				
Release object freely	X	X	X	X
Release 1-inch object into container		X	X	X
Stack 1-inch blocks*		2–6 blocks	9–10 blocks	10 blocks
Release tiny object into small hole		X	X	X
Throw small ball at least 3 feet			X	X
IN-HAND MANIPULATION				
Manipulate object between two hands	X	X	X	X
Use finger-to-palm translation, small object[†]		X	X	X
Use palm-to-finger translation				
One object[†]		2 yr	X	X
Two to three objects[†]		2 yr	X	X
With coin			X	X
Unscrew bottle top		2 yr	X	X
Use shift to separate magazine pages or cards			X	X
Roll piece of clay into a ball[‡]			X	X
Pick up marker or crayon using rotation			4 yr	X
Shift on marker or pencil			5 yr	X
Rotate pencil to use eraser and back				X
BILATERAL SKILLS				
Hold or carry large ball with two hands	X	X	X	X
Stabilize paper during coloring or writing			X	X
Hold paper during scissors use			X	X
Manipulate paper during scissors use				X
TOOL USE				
Use scissors to cut				
Line			3 yr	X
Simple shapes			4 yr	X
Complex shapes				X
Scribble with marker	X			
Copy appropriate forms		X		X
Handwriting appropriate for grade				X

*Block stacking allows for assessment of arm stability in space, spatial orientation of the objects, and controlled finger extension. Voluntary release of objects other than blocks may be used. Screening should include placement of objects when arm is not supported and placement that requires precision.
[†]An object that is not flat should be used, such as small pieces of cereal (appropriate for children younger than 3 years or those who still mouth objects), small beads, or small pegs.
[‡]A piece of clay approximately 1/4 inch thick and 1 inch in diameter is placed in the palm of the child's hand. The child is asked to form the clay into a ball without using the other hand or the table surface. Palm-to-finger translation, finger-to-palm translation, simple rotation, and sometimes complex rotation may be observed.

evaluated so that the characteristics of the problem and the situations in which the child's performance is optimal can be carefully delineated. When determining the child's performance in the area of hand skills and potential reasons for any problems, the occupational therapist often uses a variety of standardized and nonstandardized assessments. All children should receive an assessment of hand skills in activities such as dressing, eating, hygiene skills, school activities, and play activities. Completion of a parent interview is helpful in determining persistent concerns and priorities. Wilson,

BOX 10-2 Problem: Inability to Engage Effectively in Constructive Play (Performance Problems, Body Function Factors, and Causes)

1. Lacks in-hand manipulative skills
   a. Unstable wrist in neutral position or extension, uses wrist flexion; possible causes:
      (1) Decreased tone in wrist extensors
      (2) Increased tone in wrist flexors
   b. Unstable metacarpophalangeal (MCP) joints; possible causes:
      (1) Poor co-contraction in finger joints
      (2) Increased pull of extensor digitorum
   c. Inability to identify finger being touched because of decreased tactile discrimination
   d. Lack of midrange movements of finger joints; possible causes:
      (1) Decreased proprioception
      (2) Poor co-contraction of MCP and interphalangeal (IP) flexors and extensors
      (3) Tightness in intrinsics and long finger flexors

2. Breaks materials, often by dropping and crushing them
   a. Inability to sustain finger pad grasp; possible causes:
      (1) Poor tactile or proprioceptive awareness
      (2) Poor co-contraction of muscle groups
   b. Excessive finger flexion in grasp; possible causes:
      (1) Poor proprioceptive awareness of size and weight of object
      (2) Increased finger flexor tone
      (3) Associated reactions
      (4) Inactivity in intrinsics
   c. Ineffective bilateral handling; possible causes:
      (1) Unstable grasp because of poor wrist extension caused by increased flexor tone
      (2) Overflow in one upper extremity
      (3) Learned nonuse

Kaplan, Crawford, Campbell, and Dewey have developed a Developmental Coordination Disorder Questionnaire for parents.[147]

Analysis of the identified hand skills problem involves administration of specific assessments or scales that define the basis of the problem and the extent of the impairment. A sample analysis of an occupational performance problem in the area of constructive play that is at least partly caused by hand skill difficulties is presented in Box 10-2. In this example the therapist has identified two main performance problems: lack of ability to manipulate materials after grasp and breakage of materials being handled ("manipulates" and "calibrates"[1]). The therapist then attempts to determine how sensory functions, neuromusculoskeletal and movement-related functions, and mental functions contribute to this performance limitation. Muscle and movement functions associated with this problem may include difficulties with wrist and MCP joint stability, limited midrange movement control, lack of isolated finger movement, and excessive use of flexion. Based on evaluation findings and the therapist's frames of reference, specific impairments are identified.

The following outline presents examples of tools and methods used in comprehensive evaluation to assess the underlying impairments associated with hand skill difficulties and delays.

1. Measurement of active and passive ROM (especially important for children who have weakness or increased muscle tone)
2. Evaluation of strength
   - Muscle testing (general and/or specific)
   - Grip and pinch strength testing
3. Evaluation of tactile functioning using standard assessment of tactile discrimination or two-point discrimination and finger identification with vision occluded
4. Assessment of postural alignment and postural stability, including stability and mobility of the hand
5. Administration of a standardized general developmental test that includes a fine motor section for young children (see Appendix 7-A)
   - Hawaii Early Learning Profile (HELP)
   - Bayley Scales of Infant and Toddler Development (3rd Ed.): Motor Scale
6. Administration of a developmental motor test
   - PDMS-2 Fine Motor Scale
   - Bruininks-Oseretsky Test of Motor Proficiency (BOT-2)
7. Administration of a test of fine motor skills for older children and adolescents
   - Purdue Pegboard Test
   - BOT-2
   - Movement Assessment Battery for Children
   - The Melbourne Assessment of Unilateral Upper Limb Function
   - The QUEST
   - Test of In-Hand Manipulation
8. Classification of manual skills to document outcomes
   - The Manual Ability Classification System (MACS)
9. Administration of a visual-motor integration test
   - Preschool Visual Motor Integration Assessment (PVMIA)
   - Test of Visual-Motor Skills (TVMS)
   - Developmental Test of Visual-Motor Integration (VMI)
10. Assessment of hand skills in prevocational or work tasks (important for adolescents)

GUIDELINES FOR INTERVENTION

Setting Goals

Several factors affect the types of goals developed in the area of hand skills and in other areas of the child's functioning: the child's occupational performance problems, the contexts in which the skills are needed, the types of problems in the hand skill area, the therapist's frame of reference, and the setting in which services are to be provided. For some children, developmental sequences of skills influence the selection of goals, but for the child with a motor disability, other factors will affect the goals established and the strategies selected for intervention. These factors include the types of occupational performance skills the child needs, the complexity and severity of the child's problems, and the human and nonhuman resources available to support the intervention program.

A child's goals generally are developed through a process of child/adolescent, family, and professional collaboration. The Perceived Efficacy and Goal Setting System[100] is helpful in setting goals with children who are functioning at approximately the 6- to 9-year-old level.

Overall, the therapist must be realistic in the number and types of goals to recommend relative to other goals for the child. In addition, the therapist must consider hand skill goals that are feasible for the child to accomplish. Such goals may be limited for children with severe disabilities. In all cases the therapist must link hand skill goals to the child's ability to engage in occupational activities more effectively. For some children the most appropriate focus of intervention is the development of skills in using adaptive equipment and strategies for accomplishing skills needed in activities of daily living. For children who show readiness to develop better quality or more complex hand skills, intervention can focus on acquisition of these skills. Factors to consider in planning intervention for hand skills problems are discussed in the following sections.

Considering Roles of the Occupational Therapy Assistant and Others in Intervention

Clearly the occupational therapist has a key role in evaluation, goal setting, and intervention planning for a child or adolescent with hand skill problems that are affecting functioning in daily life skills. However, others have a significant role as well. Typically not only is a parent/caregiver and/or a teacher involved in noting concerns relative to hand skills, but the child or adolescent, parent/caregiver, and other professionals need to identify their roles relative to intervention. In addition to parents/caregivers, teachers often have a key role. In fact, in some schools, the occupational therapist has predominantly a consultant role and the teacher is the primary interventionist.[8] However, although teachers indicate a high level of receptivity to input and recommendations from the occupational therapist in helping children with hand skill difficulties, they may have limited knowledge of the role of the occupational therapist[76] and/or want a higher level of input than periodic consultation for these children.[8]

In general, teachers and parents/caregivers can be provided with specific activities (classroom or games or selected tasks that work well within daily living skills) that allow for repetition of skills that the child or adolescent is able to show with simple cuing or with particular materials. Thus, it is preferable for the occupational therapist to provide activities that allow for practice of skills, but not to expect these individuals to determine how to vary or adapt an activity to elicit a better response from the child or adolescent.

The occupational therapist and the occupational therapy assistant can be an excellent team in providing both direct and consultative intervention in the area of hand skills. When a child has complex problems and/or is highly inconsistent in performance, intervention by the occupational therapist who is continually assessing and modifying the intervention strategies is generally preferable. When a child has less variability or when the child is ready to make incremental gains in motor skills or to use motor skills within graded functional activities, often the occupational therapy assistant can provide highly appropriate intervention with grading of activities in response to changes in child performance.

Sequencing of Intervention Sessions

When the therapist provides direct services to improve hand and arm function, he or she usually carries out in the following sequence:

1. Preparation
   - Positioning of the child
   - Attending to postural tone issues
   - Improving postural control (pelvis, shoulder, head)
   - Improving muscle strength
2. Development of hand skills
   - Promoting isolated arm and hand movements, such as external rotation, supination, and wrist extension
   - Enhancing reach, grasp, carry, and release skills
   - Enhancing in-hand manipulation skills
   - Facilitating bilateral hand use skills
   - Generalizing skills (integration of hand skills into functional activities)

Not all children need all the steps in this sequence. In addition, intervention for all areas is rarely done in one session.

Preparation for Hand Skill Development

Many children require preparation of the total body in each treatment session before the therapist can begin intervention for specific hand skill problems. In addition to intervention to improve motor function, the therapist should pay specific attention to the child's sensory functioning. The therapist can provide tactile and proprioceptive input to the arms and hands to enhance sensory awareness and discrimination. Lotion, toys, the child's own clothing or, preferably, active movements of the child's hands, with or without assistance, can provide stimuli. Children have greater tactile sensitivity when performing an activity that involves active touching rather than being touched.[67] The therapist should also encourage visual awareness of the hands with tactile and proprioceptive input.

Positioning the Child

In selecting the positioning of the therapist and the child for fine motor intervention, the therapist must consider the optimal position for eliciting the particular skills desired in that child and the position in which the child will use the skills. When these positions are different, the therapist must consider whether to use only one position at this time and introduce the other position later or to use both positions concurrently. For example, the child may be able to bring both hands to midline and to reach with the greatest elbow extension in the side-lying position. However, for functional use the child may need to be able to contact a switch on a surface while in an adapted sitting position. In an intervention session the therapist initially may work with the child in the side-lying position, then move to a supported sitting position to help the child generalize the skills to a functional position. Eventually the therapist may work with the child primarily in a supported sitting position. The therapist almost always needs to specifically address carryover of skills across positions with the child, often through activities developed collaboratively with the parents or the teacher.

The therapist can use certain body positions to elicit specific hand skills. The supine position is effective for working with children on arm movements and visual regard of the hands during movement. The prone position on the forearms is appropriate for addressing shoulder stability and co-contraction in 90-degree elbow flexion, dissociation of the two sides of the body during weight bearing on one arm while manipulating with the other, gross bilateral manipulation of objects, and visual regard of the hands. Side-lying can be an effective position for encouraging unilateral arm movement to bat at an object and for hand-to-hand play. Visual regard of the hands and objects is difficult to address in the side-lying position.

Sitting at a table is often the position in which children are most likely to use fine motor skills. For optimal hand use, children need a stable chair with adequate foot support. Even young children without motor disabilities benefit from sitting in furniture that fits appropriately. Smith-Zuzovsky and Exner found that typical young children had significantly better in-hand manipulation skills when seated in chairs and at a table fitted to them (Figure 10-16) than when seated in chairs and at a table that were slightly too large.[125] These workers suggest that appropriately fitted furniture may enhance hand function by means of its effect on proximal stability and/or by allowing the child to focus more on the manipulative tasks and less on postural readjustments. A study by Wingrat and Exner supported the theory that classroom chair size affects posture and attention.[149] They found that typical young children's sitting posture and on-task classroom behaviors were enhanced when they were in chairs appropriate to their size compared with their performance when seated in standard but slightly too large classroom chairs.

For children with disabilities, seated positioning for hand function activities requires specific attention. The therapist should not expect a child who cannot yet sit independently to work on sitting stability while working on hand skills. Such children need adaptations for sitting (e.g., lateral supports and chest straps) when working on hand skills. A tray or table surface should be a work surface rather than a support surface. The table or tray should be only slightly above elbow height, because a lower table promotes use of body flexion and a higher surface promotes use of abduction and internal rotation of the arms. The therapist also may provide activities with the child sitting on the floor or in a chair without a table, particularly when working on reaching skills or gross bilateral skills. Enhancement of hand function based on body position was illustrated in the study by Savalsbergh and colleagues. Their study of ball catching in 9- and 10-year-old children illustrated the significantly greater difficulty exhibited by less skilled children when they were standing than when they were sitting. Children who had good catching skills were not affected by the change in body position, thus illustrating their ability to combine a greater postural challenge with timed arm-hand movements.

For children with mild to moderate motor involvement, standing may be an appropriate position for treatment of some hand skills. Many daily living skills that rely on hand skills are most commonly done while standing, such as brushing the teeth, zipping and buttoning clothing, shaving, applying makeup, and cooking. For children who have substantial difficulties with standing, the therapist should use this position only after the child has mastered the skills in a sitting position.

Improving Postural Tone and Control

The child with increased tone throughout the body may need overall inhibition of tone before participating in hand skill activities. Slow rotary movements using small ranges of motion between internal and external shoulder rotation and between forearm pronation and supination can help inhibit tone. Upper extremity weight bearing is particularly useful as a treatment technique for improving postural control and improving stability in the scapulohumeral area. The therapist can also use upper extremity weight bearing to encourage the child to maintain elbow co-contraction and some degree of wrist extension while engaging in slight weight shifting.[12,32] The therapist provides proprioceptive input during weight bearing. For most children the primary focus is on helping the child increase overall stability rather than concentrating on achieving full elbow, wrist, or finger extension. The therapist can carry out weight-bearing activities with the child in the prone position on the forearms, the prone position on extended arms, the side-sitting position, or the long-sitting position, depending on the child's skill level.[12]

For the child who has tightness in wrist flexion, a position of upper extremity weight bearing on hands with the arms extended often is difficult, if not impossible, to achieve. The most appropriate positions for these children to use for weight bearing include prone on the forearms and side-lying. The therapist can help the child position the wrists in neutral position, and some therapists use splints during weight bearing to assist with wrist and hand positioning.[81]

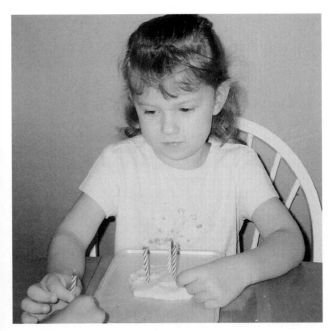

FIGURE 10-16   This child is seated at a table that is an appropriate height for tabletop activities. She can effectively place her arms on the surface without elevating her shoulders. Arm support on the surface, elbow flexion, and handing her the candles in a vertical position rather than having her grasp them from a table surface encourages the child's use of forearm supination and fingertip control during grasp and placement of the candles on the clay birthday cake.   (Courtesy Kanji Takeno, Towson University.)

Finger flexion is permitted during weight bearing as long as the thumb is not in an abnormal position. If the child's thumb is tightly adducted and flexed, the therapist should use handling techniques before weight bearing. The therapist can use his or her own hand to provide firm pressure over the first metacarpal joint and relax the child's hand through slow, small, rotary, and flexion-extension movements. Children with mildly and moderately increased tone often can work toward maintaining full finger extension during weight bearing.

Using a multiple-baseline single-subject design, Barnes found that children with cerebral palsy demonstrated increased use of wrist extension and finger extension after upper extremity weight bearing.[5-7] The weight bearing increased wrist extension during these activities but did not affect grasp and voluntary release quality and skill. Kinghorn and Roberts, who conducted a single-subject study of weight bearing with splinting for a child with cerebral palsy, did not find significant changes in objective measures of tone, positioning, or function.[81] However, family members reported improved functioning.

Improving Muscle Strength

Interventions to increase strength may improve skilled hand use in children with certain disabilities. Focus on strength needs to be addressed carefully in children with tone problems, because a primary focus on strength would diminish focus on coordination, which seems to be the primary problem in these children. Damiano and Abel reported on the use of strength training to support functioning in children with cerebral palsy.[31] They researched strengthening for walking and found that the children they assessed had marked muscle weakness. With a controlled program of strengthening, the children's strength improved, as did the quality of some components of walking. However, caution is required in applying these results to hand skills, because strengthening programs to enhance arm and hand function of children with cerebral palsy have not yet been researched.

In another study that focused on strengthening, Weaver, Gardner, Triolo, and Betz used neuromuscular electrical stimulation (NMES) with toddlers who had arthrogryposis that significantly affected their arm and finger strength and movement.[143] The NMES resulted in several positive changes in functions of the fingers, including greater ROM at the various finger joints. Associated changes in the developmental level of the children's grasp patterns occurred as well, resulting in the use of a more radial and distal grasp rather than an ulnar-palmar pattern. The authors suggest that NMES may be a positive addition to other interventions for this population.

Development of Hand Skills

The interventions described in this section apply and integrate four models of practice or frames of reference: neurodevelopmental treatment, developmental, motor learning, and biomechanical. *Neurodevelopmental treatment* frame of reference focuses on understanding and improving the child's impairments in postural tone, postural control, and stability and mobility.[122] The intervention activities focus on providing adequate support and helping the child develop dissociated and coordinated patterns of movement. *Developmental* theories give us a frame of reference to describe the sequences of skills that children develop (e.g., the progression from palmer grasp to a

pincer grasp pattern). This frame of reference suggests that tasks should be presented in a sequential order and that children achieve increasingly more difficult skills in a specific developmental sequence.

When therapists use *motor learning* theory, they focus on how the child learns specific motor skills. The occupational therapist assists the child in acquiring motor skills through structure and feedback and provides him or her with structured practice to refine the skills. The therapist selects a specific type of practice and feedback based on the child's level of performance and response to intervention. Sullivan, Kantak, and Burtner presented a clear example of research with children based on motor learning theory.[132] In their study, different frequencies of feedback were provided during a task involving arm movements. The authors found that children use feedback in a manner different from that of adults and require longer periods of practice. Chapter 9 provides additional description of motor learning theory.

The *biomechanical* frame of reference is used primarily to assess and provide intervention activities that improve a child's range of motion, strength, or endurance. Biomechanical approaches focus on postural alignment, joint stability and relationships, and musculoskeletal problems. Biomechanics helps the therapist understand the principles involved in tenodesis grasping patterns and the relationship of intrinsic and extrinsic muscle control for grasp and in-hand manipulation patterns.

When addressing hand skill development in children, the therapist must select activities that are interesting and appropriately challenging to the child. To support skill development, the therapist must be able to repeat these activities. Eliasson stated specifically that "practice or repetition is an important part of the learning process" (p. 50).[40] She defines learning as evidenced through "relatively consistent performance and retention of the task" (p. 50).[40] Therefore, eating activities and toys and games with many pieces can be particularly useful and enjoyable. Engaging in play while addressing hand skills can have important benefits, including motivating the child to engage in activities repeatedly and building his or her play repertoire.[29,137] Recent research suggests that the use of cognitive strategies to encourage awareness of elements of task performance may be helpful for enhancing the performance of children with developmental coordination disorders (Research Note 10-2).[17,98] Eliasson provides an excellent summary of a wide range of approaches to hand skill interventions for children with cerebral palsy, citing key research references as a basis for each of the approaches.

Promoting Isolated Arm and Hand Movements

The therapist may choose to address specific movements in the upper extremity apart from specific hand skills. For example, the therapist may assist the child in using elbow flexion-extension, supination-pronation, or wrist flexion-extension movements before integrating these movements into reaching, grasping, or releasing patterns. Helping children generalize the movement patterns they have practiced and learned into a functional activity is an important aspect of motor learning theory. Such an approach is most successful with children who can follow verbal instructions and participate actively in working on specific hand skills. The therapist can use games or songs to practice the use of these movements. The therapist

RESEARCH NOTE 10-2

Miller, L. T., Polatajko, H. J., Missiuna, C., Mandich, A. D., & Macnab, J. J. (2001). A pilot trial of a cognitive treatment for children with developmental coordination disorder. Human Movement Science, 20, 183-210.

ABSTRACT

A positive impact on daily life skills is the desired outcome from occupational therapy intervention with children who have developmental coordination disorder. This study was designed to assess the effectiveness of the Cognitive Orientation to (daily) Occupational Performance (CO-OP) as compared with a program reflecting treatment approaches and strategies most commonly used with this population of children (Contemporary Treatment Approach). This study was conducted as a clinical trial in which 7- to 12-year-old children were randomly assigned to groups, yielding 10 per group, with approximately twice as many boys as girls in each of the two groups. The children were assessed with a variety of cognitive and motor instruments to verify their diagnosis of DCD and to rule out other key interfering factors that could influence the intervention. Measures used to assess the effectiveness of the two types of intervention included interviews of the child and parent/caregiver, a qualitative assessment of performance of child-selected tasks. Other tests/measures were included to assess how performance changes may be generalized to other skills. Intervention consisted of 10 individual therapy sessions of just slightly less than 1 hour each. In the CO-OP treatment, children selected their goals and were taught to use a strategy of (1) identifying their goal, (2) determining a plan, (3) performing the task, and (4) evaluating how they did. In the Contemporary Treatment Approach multiple strategies were used, based on the therapist's determination of strategies believed to be effective. A key element was therapist selection of goals and activities and therapist-provided guidance in skill learning within the treatment. Both groups of children showed improvements on a number of measures, but those in the CO-OP treatment group were found to have a significant improvement in the skills, particularly with the goals set, and in sustaining the improvement at time of follow-up testing approximately 9 to 10 months after conclusion of the intervention. They also appeared to be more likely to show changes in skills not specifically addressed in the intervention. However, it should be noted that the CO-OP group had a significantly higher mean score on a vocabulary/verbal test given prior to treatment.

IMPLICATIONS FOR PRACTICE

- School-age children with DCD appear to be able to effectively identify goals to address in intervention, selecting goals that are meaningful to their daily life occupations.
- These children demonstrated the ability to learn to use a cognitive strategy for approaching an occupational task with motor components within a 10-session intervention (approximately 8 to 9 hours of intervention time). Having good verbal skills may have contributed to the success of this intervention.

- Once the children learned the cognitive strategy of goal-plan-do-check and could talk themselves through this strategy with therapist guidance, the children also appeared to be effective in using this strategy to enhance their performance on a number of activities involving motor skills.
- Children who received the Contemporary Treatment Approach also showed changes in a number of skill areas, including performance of occupational tasks targeted in the intervention. Since the children in this group had a higher initial mean score on the Canadian Occupational Performance Measure performance and satisfaction scales and the post-test scores of both groups were similar, it is difficult to determine if a ceiling effect may have influenced the amount of change feasible in the time frame of the study.
- On the basis of the findings of this study, therapists can be encouraged to actively involve children in selecting goals for intervention and, where feasible, encourage children to systematically determine goals for a session, identify strategies that may help to reach those goals, and evaluate the outcome of their strategies.

needs to emphasize specific movements and, in the same treatment session, use them in a functional context.

Supination control is one of the areas of greatest difficulty for children with disabilities, particularly those with tone problems. Abnormal posturing at the trunk, shoulder, elbow, or wrist often compensates for difficulties in initiating or sustaining forearm supination. Supination is easiest to use when the elbow is fully flexed and most difficult to use with full elbow extension. The therapist therefore can use activities that position the elbow in greater than 90° of flexion to facilitate supination. Examples of such activities include finger feeding, holding a kaleidoscope, and putting lotion on the face.

If the child can initiate supination but has poor control of this pattern, he or she can benefit from activities with the elbow held in 90° of supination with the forearm stabilized on a surface and an object presented vertically (see Figure 10-16). Gradually the therapist moves materials to encourage the child to use more elbow extension while maintaining the supinated position. Children with more severe involvement may be able to achieve only about 30° of supination, the minimum amount needed to handle materials on a table effectively. The therapist should encourage children with less motor impairment to obtain and use at least 90° of supination to accomplish functional activities such as drinking, eating with utensils, or turning a doorknob. Supination is critical for successful, smooth use of in-hand manipulation skills. In these activities it also is helpful to facilitate supination in the nonpreferred arm so that that hand can stabilize materials more effectively.

Enhancement of Reach and Carry Skills

Problems

Children with neuromotor disabilities exhibit typical problems in reach that limit range and control. Examples of problems in reach are:

- Use of abduction and internal rotation to initiate reach

- Use of shoulder elevation and lateral trunk flexion to increase the height of the arm for reaching and carrying
- Inability to coordinate the degree of hand opening or the hand position with the timing of the reach
- Difficulty maintaining an upright body posture when reaching or carrying forward or across the midline

Goals

Presented next are examples of goals the therapist can use for children with a variety of levels of disability. The goals are in approximate order of difficulty, although difficulty using any one pattern can vary with the individual child. All of the goals are associated with increasing the child's independence in morning hygiene skills. Some children may attain more limited independence in morning hygiene activities. Sample applications of the specific objects that could be the focus of the goals are indicated in parentheses. The goals are that the child will:

1. Maintain visual regard of the (soap, faucet handle, comb) while making hand contact
2. Bring the hand into contact with hygiene items (soap, toothpaste, towel) presented in various planes
3. Attain and carry hygiene items needed (soap, toothpaste, toothbrush, comb) located near the body but in various planes while sustaining sufficient finger extension to allow for grasp
4. Pick up objects (a towel, a large plate or pan) presented at midline by reaching with both hands together (forearm may be pronated)
5. Attain and carry large objects (e.g., a towel) in a variety of locations using both hands and incorporating appropriate forearm positioning
6. Attain and carry hygiene items (toothbrush, toothpaste, shampoo bottle, safety razor) using appropriate hand positioning for grasp combined with a mature reaching pattern
7. Pick up and place items (toothbrush, washcloth, makeup items) in various locations on a bathroom sink or counter, crossing the midline with an erect trunk posture and humeral external rotation, elbow extension, and forearm supination to midposition
8. Attain items from all levels in a cabinet or closet (including reaching above the head) with control

Intervention Strategies

When the child initiates little movement or is unable to open the hand during arm movement, the primary focus of intervention is on controlled initiation of arm movements. This includes using various types of arm movements and being able to place and hold the arm to allow for contact with objects. This type of reaching goal is a priority for children with extremely limited movement control or strength and those with a degenerative disease process that results in skill regression. These movements are important for contact with others, and the child can use them to activate switches for toys and electronic equipment.

To facilitate arm movements and contact with objects, the therapist must identify the best position to promote postural stability and visual regard. The most commonly used position is sitting, with attention given to head and trunk control, visual regard, and visual tracking. However, the therapist also can use the supine and side-lying positions effectively.

Children with severe motor involvement need toys and materials that are easy to activate and that have no "failure" elements. Such items include play foam, beans, rice, musical toys activated by light touch, and soap bubbles. The therapist usually can obtain the best results through proximal handling at the shoulders and upper arms while assisting the child with movements of either or both arms. The emphasis initially is on general arm movement, then on hand and arm placement, and finally on finger extension during arm movement as a precursor for reach with grasp.

When children are able to contact objects with some control, the therapist should introduce structured activities to assist the child in using elements of a more mature reaching pattern. Gradually these elements are combined to promote a smooth, direct reach. The therapist needs to determine the placement of objects in relation to the child's body so that the child can use the best reaching pattern possible. From that position the therapist can begin to vary object placement and orientation. For example, because presentation of objects at shoulder height often results in the child reaching with internal rotation and elbow flexion, initial presentation of objects at a level below the child's shoulder may facilitate the use of shoulder flexion and neutral rotation. Gradually the therapist can raise objects higher as the child develops more control. The therapist can use activities that require lateral reaching with shoulder abduction and slight external rotation before encouraging reaching with shoulder flexion. Box 10-3 includes a sequence of promoting reach and grasp while encouraging use of shoulder flexion or neutral or external rotation at the shoulder and elbow extension.

The therapist should also encourage the child to reach behind his or her body, combining humeral hyperextension with controlled internal rotation and various elbow positions. Many children have difficulty with this posterior reaching pattern, which is required in dressing and other daily living skills. Some children can use neutral to slight external shoulder rotation in combination with humeral flexion if the therapist

---

BOX 10-3 Typical Sequence of Reaching Patterns Used to Enhance Shoulder Flexion, Neutral Rotation, and Elbow Extension*

1. Present objects lateral to the child's leg: motion is slight shoulder flexion, elbow is extended (if possible).
2. Increase height of object, still with object presented lateral to child's leg.
3. Increase height, with object aligned with child's shoulder, at arm's length: motion is shoulder flexion with neutral rotation.
4. Use activities that require lateral reaching with shoulder abduction and slight external rotation, beginning low and gradually raising the height of the object presented.
5. Gradually move the object toward midline but at arm's length: monitor to encourage external rotation.
6. Move object to opposite side to encourage crossing the midline.
7. Present object above the child's head, encourage a lateral, midline, and across midline reach.

*The child generally is in a seated position.

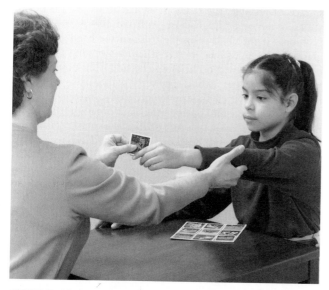

FIGURE 10-17 Facilitation is provided to prompt use of slight humeral external rotation and forearm supination. The object is held vertically to assist this reaching pattern. A lotto card game is used to engage the child and allow for repetition of the pattern. (Courtesy Kanji Takeno, Towson University.)

provides them with a minimal amount of handling at the humerus or elbow and appropriate object orientation (Figure 10-17). However, if such handling techniques are required for a child to use a mature reaching pattern, the therapist should present objects somewhat to the side or in front of the shoulder initially and then gradually toward the midline. To encourage reaching that incorporates neutral to slight external rotation of the shoulder and forearm supination, the therapist should orient the objects vertically. Horizontal orientation of an object encourages the use of forearm pronation.

To carry an object, the child must be able to vary all joint positions in the arm while sustaining grasp. Generally the child maintains wrist extension with sustained finger flexion when carrying or lifting an object to place it. The therapist should be especially attentive to the child's use of compensatory trunk movements and to difficulty dissociating arm and trunk movements. If these are present, the child may need intervention to improve sustained trunk control in the midline and trunk rotation with arm movements. The use of adapted equipment to support the trunk in a symmetric, erect posture is helpful for many children. The therapist also may need to stabilize the shoulder to prevent scapular elevation.

The therapist can use facilitation of arm movements in a manner similar to that described for reaching to encourage carrying patterns of shoulder rotation, graded elbow movements, and forearm supination. Most children with increased tone or stability problems have more difficulty carrying small or thin objects. Use of objects that are larger in diameter, such as those adapted with built-up handles, can promote wrist extension and management of objects during carrying.

Children with muscle weakness can more effectively reach and carry objects when they can use a table or tray surface at or slightly above elbow height. The therapist can use mobile

arm suspension systems to support and assist the child who has muscle strength rated as fair-minus or less.

The therapist should provide objects that have high color contrast or bright, solid colors to children with visual impairment. In cases of severe visual impairment, objects can combine both auditory stimuli and varied textures. If the child has not developed the ability to search for objects, the therapist should provide materials in a confined space or tied to strings so that the child can easily retrieve them when they are dropped.

Enhancement of Grasp Skills

Problems

The following are problems in the development of effective grasp, some of which are illustrated in Figure 10-18:
- Fisting or finger flexion that prevents hand opening
- Wrist flexion (often with ulnar deviation) in combination with finger extension
- Excessive forearm pronation, which interferes with the use of radial finger grasp patterns
- Thumb adduction in grasps that should use opposition, often with MCP or IP flexion
- Inability to use thumb abduction and adduction with MCP and IP extension

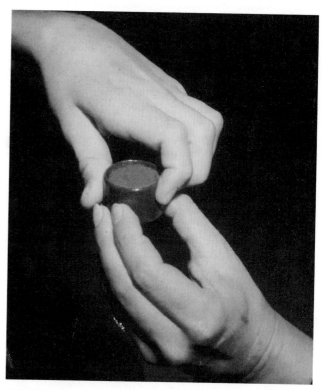

FIGURE 10-18 When this child combines reach with grasp, he demonstrates significant difficulties with effective hand positioning. Note the slight wrist flexion, the thumb adduction with IP joint extension, and the finger MCP joint hyperextension with IP flexion that he uses in an attempt to achieve stability with this grasp. The arm positioning in abduction and internal rotation (not shown) contribute to use of this grasp pattern.

- Inability to initiate or sustain thumb opposition
- Inability to use grasp patterns that involve control of the intrinsic finger muscles
- Inability to vary grasp in accordance with object characteristics and activity demands

Goals

Presented next are examples of goals that can be used for children with a variety of levels of disability. The goals are in approximate order of difficulty, although difficulty using any one pattern can vary with the individual child. Some children may develop grasp only up to one of the lower levels identified here, whereas others may be able to attain the higher level skills. To illustrate how the goals associated with grasp may be integrated with occupations of the child or adolescent, sample occupations (in parentheses) are identified for each grasp. The goals are that the child will:

1. (Put on clothing, pick up a towel, play a game with large game pieces) using a sustained grasp with the arm in a variety of positions.
2. (Hold hard finger foods, pick up clothing, play with a car set) using a finger surface grasp on a variety of objects.
3. (Eat finger foods, use manipulative objects in math activities, play a game with small pieces, do a puzzle) using a finger pad grasp with thumb opposition on small objects.
4. (Prepare a meal, perform dressing tasks, perform hygiene tasks) using an opposed thumb and fingertip grasp pattern in accordance with object shapes and characteristics.
5. (Use a key to open a door, build with construction toys) using an effective lateral pinch grasp pattern.
6. (Handle computer materials such as paper and disks and file papers in folders; eat a cracker or sandwich) using finger pads to hold thin, flat objects.
7. (Brush the teeth, use a knife, comb the hair, and use a safety razor) using a power grasp.

Intervention Strategies

For children with delays and functional difficulties in grasp, the therapist needs to match preparation techniques, such as positioning, handling, or strengthening, to the child's problem. Some children fist their hands or refuse to grasp objects because of tactile hypersensitivity, which also can influence the ability to maintain grasp. If this problem is present, grading tactile input from well tolerated to more difficult to tolerate is helpful. Initially, the child best tolerates firm objects with smooth surfaces and contours.

Tactile discrimination problems can contribute to grasp problems. Poor discrimination can affect dynamic use of grasp patterns and regulation of pressure in grasp. Problems with regulating pressure are seen as the child either holding objects with excessive force or dropping objects. Most children benefit from graded sensory input and attention to sensory discrimination as part of the intervention for grasp skills. Having the child actively explore the sizes, shapes, and textures of objects can precede emphasis on grasp in a treatment session.

In planning intervention that addresses grasp problems, the therapist, when selecting objects, should keep in mind the child's interests, sensory needs, and motor skills. Properties to consider include the size, shape, color, weight, and texture of objects.

Children with Severe Disabilities

Children with severe disabilities need to develop an effective palmar grasp and, if possible, grasp patterns using the finger surface. If possible, the therapist should stress the abilities to initiate grasp and sustain grasp with the arm in a variety of positions. If the child is unable to open the hand readily for grasp, the therapist may explore whether changing the child's body position would be helpful. The side-lying position may reduce stress on overall body posture and may make it possible for the child to open the hand more easily. In supported sitting, the child may find opening the hand easier if the therapist places an object below the seat of the chair and lateral to the child's body. Boehme described other handling techniques that may assist the child with hand opening.[12] The therapist should follow these techniques with movement of the open hand across objects and surfaces as a way of increasing the child's sustained hand opening and object interaction.

For the child who can independently open the hand but who shows wrist flexion with grasp, the therapist can emphasize wrist extension with grasp by positioning objects above the table surface or at chest height. Once the child can sustain wrist extension, the therapist can assist or encourage him or her to move the arm while maintaining grasp of an object. Sample activities using this skill include using a small stick to hit a suspended balloon or to break soap bubbles blown by the therapist, touching pictures on a wall or mirror with a stick, or holding onto clothing items while they are pulled up or down.

The child with a severe disability can wear a splint or other orthotic device during treatment and at other times of the day. Splinting techniques that may be useful in supporting hand function during treatment are described later in this chapter. Burtner et al. found that dynamic splints had a significant positive effect on grip over a static splint or no splint in a study that compared children with spastic cerebral palsy and typical children.[15] Of note was a finding of compensatory movements at the shoulder when these children wore a static splint during grasp activities.[15]

In addition to the above strategies, many children need adaptations of materials to support their performance of activities at home, school, and play. Use of standard materials may not be possible. Built-up handles that accommodate a palmar grasp pattern and larger objects, such as game pieces and blocks, may be used instead of smaller ones. Adapted page turners for books, switches for toys, and computer adaptations may be necessary to give the child some independence in play and school activities.

Children with Moderate Disabilities

Children with moderate disabilities are able to grasp but have difficulty with functional use of a variety of grasp patterns. They have problems in forearm control, wrist extension, thumb opposition, and control of the MCP and IP joints (see Figure 10-18). Grasp may be initiated with wrist flexion. Grasp goals for these children usually are designed to address the use of opposed grasp patterns and grasp patterns in which the hand effectively accommodates to objects.

The occupational therapist selects specific object shapes, sizes, and textures to develop opposed grasp patterns. The therapist selects activities that are age appropriate, interesting, and meaningful to the child and have elements the child can repeat. Games and imaginary play materials can provide opportunities for repetitive presentation of objects to the child. The child can use opposed grasps with medium-sized, small, and tiny objects. Children often can demonstrate better thumb and finger control with small or medium-sized objects that have well-defined edges. Tiny objects require too much precision, such that the child often resorts to a more primitive grasping pattern. In fact, skill in using a pincer grasp usually is less critical for the child's functional performance of daily life tasks than skill in using and varying a three-finger opposed grasp pattern. Once the child begins to acquire an opposed grasp pattern, the therapist can vary the objects by size, shape, texture, and weight.

The research findings of Case-Smith et al. support the clinical observation that object characteristics are important in eliciting specific grasp patterns, particularly when these patterns are emerging.[25] To help the child develop an opposed grasp pattern, the therapist can begin working on grasp alone rather than reach and grasp. The child's arm should be well stabilized when objects are presented. Having the wrist in a neutral or slightly extended position is critical; if appropriate, the therapist can stabilize the volar surface of the child's forearm on the table surface and give support over the dorsum of the forearm. The therapist should present objects in line with the shoulder and not at midline, because midline positioning has a tendency to encourage the use of pronation. With objects presented in line with the shoulder, neutral rotation of the humerus is encouraged (versus internal rotation) and slight forearm supination is likely to occur. The therapist holds the object with the fingers and presents the object directly to the child's fingers (Figure 10-19, *A*). After grasp, the child

carries the object to a nearby container or surface. Practice of this strategy for grasp, carry, and release using a variety of objects is needed for the child to integrate this skill.

Once the child is able to use this pattern well, the therapist can move to the next skill level. At this level the therapist places the object in his or her cupped hand (just under the child's hand and in line with the child's shoulder), so that the object is stable, and asks the child to grasp the object (Figure 10-19, *B*). When the therapist uses this strategy, the child needs to use more internal stability of the arm and some degree of prepositioning of the fingers before grasp.

As the child develops skill in grasping from the therapist's hand, the therapist can begin to place an object on the table surface. As at the prior two levels, the object is in line with the child's shoulder, not at midline. The therapist may need to stabilize the object or place it on a nonskid surface for the child who does not have sufficient arm stability to grasp without unintentionally moving the object.

After the child is able to grasp from the table surface with the object in line with the shoulder, the therapist can begin to move the object further away on the table surface, above the table surface, and closer to midline. In this way the therapist is structuring activities to combine reach with grasp. This requires the child to stabilize the arm in space while controlling finger movements. The therapist may use a variety of these object placements in a therapy session to elicit the

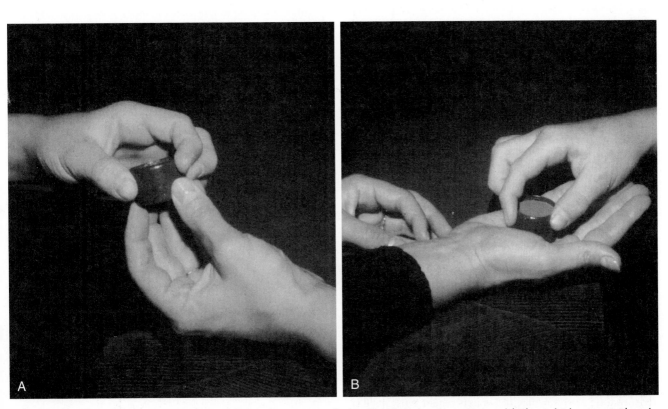

FIGURE 10-19   A, The child shows the ability to use a controlled radial-digital grasp pattern with the wrist in a neutral position, thumb opposition, and appropriate finger flexion when he is not asked to combine reach with grasp. Note that the therapist's presentation of the object helps ensure that the child will grasp the object with his fingertips. Her grasp also ensures that the object remains stable while the child initiates the grasp pattern. **B,** The child practices grasping from the therapist's hand. His arm is stabilized on his leg during this grasp. The therapist's hand provides some degree of stability to prevent the object from moving during initiation of grasp.

child's best skills. Different object placements may be needed with various sizes and shapes of objects.

Using principles of motor learning theory, the therapist systematically varies object placement and the size and weight of objects during intervention activities. Varying the input enables the child to develop more adaptable, flexible skills that can be generalized to a variety of situations. Duff and Gordon noted that 7- to 14-year-old children with hemiplegic cerebral palsy were able to demonstrate anticipatory control (i.e., the ability to adjust the force needed to lift an object) with novel objects, given the ability to practice these grasp-lift patterns.[37] Their findings suggest that these children can develop an awareness of the object properties and the adjustment in force needed by practicing grasping and lifting objects of similar size but different weights. In addition, this ability can be achieved through practice of several grasp-lift repetitions with objects that have the same weight followed by repetitions with objects that have a different weight, or the weights of the objects can be varied randomly in a practice session.[37] The therapist can assess the type of repetition that seems to have the most positive effect for a particular child. Further study is needed to determine children's retention of these skills over time. Gordon, Charles, and Steenbergen also found that children with cerebral palsy improved in their adjustment of the force necessary to lift an object via experiences with the opposite hand.[60] They were able to anticipate the force after using either the involved hand or the noninvolved hand. Thus, therapists should consider presenting objects for grasp to both hands, even if one is more impaired—and thus receiving more focus in therapy.

Children with Mild Disabilities

Children with mild disabilities typically have difficulty with small ranges of movement in supination and wrist extension. Sustained control with the intrinsic muscles of the hand may be difficult for these children to achieve. Fingertip control in grasp often is poor, as is the ability to control the palmar arches and to achieve radial-ulnar dissociation of movements within the hand. Some children substitute use of the middle finger for the index finger in attempting a pincer grasp (Figure 10-20); typical children may use this pattern occasionally, but children with tone problems (high or low) tend to use it frequently because of instability with the index finger and/or difficulty controlling the thumb in true opposition. Thus the thumb aligns more directly with the middle finger. This pattern can be functional for activities with tiny objects, but if the index finger cannot be used effectively with the middle finger, stable three-jaw chuck grasp patterns are not available for the child.

Goals for grasp skills for these children usually focus on the use of a variety of grasp patterns, with accommodation of the grasp pattern to the object characteristics. These patterns include use of an effective pincer grasp and lateral pinch grasp pattern; use of a grasp with MCP flexion and IP extension to hold thin, flat objects; and/or use of a power grasp on a variety of tools in daily living tasks. The standard and lateral pinch patterns and the grasp for thin, flat objects require wrist stability and use of the intrinsic muscles.

The therapist can use a variety of treatment strategies with children who are working on these skills, including verbal cueing and structuring of activities to elicit intrinsic muscle activity. Sample activities include holding all fingers in adduction and extension while rolling out clay, using finger abduction

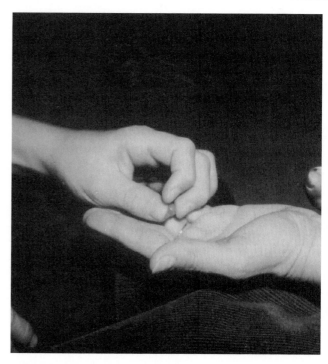

FIGURE 10-20 The child uses a substitution for a standard pincer grasp or tip pinch. Note that with slight adduction of the thumb, the pad of the thumb is more aligned with the middle finger than the index finger. The index finger is slightly too flexed to participate in the grasp.

to stretch rubber bands placed around two or more fingers, playing finger games that require isolation and small ranges of finger movements, holding or hiding objects in a cupped hand, and squeezing clay or other objects between the pad of the thumb and the pads of one or more fingers.

Development of a power grasp relies on the development of radial-ulnar dissociation and the ability to extend the index finger and thumb during ulnar finger flexion. Emphasis on radial-ulnar dissociation in the hand and on grasp with MCP flexion and IP extension is helpful as a precursor to the power grasp pattern. To address radial-ulnar dissociation, the therapist structures activities in which the child holds two objects in one hand and releases one at a time; holds an object in the ulnar side of the hand with the ring and little fingers while grasping and releasing with the radial fingers and thumb; and engages in activities that develop finger-to-palm translation with stabilization skills. In addressing the power grasp in functional activities, the therapist carefully selects the type of tool the child handles. Tools that have a narrow surface for index finger contact are particularly difficult for children to control. The therapist can use verbal cues, stickers, or dots on the handles of the tools to encourage appropriate finger placement. The child may need built-up handles to facilitate performance initially.

Enhancement of Voluntary Release Skills

Problems

Therapists usually combine treatment for voluntary release problems with intervention for grasp. Children who have difficulty releasing objects may exhibit the following:

- Fisting and tight finger flexion
- Difficulty with sustained arm position during object placement and release
- Difficulty combining wrist extension with finger extension
- Inability to use slight forearm supination to allow for release in small areas or near other objects and with visual monitoring of the placement
- Overextension of the fingers in release, limiting control of specific object placement

In their study of 7- to 13-year-old children with hemiplegic cerebral palsy, Eliasson and Gordon reported specific difficulties with both the placement phase and the release phase of object voluntary release.[43] The children's replacement "is abrupt," they said, "and their force coordination is impaired, resulting in a prolonged and uncoordinated release of the grasp" (p. 232).[43]

Goals

Presented next are examples of goals the therapist can use for children with a variety of levels of disability. These goals specifically define the size of an area in which the child can release the object (e.g., into a container with a 4-inch opening) or the height of a surface on which the child can release the object (e.g., a stack of six cubes). The following goals incorporate these commonly used measures of voluntary release skill. The goals are in approximate order of difficulty, although difficulty using any one pattern can vary with the individual child. The therapist should integrate these goals with the child's functional goals. The goals are that the child will:

1. Release objects into a container placed on the floor (e.g., pick up toys to put away [hard objects may be easier to use than soft objects]).
2. Release objects into a container placed on a table surface with the container at arm's length from the child's body to encourage wrist extension with finger extension (e.g., put objects into and take them out of a container).
3. Release objects into a container at the midline while using wrist extension (e.g., put pens and pencils into a basket after a group activity).
4. Release tiny objects into a container with a small opening (e.g., put nails or screws into a container after a project or put beads into a container for a beaded art project).
5. Place objects within 1 inch of other objects without making other objects move or fall (e.g., place game board pieces during a game, set the table with utensils).
6. Release unstable, lightweight objects while keeping them in an upright position (e.g., place objects on a desk at school and paper cups on the lunch table).
7. Release objects without visual monitoring (e.g., put a tooth-brush into a container, pencils into a container, paper on a desk).

Intervention Strategies

Intervention focuses on one or more of the following areas, depending on the child's problems: hand opening for object release, arm placement and stability for release, and accuracy of object placement. Releasing patterns correlate with grasping patterns. A child who uses a palmar grasp will use full finger extension to release the object. A child who uses a pincer grasp can use voluntary release with good control of the intrinsic muscles as balanced with the extrinsic muscles.

When the child shows excessive finger flexion (fisting), initial treatment for voluntary hand opening focuses on the child's ability to move the arm while maintaining some finger extension. Splinting may be helpful in supporting the child's wrist or facilitating increased wrist and finger extension. In children with fisting, asking the child to place the object into a container increases the child's fisting. Some children have success releasing to the side of their body because movement away from the midline decreases the pronation-flexion posturing, thus increasing the hand fisting.

If the child can accomplish this level of voluntary release, he or she can attempt release of large and medium-sized objects into a container with a large opening that is placed on the floor. For some children, transfer of objects from hand to hand is a reasonable strategy for encouraging release with object stabilization.

Children who can voluntarily open their hands but who use tenodesis patterns may benefit from intervention to increase voluntary finger extension while maintaining the wrist in a neutral position. For some children, structured activities and handling are effective; other children benefit from wearing a dorsal wrist splint. A therapist can have the child wear a splint during part of the therapy session and encourage finger extension through a variety of activities, including voluntary release. The child can practice similar activities after splint removal.

Children who use wrist flexion with voluntary release may benefit from structured activities in which a container for objects is placed slightly lateral to the child's midline and at a sufficient distance from the child's body that the child needs to extend the elbow (Figure 10-21). This level of control is

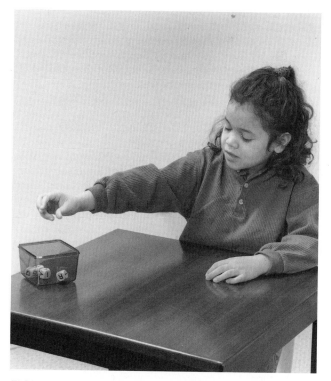

FIGURE 10-21 Positioning materials to elicit elbow extension during release encourages the child's use of wrist extension. (Courtesy Kanji Takeno, Towson University.)

similar to that of an infant who releases objects with the arm held in a total extension pattern. Over time, the therapist can move the target containers closer to the child's body, requiring gradually increasing elbow flexion with wrist extension for release of objects. Sometimes the therapist can facilitate this pattern if he or she sets the containers at an angle. Once the child can release medium-sized objects into a container at the midline while maintaining wrist extension to at least a neutral position, the therapist can reduce the size of the container opening.

Children with overextension of the fingers during voluntary release may benefit from activities described previously that address the development of intrinsic muscle control. They also may need intervention to improve somatosensory awareness of their hands. Activities for these children often incorporate the use of lightweight materials and objects that vary in size and stability. Verbal cueing of the child to attend to object and hand placement and graded activities to facilitate increasing accuracy and visual monitoring of materials are often helpful. Also, Gordon et al. observed that tasks that required increased accuracy (including object placement on a relatively unstable surface) could be used to encourage children with hemiplegia to slow their movements.[65] Instruction was helpful to the children in encouraging faster movements.[63] On the basis of findings from their studies, these researchers suggested that different speeds be used during voluntary release activities and that "practicing release tasks with the noninvolved hand first or practicing with bimanual tasks may enhance performance and should be studied" (p. 247).[63] In addition, the work of Eliasson and Gordon suggests that repetition of object release in which the object's weight remains constant over a number of trials allows children with hemiplegic cerebral palsy to learn to adjust the release of grasp.[43] These findings provide support for the use of activities for voluntary release in which repetition and timing can be adjusted. Games of various types are often very effective for this purpose and are selected for the child's cognitive level as well as the motor level.

Enhancement of In-Hand Manipulation Skills

Problems

Children who have difficulty with in-hand manipulation skills drop objects, use surfaces for support during manipulation, or are slow in the execution of skills.[45] Case-Smith found empirical support for these problems in her study of children with and without fine motor delays.[20] These problems are associated with tactile problems.[19] Praxis and motor control problems, particularly of the intrinsic muscles, also may be a major cause of limited in-hand manipulation skill development. Attentional and cognitive problems contribute to these problems in some children. Problems that limit in-hand manipulation include the following:

- Limited finger isolation and control
- Inability to effectively cup the hand to hold objects in the palm
- Inability to hold more than one object in the hand at the same time
- Insufficient stability for controlling object movement at the finger pads, resulting in objects being dropped frequently

Goals

Presented next are examples of goals the therapist can use for children with a variety of levels of in-hand manipulation skill. The goals are in approximate order of difficulty, although difficulty using any one pattern can vary with the individual child. The activities, including additional examples in parentheses, require specific in-hand manipulation skills. The goals are that the child will:

1. Move coins (move finger foods) into the palm of the hand by demonstrating finger-to-palm translation.
2. Move several coins (move pieces of finger foods) into the palm of one hand by using finger-to-palm translation with stabilization skills.
3. Adjust coins for placement into a bank (adjust playing cards for a game) using shift skills.
4. Adjust eating utensils (adjust a toothbrush while cleaning the teeth) using simple rotation skills.
5. Eat small finger foods (setup/clean up a game board) using palm-to-finger translation (and palm-to-finger translation with stabilization).
6. Play with a building set (put caps onto markers) using simple rotation with stabilization skills.
7. Erase with a pencil (handle containers or lids) using complex rotation skills.

Intervention Strategies

The therapist's assessment of the causes of the child's problems and the therapist's determination of the child's potential for acquiring specific in-hand manipulation skills influence intervention goals and strategies. Many children with moderate and severe disabilities who lack the necessary prerequisite skills cannot develop in-hand manipulation skills. Children with mild disabilities usually can develop at least lower level in-hand manipulation skills.

Specific activity suggestions are given in Box 10-4. Suggestions for strategies therapists can use with children with different levels of skills are discussed next. Exner provides additional information on treatment of in-hand manipulation skills.[48]

Children with No In-Hand Manipulation Skills

The therapist may encourage the child with no in-hand manipulation skills or only finger-to-palm translation to manipulate objects between the two hands and use support surfaces to assist in object manipulation. Use of these strategies can help the child begin to move the fingers actively over object surfaces. The therapist can use objects such as cubes that have pictures on all sides, kaleidoscopes, and textured toys. When the child can effectively move the fingers over objects, the therapist can introduce finger-to-palm translation activities in the context of "hiding the object" games using various objects. Finger isolation games can be useful, and the therapist should incorporate the thumb into these activities. The child should be assisted in developing and functionally using a variety of grasp patterns, including those that combine flexion at the MCP joints with extension at the IP joints. The therapist can use tactile discrimination and proprioception activities to enhance awareness of fingers and areas of the palm of the hand.

Children with Beginning In-Hand Manipulation Skills

Children who can use finger-to-palm translation and beginning simple rotation, or shift, or palm-to-finger translation skills can work on refining these skills, expanding their repertoire of skills used without stabilization, and beginning their

BOX 10-4 In-Hand Manipulation Activities

PREPARATION ACTIVITIES

1. Activities involving general tactile awareness
   - Using crazy foam
   - Using shaving cream
   - Applying hand lotion
   - Finger painting
2. Activities involving proprioceptive input
   - Weight bearing (e.g., wheelbarrow, activities on a small ball)
   - Pushing heavy objects (e.g., boxes, chairs, benches)
   - Pulling (e.g., tug-of-war)
   - Pressing different parts of the hand into clay
   - Pushing fingers into clay or therapy putty
   - Pushing shapes out of perforated cardboard
   - Tearing open packages or boxes
   - Playing clapping games
3. Activities involving regulation of pressure
   - Tearing edges off computer paper
   - Rolling clay into a ball
   - Squeezing water out of a sponge or washcloth
   - Pushing snaps together
4. Activities involving tactile discrimination
   - Playing finger games and singing songs
   - Playing finger identification games
   - Discriminating among objects with the objects stabilized
   - Discriminating among shapes with the shapes stabilized
   - Writing on the body and identifying the shape, letter, or object drawn
   - Discriminating among textures

SPECIFIC IN-HAND MANIPULATION ACTIVITIES

1. Translation (fingers to palm)
   - Getting a coin out of a change purse
   - Hiding a penny in the hand (magic trick)
   - Crumpling paper
   - Picking up a small piece of food and bringing it into the palm
2. Translation (fingers to palm with stabilization)
   - Getting two or more coins out of a change purse, one at a time
   - Taking two or more chips off a magnetic wand, one at a time
   - Picking up pegs or paper clips one at a time and holding two or more in the hand at one time
   - Picking up several utensils one at a time and holding two or more in the hand at one time
3. Translation (palm to fingers)
   - Moving a penny from the palm to the fingers
   - Moving a chip to the fingers to put on a magnetic wand
   - Moving an object to put it into a container
   - Moving a food item to put it in the mouth
4. Translation (palm to fingers with stabilization)
   - Holding several chips to put on a wand, one at a time
   - Handling money to put it into a coin bank or soda machine
   - Putting one utensil down when holding several
   - Holding several game pieces (chips, pegs, or markers)
5. Shift
   - Turning pages in a book
   - Picking up sheets of paper, tissue paper, or dollar bills
   - Separating playing cards
   - Stringing beads (shifting string and bead as string goes through the bead)
   - Shifting a crayon, pencil, or pen for coloring or writing
   - Shifting paper in the nonpreferred hand while cutting
   - Playing with Tinker Toys (long, thin pieces)
   - Moving a cookie while eating
   - Adjusting a spoon, fork, or knife for appropriate use
   - Rubbing paint, dirt, or tape off the pad of a finger
6. Shift with stabilization
   - Holding a pen and pushing the cap off with the same hand
   - Holding chips while flipping one out of the fingers
   - Holding fabric in the hand while attempting to button or snap
   - Holding a key ring with the keys in hand, shifting one for placement in a lock
7. Simple or complex rotation (depending on object orientation)
   - Removing or putting on a small jar lid
   - Putting on or removing bolts from nuts
   - Rotating a crayon or pencil with the tip oriented ulnarly (simple rotation)
   - Rotating a crayon or pencil with the tip oriented radially (complex rotation)
   - Removing a crayon from the box and preparing it for coloring
   - Rotating a pen or marker to put the top on it
   - Rotating toy people to put them in chairs, a bus, or a boat
   - Rotating a puzzle piece for placement in the puzzle
   - Feeling objects or shapes to identify them
   - Handling construction toy pieces
   - Turning cubes that have pictures on all six sides
   - Constructing twisted shapes with pipe cleaners
   - Rotating a toothbrush or eating utensils during use
8. Simple or complex rotation with stabilization
   - Handling parts of a small-shape container while rotating the shape to put it into the container
   - Holding a key ring with keys, rotating the correct one for placement in the lock

ability to stabilize objects in the ulnar side of the hand while manipulating with the radial fingers.

Object selection for in-hand manipulation skills with these children is important. Objects that do not roll and that are small (not tiny) are often the easiest for the child to handle. Examples are dice-sized cubes, nickels, game pieces, and other small toys. With larger objects, the child must involve all fingers in the manipulation and must use more hand expansion; therefore, these objects are more difficult for the child to handle. With tiny objects, the child must have excellent tactile discrimination and fingertip control, which also makes these objects more difficult to handle than small objects.

The therapist structures the presentation of objects to assist the child in using a particular in-hand manipulation skill and often cues the child in the use of the skill. In a study of preschool children without disabilities who had emerging in-hand manipulation skills, Exner found that use of verbal cues or demonstration of skills had a positive effect on the children's scores (as a group).[46] However, children with lower scores showed more improvement with cues than children with higher scores. These findings suggest that verbal cueing may be an important component of intervention for in-hand manipulation skills. The Cognitive Orientation to Occupational Performance (CO-OP) approach encourages the therapist to provide verbal cues and the child to select his or her own goals and strategies and to talk his or her way through an activity as a method of increasing coordination and motor planning.

In addressing palm-to-finger translation, the therapist first places the object on the middle phalanx of the child's index finger. When the child is able to move the object from this position out to the pads of the fingers, the therapist places the object on the volar surface of the proximal phalanx of the index finger. Later the therapist places the object in the palm of the child's hand to promote thumb isolation and control to move the object.

The therapist can structure simple rotation skills by placing the object in the child's hand (in a radial grasp pattern) and asking the child to turn it upright (Figure 10-22). Pegs and peglike objects (e.g., candles and objects that look like little people) can be helpful in developing these skills.

Finger-to-palm translation with stabilization is the one skill with stabilization that is likely to be feasible for these children. This child often can facilitate this skill during finger-feeding activities and in play with coins. The therapist first encourages the child to hold one object in the hand while picking up and hiding another. After the child can manage two objects, the therapist can progress to using three or more objects.

Children with Basic In-Hand Manipulation Skills

For children with basic in-hand manipulation skills, the therapist emphasizes the development of complex rotation skills (Figure 10-23) and the use of stabilization with the other skills. The therapist introduces small and medium-sized objects and emphasizes use of the skills in a variety of functional activities, including dressing, hygiene, and school tasks. The child

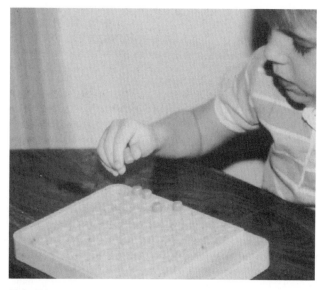

FIGURE 10-22 The peg has been placed in the child's hand upside down to encourage rotation prior to placement in the game board.

practices combinations of skills, such as finger-to-palm translation, palm-to-finger translation, and simple rotation. The therapist also can stress speed of skill use by timing skills and reporting the speed to the child. Children who are working at this level of skill typically respond well to verbal cueing for strategies to use in performing skills and to feedback about the effectiveness and speed of their skills. Eliasson, Bonnier, and Krumlinde-Sundholm studied the impact of practice of shift skills with a pen by adolescents who have cerebral palsy.[41] Eight of the nine adolescents showed improvements in use of this skill after a 2-week period of daily practice and retention of the skill 5 months later by five of the adolescents. Three adolescents had some loss of skill at the 5-month time period; however, none returned to their original performance level. The only adolescent to show no change with intervention had a 0 score (of 8) on the initial assessment, but three other children with initial performance at this level did show improvement in in-hand manipulation skills.

Facilitation of Bilateral Hand Use Skills

Problems

Difficulties with bilateral hand use result from a combination of problems, of which motor factors are only one component. Some children with significant cognitive delays cannot attend to two objects simultaneously; therefore, reciprocal hand use or stabilization with one hand combined with object handling by the other hand is challenging and may not be possible. Children may exhibit deficits in integration of the two body sides, and some children have impaired sensation with a lack of attention to one body side. Lack of bilateral motor experience, as with hemiplegia or after brachial plexus injuries, can cause children to approach all tasks in a one-handed manner. Other problems may include the following:

- The child cannot effectively sustain both hands at the midline.
- The child has difficulty using supination during bilateral activities.
- The child has overflow movements and associated reactions in one upper extremity when using the other.

Goals

Presented next are examples of goals the therapist can use for children with a variety of levels of disability. These goals fit the categories of gross symmetrical bilateral skills, stabilizing or manipulating with one hand while manipulating with the other hand, and bilateral simultaneous manipulation. The goals are listed in increasing level of difficulty, consistent with a developmental approach. This progression in skills may not be appropriate for children with significant weakness or motor problems on one body side. The goals are that the child will:

1. Push large objects using both hands together.
2. Lift and carry large objects using both hands.
3. Lift and carry medium-sized objects using both hands.
4. Color (write), demonstrating the ability to stabilize. materials on a table surface with one open hand while the other hand manipulates materials.
5. Hold the handle of a small pan while pretending to cook (hold the edge of a puzzle box while putting pieces away, hold the handle of a small bucket while filling with water), demonstrating the ability to stabilize materials using a palmar grasp while the other hand manipulates materials.

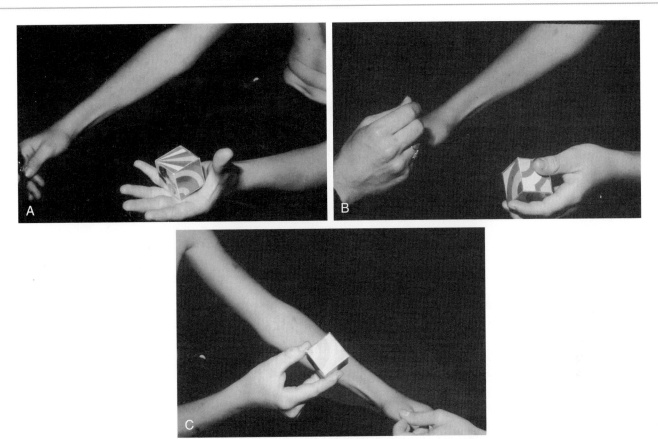

FIGURE 10-23   A, The child is forming a picture with a set of puzzle blocks. He is encouraged to find the side of the block that fits the design being constructed. The therapist has placed the correct side of the block against the palm of his hand so that he must use complex rotation to find it. **B,** Prior to using the in-hand manipulation skill of complex rotation, the child must use palm-to-finger translation to move the block toward the distal finger surface. In that process the block begins to be turned. **C,** Having identified the correct side, the child shifts the object out to the pads of the fingers prior to placement with the other blocks.

6. Hold a cup while pouring liquid into it (hold a slice of bread while spreading butter on it, hold a marker box while putting the markers away), demonstrating the ability to stabilize materials using a variety of grasp patterns while the other hand manipulates materials (Figure 10-24, *A*).
7. Button (tie shoes, fix hair, complete a mechanical project), demonstrating the ability to manipulate objects with both hands simultaneously (Figure 10-24, *B*).

Treatment goals vary depending on the severity of the child's disability and the level of skills the child is expected to acquire. The therapist must consider the child's need and potential for gross symmetrical hand use, stabilizing with one hand while manipulating with the other, and bilateral simultaneous manipulation.

Intervention Strategies

Children with Severe Disabilities

Intervention for the child with significantly increased tone or marked asymmetry focuses on promoting the child's ability to stabilize materials with the more involved hand while manipulating with the more proficient hand. Activities that require stabilization with grasp are often easier for these children than are symmetrical bilateral skills or stabilization without grasp. However, the child can accomplish stabilization without grasp as long

as he or she can use the hand in a fisted position with the wrist in neutral to slight extension. Activities that elicit symmetrical bilateral hand use can increase awareness of one arm to increase movement and/or control of that arm. Simultaneous bilateral manipulation skills usually are inappropriate for these children unless the therapist can use adaptations.

Special handling techniques can promote the child's ability to stabilize objects while manipulating them or to use gross bilateral skills. The therapist can sit behind the child and stabilize both shoulders to help the child bring and keep both hands at the midline. The therapist should also encourage trunk rotation so that the child can cross the midline effectively.

Toys and materials selected for bilateral activities must require both hands to be used, particularly in the early phases of treatment. Initially the child may be more successful with gross bilateral skills if he or she can sustain grasp and keep the forearms pronated, such as in holding a stick horizontally to hit a balloon. Expecting bilateral hand use to occur with the forearms in supination to midposition may be far too difficult for the child.

For the child who is working on stabilizing with one hand while manipulating with the other, presenting objects on a slippery surface may require the child to use one hand as a

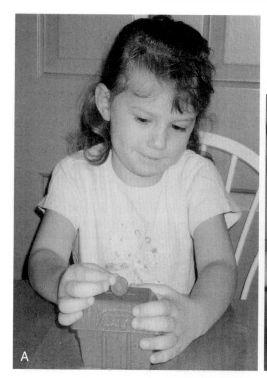
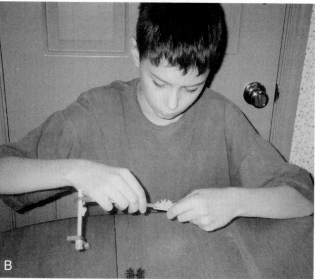

FIGURE 10-24   **A,** This child shows the bilateral skill of stabilizing with a refined grasp with her left hand while placing a penny in the bank with her right hand. Note the appropriate use of force in holding both objects. **B,** Bilateral manipulation occurs with both hands in this construction activity. The child uses modifications of the power grasp with different forearm positions on the right and left while connecting two parts of the toy.

stabilizer. Objects that have handles are useful when the therapist is working on stabilization with grasp. Activities that are simple for the manipulating hand can allow the child to focus on the role of the stabilizing hand. Usually the therapist places materials for bilateral skill development at the midline. However, the therapist and the child should explore other positions if midline positioning is not optimal.

If a child cannot successfully stabilize materials and does not show potential for this skill in the near future, the therapist should consider adaptations. Nonskid surfaces and other devices can assist in stabilization of materials for table activities.

Children with Moderate Disabilities

Intervention for children with low tone or some degree of involuntary movement can approximate the normal sequence of bilateral hand skill development. Therapy initially focuses on improving symmetry and stability and proceeds through developing the child's skills in stabilizing with and without grasp. Children at this skill level may benefit from working on a slightly unstable surface to prompt spontaneous stabilization of materials during manipulation. The child may need adaptations for certain highly demanding activities (e.g., handwriting) in which one hand must be an effective stabilizer. Generally, simultaneous bilateral manipulation is not feasible for these children.

Children with Mild Disabilities

Children with mild disabilities may require further refinement of gross symmetrical bilateral skills and stabilizing with one hand while manipulating with the other. These children can also develop or improve their simultaneous bilateral manipulation skills. To enhance development of simultaneous bilateral manipulation skills, the therapist carefully selects, grades, and structures a variety of activities that elicit these skills. The therapist may also use functional activities of daily living to facilitate development of these skills.

Children with Muscle Weakness

Children with muscle weakness can often manage simultaneous manipulation activities well because little hand strength and movement of the arms against gravity are required. These children often need assistance or adaptations to develop the ability to stabilize materials with one hand because this demands more strength in the stabilizing arm. The child may be able to accomplish gross symmetrical bilateral skills only on table surfaces that provide arm support.

Group Intervention for Children with Hand Skill Problems

Often occupational therapy intervention for children with hand skill problems is provided on an individual basis. However, small group intervention can have many benefits and may be considered at the least as a supplement to individual intervention. In a study comparing individual and group intervention using the same types of activities with children with spastic diplegia, Bumin and Kayihan found that children improved significantly in both types of intervention.[14]

Small group intervention can allow for focus on a number of skills in addition to sensory and motor factors. The social context of the small group allows children to observe and learn from one another and to practice leadership skills, depending on the opportunities created by the therapist. In addition, small groups support turn-taking and communication skills. Many children are more willing to engage in repetition of actions (which is very beneficial for some hand skills) in a gamelike atmosphere in a small group than in an individual session with a therapist. In addition, some games benefit from having more players than just the child and the therapist.

In structuring small group therapy sessions that focus on enhancing the development of hand skills, the therapist should consider the cognitive and interactional skills of the children as well as their hand skill problems. However, sessions that use play/leisure- or work-based activities are particularly amenable to modification for inclusion of other children. In contrast, intervention that focuses on improved use of hand skills in activities of daily living often is more appropriately carried out in individual sessions.

Generalization of Skills into Functional Activities

Most children do not readily generalize skills from isolated activities to everyday life activities without assistance. The therapist therefore should present activities to the child who has hand or arm function problems in a meaningful context and should seek ways in which the child can practice specific fine motor skills in everyday activities. For example, the child can carry out reaching program activities during dressing and hygiene training or while playing with a toy that has many different parts. The therapist can incorporate grasp activities into independent eating and vocational readiness tasks. The child can facilitate in-hand manipulation by using materials from a pencil or crayon box or by building with construction toys. The therapist can structure voluntary release into a game that uses moveable pieces. The child can develop bilateral hand use through meal preparation activities, play, and schoolwork. Many other combinations are possible to help the child develop mature hand or arm function, with increasing competence in daily life activities. Therapists should help the child and family link and apply the child's newly developed hand skills to occupational performance and social participation. Parents of children with mild motor problems (developmental coordination disorder) report a substantial negative impact on their children's activities of daily living.[92] Mandich, Polatajko, and Rogers emphasize that children need to have the opportunity to choose the activity-oriented goals for their intervention. These goals are often important to supporting the children's involvement in social settings. The occupational therapist should be mindful of how intervention activities match the child's goals and help the child generalize new skills to his/her valued daily living and social activities.

RESEARCH ON INTERVENTION FOR HAND SKILL PROBLEMS

Studies on the efficacy of fine motor and hand skill intervention in children increasingly are providing information that is useful in the determination of intervention strategies and the planning of occupational therapy programs. However, currently almost all studies have looked at the short-term benefits of intervention. Longer-term and longitudinal studies are beginning to emerge.

A study by Heathcock, Lobo, and Galloway with full-term and preterm infants involved caregiver-provided interventions performed for approximately 75 to 100 minutes per week for 8 weeks.[69] They found that the infants who received intervention in which reach and hand contact with objects were facilitated demonstrated a significant positive difference in these skills when compared to infants who were provided with a social intervention. The motor intervention was identified as affecting frequency and consistency of these skills as well as some aspects of quality. Thus, although certain elements of the preterm infants' reach and object contact skills were noted to differ from the full-term infants, the motor intervention had a positive effect. It should be noted that outcomes were assessed during the intervention; retention of these improvements after the intervention concluded was not reported.

Case-Smith has conducted a number of studies designed to assess the effectiveness of school-based occupational therapy on improvement in children's hand skills. In a study designed to assess the outcomes of occupational therapy programs for 26 preschool-age children who were treated during one school year, Case-Smith found that the children showed significant change in several aspects of fine motor skills, including in-hand manipulation skills, motor accuracy, and tool use.[21] In addition, the children showed significant improvement in their self-care skills. In a follow-up study with a larger group of preschool-age children with problems and a group of children without problems, Case-Smith et al. compared children who received services with those without problems.[25] The children who received services made significant progress in the areas of in-hand manipulation skills and motor accuracy. The researchers also found that more consultation was significantly associated with the children's improvement in some fine motor skills.

A subsequent study by Case-Smith included 38 children of elementary school age (7 to 10 years old) who had handwriting difficulties.[22] Data were collected regarding the children's in-hand manipulation skills as well as their handwriting skills. As a group, the 29 children who had received occupational therapy services across the school year (i.e., a 7-month period) showed more improvement in in-hand manipulation speed than the group of 9 children who did not receive occupational therapy. The occupational therapists who provided the services to these children reported that they included object manipulation activities in their weekly 30-minute treatment sessions with the children. This study, as well as Case-Smith's 1998 study, is particularly valuable in supporting intervention for in-hand manipulation problems in children in that even in studies in which the intervention was not highly controlled (in which different therapists provided treatment activities that varied based on the child's needs), in-hand manipulation skills have been shown to improve. Such studies suggest that children with mild involvement can make significant changes in these skills with occupational therapy intervention. Further studies are needed to determine more specifically the impact of such improvement on occupational performance in the children.

A study by Schoemaker, Niemeijer, Reynders, and Smits-Engelsman similarly supports intervention for children with mild disabilities.[120] Children with developmental coordination disorder were placed in a treatment group (n = 10) or a control group (n = 5). The experimental group received 18 treatment sessions of "a task-oriented treatment program based upon recent insights from motor control and motor learning research," and the control group did not receive treatment (p. 155).[120] The children who received treatment improved significantly in handwriting quality and in dexterity and ball skills performance on the Movement Assessment Battery for Children (ABC). The authors noted that some of the changes were quite substantial and seemed to be related to whether a skill was practiced or not. Although no follow-up data were reported, this approach seems to be worthy of further study in children with DCD as well as other types of motor coordination difficulties.

In 2001, Mandich, Polatajko, Macnab, and Miller presented a critical analysis of the research available at that time related to effectiveness of interventions for children with DCD, particularly "focusing on the extent to which treatments improve the child's motor performance in daily activities such as bike riding, shoe tying, handwriting, and hitting a baseball" (p. 54).[91] Functional skills such as these are often identified by both children and parents as problematic and areas of desired improvement. The literature they analyzed included studies in which intervention focused on (1) identified underlying problems ("bottom-up approaches") such as sensory integration, process-oriented treatment (which focuses on kinesthesia in interventions), perceptual-motor training, and combined approaches, or (2) interventions that focus more directly on the task/skill desired such as task-specific intervention and cognitive approaches. They conclude that

> ... although the bottom up approaches have a long tradition, the empirical data do not convincingly support their effectiveness in improving the motor skills of children with DCD, nor do they support the assumed relationship between underlying processes and functional performance... [in contrast] early evidence for the use of top down approaches with a DCD population, and collateral evidence from other populations, suggests that these approaches may be very effective in teaching specific tasks and in improving the functional performance of children with DCD (p. 65).[91]

Generalization of skills learned via these approaches need further study. They concluded that use of motor learning theories with functional skills may be a strategy that will be useful with children who have DCD.

Miller, Polatajko, Missiuna, Mandich, and Macnab presented the findings of their pilot study using CO-OP with this population (see Research Note 10-2).[98] CO-OP emphasizes problem-solving strategies and guided discovery of child- and task-specific strategies. The child identifies the specific occupational tasks to be learned and then discovers and practices strategies for performing the task. As Candler and Meeuwsen noted, "Children with developmental coordination disorder can implicitly recognize and respond to environmental cues important to task performance" (p. 434).[17] These children do not necessarily benefit from highly specific cueing of their performance.

In Europe an intensive approach to treatment, referred to as *conductive education*. is used with some children who have cerebral palsy. This approach is described as "a combined therapeutic and pedagogic program"[11] with a focus on engagement in specific tasks, use of rhythmic speech, application of

specific hand skills in daily activities, and group activities with other children. In the study by Blank et al., children participated in the conductive education program 7 hours a day for 4 weeks on three occasions within a 9-month period.[11] The other form of intervention was considered standard with a minimum of 2 hours of therapy weekly. The authors found that both the preferred and nonpreferred hands showed more improvement in coordinated hand use and independent living skills that rely on hand use than in basic hand functions and that these positive changes were noted by parents as well. Although this model was shown to be effective in this study of 64 children, it is an extremely intensive program that is not readily available either in terms of personnel trained in this approach and/or in the opportunity to participate in a program requiring such intensive involvement.

Research of children with more substantial motor disabilities has documented evidence of intervention effects (e.g., see the review by Boyd, Morris, and Graham[13]). Fedrizzi, Pagliano, Andreucci, and Oleari conducted a longitudinal study with 31 children with spastic hemiplegia in which they assessed the children for grip skill and use of the more involved hand in bilateral activities.[52] From the time of the initial referral to age 4, the children received individual therapy two or three times a week, then from 4 to 7 years of age the children received small group treatment (three or four children per group). Therapy focused on improvement of hand skills through the use of motor learning principles in play and activities of daily living. These authors' findings support intervention focused on use of the hemiplegic hand in functional activities for these children. In fact, the greatest improvements in grasp were found to occur during the years of small group treatment (ages 4 to 7). However, this change may have been due to developmental readiness for improvement in grasp at that time; further study would be needed to determine whether the change was associated with the specific treatment. The authors noted that the more involved hand was more impaired in spontaneous bilateral activities than when used alone in grasping skills. The children in their study with the most severe motor disabilities (a small number of children) tended to deteriorate in grasp skill as they approached adolescence. These authors recommended monitoring of children with more severe involvement in this age group to determine the need for continued intervention.

Constraint-Induced Movement Therapy for Children with Hemiplegic Cerebral Palsy

Children with hemiplegic cerebral palsy demonstrate limitations in bilateral hand use.[52] Sterr, Freivogel, and Schmalohr documented differences in available movement/skill versus spontaneous use in children and young adults with hemiplegia.[131] They found that although these individuals were able to use their involved hand, they tended not to do so and that they believed they had more ability to use their hands than they actually demonstrated. Therapists therefore have often sought a variety of strategies to increase spontaneous use of the involved hand.

Taub's research has provided the basis for clinical application of constraint-induced movement therapy, which is now used with adults and children with hemiplegia in a number of clinical settings.[134] A key characteristic of this therapy is the use of some method of restraint of the less involved arm and hand to promote use of the more involved arm and hand. Implementation of this intervention with children varies in the method used to restrict movement in the less involved arm and hand, in the amount of intervention provided during the restriction of movement, and the number of days or weeks of restriction. Some researchers report using a splint on the less involved hand[30,59]; others report using casting of the less involved arm and hand.[35,145] In the studies (which may reflect clinical practice models), some children were provided with no additional specific intervention,[30,145] others received additional therapy sessions during the days of restricted movement of the less involved hand,[59] and still others received 6 hours of intervention per day during the casting.[35] The most common time frame reported in the research studies was 3 to 4 weeks.[30,35,145] The one factor that appeared to be relatively constant in implementation of this intervention is restriction of the less involved hand for at least 6 waking hours a day.

Crocker and others used a single case study to evaluate the effectiveness of this approach with a 2-year-old child.[30] Outcomes immediately after splinting and 2 weeks later included more arm-hand use with better quality, as demonstrated in play, finger feeding, and PDMS Fine Motor Test results. Six months later, additional improvement was noted.

Glover et al. assessed constraint-induced movement therapy in a 19-month-old child.[59] Changes noted were significant in frequency of arm-hand use, accuracy of movements, and strength. Spontaneous use in bilateral activities and quality of reaching and voluntary release were evident, but grasp was not substantially improved. Although spasticity was diminished immediately on discontinuation of the constraint-induced movement program, it did return gradually. At 2½ months after intervention, spontaneous use remained improved.

Another case study to assess constraint-induced movement therapy was conducted by DeLuca et al. with a 15-month-old girl.[35] In this study, the researchers provided a second session of this therapy 5 months after the end of the first session. Positive changes in the child's arm-hand use and major changes in the spontaneity of her use of the more involved hand resulted. She showed significant improvement in occupational performance activities appropriate for her age.

A group comparison study of constraint-induced movement therapy in children between the ages of 1 and 8 years was conducted by Willis et al.[145] Using a cross-over design, half of the children received casting and intervention for a month, then after a 6-month period the other half received casting and intervention. During each of the study time periods, the children who were casted improved approximately 10 points more on the PDMS than those who were not casted. All parents of the children casted also documented improvement.

Constraint-induced movement therapy, therefore, seems to be a potential adjunct to other interventions for children with asymmetric motor involvement due to CNS dysfunction. All children studied showed improvement in one or more aspects of neuromusculoskeletal and movement-related functions, performance skills, and occupational performance. However, some authors noted the parents' concern, at least initially, with the constraint regarding the loss of independence in activities they previously could accomplish since the children were unable to use their preferred hand[35] and because of the children's level of frustration.[59] However, the parents also

noted substantial improvements in their children's functioning as a result of participation in this type of intervention. Therefore psychosocial support for the parents and the child seems imperative with constraint-induced movement therapy.

In response to some of the aforementioned concerns, Gordon, Charles, and Wolf have modified the constraint-induced movement therapy protocol for children over time, with a commitment to making it as child-friendly as possible.[61] Rather than a cast, a sling is used in their studies. The intensive intervention includes activities for the involved arm and hand during 10 of 12 consecutive days. Activities are selected to allow for progressive shaping of responses and multiple repetitions of each movement pattern. Their program has been used with 37 children in the 4- to 14-year-old age range and is conducted in small groups. In addition to describing the program, they include information regarding consideration of other factors and assessment of outcomes. Hart outlines key issues to be addressed in subsequent studies of this approach with children.[68] In all cases the intervention has been found to be effective, suggesting that intensive intervention focused on graded approaches to building hand skills yield results that are sustained over time. Although the children in these studies continue to have difficulties with hand use, their function after this intervention is demonstrably improved (Table 10-2).

SPLINTING

Splinting is often a component of occupational therapy intervention for children with hand function problems. Children who have one or more of the following problems may benefit most:

- Sustained abnormal posturing
- Increased tone or markedly decreased tone
- Limitations in movement of the hand
- Limitations in functional skills secondary to problems with hand functions

Children with severe motor disability associated with CNS dysfunction may benefit from splinting to reduce tone or improve mobility and functional skills. The child with minimal involvement secondary to CNS damage may have more difficulty with thumb use than with wrist or finger control. This child may need a thumb splint to diminish flexor muscle tone or to provide thumb MCP stability so that function is enhanced.

This section presents an overview of splinting for children with disabilities. Gabriel and Duvall-Riley provide additional information on the selection of splints and more specific details about construction of a wide variety of splints for children.[56]

Precautions and Indications for Splint Use

Precautions for splint use are always in order, particularly for nonverbal children who may have poor sensation. These factors make them vulnerable to skin irritation and pressure problems. Children may be unable to report sensory problems during or after splint application; therefore the therapist must carefully instruct the child's parents regarding the wearing schedule, possible problems, and postural changes to note.

Static splints generally are worn for shorter periods than splints that allow hand movement. Initially children may tolerate

TABLE 10-2 Evidence Table and Research Summary: Constraint-Induced Movement Therapy (CIMT) & Hand-Arm Bimanual Intensive Training (HABIT)

Study	Number of Children and Age	Type of Study	Method of constraint	Constraint wearing intensity	Findings
Gordon et al. (2008)	2, 1–3 yr	Single-case design	Forearm splint	CONSTRAINT: 8-24 hr/day for 2-6 weeks THERAPY: 5-7 2-hr sessions/week	Observed improvements in: • spontaneous use • speed of movement • range of movement • accuracy and success of play in affected arm
Elisasson, Bonnier, & Krumlinde-Sundholm (2003)	9, 13–18 yr	Cohort	Glove splint	CONSTRAINT: 7 hr/day for 10 days THERAPY: All day at summer camp	Measured improvements in: • upper limb coordination 1 mo (p < .01); 5 mo (p < .05) • dexterity 1 mo (p < .01); 5 mo (p < .01) • motor skills 1 mo (p < .05); .5 mo (NS) • manipulation 1 mo (p < .05); 5 mo (p < .05) • task performance (p < .01); 5 mo (not tested)
Willis, Morello, Davie, Rice, & Bennet (2002)	12, 1–8 yr	Cross-over	Plaster cast (below elbow)	CONSTRAINT: 24 hr/day for 4 weeks THERAPY: 1-4 hrs/wk	Measured improvements in: • arm movement 1 mon (p < .0001); 6 mo (p < .05)
Charles, Lavinder, & Gordon (2001)	3, 9–13 yr	Single-case design	Sling	CONSTRAINT: 6 hr/day for 2 weeks	Measured improvement in: • hand function • dexterity • sensation Observed improvement in: • functional achievement No change in finger tip force coordination
Pierce, Daly, Gallagher, Gershkoff, & Schaumburg (2002)	1, 12 yr	Single-case design	Mitt	CONSTRAINT: 1 hr/day THERAPY: 4 hr/wk for 3 weeks	Measured improvements in: • speed on 13/15 items (37.5% improvement) • grip strength • movement 8/16 items • self-reported improvement: function, e.g., remote control
DeLuca, Echols, Ramey, & Taub (2003)	1, 15 mo old	Single-case design	Plastercast (shoulder to finger tips)	CONSTRAINT: 2 hr/day for 3 weeks THERAPY: plus 6 hr/day training and 4 hr/wk therapy	Measured improvement in movement, Peabody, score increased from 43 to 62. No statistics on measures available
Taub, Ramey, DeLuca, & Echols (2004)	18, 7 mo–8 yr	Randomized control trial	Plaster cast	CONSTRAINT: 24 hr/day for 3 weeks THERAPY: plus 6 hr/day therapy	Measured improvement in: • net gain of 7.0 new motor patterns and major classes of functional activity not previously observed. • significant gains in mean amt of quality of movement at home • increases in unprompted use of the more affected arm

Study	N, age	Design	Restraint/Intervention	Dosage	Measured improvement
Eliasson, Krumlinde-Sundholm, Shaw, & Wang (2005)	41, 18 mo–4 yr	Cohort	Restraint glove	CONSTRAINT: 2 hr/day for 2 mo	Measured improvement in: • reaching • movement of upper arm • stabilizing by weight
Gordon, Chinnan, & Charles (2007)	20, 3 yr 6 mo–15 yr 6 mo	Randomized controlled trial	Hand-arm bimanual intensive therapy (HABIT)	(HABIT): 6 hr/day for 10 days	Measured improvement in: • bimanual items on the BOTMP • Improved score on Assistive Hand Assessment
Charles, Wolf, Schneider, & Gordon (2006)	22, 4–8 yr	Cohort	Sling in non-involved upper limb	CONSTRAINT: 6 hr/day for 10–12 consecutive days	Measured improvement in: • improved movement efficacy and dexterity • No change in strength, sensibility, or muscle tone.
Gordon, Charles, & Wolf (2005)	37, 4–14 yr	Cohort	Sling in non-involved upper limb (90% of waking hours)	CONSTRAINT: 6 hr/day for 10 days	Measured improvements in: • N/A (article does not discuss improvements as its central focus is the adaptation of CIMT for children) • demonstrated successful adaptation of CIMT for children 4–14 yr with hemiplegic CP
Gordon et al. (2008)	16, 8 mo–13 yr	Randomized controlled trial	CIMT (Mitt) HABIT (no restraint)	CIMT or HABIT 6 hrs/day for 10–12 days consecutively	Measured improvements in: • Jebsen-Taylor Hand Test of Hand Function • Assisting Hand Assessment (AHA) • % of time affected UE used • improvements similar between groups pretest-posttest on all measures (p < .05) • 13–16% decrease in time to complete Jebsen • 8% increase in AHA • 15% increase in affected hand use • amount of improvement dependent not on restraint but on intensity

Charles, J. R., Lavinder, G., & Gordon, A. M. (2001). Effects of constraint-induced therapy on hand function in children with hemiplegic cerebral palsy. *Pediatric Physical Therapy, 13*(2), 68-76; Charles, J. R., Wolf, S. L., Schneider, J. A., & Gordon, A. M. (2006). Efficacy of a child-friendly form of constraint-induced movement therapy in hemiplegic cerebral palsy: a randomized control trial. *Developmental Medicine & Child Neurology, 48*(8), 635-642; DeLuca, S. C., Echols, K., Ramey, S. L., & Taub, E. (2003). Pediatric constraint induced movement therapy for a young child with cerebral palsy: Two episodes of care. *Physical Therapy, 83*, 1003-1013; Eliasson, A. C., Krumlinde-Sundholm, L., Shaw, K., & Wang, C. (2005). Effects of constraint-induced movement therapy in young children with hemiplegic cerebral palsy: an adapted model. *Developmental Medicine & Child Neurology, 47*(4), 266-275; Eliasson, A. C., Bonnier, B., & Krumlinde-Sundholm, L. (2003). Clinical experience of constraint induced movement therapy in adolescents with hemiplegic cerebral palsy: a day camp model. *Developmental Medicine & Child Neurology, 45*(5(99)), 18; Gordon, A. M., Charles, J. R., & Wolf, S. L. (2005). Methods of constraint-induced movement therapy for children with hemiplegic cerebral palsy: development of a child-friendly intervention for improving upper-extremity function. *Archives of Physical Medicine & Rehabilitation, 86*(4), 837-844; Gordon, A. M., Chinnan, A., & Charles, J. R. (2007). Efficacy of a hand-arm bimanual intensive therapy (HABIT) in children with hemiplegic cerebral palsy: a randomized control trial. *Developmental Medicine & Child Neurology, 49*, 830-838; Gordon, A. M., Chinnan, A., Gill, S., Petra, E., Hung, Y. C., & Charles, J. R. (2008). Both constraint-induced movement therapy and bimanual training lead to improved performance of upper extremity function in children with hemiplegia. *Developmental Medicine & Child Neurology, 50*(12), 957-958; Pierce, S. R., Daly, K., Gallagher, K. G., Gershkoff, A. M., & Schaumburg, S. W. (2002). Constraint induced therapy for a child with hemiplegic cerebral palsy: A case report. *Archives of Physical Medicine & Rehabilitation, 83*, 1462-1463; Taub, E., Griffin, A., Nick, J., Gammons, K., Uswatte, G., & Law, C. R. (2007). Pediatric CI therapy for stroke-induced hemiparesis in young children. *Developmental Neurorehabilitation, 10*(1), 3-18; Taub, E., Ramey, S. L., DeLuca, S., & Echols, K. (2004). Efficacy of constraint-induced movement therapy for children with cerebral palsy with asymmetric motor impairment. *Pediatrics, 113*(2), 305-312; and Willis, J. K., Morello, A., Davie, A., Rice, J. C., & Bennet, J. T. (2002). Forced use treatment of childhood hemiparesis. *Pediatrics, 110*(1), 94-96.
Courtesy Sandra Rogers.

wearing a splint for only 5 to 10 minutes. Usually the therapist can gradually increase these periods. If the child has increased tone, maximum wearing time for a static splint is usually 6 to 8 hours per day. However, if splints allow some hand movement and the therapist uses them to aid accomplishment of functional activities, the child may tolerate them for additional hours.

Children generally wear night splints all night, but they should spend at least a part of each 24-hour period without the splints. Not all children with increased tone need night resting splints. In many cases their hands are more relaxed during sleep, and their parents can arrange their arms and hands in neutral position. Children who have neutral positioning at night generally are at less risk for the development of contractures. However, the child who shows abnormal hand posturing during the day but not at night may require daytime splint application to increase function.

Boehme noted that some children have learned to use abnormal patterns of wrist flexion and ulnar deviation or thumb adduction to accomplish their daily activities.[12] If a splint inhibits this pattern, the child may compensate by using another abnormal position of the hand or arm. Therefore before the therapist applies a splint, he or she must determine whether functional skill patterns that the child is using will be lost. Often the therapist needs to increase the frequency of intervention sessions when children are wearing splints so that they can develop better patterns of hand use.

Types of Splints Used with Children

Splints are categorized as those that allow hand movement and those that do not. *Static splints* include resting pan splints, other volar and dorsal full hand and wrist splints, spasticity reduction splints, and thumb positioning splints. *Dynamic splints* assist the child with a particular wrist, finger, or thumb movement. A *neurophysiologically based* splint may provide stimulation to the hand or arm or assist with stabilization of one or more joints during hand or arm activities.

Doubilet and Polkow[36] and Snook[129] reported case studies suggesting that *spasticity reduction splints* help decrease tone in adults. McPherson examined the effectiveness of Snook's spasticity reduction splint in five adolescents with severe disabilities.[96] Splint-wearing time was gradually increased from 15 minutes the first day to 2 hours daily by the fourth week. The outcome measure was passive muscle tone at the wrist, which was documented on a daily basis through use of a scale that measured pounds of force when the individual assumed wrist flexion. During the 4 weeks of splint application, the subjects' wrist tone decreased significantly. When they did not wear the splints for a week, their tone increased again.

When the therapist applies spasticity reduction splints, he or she should take care to control the thumb MCP joint. Distal force on the thumb can result in stretching or even rupture of the ulnar collateral ligament of the thumb's MCP joint[109] and subluxation of the MCP joint. Because children with spasticity usually demonstrate marked thumb adduction, distal control of the thumb moves the MCP and IP joints into hyperextension; therefore control at the carpometacarpal (CMC) joint is needed to abduct and extend the first metacarpal CMC joint.

Resting pan splints may provide more support to and control of the thumb than some of the spasticity reduction devices. However, the therapist should plan and monitor splints carefully

for reactions at the wrist and fingers. Children with increased tone may not tolerate the classic position for a resting hand splint, in which the wrist is in 20° to 30° of extension and the fingers are in slight flexion. The child with moderately increased tone may have more tolerance for a resting splint that holds the wrist in neutral position and the fingers in slight flexion. However, if flexor spasticity is severe, splinting that begins with the wrist in marked flexion and emphasizes slightly increased finger extension (out of full fisting) may be most effective. Initially the therapist should stabilize the wrist position in just slightly more extension than the child normally achieves. The therapist then adjusts or reconstructs splints to position the wrist, thumb, and fingers. In general, the therapist increases extension at only the wrist *or* fingers at one time to prevent the occurrence of flexion or extension deformities in the fingers.

The therapist may use other *volar splints,* such as the wrist support splint, with children who respond to control of wrist flexion but who do not need or cannot tolerate positioning of the fingers or thumb simultaneously. Wrist support splints allow the child to use the hand to perform functional activities, and the therapist may adjust them periodically to promote a progression of controlled finger extension during activities. The volar wrist splint should control ulnar deviation.

Controversy regarding the use of dorsal versus volar static splints is long-standing and has yet to be resolved. From a functional perspective, dorsal splints are most effective with children with muscle weakness or mild to moderately increased tone. The therapist uses the dorsal splint shown in Figure 10-25, *A,* on children with high tone and on those with low tone to hold the wrist in a neutral position. The splint provides support to the palmar arch. Although the child cannot use extreme wrist flexion, the therapist may use a small degree of wrist flexion in functional activities. Because no splint material contacts the volar surface of the hand and forearm, this splint interferes less with controlled arm use on a surface than a volar splint would. Children have responded favorably to this splint. However, dorsal static splints have limited use in controlling abnormal finger position in children with CNS deficits.

The therapist uses thumb splints when a child has difficulty with thumb control but can adequately coordinate movements in other parts of the wrist and hand or when thumb control is the greatest problem. Exner and Bonder reported a study of short opponens thumb splint use with 12 children who had cerebral palsy with spastic hemiplegia.[49] These splints controlled the thumb over the first metacarpal joint and extended onto the distal phalanx (Figure 10-25, *B*). The researchers used the splints 8 hours daily for 6 weeks. After this program, two children showed improvement in bilateral hand use and three children showed improved grasp. Some children found that wearing the splints on the nonpreferred hand interfered with stabilization of materials that could not be grasped. In clinical use, the splint is beneficial in improving children's functional use of their hands.

The therapist can use a soft splint to enhance thumb control in children with mildly increased tone. Neoprene and Neoplush are commonly used materials for soft splints. Use of the opponens splint pattern described previously is suitable when higher tone is present (Figure 10-25, *B*). The McKie splint (Figure 10-25, *C*) is a soft thumb splint designed specifically for use with children.[95] In a small study of four young children with cerebral palsy, this splint was found to have a positive effect on

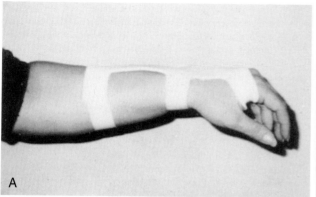

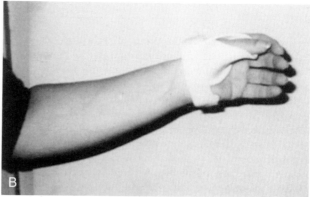

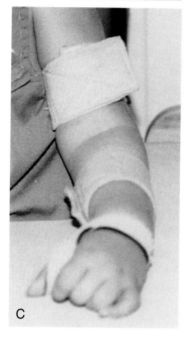

FIGURE 10-25 **A,** Dorsal splint to support the wrist in extension for stability or to control a mild to moderate pull into flexion. The hand section can be molded to support the palmar arch. **B,** Short opponens thumb splint made of a thermoplastic material. A similar design can be made with Neoplush. **C,** A Neoplush thumb splint is worn with orthokinetic cuffs on the forearm and upper arm. Both orthokinetic cuffs are designed to promote extension and inhibit flexion. The active area of the cuff on the forearm is over the wrist and finger extensors. The active area on the cuff on the upper arm is over the triceps.

grasp and supination. The author noted that the children also showed improvement in use of the hand in play activities.

Gabriel and Duvall-Riley reported on the use of a weight-bearing splint for children who need additional wrist and/or finger-thumb support to allow for more effective weight bearing.[56] This splint is usually designed to extend from the forearm to the fingertips. It positions the child's wrist in approximately 90° of wrist extension and the fingers in appropriate extension. The child wears this splint only during weight-bearing activities.

Other orthotic devices are available for children with increased tone or contractures. The positioning to prevent loss of range in children who have suffered head injuries is particularly important during extensive comatose, semicomatose, and recovery periods. The therapist uses inflatable air (pneumatic) splints[72] to decrease tone, maintain and increase joint range, and stimulate somatosensory function.

Some therapists use casting with children who exhibit spasticity and contractures secondary to cerebral palsy or head injury.[71,151,152] Casting may be used with children in an effort to enhance ROM and/or movement quality.[135] Tona and Schneck conducted a single-subject study using upper extremity casting.[138] Their findings were positive regarding the

effectiveness of the approach for that child. Law et al. conducted a well-designed group experimental study to determine the effects of standard occupational therapy treatment on young children's use of hand skills compared to an intervention program with upper extremity casting and intensive neurodevelopmental treatment.[86] The study was conducted over a 10-month period. The children in the study appeared to benefit as much from standard occupational therapy treatment as from the more intensive treatment coupled with casting. Casting of the arm and hand may be useful for decreasing tone, increasing ROM, or enhancing movement, but these changes may not result in improved occupational performance. Changes in these areas, as well as the changes in biomechanical areas, need to be assessed in research studies.

Teplicky, Law, and Russell emphasized the need for additional research on the question of hand splinting in children who have suffered a traumatic head injury as well as those with cerebral palsy.[135] In particular, they noted that although a number of studies have been reported in the literature, replication studies have not been conducted. Studies with groups of children and studies that replicate current findings are needed to support clinical decision making regarding splinting and casting in children.[135]

SUMMARY

This chapter presented a description of the components of hand and arm function that are instrumental in the performance of play, self-maintenance, and school functions. Factors that influence the development of hand function and types of problems in hand and arm use were discussed. The normal sequences of development for basic skills of reach, carry, grasp, and release, as well as advanced functions of in-hand manipulation and bilateral hand use, were reviewed. Intervention strategies for development of various hand skills were described, as were appropriate uses of splinting with children. The therapist should always frame assessment of and intervention for hand and arm function problems in the context of the child's daily environments and his or her play, school, and activities of daily living.

REFERENCES

1. American Occupational Therapy Association (AOTA). (2008). Occupational therapy practice framework: Domain and process. *American Journal of Occupational Therapy, 62,* 625-683.
2. Arnould, C., Penta, M., & Thonnard, J. L. (2007). Hand impairments and their relationship with manual ability in children with cerebral palsy. *Journal of Rehabilitative Medicine, 39,* 708-714.
3. Ayres, A. J. (1958). Ontogenetic principles in the development of arm and hand function. *American Journal of Occupational Therapy, 8,* 95-99.
4. Ayres, A. J. (1989). *Sensory Integration and Praxis Tests manual.* Los Angeles: Western Psychological Services.
5. Barnes, K.J. (1986). Improving prehension skills of children with cerebral palsy: A clinical study. *Occupational Therapy Journal of Research, 6*(4), 227-239.
6. Barnes, K.J. (1989). Direct replication: Relationship of upper extremity weight bearing to hand skills of boys with cerebral palsy. *Occupational Therapy Journal of Research, 9,* 235-242.
7. Barnes, K. J. (1989). Relationship of upper extremity weight bearing to hand skills of boys with cerebral palsy. *Occupational Therapy Journal of Research, 9,* 143-154.
8. Bayona, C. L., McDougall, J., Tucker, M., Nichols, M., Mandich, A. (2006). School-based occupational therapy for children with fine motor difficulties: Evaluating functional outcomes and fidelity of services. *Physical & Occupational Therapy in Pediatrics, 26*(3), 90-110.
9. Beckung, E., Steffenburg, U., & Uvebrant, P. (1997). Motor and sensory dysfunctions in children with mental retardation and epilepsy. *Seizure, 6,* 43-50.
10. Bertenthal, B., & Von Hofsten, C. (1998). Eye, head and trunk control: The foundation for manual development. *Neuroscience and Biobehavioral Reviews, 22,* 515-520.
11. Blank, R., Von Kries, R., Hesse, S., & Von Voss, H. (2008). Conductive education for children with cerebral palsy: Effects on hand motor functions relevant to activities of daily living. *Archives of Physical and Medical Rehabilitation, 89,* 251-259.
12. Boehme, R. H. (1988). *Improving upper body control: An approach to assessment and treatment of tonal dysfunction.* Tucson, AZ: Therapy Skill Builders.
13. Boyd, R. N., Morris, M. E., & Graham, H. K. (2001). Management of upper limb dysfunction in children with cerebral palsy: A systematic review. *European Journal of Neurology, 8*(Suppl. 5), 150-166.
14. Bumin, G., & Kayihan, H. (2001). Effectiveness of two different sensory integration programmes for children with spastic diplegic cerebral palsy. *Disability and Rehabilitation, 23* 394-399.
15. Burtner, P. A., Poole, J. L., Torres, T., Medora, A. M., Abevta, R., Keene, J., et al. (2008). Effect of wrist hand splints on grip, pinch, manual dexterity, and muscle activation in children with spastic hemiplegia: A preliminary study. *Journal of Hand Therapy, 21*(1), 36-42.
16. Bushnell, E. W., & Boudreau, J. P. (1999). Exploring and exploiting objects with the hands during infancy. In K. J. Connolly (Ed.), *The psychobiology of the hand* (pp. 144-161). London: Cambridge University Press.
17. Candler, C., & Meeuwsen, H. (2002). Implicit learning in children with and without developmental coordination disorder. *American Journal of Occupational Therapy, 56,* 429-435.
18. Carlier, M., Doyen A.-L., & Lamard, C., (2006). Midline crossing: Developmental trend from 3 to 10 years of age in a preferential card-reaching task. *Brain and Cognition, 61*(3), 255-261.
19. Case-Smith, J. (1991). The effects of tactile defensiveness and tactile discrimination on in-hand manipulation. *American Journal of Occupational Therapy, 45,* 811-818.
20. Case-Smith, J. (1993). Comparison of in-hand manipulation skills in children with and without fine motor delays. *Occupational Therapy Journal of Research, 13,* 87-100.
21. Case-Smith, J. (1996). Fine motor outcomes in preschool children who receive occupational therapy services. *American Journal of Occupational Therapy, 50,* 52-61.
22. Case-Smith, J. (2002). Effectiveness of school-based occupational therapy intervention on handwriting. *American Journal of Occupational Therapy, 56,* 17-25.
23. Case-Smith, J., Bigsby, R., & Clutter, J. (1998). Perceptual-motor coupling in the development of grasp. *American Journal of Occupational Therapy, 52,* 102-110.
24. Case-Smith, J., Fisher, A. G., & Bauer, D. (1989). An analysis of the relationship between proximal and distal motor control. *American Journal of Occupational Therapy, 43,* 657-662.
25. Case-Smith, J., Heaphy, T., Marr, D., Galvin, B., Koch, V., & Ellis, M. G., et al. (1998). Fine motor and functional outcomes in preschool children. *American Journal of Occupational Therapy, 52,* 788-796.
26. Connolly, K., & Dalgleish, M. (1989). The emergence of a tool-using skill in infancy. *Developmental Psychology, 25,* 894-912.
27. Cooper, J., Majnemer, A., Rosenblatt, B., & Birnbaum, R. (1995). The determination of sensory deficits in children with hemiplegic cerebral palsy. *Journal of Child Neurology, 10,* 300-309.
28. Corbetta, D., & Mounoud, P. (1990). Early development of grasping and manipulation. In C. Bard, M. Fleury, & L. Hay (Eds.), *Development of eye-hand coordination across the life span* (pp. 188-213). Columbia, SC: University of South Carolina Press.
29. Couch, K. J., Dietz, J. C., & Kenny, E. M. (1998). The role of play in pediatric occupational therapy. *American Journal of Occupational Therapy, 52,* 111-117.
30. Crocker, M. D., MacKay-Lyons, M., & McDonnell, E. (1997). Forced use of the upper extremity in cerebral palsy: A single case design. *American Journal of Occupational Therapy, 5,* 824-833.
31. Damiano, D., & Abel, M. F. (1998). Functional outcomes of strength training in spastic cerebral palsy. *Archives of Physical Medicine and Rehabilitation 79,* 119-125.
32. Danella, E., & Vogtle, L. (1992). Neurodevelopmental treatment for the young child with cerebral palsy. In J. Case-Smith & C. Pehoski (Eds.), *Development of hand skills in the child* (pp. 91-110). Rockville, MD: American Occupational Therapy Association.
33. Davies, P. L., & Rose, J. D. (2000). Motor skills of typically developing adolescents: Awkwardness or improvement? *Physical & Occupational Therapy in Pediatrics, 20*(1), 19-42.

34. Dellatolas, G., De Agostini, M., Curt, F., Helgard, K., Letierce, A., & Maccario, J., et al. (2003). Manual skill, hand skill asymmetry, and cognitive performances in young children. *Laterality, 8*(4), 317-338.

35. DeLuca, S. C., Echols, K., Ramey, S. L., & Taub, E. (2003). Pediatric constraint-induced movement therapy for a young child with cerebral palsy: Two episodes of care. *Journal of the American Physical Therapy Association, 83*, 1003-1013.

36. Doubilet, L., & Polkow, L. S. (1977). Theory and design of a finger abduction splint for the spastic hand. *American Journal of Occupational Therapy, 31*, 320-322.

37. Duff, S. V., & Gordon, A. M. (2003). Learning of grasp control in children with hemiplegic cerebral palsy. *Developmental Medicine and Child Neurology, 5*, 746-757.

38. Edwards, S. J., Buckland, D. S., McCoy-Powlen, J. D. (2002). *Developmental and functional hand grasps.* Thoroughfare, NJ: SLACK.

39. Eliasson, A. C. (2005). Improving the use of hands in daily activities aspects of the treatment of children with cerebral palsy. *Physical and Occupational Therapy in Pediatrics, 25*(3), 37-60.

40. Eliasson, A. C. (2005). Normal and impaired development of force control in precision grip, In A. Henderson & C. Pehoski (Eds.), *Hand function in the child* (pp. 45-62). St. Louis: Mosby.

41. Eliasson, A. C., Bonnier, B., & Krumlinde-Sundholm, L. (2003). Experience of forced use of upper extremity in adolescents with hemiplegic cerebral palsy: A day camp model. *Developmental Medicine and Child Neurology, 45*, 357-359.

42. Eliasson, A. C., Forssberg, H., Hung, Y.-C., & Gordon, A. M. (2006). Development of hand function and precision grip control in individuals with cerebral palsy: A 13-year follow-up study. *Pediatrics, 118*(4), 1-17.

43. Eliasson, A. C., & Gordon, A. M. (2000). Impaired force coordination during object release in children with hemiplegic cerebral palsy. *Developmental Medicine and Child Neurology, 42*, 228-234.

44. Elliott, J. M., & Connolly, K. J. (1984). A classification of manipulative hand movements. *Developmental Medicine and Child Neurology, 26*, 283-296.

45. Exner, C. E. (1990a). In-hand manipulation skills in normal young children: A pilot study. *Occupational Therapy Practice, 1*(4), 63-72.

46. Exner, C. E. (1990b). The zone of proximal development in in-hand manipulation skills of nondysfunctional 3- and 4-year-old children. *American Journal of Occupational Therapy, 44*, 884-891.

47. Exner, C. E. (1992). In-hand manipulation skills. In J. Case-Smith & C. Pehoski (Eds.), *Development of hand skills in the child* (pp. 35-45). Rockville, MD: American Occupational Therapy Association.

48. Exner, C. E. (1995). Remediation of hand skill problems in children. In A. Henderson & C. Pehoski (Eds.), *Hand function in the child.* St. Louis: Mosby.

49. Exner, C. E., & Bonder, B. R. (1983). Comparative effects of three hand splints on the bilateral hand use, grasp, and arm-hand posture in hemiplegic children: A pilot study. *Occupational Therapy Journal of Research, 3*, 75-92.

50. Fagard, J., & Jacquet, A. Y. (1989). Onset of bimanual coordination and symmetry versus asymmetry of movement. *Infant Behavior and Development, 12*, 229-236.

51. Fagard, J., & Lockman, J. J. (2005). The effect of task constraints on infants' (bi)manual strategy for grasping and exploring objects. *Infant Behavior & Development, 28*, 305-315.

52. Fedrizzi, E., Pagliano, E., Andreucci, E., & Oleari, G. (2003). Hand function in children with hemiplegic cerebral palsy: Prospective follow-up and functional outcome in adolescence. *Developmental Medicine and Child Neurology, 45*, 85-91.

53. Flapper, B. C. T., Houwen, S., & Schoemaker, M. M. (2006). Fine motor skills and effects of methylphenidate in children with attention-deficit-hyperactivity disorder and developmental coordination disorder. *Developmental Medicine & Child Neurology, 48*, 165-169.

54. Fliers, E., Rommelse, N., Vermeulen, S. H. H. M., Altink, M., Buschgens, C. J. M., Faraone, et al. (2008). Motor coordination problems in children and adolescents with ADHD rated by parents and teachers: Effects of age and gender. *Journal of Neural Transmission, 114*, 211-220.

55. Folio, R. M., & Fewell, R. (2000). *Peabody Developmental Motor Scales—Revised.* Chicago, IL: Riverside.

56. Gabriel, L., & Duvall-Riley, B. (2000). Pediatric splinting. In B. Coppard (Ed.), *Introduction to splinting: A critical reasoning & problem solving approach* (pp. 396-443). San Diego, CA: Technical Books.

57. Gesell, A., & Amatruda, C. S. (1947). *Developmental diagnosis.* New York: Harper & Row.

58. Gillberg, C., & Kadesjo, B. (2003). Why bother about clumsiness? The implications of having developmental coordination disorder (DCD). *Neural Plasticity, 10*(1-2), 59-68.

59. Glover, J. E., Mateer, C. A., Yoell, C., & Speed, S. (2002). The effectiveness of constraint-induced movement therapy in two young children with hemiplegia. *Pediatric Rehabilitation, 5*, 125-131.

60. Gordon, A. M., Charles, J., & Steenbergen, B. (2006). Fingertip force planning during grasp is disrupted by impaired sensorimotor integration in children with hemiplegic cerebral palsy. *Pediatric Research, 60*, 587-591.

61. Gordon, A. M., Charles, J., & Wolf, S. L. (2008). Methods of constraint-induced movement therapy for children with hemiplegic cerebral palsy: Development of a child-friendly intervention for improving upper-extremity function. *Archives of Physical and Medical Rehabilitation, 86*, 837-844.

62. Gordon, A. M., & Forssberg, H. (1997). Development of neural mechanisms underlying grasping in children. In K. J. Connolly & H. Forssberg (Eds.), *Neurophysiology and neuropsychology of motor development* (pp. 214-231). London: MacKeith Press.

63. Gordon, A. M., Lewis, S. R., Eliasson, A. C., & Duff, S. V. (2003). Object release under varying task constraints in children with hemiplegic cerebral palsy. *Developmental Medicine and Child Neurology, 45*, 240-248.

64. Gordon, A. W., & Duff, S. V. (1999). Relation between clinical measures and fine manipulative control in children with hemiplegic cerebral palsy. *Developmental Medicine and Child Neurology, 41*, 586-591.

65. Graham, S., Berninger, V., Weintraub, N., & Shafer, W. (1998). The development of handwriting fluency and legibility in grades 1 through 9. *Journal of Educational Research, 92*, 42-52.

66. Hanna, S. E., Law, M. C., Rosenbaum, P. L., King, G. A., Walter, S. D., Pollock, N., et al. (2003). Development of hand function among children with cerebral palsy: Growth curve analysis for ages 16 to 70 months. *Developmental Medicine and Child Neurology, 45*, 448-455.

67. Haron, M., & Henderson, A. (1985). Active and passive touch in developmentally dyspraxic and normal boys. *Occupational Therapy Journal of Research, 5*, 101-112.

68. Hart, H. (2005). Can constraint therapy be developmentally appropriate and child-friendly? *Developmental Medicine & Child Neurology, 47*, 363.

69. Heathcock, J. C., Lobo, M., & Galloway, J. C. (2008). Movement training advances the emergence of reaching in infants born at less than 33 weeks of gestational age: A randomized clinical trial. *Physical Therapy, 88*, 310-322.

70. Henderson, A. (2005). Self-care and hand skill. In A. Henderson & C. Pehoski (Eds.), *Hand function in the child* (pp. 193–216). St. Louis: Mosby.

71. Hill, J. (1994). The effects of casting on upper extremity motor disorders after brain injury. *American Journal of Occupational Therapy, 48,* 219-224.

72. Hill, S. G. (1988). Current trends in upper extremity splinting. In R. Boehme (Ed.), *Improving upper body control* (pp. 131-164). Tucson, AZ: Therapy Skill Builders.

73. Hirschel, A., Pehoski, C., & Coryell, J. (1990). Environmental support and the development of grasp in infants. *American Journal of Occupational Therapy, 44,* 721-727.

74. Huang, F., Gillespie, R. B., Kuo, A. (2007). Visual and haptic feedback contribute to tuning and online control during object manipulation. *Journal of Motor Behavior, 39*(3), 179-193.

75. Humphry, R., Jewell, K., & Rosenberger, R. C. (1995). Development of in-hand manipulation and relationship with activities. *American Journal of Occupational Therapy, 49,* 763-774.

76. Jackman, M., & Stagnitti, K. (2007). Fine motor difficulties: The need for advocating for the role of occupational therapy in schools. *Australian Occupational Therapy Journal, 54,* 168-173.

77. Jeannerod, M. (1994). The hand and the object: The role of posterior parietal cortex in forming motor representations. *Canadian Journal of Physiology and Pharmacology, 72,* 535-541.

78. Johansson, R. S., & Westling, G. (1988). Coordinated isometric muscle commands adequately and erroneously programmed for the weight during lifting tasks with precision grip. *Experimental Brain Research, 71,* 59-71.

79. Kellor, R., Silberberg, I., & Cummings. (1971). Hand strength and dexterity. *American Journal of Occupational Therapy, 25,* 77-83.

80. Kenney, W. E. (1963). Certain sensory defects in cerebral palsy. *Clinical Orthopedics, 27,* 193-195.

81. Kinghorn, J., & Roberts, G. (1996). The effect of an inhibitive weight-bearing splint on tone and function: A single case study. *American Journal of Occupational Therapy, 50,* 807-815.

82. Krumlinde-Sundholm, L., & Eliasson, A. C. (2002). Comparing tests of tactile sensibility: Aspects relevant to testing children with spastic hemiplegia. *Developmental Medicine and Child Neurology, 44,* 604-612.

83. Kuhtz-Buschbeck, J. P., Stolze, H., Golge, M., & Ritz, A. (2003). Analyses of gait, reaching, and grasping in children after traumatic brain injury. *Archives of Physical and Medical Rehabilitation, 84,* 424-430.

84. Kuhtz-Buschbeck, J. P., Stolze, H., Johnk, K., Boczek-Funcke, A., & Illert, M. (1998). Development of prehension movements in children: A kinematic study. *Experimental Brain Research, 122,* 424-432.

85. Kunde, W., & Weigelt, M. (2005). Goal congruency in bimanual object manipulation. *Journal of Experimental Psychology: Human Perception and Performance, 31*(1), 145-156.

86. Law, M., Russell, D., Pollock, N., Rosenbaum, P., Walter, S., & King, G. (1997). A comparison of intensive neurodevelopmental therapy plus casting and a regular occupational therapy program for children with cerebral palsy. *Developmental Medicine and Child Neurology, 39,* 664-670.

87. Lawrence, D. G., & Kuypers, H. G. (1986). The functional organization of the motor system in monkey. I and II. *Brain, 91,* 1-36.

88. Lee-Valkov, P. M., Aaron, D. H., Eladoumikdachi, F., Thornby, J., & Netscher, D. T. (2003). Measuring normal hand dexterity values in normal 3-, 4-, and 5-year-old children and their relationship with grip and pinch strength. *Journal of Hand Therapy, 16,* 22-28.

89. Link, L., Lukens, S., & Bush, M. A. (1995). Spherical grip strength in children 3 to 6 years of age. *American Journal of Occupational Therapy, 49,* 318-326.

90. Long, C., Conrad, P. W., Hall, E. A., & Furler, S. L. (1970). Intrinsic-extrinsic muscle control of the hand in power grip and precision handling. *Journal of Bone and Joint Surgery, 52,* 853-913.

91. Mandich, A. D., Polatajko, H. J., Macnab, J. J., & Miller, L. T. (2001). Treatment of children with developmental coordination disorder: What is the evidence? *Physical & Occupational Therapy in Pediatrics, 20*(2/3), 51-68.

92. Mandich, A. D., Polatajko, H. J., & Rodger, S. (2003). Rites of passage: Understanding participation of children with developmental coordination disorder. *Human Movement Science, 22,* 583-595.

93. Mathiowetz, V., Weimer, D. M., & Federman, S. M. (1986). Grip and pinch strength: Norms for 6- to 19-year-olds. *American Journal of Occupational Therapy, 40,* 705-711.

94. McHale, K., & Cermak, S. A. (1992). Fine motor activities in elementary school: Preliminary findings and provisional implications for children with fine motor problems. *American Journal of Occupational Therapy, 46,* 898-903.

95. McKie, S. (2003). *Grasp study: spastic cerebral palsy.* Retrieved December 22, 2008, from http://www.mckiesplints.com/research1.htm

96. McPherson, J. J. (1981). Objective evaluation of a splint designed to reduce hypertonicity. *American Journal of Occupational Therapy, 35,* 189-194.

97. Meyer, A., & Sagvolden, T. (2006). Fine motor skills in South African children with symptoms of ADHD: Influence of subtype, gender, age, and hand-dominance. *Behavioral and Brain Functions, 2*(1), 2-33.

98. Miller, L. T., Polatajko, H. J., Missiuna, C., Mandich, A. D., & Macnab, J. J. (2001). A pilot trial of a cognitive treatment for children with developmental coordination disorder. *Human Movement Science, 20,* 183-210.

99. Missiuna, C., Moll, S., King, S., King, G., & Law, M. (2007). A trajectory of troubles: Parents' impressions of the impact of developmental coordination disorder. *Physical & Occupational Therapy in Pediatrics, 27*(1), 81-101.

100. Missiuna, C., Pollack, N., & Law, M. (2004). *The Perceived Efficacy and Goal Setting System.* San Antonio, TX: PsychCorp.

101. Monfraix, C., Tardieu, G., & Tardieu, C. (1961). Disturbances of manual perception in children with cerebral palsy. *Developmental Medicine and Child Neurology, 22,* 454-464.

102. Myers, C. A. (1992). Therapeutic fine motor activities for preschoolers. In J. Case-Smith & C. Pehoski (Eds.), *Development of hand skills in the child* (pp. 47-59). Rockville, MD: American Occupational Therapy Association.

103. Napier, J. R. (1956). The prehensile movements of the human hand. *Journal of Bone Joint Surgery, 38B,* 902-913.

104. Oliveira, M. A., Shim, J. K., Loss, J. F., Petersen, R. D. S., Clark, J. E. (2006). Effect of kinetic redundancy on hand digit control in children with DCD. *Neuroscience Letters, 410,* 42-46.

105. Pehoski, C. (1992). Central nervous system control of precision movements of the hand. In J. Case-Smith & C. Pehoski (Eds.), *Development of hand skills in the child* (pp. 1-11). Rockville, MD: American Occupational Therapy Association.

106. Pehoski, C. (2005). Cortical control of hand-object interaction. In A. Henderson & C. Pehoski (Eds.), *Hand function in the child* (pp. 3-20). St. Louis: Mosby.

107. Pehoski, C., Henderson, A., & Tickle-Degnen, L. (1997a). In-hand manipulation in young children: Rotation of an object in the fingers. *American Journal of Occupational Therapy, 51,* 544-552.

108. Pehoski, C., Henderson, A., & Tickle-Degnen, L. (1997b). In-hand manipulation in young children: Translation movements. *American Journal of Occupational Therapy, 51,* 719-728.

109. Phelps, R. E., & Weeks, P. M. (1976). Management of thumb-in-palm web space contracture. *American Journal of Occupational Therapy, 30,* 543-556.

110. Piek, J. P., Dyck, M. J., Nieman, A., Anderson, M., Hay, D., Smith, L. M., et al. (2004). The relationship between motor coordination, executive functioning and attention in school age children. *Archives of Clinical Neuropsychology, 19,* 1063-1076.

111. Pont, K., Wallen, M., Bundy, A., & Case-Smith, J. (2008). Reliability and validity of the Test of In-Hand Manipulation in children ages 5 to 6 years. *The American Journal of Occupational Therapy, 62,* 384-392.

112. Provost, B., Heimerl, S., & Lopez, B. R. (2007). Levels of gross and fine motor development in young children with autism spectrum disorder. *Physical & Occupational Therapy in Pediatrics, 28*(3), 21-36.

113. Ramsey, D. S., & Weber, S. (1986). Infant's hand preference in a task involving complementary roles for the two hands. *Child Development, 57,* 300-307.

114. Rao, A. K. (2005). Cognition and motor skills. In A. Henderson & C. Pehoski (Eds.), *Hand function in the child* (pp. 101-115). St. Louis: Mosby.

115. Reiersen, A. M., Constantino, J. N., & Todd, R. D. (2008). Co-occurrence of motor problems and autistic symptoms in attention deficit/hyperactivity disorder. *Journal of the Academy of Child and Adolescent Psychiatry, 47*(6), 662-672.

116. Reiersen, A. M., & Todd, R. D. (2008). Co-occurrence of ADHD and autism spectrum disorders: Phenomenology and treatment. *Expert Review of Neurotherapeutics, 8*(4), 657-669.

117. Rosblad, B. (2005). Reaching and eye-hand coordination. In A. Henderson & C. Pehoski (Eds.), *Hand function in the child* (pp. 89-100). St. Louis: Mosby.

118. Ruff, H. A. (1980). The development of the perception and recognition of objects. *Child Development, 51,* 981-992.

119. Ruff, H. A., McCarton, C., Kurtzber, D., & Vaughan, H. G., Jr., (1984). Preterm infants' manipulative exploration of objects. *Child Development, 55,* 1166-1173.

120. Schneck, C., & Battaglia, C. (1992). Developing scissors skills in young children. In J. Case-Smith & C. Pehoski (Eds.), *Development of hand skills in the child* (pp. 79-89). Rockville, MD: American Occupational Therapy Association.

121. Schneiberg, S., Sveistrup, H., McFadyen, B., McKinley, P., & Levin, M. (2002). The development of coordination for reach-to-grasp movements in children. *Experimental Brain Research, 146*(2), 142-154.

122. Schoen, S., & Anderson, J. (1999). Neurodevelopmental treatment frame of reference. In P. Kramer & J. Hinojosa (Eds.), *Frames of reference for pediatric occupational therapy* (pp. 49–86). Baltimore: Williams & Wilkins.

123. Sheridan, M. D. (1975). *From birth to five years: Children's developmental progress.* Atlantic Highlands, NJ: Humanities Press.

124. Smith, R. O., & Benge, M. W. (1985). Pinch and grasp strength: Standardization of terminology and protocol. *American Journal of Occupational Therapy, 39,* 531-535.

125. Smith-Zuzovsky, N., & Exner, C. E. (2004). The effect of seated positioning quality on typical 6- and 7-year-old children's object manipulation skills. *American Journal of Occupational Therapy, 58,* 380-388.

126. Smits-Engelsman, B. C., Westenberg, Y., & Duysens, J. (2003). Development of isometric force and force control in children. *Cognitive Brain Research, 17,* 68-74.

127. Smits-Engelsman, B. C., Wilson, P. H., Westenberg, Y., & Duysens, J. (2003). Fine motor deficiencies in children with developmental coordination disorder and learning disabilities: An underlying open-loop control deficit. *Human Movement Science, 22,* 495-513.

128. Smyth, M. M., & Mason, U. C. (1997). Planning and execution of action in children with and without developmental coordination disorder. *Journal of Child Psychology and Psychiatry, 38*(8), 1023-1037.

129. Snook, J. H. (1979). Spasticity reduction splint. *American Journal of Occupational Therapy, 33,* 648-651.

130. Steenbergen, B., Verrel, J., & Gordon, A. M. (2007). Motor planning in congenital hemiplegia. *Disabilities and Rehabilitation, 29*(1), 13-23.

131. Sterr, A., Freivogel, S., & Schmalohr, D. (2002). Neurobehavioral aspects of recovery: Assessment of the learned nonuse phenomenon in hemiparetic adolescents. *Archives of Physical Medicine and Rehabilitation, 83,* 1726-1731.

132. Sullivan, K., Kantak, S. S., & Burtner, P. A. (2008). Motor learning in children: Feedback effects on skill acquisition. *Physical Therapy, 88*(6), 720-732.

133. Summers, J., Dawne, L., Dewey, D. (2008). Activities of daily living in children with developmental coordination disorder: Dressing, personal hygiene, and eating skills. *Human Movement Science, 27,* 215-229.

134. Taub, E., Aswatte, G., & Pidiki, R. (1999). Constraint-induced movement therapy: A new family of techniques with broad application to physical rehabilitation-a clinical review. *Journal of Rehabilitation Research and Development, 36,* 237-251.

135. Teplicky, R., Law, M., & Russell, D. (2002). The effectiveness of casts, orthoses, and splints for children with neurological disorders. *Infant and Young Children, 15*(1), 42-50.

136. Thelen, E., Corbetta, D., Kamm, K., Spencer, J. P., Schneider, K., & Zernicke, R. F. (1993). The transition to reaching: Mapping intention and intrinsic dynamics. *Child Development, 64,* 1058-1098.

137. Tobias, M. V., & Goldkopf, I. M. (1995). Toys and games: Their role in hand development. In A. Henderson & C. Pehoski (Eds.), *Hand function in the child* (pp. 223-254). St. Louis: Mosby.

138. Tona, J. L., & Schneck, C. M. (1993). The efficacy of upper extremity inhibitive casting: A single-subject pilot study. *American Journal of Occupational Therapy, 47,* 901-910.

139. Twitchell, T. E. (1965). The automatic grasping responses of infants. *Neuropsychologics, 3,* 247-259.

140. Verdonck, M. C., & Henneberg, M. (1997). Manual dexterity of South African children growing in contrasting socioeconomic conditions. *American Journal of Occupational Therapy, 51,* 303–306.

141. Von Hofsten, C. (1982). Eye-hand coordination in the newborn. *Developmental Psychology, 18*(3), 450-461.

142. Von Hofsten, C. (1991). Structuring of early reaching movements: A longitudinal study. *Journal of Motor Behavior, 23*(4), 280-292.

143. Weaver, S., Gardner, E. R., Triolo, R. J., & Betz, R. R. (1990). Improvement of hand function in children with arthrogryposis following neuromuscular electrical stimulation (NMES): A preliminary report. *Journal of the Association of Children's Prosthetic-Orthotic Clinics, 25*(2), 32.

144. Weiss, M. W., & Flatt, A. E. (1971). Functional evaluation of the congenitally anomalous hand. II. *American Journal of Occupational Therapy, 25,* 139-143.

145. Willis, J. K., Morello, A., Davie, A., Rice, J. C., & Bennett, J. T. (2002). Forced-use treatment of childhood hemiparesis. *Pediatrics, 110,* 94-96.

146. Wilson, B., & Trombly, C. A. (1984). Proximal and distal function in children with and without sensory integrative dysfunction: An EMG study. *Canadian Journal of Occupational Therapy, 51,* 11-17.

147. Wilson, B. N., Kaplan B. J., Crawford, S. G., Campbell, A., & Dewey, D. (2000). Reliability and validity of a parent questionnaire on childhood motor skills. *American Journal of Occupational Therapy, 54*(5), 484-493.

148. Wilson, P. H., Maruff, P., Ives, S., & Currie, J. (2001). Abnormalities of motor and praxis imagery in children with DCD. *Human Movement Science, 20,* 135-159.

149. Wingrat, J., & Exner, C. E. (2005). The impact of school furniture on fourth grade children's on-task and sitting behavior in the classroom: A pilot study. *Work, 25*, 263-272.

150. Wisdom, S., Dyck, M., Piek, J., Hay, D., & Hallmayer, J. (2007). Can autism, language and coordination disorders be differentiated based on ability profiles? *European Child and Adolescent Psychiatry, 16*(3), 178-186.

151. Yasukawa, A., & Hill, J. (1988). Casting to improve upper extremity function. In R. Boehme (Ed.), *Improving upper body control* (pp. 165-188). Tucson, AZ: Therapy Skill Builders.

152. Yekutiel, M., Jariwala, M., & Stretch, P. (1994). Sensory deficit in the hands of children with cerebral palsy: A new look at assessment and prevalence. *Developmental Medicine and Child Neurology, 36*, 619-624.

153. Yim, S. Y., Cho, J. R., & Lee, I. Y. (2003). Normative data developmental characteristics of hand function for elementary school children in Suwon area of Korea: Grip, pinch, and dexterity study. *Journal of Korean Medical Science, 18*, 552-558.

11

Sensory Integration

L. Diane Parham • Zoe Mailloux

Ayres Sensory
  Integration® (ASI)
Sensory nourishment
Adaptive responses
Neural plasticity
Sensory processing
Sensory modulation

Underresponsiveness
Sensory registration
Sensation seeking
Overresponsiveness
Sensory discrimination
Praxis
Dyspraxia

OBJECTIVES

1. Explain the neurobiological concepts that are basic to an individual's sensory integrative function.
2. Explain the link between sensory input from the environment and the child's adaptive response.
3. Describe the development of sensory integration from prenatal life through childhood.
4. Explain the clinical picture and hypothesized basis for problems in sensory modulation and sensory discrimination.
5. Describe atypical vestibular-bilateral functions and the types of behaviors that children with these problems often demonstrate.
6. Define developmental dyspraxia, and identify examples of behaviors that might be observed in a child with this problem.
7. Relate the Ayres Sensory Integration® (ASI) approach to childhood occupations and to the Occupational Therapy Practice Framework.
8. Discuss the evaluation of sensory integration within varying contexts such as home and school.
9. Identify and describe tests, interviews, and instruments used to evaluate sensory integration.
10. Describe ASI intervention and discuss the disadvantages and benefits of using such an intervention approach.
11. Explain some considerations for determining whether ASI may be an appropriate frame of reference for an individual child.
12. Describe specific skill training, group programming, and consultative interventions (such as activity or environmental modifications), including the benefits and limitations of using these approaches in conjunction with or instead of ASI intervention.
13. Identify the expected outcomes of an occupational therapy program using ASI intervention.
14. Discuss published research related to the effectiveness of ASI intervention.
15. Identify some of challenges when evaluating the effectiveness of ASI intervention.

The term *sensory integration* holds special meaning for occupational therapists. In some contexts it is used to refer to a particular way of viewing the neural organization of sensory information for functional behavior. In other situations this term refers to a clinical frame of reference for the assessment and treatment of people who have functional disorders in sensory processing. Both of these meanings originated in the work of A. Jean Ayres, an occupational therapist and psychologist whose brilliant clinical insights and original research revolutionized occupational therapy practice with children.

Ayres' ideas ushered in a new way of looking at children and understanding many of the developmental, learning, and emotional problems that arise during childhood. Her innovative practice and groundbreaking research met a tremendous amount of resistance within the profession when introduced in the late 1960s and 1970s. Today, the treatment methods that she pioneered continue to be questioned and investigated, but there is little doubt that her perspective has had a profound influence on occupational therapy practice. The presence of sensory integration concepts in nearly all of the chapters of this book attests to the extent to which these ideas have affected the thinking of pediatric occupational therapists. Furthermore, the research base of the sensory integration approach to practice is extensive.

This chapter provides an in-depth orientation to this fascinating aspect of occupational therapy practice. The reader will gain a general sense of how sensory integration as a brain function is related to everyday occupations. Following is a description of how sensory integration is manifested in typically developing children and in relation to the daily life problems of children who experience difficulty with sensory integration. The history of research on sensory integration problems is reviewed to give the reader a perspective on how this field came into being, what the major constructs are, and how they have changed—and continue to change—over time. Sensory integration, as an intervention approach developed by Ayres, is now trademarked through the Franklin B. Baker/A. Jean Ayres Baker Trust as *Ayres Sensory Integration*® (ASI).[130]

According to the trademark document, ASI encompasses the theory, assessment methods, patterns of sensory integration and praxis problems, and intervention concepts, principles, and techniques developed by Ayres.[129] In this chapter, ASI is described with respect to different types of sensory integration problems encountered by children, methods of clinical assessment, and characteristics of both direct and indirect modes of intervention, with emphasis on the principles of individual ASI intervention. Effectiveness research on individual ASI intervention is presented and case examples of children who have been helped by occupational therapists using an ASI approach are provided.

SENSORY INTEGRATION IN CHILD DEVELOPMENT

One of the most distinctive contributions that Ayres made to understanding child development was her focus on sensory processing, particularly with respect to the proximal senses (vestibular, tactile, and proprioceptive). From the sensory integration viewpoint, these senses are emphasized because they are primitive and primary; they dominate the child's interactions with the world early in life. The distal senses of vision and hearing are critical and become increasingly more dominant as the child matures. Ayres believed, however, that the body-centered senses are a foundation on which complex occupations are scaffolded. Furthermore, when Ayres began her work, the vestibular, tactile, and proprioceptive senses were virtually ignored by scholars and clinicians who were interested in child development. She devoted her career to studying the roles that these previously forgotten senses play in development and in the genesis of developmental problems of children.

Ayres' basic assumption was that brain function is a critical factor in human behavior.[11] She reasoned, therefore, that knowledge of brain function and dysfunction would give her insight into child development and would help her understand the developmental problems of children. However, Ayres also had a pragmatic orientation that sprang from her professional background as an occupational therapist. She was concerned particularly with how brain functions affected the child's ability to participate successfully in daily occupations. Consequently, her work represents a fusion of neurobiological insights with the practical, everyday concerns of human beings, particularly children and their families.

As Ayres developed her ideas about sensory integration, she used terms such as *sensory integration, adaptive response,* and *praxis* in ways that reflected her orientation. A glossary of terms that are commonly used within the framework of sensory integration theory is presented on the Evolve website. It may be helpful to the reader to refer to these definitions frequently while reading this chapter.

Ayres coined some of these terms, whereas other terms were drawn from the literature of other fields. When Ayres borrowed a term from another field, however, she imparted a particular meaning to it. For example, Ayres did not use the term *sensory integration* to refer solely to intricate synaptic connections within the brain, as neuroscientists typically do. Rather, she applied it to neural processes as they relate to functional behavior. Hence, her definition of sensory integration is the "organization of sensation for use" (p. 5).[1] It is the inclusion of the final clause "for use" that is Ayres' hallmark, because it ties sensory processing to the person's occupation.[5]

Ayres introduced a new vocabulary of sensory integration theory and synthesized important concepts from the neurobiologic literature to organize her views of child development and dysfunction. Many of these ideas were first published in her classic book *Sensory Integration and Learning Disorders.*[11] Later she wrote a book for parents, *Sensory Integration and the Child,*[18,22] outlining the behavioral changes that can be observed in a child as sensory integration develops. Major points made in these books regarding neurobiologic concepts in relationship to development and the ontogeny of sensory integration are presented in the following section.

NEUROBIOLOGICALLY BASED CONCEPTS

Sensory Support for Development and Brain Function

Sensory input is necessary for optimal brain function. The brain is designed to constantly take in sensory information, and it malfunctions if deprived of it. Sensory deprivation experiments conducted in the 1950s and 1960s made it clear that without an adequate inflow of sensation, the brain generates its own input in the form of hallucinations and subsequently distorts incoming sensory stimuli.[145] If adequate sensory stimulation is not available at critical periods in development, brain abnormalities and resulting behavioral disorders result.[74,77,79] It is now well established that persistent, serious impairments in cognitive, social, and emotional functioning often result when infants and young children are institutionalized in environments that are impoverished with respect to availability of a wide range of sensory experiences, the presence of a nurturing caregiver, and opportunities for sensory-motor exploration.[29,47,56,122]

Ayres considered sensory input to be *sensory nourishment* for the brain, just as food is nourishment for the body.[18] Wilbarger, a colleague of Ayres, built on this concept with the *sensory diet,* designed to provide individualized sensory experiences for the child with sensory integrative dysfunction.[152] The therapeutic sensory diet provides an optimal combination of sensory-based activities at the appropriate intensities for a specific child. For most typically developing children, the sensory diet does not require conscious monitoring by caregivers. The environment continuously "feeds" the child a variety of nourishing sensations in the flow of everyday life.

As critical as input is to the developing brain, the mere provision of sensory stimulation is limited in value. Too much stimulation can generate stress that is detrimental to brain development and may reduce the person's subsequent ability to cope with stress.[72] To have an optimal effect on development, learning, and behavior, the sensory input must be actively organized and *used* by the child to act on and respond to the environment.

Adaptive Response

A child does not passively absorb whatever sensations come along. Rather the child actively selects the sensations most useful at the time and organizes them in a fashion that facilitates accomplishing goals. This is the process of *sensory integration*. When this process is going well, the child organizes a successful, goal-directed action on the environment, which is called an *adaptive response*. When a child makes an adaptive response, he or she successfully meets some challenge presented in the environment. The adaptive response is possible because the brain has been able to efficiently organize incoming sensory information, which then provides a basis for action (Figure 11-1).

Adaptive responses are powerful forces that drive development forward. When a child makes an adaptive response that is more complex than any previously accomplished response, the brain attains a more organized state and its capacity for further sensory integration is enhanced. Thus, sensory integration leads to adaptive responses, which in turn result in sensory integration that is more efficient.

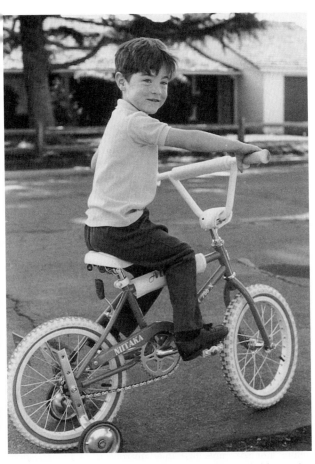

FIGURE 11-1 Adaptive responses help the child acquire skills such as riding a bicycle. Although training wheels reduce the challenge for this boy, his nervous system must integrate vestibular, proprioceptive, and visual information adequately for him to successfully steer the bicycle while it is moving. (Courtesy Shay McAtee.)

Ayres provides the example of learning to ride a bicycle to illustrate this process.[18] The child must integrate sensations, particularly from the vestibular and proprioceptive systems, to learn how to balance on the bicycle. The senses must accurately and quickly detect when the child begins to fall. Eventually, perhaps after many trials of falling, the child integrates sensory information efficiently enough to make the appropriate weight shifts over the bicycle to maintain balance. This is an adaptive response, and once made, the child is able to balance more effectively on the next attempt to ride the bike. The child's nervous system has changed, so the child is now more adept at bicycle riding.

In making adaptive responses, the child is an active doer, not a passive recipient. Adaptive responses come from within the child. No one can force a child to respond adaptively, although a situation may be set up that is likely to elicit adaptive responses from the child. For typically developing children and for most children with disabilities, there is an innate drive to develop sensory integration through adaptive responses. Ayres called this *inner drive* and speculated that it is generated primarily by the limbic system of the brain, a structure known to be critical in both motivation and memory.[18] Ayres designed therapeutic activities and environments to engage the child's inner drive (elicit adaptive responses) and, in so doing, advance sensory integrative development and the child's occupational competence.

Neural Plasticity

It is thought that when a child makes an adaptive response, change occurs at a neuronal synaptic level. This change is a function of the brain's neural plasticity. *Plasticity* is the ability of a structure and concomitant function to be changed gradually by its own ongoing activity.[11] It is well established in the neuroscientific literature that when organisms are permitted to explore interesting environments, significant increases in dendritic branching, synaptic connections, synaptic efficiency, and size of brain tissue result.[79] These changes are most dramatic in a young animal and probably represent a major mechanism of brain development,[74] although it is clear that such manifestations of plasticity are characteristic of optimal brain functioning throughout the lifespan.[27,55,88]

Studies of the effects of enriched environments on animals indicate that the essential ingredient for positive brain changes is that the organism actively interacts with a meaningful and challenging environment.[31,79] Passive exposure to sensory stimulation does not produce these same positive changes.[55,59] It can be hypothesized from these findings that adaptive responses activate the brain's neuroplastic capabilities. Furthermore, the brain's plasticity makes it possible for an adaptive response to increase the efficiency of sensory integration at a neuronal level.

Central Nervous System Organization

Ayres looked to the organization of the central nervous system (CNS) for clues to how children organize and use sensory information and how sensory integration develops over time.[11] At the time that she was developing her theory, *hierarchic* models of the CNS dominated thinking in the neurosciences.

Hierarchic models view the nervous system in terms of vertically arranged levels, with the spinal cord at the bottom, the cerebral hemispheres at the top, and the brainstem sandwiched in between. These levels are interdependent yet reflect a trend of ascending control and specialization. Thus, the cerebral cortex at the top of the hierarchy is highly specialized and analyzes precise details of sensory information. Ordinarily the cortex assumes a directive role over lower levels of the hierarchy. For example, the cortex may command lower centers to "ignore" certain stimuli deemed unimportant. This process is called *descending inhibition* and is critical in enabling higher brain functions to work efficiently.[11] The lower levels of the CNS, however, have functions that are more diffuse and primitive, less specialized, and yet potentially more pervasive in influence compared with those of the higher levels. One of the important responsibilities of the lower levels is to filter and refine sensory information before relaying organized sensory messages upward to the cerebral cortex. Thus, cortical centers depend on lower centers for the receipt of essential, well-organized sensory information to analyze in preparation for the planning of action. According to hierarchic views, the higher levels of the CNS superimpose functions that are more sophisticated on the lower levels, but these do not replace the important lower level functions.[11]

Ayres believed that critical aspects of sensory integration are seated in the lower levels of the CNS, particularly the brainstem and thalamus.[11] Most of the CNS processing of vestibular information occurs in the brainstem, and much somatosensory processing takes place there and in the thalamus. One of the basic tenets of Ayres's theory is that, because of the dependence of higher CNS structures on lower structures, increased efficiency at the levels of the brainstem and thalamus enhance[5] higher order functioning.[11] This view varies from traditional neuropsychology and education models, which have tended to emphasize the direct study and remediation of high-level, cortically directed skills such as reading and writing. However, newer models of education have considered "readiness" for academics and the importance of other modes such as "kinesthetic" learning.[60,141]

In adopting a hierarchic view of the CNS, Ayres also assumed that the CNS develops hierarchically from bottom to top, with spinal and brainstem structures maturing before higher level centers.[11] At the time that Ayres was developing her theory, this was somewhat speculative, although generally accepted by neuroscientists. In research conducted in more recent years, the use of positron electron tomography (PET) scans on infants has provided direct support for the notion that brain development proceeds in a bottom-to-top direction.[48]

The hierarchic approach to CNS functioning and development led Ayres to emphasize the more primitive vestibular and somatosensory systems in her work with young children. These systems mature early and are seated in the lower CNS centers (particularly the brainstem, cerebellum, and thalamus). Using the logic of hierarchy, Ayres reasoned that the refinement of primitive functions, such as postural control, balance, and tactile perception, provides a sensorimotor foundation for higher-order functions, such as academic ability, behavioral self-regulation, and complex motor skills (e.g., those required in sports). Thus, she viewed the developmental process as one in which primitive body-centered functions serve as building blocks upon which complex cognitive and social skills can be scaffolded. This view undergirds a basic premise of the therapy approach that she developed: enhancing lower-level functions related to the proximal senses might have a positive influence on higher-level functions.

On some points Ayres departed from a strictly hierarchic view of the CNS.[11] For example, she noted that each level of the CNS can function as a self-contained sensory integration system. Therefore, the brainstem can independently direct some sensorimotor patterns without being directed by the higher level cortex. Furthermore, the sensory integrative process involves the brain working as a whole, not simply as a series of hierarchically controlled messages, as rigid hierarchic models might suggest. These ideas are more consistent with the view of some contemporary biologists that the brain is a *heterarchic* system. A heterarchy is a system in which different parts may assume the controlling role in different situations; control does not always flow in a top-down direction.[135] Ayres was ahead of her time in suggesting that the brain does not operate exclusively as a hierarchy but has holistic characteristics. These heterarchic notions strengthened her view that functions considered primitive were worthy of serious consideration in therapy.

SENSORY INTEGRATIVE DEVELOPMENT AND CHILDHOOD OCCUPATIONS

Ayres believed that the first 7 years of life is a period of rapid development in sensory integration.[18] She drew this conclusion not only from her many years of observing children, but also from research in which she gathered normative data on tests of sensory integration.[11] By the time most children reach 7 or 8 years of age, their scores on standardized tests of sensory integrative capabilities reflect almost as much maturity as an adult's.

Development, from a sensory integrative standpoint, occurs as the CNS organizes sensory information and adaptive responses with increasing degrees of complexity. Sensory integration, of course, enables adaptive responses to occur, which in turn promote the *development of sensory integration* and the emergence of occupational engagement and social participation.[114,146] As this process unfolds in infancy, the developing child begins to attach meaning to the stream of sensations experienced. The child becomes increasingly adept at shifting attention to what he or she perceives as meaningful, tuning out that which is irrelevant to current needs and interests. As a result, the child can organize play behavior for increasing lengths of time and gains control in the regulation of emotions.

Inner drive leads the child to search for opportunities in the environment that are "just right challenges." These are challenges that are not so complex that they overwhelm or induce failure, nor so simple that they are routine or uninteresting. The just right challenge is one that requires effort but is accomplishable. Because there is an element of challenge, a successful adaptive response engenders feelings of mastery and a sense of oneself as a competent being.

It is fascinating to watch this process unfold. Most children require no adult guidance or teaching to acquire basic developmental skills such as manipulating objects, sitting, walking, and climbing. Little, if any, step-by-step instruction is needed to learn daily occupations such as playing on playground equipment, dressing and feeding oneself, drawing and painting, and constructing with blocks. These achievements seem to just happen. They are the product of an active nervous system busily organizing sensory information and searching for challenges that bring forth more complex behaviors, all shaped within the context of a world saturated with sociocultural expectations and meanings.[114]

In this section, developmental hallmarks of sensory integration are identified and connected to the occupational achievements of childhood. The proximal senses dominate early infancy and continue to exert their influence in critical ways as the visual and auditory systems gain ascendancy. Although there is some variability across children in the sequence in which developmental achievements unfold during the first year of life, this variability becomes increasingly apparent after this first year. By kindergarten age, skills vary tremendously among children because of differences in environmental opportunities, familial and cultural influences, personal experiences, and genetic endowment. It is important to keep in mind that, throughout development, sensory integrative processes contribute to the child's construction of his or her identity, but many other influences are powerful as well—the family and cultures that shape the child's occupational routines, the interpretations given to the child's behaviors by others, the child's talents and abilities, and even chance events that carry special meaning to the child.[114]

Prenatal Period

The first known responses to sensory stimuli occur early in life, at approximately 5½ weeks after conception.[78] These first responses are to tactile stimuli. Specifically, they involve reflexive avoidance reactions to a perioral stimulus (e.g., the embryo bends its head and upper trunk away from a light touch stimulus around the mouth). This is a primitive protective reaction. It is not until about 9 weeks' gestational age that an approach response (moving of the head toward the chest) occurs,[78] probably as a function of proprioception.

The first known responses to vestibular input in the form of the Moro reflex also appear at about 9 weeks after conception. The fetus continues to develop a repertoire of reflexes such as rooting, sucking, Babkin, grasp, flexor withdrawal, Galant, neck righting, Moro, and positive supporting in utero that are fairly well established by the time of birth. Thus, when the time comes to leave the uterus, the newborn is well equipped with the capacity to form a strong bond with a caregiver and to actively participate in the critical occupation of nursing. These innate capacities require rudimentary aspects of sensory integration that are built into the nervous system. However, even in this earliest period of development, environmental influences, such as maternal stress, can have a significant impact on the quality of sensory integrative development. For example, Schneider and her colleagues found that infant rhesus monkeys born to mothers who had experienced stress in early pregnancy had signs of diminished responses to vestibular input, such as impaired righting responses, weak muscle tone, and attenuated postrotary nystagmus.[138,139]

Neonatal Period

Touch, smell, and movement sensations are particularly important to the newborn infant, who uses these to maintain contact with a caregiver through nursing, nuzzling, and cuddling. Tactile sensations, especially, are critical in establishing a primary attachment relationship with a caregiver and fostering feelings of security in the infant. This is just the beginning of the important role that the tactile system plays in a person's emotional life because it is directly involved in making physical contact with others (Figure 11-2). Proprioception is also critical in the mother–infant relationship, enabling the infant to mold to the adult caregiver's body in a cuddly manner. The phasic movements of the infant's limbs generate additional proprioceptive inputs. Together, all of these tactile and proprioceptive inputs set the stage for the eventual development of body scheme (the brain's map of the body and how its parts interrelate).

The vestibular system is fully functional at birth, although refinement of its sensory integrative functions, particularly its integration with visual and proprioceptive systems, continues through childhood. Of all the sensory systems, the vestibular system is the first to mature.[98] Most caregivers who use rocking and carrying to soothe and calm the infant instinctively appreciate the influence of vestibular stimuli on the infant's arousal level. Ayres pointed out that sensations such as these, which make a child contented and organized, tend to be integrating for the child's nervous system.[18]

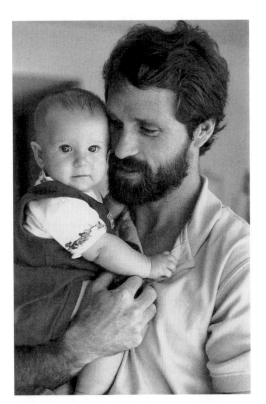

FIGURE 11-2 Tactile sensations play a critical role in generating feelings of security and comfort in the infant and are influential in emotional development and social relationships throughout the lifespan. (Courtesy Shay McAtee.)

Experiences that activate the vestibular sense have other integrating effects on the infant as well. Being lifted into an upright position against the caregiver's shoulder is known to increase alertness and visual pursuit.[70] While being held in such a position, the young infant's vestibular system detects the pull of gravity and begins to stimulate the neck muscles to raise the head off the caregiver's shoulder. This adaptive response reaches full maturation within 6 months. In the first month of life, head righting may be minimal and intermittent with much wobbling, but it will gradually stabilize and become firmly established as the baby assumes different positions (first when the baby lies in a prone position and later in the supine position).

The visual and auditory systems of the newborn are immature. The newborn orients to some visual and auditory inputs and is particularly interested in human faces and voices, although meaning is not yet attached to these sensations. Visually the infant is attracted to high-contrast stimuli, such as black-and-white designs, and the range of visual acuity for most stimuli is limited to approximately 10 inches. The infant's visual acuity and responsiveness to visual patterns expand dramatically over the first few months of life.[98] During this time the infant begins to use eye contact to relate to the caregiver, further strengthening the bond between them.

Stimulation in each of the sensory systems potentially affects the infant's state of arousal. The infant's capacity to behaviorally adapt to changing sensations is another important aspect of sensory integrative development—the development of self-regulation. It is relatively easy to overstimulate young infants, for example, with changes in water temperature, changes in body position, or an increase in auditory or visual stimuli.[136] However, as sensory integration develops, the older child is better able to self-regulate his or her responses to changing stimuli by initiating behaviors that will be calming and soothing (such as thumb sucking or cuddling with a favorite blanket) or exciting and energizing (such as jumping or singing).[124] This process of self-regulation begins in the neonatal period and develops throughout early childhood.

First 6 Months

By 4 to 6 months of age, a shift occurs in the infant's behavioral organization. The sensory systems have matured to the extent that the baby has much greater awareness and interest in the world, and developing vestibular-proprioceptive-visual connections provide the beginnings of postural control. During the first half of the first year, the infant begins to show a strong inner drive to rise up against gravity (Figure 11-3), and this drive is evident in much of the baby's spontaneous play. Body positions during the first 6 months characteristically involve the prone position, with gradually increasing extension from the neck down through the trunk as the arms gradually bear more weight to help push the chest off the floor. By 6 months of age, many infants spend a great deal of time in the prone position with full active trunk extension, and most are able to sit independently, at least if propped with their own hands. These body positions usually are the infant's preferred positions for play and are reflect the maturing of the lateral vestibulospinal tract. Head control is well established by 6 months of age and provides a stable base for control of eye muscles. This, of course, reflects the growing

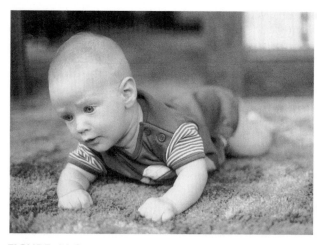

FIGURE 11-3 Strong inner drive to master gravity is evident in this infant's efforts to lift his head and shoulders off the floor. This is an early form of the prone extension posture. (Courtesy Shay McAtee.)

integration of vestibular, proprioceptive, and visual systems, which becomes increasingly important in providing a stable visual field as the baby becomes mobile.

Somatosensory achievements at this time are particularly evident in the infant's hands. The infant uses tactile and proprioceptive sensations to grasp objects, albeit with primitive grasps. Touch and visual information are integrated as the baby begins to reach for and wave or bang objects. The infant has a strong inner drive to play with the hands by bringing them to midline while watching and touching them. Connections between the tactile and visual systems pave the way for later hand–eye coordination skills. Midline hand play is a significant milestone in the integration of sensations from the two sides of the body.

By now, neonatal reflexes no longer dominate behavior; the baby is beginning to exercise voluntary control over movements during play. The earliest episodes of motor planning occur as the infant works to produce novel actions. This becomes evident as the infant handles objects and begins to initiate transitions from one body position to another, as in rolling from prone position to supine. Although reflexes play a role in such actions (such as grasp and neck righting reflexes), the infant's actions have a goal-directed, volitional quality and are not stereotypically reflex bound. The emergence of intentionality is a marker of the beginning of occupational engagement.

Second 6 Months

Another major transition occurs during the latter half of the first year. Infants become mobile in their environments, and by the first birthday they can willfully move from one place to another, many walking while others creep or crawl. These locomotor skills are the product of the many adaptive responses that have gone before, resulting in increasingly more sophisticated integration of somatosensory, vestibular, and visual inputs.

As the infant explores the environment, greater opportunities are generated for integrating a variety of complex sensations, particularly those responsible for developing body scheme and spatial perception. The child learns about environmental space and about the body's relationship to external space through sensorimotor experiences.

During the second 6 months after birth, tactile perception becomes further refined and plays a critical role in the child's developing hand skills. The infant relies on precise tactile feedback in developing a fine pincer grasp, which is used to pick up small objects. Proprioceptive information is also an important influence in developing manipulative skills, and now the baby experiments with objects using a variety of actions. These somatosensory-based adaptive responses contribute to development of motor planning ability. Further development of midline skills is also apparent as the baby easily transfers objects from one hand to the other and may occasionally cross the midline while holding an object.

Through the first year, auditory processing plays a significant role in the infant's awareness of environment, especially the social environment. Auditory information is integrated with tactile and proprioceptive sensations in and around the mouth as the infant vocalizes. The fruits of this process begin to blossom in the latter half of this first year, when the infant begins to experiment with creating the sounds of the language used by caregivers. Vocalizations such as consonant–vowel repetitions ("baba" and "mamama") are common. Parents often attach meaning to these infant vocalizations and strongly encourage them, thus leading the infant also to attach meaning to these sounds. By their first birthday, many infants have a small vocabulary of words or wordlike sounds that they use meaningfully to communicate desires to caregivers.

Another major landmark toward the end of the first year is beginning independence in self-feeding. This complex achievement requires refined somatosensory processing of information from the lips, the jaw, and inside the mouth to guide oral movements in the chewing and swallowing of food. Taste and smell sensations are also integral to this process, but self-feeding involves more than the mouth. All of the acquired sensory integrative milestones involving hand–eye coordination are important to self-feeding. The infant at this period of life uses the fingers directly to feed him or herself and to explore the textures of foods. At this stage, use of a utensil such as a spoon is not very functional and is messy because motor planning skills have not progressed to the point that the child can manipulate the utensil successfully. However, many infants begin to demonstrate a drive to use the spoon in self-feeding by the end of the first year. For many contemporary American infants, use of a spoon is the first real experience in using a tool (Figure 11-4).

The occupation of dining, then, begins to emerge in infancy as sensory integrative abilities mature, allowing the child to engage in self-feeding. As an occupation, dining in its fullest sense goes far beyond the physical, sensorimotor act of feeding. Dining usually takes place within a social context, whether at a family dinner at home or in a formal restaurant, so social standards for acceptable behavior and etiquette become increasingly important as the child develops. Furthermore, partaking in a meal and sharing certain types of food gradually come to take on powerful symbolic meanings. The sensory integrative underpinnings of the dining experience influence how the child experiences mealtimes and how others view the child as a dining partner, thus playing a role in shaping the social and symbolic aspects of this vitally important occupation.

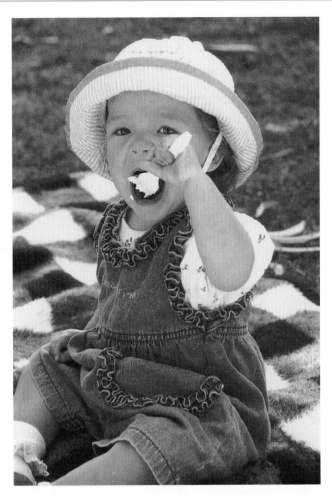

FIGURE 11-4 Because somatosensory processing and visual-motor coordination strongly influence self-feeding skills, sensory integration is an important contributor to the development of dining, a fundamental occupation. (Courtesy Shay McAtee.)

Second Year

As the child moves into the second year, the basic vestibular-proprioceptive-visual connections that were laid down earlier continue to refine, resulting in growing finesse in balance and fluidity of dynamic postural control. Discrimination and localization of tactile sensations also become much more precise, allowing for further refinement of fine motor skills.

Increasingly complex somatosensory processing contributes to the continuing development of body scheme. Ayres hypothesized that as body scheme becomes more sophisticated, so does motor planning ability.[11] This is because the child draws on knowledge of how the body works to program novel actions (Figure 11-5). Throughout the second year, the typically developing toddler experiments with many variations in body movements. Imitation of the actions of others contributes further to the child's movement repertoire. In experiencing new actions, the child generates new sensory experiences, thus building an elaborate base of information from which to plan future actions.

While motor planning ability becomes increasingly more complex in the second year, another aspect of praxis, ideation,

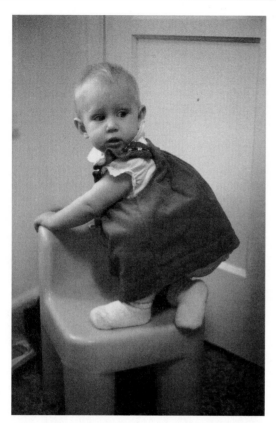

FIGURE 11-5 As motor planning develops during the second year of life, the infant experiments with a variety of body movements and learns how to transition easily from one position to another. These experiences are thought to reflect the development of body scheme. (Courtesy Shay McAtee.)

begins to emerge. Ideation is the ability to conceptualize what to do in a given situation. Ideation is made possible by the cognitive ability to use symbols, first expressed gesturally and then vocally during the second year of life.[35] Symbolic functioning enables the child to engage in pretend actions and to imagine doing actions, even actions that the child has never before done. By the end of the second year, the toddler can join several pretend actions in a play sequence.[102] Furthermore, the 2-year-old child demonstrates that he or she has a plan before performing an action sequence, either through a verbal announcement or through a search for a needed object.[102] Thus, a surge in practic development occurs in the second year as the child generates many new ideas for actions and begins to plan actions in a systematic sequence.

The burgeoning of praxis abilities plays an important role in the development of self-concept. Infant psychiatrist Daniel Stern suggests that the sense of an integrated core self begins in infancy as an outcome of the volition and the proprioceptive feedback involved in motor planning.[147] The consequences of the child's voluntary, planned actions add to the developing sense of self as an active agent in the world. As praxis takes giant leaps during the second year, so does this sense of self as an agent of power. The child feels in command of his or her own life when sensory integration allows the child to move freely and effectively through the world.[18]

Third through Seventh Years

The child's competencies in the sensorimotor realm mature in the third through seventh years of life, which Ayres considered a crucial period for sensory integration because of the brain's receptiveness to sensations and its capacity for organizing them at this time.[18] This is the period when sensorimotor functions become consolidated as a foundation for higher intellectual abilities. Although further sensory integrative development can and usually does occur beyond the eighth birthday, the changes that take place are likely to be more limited than those that occurred earlier.

In the third through seventh years, children have strong inner drives to produce adaptive responses that not only meet complicated sensorimotor demands but also sometimes require interfacing with peers. The challenges posed by children's games and play activities attest to this complexity. In the visual-motor realm, sophistication develops through involvement in crafts, drawing and painting, constructional play with blocks and other building toys, and video games (Figure 11-6). Children are

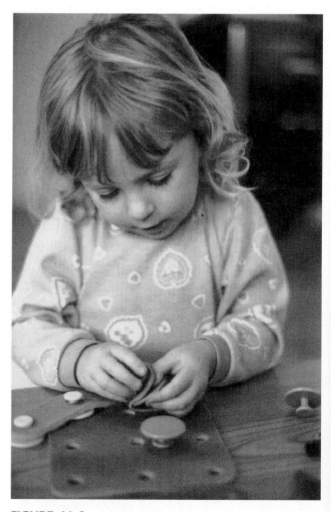

FIGURE 11-6 Adaptive responses involved in this activity require precise tactile feedback and sophisticated praxis. During activities such as this one, the preschooler becomes adept at handling tools and objects that are encountered in daily occupations throughout life. (Courtesy Shay McAtee.)

driven to explore playground equipment by swinging, sliding, climbing, jumping, riding, pushing, pulling, and pumping. Toward the end of this period they enthusiastically grapple with the motor-planning challenges posed by games such as jump rope, jacks, marbles, and hopscotch. It is also during this period that children become expert with cultural tools such as scissors, pencils, zippers, buttons, forks and knives, pails, shovels, brooms, and rakes (Figure 11-7). Many children begin to participate in occupations that present sensorimotor challenges for years to come, such as soccer, softball, karate, gymnastics, playing a musical instrument, and ballet. Furthermore, children develop the ability to organize their behavior into more complex sequences over longer time frames. This makes it possible for them to become more autonomous in orchestrating daily routines, such as getting ready for school in the morning, completing homework and other school projects, and performing household chores.

As children participate in these occupations, they must frequently anticipate how to move in relation to changing environmental events by accurately timing and sequencing their actions.[39] This is particularly challenging in sports when peers, with their often unpredictable moves, are involved. Their bodies are challenged to maintain balance through dynamic changes in body position. In fine motor tasks, children must efficiently coordinate visual with somatosensory information to guide eye and hand movements with accuracy and precision while maintaining a stable postural base.

Children meet these challenges with varying degrees of success. Some are more talented than others with respect to sensory integrative abilities, but most children eventually achieve a degree of competency that allows them to fully participate in the daily occupations that they are expected to do and wish to do at home, in school, and in the community. Furthermore, most children experience feelings of satisfaction and self-efficacy as they master occupations that depend heavily on sensory integration.

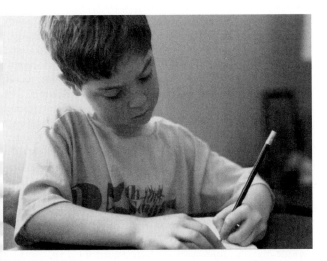

FIGURE 11-7 By the time a child reaches school age, sensory integrative capacities are almost mature. The child now can devote full attention to the demands of academic tasks because basic sensorimotor functions, such as maintaining an upright posture and guiding hand movements while holding a tool, have become automatic. (Courtesy Shay McAtee.)

WHEN PROBLEMS IN SENSORY INTEGRATION OCCUR

Unfortunately, not every child experiences competency in sensory integration. When some aspect of sensory integration does not function efficiently, the child may experience stress in the course of everyday occupations because processes that should be automatic or accurate are not. It may be stressful, for example, to simply maintain balance when sitting in a chair, to get dressed in the morning before school, to attempt to play jump rope, or to eat lunch in a socially acceptable manner. The child is aware of these difficulties and becomes frustrated by frequent failure when confronted with ordinary tasks that come easily for other children. Many children with sensory integrative problems develop a tendency to avoid or reject simple sensory or motor challenges, responding with refusals or tantrums when pushed to perform. If this becomes a long-term pattern of behavior, the child may miss important experiences, such as playing games with peers, which are critical in building feelings of competency, mastering a wide repertoire of useful skills, and developing flexible social strategies. Thus, the capacity to participate fully in the occupations that the child wants to do and needs to do is compromised.

Often behavioral, social, academic, or motor coordination concerns are cited when a child with a sensory integrative dysfunction is referred for occupational therapy. The occupational therapist needs to evaluate whether a sensory processing problem may underlie these concerns. The therapist then must decide on a course of action to help the child move toward the goal of greater success and satisfaction in doing meaningful occupations. These challenges to the therapist—to identify a problem that may be hidden and to figure out how to best help the child—were the challenges to which Ayres devoted most of her career.

As mentioned previously, Ayres turned to the neurobiologic literature to give her insight into understanding children's learning and behavior problems. Ayres also took on the responsibility of conducting research to develop her theory of sensory integration. In doing so, she produced a diagnostic system for clinical evaluation of children through the use of standardized tests. She also conducted research that was designed to evaluate the effectiveness of her treatment methods. After each study, Ayres returned to her theory to revise and refine it in light of research findings. While she was doing this, she maintained a private practice; thus, she had many years of firsthand, clinically based experience on which to ground her theoretical work.

The following sections examine the research that Ayres conducted to identify different types of sensory integrative dysfunction in children. The general categories of sensory integrative problems that concern clinicians today, based on research findings and clinical experience, are discussed. The field of sensory integration continues to be a dynamic field that changes as research generates new findings and as experiences of clinicians generate new ways of interpreting those findings.

RESEARCH BASE FOR SENSORY INTEGRATIVE PROBLEMS

Throughout her professional career, Ayres was guided by her keen observation skills and her search to reach a deeper understanding of the clinical problems that she encountered in practice.

To begin answering the questions that arose as she worked with children, Ayres initiated the process of developing standardized tests of sensory integration during the 1960s. She originally developed these tests solely as research tools to aid in theory development. At the time, she was working with children with learning disabilities, many of whom she suspected had covert difficulties processing sensory information, and she sought to uncover the nature of whatever sensory integrative difficulties might exist. It was after her initial efforts at research using her tests that other therapists asked to have access to the tests, instigating their publication by Western Psychological Services.

The first group of tests Ayres created was published as the Southern California Sensory Integration Tests (SCSIT).[12] These were later revised and renamed the Sensory Integration and Praxis Tests (SIPT).[21] Normative data were collected on a regional scale for the SCSIT and on a national scale for the SIPT. The tests were designed to measure aspects of visual, tactile, kinesthetic, and vestibular sensory processing as well as motor planning abilities.

Using first the SCSIT and later the SIPT with samples of children, Ayres used a statistical procedure called *factor analysis* to develop a typology of sensory integrative function and dysfunction. Tables 11-1 and 11-2 summarize results of her factor analytic studies, along with results of several studies conducted by other researchers. In factor analysis, sets of test scores are grouped according to their associations with one another. The resulting groups of associated test scores are called *factors*. Ayres interpreted the factors that emerged from her studies as representative of neural substrates underlying learning and behavior in children. For example, in her 1965 study, Ayres found that the tactile tests correlated highly with the motor planning tests, forming a factor.[5] She hypothesized that there is an ability called *motor planning* that depends on somatosensory processing and influences one's interactions with the physical world. *Apraxia* is the term she used to identify a disorder in this ability. In her later work, she subsumed the notion of motor planning under the construct of praxis and replaced the term *apraxia* with *dyspraxia* when referring to children.

In her last set of analyses with the SIPT, just before her death in 1988, Ayres used both factor analysis and another statistical technique called *cluster analysis*, which groups together children with similar SIPT profiles (see Table 11-1). This approach was used to further carve out diagnostic groupings of children that might be useful clinically. Today, consideration of both factor analysis and cluster groupings is a critical component in the interpretation of a child's SIPT scores.

Through the years as Ayres conducted her studies with different groups of children, she continually revisited her theory, bringing along new hypotheses based on new research results. Of particular interest were the patterns that recurred despite being generated from different samples of children. Among the most consistent findings was that children who had been identified as having learning or developmental problems often displayed difficulties in more than one sensory system. Ayres interpreted this finding in light of the neurobiologic literature on intersensory integration, which indicates that the sensory systems tend to function synergistically with each other rather than in isolation.[11] Thus, the idea of intersensory integration as critical to human function became one of the major tenets of sensory integration theory.

Another finding, which emerged in early studies and in later SIPT studies, was that some patterns of scores were seen only in groups of children who had been identified as having disorders. In other words, some factors were not evident in typically developing children at any age. This led to the proposal that the sensory integrative problems associated with these particular patterns were representative of neural dysfunction rather than developmental lag.

Yet another recurrent pattern was a relationship between tactile perception and praxis scores. This association appeared repeatedly in her studies and led Ayres to theorize that the tactile system contributes importantly to the development of efficient practic functions. The robustness of this finding across many studies influenced Ayres to emphasize the relationship between the tactile system and praxis, a relationship that has become a cornerstone of sensory integration theory.

Throughout her research, several patterns emerged that Ayres suspected were related to a discrete involvement of cortical rather than brainstem or intersensory dysfunction. Ayres came to view these types of problems as different than those classified as sensory integrative disorders and less likely to be responsive to the treatment techniques that she was developing. An example is the association of low Praxis on Verbal Command scores with high postrotary nystagmus scores. Praxis on Verbal Command is the only test on the SIPT with a strong language comprehension component. Postrotary nystagmus is a test that may reflect cortical dysfunction if scores are extremely high. In this example, it is hypothesized that an underlying cortical dysfunction, possibly involving the left hemisphere (where language centers are located), is responsible for the pattern of scores. Ayres did not view this particular pattern as a sensory integrative dysfunction, although it might be detected by her tests.

In spite of small sample sizes, Ayres found similar factors across multiple studies (see Tables 11-1 and 11-2). Many of these findings were replicated by Mulligan (1998) in a confirmatory factor analytic study of more than 10,000 children. Mailloux, Mulligan, Smith Roley, et al. found a very close replication of the same factors identified by Ayres.[96] In a study of children with suspected sensory integrative problems, factors emerged that reflected associations among (1) visual and tactile perception with praxis, (2) vestibular and proprioceptive processing with bilateral functions, (3) attention and tactile defensiveness, and (4) visual and tactile discrimination. The robustness of some of these findings across many studies strengthens the hypothesis that they reflect underlying patterns of function.

Ayres conducted her factor and cluster analyses to shed light on the types of sensory integrative dysfunctions that children experience, yet she did not view the resulting typologies as specific diagnostic labels to pin on individual children. Rather, the typologies were seen as general patterns exhibited time after time by groups of children who were struggling in school or with some other aspect of behavior or development. They provide the therapist with relevant information to consider when conducting clinical assessments. They do not provide prefabricated slots in which to fit children. Ultimately, the important job of interpreting an individual child's pattern of scores in relation to his or her unique life situation lies in the purview of the therapist's judgment, using research, training, and experience to guide decision making.

Text continued on page 343

TABLE 11-1 Purpose, Methods, Results, and Contributions of Studies of Sensory Integrative Patterns

Author	Purpose	Instruments	Hypothesis	Analysis	Subjects	Results	Contributions to Theory
Ayres (1965)	Identify relationships among sensory perception, motor performance, laterality in normal children and children with perceptual problems. Establish construct and discriminant validity	Early versions of the SCSIT, additional perceptual-motor and laterality tests, also freedom from hyperactivity and tactile defensiveness.	Test results would identify factors for children with and without dysfunction. Normal and dysfunctional children will demonstrate different factors.	Thirty-three tests. Two behavioral parameters. Analysis of difference between group means. Q- and R-technique factor analysis.	n = 100 dysfunctional n = 50 normal Dysfunctional children had learning or behavioral disorders.	Tests discriminated between normal and dysfunctional groups. Five patterns detected: apraxia, dysfunction form and space perception, deficit bilateral integration, visual figure-ground perception, tactile defensiveness	Established discriminant validity of early versions of SCSIT. Most children demonstrated more than one factor; therefore factors related. Sensory integration: Clusters were not by sensory systems. Praxis and tactile functions linked. Tactile defensiveness, hyperactivity, distractibility linked. Cognitive aspects deemphasized. Eye-hand agreement not discriminative. Empirical support for syndromes.
Ayres (1966a)	Explore perceptual-motor relationships in a normal sample and compare with prior studies. Establish construct validity.	Frostig tests, early versions of the SCSIT. Also freedom from hyperactivity and tactile defensiveness.	That factors would emerge.	Seventeen tests. R-technique factor analysis (simplified matrix).	n = 92 Formed normal distribution, 10% abnormal, three with mild cerebral palsy.	Praxis accounted for most variance. Motor planning, kinesthesia, tactile functions, motor accuracy, bilateral coordination. Visual perception factor: Ayres Space Test, Frostig.	More support for praxis syndrome. Visual component without motor element. Perceptual-motor functions correlate as a whole in normative sample. Kinesthesia closer to tactile than visual perception as in prior study.

Continued

TABLE 11-1 Purpose, Methods, Results, and Contributions of Studies of Sensory Integrative Patterns—Cont'd

Author	Purpose	Instruments	Hypothesis	Analysis	Subjects	Results	Contributions to Theory
Ayres (1966b)	Provide an understanding of whether syndromes represent dysfunction or developmental lag. Establish construct validity.	Nearly the same as in Ayres, 1966a.	That variation in perceptual-motor abilities would be small in a group of typical children.	Sixteen tests Two behavioral parameters. R-technique factor analysis.	n = 64 Adopted, all normal on Gesell.	Visual motor ability accounted for most variation. Praxis and tactile perception were least variable. Hyperactivity, distractibility, tactile defensiveness factor. Factors weak because of lack of variance in performance of normal children.	Suggested that low scores in praxis and tactile perception represent developmental deviation, not delay. Little systematic variation when tests given to normal children. Tactile defensiveness: Hyperactivity may have a maturational component.
Ayres (1969)	Provide an in-depth analysis of dysfunctional patterns in children with learning handicaps. Establish construct validity.	Sixty-four tests and observations: SCSIT, psycho-linguistic, intelligence, auditory, postural-ocular reactions, academic achievement.	Brain functions involve several levels and will cluster accordingly.	Q-technique factor analysis.	n = 36 Educationally handicapped children.	Five factors identified: auditory language, sequencing; postural and bilateral integration; right hemisphere dysfunction; apraxia; tactile defensiveness.	Hints to left hemisphere dysfunction.
Ayres (1971)	Identify predictors of severity of sensory integrative syndromes.	Forty-eight tests and observations: SCSIT, psycholinguistic, intelligence, eye-hand usage, postural responses.	That predictive equations would emerge.	Ten-step regression equations for each syndrome calculated.	n = 140 Educationally handicapped children.	Presence of more than one type of disorder was the norm. Prone extension best predictor of postural-bilateral integration. Imitation of postures best predictor of praxis.	Somatosensory and praxis linked again. Elucidated best predictors of syndromes. As many children may have apraxia as have postural and bilateral coordination problems.
Ayres (1972)	Further analyze and refine factors. Establish construct validity	Same as above.	That similar factors as presented previously would emerge.	R-technique factor analysis.	n = 148 Educationally handicapped children.	Six factors identified: form and space perception; auditory language; postural ocular; motor planning; reading, spelling, and IQ; hyperactivity, tactile perception.	Further confirmed left hemisphere dysfunction. Reconfirmed syndromes found in other samples of learning-disabled children.

Study	Purpose	Tests	Question/Hypothesis	Sample	Analysis	Findings	Contribution
Ayres (1977)	Further analyze interrelationships (add SCPNT) so that differential diagnosis can be further refined.	SCSIT SCPNT, postural-ocular and lateralization measures, dichotic listening, ITPA, intelligence, academic achievement. Flowers-Costello (auditory).	That clusters would continue to be refined.	n = 128 Learning-disabled children.	Series of R-technique factor analyses (not all measures entered each time).	Five major domains identified: somatosensory-motor planning; auditory-language; postural-ocular, eye-hand coordination, postrotary nystagmus.	Further elucidated nature of interhemispheric integration. Role of vestibular system clarified.
Ayres, Mailloux, & Wendler (1987)	Continue to attempt to differentiate types of sensory integration dysfunction. New praxis tests as well as many of the tests that had been used in past studies.	SCSIT, SCPNT, selected ITPA test, sentence repetition. Clinical observation of prone extension, supine flexion, ocular pursuits. Preliminary versions of newly designed praxis tests: Sequencing Praxis, Praxis on Verbal Command, Oral Praxis, block-building test.	Is praxis a unitary function? Would computer-generated clusters match those that had been identified clinically and through factor analysis?	n = 182 Learning or behavior disorders.	Screen plot factor analyses, correlation coefficients. Comparison of test profiles of children with diagnoses. Use of computer-generated clusters.	Praxis tests were related with one another. Visual tests correlated with tactile tests. Somatovisual-practic factor identified. Tactile scores and praxis related; short duration postrotary nystagmus; statistical association with praxis.	Suggestion of a general somatopractic function. Further verified close association of tactile score and praxis. Computer-generated clusters were not meaningful.
Ayres (1989)	Factor analyses: to clarify the nature of the constructs measured by the Sensory Integration and Praxis Tests (SIPT).	SIPT (17 tests).	That factors related to those of the SCSIT would emerge.	Three analyses: n = 1750. Normative sample. n = 125 Learning or sensory integrative disorders. n = 293 Combined sample of learning or sensory integrative disorders and matched children from normative sample.	Principal components analysis.	Visuopraxis and somatopraxis factors emerged in all three analyses. Bilateral integration and sequencing factor and praxis on verbal command factor seen only in dysfunctional sample. Other factors related to vestibular and somatosensory processing identified.	Expanded understanding of vestibular-bilateral disorders to include sequencing element. Somatopraxis factor reinforced previous findings linking tactile perception and praxis. Visuopraxis factor provided support for previous visual-motor linkages.

Continued

TABLE 11-1 Purpose, Methods, Results, and Contributions of Studies of Sensory Integrative Patterns—Cont'd

Author	Purpose	Instruments	Hypothesis	Analysis	Subjects	Results	Contributions to Theory
Ayres (1989)	Cluster analyses: to assist in identifying children in need of different types of remediation or services.	SIPT (17 tests).	That meaningful diagnostic groupings would emerge.	Agglomerative cluster analysis, Ward's method.	n = 293 Same sample as above, combined dysfunctional and normative.	Six cluster groups identified: low average bilateral integration and sequencing, generalized sensory integrative dysfunction, visuo- and somatodyspraxia, low average sensory integration and praxis, dyspraxia on verbal command, high average sensory integration and dysfunction.	Children with and without dysfunction can be differentiated on the basis of SIPT profiles. Identified specific SIPT profile that may be characteristic of left hemisphere dysfunction.
Mulligan (2000)	To explore subgroupings of children referred for SIPT testing and to provide information about the validity of the six cluster groups identified in the SIPT manual.	SIPT.	That cluster groups similar to those identified by Ayres (1989) would emerge.	Agglomerative cluster analysis, Ward's method.	n = 1961 children assessed with the SIPT between 1989 and 1993.	Five cluster groups identified: generalized sensory integration dysfunction and dyspraxia–severe, generalized sensory integration dysfunction and dyspraxia–moderate, low average bilateral integration and sequencing, average sensory integration and praxis.	Demonstrated many similarities with Ayres's cluster analysis, with some differences. Supports evidence of dyspraxia, bilateral integration and sequencing deficit, dyspraxia on verbal command, and more general dyspraxia. More helpful in identifying degree of dysfunction rather than type, as this sample did not include a normative sample as did Ayres's analysis.
Parham (1998)	To examine whether sensory integrative measures are predictive of school achievement, when intelligence and other factors are taken into account, concurrently and over a 4-year period.	SIPT, converted into 3 factor scores: praxis, visual perception, and somato-sensory. Intelligence, reading, and math achievement. Socioeconomic status.	That sensory integrative performance at ages 6–8 years is related to achievement concurrently and predictively 4 years later. That sensory integrative performance at ages 10–12 is not related to achievement.	Multiple regression analyses.	n = 91, of whom 43 were identified as learning disabled. Children were 6–8 years old initially, 10–12 years old at follow-up.	When controlling for IQ sensory integration: at ages 6–8 significantly correlated with math, but not reading; at ages 6–8 significantly predicted math and reading 4 years later; at ages 10–12 significantly predicted math and reading at same age. Strong relationships between praxis and math achievement identified.	Supported the hypothesis that sensory integration, especially praxis, is related to achievement when taking IQ into account. Sensory integration continues to contribute to achievement at middle school age.

Study	Purpose	Measures	Hypothesis	Analysis	Sample	Results	
Mailloux, Mulligan, Roley, et al. (In preparation)	Explore relationships among modulation measures; examine low and high PRN as separate measures.	18 test scores from the SIPT; subtests for directionality, laterality and crossing midline; SPM items measuring sensory over responsiveness; parent report of problems in attention.	Low PRN & measures of directionality, laterality and crossing midline would be associated with measures of vestibular bilateral integration; SPM items measuring sensory over-responsiveness would be more related to attention than other sensory or practic functions.	Exploratory factor analyses using Varimax and Promax rotations.	273 children from a retrospective clinical sample. PRN scores fell primarily in the low to average range.	Four factors: visuo- and somatodyspraxia, vestibular bilateral integration and sequencing, tactile defensiveness and attention, tactile and visual discrimination.	Low PRN is related to vestibular and bilateral integration functions; tactile defensiveness is more strongly related to attention problems than to perception measures or praxis; measures of directionality, laterality and crossing midline and modulation items other than for tactile defensiveness were not significant on factors

CFA, Confirmatory factor analysis; *ITPA*, Illinois Test of Psycholinguistic Abilities; *SCPNT*, Southern California Postrotary Nystagmus Test; *SCSIT*, Southern California Sensory Integration Test; *SIPT*, Sensory Integration and Praxis Tests; *SEM*, structural equation modeling.

Ayres, A. J. (1965). Patterns of perceptual-motor dysfunction in children: a factor analytic study. *Perceptual and Motor Skills, 20,* 335-368.

Ayres, A. J. (1966a). Interrelationships among perceptual-motor functions in children. *American Journal of Occupational Therapy, 20,* 68-71.

Ayres, A. J. (1966b). Interrelations among perceptual-motor abilities in a group of normal children. *American Journal of Occupational Therapy, 20,* 288-292.

Ayres, A. J. (1969). Deficits in sensory integration in educationally handicapped children. *Journal of Learning Disabilities, 2*(3), 44-52.

Ayres, A. J. (1971). Characteristics of types of sensory integrative dysfunction. *American Journal of Occupational Therapy, 25,* 329-334.

Ayres, A. J. (1972). Types of sensory integrative dysfunction among disabled learners. *American Journal of Occupational Therapy, 26,* 13-18.

Ayres, A. J. (1977). Cluster analyses of measures of sensory integration. *American Journal of Occupational Therapy, 31,* 362-366.

Ayres, A. J., Mailloux, Z., & Wendler, C.L.W. (1987). Development apraxia: is it a unitary function? *Occupational Therapy Journal of Research, 7,* 93-110.

Ayres, A. J. (1989). *Sensory Integration and Praxis Tests manual.* Los Angeles: Western Psychological Services.

Mailloux, Z., Mulligan, S., & Roley, S. S., et al. (2009). *Verification and clarification of patterns of sensory integrative dysfunction* (manuscript in progress).

Mulligan, S. (2000). Cluster analysis of scores of children on the Sensory Integration and Praxis tests. *Occupational Therapy Journal of Research, 20,* 256-270.

Parham, L. D. (1998). The relationship of sensory integrative development to achievement in elementary students: Four-year longitudinal patterns. *Occupational Therapy Journal of Research, 18,* 105-127.

TABLE 11-2 Factors and Clusters Identified in Research

Author and Date of Study	Somatodyspraxia	Visual Perception & Visuomotor/Visuopraxis	Vestibular, Postural, and Bilateral Integration	Auditory Language Functions	Somatosensory Perception	Tactile Defensiveness and Attention	Other Findings
Ayres (1965)	Tactile tests Motor planning (imitation of posture, motor accuracy) Eye pursuits	Frostig tests Kinesthesia Manual form Perception Ayres' Space Test	Right-left discrimination Avoidance crossing midline Rhythmic activities	Not tested	No specific factor	Hyperactive/ distractible behavior and tactile defensiveness	Figure-ground a separate factor Eye-hand agreement not related to perceptual-motor dysfunction
Ayres (1966a)	Accounted for most variance Motor planning Tactile and kinesthesia Motor accuracy Figure-ground Frostig tests	Figure-ground Frostig spatial relations Ayres' Space Test		Not tested	No specific factor	Low association of tactile defensiveness with praxis factor	Identified two main factors in normal sample: general perceptual-motor (somatosensory and motor) and visual perception
Ayres (1966b)	Frostig tests	Frostig tests Ayres' Space Test Motor accuracy Figure-ground	Integration two sides of body and tactile perception	Not tested	No specific factor	Tactile defensiveness and hyperactivity; may be a maturational factor involved	Visual-motor ability accounted for most variation in normal children Poor motor planning—tactile perception not seen in normal children
Ayres (1969)	Tactile Motor planning	Most SCSIT; visual tests not included in analysis Possible right hemisphere dysfunction: eye movement deficits, better right- than left-sided function	Bilateral integration Postural reactions Reading and language problems	Possible left hemisphere dysfunction: auditory-language Reading achievement Auditory and visual-motor sequencing	No specific factor	Tactile defensiveness, hyperactivity, and attention related to each other, but not a distinct factor	

Ayres (1972)	Motor planning Hyperactivity Tactile defensiveness (more emphasis on motor than tactile)	Poor praxis related to hyperactivity and tactile defensiveness	Poor ocular control Excessive residual primitive postural responses Relatively good left-hand coordination	Auditory language Intelligence	Tactile perception and hyperactivity formed a factor separate from praxis	Tactile defensiveness and hyperactivity loaded with praxis	Reading-spelling load together Motor accuracy highly associated with all parameters
Ayres (1977)	*Analysis 5:* imitation of postures Composite tactile Kinesthesia	*Analysis 3:* four SCSIT visual tests Manual form Perception	*Analysis 5:* prone extension Composite postural Flexion posture Composite tactile Kinesthesia Bilateral integration symptom did not load	*Analysis 5:* composite language (ITPA) Dichotic listening Flowers-Costello (auditory)	No specific factor	Not studied	Visual tests have strong cognitive component (loaded with IQ on Analysis 2) SVCU associated with lateralization indices Motor accuracy loaded separately on all
Ayres (1989)	Somatopraxis factor (Oral Praxis, Postural Praxis, Graphesthesia) Visuo- and somatodyspraxia cluster	Visuopraxis factor (Constructional Praxis, Design Copying, Space Visualization, Figure-Ground)	Bilateral integration and sequencing factor (Sequencing Praxis, Bilateral Motor Coordination, Standing and Walking Balance) Low average bilateral integration and sequencing cluster	Praxis on verbal command factor Dyspraxia on verbal command cluster (high Postrotatory Nystagmus with low Praxis on Verbal Command)	Somatosensory perception factor	Not studied	High-functioning group identified within normative sample Generalized dysfunction group identified within group with learning disorders and sensory integrative dysfunction

Continued

TABLE 11-2 Factors and Clusters Identified in Research—Cont'd

Author and Date of Study	Somatodyspraxia	Visual Perception & Visuomotor/ Visuopraxis	Vestibular, Postural, and Bilateral Integration	Auditory Language Functions	Somatosensory Perception	Tactile Defensiveness and Attention	Other Findings
Mulligan (1998)	Dyspraxia (Oral Praxis, Postural Praxis, and Praxis on Verbal Command); also suggests generalized function underlying all other factors	Visual Perceptual Deficit (Design Copying, Constructional Praxis, Space Visualization, Manual Form Perception, Figure Ground Perception)	Bilateral integration and sequencing deficit (Sequencing Praxis and Bilateral Motor Coordination)	Not tested	Tactile tests and Kinesthesia	Not studied	
Mailloux, Mulligan, Roley, et al., (manuscript in preparation)	Some somatopraxis tests seen within the visuopraxis factor	Visuopraxis formed a distinct factor	PRN included as part of a bilateral integration and sequencing factor)	Not tested	Tactile perception loaded with visual perception	Tactile defensiveness items loaded with signs of attention problems	

ITPA, Illinois Test of Psycholinguistic Abilities; *SCSIT*, Southern California Sensory Integration Test; *SVCU*, Space Visualization Contralateral Use.

Ayres, A.J. (1965). Patterns of perceptual-motor dysfunction in children: A factor analytic study. *Perceptual and Motor Skills, 20*, 335-368.

Ayres, A.J. (1966a). Interrelationships among perceptual-motor functions in children. *American Journal of Occupational Therapy, 20*, 68-71.

Ayres, A.J. (1966b). Interrelations among perceptual-motor abilities in a group of normal children. *American Journal of Occupational Therapy, 20*, 288-292.

Ayres, A.J. (1969). Deficits in sensory integration in educationally handicapped children. *Journal of Learning Disabilities, 2*(3), 44-52.

Ayres, A.J. (1972). Types of sensory integrative dysfunction among disabled learners. *American Journal of Occupational Therapy, 26*, 13-18.

Ayres, A.J. (1977). Cluster analyses of measures of sensory integration. *American Journal of Occupational Therapy, 31*, 362-366.

Ayres, A.J. (1989). *Sensory Integration and Praxis Tests manual.* Los Angeles: Western Psychological Services.

Mailloux, Z., Mulligan, Smith, Roley (in prep).

Mulligan, S. (1998). Patterns of sensory integration dysfunction: A confirmatory factor analysis. *American Journal of Occupational Therapy, 52*, 819-828.

Mulligan, S. (2000). Cluster analysis of scores of children on the Sensory Integration and Praxis tests. *Occupational Therapy Journal of Research, 20*, 256-270.

SENSORY INTEGRATIVE PROBLEMS

The results of research, combined with the experiences of clinicians and the work of scholars in the field, have generated many different ways of conceptualizing sensory integrative problems over the past 30 years. The complexity of this domain can be daunting for the novice therapist, but is also a reflection of the growth in knowledge in this field. The terms *sensory integrative disorder, sensory integrative dysfunction,* and *sensory integrative problems* do not refer to one specific type of difficulty but describe a heterogeneous group of problems that are thought to reflect subtle neural differences involving multisensory and motor systems.

Most discussions of sensory integrative problems assume normal sensory receptor function. In other words, sensory integrative problems involve central, rather than peripheral, sensory functions. This assumption has been supported in several well-designed studies. For instance, Parush, Sohmer, Steinberg, and Kaitz found that the somatosensory-evoked potentials of children with attention deficit–hyperactivity disorder (ADHD) differ from those of typically developing children with respect to indicators of central tactile processing but not peripheral receptor responses.[119] Many of the children with ADHD in this study were also identified as having tactile defensiveness, a sensory integrative problem. In another study, researchers found that children with learning disabilities, compared with nondisabled children, had impaired postural responses involving central integration of vestibular, proprioceptive, and visual inputs, whereas measures of peripheral receptor functions were normal.[142] Thus, when sensory integrative problems involving the vestibular system are discussed, these problems are generally thought to be based within CNS structures and pathways (i.e., the vestibular nuclei and its connections) rather than the vestibular receptors (i.e., the semicircular canals, utricle, or saccule).[159] In this chapter, the discussions of sensory integrative problems assume that peripheral function is normal.

As noted previously, different conceptualizations of sensory integrative problems have been generated over the years. Although perfect consensus on how to categorize these problems does not exist, clearly there are recurring themes across authors. Distinct but overlapping taxonomies of sensory integrative problems include, for example, those of Bundy and Murray[39] and Kimball.[81] Bundy and Murray presented a taxonomic model that depicts sensory integrative dysfunction as manifested in two major ways: poor sensory modulation and poor praxis.[39] Miller, Anzalone, Lane, Cermak, and Osten proposed a nosology of Sensory Processing Disorders (SPD) that includes three main types of disorder: sensory modulation disorder, sensory-based motor disorder, and sensory discrimination disorder.[105] Subtypes within their category of sensory modulation disorder are overresponsivity, underresponsivity, and sensory seeking. Subtypes within their sensory-based motor disorder category include postural disorders and dyspraxia.

For the purposes of this chapter, sensory integrative problems are divided into four general categories:

1. Sensory modulation problems
2. Poor sensory discrimination and perception
3. Problems related to vestibular-proprioceptive functions
4. Difficulties related to praxis

These four categories are used here because they are consistent with the research data available at this time. Although variations were reported across studies, these patterns emerged in research on different samples of children over many decades. This research indicated that the patterns are interrelated and often coexist in individual children. When planning intervention, occupational therapists need to carefully analyze assessment data to discern whether one or more specific patterns of sensory integration problems seem to be affecting an individual child's participation in activities. Each of the main categories of sensory integration problems is presented in the next section.

Sensory Modulation Problems

Modulation refers to CNS regulation of its own activity.[18] The term *sensory modulation* refers to the tendency to generate responses that are appropriately graded in relation to incoming sensory stimuli, rather than underreacting or overreacting to them. Cermak[45] and Royeen[131] hypothesized that there is a continuum of sensory responsivity, with hyporesponsivity at one end and hyperresponsivity at the other. An optimal level of arousal and orientation lies in the center of the continuum (Figure 11-8). This is where most activity falls for most individuals, although everyone experiences fluctuations across this continuum of sensory responsivity in the course of a day. In the continuum model, dysfunction is indicated when the fluctuations within an individual are extreme or when an individual tends to function primarily at one extreme of the continuum or the other. The individual who tends to function at the extremely underresponsive end of the continuum may fail to notice sensory stimuli that would elicit the attention of most people. This characteristic often is identified as a problem in sensory registration. At a less severe degree of underresponsiveness, the individual notices sensory stimuli, but is slow to respond or seems to crave intense sensory input. At the opposite extreme of the continuum is the overresponsive individual with sensory defensiveness. This person is overwhelmed and overstressed by ordinary sensory stimuli.

Originally, Ayres thought of sensory registration problems as different in nature from sensory modulation problems such as tactile defensiveness.[18] Soon after she introduced the concept of sensory registration, however, other experts in the field of sensory integration suggested that sensory registration and tactile defensiveness might be related through common

Failure to orient   Optimal arousal   Overorientation

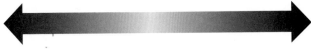

HYPORESPONSIVITY   **HYPERRESPONSIVITY**
Sensory registration   Sensory defensiveness
problem

FIGURE 11-8 Continuum of sensory responsivity and orientation. (Modified from Royeen, C. B., & Lane, S. J. [1991]. Tactile processing and sensory defensiveness. In A. G. Fisher, E. A. Murray, & A. C. Bundy [Eds.], *Sensory integration: Theory and practice.* Philadelphia: F.A. Davis.)

underlying neural functions.[66,134] This idea contributed to the continuum model. Experts soon found that this simple continuum model did not adequately address the complexity of child behaviors, however. For example, Royeen and Lane hypothesized that the relationship between underresponsiveness and overresponsiveness may be circular instead of linear, because a child who is extremely defensive may be overloaded to the point of shutting down and becoming underresponsive.[134] Previously, we have criticized the continuum model as overly simplistic because sensory modulation very likely is influenced by the individual's history of personal experiences and interpretation of the situation, as well as interactions among multiple neural systems.[117] Furthermore, individuals who are unusually underresponsive to input from one sensory system may tend to be overresponsive in another system. For example, a child may be overresponsive to touch, but at the same time be underresponsive to vestibular sensations. The continuum model does not account for this phenomenon.

Dunn presented a conceptual model that takes into account the potential roles of various neural processes in generating patterns of underresponsiveness and overresponsiveness (Figure 11-9).[61,63] In her model, four main patterns represent individual differences in sensory responding: low registration, sensation seeking, sensitivity to stimuli, and sensation avoiding. Dunn hypothesized these patterns emerge from individual differences in the neural processes of habituation, sensitization, threshold, and maintenance of homeostasis. The person who falls in the low-registration quadrant of the model is underresponsive due to a high threshold for reactivity and therefore needs to have a high level of intensity in environmental stimuli in order to notice and attend. The person who falls in the sensation-seeking quadrant is also considered underresponsive with a high threshold but expresses this behaviorally by actively seeking out intense sensory input. The sensory sensitivity and sensation-avoiding quadrants represent overresponsive patterns. Individuals who fall in the sensory sensitivity quadrant have heightened awareness of, and are distracted by, sensory stimuli due to a low threshold, but they tend to passively cope with these sensations. In contrast, those who are sensation-avoiding not only have heightened awareness of sensory stimuli but actively attempt to avoid the ordinary sensations that they experience as noxious. One of the most important contributions of this model is that it can be used to consider what kinds

of work and play or leisure environments present an optimal match for an individual's sensory modulation characteristics.[63]

In another model that addresses the complexity of sensory modulation, Miller, Reisman, McIntosh, and Simon differentiate between physiologic and behavioral elements of what they call *sensory modulation disorders* (SMDs).[107] Their ecologic model includes both external and internal dimensions affecting sensory modulation (Figure 11-10). External dimensions identified are culture, environment, relationships, and tasks, whereas internal dimensions are sensory processing, emotion, and attention. The external dimensions highlight the importance of context, whereas the internal dimensions focus on enduring differences among individuals. In this model, external and internal dimensions are interlinked through multidirectional, rather than linear, relationships and must be viewed together to design interventions for children with SMDs.

These models of sensory modulation help us to organize the complex information relevant to understanding children with difficulties in overresponding or underresponding to sensory information in everyday situations. Many unanswered questions about modulation remain. For example, some research indicates that many children frequently demonstrate behavioral characteristics of both underresponding and overresponding, often within the same sensory system.[86] This may be particularly the case for children with autism.[87,148] Existing models do not yet do an adequate job of explaining these phenomena. Nevertheless, these models are important because they provide a foundation upon which research programs can be built to explicate the complex issues that are involved. Today, research on patterns of sensory modulation and their manifestations in everyday activities is an area of focused investigation in occupational therapy.[28,67,107] In addition, the relationship between physiologic measures and patterns of behavior that characterize sensory modulation problems continues to be explored—for example, through studies of brain electrical activity[57] and autonomic responses[106,137] to sensory input.

Although there remains much to learn about sensory modulation, a general consensus exists among sensory integration experts regarding the behaviors that characterize different kinds of sensory modulation difficulties. These behaviors are described next.

Sensory Registration Problems

As noted previously in this chapter, sensory integration is the "organization of sensory input for use" (p. 184).[18] However, before sensory information can be used functionally, it must be registered within the CNS. When the CNS is working well, it knows when to "pay attention" to a stimulus and when to "ignore" it. Most of the time, this process occurs automatically and efficiently. For example, a student may not be aware of the noise of traffic outside the window of a classroom while listening to a lecture, instead focusing attention on the sound of the lecturer's words. In this situation, the student registers the auditory stimuli generated by the lecturer but not the stimuli generated by the traffic. The process of sensory registration is critical in enabling efficient function so that people pay attention to those stimuli that enable them to accomplish desired goals. Simultaneously, if the process is working well, energy is not wasted attending to irrelevant sensory information.

Thresholds/Reactivity	Responding/Self-Regulation Strategies	
	Passive	Active
High	Low Registration	Sensory Seeking
Low	Sensory Sensitivity	Sensory Avoiding

FIGURE 11-9 Dunn's Model of Sensory Processing. (Adapted from Dunn, W. [1997]. The impact of sensory processing abilities on the daily lives of young children and families: A conceptual model. *Infants and Young Children*, 9[4] 23-25.)

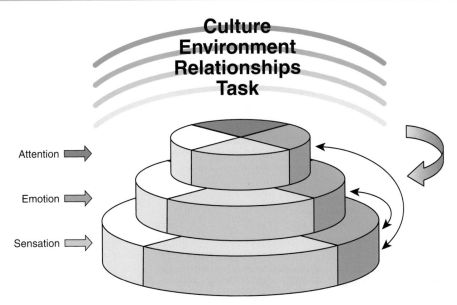

FIGURE 11-10 Miller et al.'s (2001) Ecological Model of Sensory Modulation. *Light shading,* underresponsivity; *medium shading,* normal responsivity (a match between the external and internal dimensions); *dark shading,* overresponsivity; *darkest shading,* lability, severe overresponsivity alternating with severe underresponsivity. (The Ecological Model of Sensory Modulation. Note. From Roley, S. S., Blanch, E. I., Scharr, R. C. (2001). *Understanding the nature of sensory integration with diverse populations* (p. 61). Austin, TX: PRO-ED. Copyright 2001 by PRO-ED, Inc., Reprinted with permission.)

Traditionally, occupational therapists, beginning with Ayres,[18] have used the term *sensory registration problem* to refer to the difficulties of the person who frequently fails to attend to or register relevant environmental stimuli. This kind of problem is often seen in individuals with autism, but it may also be seen in other individuals with developmental problems. When a sensory registration problem is present, the child often seems oblivious to touch, pain, movement, taste, smells, sights, or sounds. Usually more than one sensory system is involved, but for some children one system may be particularly affected. Sometimes the same child who does not register relevant stimuli may be overfocused on irrelevant stimuli; this is commonly seen with autism. It is also common for children with severe developmental problems, such as autism, to lack sensory registration in some situations but react with extreme sensory defensiveness in other situations.

Safety concerns are frequently an important issue among children with sensory registration problems. For example, the child who does not register pain sensations has not learned that certain actions naturally lead to negative consequences, such as pain, and therefore may not withdraw adequately from dangerous situations. Instead of avoiding situations likely to result in pain, the child may repeatedly engage in activities that may be injurious, such as jumping from a dangerous height onto a hard surface or touching a hot object. Other children with sensory registration problems may not register noxious tastes and smells that warn of hazards. Similarly, sights and sounds such as sirens, flashing lights, firm voice commands, and hand signals or signs that are meant to warn of perils go unheeded if not registered.

This can be a life-endangering problem in some circumstances (e.g., when a child steps in front of a moving car).

A sensory registration problem interferes with the child's ability to attach meaning to an activity or situation. Consequently, in severe cases, the child lacks the inner drive that compels most children to master ordinary childhood occupations (e.g., the child who is generally unmotivated to engage in play activities or to practice skills). Therefore the long-term effects on the child's development can be profound.

Sensation-Seeking Behavior

Some children register sensations, but may be "underresponsive" to the incoming stimuli. These children seem to seek intense stimulation in the sensory modalities that are affected. The child who is hyporesponsive to vestibular stimuli may seek large quantities of intense stimulation when introduced to suspended equipment in a clinic setting. This child registers the vestibular sensations and usually shows signs of pleasure from the sensations, but the input does not affect the nervous system to the extent that it does for most other children. The underresponsive child may not become dizzy or show the expected autonomic responses to stimulation that is so intense it would be overwhelming for most peers. This is called *hyporesponsivity* because it refers to the underlying mode of sensory processing rather than to observable motor behavior. Although the child may appear to be active motorically, the child is not reacting to intense vestibular stimuli to the degree that most children do. In everyday settings, these children often appear to be restless, motorically driven, and thrill seeking.

Some children seem to seek greater than average amounts of proprioceptive input. Typically these children often seek active resistance to muscles, deep touch pressure stimulation, or joint compression and traction (e.g., by stomping instead of walking; intentionally falling or bumping into objects, including other people; or pushing against large objects). They may tend to use strong ballistic movements such as throwing objects forcefully. Some of these children may not seem to register the positions of body parts unless intense proprioceptive stimulation is present.

Some children who seek large amounts of proprioceptive input demonstrate signs of tactile defensiveness or gravitational insecurity. Because proprioception is thought to have an inhibitory effect on tactile and vestibular sensations, these children may be seeking increased proprioceptive input in order to help themselves modulate the overwhelming touch and movement sensations that they often experience.

The behaviors generated by sensation-seeking children may be disruptive or inappropriate in social situations. Safety issues frequently are of paramount concern, and often these children are labeled as having social or behavioral problems. A challenge for the occupational therapist working with these children may be to identify strategies by which they can receive the high levels of stimulation that they seek without being socially disruptive, inappropriate, or dangerous to themselves or others.

Overresponsiveness

At the opposite end of the sensory modulation continuum are problems associated with overresponsiveness, sometimes called *hyperresponsivity* or *sensory defensiveness*. The child who is overresponsive is overwhelmed by ordinary sensory input and reacts defensively to it, often with strong negative emotion and activation of the sympathetic nervous system. This condition may occur as a general response to all types of sensory input, or it may be specific to one or a few sensory systems.

The term *sensory defensiveness* was first introduced by Knickerbocker[84] and later used by Wilbarger and Wilbarger[152] to describe sensory modulation disorders involving multisensory systems. Sensory modulation problems include overreactions to touch, movement, sounds, odors, and tastes, any of which may create discomfort, avoidance, distractibility, and anxiety. Most of the research-based and clinical knowledge regarding overresponsiveness is related to the tactile and vestibular systems.

Tactile Defensiveness

Tactile defensiveness involves a tendency to overreact to ordinary touch sensations.[4,11,18] It is one of the most commonly observed sensory integrative disorders involving sensory modulation. Individuals with tactile defensiveness experience irritation and discomfort from sensations that most people do not find bothersome. Light touch sensations are especially likely to be disturbing. Common irritants include certain textures of clothing, grass or sand against bare skin, glue or paint on the skin, the light brush of another person passing by, the sensations generated when having one's hair or teeth brushed, and certain textures of food. Common responses to such irritants include anxiety, distractibility, restlessness, anger, throwing a tantrum, aggression, fear, and emotional distress.

Common self-care activities such as dressing, bathing, grooming, and eating are often affected by tactile defensiveness. Classroom activities such as finger painting, sand and water play, and crafts may be avoided. Social situations involving close proximity to others, such as playing near other children or standing in line, tend to be uncomfortable and may be disturbing enough to lead to emotional outbursts. Thus, ordinary daily routines can become traumatic for children with tactile defensiveness and for their parents. Teachers and friends are likely to misinterpret the child with tactile defensiveness as being rejecting, aggressive, or simply negative.

It is difficult for individuals with tactile defensiveness to cope with the fact that others do not share their discomforts and may actually enjoy situations that they find so upsetting. For a child with this disorder, who may not be able to verbalize or even recognize the problem, the accompanying feelings of anxiety and frustration can be overwhelming and the influence on functional behavior is likely to be significant.

An occupational therapist working with a child who is tactually defensive must become aware of the specific kinds of tactile input that are aversive and the kinds that are tolerated well by that particular child. Usually light touch stimuli are aversive, especially when they occur in the most sensitive body areas such as the face, abdomen, and palmar surfaces of the upper and lower extremities. Generally, tactile stimuli that are actively self-applied by the child are tolerated much better than stimuli that are passively received, as when being touched by another person. Tactile stimuli may be especially threatening if the child cannot see the source of the touch. Most individuals with tactile defensiveness feel comfortable with deep touch stimuli and may experience relief from irritating stimuli when deep pressure is applied over the involved skin areas.

Knowledge of these characteristics of tactile defensiveness helps the occupational therapist identify strategies that help the child and others who interact with the child to cope with this condition. For example, the occupational therapist may recommend to the teacher that if the child needs to be touched, it should be done with firm pressure in the child's view, rather than with a light touch from behind the child.

Gravitational Insecurity

Gravitational insecurity is a form of overresponsiveness to vestibular sensations, particularly sensations from the otolith organs, which detect linear movement through space and the pull of gravity.[18] Children with this problem have an insecure relationship to gravity characterized by excessive fear during ordinary movement activities. The gravitationally insecure child is overwhelmed by changes in head position and movement, especially when moving backward or upward through space. Fear of heights, even those involving only slight distances from the ground, is a common problem associated with this condition.

Children who display gravitational insecurity often show signs of inordinate fear, anxiety, or avoidance in relation to stairs, escalators or elevators, moving or high pieces of playground equipment, and uneven or unpredictable surfaces. Some children are so insecure that only a small change from one surface to another, as when stepping off the curb or from the sidewalk to the grass, is enough to send them into a state of high anxiety or panic.

Common reactions of children with gravitational insecurity include extreme fearfulness during low-intensity movement or when anticipating movement and avoidance of tilting the head in different planes (especially backward). They tend to move slowly and carefully, and they may refuse to participate in many gross motor activities. When they do engage in movement activities such as swinging, many of these children refuse to lift their feet off the ground. When threatened by simple motor activities, they may try to gain as much contact with the ground as possible or they may tightly clutch a nearby adult for security. These children often have signs of poor proprioception in addition to the vestibular overresponsiveness. May-Benson and Koomar developed a Gravitational Insecurity (GI) Assessment and found that scores on this standardized tool, which involves activities such as performing a backward roll and stepping off a chair with eyes closed, significantly discriminated between children with gravitational insecurity and typical children.[101]

Playground and park activities are often difficult for children with gravitational insecurity, as are other common childhood activities such as bicycle riding, ice skating, roller skating, skateboarding, skiing, and hiking. Ability to play with peers and to explore the environment is therefore significantly affected. Functioning in the community may also be affected when the child needs to use escalators, stairs, and elevators.

A distinction may be made between gravitational insecurity and a similar condition called *postural insecurity*. Postural insecurity was the term Ayres originally used to refer to all children with fears related to movement. Later, however, she hypothesized that some children moved slowly and displayed fears of movement not because of a hyperresponsivity to vestibular input but because they lacked adequate motor control to perform many activities without falling. The fears of these children, then, seemed to be based on a learned, realistic appraisal of their motor limitations. The term *posturally insecure* is used to refer to these children.

Often it is difficult to discern whether a child's anxiety is based on sensory overresponsivity or limited motor control because these two conditions can, and often do, coexist in the same child. Sometimes, however, the distinction is clear. Children with mild spastic diplegia, for example, commonly have postural but not gravitational insecurity. These children typically (and appropriately) react with anxiety when faced with a minimal climbing task; however, they may show pleasure at receiving vestibular stimulation, including having the head radically tilted in different planes so long as they are securely held and do not have to rely on their own motor skills to maintain a safe position.

Overresponsiveness in Other Sensory Modalities

Hyperresponsivities in other sensory systems can also have a significant influence on a person's life. For example, overreactions to sounds, odors, and tastes are often problematic for children with heightened sensitivities. These types of problems, like overresponsiveness to touch and movement, may create discomfort, avoidance, distractibility, and anxiety. Most people interpret the raucous sounds found at birthday parties, parades, playgrounds, and carnivals as happy sounds, but these can be overwhelming to a child with auditory defensiveness. A visually busy and unfamiliar environment may evoke an unusual degree of anxiety in a child with visual defensiveness. Similarly, the variety of tastes and odors encountered in some environments may be disturbing to a child with overresponsivity in these systems.

Sensory Discrimination and Perception Problems

Sensory discrimination and perception allow for refined organization and interpretation of sensory stimuli. Some types of sensory integrative disorders involve inefficient or inaccurate organization of sensory information (e.g., difficulty differentiating one stimulus from another or difficulty perceiving the spatial or temporal relationships among stimuli). A classic example involving the visual system is that of the older child with a learning disability who persists in confusing a *b* with a *d*. A child with an auditory discrimination problem may be unable to distinguish between the sounds of the words *doll* and *tall*. A child with a tactile perception problem may not be able to distinguish between a square block and a hexagonal block using touch only, without visual cues.

Some children with perceptual problems have no difficulty with sensory modulation. However, modulation problems often coexist with perceptual problems. It makes sense that these two types of problems are associated. A child who often does not register stimuli probably has a deficit in perceptual skills because of a lack of experience interacting with sensory information. Conversely, the child who has sensory defensiveness may exert a lot of energy trying to avoid certain sensory experiences. Defensive reactions may make it difficult to attend to the detailed features of a stimulus and thereby may impede perception.

Discrimination or perception problems can occur in any sensory system. They are best detected by standardized tests, except in the case of proprioception, which is difficult to measure in a standardized manner. Discrimination or perception problems can occur in any sensory system. They are best detected by standardized tests, except in the case of proprioception, which is difficult to measure in a standardized manner. Although most factor analytic studies of the SIPT test scores revealed patterns that linked sensory perception with motor functions, certain patterns reflected specific sensory perception factors (e.g., a visual form and space perception factor or a tactile perception factor, as well as a somatosensory perception factor). Professionals in many fields, such as neuropsychology, special education, and speech language pathology, are trained to evaluate perceptual problems, and their focus usually is on the visual and auditory systems. In contrast, occupational therapists are unique in their understanding of the functional relevance of lesser known areas of sensory perception such as tactile, kinesthetic, and vestibular sensory processing.

Tactile Discrimination and Perception Problems

Poor tactile perception is one of the most common sensory integrative disorders. Children with this disorder have difficulty interpreting tactile stimuli in a precise and efficient manner. For example, they may have difficulty localizing precisely where an object has brushed against them or using stereognosis to manipulate an object that is out of sight. Fine motor skills are likely to suffer when a tactile perception problem is present, especially if tactile defensiveness is also present.[44]

As discussed previously, the tactile system is a critical modality for learning during infancy and early childhood. Tactile exploration using the hands and mouth is particularly important. If tactile perception is vague or inaccurate, the child is at a disadvantage in learning about the different properties of objects and substances. It may be difficult for a child with such problems to develop the manipulative skills needed to efficiently perform tasks such as connecting pieces of constructional toys, fastening buttons or snaps, braiding hair, or playing marbles. Inadequate tactile perception also interferes with the feedback that is normally used to precisely guide motor tasks such as writing with a pencil, manipulating a spoon, or holding a piece of paper with one hand while cutting with the other.

Tactile perception is associated with visual perception[24]; thus, it is fairly common to see children with problems in both of these sensory systems. Not surprisingly, these children tend to have concomitant problems with hand–eye coordination. A discrete somatosensory perception factor emerged as a pattern in analyses of the SIPT,[21] but a more striking finding in the factor analytic studies of sensory integration tests over many decades was the link between tactile perception and motor planning, which recurred in many different studies.[5-7,9,10,16,24,111] These findings led Ayres to hypothesize that tactile perception is an important contributor to the ability to plan actions. She speculated that the tactile system is responsible for the development of body scheme, which then becomes an important foundation for praxis.

Ordinarily, tactile perception operates at such an automatic level that, when it is impaired, compensation strategies take a great deal of energy. An example of this is that of the child who cannot make the subtle manipulations needed to fasten a button without looking at it. Because this child needs to use compensatory visual guidance, the task of buttoning, which is usually performed rapidly and automatically, becomes tedious, tiring, and frustrating. The necessity of using such compensatory strategies throughout the day tends to interrupt the child's ability to focus on the more complex conceptual and social elements of tasks and situations.

Proprioception Problems

Another type of perceptual problem involves proprioception, which arises from the muscles and joints to inform the brain about the position of body parts. This is a difficult area to research because direct standardized measures of proprioception are not available. However, the experience of many master clinicians suggests that many children have serious difficulties interpreting proprioceptive information.

Children who do not receive reliable information about body position often appear clumsy, distracted, and awkward. As with poor tactile perception, these children must often rely on visual cues or other cognitive strategies (e.g., use of verbalizations) to perform simple aspects of tasks, such as staying in a chair or using a fork correctly. Other common attributes of children with poor proprioception include using too much or too little force in activities such as writing, clapping, marching, or typing. Breaking toys, bumping into others, and misjudging personal space are other consequences of poor proprioception that which have strong social implications.

Many children thought to have proprioception problems seek firm pressure to their skin or joint compression and traction. These sensation-seeking behaviors may be an attempt to gain additional feedback about body position, or they may reflect a concomitant hyporesponsiveness to tactile and proprioceptive sensations. In any case, if these behaviors are done in socially inappropriate ways or at inopportune times, such as leaning on another child during circle time or hanging from a doorway at school, the child's behavior may be misinterpreted as being willfully disruptive.

Visual Perception Problems

Visual perception is an important factor in the competent performance of many constructional play activities and fine motor tasks. Early factor analyses of sensory integration test scores revealed a form and space perception factor. Tests are available to measure figure-ground perception, spatial orientation, depth perception, and visual closure, to name just a few of the many aspects of visual perception that have been of concern to professionals in many disciplines.

Problems with visual perception are commonly seen in children with sensory integrative disorders, particularly when poor tactile perception or dyspraxia is present.[21,24] Whereas some children have only a specific visual perception problem without any other sign of a sensory integrative dysfunction, many others have difficulties in visual perceptual abilities as a component of broader sensory integration difficulties. Henderson, Pehoski, and Murray point out the many relationships between visual spatial abilities and functions such as grasp, balance, locomotion, construction, and cognition.[73] As these authors note, low scores on tests of visual perception can occur for a variety of reasons and in some cases will represent a problem that therapists would not view as reflective of a sensory integrative issue.

A sensory integrative treatment approach, as described later in this chapter, may be appropriate for the child who demonstrates visual perception problems along with other indicators of sensory integrative difficulties, such as poor tactile perception or praxis. A sensory integration approach may not be appropriate for children who show discrete visual perceptual problems. When other sensory integration issues are not present or have been resolved with intervention, the occupational therapist may choose to work with the child using another treatment approach, such as visual perception training, use of compensatory strategies, or skill training in specific activities.

Other Perceptual Problems

Many other dimensions of perception and sensory discrimination exist. For example, perception of movement through space involves the integration of vestibular, proprioceptive, and visual integration and may be affected in children with vestibular-proprioceptive problems. Auditory perception is an important function that may, when impaired, contribute to sensory integrative disorders in some children. Central auditory processing disorders recently have received increasing attention in the literature, and some authors have suggested that more attention should be given to the role of the auditory system in the sensory integration literature.[41] However, since so much of the function of the auditory system is related to the functions of hearing, speech, and language, this area of study in sensory integration may be most appropriately pursued in collaboration with speech–language pathologists and audiologists. Although auditory perception problems are not usually considered to be a type of sensory integrative dysfunction when seen in isolation, difficulties with auditory perception and language development often coexist with signs of sensory integrative dysfunction. The relationship between these processes warrants further research.

Vestibular-Proprioceptive Problems

In her research, Ayres identified a pattern of problems thought to reflect inefficient central vestibular processing. Clinical signs related to this type of problem involve the motor functions that are outcomes of vestibular processing, such as poor equilibrium reactions and low muscle tone, particularly of the extensor muscles, which are strongly influenced by the vestibular system. These disorders are assessed using informal and formal clinical observations and standardized test scores.

Different names have been applied to vestibular processing problems at different points in time because of the changing patterns of research findings. In her early factor analytic studies, Ayres identified a linkage between postural-ocular mechanisms and integration of the two sides of the body. Clinically, she called the related dysfunction a disorder in *postural and bilateral integration*, and she noted that it often occurred in children with learning disabilities, especially those with reading disorders.[11] Additional problems commonly seen in this disorder include low muscle tone, immature righting and equilibrium reactions, poor right-left discrimination, and lack of clearly defined hand dominance.

Later in the 1970s, Ayres included the Southern California Postrotary Nystagmus Test (SCPNT) in her research as a more specific measure of vestibular processing.[14] This test continues to be used and is part of the SIPT. Based on analysis of SCPNT scores, Ayres identified a vestibular processing component to the postural and bilateral integration (PBI) disorder.[17] At this point she replaced the old PBI concept with the term *vestibular-bilateral integration (VBI)* disorder. One of the main characteristics of this problem was depressed postrotary nystagmus scores, suggesting inefficient central processing of vestibular input. Also characteristic were other signs of vestibular-related dysfunction, such as low muscle tone, postural-ocular deficits, and diminished balance and equilibrium reactions. In addition, poor bilateral coordination was implicated in VBI disorder.

Factor and cluster analyses using the SIPT led to further evolution of the concept of vestibular processing disorders. The SIPT studies identified a *bilateral integration and sequencing (BIS)* factor characterized by poor bilateral coordination and difficulty sequencing actions, which Ayres proposed was influenced primarily by vestibular functioning.[21] Building on Ayres ideas, Fisher suggested that poor vestibular-proprioceptive processing is the basis for a type of sensory integrative dysfunction characterized by poor bilateral integration and sequencing.[68] She used the term *vestibular-proprioceptive* to emphasize that these two sensory systems work so closely together that their functions are intertwined.

In addition, Fisher introduced an interesting new concept in relation to the BIS pattern: the notion of *projected action sequences*.[68] To perform a projected action sequence, the child anticipates how to move as his or her spatial relationship to the environment changes, as when running to kick a ball or catching a moving ball. Fisher suggested that difficulty with projected action sequences is related to poor vestibular-proprioceptive processing, and, furthermore, that such deficits are a form of motor planning disorder. Thus, Fisher proposed a formal link between vestibular processing and praxis through the production of bilateral and sequenced movements.

Following Fisher's work, other experts recently addressed the BIS pattern as a mild form of praxis disorder that generally is associated with vestibular-proprioceptive difficulties and characterized by problems with bilateral coordination as well as anticipatory actions.[39,85,125] These authors also acknowledged that there may be a subset of children with BIS problems who do not have sensory integrative difficulties, in much the same way that children with isolated visual or auditory perception problems are not thought to have a sensory integration disorder.

Despite the variety of ways that have been used to describe vestibular-proprioceptive problems, certain classic clinical signs are common to all. In general, many children with these problems do not have a severe level of dysfunction, so the problem is easy to overlook. These children often exhibit poor equilibrium reactions, lower than average muscle tone (particularly in extensor muscles), poor postural stability, a tendency toward slouching, and difficulty in keeping the head upright. Inefficiency of the vestibularocular pathways may adversely affect function in directing head and eye movements while moving, as when watching a rolling soccer ball while running to kick it. Impaired balance and equilibrium reactions are likely to affect competence in performing activities such as bicycle riding, roller-skating, skiing, and playing games like hopscotch. Poor bilateral integration interferes with these activities as well. In addition, poor bilateral integration makes activities such as cutting with scissors, buttoning a shirt, or doing jumping jacks especially challenging. Bilateral integration difficulties are sometimes manifested in delays in body midline skill development, such as hand preference, spontaneous crossing of the body midline, and right-left discrimination. Neural connections between the vestibular centers in the brainstem and the reticular activating system also put children with vestibular processing disorders at risk for problems with attention, organization of behavior, communication, and modulation of arousal.

Praxis Problems

Praxis is the ability to conceptualize, plan, and execute a non-habitual motor act.[18] Problems with praxis are often referred to as *dyspraxia*. When the term *dyspraxia* is used in regard to children, it usually refers to a condition characterized by difficulty with praxis that cannot be explained by a medical diagnosis or developmental disability and that occurs despite ordinary environmental opportunities for motor experiences. When Ayres originally wrote about dyspraxia, she used the term *developmental apraxia*.[11] However, because the term *apraxia* is often associated with brain damage in adults, she later replaced this term with *developmental dyspraxia*.[18,20] The prefix *developmental* implies that the condition emerges in early childhood development and is not the result of traumatic injury.

As noted previously, Ayres was struck with the relationship between tactile perception and praxis that emerged in study after study. She hypothesized that good tactile perception contributes to development of an accurate and precise body scheme, which serves as a reservoir of knowledge to be drawn on in planning new actions. Her interest in praxis appeared to grow over time, as is evident in the number of praxis tests included in the SIPT as opposed to the older SCSIT. When Ayres discussed praxis in relation to her SIPT studies, she introduced the idea that praxis problems may be manifested in different forms, not all of which are sensory integrative in nature.[21] She coined the term *somatopraxis* to refer to the aspect of praxis that is sensory integrative in origin and grounded in somatosensory processing. At the same time she introduced the term *somatodyspraxia* to refer to a sensory integrative deficit that involves poor praxis and impaired tactile and proprioceptive processing. By definition, somatodyspraxia involves a disorder in tactile discrimination and perception. Cermak noted that not all children with developmental dyspraxia demonstrate poor tactile perception.[47] The term *somatodyspraxia* applies only to those who do.

The child with somatodyspraxia typically appears clumsy and awkward. Novel motor activities are performed with great difficulty and often result in failure. Transitioning from one body position to another or sequencing and timing the actions involved in a motor task may pose a great challenge. These children typically have difficulty relating their bodies to physical objects in environmental space. They often have difficulty accurately imitating actions of others. Directionality of movement may be disturbed, resulting in unintentional breakage of toys when the child forcefully pushes an object that should be pulled. Many of these children have difficulties with oral praxis, which may affect eating skills or speech articulation.

Some children with dyspraxia have problems with *ideation* (i.e., they have difficulty generating ideas of what to do in a novel situation). When asked to simply play, without being given specific directions, these children may not initiate any activity or they may initiate activity that is habitual and limited or seems to lack a goal. Typical responses may include are to wander aimlessly; to perform simple repetitive actions such as patting or pushing objects around; to randomly pile up objects with no apparent plan; or for the more sophisticated child, to wait to observe others doing an activity and then imitate them rather than initiating an activity independently. May-Benson expanded on the role of ideation in praxis, highlighting the role of language and the social environment and reviewing the neuroanatomic foundations for this important function.[99]

For children with dyspraxia, skills that most children attain rather easily can be excessively challenging (e.g., donning a sweater, feeding oneself with utensils, writing the alphabet, jumping rope, completing a puzzle). These skills can be mastered only with high motivation on the part of the child, coupled with a great deal of practice, far more than most children require. Participation in sports is often embarrassing and frustrating, and organization of schoolwork may be a problem of particular concern. Children who have somatodyspraxia and are aware of their deficits often avoid difficult motor challenges and may attempt to gain control over such situations by assuming a directing or controlling role over others.

Praxis is best evaluated using the SIPT, which is sensitive to difficulties in this area. However, parent interview and informal observations provide critical pieces in the assessment process. These are essential in evaluating ideation because currently available standardized tests on large normative samples are extremely limited in their measurement of this aspect of praxis. The new Test of Ideational Praxis is promising as a standardized, objective means for assessing ideation.[100]

Secondary Problems Related to Sensory Integrative Difficulties

As already shown, sensory integration difficulties often impose some limitation on the quality of the child's participation in occupations that he or she wants or needs to do as a member of a family, classroom, or community. How others respond to the child's struggles may have a powerful effect on the child's developing competence. In addition, the child's willingness to grapple with challenging experiences will influence his or her occupational life over the years.[114] Unfortunately, a number of secondary problems often arise in conjunction with sensory integration problems. These secondary problems may actually have a more powerful impact on the child's life outcomes than the original sensory integration difficulty. In some cases, what started out as a minor sensory integration difficulty can become magnified into a major barrier to life satisfaction. Following is an explanation of several of these indirect, but significant, influences on the child and family.

First, sensory integrative dysfunction is an "invisible" disability (i.e., not directly and easily detected by the casual observer) that is easily misinterpreted. Sensory integrative disorders can fluctuate in severity from one time to another within the same child. Moreover, the severity of dysfunction and the ways in which dysfunction is expressed vary tremendously from one individual to another. This variability makes it difficult to predict which situations cause problems for a particular child, how much discomfort results, and when distress is likely to occur. Parents and teachers of children with these disorders often find the unpredictability of the child's behavior to be frustrating and difficult to understand. As a result, sensory integrative problems are frequently misinterpreted as purely behavioral or psychological issues. Consequently, the child may be punished or responded to inappropriately, which may lead to chronic feelings of hopelessness as the child develops a self-view as bad or incapable.

A second indirect effect of sensory integrative dysfunction on the child's life is its negative influence on skill development secondary to limited participation in childhood occupations. The child who avoids finger painting because of tactile defensiveness or who rarely attempts climbing on the jungle gym because of dyspraxia misses more than these singular experiences. The child also misses experiences that hone underlying functions such as tactile discrimination, hand strength and dexterity, shoulder stability, balance and equilibrium, hand-eye coordination, bilateral coordination, ideation, and motor planning. If the child misses a substantial amount of such experiences over time, the gap between the child's sensorimotor skills and the skills of peers may grow.

In addition to interference with the development of sensorimotor functions, interactions important to the development of communication and social skills may not occur. Thus, some children with sensory integrative disorders may lack the ability to play successfully with peers partly because they have not been able to participate fully in the play occupations in which sensory, motor, cognitive, and social skills emerge and develop. The fear, anxiety, or discomfort that accompanies many everyday situations is also likely to work against the expression of the child's inner drive toward growth-inducing experiences. Therefore lack of experience and diminished drive to participate compound the direct effects of a sensory integrative disorder. Consequently, the development of competence in many domains of development may be seriously compromised.

A third indirect effect of sensory integrative problems is the undermining of self-esteem and self-confidence over time. Children with sensory integrative problems are often aware of their struggles with commonplace tasks, so it is natural for them to react with frustration. Frustration is likely to mount as the child observes peers mastering these same tasks effortlessly. Chronic frustration can negatively affect and detract from the child's feelings of self-efficacy. Instead, the child may develop feelings of helplessness. This leads to further limitations in the child's experiences because the child becomes less likely to attempt challenging activities.

ASSESSMENT OF SENSORY INTEGRATIVE FUNCTIONS

Assessment of sensory integration, like all other areas addressed in occupational therapy, requires a multifaceted approach because of the need to understand presenting problems, not only in relation to the individual who is being assessed but also with respect to the family and environments in which that individual participates. Assessment by the occupational therapist begins with a general exploration of the occupations of the child and family, focusing on their concerns and hopes in relation to the child's strengths and challenges in routine activities. A variety of tools are needed to help the therapist detect problems in sensory integration, to understand the nature and scope of these difficulties, and to decide whether intervention should be recommended. Assessment tools employed by occupational therapists using a sensory integration perspective include interviews and questionnaires, informal and formal observations, standardized tests, and consideration of services and resources available to and appropriate for the family. Roley[127] provided an excellent discussion of how this process of assessment is consistent with the guidelines laid out in the Occupational Therapy Practice Framework.[1]

Interviews and Questionnaires

The need for an occupational therapy assessment of sensory integration usually arises when a parent, teacher, physician, or other person who knows the child notices problems that the child is experiencing that are not easily explained by other conditions or considerations. The referral source, family members, and others who work with the child may all be valuable sources of information through interview or questionnaire (Figure 11-11). This initial phase of evaluation identifies the presenting problems, or main concerns, about the child and begins the process of determining whether sensory integration difficulties might account for the concerns about the child.

The initial interview with the parent, teacher, or other referral source provides an opportunity for the therapist to gather important information about signs of sensory integration problems that may be present. For example, the teacher may report that the child is always fighting while standing in line and cannot seem to stay seated during reading circle time. Further questioning by the therapist may disclose signs of tactile defensiveness that might explain the child's behavior but were not considered by the teacher, who is unfamiliar with this condition. A parent may be able to provide critical information about the child's development, which may be helpful in identifying early signs of sensory integrative dysfunction. For instance, parents may have noticed that specific tasks, such as cutting with scissors or pedaling a tricycle, were especially difficult for the child.

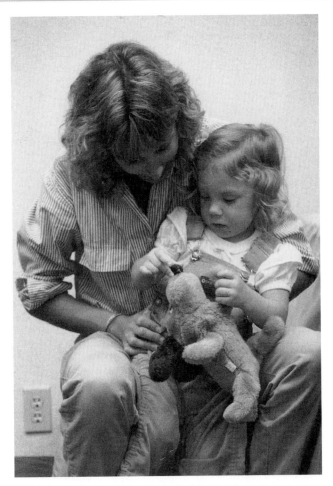

FIGURE 11-11 Because parents know their child better than anyone else, they are invaluable sources of information to the therapist, especially in beginning phases of the assessment process.   (Courtesy Shay McAtee.)

Since difficulty coordinating the two sides of the body is common when vestibular processing difficulties are present, this type of information can inform the therapist about additional observations and tests needed. Another important role of the interview is to uncover alternative explanations of the child's difficulties that may rule out sensory integration problems, such as when a recent emotional crisis (e.g., a divorce or death) coincides with the onset of problems. Miller and Summers provided examples of the kinds of questions to ask in a parent interview.[108]

Questionnaires, checklists, and histories given by caregivers and other adults who know the child well are other means for gathering information that aid in identifying presenting problems, estimating how long they have been a concern, and clarifying the priorities of the family. One such instrument is a sensory history or similar questionnaire. Originally developed by Ayres as an unpublished questionnaire, this type of instrument asks parents questions regarding specific child behaviors indicative of sensory integrative dysfunction, and parents respond by rating the child using a Likert-style scale. These types of questionnaires were subsequently developed using normative samples to produce reliable and valid scores.

The Sensory Profile[62] and the Sensory Processing Measure (SPM)[116] are two sensory questionnaires used extensively in pediatric occupational therapy. The Sensory Profile is available in versions for parents of infants and toddlers[64] and of children in early and middle childhood,[62] as well as for self-reports of adolescents and adults.[36] Additionally, a Sensory Profile School Companion is available for teacher report of child behavior at school.[65] The SPM has two forms, Home[115] and Main Classroom,[109] that are standardized on the same sample of 5- to 12-year-old children and can furnish a score that aids the therapist in discerning whether a child's sensory issues are manifested differently in the contexts of home versus school. In addition, the SPM contains separate rating scales for school personnel other than the main teacher, such as art teacher, music teacher, or bus driver.

An additional way to gather information in the initial phases of assessment is through review of records, including previous reports from other professionals as well as educational and medical histories. It is useful to talk with the child directly when possible. Royeen and Fortune developed a child questionnaire for the assessment of tactile defensiveness, called the Touch Inventory for Elementary School–Aged Children (TIE).[133,134] Children with sufficient verbal skills to discuss their own abilities, perceptions, and difficulties can sometimes provide invaluable insight into their condition through such a questionnaire-based interview. The Alert Program, a group intervention program for older children and adults, includes a self-assessment of sensory preferences that can be adapted for assessment of younger children to help them identify and communicate their characteristic sensory responses.[154]

The information garnered through the initial interview process is used to decide whether further assessment is warranted and, if so, which evaluation procedures are most appropriate. This information is also critical in interpreting the final pool of information gathered through assessment and in prioritizing goals for the child in light of the main concerns of the family.

Informal and Formal Observations of the Child

Direct observation of the child is essential to the evaluation of sensory integration. Informal observations, clinical observations, and standardized testing are commonly used.

Informal Observations

Informal observation of the child in natural settings, such as a classroom, playground, or home, is informative and helpful whenever feasible. Informal observation will influence the conclusion as to whether a sensory integrative disorder is present and will, perhaps more importantly, indicate how the child's difficulties are interfering with daily occupations. For example, an experienced therapist can often detect signs of poor body awareness by observing the child at school. Such signs may include exerting too much pressure on a pencil, standing too close to classmates in line, poor foot placement when climbing on a jungle gym, or sitting in an ineffective position in a chair while doing class assignments. Teachers may not necessarily report these behaviors to the therapist if they perceive them as typical signs of inattentiveness or clumsiness.

Informal observation of the child in the clinical setting can also be useful in showing how the child responds to situations that are novel or unpredictable. A child with dyspraxia may have a great deal of difficulty problem-solving how to mount an unfamiliar climbing structure in the clinic, even though performance is adequate on similar tasks at home or at school, where the child has practiced them. The novelty of the clinical therapy room elicits responses from children that may be diagnostically relevant. For children with good ideation and sensory processing abilities, the endless opportunities afforded by sensory integration equipment in the clinic can be exhilarating. For the child with a disorder like dyspraxia, the same environment may be confusing, puzzling, or frustrating. A child with gravitational insecurity may be terrified by the prospect of equipment that moves, whereas a child with autism may be distressed by the clinic environment because of its unpredictability and discrepancy from familiar settings. Parham has provided some guidelines for organizing informal observations in the clinic, with special attention to issues related to praxis.[113] Although her suggestions are focused on the assessment of preschoolers, they can also be applied to older children and may be particularly helpful in evaluating older children who are unable to cooperate with standardized testing. Roley[128] and Windsor, Roley, and Szklut[158] provide additional guidelines for assessing praxis through informal observations.

Clinical Observations

Formal observations that are highly structured and similar to test items are often used in an occupational therapy assessment of sensory integration. Usually referred to as *clinical observations,* these typically involve a set of specific procedures that allow the therapist to observe signs of nervous system integrity that are associated with sensory integrative functioning. Ayres included measures of such formal observations in her factor analytic studies, along with standardized tests.[5-9,13,16] She also developed a set of clinical observations that she used in clinical practice. These unpublished, nonstandardized evaluation tools were intended to supplement standardized test scores and subsequently were revised, expanded upon, and studied by many other therapists over the years.[32,38,157] Examples of some of the most commonly used clinical observations are presented in Box 11-1.

One of the difficulties in using clinical observations as an assessment tool is that often the administration and scoring criteria have not been standardized. This means that they are administered using different procedures from one clinician to another. Furthermore, most of them lack normative data to aid in interpretation of the scores obtained. Some, but not all, clinical observations are supported by research using standardized administration to inform interpretation.[71,91,100,101,157]

Occupational therapists must rely on the information from these studies, as well as their personal expertise and judgment, to interpret the results of clinical observations. Without the requisite data in hand, occupational therapists are cautioned to avoid overinterpretation of clinical observations in light of the lack of standardized procedures and inadequate information regarding expected performance across age, gender, and other demographically related groups.

Most clinical observations address motor functions that may be strongly affected by conditions other than sensory

BOX 11-1   Examples of Commonly Used Clinical Observations

Crossing body midline: A movement that has a tendency to occur when using the hand to reach for or manipulate an object in contralateral space. This tendency typically emerges during toddlerhood and early childhood and is related to the development of hand preference. Delays in midline crossing may be related to inadequate hand preference and bilateral integration.

Equilibrium reactions: Automatic postural and limb adjustments that occur when the body's center of gravity shifts its base of support. These adjustments serve to restore the body's center of gravity over its base of support so that balance is maintained or restored. Difficulties with equilibrium reactions are associated with vestibular processing problems.

Muscle tone: The readiness of a muscle to contract. Force with which a muscle resists being lengthened.

Prone extension: Ability to assume and hold an "airplane" position (neck, upper body, and hips extended to lift head, arms, and legs off the floor) while lying prone. Difficulty maintaining this position for 30 seconds is related to inefficient vestibular processing in children 6 years of age and older.

Supine flexion: Ability to assume and hold a curled position (neck, upper body, hips, and knees flexed so that knees are drawn close to the head) while lying supine. Difficulty maintaining this position for 30 seconds is related to poor praxis in children 6 years of age and older.

TABLE 11-3   Functions Measured by the Sensory Integration and Praxis Tests

Function	Description
Space visualization	Motor-free visual space perception; mental manipulation of objects
Figure-ground perception	Motor-free visual perception of figures on a rival background
Manual form perception	Identification of block held in hand with visual counterpart or with block held in other hand
Kinesthesia	Somatic perception of hand and arm position and movement
Finger identification	Tactile perception of individual fingers
Graphesthesia	Tactile perception and practic replication of designs
Localization of tactile stimuli	Tactile perception of specific stimulus applied to arm or hand
Praxis on verbal command	Ability to motor-plan body postures on the basis of verbal directions without visual cures
Design copying	Visuopractic ability to copy simple and complex two-dimensional designs, and the manner or approach one uses to copy designs
Constructional praxis	Ability to relate objects to each other in three-dimensional space
Postural praxis	Ability to plan and execute body movements and positions
Oral praxis	Ability to plan and execute lip, tongue, and jaw movements
Sequencing praxis	Ability to repeat a series of hand and finger movements
Bilateral motor coordination	Ability to move both hands and both feet in a smooth and integrated pattern
Standing and walking balance	Static and dynamic balance on one or both feet with eyes opened and closed
Motor accuracy	Hand-eye coordination and control of movement
Postrotary nystagmus	Central nervous system processing of vestibular input assessed through observation of the duration and integrity of a vestibulo-ocular reflex

From Mailloux, Z. (1990). An overview of the Sensory Integration and Praxis Tests. *American Journal of Occupational Therapy, 44,* 589-594.

integration problems. Therefore, the therapist must use sound clinical reasoning with advanced knowledge of sensory integration theory in order to appropriately interpret these observations.

Standardized Testing

Occupational therapists frequently use standardized tests to evaluate sensory integration. Although several tests are available that contribute incidental information regarding sensory integrative functions, the SIPT protocol is the only set of standardized tests designed specifically for in-depth evaluation of sensory integration. The SIPT evolved from a series of tests that Ayres developed in the 1960s[3,4,6,7,18] and later published as the SCSIT[12] and the SCPNT.[14] The standardization process used in the development of the SIPT was rigorous, involving normative data on approximately 2000 children in North America and extensive reliability and validity studies.[21] Its 17 tests measure tactile, vestibular, and proprioceptive sensory processing; form and space perception and visuomotor coordination; bilateral integration and sequencing abilities; and praxis.[25] A list of the 17 tests and the functions measured by each is presented in Table 11-3.

The SIPT protocol requires about 1½ to 2 hours to administer and another 30 to 45 minutes to score. Raw scores may be translated into standard scores by the therapist using a computer diskette available from the publisher. Alternatively, raw scores may be sent to the publisher, Western Psychological Services, for an analysis using the normative data. After normative scores are obtained, the therapist critically examines them to determine if patterns of sensory integrative dysfunction are evident. Not only are patterns of test scores scrutinized, but also the therapist's observations of child behavior during testing are considered in interpreting test scores. Finally, test scores and test behaviors are integrated with all other sources of information from the assessment in reaching a conclusion regarding the status of sensory integrative functioning.

Like all standardized tests, the SIPT protocol is administered with adherence to standardized procedures (Figure 11-12). Specialized training is required for administration and interpretation. This tool is a complex set of tests and, unlike most

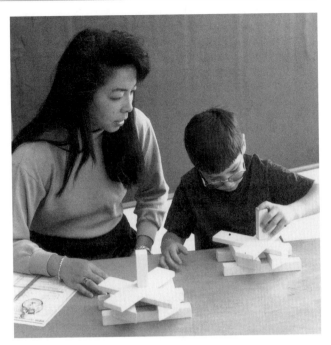

FIGURE 11-12 The Constructional Praxis Test is 1 of 17 tests of the Sensory Integration and Praxis Tests (SIPT). The SIPT must be administered individually with strict adherence to standardized procedures. (Courtesy Shay McAtee.)

published tests, cannot be self-taught by simply reading the manual. In addition to formal training for the SIPT, it is strongly recommended that therapists practice administration of the tests with children who do not have any known problems and with children who have recognized difficulties. With this experience and training, the therapist can administer the tests in a manner that produces reliable scores while allowing for observation of behaviors that provide additional information about the child's sensory integration and praxis abilities.

Other pediatric tests include items or subtests from which inferences regarding sensory integration may be drawn. For example, the Miller Function & Participation Scales includes tests of praxis, visual-motor integration, figure–ground perception, and some vestibular functions.[104] A number of tests, such as the Bruininks-Oseretsky Test of Motor Proficiency, (BOT-2),[37] measure aspects of fine and gross motor skills (such as bilateral coordination) that are related to sensory integrative functions. Other tests, such as the Developmental Test of Visual Motor Integration,[30] provide specific information related to visual-perceptual and perceptual-motor skills.

Some tests geared toward the broader evaluation of occupation, such as the School Function Assessment (SFA)[54] or the Social Participation Scale of the SPM,[116] are useful for identifying the extent to which sensory integrative disorders may be affecting the child's participation in occupations within specific settings. For the child with suspected sensory integrative problems, tests such as the SFA are most effectively used along with specific measures of sensory integration. When combined, these tests identify the functional problems to target in intervention and the reasons for the child's difficulties.

Consideration of Available Services and Resources

In addition to the information that is gathered about the child, an occupational therapy assessment of sensory integration takes into consideration the services and resources that are available to the child and family. Information regarding the type of services that the child is currently receiving, how he or she is responding to these services, and what services, programs, and resources are available to the child need careful consideration in light of the purpose and findings of the evaluation before recommendations can be formulated. For example, an occupational therapist may be asked to provide a reevaluation of a child who has been receiving occupational therapy for several years. If the child continues to demonstrate significant sensory integrative problems and has shown a diminishing response to treatment using a sensory integration approach, the recommendations would be different from those for a child no longer showed evidence of a significant sensory integrative problem.

Similarly, a child who lives in an area where no occupational therapists are qualified to provide sensory integration intervention needs a different program recommendation from that for a child who has easy access to this type of service. Understanding family aspirations and values, as well as resources, such as funding, transportation, time, and caregivers, is also critical in identifying the types of services that will be most helpful to the child and family. These issues are as important to the assessment process as the child factors that are addressed in a sensory integration evaluation.

Interpretation of Assessment Findings

Once all of the information from interviews, questionnaires, informal and formal observations, standardized tests, and consideration of available services and resources has been collected, the occupational therapist must integrate and interpret these data to reach meaningful conclusions and appropriate recommendations for the individual child. Conclusions and recommendations are framed with an overriding consideration of the occupations of the child and family and the contexts that influence occupational engagement.[1,127] Burke, Schaaf, and Hall advocate the strategy of creating a narrative, or story, to form an integrated understanding of the child and family in order to focus assessment and intervention planning on issues that are most meaningful and important to them.[40] In using such a future-oriented, top-down approach, the therapist not only generates a picture of the child and family in the present, but also imagines how changes might unfold over the next few years.[114] Therapists use research as well as training and experience to formulate conclusions and recommendations. (See Research Note 11-1 for an example of research that can inform interpretation of how assessment data relate to a child's academic functioning in school.)

One of the important steps in interpretation of assessment findings is to evaluate whether a sensory integrative problem may contribute to the occupational challenges of the child. To do this, data are classified into categories that either support or refute the presence of particular types of sensory integrative problems. After a detailed analysis of the constellation of assessment findings, a hypothesis is generated as to whether

RESEARCH NOTE 11-1

Parham, L. D. (1998). The relationship of sensory integrative development to achievement in elementary students: Four-year longitudinal patterns. Occupational Therapy Journal of Research, 18, 105-127.

OBJECTIVES. The objective of the study was to examine the relationship between sensory integrative development and academic achievement in math and reading in elementary school children across a 4-year period, while statistically controlling for other influences on achievement.

METHOD. A total of 67 children participated, 32 of whom had previously been identified as having learning disabilities. The remaining 35 children had no history of learning problems. Children completed the Sensory Integration and Praxis Tests, as well as intelligence and achievement tests. Demographic information was gathered from parents. Data were gathered prospectively in two data collection waves: first when the children were 6 to 8 years old, and 4 years later, when they were 10 to 12 years old.

RESULTS. Sensory integration measures significantly predicted math scores contemporaneously when the children were 6 to 8 years old as well as 4 years later, while controlling for intelligence, socioeconomic status, and other variables. Praxis in particular was a strong predictor of math achievement. Sensory integration measures did not predict reading at ages 6 to 8, after controlling for intelligence and socioeconomic status. However, praxis and visual perception did predict reading 4 years later, after controlling for other factors.

CONCLUSION. Sensory integration difficulties place a young child at risk for achievement problems in school, even when intellectual ability and socioeconomic status are high. Praxis difficulties may especially place a child at risk for problems with math achievement from elementary to middle school years.

IMPLICATIONS FOR PRACTICE

Therapists can use this study to advocate that children who have documented SI problems receive support to maximize their academic achievement in school, because Sensory integration problems place them at risk. This study did not examine intervention effectiveness, so other sources of information must be used to make decisions about what kinds of interventions or support are appropriate for specific children.

a sensory integrative problem appears to be present and, if so, what type it appears to be.

As in any aspect of occupational therapy, it is critical to relate the assessment findings to the presenting problems and initial concerns of the family or referral source. For example, an assessment may uncover signs of tactile defensiveness in a child described by the parents as destructive and impulsive. The evaluating therapist explains how tactile defensiveness may be related to the child's behavior problems. Because sensory integrative problems are not always recognized and understood, the therapist includes an explanation of how the assessment findings are linked to the daily life experiences and occupations of the child and family.[94]

If an assessment leads to a recommendation for intervention, it generally includes an estimate of the duration of time that the child should receive therapy, some indication of prognosis, and a statement regarding expected areas of change. The anticipated gains can be further clarified through the establishment of specific goals and objectives. Writing and explaining goals will provide the occupational therapist with an opportunity to illuminate the ways in which the identified sensory integration issues intersect with the presenting problems and desired functional outcomes.[94] Regardless of the types of goals that are written, goals are established in a manner that is culturally relevant for the family and considers the needs and wishes of the individual child.

The format in which goals are specified is often a function of the setting in which therapy is delivered. For example, a school district may include certain types of goals as part of an individualized education plan, whereas a hospital setting may require medically related outcomes. Goal attainment scaling is a specific method for writing goals that are individualized and then quantified to allow for comparison of outcomes across a large group of children.[95] In this process, individualized goals are carefully placed on a standard scale that allows for quantitative comparison of changes across dissimilar outcomes (e.g., the amount of change in pumping a swing in comparison with the amount of change in tolerance of food textures). Although this method was developed for outcomes research, it may be useful in documenting intervention effectiveness across a large group of children for purposes of program evaluation.

INTERVENTIONS FOR CHILDREN WITH SENSORY INTEGRATIVE PROBLEMS

Planning an occupational therapy program for a child with a sensory integrative problem requires the same careful analysis used in applying any theoretical framework in clinical practice. The constellation of child and family characteristics is analyzed in relation to the occupations of the individuals involved. Intervention is designed to focus on engagement in occupation in order to support the participation of the child in the everyday contexts of his or her life.[1] When a sensory integration approach is used in occupational therapy, the unique ways in which sensory integrative problems affect engagement and participation in the occupations of the particular child and his or her family provide the cornerstone upon which decisions regarding treatment are made.[127] Intervention is continually planned and evaluated in relation to the occupations that the child wants and needs to do in the contexts of home, school, and community.

The assessment process helps the therapist decide whether any intervention is recommended and, if so, in what format: individual therapy, group sessions, or collaborative consultation with parents and teachers. Regardless of the form in which intervention is delivered, theory-based concepts regarding the nature of sensory integration are applied whenever a sensory integration approach is selected. Guiding principles of the ASI approach are summarized in Box 11-2.[11,18,19] The key ideas behind these principles were introduced previously in this chapter in the sections on sensory integrative development and problems.

Therapists who plan interventions for children with sensory integrative problems are responsible for developing their professional expertise through advanced training, mentorship, and review of the research literature. The field of sensory integration is a complex, specialized area of occupational therapy practice that demands that the therapist synthesize information from many sources. Because it is a dynamically changing field of practice, it is important that the therapist stay abreast of research evidence, as well as of new developments in sensory integration theory and practice, to guide practice decisions. These sources of information, in combination with the unique situation of the child and family being helped, all influence the decision of whether to intervene and, if so, how.

In this section, four of the primary methods of occupational therapy intervention for children with sensory integrative problems are described: (1) individual ASI intervention to improve underlying sensory integration abilities, (2) individual skill development training, (3) group skill development intervention, and (4) consultation, including modifications of activities, routines, and environments at home and in school. These forms of intervention are often used in combination with each other, rather than as the sole service delivery method. With careful consideration on the part of the therapist, interventions based on other theoretical frameworks and treatment models may be used along with those discussed in the following sections of this chapter. The therapist must be mindful that if the intervention strategies being combined are not compatible owing to contradictory underlying principles, intervention effectiveness may be reduced. Therefore, although selection of a combination of intervention approaches is often desirable, it must be done with care.

Individual *Ayres Sensory Integration*® (ASI) *Intervention*

Individual occupational therapy using Ayres Sensory Integration® (ASI) intervention is the most intensive form of occupational therapy available for children with sensory integration problems. The term *Ayres Sensory Integration*® (ASI) was trademarked by the Franklin B. Baker/J. Jean Ayres Baker Trust, "for the purpose of protecting and promoting Dr. Ayres' body of work and to assist in differentiation of this approach from others that might share some similar terminology or techniques."[129]

In this chapter, the term ASI intervention refers to the kind of individual occupational therapy that Ayres developed specifically to remediate sensory integrative problems in children.[130] In this intervention, the therapist presents activity challenges that are individually tailored to improve the specific sensory integration problems affecting the child's performance. This intervention is designed to help a child gain improved sensory integrative capabilities when problems with sensory integration are interfering with the child's occupations at home, in play, at school, or in the community (Case Study 11-1). Although Ayres originally designed this therapy for children with learning disabilities,[11] she and many other expert practitioners have used this kind of intervention, along with specific skill training and consultation, to help children with other disabilities, including autism.[93,97]

In designing this specialized form of occupational therapy, Ayres was influenced by the neurobiologic literature, which shows that the nervous system has plasticity or changeability. Plasticity is particularly characteristic of the developing young child. This led Ayres to hypothesize that the neural systems that impair function may be remediable, especially in the young child. Accordingly, she set out to design therapy that capitalized on the plasticity of the nervous system to remediate sensory integrative dysfunction. This is *not* to say that ASI intervention cures conditions such as learning disability, autism, or developmental delays. Rather, the intent is to improve the efficiency with which the nervous system interprets and uses sensory information for functional use. Therefore ASI is aimed at promoting underlying capabilities to the greatest degree possible.

ASI intervention has several defining characteristics. It is applied on an *individual* basis because the therapist must adjust therapeutic activities moment by moment in relation to the individual child's interest in the activity or response to a specific challenge or sensory experience.[49,81,85] This requires the therapist to continually focus attention on the child while being mindful of opportunities in the environment for eliciting adaptive responses. The therapist's decisions regarding how and when to intervene involve a delicate interplay between the therapist's judgment regarding the potential therapeutic value of an activity and the child's motivation to do the activity. The therapist does not use a "cookbook" approach in providing this therapy (e.g., by entering the therapy situation with a predetermined schedule of activities that the child is required to follow). Rather, the therapist enters into a relationship with the child that fosters the child's inner drive to actively explore the environment and to master challenges posed by the environment.

Intervention involves a *balance between structure and freedom*,[11,18] and its effectiveness is contingent on the proficiency of the therapist in making judgments regarding when to step in to provide structure and when to step back and allow the child to choose activities. The therapist's job is to create an environment that evokes increasingly complex adaptive responses from the child. To accomplish this, the therapist respects the child's needs and interests while structuring opportunities to help the child successfully meet a challenge. An example is a child who needs to develop more efficient righting and equilibrium reactions and chooses to sit and swing on a platform swing. The therapist may allow the child to swing awhile to become accustomed to the vestibular sensations. Once the child seems comfortable,

CASE STUDY 11-1   Karen

HISTORY

Karen was born after a full-term pregnancy complicated by gestational diabetes. Labor, which was induced at 40 weeks, was prolonged, and it was believed that Karen broke her right collarbone during delivery. Karen achieved her early motor and language milestones within average age ranges. However, she was described as an irritable baby who had difficulty breast feeding, startled easily, and could be calmed only by swinging. Karen attended a parent cooperative child development program as a toddler, and at 4 years of age she was eligible for a special education preschool program through her school district. She has not been given any specific medical or educational diagnosis.

REASON FOR REFERRAL

Karen's mother expressed concern about Karen's fine and gross motor skills to a neurologist, who referred Karen for an occupational therapy assessment when she was 4 years of age. When asked why she was seeking an evaluation for Karen, her mother wrote, "Up until recently I had been very patiently waiting for normal development to occur (for example, handedness, fine motor). The school psychologist feels that this still may occur, but I am convinced that something isn't right. Karen's increasing frustration and decreasing belief in herself prompted me to seek evaluations. While a part of me wishes to have a 'normal child,' the other part will be relieved to find that the child I have had so many doubts about since infancy does indeed have some behaviors and actions that are unusual."

EVALUATION PROCEDURE

The Sensory Integration and Praxis Tests (SIPT) were administered in one testing session. Karen was also observed in a clinical therapy setting and at home. In addition, Karen's mother was interviewed, and she completed a developmental and sensory history on which she provided detailed accounts of Karen's early and current sensorimotor, language, cognitive, social, and self-care development.

EVALUATION RESULTS

On the SIPT, Karen scored below average for age expectations on 7 of 17 tests. This profile was generated through computer scoring by the test publisher. The unit of measure represented by the scores is a statistical measure called a *standard deviation*, which represents how different the child's score is from that of an average child of the same age. The closer a child's score is to 0 on the horizontal axis, the closer to average is the child's performance on that test. Karen's scores are plotted as solid squares that are connected by a dark line on the computer-generated profile. Scores falling below -1.0 on the horizontal axis are considered to be possibly indicative of dysfunction.

One of Karen's scores was low on a motor-free visual perception test (space visualization), and it was noted that she had difficulty fitting a geometric form into a puzzle board during this test. Her mother reported that Karen knew colors at 18 months of age but had trouble learning shapes.

However, she was reported to have a strong visual memory for roads, signs, and faces. These findings suggested difficulty with spatial orientation of objects but relative strengths in visual memory.

Karen had several low scores and showed signs of difficulty performing on several of the tests of somatosensory and vestibular processing. A low score on finger identification suggested inefficient tactile feedback involving the hands. This was corroborated by observations of poor manipulative skills during activities such as buttoning and using utensils. She was also observed to have signs of tactile defensiveness, also corroborated by her mother's report. Her low score on Kinesthesia, as well as her difficulty in exerting the appropriate amount of pressure on a pencil and in positioning her body for dressing, suggested problems with proprioceptive feedback. Karen's lowest score on the SIPT was on the Postrotary Nystagmus test (-2.2 standard deviations). This low score, as well as below-average scores on Standing and Walking Balance, observations of poor functional balance in dressing and playground activities, a tendency not to cross her body midline, poor bilateral coordination in activities such as cutting, and reports that she never appeared to get dizzy, pointed to the probability of vestibular processing problems.

Karen showed above-average performance on a praxis test on which she could rely on verbal directions. However, tests of motor planning that were more somatosensory dependent (Oral Praxis and Postural Praxis) were substantially more difficult for her. Karen was unable to ride a tricycle, pump a swing, or skip. She had extreme difficulty planning her movements to dress herself or even to let someone else dress her. She also had a great deal of difficulty using utensils during eating and often choked on food and drinks. Writing skills were particularly difficult for Karen, and her lack of hand preference, immature grasp, and hesitancy to cross her midline hampered her attempts at drawing or writing.

Karen was reported to be a social child who was liked by adults and younger peers. However, her mother worried that she did not seem able to "pick up on the hints and unwritten rules of her peers" and was "definitely starting to march to her own beat." She noticed increasing signs of frustration that she thought were beginning to impinge on Karen's willingness to participate with peers.

Overall, the evaluation results suggested deficits in sensory processing of some aspects of visual, tactile, proprioceptive, and vestibular sensory information. These difficulties were seen as related to somatodyspraxia, poor balance and bilateral integration, difficulties with specific gross and fine motor skills, and emerging concerns around socialization. Karen's strengths included age-appropriate cognitive and language skills, good ability to motor plan actions using verbal directions, and an exceptionally supportive and involved family.

RECOMMENDATION

Based on the evaluation results and a meeting of Karen's IEP team, who met shortly after the assessment, it was recommended that Karen receive individual occupational therapy

Continued

RECOMMENDATION—CONT'D

using a sensory integration approach to enhance foundational sensory and motor processes. Because of her significant sensory integrative problems and need for a specialized approach, the therapy was recommended to initially occur in a setting equipped for *Ayres Sensory Integration®* (ASI) intervention.

OCCUPATIONAL THERAPY PROGRAM

In the first 6 months of individual occupational therapy, an ASI approach was used that included individualized, carefully selected therapeutic activities aimed at enhancing visual, tactile, proprioceptive, and vestibular sensory processing. As part of her intervention program, Karen's therapist provided her with graded challenges to praxis, bilateral coordination, and balance.

After 6 months of therapy, Karen has shown decreasing tactile defensiveness, a reduced tendency to choke on food, acquisition of the ability to ride a tricycle, and an improved ability to plan new or unusual motor actions. Although these are significant gains for Karen, she continues to exhibit substantial difficulties with many aspects of sensory processing, general motor planning ability, and many age-appropriate fine and gross motor skills. If she continues to respond to occupational therapy using an ASI approach, it is expected that by the beginning of the next school year (in about 6 months), she will have improved in basic sensory and motor functions to the extent that some specific skill training will become more appropriate. It is likely that at that time some therapy will occur at school with the introduction of a consultation program for her teacher. Her parents have already begun a home program, which appears to support the gains she is making through direct services. Karen's young age and initial positive response to therapy make her an optimal candidate for application of the sensory integration approach, and her long-term outlook is excellent.

---

the therapist steps in to jiggle the swing to stimulate the desired responses. However, if the child responds to this challenge with signs of anxiety or fear, the therapist needs to intervene quickly to help the child feel safer. For example, the therapist might set an inner tube on the swing to provide a base to stabilize the lower part of the child's body and increase feelings of security while the child's upper body is free to make the required righting reactions. Therapeutic activities thus emerge from the interaction between therapist and child. Such individualized treatment can be fully realized only with one-to-one interaction between therapist and child (Figure 11-13).

The emphasis on the *inner drive* of the child is another key characteristic of ASI intervention.[11,18,49,85] Self-direction on the part of the child is encouraged because therapeutic gains are maximized if the child is fully invested as an active participant. However, this is not to say that the child is permitted to engage in free play with no adult guidance. The optimal therapy situation is one in which a balance is struck between the structure provided by the therapist and some degree of freedom of choice on the part of the child.[11,19] Drawing on the child's interests and imagination is often key to encouraging greater effort on a difficult task or staying with a challenging activity for a longer time. However, because children with sensory integrative problems do not always demonstrate inner drive toward growth-inducing activities, it is often necessary to modify activities and to find ways to entice such children toward interaction. A relatively high degree of directedness often is needed when working with children with autism or other children whose inner drive is limited. Occasionally a therapist may use a high degree of directedness within the context of a particular activity to show a child that the challenging activity is possible not only to achieve, but also to enjoy.

Related to inner drive is another key feature of ASI intervention—the valuing of *active participation*, rather than passive participation, on the part of the child. Because the

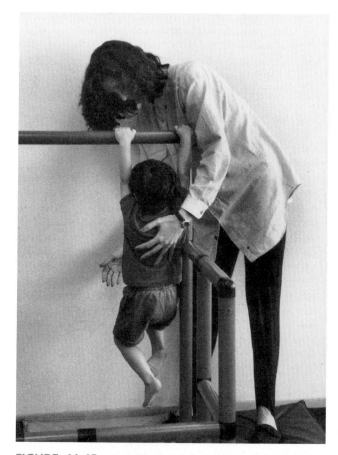

FIGURE 11-13 Individual ASI intervention requires the therapist to attend closely to the child on a moment-by-moment basis to ensure that therapeutic activities are individually tailored to changing needs and interests of the child. (Courtesy Shay McAtee.)

brain responds differently and learns more effectively when an individual is actively involved in a task rather than merely receiving passive stimulation, it is considered optimal for a child to be an active participant to the greatest degree possible. For example, sensory integration theory posits that a child experiences a greater degree of integration from pumping a swing or pulling on a rope to make it go than from being swung passively.

Maximal active involvement generally takes place when therapeutic activities are at just the right level of complexity, at which the child not only feels comfortable and nonthreatened but also experiences some challenge that requires effort. The course of therapy usually begins with activities in which the child feels comfortable and competent and then moves toward increasing challenges. For example, for children with gravitational insecurity, therapy usually begins with activities close to the ground and with close physical support from the therapist to help the child feel secure. Gradually, over weeks of therapy, activities that require stepping up on different surfaces and moving away from the floor are introduced as the therapist subtly withdraws physical support. Introducing just the right level of challenge, while respecting the child's need to feel secure and in control, is a key to maximizing the child's active involvement in therapy (Figure 11-14).

However, there are situations in which passive stimulation is needed to help prepare a child for more complex or challenging activities. For example, the child with autism may show improved sensory registration after receiving passive linear vestibular stimulation.[144] The improved registration means that the child has greater awareness of the environment, and thus the passive stimulation is a stepping stone toward active involvement in an activity. Another example is the use of passive tactile stimulation as a means for reducing tactile defensiveness.[11,153] However, this aspect of therapy is seen as a limited component of a sensory integrative treatment program and then only as a step toward facilitating more active participation.

Another key characteristic of ASI intervention is the *setting* in which it takes place. The provision of a special therapeutic environment is an important aspect of this kind of intervention and has been described in detail by other authors.[143,150] Based on the research that shows that brain structure and function are enhanced when animals are permitted to actively explore an interesting environment,[79] a sensory-enriched environment is designed to evoke active exploration on the part of the child. The clinic that is designed for ASI intervention contains large activity areas with an array of specialized equipment. The availability of suspended equipment is a hallmark of this treatment approach.[49,85] Suspended equipment provides rich opportunities for stimulating and challenging the vestibular system. In addition, equipment and materials are available that provide a variety of somatosensory stimuli, including tactile, vibratory, and proprioceptive. Mats and large pillows are used for safety. Overall, this special environment provides the child with a safe and interesting place in which to explore his or her capabilities. At the same time it provides the therapist with a tool kit for creating sensory experiences that are enticing and for gently guiding the child toward activities that challenge perception, dynamic postural control, and motor planning (Figure 11-15).

Because of the prominence of vestibular based activities in the environments in which ASI is applied, a few cautionary words are in order regarding this powerful tool. Activation of the vestibular system, most often in the form of linear movement, is commonly introduced early in the course of treatment for many children because it is believed to have an organizing effect on other sensory systems.[11,18,19] However, it can have a highly disturbing and disorganizing effect on the child if used carelessly. Vestibular system activation may produce strong autonomic responses, such as blanching and nausea. It directly influences the arousal level and, if not regulated carefully, may produce hyperactive, distractible states or lethargic, drowsy states. ASI intervention emphasizes active participation on the part of the child; therefore, vestibular stimulation is not

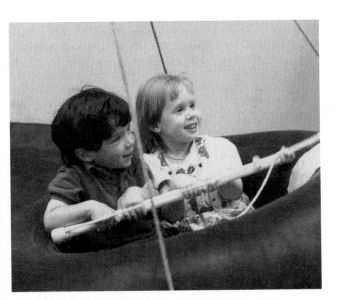

FIGURE 11-14 Rather than passively imposing vestibular input on the child, classic sensory integration treatment emphasizes active participation and self-direction of the child. (Courtesy Shay McAtee.)

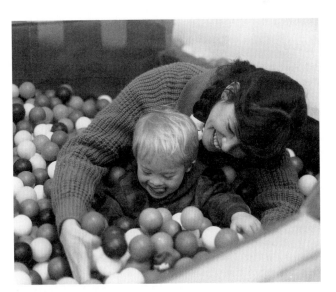

FIGURE 11-15 The setting in which classical sensory integration treatment takes place provides a variety of sensory experiences. Immersion in a pool of balls presents challenges to sensory modulation. (Courtesy Shay McAtee.)

passively imposed on the child. Rather, the child is allowed to initiate and actively participate in vestibular activities as much as possible, with the therapist stepping in to help modulate it when indicated. For example, if a child is actively rotating while sitting in a tire swing and begins to exhibit mild signs of autonomic activation, the therapist may intervene. The therapist may reduce the intensity of the swinging by guiding the child to shift to slow linear swinging or by offering the child a trapeze to pull to increase the amount of proprioceptive input. Proprioceptive input is believed to have an inhibiting effect on vestibular input, as indicated by results of animal research.[69] Therefore, knowledge of the effects of vestibular stimulation and its interactions with other sensory systems is critical in this treatment approach. Responsible use of vestibular-based activities absolutely requires advanced training in sensory integration.

To summarize the key features of ASI intervention, therapeutic activities are neither predetermined nor are they simply free play. The flow of the treatment session results from a collaboration between the therapist and child in which the therapist encourages and supports the child in a way that moves the child toward therapeutic goals. This all takes place within a special environment that is safe yet challenging. The use of special equipment and powerful sensory modalities requires that the therapist have special training well beyond the entry level of practice in occupational therapy.

ASI intervention can be intensive and long term. Although treatment schedules vary, a typical schedule involves two sessions per week, each lasting 45 minutes to 1 hour. A typical course of therapy lasts for about 2 years. Most experts agree that at least 6 months of therapy is needed to detect results.

After Ayres developed ASI intervention,[11,18] her colleagues and students continued to further develop and expand on her intervention concepts. Koomar and Bundy provided a particularly thorough description of the application of sensory integration procedures for specific types of sensory integrative disorders.[85] Holloway has imported ASI concepts into the neonatal intensive care unit (NICU), where the treatment principles are used to help young infants when their developing nervous systems are most plastic.[76] Others have adapted ASI intervention to address the needs of infants and toddlers who are developmentally at risk,[136] as well as the needs of children with visual impairments,[126] cerebral palsy,[33] environmental deprivation,[47] and fragile X syndrome.[75]

Application of the ASI approach requires advanced study and training. Koomar and Bundy advocated a mentorship process as the best preparation for learning how to clinically apply sensory integration principles.[85] Ayres also advocated this and established a 4-month course in which therapists receive both didactic instruction and intensive hands-on experience treating children under close supervision. Ayres believed that this level of intensity was required to master the sensory integration approach. Because of the highly specialized and complex nature of the classical sensory integration approach, it is important that occupational therapists gain mentored experience in this area before independently engaging in this form of practice.

In addition, ongoing study and discussion with peers are highly recommended to hone clinical expertise in this area after acquiring advanced training. Although ASI intervention as described here occurs within specialized therapy centers, many of the concepts can be applied in other settings as well.

School-based occupational therapists have found ways to incorporate the central principles of ASI into the educational setting, including bringing specialized equipment into classrooms and playgrounds in ways that help to organize and prepare a child for learning. Successful therapy programs frequently involve helping families to understand and use the sensory integrative concepts that support and facilitate their children's success by developing activities at home and identifying resources within the community that reinforce the experiences emphasized during therapy.[120]

Training in Specific Skill Development

Although ASI intervention is focused on improving foundational neural functions that allow a wide range of capabilities and skills to emerge, therapists will often want to help a child and family to develop specific skills or short-term coping strategies to deal immediately with the special challenges posed by sensory integration problems. For example, a child with poor proprioceptive feedback may need to keep up with handwriting exercises assigned in class. Application of individual ASI intervention would aim to help the child develop better body awareness that eventually will help not only with writing but also with catching, throwing, cutting, buttoning, and many other proprioception-dependent skills. However, because of everyday classroom stress from the demands of handwriting, the child may not be able to afford to wait for these generalized capabilities to develop through sensory integrative treatment. For this child, specific handwriting training may be used to help develop better handwriting skills, despite poor proprioceptive feedback. When working on specific skill development, the occupational therapist can still be mindful of the guiding principles of sensory integration theory (see Box 11-2). For example, it is optimal to involve self-direction and active participation as much as possible. This might be accomplished with the child in this example by having the child write stories related to individual interests and experiences. In addition, handwriting exercises that require active movement are expected to accomplish more than those dependent on passive guidance of the child's hand. The therapist's ability to read the child's responses to writing activities helps ensure that the activities remain motivating and appropriately challenging.

Group Intervention

The occupational therapist working with a group of children cannot provide the same level of vigilance to individual responses that takes place during individual therapy. Therefore, some of the highly individualized applications of ASI intervention cannot be used within a group, nor can the therapist give the close guidance that is finely tuned to the individual child's needs every moment of the treatment session. Again, however, the principles of ASI outlined in Box 11-3 are important concepts to incorporate into the group format as much as possible.

Working with children in a group provides the opportunity to observe some of the ways in which sensory integrative problems disrupt participation in a social context (Figure 11-16). Some problems emerge only in a group situation and may not be evident during individual therapy. For example, tactile defensiveness may not be apparent in the safe constraints of individual therapy but may become obvious as a child tries to

BOX 11-3   Expected Outcomes of *Ayres Sensory Integration*® (ASI®) Intervention

1. Increase in the frequency or duration of adaptive responses
2. Development of increasingly more complex adaptive responses
3. Improvement in gross and fine motor skills
4. Improvement in cognitive, language, and academic performance
5. Increase in self-confidence and self-esteem
6. Enhancement of occupational engagement and social participation
7. Enhancement of family life

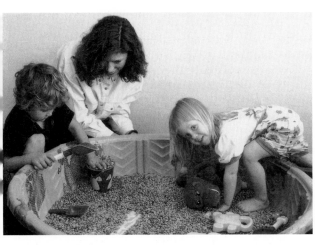

FIGURE 11-16 Group programs provide opportunities for children with sensory integrative disorders to develop coping skills that help them function in social context with peers. (Courtesy Shay McAtee.)

participate within a group of people who are brushing by in an unpredictable manner. Observing how the group dynamic affects the child can help the therapist know what aspects of the classroom, playground, park, or after-school activities are likely to pose a threat or challenge (Case Study 11-2).

In some situations, external variables such as funding limitations, availability of staff, or organizational policies create the need for children to receive therapy in a group setting. It is important that occupational therapists make recommendations based primarily on the needs of the children being served, taking into consideration such outside factors, rather than allowing the external factors to dictate the type of intervention that is provided. It is also important to differentiate between what can be accomplished within a group versus an individual therapy session. Because group programs do not permit the same degree of intensive, individualized work, they are not expected to lead to the same outcomes.

An especially innovative application of sensory integration concepts to groups is reflected in the work of Williams and Shellenberger.[154] Through a group format, their Alert Program helps children learn to recognize how they feel when their levels of alertness change throughout the day, to identify

the sensorimotor experiences that they can use to change their level of alertness, and to monitor their arousal levels in a variety of settings. Another application of ASI concepts to groups is the work of Piantanida and Baltazar, who present a variety of sensory integration–based group activities for developing appropriate social skills.[121]

To apply sensory integration principles to a group program, an occupational therapist should be familiar enough with sensory integration theory to understand precautions and general effects of various sensory and motor activities. Experience and training in working with groups, including how to maintain the attention of children in a group, how to address varying skill and interest levels, and how to deal with behavioral issues, are also recommended for occupational therapists applying ASI principles in group programs.

Consultation on Modification of Activities, Routines, and Environments

Sensory integrative problems are complex and are often misinterpreted as behavioral, psychological, or emotional in origin. Helping family members, teachers, and others to understand the nature of the problem can be a powerful means toward helping the child. Providing information to those who are in ongoing contact with the child and developing strategies through collaboration with them are important ways in which the therapist can indirectly intervene to influence the child's life positively across a variety of settings. Indirect intervention in the form of consultation is often critical for success in a comprehensive occupational therapy program for the child with sensory integration challenges.

Although many sensory integration concepts are not familiar to family members, teachers, or other professionals, once they are explained in everyday terms, a new understanding of the child often ensues. Cermak aptly referred to this process as *demystification*.[47] Parents commonly express relief at finally having a name for behaviors that they have observed, and they may experience release from feeling that they have caused these problems through a maladaptive parenting style. Teachers also may appreciate having an alternative way to view child behaviors, especially when this new perspective is coupled with the application of strategies that promote responses from the child that are more productive.

Helping those around the child understand their own sensory integrative processes is sometimes a good way to make these new concepts more meaningful. Williams and Shellenberger use this tactic when introducing their Alert Program to promote optimal states of organization and levels of alertness.[154] They encourage the adults being trained to administer the program to develop awareness and insight into their own sensorimotor preferences. This first step in initiating consultation is to help the significant adults in the child's life better understand sensory integration in general and in relation to the specific child. This can be achieved through several avenues, including parent/teacher conferences, experiential sessions, lecture and discussion groups, professional in-services, and ongoing education programs. Whatever format is used, it is likely that the greater the understanding of the basic concepts of sensory integration, the greater the openness and willingness to address these problems (Figure 11-17).

CASE STUDY 11-2   Drew

HISTORY

Drew was diagnosed with autism (high functioning) when he was 7 years of age. His mother is Korean, and his father is American. All of Drew's early developmental milestones were attained within normal limits, except for language acquisition. He did not speak any words until 2 years of age, and by 3 years of age his family was concerned about his development because of delayed language skills. Drew attended an English-language preschool at 3 years of age and then a Korean-language preschool. (His family speaks both Korean and English at home.) He was asked to leave the second preschool because of aggressive behavior. At 4 years of age, Drew attended a private special education school where he received speech therapy and participated in a language-intensive playgroup. When Drew reached kindergarten age, he was enrolled in public special education programs, where he attended specialized classrooms for speech and language disorders, autism, and multiple handicaps.

REASON FOR REFERRAL

Drew initially was referred by the state regional center for developmental disabilities to an occupational therapy private practice for evaluation when he was nearly 8 years of age. His regional center counselor thought that Drew had signs of a sensory integrative disorder, and he believed that Drew might benefit from occupational therapy. Drew's mother reported that her main concerns for Drew were related to his poor socialization skills, his limited ability to play with games and toys, and his tendency to become easily frustrated.

EVALUATION PROCEDURE

Although the Sensory Integration and Praxis Tests (SIPT) were attempted during the initial occupational therapy assessment, Drew was unable to follow the directions or attend to the tests sufficiently to obtain reliable scores. Therefore, his occupational therapy evaluation consisted of a parent interview, including completion of a developmental and sensory history, and observation of Drew in a clinical therapy setting. At the time of assessment it was not possible to interview Drew's teacher. However, Drew's mother, who often observed him in the classroom, provided information about his performance at school.

EVALUATION RESULTS

Drew demonstrated inefficiencies in sensory processing in a number of sensory systems. During the assessment, signs of inconsistent responses to tactile input were evident. For example, Drew demonstrated a complete lack of response to some stimuli such as a puff of air on the back of his neck or the light touch of a cotton ball applied to his feet when he was not visually attending. However, he withdrew in an agitated fashion when the therapist attempted to position him. His mother reported that he showed extreme dislike for certain textures of food and clothing and that he disliked being touched. She also stated that he seemed to become irritated by being near other children at school and sometimes pinched or pushed peers who came close to him. Drew also appeared easily overstimulated by

extraneous visual and auditory stimuli. His mother stated that he often covered his ears at home when loud noises were present and that at school he sometimes seemed confused as to the direction of sounds. He was observed to pick up objects and look at them very closely, and he appeared to rely on his vision a great deal to complete tasks. In response to movement, he enjoyed swinging slowly but became fearful with an increase in velocity. His mother stated that he often became fearful at the park when climbing.

Drew's balance was observed to be poor, and his equilibrium reactions were inconsistent. He also had trouble positioning himself on various pieces of equipment, showing poor body awareness. During the assessment he appeared to seek touch-pressure stimuli, including total body compression. He was reported to jump a great deal at home and at school. These types of proprioception-generating actions appeared to have a calming effect on Drew.

In the areas of praxis, Drew was able to imitate positions and follow verbal directions to complete motor actions, but he had a great deal of difficulty initiating activities on his own or attempting something that was unfamiliar to him. He also had difficulty timing and sequencing his actions. His mother reported that he tended not to participate in sports or in park activities and that he had trouble throwing, catching, and kicking balls. Drew was able to complete puzzles, string beads, and write his name; however, bilateral activities such as cutting and pasting were difficult for him.

Socially, Drew demonstrated poor eye contact and tended to use repetitive phrases that he had heard in the past. His mother stated that he wanted to play with peers but found it hard to make friends. Drew was independent in all self-care skills, except for tying shoes and managing some fasteners.

Based on an interview and questionnaire with Drew's mother, as well as observation of Drew in a clinical therapy setting, it was determined that he displayed irregularities in sensory processing, including hypersensitivity to some aspects of touch, movement, visual, and auditory stimuli. He also demonstrated difficulty with position sense, balance, bilateral integration, and the ideation, timing, and sequencing aspects of praxis. These difficulties were thought to interfere with Drew's ability to play purposefully with toys and to participate in age-appropriate games and sports. These problems, in combination with his language delays, were interfering significantly with his social skills and his ability to make friends, and they were increasing his tendency to become frustrated, all of which were the major concerns of his parents.

RECOMMENDATION

Individual occupational therapy was recommended to address Drew's sensory integration problems and the development of specific fine and gross motor skills. Because socialization issues were such a major concern for Drew's family and were interfering with his performance at school, the evaluating therapist also recommended that Drew participate in an after-school group occupational therapy program to facilitate the acquisition of social skills.

CASE STUDY 11-2 Drew—cont'd

OCCUPATIONAL THERAPY PROGRAM

Drew received individual and group occupational therapy in a therapy clinic for 1 year. The individual therapy involved a combination of *Ayres Sensory Integration*® (ASI) intervention and a specific skill development approach. During this time, Drew demonstrated significant gains in sensory processing with no further significant signs of tactile defensiveness or fear of movement activities. Motor planning of novel actions improved but continued to be of some concern for Drew. He did make notable gains in being able to catch and throw a ball and in writing and scissors skills. Through the group occupational therapy program, Drew became able to initiate and maintain interaction with peers, share objects, and play cooperatively with some assistance and structure from adults.

After this year of clinically based individual and group occupational therapy, it was recommended that individual therapy be continued at school. The focus of this occupational therapy program was to help Drew apply his improved sensorimotor and social skills in the natural context of school. Through a combination of direct service and consultation, several activities and adaptations were made to facilitate his performance at school. Because the initial year of intensive therapy using an ASI approach had helped Drew tolerate and respond appropriately to sensory information and because he had developed many of the specific skills that he needed in the classroom during individual therapy, he was much better able to focus on the demands expected of him at school at that time. By the end of the school year, Drew's occupational therapist recommended that occupational therapy be discontinued because she believed that his teacher would be able to continue to help him in the areas that had been addressed through the consultation program.

However, when the individualized educational program (IEP) team met to discuss Drew's transition to a new school, they had significant concerns about the possibility of Drew's regressing in a new setting, where he would need to adjust to many different routines. The IEP team requested that occupational therapy continue to ensure a smooth transition for Drew and to put in place a plan that would continue to help him develop socially.

When school resumed in the fall, the occupational therapist had arranged a "big buddy" program with a local high school. Two high school seniors worked with Drew as part of a social service assignment during recess for the fall semester. The occupational therapist trained the high school students to carry out a socialization program aimed at helping Drew feel comfortable with a new set of peers. Drew seemed to look up to the high school students and responded well to the "big buddy" program.

By the end of the fall semester in the new school, Drew played cooperatively with peers, interacting independently and communicating appropriately. His occupational therapy program was formally discontinued at this time, although the occupational therapist continued to check in with Drew's teacher when at his school site to work with other children. No additional intervention has been needed, but the option for further consultation or direct intervention is available should the need arise.

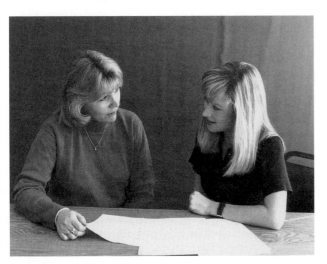

FIGURE 11-17 Consultation in school involves joint problem solving between the occupational therapist and the teacher. (Courtesy Shay McAtee.)

Perhaps the most important component of any consultation program is providing guidance for identifying, preventing, and coping with the challenges in everyday life that stem from the sensory integrative problems. Sometimes specific activities can be suggested that will help a child to prepare for a challenging task. For example, a child who has tactile defensiveness may be better able to tolerate activities such as finger painting or sand play if some desensitization techniques, such as applying firm touch-pressure to the skin, are used just before the activity. Modifying the activity might involve providing tools to use with the paint or sand to give the child a ready "break" from the unpleasant sensation. A home program that includes gradual introduction of tactile sensation in a safe place, such as the bathtub, can also help to lessen reactions. The therapist can also promote success in activities by suggesting individualized ways to help a child through difficult tasks. For example, some children with dyspraxia are likely to be more successful in completing a novel task when they receive verbal directions, whereas others respond optimally to visual demonstrations, and still others need physical assistance with the motion. Determining which method or combination of methods is most likely to help the individual child can assist adults in facilitating success.

Making adjustments in the environment can be especially important in the school setting since children spend large amounts of time in this environment. For example, children with autism are often highly affected by the sensory characteristics of their environments. Finding ways to manage sound, lighting, contact with other people, environmental odors, and visual distractions in the classroom, playground, cafeteria, and assembly rooms can make an important difference in attention, behavior, and, ultimately, performance. Dunn's work has led to a deeper understanding of how the sensory aspects of ordinary environments affect individuals who have the various sensory modulation styles that are depicted in her model (see Figure 11-9).[61,63] Because individual differences in sensory processing tend to be lifelong tendencies, Dunn emphasizes how important it is for a person to learn to construct daily routines and manipulate sensory aspects of work and play environments in order to live as comfortably and successfully as possible.[63] Consultation to develop the family's insight into a child's sensory characteristics, or to foster the child's own insight, along with ideas for home and community-based activities, may be critical to intervention.

Procedures or techniques that require advanced training of an occupational therapist should not be recommended for parents and other professionals. For example, an appropriate consultation program never attempts to train a parent or teacher to provide individual therapeutic activities that require advanced training for monitoring the child's response. Therapists should also be familiar enough with the child to be aware of any precautions that might apply before they make any suggestions. For example, some children display delayed responses to vestibular stimulation and can become overstimulated or lethargic hours after engaging in activities involving this type of sensation. Some sensory integrative techniques can lead to adverse reactions and must be used with care. Consultation services, environmental modifications, and home programs are meant to supplement, not replace, direct intervention. Used appropriately, they provide effective avenues for supporting the child, as well as family members, teachers, and other professionals who share in the efforts to help the child succeed.

The same therapist qualifications needed to provide individual ASI intervention are desirable in using consultation because the therapist needs to be able to predict what the child's likely responses will be to various activities and situations, given the characteristics of the child's sensory integrative difficulties. In addition, the therapist should be well enough versed in sensory integration concepts to be able to explain them in simple yet meaningful terms. Also, it is imperative that the therapist have excellent communication skills and respect for the various people and environments that are involved. Bundy provided an excellent description of the communication process involved in a good consultation program.[38]

Expected Outcomes of Occupational Therapy

As discussed previously, occupational therapy is not expected to "cure" sensory integrative problems. Rather, occupational therapy aims to improve the child's health and quality of life through engagement in meaningful and important occupations or activities. To accomplish this with a child who has sensory integrative problems, the occupational therapist may aim to improve sensory integrative functions through direct remediation via ASI intervention, to minimize the effects of the problems by teaching the child specific skills and strategies, and by consulting with parents and teachers to plan modifications of activities, routines, and environments. Often remediation, skill training, and consultation are thoughtfully combined in an intervention plan that is tailored to the particular needs of the child and family.

The goals and objectives that are formulated as part of a child's intervention plan target specific occupations in which positive changes are expected. These goals and objectives can be conceptualized as falling under the traditional occupational categories of work, rest, play, and self-care. For example, a toddler who tends to be overstimulated much of the time because of severe sensory modulation problems may consequently have difficulty falling asleep and staying asleep. One result of this situation is sleep deprivation, which aggravates defensiveness and behavior problems. A goal addressing the occupational domain of rest may be for the child to acquire more predictable sleep patterns with adequate amounts of sleep. A corresponding behavioral objective might be that the child will take a midday nap of at least 1 hour for 3 days per week. The intervention could involve direct remediation to reduce the sensory defensiveness as well as parent consultation on strategies such as calming activities, a very predictable activity schedule including a specific rest time ritual, and creation of an arousal-reducing environment after lunch (e.g., lights dimmed and noise reduced and screened with rhythmic sounds or "white noise").

Sometimes specific behavioral objectives that address performance skills are appropriate as a way to monitor progress toward the desired changes in daily occupations. Goals can be conceptualized as falling into seven general categories of expected outcomes that address performance skills and patterns, as well as occupational engagement. These outcomes are summarized in Box 11-3; more detailed descriptions of each category follow.

Increase in the Frequency or Duration of Adaptive Responses

As discussed in the introduction of this chapter, adaptive responses occur when an individual responds to environmental challenges with success. Application of ASI principles helps the therapist envision how to create opportunities for the child to make adaptive responses. This may be accomplished through systematic use of sensory input to promote organization within the child's nervous system. Ensuring that the sensory inputs inherent in activities are organizing rather than disorganizing and integrating rather than overwhelming requires careful monitoring on the part of the therapist, who must be sensitive to the child's response to each aspect of an activity and to each type of sensory input involved. The ASI intervention approach intensively focuses on the child's demonstration of higher level adaptive responses. However, specific skill training, group intervention, and consultation services may also boost the frequency and duration of adaptive responses by changing the child's everyday environments in ways that enable the child to make adaptive responses more easily.

Increasing the duration and frequency of adaptive responses is an important outcome of sensory integration because functional behavior and skills are developed by mastering simple adaptive responses. For example, a child who has difficulty staying with an activity for more than a few seconds tends to shift from one activity to another. A desirable outcome for that child might be to stay for a longer time with a simple activity, such as swinging, in a therapy environment. Achievement of this simple adaptive response may eventually contribute to the functional behavior of staying with the reading circle in the school classroom for the required amount of time, despite the many distractions and cognitive challenges imposed by this occupation.

Development of Increasingly More Complex Adaptive Responses

Adaptive responses can vary in complexity, quality, and effectiveness.[19] A simple adaptive response might be simply holding onto a moving swing. A more complex adaptive response involving timing of action might be releasing grasp on a trapeze at just the right moment to land on a pillow. Over time, effective ASI intervention is expected to enable the child to make adaptive responses that are more complex. This outcome is based on the assumption that sensory integrative procedures promote more efficient organization of multisensory input at primitive levels of functioning, which in turn is expected to enhance functions that are more complex. The result is an improvement in the child's ability to make judgments about the environment, what can be done with objects, and what specific actions need to be taken to accomplish a goal.[19]

Although repetition of a familiar activity may be important while a child is assimilating a new skill and may be useful in helping a child get ready for another, more challenging activity, development of increasingly more complex abilities occurs only when tasks become slightly more challenging than the child's previous accomplishments. Presenting activities slightly above the child's current skills levels is one of the main tenets of ASI intervention. Because of the high degree of personal attention continuously given to the child during this kind of therapy, a fine gradient of complexity can be built into therapeutic activities while simultaneously ensuring that the child experiences success and a growing sense of "I can do it!"

Group programs, compared with individual therapy, tend to place greater demands on children for several reasons, including limited opportunity for individualization of activities, the presence of other children with their unpredictable behaviors, and reduced opportunity for direct assistance from the therapist. Thus, a limitation posed by group programs is that challenges imposed on the group may at times be too great for an individual child, leading to frustration and failure. The therapist who provides a group program needs to be alert to the potential for this undesirable effect and strive to avoid it as much as possible. Whatever format for intervention is used, the therapist uses activity analysis, assessment information, ongoing observations, and knowledge of child development to ensure that the program engages the child's inner drive as much as possible to draw forth increasingly more complex interactions within the clinical, school, home, or community environments.

Improvement in Gross and Fine Motor Skills

The child who makes consistent and more complex adaptive responses shows evidence of improved sensory integration. Moreover, this child meets new challenges with greater self-confidence. A net result of these gains frequently is greater mastery in the motor domain. An example is the child with a vestibular processing problem who exhibits greater competency and interest in playground activities and sports after individual ASI intervention, even though these activities were not practiced during therapy. Motor skills may be among the earliest complex skills to show measurable change in response to an ASI approach, probably because of the extent of the motor activity inherent in this intervention approach. Skill training, group intervention, or consultation for children with sensory integrative problems should result in improvement of specific motor skills if these are targeted by the intervention. For example, if a skill-training approach to handwriting is used to help a child with poor somatosensory perception, specific gains in handwriting performance should follow if the intervention is successful.

Improvement in Cognitive, Language, or Academic Performance

Although cognitive, language, and academic skills are not usually the specific objectives of sensory integration–based occupational therapy, improvement in these domains has been detected in some effectiveness studies involving the provision of ASI intervention.[10,15,17,23,42,92,123,151] Application of ASI therapeutic procedures is thought to generate broad-based changes in these areas secondary to enhancement of sensory modulation, perception, postural control, or praxis.[18,19,43] For example, a child with autism may be helped through a sensory integrative approach to respond in a more adaptive way to sights, sounds, touch, and movement experiences that initially were disturbing. This improvement in sensory modulation may lead to a better ability to attend to language and academic tasks; thus, improvement in these areas may follow. A child who has a vestibular processing disorder may improve in postural control and equilibrium, freeing the child to more efficiently concentrate on academic material without the distraction of frequent loss of sitting balance or loss of place while copying from the blackboard. This child's vestibular-related improvements are also likely to have a positive effect on playground and sports activities because effects of classic sensory integration treatment are expected to generalize to a wide range of outcome areas.

Occupational therapy aimed at developing specific skills such as improved handwriting also may free the child to focus on the conceptual aspects of academic tasks rather than the perceptual-motor details of how to write letters on a page or how to keep a sentence on a printed line. For such interventions, effects on outcome skills tend to be limited to the specific task of concern. Similarly, consultation programs may enhance language, cognitive, or academic skills by providing strategies for reducing the effect of sensory integrative disorders on these functions. For instance, helping a teacher understand how best to seat a child in class (such as in a beanbag chair versus a firm wooden chair or in the front corner of the room near the teacher's desk) may help reduce the negative effects of a sensory integrative problem by making it easier for the child to attend to instruction in the classroom.

Increase in Self-Confidence and Self-Esteem

Ayres asserted that enhanced ability to make adaptive responses promotes self-actualization by allowing the child to experience the joy of accomplishing a task that previously could not be done.[18] The outcome of therapy that encourages successful, self-directed experiences is a child who perceives the self as a competent actor in the world. Individual and group programs and direct and indirect services all can be geared to helping the child master the activities that are personally meaningful and essential to success in the world of everyday occupations. Mastery of such activities is expected to result in feelings of personal control that, in turn, lead to increased willingness to take risks and to try new things.[18] For example, a child with gravitational insecurity may experience not only fear responses to climbing and movement activities, but also feelings of failure and frustration at not being able to participate in the play of peers. In such a case, an increase in self-confidence and comfort in one's physical body is often accompanied by a general boost in feelings of self-efficacy and worth. Cohn, Miller, and Tickle-Degnen noted that parents' perceptions of the benefits of occupational therapy using a sensory integrative approach included a reconstruction of self-worth, in addition to improvement in abilities and activities.[53] Parents in this study perceived that this intervention enabled their children to take more risks and to try new things, thus opening the door to greater possibilities.

Enhanced Occupational Engagement and Social Participation

Occupational therapy programs that address sensory integrative problems encourage the child to organize his or her own activity, particularly in the ASI intervention approach. As the child develops general sensory integrative capabilities and improved strategies for planning action, gains are seen in relation to the ability to master self-care tasks, to cope with daily routines, and to organize behavior more generally.[18] As a result, the child often is able to participate more fully in the occupations that are typical for his or her peers, a broad but critically important outcome for social participation. For example, intervention may help the child who is overly sensitive to touch or movement to deal with sensations in a more adaptive manner. As a result, the child approaches and engages in the challenges of everyday occupations, such as getting himself or herself ready for school in the morning, sharing a table with others in the school cafeteria, behaving appropriately in the classroom, and playing with friends on the playground with greater security and confidence. As noted previously, Cohn et al. reported that parents viewed their children as more willing to try new experiences following intervention, thus enhancing their opportunities for social participation.[53] Not only is participation in daily occupations performed with greater competency and satisfaction, but relationships with others are likely to become more comfortable and less threatening. Group therapy programs are ideal arenas in which the increases in self-confidence made in individual therapy can be tried out in the more challenging context of a social setting. Gains in occupational engagement and social participation are among the most significant of intervention outcomes.

Enhanced Family Life

When children with sensory integrative problems experience positive changes during intervention, their lives and the lives of other family members may be enhanced. One possible by-product of intervention based on ASI principles is that parents gain a better understanding of their children's behavior and begin to generate their own strategies for organizing family routines in a way that supports the entire family system. This kind of change can be particularly powerful for parents of children with autism, whose perceptions of child behaviors may be reframed as they become familiar with the sensory integrative perspective. For example, behavior that is interpreted as bizarre, such as insisting on wearing rubber bands on the arms, may be reframed as a meaningful strategy that the child uses to obtain deep pressure input for self-calming.[2] Instead of viewing the behavior as a frustrating, pathologic sign that should be eliminated, reframing may lead the parents to explore other ways that they could provide the child with the deep pressure experiences that he or she seeks. Thus, an important outcome of sensory integrative intervention may include changes in parents' understanding of the child, leading to new coping strategies and alleviation of parental stress.[52] In her studies of parental perspectives, Cohn has found that an important outcome of the sensory integrative approach is that parents tend to "reframe" their view and expectations of their children in a positive manner.[50,51]

Measuring Outcomes

Because every child with a sensory integrative problem is unique, the expected outcomes of occupational therapy using an ASI approach are individualized and diverse. Outcomes are sometimes measured using standardized tests. In fact, some of the SIPT tests (e.g., Design Copying, Standing and Walking Balance, and most of the praxis tests) are good measures of change because of their strong test–retest reliability, in addition to being relevant to concerns that are commonly voiced by parents and teachers. However, standardized tests often do not address key occupational issues.

Goal attainment scaling (GAS) is an alternative to standardized tests that addresses the uniquely individualized nature of expected outcomes of ASI. The GAS method was developed in the mental health arena as a program evaluation tool to facilitate patient participation in the goal-setting process.[83] GAS provides a means to prioritize goals that are specifically relevant to individuals and their families and to quantify the results using a standard metric that allows comparison of achievement across different types of goals. This process also captures functional and meaningful aspects of an individual's progress that are often challenging to assess using available standardized measures. For this reason, GAS is an attractive methodology for measuring change during occupational therapy, and it has now been successfully applied in occupational therapy effectiveness research in a variety of settings, including rehabilitation,[80,110] school systems,[58,82] and mental health programs.[90,140] This approach seems promising for capturing the diverse changes that are reported following ASI intervention programs.[95] Case examples demonstrating how GAS has been applied to measure outcomes of ASI-based occupational therapy are described by Miller and Summers.[108] In a randomized, controlled clinical trial, GAS detected significant improvements among children who received ASI intervention, compared to children receiving alternative conditions.[106]

Research on Effectiveness of Intervention

Therapists who wish to use an ASI approach in practice need to keep up to date on research in this field to ensure that intervention is informed by the growing knowledge base. Research on the effectiveness of ASI-based interventions is particularly critical to evidence-based practice in this specialty area.

In a meta-analysis of experimental research on sensory integrative treatment, Vargas and Camilli analyzed 16 studies comparing sensory integrative treatment with no treatment and 16 studies comparing sensory integrative treatment with alternative treatments.[149] These included studies of adults as well as studies in which the descriptions of intervention were inconsistent with ASI principles. A significant overall average effect size of 0.29 was found for sensory integrative treatment compared with no treatment, indicating an advantage for children receiving the treatment. The largest effect sizes were found for psychoeducational and motor outcome measures. However, older studies had a significantly higher effect size than more recent studies, which did not have a significant effect size when considered by themselves. The average effect size for sensory integrative treatment compared with alternative treatments was 0.09, a quite small effect, and the sensory integrative treatments did not differ significantly from alternative treatments in effect size.

The decline in effect size of sensory integrative treatment studies over the years is puzzling. The authors of the meta-analysis suggest that the reason for this finding may lie in some unidentified difference in treatment implementation, or with selection and assignment of participants to experimental and control groups in the older studies versus the more recent ones.[149] They point out that, in general, the studies examined sensory integration intervention in isolation and therefore do not represent the ways that sensory integration is implemented clinically, which usually involve incorporation of other treatment methods in addition to those that adhere to ASI principles. Another plausible explanation not explored by these authors is that, although the studies included in this meta-analysis all claimed to study intervention based on the work of Ayres, the interventions delivered in the studies were not all consistent with the core elements and key therapeutic strategies of ASI. This limitation is called a problem with fidelity, discussed further on.

After examining the effectiveness research on sensory integration, both Miller[103] and Mulligan[112] concluded that the effectiveness of sensory integration–based occupational therapy is neither proved nor unproved. This is because all of the existing studies that support the effectiveness of sensory integration intervention, as well as those that do not support its effectiveness, are flawed. Randomized, controlled clinical trials are considered to yield valid results only if they adhere to four standards: replicable intervention, homogeneous sample, sensitive and relevant outcome measures, and rigorous methodology.[34]

Many studies used unclear or unsound methods to identify who is to receive sensory integration treatment. This created the possibility that some children who do not have sensory integrative dysfunction were inappropriately assigned to this treatment. An exemplary pilot study with respect to selection of participants is the small randomized, controlled clinical trial conducted by Miller, Coll, and Schoen, who focused on effectiveness of ASI intervention for children with sensory modulation disorders (Research Note 11-2).[106] These researchers carefully selected children using behavioral and physiologic measures to confirm the presence of sensory modulation disorder and then randomly assigned each child to one of three

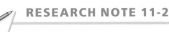

RESEARCH NOTE 11-2

Miller, L. J., Coll, J. R., & Schoen, S. A. (2007). A randomized controlled pilot study of the effectiveness of occupational therapy for children with sensory modulation disorder. American Journal of Occupational Therapy, 61, *228-238.*

OBJECTIVES. This was a pilot randomized controlled trial (RCT) of the effectiveness of occupational therapy using a sensory integration approach (OT-SI) with children who had sensory modulation disorders (SMDs). The primary objectives of the study were to evaluate the effectiveness of OT-SI compared with an alternative treatment and no treatment and to use study results to estimate desirable sample size for a larger multisite study.

METHOD. Twenty-four children with SMD were randomly assigned to one of three treatment conditions; OT-SI, Activity Protocol (a tabletop play activity program), and No Treatment. SMD was confirmed with behavioral and physiologic measures that indicated overresponsiveness. Pretest and posttest measures of behavior, sensory and adaptive functioning, and physiology were administered.

RESULTS. The OT-SI group, compared with the other two groups, made significant gains on goal attainment scaling and on the Attention subtest and the Cognitive/Social composite of the Leiter International Performance Scale-Revised. In addition, children receiving OT-SI demonstrated changes in the hypothesized directions, compared with the control groups, on the Short Sensory Profile, Child Behavior Checklist, and electrodermal reactivity.

CONCLUSION. Findings suggest that OT-SI may be effective in improving the functioning and participation of children with sensory modulation difficulties, such as tactile or auditory overresponsiveness.

IMPLICATIONS FOR PRACTICE

This study indicates that occupational therapy using a sensory integration approach may be an appropriate choice of intervention for children with sensory modulation problems involving overresponsiveness, when the therapist has adequate clinical assessment data to confirm the presence of these problems. Expected outcomes may include improvements in attention and social participation and achievement of individualized family goals for the child in daily life.

conditions: individual ASI intervention, an alternative tabletop activity program, or a passive placebo condition. Results showed that children who had received ASI intervention had better outcomes than children in the other conditions, and that some of their gains were statistically significant, specifically in Goal Attainment Scaling measures, as well as measures of attention and cognitive/social functioning.

Another common flaw is lack of fidelity. *Fidelity* refers to the extent to which the intervention provided in a study is faithful to the key elements of the intervention approach. Sometimes investigators use a rigid or very limited treatment protocol in an effort to ensure that the sensory integration treatment is well defined and adheres to strict criteria. Although the purpose of this strategy is laudable (i.e., to ensure that the treatment is replicable), it may result in an intervention that lacks fidelity to the core elements of the sensory integration approach. This is because a rigid treatment protocol is incompatible with the highly individualized, child-centered, fluid nature of ASI intervention; therefore, any results obtained do not represent the effects of ASI intervention. On the other hand, if treatment guidelines are too vague, or are not checked systematically during the delivery of the intervention, one cannot trust that the intervention was delivered in a consistent manner across the participants and across the intervention period of the study.

To examine fidelity in sensory integration research, Parham et al. conducted a systematic review of 61 separate published studies that purportedly evaluated the effectiveness of sensory integration–based occupational therapy.[116] Of the 61 studies, 34 provided this intervention to participants in the age range for which it was developed, preschool through elementary school age, without combining it with a non–sensory integration intervention. These 34 studies were analyzed for whether their descriptions of intervention adhered to key elements of ASI intervention that the authors and collaborating clinicians had extracted from the sensory integration literature. Results showed that only one of the key elements, "presents sensory opportunities," was described in the majority of studies. More than one third of the studies contained sensory integration intervention descriptions that were contrary to one of the key elements, "collaborates with child on activity choice." This is because, in these studies, the specific activities to be used in the intervention were determined by the researcher or the treating therapist prior to provision of intervention, rather than emerging from the interactions between child and therapist. Moreover, only one study used a quantifiable instrument to measure fidelity of intervention, and this instrument documented use of activities and equipment rather than the process of intervention. Parham et al. concluded that the effectiveness of sensory integration intervention cannot yet be made with confidence due to the lack of intervention fidelity in this research.[116] To address this fidelity problem, a national network of occupational therapy researchers and practitioners, the Sensory Integration Research Collaborative (SIRC), developed a reliable and valid instrument, the Sensory Integration Fidelity Measure, to be used in research on ASI intervention.[118] This instrument contains ratings of the structural background aspects of intervention, such as therapist qualifications and equipment, as well as ratings of the process of therapy (i.e., the therapeutic strategies used by the intervener during a therapy session), that reflect the core elements of ASI intervention.

Another common problem in sensory integration outcomes research is related to selection of outcome measures. Often children's responses to ASI intervention are as individualized as the intervention strategies, making it difficult, perhaps impossible, for the researcher to select tests and other measurements that target the precise areas of gain for individual children. Moreover, it is likely that children with different types of sensory integrative problems respond to this treatment with different kinds of gains. For example, children with tactile defensiveness are likely to show gains in outcome domains different from those in which children with vestibular processing difficulties made progress; yet almost all of the research studies lump children together with sensory integrative problems as if they should have similar responses to a standard treatment. This certainly was not Ayres's view, because she spent considerable effort attempting to identify subgroups of children with sensory integrative problems who might differ from one another with respect to degree and type of responsiveness to intervention.[10,17,26] It is hoped that researchers who conduct future effectiveness studies will become more sensitive to this important issue.

Another important issue that is rarely addressed is the maintenance of long-term gains after completion of a period of ASI-based occupational therapy is completed. An encouraging finding reported by Wilson and Kaplan suggests that children who receive sensory integration intervention may obtain long-term benefits that are not obtained by children who receive other interventions.[155] These researchers retested children who had participated in an earlier randomized, controlled clinical trial comparing sensory integration intervention with tutoring. Although no significant differences in outcomes were found between the two intervention groups in the original study,[156] at follow-up 2 years later, only the children who had received the sensory integration treatment maintained the gross motor gains that they had made after intervention. Maintenance of intervention gains is a critical issue that has an influence on cost-effectiveness questions. Replication of Wilson and Kaplan's findings[155] using the Sensory Integration Fidelity Measure to document the intervention would make an important contribution to understanding the extent to which gains after sensory integration treatment can be maintained.

Although group experimental treatment designs are considered to be the gold standard of effectiveness studies, other research designs examining treatment outcomes also make valuable contributions to an understanding of the potential effects of sensory integration intervention. Single system research has been particularly useful in revealing individual differences in responses to sensory integrative treatment. In this kind of research, a child serves as his or her own control and is monitored repeatedly before intervention (the baseline phase) and during intervention. An advantage to this approach is that behavioral outcomes can be highly individualized and tracked over time to provide a snapshot of each child's response to intervention. An example of this type of research is the study conducted by Linderman and Stewart on two preschoolers with pervasive developmental disorders. The researchers measured three behavioral outcomes for each child.[89] Each outcome was observed in the child's home and was tailored to address functional issues for each child (e.g., response to holding and hugging for one child and functional communication during mealtime for the other). Results indicate significant improvements between baseline and intervention phases for five of the six outcomes measured.

A great deal of investigation remains to be done to explore questions regarding effectiveness of interventions based in ASI. It would be particularly beneficial to be able to better predict who will best respond to individual ASI intervention and who may be better served by other interventions. The effectiveness of combining individual ASI intervention with other ASI-informed interventions, such as specific skill training, group programs, or consultation, is another area in need of research, particularly because such intervention combinations are typically done in clinical practice. The kinds of outcomes likely to proceed from various treatment approaches and the timeframes in which those outcomes can be expected to emerge deserve close examination in effectiveness studies. Long-term maintenance of gains, particularly of those related to outcomes that are measures of social participation, is a particularly important question that should be addressed in research. Finally, studies need to explore which intervention outcomes are most meaningful to the families of children with sensory integration problems to ensure that intervention programs are responsive to the needs of the people served.

REFERENCES

1. American Occupational Therapy Association. (2008). Occupational therapy practice framework: Domain and process. (2nd ed). *American Journal of Occupational Therapy, 62,* 625-668.

2. Anderson, E. L. (1993). *Parental perceptions of the influence of occupational therapy utilizing sensory integrative techniques on the daily living skills of children with autism.* Unpublished master's thesis. Los Angeles: University of Southern California.

3. Ayres, A. J. (1963). The Eleanor Clark Slagle Lecture. The development of perceptual-motor abilities: A theoretical basis for treatment of dysfunction. *American Journal of Occupational Therapy, 17,* 221-225.

4. Ayres, A. J. (1964). Tactile functions: Their relation to hyperactive and perceptual motor behavior. *American Journal of Occupational Therapy, 18,* 6-11.

5. Ayres, A. J. (1965). Patterns of perceptual-motor dysfunction in children: A factor analytic study. *Perceptual and Motor Skills, 20,* 335-368.

6. Ayres, A. J. (1966). Interrelations among perceptual-motor abilities in a group of normal children. *American Journal of Occupational Therapy, 20,* 288-292.

7. Ayres, A. J. (1966). Interrelationships among perceptual-motor functions in children. *American Journal of Occupational Therapy, 20,* 68-71.

8. Ayres, A. J. (1969). Deficits in sensory integration in educationally handicapped children. *Journal of Learning Disabilities, 2*(3), 44-52.

9. Ayres, A. J. (1971). Characteristics of types of sensory integrative dysfunction. *American Journal of Occupational Therapy, 25,* 329-334.

10. Ayres, A. J. (1972). Improving academic scores through sensory integration. *Journal of Learning Disabilities, 5,* 338-343.

11. Ayres, A. J. (1972). *Sensory integration and learning disorders.* Los Angeles: Western Psychological Services.

12. Ayres, A. J. (1972). *Southern California Sensory Integration Tests.* Los Angeles: Western Psychological Services.

13. Ayres, A. J. (1972). Types of sensory integrative dysfunction among disabled learners. *American Journal of Occupational Therapy, 26*(1), 13-18.

14. Ayres, A. J. (1975). *Southern California Postrotary Nystagmus Test.* Los Angeles: Western Psychological Services.

15. Ayres, A. J. (1976). *The effect of sensory integrative therapy on learning disabled children: The final report of a research project.* Los Angeles: Center for the Study of Sensory Integrative Dysfunction.

16. Ayres, A. J. (1977). Cluster analyses of measures of sensory integration. *American Journal of Occupational Therapy, 31*(6), 362-366.

17. Ayres, A. J. (1978). Learning disabilities and the vestibular system. *Journal of Learning Disabilities, 11*(1), 30-41.

18. Ayres, A. J. (1979). *Sensory integration and the child.* Los Angeles: Western Psychological Services.

19. Ayres, A. J. (1981). *Aspects of the somatomotor adaptive response and praxis.* [Audiotape]. Pasadena, CA: Center for the Study of Sensory Integrative Dysfunction.

20. Ayres, A. J. (1985). *Developmental dyspraxia and adult-onset apraxia.* Torrance, CA: Sensory Integration International.

21. Ayres, A. J. (1989). *Sensory Integration and Praxis Tests manual.* Los Angeles: Western Psychological Services.

22. Ayres, A. J. (2004). *Sensory integration and the child* (2nd ed.). Los Angeles: Western Psychological Services.

23. Ayres, A. J., & Mailloux, Z. (1981). Influence of sensory integration procedures on language development. *American Journal of Occupational Therapy, 35*(6), 383-390.

24. Ayres, A. J., Mailloux, Z., & Wendler, C. L. W. (1987). Developmental apraxia: Is it a unitary function? *Occupational Therapy Journal of Research, 7,* 93-110.

25. Ayres, A. J., & Marr, D. (1991). Sensory Integration and Praxis Tests. In A. G. Fisher, E. A. Murray, & A. C. Bundy (Eds.), *Sensory integration: Theory and practice* (pp. 203-250). Philadelphia: F.A. Davis.

26. Ayres, A. J., & Tickle, L. (1980). Hyperresponsivity to touch and vestibular stimuli as a predictor of positive response to sensory integration procedures in autistic children. *American Journal of Occupational Therapy, 34,* 375-381.

27. Bach-Y-Rita, P. (1981). Brain plasticity. In J. Goodgold (Ed.), *Brain plasticity.* St. Louis: Mosby.

28. Baranek, G. T., Foster, L. G., & Berkson, G. (1997). Sensory defensiveness in persons with developmental disabilities. *Occupational Therapy Journal of Research, 17,* 173-185.

29. Beckett, C., Maughan, B., Rutter, M., Castle, J., Colvert, E., Groothues, C., et al. (2006). Do the effects of early severe deprivation on cognition persist into early adolescence? Findings from the English and Romanian Adoptees Study. *Child Development, 77,* 696-711.

30. Beery, K. E., & Beery, N. A. (2006). *The Developmental Test of Visual-Motor Integration* (5th ed.). San Antonio, TX: Psychological Corporation.

31. Bennett, E. L., Diamond, M. C., Krech, D., & Rosenzwieg, M. R. (1964). Chemical and anatomical plasticity of brain. *Science, 146,* 610-619.

32. Blanche, E. I. (2002). *Observations based on sensory integration theory.* Torrance, CA: Pediatric Therapy Network.

33. Blanche, E., & Schaaf, R. (2001). Proprioception: A cornerstone of sensory integrative intervention. In S. S. Roley, E. I. Blanche, & R. C. Schaaf (Eds.), *Understanding the nature of sensory integration with diverse populations* (pp. 385-408). San Antonio, TX: Therapy Skill Builders.

34. Boruch, R. F. (1997). *Randomized experiments for planning and evaluation: A practical guide.* Thousand Oaks, CA: Sage.

35. Bretherton, I., Bates, E., McNew, S., Shore, C., Williamson, C., & Beeghly-Smith, M. (1981). Comprehension and production of symbols in infancy: An experimental study. *Developmental Psychology, 17,* 728-736.

36. Brown, C., & Dunn, W. (2002). *Adolescent/Adult Sensory Profile.* San Antonio, TX: The Psychological Corporation.

37. Bruininks, R. H., & Bruininks, B. (2006). *Bruininks-Oseretsky Test of Motor Proficiency examiner's manual.* Circle Pines, MN: American Guidance Service.

38. Bundy, A. C. (2002). Using sensory integration theory in schools: Sensory integration and consultation. In A. C. Bundy, S. J. Lane, & E. A. Murray (Eds.), *Sensory integration: Theory and practice* (2nd ed., pp. 309-332). Philadelphia: F.A. Davis.

39. Bundy, A. C., & Murray, E. A. (2002). Sensory integration: A. Jean Ayres' theory revisited. In A. C. Bundy, S. J. Lane, & E. A. Murray (Eds.), *Sensory integration: Theory and practice* (2nd ed., pp. 141-165). Philadelphia: F.A. Davis.

40. Burke, J. P., Schaaf, R. C., & Hall, T. B. L. (2008). Family narratives and play assessment. In L. D. Parham & L. S. Fazio (Eds.), *Play in occupational therapy for children* (2nd ed., pp. 195-215). St. Louis: Mosby.

41. Burleigh, J. M., McIntosh, K. W., & Thompson, M. W. (2002). Central auditory processing disorders. In A. C. Bundy, S. J. Lane, & E. A. Murray (Eds.), *Sensory integration: Theory and practice* (2nd ed., pp. 141-165). Philadelphia: F.A. Davis.

42. Cabay, M. (1988). *The effect of sensory integration–based treatment on academic readiness of young, "at risk" school children.* Phoenix,

AZ: Annual conference of the American Occupational Therapy Association.

43. Cabay, M., & King, L. J. (1989). Sensory integration and perception: The foundation for concept formation. *Occupational Therapy in Practice, 1,* 18-27.

44. Case-Smith, J. (1991). The effects of tactile defensiveness and tactile discrimination on in-hand manipulation. *American Journal of Occupational Therapy, 45,* 811-818.

45. Cermak, S. A. (1988). The relationship between attention deficits and sensory integration disorders (Part I). *Sensory Integration Special Interest Section Newsletter, 11*(2), 1-4.

46. Cermak, S. A. (1991). Somatodyspraxia. In A. G. Fisher, E. A. Murray, & A. C. Bundy (Eds.), *Sensory integration: Theory and practice* (pp. 137-170). Philadelphia: F.A. Davis.

47. Cermak, S. A. (2001). The effects of deprivation on processing, play and praxis. In S. S. Roley, E. I. Blanche, & R. C. Schaaf (Eds.), *Understanding the nature of sensory integration with diverse populations* (pp. 385-408). San Antonio, TX: Therapy Skill Builders.

48. Chugani, H. T., & Phelps, M. E. (1986). Maturational changes in cerebral function in infants determined by 18FDG positron emission tomography. *Science, 231,* 840-843.

49. Clark, F. A., Mailloux, Z., & Parham, D. (1989). Sensory integration and children with learning disorders. In P. N. Pratt & A. S. Allen (Eds.), *Occupational therapy for children* (2nd ed., pp. 457-509). St. Louis: Mosby.

50. Cohn, E. S. (2001). From waiting to relating: Parents' experiences in the waiting room of an occupational therapy clinic. *American Journal of Occupational Therapy, 55,* 168-175.

51. Cohn, E. S. (2001). Parent perspectives of occupational therapy using a sensory integration approach. *American Journal of Occupational Therapy, 55,* 285-294.

52. Cohn, E. S., & Cermak, S. A. (1998). Including the family perspective in sensory integration outcomes research. *American Journal of Occupational Therapy, 52,* 540-546.

53. Cohn, E. S., Miller, L. J., & Tickle-Degnen, L. (2000). Parental hopes for therapy outcomes: Children with sensory modulation disorders. *American Journal of Occupational Therapy, 54,* 36-43.

54. Coster, W., Deeney, T., Haltwanger, J., & Haley, S. (1998). *School Function Assessment.* San Antonio, TX: Therapy Skill Builders.

55. Cui, M., Yang, Y., Zhang, J., Han, H., Ma, W., Li, H., et al. (2007). Enriched environment experience overcomes the memory deficits and depressive-like behavior induced by early life stress. *Neuroscience Letters, 404,* 208-212.

56. Daunhauer, L., & Cermak, S. (2008). Play occupations and the experience of deprivation. In D. Parham & L. Fazio (Eds.), *Play in occupational therapy for children* (2nd ed.). St. Louis: Mosby.

57. Davies, P. L., & Gavin, W. J. (2007). Validating the diagnosis of sensory processing disorders using EEG technology. *American Journal of Occupational Therapy, 61,* 176-189.

58. Dreiling, D. S., & Bundy, A. C. (2003). A comparison of consultative model and direct-indirect intervention with preschoolers. *American Journal of Occupational Therapy, 57,* 566-569.

59. Dru, D., Walker, J. P., & Walker, J. B. (1975). Self-produced locomotion restores visual capacity after striate lesion. *Science, 187,* 265-266.

60. Dunn, R., Dunn, K., & Perrin, K. J. (1994). *Teaching young children through their individual learning styles.* Boston: Allyn & Bacon.

61. Dunn, W. W. (1997). The impact of sensory processing abilities on the daily lives of young children and families: A conceptual model. *Infants and Young Children, 9*(4), 23-25.

62. Dunn, W. W. (1999). *Sensory Profile: User's manual.* San Antonio, TX: Psychological Corporation.

63. Dunn, W. W. (2001). The sensations of everyday life: Empirical, theoretical, and pragmatic considerations. *American Journal of Occupational Therapy, 55,* 608-620.

64. Dunn, W. W. (2002). *The Infant/Toddler Sensory Profile manual.* San Antonio, TX: Psychological Corporation.

65. Dunn, W. (2006). *Sensory Profile School Companion manual.* San Antonio, TX: Psychological Corporation.

66. Dunn, W., & Fisher, A. G. (1983). Sensory registration, autism, and tactile defensiveness. In J. Melvin (Ed.), *Occupational therapy in practice* (Vol. 1, pp. 181-182). Rockville, MD: American Occupational Therapy Association.

67. Dunn, W., Myles, B. S., & Orr, S. (2002). Sensory processing issues associated with Asperger syndrome: A preliminary investigation. *American Journal of Occupational Therapy, 56,* 97-102.

68. Fisher, A. G. (1991). Vestibular-proprioceptive processing and bilateral integration and sequencing deficits. In A. G. Fisher, E. A. Murray, & A. C. Bundy (Eds.), *Sensory integration: Theory and practice* (pp. 69-107). Philadelphia: F.A. Davis.

69. Fredrickson, J. M., Schwartz, D. W., & Kornhuber, H. H. (1966). Convergence and interaction of vestibular and deep somatic afferents upon neurons in the vestibular nuclei of the cat. *Acta Otolaryngologica, 61,* 168-188.

70. Gregg, C. L., Hafner, M. E., & Korner, A. (1976). The relative efficacy of vestibular-proprioceptive stimulation and the upright position in enhancing visual pursuit in neonates. *Child Development, 47,* 309-314.

71. Gregory-Flock, J. L., & Yerxa, E. J. (1984). Standardization of the prone extension postural test on children ages 4 through 8. *American Journal of Occupational Therapy, 38,* 187-194.

72. Gunnar, M. R., & Barr, R. G. (1998). Stress, early brain development, and behavior. *Infants and Young Children, 11*(1), 1-14.

73. Henderson, A., Pehoski, C., & Murray, E. (2002). Visual-spatial abilities. In A. C. Bundy, S. J. Lane, & E. A. Murray (Eds.), *Sensory integration: Theory and practice* (pp. 123-140). Philadelphia: F.A. Davis.

74. Hensch, T. K. (2005). Critical period plasticity in local cortical circuits. *Nature Reviews. Neuroscience, 6,* 877-888.

75. Hickman, L. (2001). Sensory integration and fragile X syndrome. In S. S. Roley, E. I. Blanche, & R. C. Schaaf (Eds.), *Understanding the nature of sensory integration with diverse populations* (pp. 385-408). San Antonio, TX: Therapy Skill Builders.

76. Holloway, E. (1998). Early emotional development and sensory processing. In J. Case-Smith (Ed.), *Pediatric occupational therapy and early intervention* (pp. 163-197). Boston: Andover Medical.

77. Hubel, D. H., & Wiesel, T. N. (1963). Receptive fields of cells in striate cortex of very young, visually inexperienced kittens. *Journal of Neurophysiology, 26,* 994-1002.

78. Salihagic-Kadic, A., Kurjak, A., Medic, M., Andonotopo, W., & Azumendi, G. (2005). New data about embryonic and fetal neurodevelopment and behavior obtained by 3D and 4D sonography. *Journal of Perinatal Medicine, 33,* 478-490.

79. Jacobs, S. E., & Schenider, M. L. (2001). Neuroplasticity and the environment. In S. S. Roley, E. I. Blanche, & R. C. Schaaf (Eds.), *Understanding the nature of sensory integration with diverse populations* (pp. 29-42). San Antonio, TX: Therapy Skill Builders.

80. Joyce, B. M., Rockwood, K. J., & Mate-Kole, C. C. (1994). Use of goal attainment scaling in brain injury in a rehabilitation hospital. *American Journal of Physical Medicine and Rehabilitation, 73*(1), 10-14.

81. Kimball, J. G. (1999). Sensory integrative frame of reference. In P. Kramer & J. Hinojosa (Eds.), *Frames of reference for pediatric occupational therapy* (pp. 169–204). Baltimore: Williams & Wilkins.

82. King, G. A., McDougall, J., Tucker, M. A., Gritzan, J., Malloy-Miller, T., Alambets, P., et al. (1999). An evaluation of functional, school-based therapy services for children with special needs. *Physical & Occupational Therapy in Pediatrics, 19*(2), 5-29.

83. Kiresuk, T. J., Smith, A., & Cardillo, J. E. (1994). *Goal attainment scaling: Applications, theory, and measurement.* Hillsdale, NJ: Lawrence Erlbaum Associates.

84. Knickerbocker, B. M. (1980). *A holistic approach to learning disabilities.* Thorofare, NJ: C.B. Slack.

85. Koomar, J. A., & Bundy, A. C. (2002). Creating direct intervention from theory. In A. C. Bundy, S. J. Lane, & E. A. Murray (Eds.), *Sensory integration: Theory and practice* (2nd ed., pp. 261-308). Philadelphia: F.A. Davis.

86. Lai, J. S., Parham, L. D., & Johnson-Ecker, C. (1999). Sensory dormancy and sensory defensiveness: Two sides of the same coin? *Sensory Integration Special Interest Section Quarterly, 22,* 1-4.

87. Lee, J. R. V. (1999). *Parent ratings of children with autism on the Evaluation of Sensory Processing (ESP)*. Unpublished master's thesis. Los Angeles: University of Southern California.

88. Lee, H. W., Shin, J. S., Webber, W. R. S., Crone, N. E., Gingis, L., & Lesser, R. P. (2009). Reorganisation of cortical motor and language distribution in human brain. *Journal of Neurology, Neurosurgery, and Psychiatry, 80,* 285-290.

89. Linderman, T. M., & Stewart, K. B. (1999). Sensory integrative-based occupational therapy and functional outcomes in young children with pervasive developmental disorders: A single-subject study. *American Journal of Occupational Therapy, 53,* 207-213.

90. Lloyd, C. (1986). The process of goal setting using goal attainment scaling in a therapeutic community. *Occupational Therapy in Mental Health, 6*(3), 19-30.

91. Magalhaes, L. C., Koomar, J., & Cermak, S. A. (1989). Bilateral motor coordination in 5- to 9-year-old children. *American Journal of Occupational Therapy, 43,* 437-443.

92. Magrun, W. M., Ottenbacher, K., McCue, S., & Keefe, R. (1981). Effects of vestibular stimulation on spontaneous use of verbal language in developmentally delayed children. *American Journal of Occupational Therapy, 35,* 101-104.

93. Mailloux, Z. (2001). Sensory integrative principles in intervention with children with autistic disorder. In S. S. Roley, E. I. Blanche, & R. C. Schaaf (Eds.), *Understanding the nature of sensory integration with diverse populations* (pp. 385-408). San Antonio, TX: Therapy Skill Builders.

94. Mailloux, Z. (2006). Goal writing. In S. Smith Roley, & R. Schaaf (Eds.), *SI: Applying clinical reasoning to practice with diverse populations* (pp. 63-70). San Antonio, TX: PsychCorp.

95. Mailloux, Z., May-Benson, T., Summers, C. A., Miller, L. J., Brett-Green, B., Burke, J. P., et al. (2007). The issue is—goal attainment scaling as a measure of meaningful outcomes for children with sensory integration disorders. *American Journal of Occupational Therapy, 61*(2), 254-259.

96. Mailloux, Z., Mulligan, S., Roley, S. S., Blanche, E., Cermak, S., Bodison, S., et al. *Verification and clarification of patterns of sensory intergrative dysfunction.* Presented April 25, 2009 American Occupational Therapy Association Annual Conference and Exhibition Houston Texas.

97. Mailloux, Z., & Roley, S. S. (2002). Sensory integration. In H. Miller-Kuhaneck (Ed.), *Autism: A comprehensive occupational therapy approach* (pp. 215-244). Rockville, MD: AOTA Press.

98. Maurer, D., & Maurer, C. (1988). *The world of the newborn.* New York: Basic Books.

99. May-Benson, T. (2001). A theoretical model of ideation in praxis. In E. Blanche, S. Roley, & R. Schaaf (Eds.), *Sensory integration and developmental disabilities* (pp. 163-181). San Antonio, TX: Therapy Skill Builders.

100. May-Benson, T. A., & Cermak, S. A. (2007). Development of an assessment for ideational praxis. *American Journal of Occupational Therapy, 61,* 148-153.

101. May-Benson, T. A., & Koomar, J. A. (2007). Identifying gravitational insecurity in children: A pilot study. *American Journal of Occupational Therapy, 61,* 142-147.

102. McCune-Nicolich, L. (1981). Toward symbolic functioning: Structure of early pretend games and potential parallels with language. *Child Development, 52,* 785-797.

103. Miller, L. J. (2003, February). Empirical evidence related to therapies for sensory processing impairments. *National Association of School Psychologist Communique, 31*(5), 34-37.

104. Miller, L. J. (2006). *Miller Function & Participation Scales.* San Antonio, TX: Pearson Education.

105. Miller, L. J., Anzalone, M. E., Lane, S. J., Cermak, S. A., & Osten, E. T. (2007). Concept evolution in sensory integration: A proposed nosology for diagnosis. *American Journal of Occupational Therapy, 61,* 135-140.

106. Miller, L. J., Coll, J. R., & Schoen, S. A. (2007). A randomized controlled pilot study of the effectiveness of occupational therapy for children with sensory modulation disorder. *American Journal of Occupational Therapy, 61,* 228-238.

107. Miller, L. J., Reisman, J., McIntosh, D. N., & Simon, J. (2001). An ecological model of sensory modulation: Performance of children with Fragile X Syndrome. In S. S. Roley, E. I. Blanche, & R. C. Schaaf (Eds.), *Understanding the nature of sensory integration in diverse populations* (pp. 57-82). San Antonio, TX: Therapy Skill Builders.

108. Miller, L. J., & Summers, C. (2001). Clinical applications in sensory modulation dysfunction: Assessment and intervention considerations. In S. S. Roley, E. I. Blanche, & R. C. Schaaf (Eds.), *Understanding the nature of sensory integration in diverse populations* (pp. 247-274). San Antonio, TX: Therapy Skill Builders.

109. Miller-Kuhaneck, H., Henry, D., & Glennon, T. (2007). *Sensory Processing Measure— Main Classroom Form.* Los Angeles: Western Psychological Services.

110. Mitchell, T., & Cusick, A. (1998). Evaluation of a client-centered pediatric rehabilitation programme using goal attainment scaling. *Australian Occupational Therapy Journal, 45,* 7-17.

111. Mulligan, S. (1998). Patterns of sensory integration dysfunction: A confirmatory factor analysis. *American Journal of Occupational Therapy, 52,* 819-828.

112. Mulligan, S. (2003). Examination of the evidence for occupational therapy using a sensory integration framework with children: Part two. *Sensory Integration Special Interest Section Quarterly, 26*(2), 1-5.

113. Parham, L. D. (1987). Evaluation of praxis in preschoolers. *Occupational Therapy in Health Care, 4*(2), 23-36.

114. Parham, L. D. (2002). Sensory integration and occupation. In A. C. Bundy, S. J. Lane, & E. A. Murray (Eds.), *Sensory integration: Theory and practice* (2nd ed., pp. 413-434). Philadelphia: F.A. Davis.

115. Parham, L. D., & Ecker, C. J. (2007). *Sensory Processing Measure–Home Form.* Los Angeles: Western Psychological Services.

116. Parham, L. D., Ecker, C., Miller-Kuhaneck, H., Henry, D., & Glennon, T. (2007). *Sensory Processing Measure manual.* Los Angeles: Western Psychological Services.

117. Parham, L.D., & Mailloux, Z. (2001). Sensory integration. In J. Case-Smith (Ed.), *Occupational therapy for children* (4th ed., pp. 329-381). St. Louis: Mosby.

118. Parham, L. D., Roley, S. S., May-Benson, T. A., Koomar, J. A., Brett-Green, B., Burke, J. P., et al. *Development of a fidelity measure for research on effectiveness of Ayres Sensory Integration® intervention.* Manuscript submitted for publication.

119. Parush, S., Sohmer, H., Steinberg, A., & Kaitz, M. (1997). Somatosensory functioning in children with attention deficit hyperactivity disorder. *Developmental Medicine and Child Neurology, 39,* 464-468.

120. Pediatric Therapy Network [producer]. (2003). *Applying sensory integration principles where children live, learn and play [motion picture].* Available from Pediatric Therapy Network, 1815 West 213th Street, Suite 100, Torrance, CA 90501.

121. Piantinada, D., & Baltazar, A. (2006). *Every child wants to play: Simple and effective strategies for teaching social skills.* Torrance, CA: Pediatric Therapy Network.

122. Provence, S., & Lipton, R. (1962). *Infants in institutions.* New York: International Universities Press.

123. Ray, T., King, L. J., & Grandin, T. (1988). The effectiveness of self-initiated vestibular stimulation in producing speech sounds in an autistic child. *Occupational Therapy Journal of Research, 8,* 186-190.

124. Reeves, G. D. (2001). From neurons to behavior: Regulation, arousal, and attention as important substrates for the process of sensory integration. In S. S. Roley, E. I. Blanche, & R. C. Schaaf (Eds.), *Understanding the nature of sensory integration in diverse populations* (pp. 89-108). San Antonio, TX: Therapy Skill Builders.

125. Reeves, G. D., & Cermak, S. A. (2002). Disorders of praxis. In A. C. Bundy, S. J. Lane, & E. A. Murray (Eds.), *Sensory integration: Theory and practice* (2nd ed., pp. 71-100). Philadelphia: F.A. Davis.

126. Roley, S. S., & Schneck, C. (2001). Sensory integration and visual deficits, including blindness. In S. S. Roley, E. I. Blanche, & R. C. Schaaf (Eds.), *Understanding the nature of sensory integration with diverse populations* (pp. 313-344). San Antonio, TX: Therapy Skill Builders.

127. Roley, S. S. (2002). Application of sensory integration using the Occupational Therapy Practice Framework. *Sensory Integration Special Interest Section Quarterly, 25*(4), 1-4.

128. Roley, S. S. (2006). Evaluating Sensory Integration Function and Dysfunction. In R. Schaaf & S. S. Roley (Eds.), *SI: Applying clinical reasoning to practice with diverse populations* (pp. 15-36) San Antonio, TX: PsychCorp.

129. Roley, S. S., Mailloux, Z., & Erwin, B. (2008). Ayres Sensory Integration. Retrieved November 16, 2008, from Sensory Integration Global Network Web Site: http://www.siglobalnetwork.org/asi.htm

130. Roley, S. S., Mailloux, Z., Miller-Kuhaneck, H., & Glennon, T. (2007). Understanding Ayres Sensory Integration®. *Occupational Therapy Practice, 12*(17), CE1–CE8.

131. Royeen, C. B. (1989). Commentary on "Tactile functions in learning-disabled and normal children: Reliability and validity considerations." *Occupational Therapy Journal of Research, 9,* 16-23.

132. Royeen, C. B., & Fortune, J. C. (1990). TIE: Touch Inventory for Elementary School–Aged Children. *American Journal of Occupational Therapy, 44,* 165-170.

133. Royeen, C. B., & Fortune, J. C. (2002). TIE: Touch Inventory for Elementary School–Aged Children. In A. C. Bundy, S. J. Lane, & E. A. Murray (Eds.), *Sensory integration: Theory and practice* (2nd ed., pp. 196-198). Philadelphia: F.A. Davis.

134. Royeen, C. B., & Lane, S. J. (1991). Tactile processing and sensory defensiveness. In A. G. Fisher, E. A. Murray, & A. C. Bundy (Eds.), *Sensory integration: Theory and practice* (pp. 108-136). Philadelphia: F.A. Davis.

135. Salthe, S. N. (1985). *Evolving hierarchical systems.* New York: Columbia University Press.

136. Schaaf, R., & Anzalone, M. (2001). Sensory integration with high risk infants and young children. In S. S. Roley, E. I. Blanche, & R. C. Schaaf (Eds.), *Understanding the nature of sensory integration with diverse populations* (pp. 385-408). San Antonio, TX: Therapy Skill Builders.

137. Schaaf, R. C., Miller, L. J., Seawell, D., & O'Keefe, S. (2003). Children with disturbances in sensory processing: A pilot study examining the role of the parasympathetic nervous system. *American Journal of Occupational Therapy, 57,* 442-449.

138. Schneider, M. L. (1992). The effect of mild stress during pregnancy on birth weight and neuromotor maturation in rhesus monkey infants *(Macaca mulatta). Infant Behavior and Development, 15,* 389-403.

139. Schneider, M. L., Clarke, A. S., Kraemer, G. W., Roughton, E. C., Lubach, G., Rimm-Kaufman, S., et al. (1998). Prenatal stress alters brain biogenic amine levels in primates. *Development and Psychopathology, 10,* 427-440.

140. Scott, A. H., & Haggarty, E. J. (1984). Structuring goals via goal attainment scaling in occupational therapy groups in a partial hospitalization setting. *Occupational Therapy in Mental Health, 4*(2), 39-58.

141. Searson, R. R., Dunn, S. J., Denig, H., Pierson, & Solomon, P. (2001). Effects of tactual and kinesthetic instructional resources on science achievement of third-grade students. In R. Dunn (Ed.), *The art of significantly increasing science achievement test scores: Research and practical applications* (pp. 3-28). New York: St. John's University's Center for the Study of Learning and Teaching Styles.

142. Shumway-Cook, A., Horak, F., & Black, F. O. (1987). A critical examination of vestibular function in motor-impaired learning-disabled children. *International Journal of Pediatric Otolaryngology, 14,* 21-30.

143. Slavik, B. A., & Chew, T. (1990). The design of a sensory integration treatment facility: The Ayres Clinic as a model. In S. C. Merrill (Ed.), *Environment: Implications for occupational therapy practice* (pp. 85-101). Rockville, MD: American Occupational Therapy Association.

144. Slavik, B. A., Kitsuwa-Lowe, J., Danner, P. T., Green, J., & Ayres, A. J. (1984). Vestibular stimulation and eye contact in autistic children. *Neuropediatrics, 15,* 333-336.

145. Solomon, P., Kubzansky, P. E., Leiderman, P. H., Mendelson, J. H., Trumball, R., & Wexler, D. (Eds.). (1961). *Sensory deprivation.* Cambridge, MA: Harvard University Press.

146. Spitzer, S., & Roley, S. S. (2001). Sensory integration revisited: A philosophy of practice. In S. S. Roley, E. I. Blanche, & R. C. Schaaf (Eds.), *Understanding the nature of sensory integration with diverse populations* (pp. 3-27). San Antonio, TX: Therapy Skill Builders.

147. Stern, D. N. (1985). *The interpersonal world of the infant.* New York: Basic Books.

148. Tomchek, S. D., & Dunn, W. (2007). Sensory processing in children with and without autism: A comparative study using the Short Sensory Profile. *American Journal of Occupational Therapy, 61,* 190-200.

149. Vargas, S., & Camilli, G. (1999). A meta-analysis of research on sensory integration treatment. *American Journal of Occupational Therapy, 53,* 189-198.

150. Walker, K. F. (1991). Sensory integrative therapy in a limited space: An adaptation of the Ayres Clinic design. *Sensory Integration Special Interest Section Newsletter, 14*(3), 1, 2, 4.

151. White, M. (1979). A first-grade intervention program for children at risk for reading failure. *Journal of Learning Disabilities, 12,* 26-32.

152. Wilbarger, P. (1984). Planning an adequate "sensory diet": Application of sensory processing theory during the first year of life. *Zero to Three,* 7-12.

153. Wilbarger, P., & Wilbarger, J. L. (1991). *Sensory defensiveness in children aged 2-12.* Denver: Avanti Educational Programs.

154. Williams, M. S., & Shellenberger, S. (1994). *"How does your engine run?" A leader's guide to the Alert Program for Self-regulation.* Albuquerque, NM: TherapyWorks.

155. Wilson, B. N., & Kaplan, B. J. (1994). Follow-up assessment of children receiving sensory integration treatment. *Occupational Therapy Journal of Research, 14,* 244-266.

156. Wilson, B. N., Kaplan, B. J., Fellowes, S., Gruchy, C., & Faris, P. (1992). The efficacy of sensory integration treatment compared to tutoring. *Physical and Occupational Therapy in Pediatrics, 12,* 1-36.

157. Wilson, B. N., Pollock, N., Kaplan, B. J., & Law, M. (2000). *Clinical Observations of Motor and Postural Skills (COMPS)* (2nd ed.). Framingham, MA: Therapro.

158. Windsor, M. M., Roley, S. S., & Szklut, S. (2001). Evaluating sensory integration and praxis within the context of occupational therapy. In S. S. Roley, E. I. Blanche, & R. C. Schaaf (Eds.), *Understanding the nature of sensory integration with diverse populations* (pp. 216-234). San Antonio, TX: Therapy Skill Builders.

159. Wiss, T. (1989). Vestibular dysfunction in learning disabilities: Differences in definitions lead to different conclusions. *Journal of Learning Disabilities, 22,* 100-101.

12 Visual Perception

Colleen M. Schneck

Visual perception
Visual-receptive component
Visual-cognitive component
Visual attention
Visual memory
Visual discrimination
Object (form) perception
Spatial perception

1. Define visual perception.
2. Describe the typical development of visual-perceptual skills.
3. Identify factors that contribute to typical or atypical development of visual perception.
4. Explain the effects of visual-perceptual problems on occupations and life activities such as activities of daily living, education, work, play, leisure, and social participation.
5. Describe models and theories that may be used in structuring intervention plans for children who have problems with visual-perceptual skills.
6. Identify assessments and methods useful in the evaluation of visual-perceptual skills in children.
7. Describe intervention strategies for assisting children in improving or compensating for problems with visual-perceptual skills.
8. Give case examples, including principles of evaluation and intervention.

Some consider vision to be the most influential sense in humans.[15] There is little argument that vision is the dominant sense in human perception of the external world; it helps the individual to monitor what is happening in the environment outside the body. Because of the complexity of the visual system, it is difficult to imagine the impact of a visual-perceptual deficit on daily living. Functional problems that may result include difficulties with eating, dressing, reading, writing, locating objects, driving, and many other activities necessary for engagement in an occupation.

Given that occupational therapists focus on individuals' participation in activities of daily living (ADLs), education, work, play, leisure, and social activities, the focus on the client factor of visual perception and its effects on performance skills, including literacy, can be critical. Literacy is embedded within all areas of occupational performance,[141] from ADLs (reading recipes) and education (taking notes in class) to social participation (reading bus schedules). The reauthorization of both the Individuals with Disabilities Education Act (IDEA, 2004) and the No Child Left Behind Act (NCLB, 2001) addresses the need to better address literacy for children in public schools. Part C of the reauthorized IDEA requires that preliteracy be addressed in the very young child. For children of any age, occupational therapists can support literacy in many ways, including providing services to improve visual perception.

Although visual perception is a major intervention emphasis of occupational therapists working with children, it is one of the least understood areas of evaluation and treatment. The information presented in this chapter reflects current knowledge of visual perception that relates to evaluation of and intervention for children. The information in this area continues to evolve as research confirms or disproves explanatory models of the visual-perceptual system.

DEFINITIONS

Visual perception is defined as the total process responsible for the reception (sensory functions) and cognition (specific mental functions) of visual stimuli. The sensory function or *visual-receptive component* is the process of extracting and organizing information from the environment, and the specific mental functions that constitute the *visual-cognitive component* provide the capacity to organize, structure, and interpret visual stimuli, giving meaning to what is seen.[102] Together these two components enable a person to understand what he or she sees, and both are necessary for functional vision. Visual-perceptual skills include the recognition and identification of shapes, objects, colors, and other qualities. Visual perception allows a person to make accurate judgments on the size, configuration, and spatial relationships of objects. The visual-receptive components are described in the *Occupational Therapy Practice Framework: Domain and Process*, 2nd Edition, under client factors of sensory functions and pain, and the visual-cognitive components are described under specific mental functions.[2]

THE VISUAL SYSTEM

Hearing and vision are the distant senses that allow a person to understand what is happening in the environment outside his or her body or in extrapersonal space. These sense organs transmit information to the brain, the primary function of which is to receive information from the world for processing and coding. The visual sensory stimuli are then integrated with other sensory input and associated with past experiences. Approximately 70% of the sensory receptors in humans are allocated to vision. The eye, oculomotor muscles and pathways, optic nerve, optic tract, occipital cortex, and associative areas of the cerebral cortex (parietal and temporal lobes) are all included in this process. It is imperative that occupational therapists gain an understanding of the neurophysiologic interactions in the central nervous system (CNS) so that they can effectively evaluate and treat children with problems in the visual system. This discussion begins with the sensory receptor, the eye.

Anatomy of the Eye

A basic understanding of the anatomy and physiology of the eye aids comprehension of its influence on perception (Figure 12-1). The eye functions to transmit light to the retina, on which it focuses images of the environment. The eye is shaped to refract light rays such that the most sensitive part of the retina receives rays at a convergent point. The *cornea* covers the front of the eye and is part of the outermost layer of the eyeball. It plays a significant part in the focusing or bending of light rays that enter the eye. Behind the cornea is the *aqueous humor,* a clear fluid; the pressure of this fluid helps both to maintain the shape of the cornea and to focus light rays. The colored part of the eye, the *iris,* with its center hole, the *pupil,* is directly behind the cornea. The iris controls the amount of light entering the eye by increasing or decreasing the size of the pupil. The light then progresses through the crystalline *lens,* which does the fine focusing for near or far vision, and through a jelly-like substance called the *vitreous humor.*

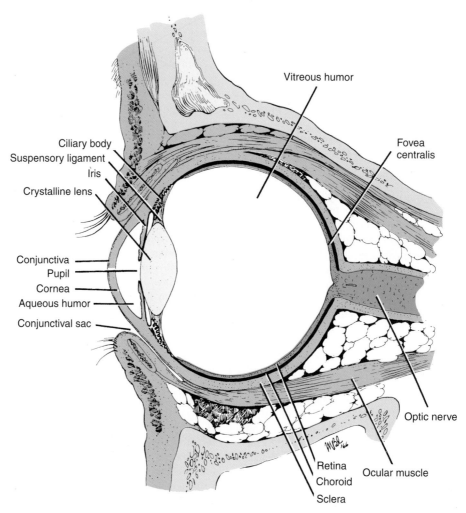

FIGURE 12-1 Cross-section of the eye. (From Ingalls, A. J., & Salerno, M. C. [1983]. *Maternal and child health nursing* [5th ed.]. St. Louis: Mosby.)

The eye has three layers: the sclera, the choroid, and the retina. The *sclera,* which is fibrous and elastic, helps hold the rest of the eye structure in place; the *choroid* is composed primarily of blood vessels that nourish the eye; and the *retina* is the innermost layer. The retinal layer is composed of receptor nerve cells that contain a chemical activated by light. The retina has three types of receptor cells: *cones,* which are used for color perception and visual acuity; *rods,* which are used for night and peripheral vision; and *pupillary cells,* which control opening (dilation) and closing (constriction) of the pupil.

The *fovea centralis,* which is located in the retina, is the point of sharpest and clearest vision. It is most responsive to daylight and must receive a certain amount of light before it transmits the signal to the optic nerve. The retina responds to spatial differences in the intensity of light stimulation, especially at contrasting border areas, and provides basic information about light and dark areas. Light stimulates the visual receptor cells in the retina, causing electrochemical changes that trigger an electrical impulse to flow to the optic nerve. The *optic nerve* (cranial nerve II) transmits the visual sensory messages to the brain for processing. This information travels to the brain in a special way. Fibers from the nasal half of each retina divide, and half of the fibers cross to the contralateral side of the brain. Fibers from the outer half of each retina do not divide; therefore, they carry visual information ipsilaterally. Thus visual information from either the left or right visual field enters the opposite portion of each retina and then travels to the same hemisphere of the brain. This organization means that even with the loss of vision in one eye, information is transmitted to both hemispheres of the brain. It also means that damage in the region of the left or right occipital cortex can cause a loss of vision, referred to as a *field cut,* in the opposite visual field.[72]

The optic nerve leads from the back of the eye to the lateral geniculate nucleus in the optic thalamus. It is here that binocular information is received and integrated at a basic level, which may contribute to crude depth perception. Information then passes from the two lateral geniculate bodies of the thalamus to the visual cortex in the occipital lobe (area 17). From the occipital cortex the refined visual information is sent in two directions via visual area 18 or 19.[109,110] Some impulses flow upward to the posterior parietal lobe, where visual-spatial processing occurs, focusing on the location of objects and their relationships to objects in space. This pathway is referred to as the *dorsal stream.* The magnocellular channel is dominant in the dorsal stream; this channel is associated with motion and depth detection, stereoscopic vision, and interpretation of spatial organization.[69] Other impulses flow downward to the inferior temporal lobe, where visual object processing takes place. Information sent here is analyzed for the specific details of color, form, and size needed for accurate object identification; the focus is on pattern recognition and detail and on remembrance of the qualities of objects. This is referred to as the *ventral stream.* The parvocellular channel is dominant in the ventral stream; this channel is thought to be important for color perception and for detailed analysis of the shape and surface properties of objects.[82]

Visual-Receptive Functions

The oculomotor system enables the reception of visual stimuli (visual-receptive process). The visual-receptive components include visual fixation, pursuit and saccadic eye movements, acuity, accommodation, binocular fusion and stereopsis, and convergence and divergence. *Visual fixation* on a stationary object is a prerequisite skill for other oculomotor responses, such as shifting the gaze between objects (scanning) or tracking. Each eye is moved by the coordinated actions of the six extraocular muscles. These are innervated by cranial nerves III, IV, and VI (oculomotor, trochlear, and abducens nerves). The oculomotor nuclei are responsible for automatic conjugate eye movements (lateral, vertical, and convergence). They also help regulate the position of the eyes in relation to the position of the head. The nuclei receive most of their information from the superior colliculus.

Two types of eye movements are used to gather information from the environment: pursuit eye movements, or tracking, and saccadic eye movements, or scanning. *Visual pursuit,* or *tracking,* involves continued fixation on a moving object so that the image is maintained continuously on the fovea. The smooth pursuit system is characterized by slow, smooth movements. Tracking may occur with the eyes and head moving together or with the eyes moving independently of the head. *Saccadic eye movements,* or *scanning,* are defined as a rapid change of fixation from one point in the visual field to another. A saccade may be voluntary, as when localizing a quickly displaced stimulus or when reading, or it may be involuntary, as during the fast phases of vestibular nystagmus. A saccadic movement is precise, although the presence of a slight overshoot or undershoot is normal.

In addition to voluntary control of eye movements, the vestibulo-ocular pathways control conjugate eye movements reflexively in response to head movement and position in space. These pathways enable the eyes to remain fixed on a stationary object while the head and body move.

In addition to the tasks of visual fixation, pursuit movements, and saccadic movements, other visual-receptive components include the following:

- *Acuity:* The capacity to discriminate the fine details of objects in the visual field. A visual acuity measurement of 20/20 means that a person can perceive as small an object as an average person can perceive at 20 feet.
- *Accommodation:* The ability of each eye to compensate for a blurred image. Accommodation refers to the process used to obtain clear vision (i.e., to focus on an object at varying distances). This occurs when the internal ocular muscle (the ciliary muscle) contracts and causes a change in the crystalline lens of the eye to adjust for objects at different distances. Focusing must take place efficiently at all distances, and the eyes must be able to make the transition from focusing at near point (a book or a piece of paper) to far point (the teacher and the blackboard) and vice versa. It should take only a split second for this process of accommodation to occur.
- *Binocular fusion:* The ability mentally to combine the images from the two eyes into a single percept. There are two prerequisites for binocular fusion. First, the two eyes must be aligned on the object of regard; this is called *motor fusion,* and it requires coordination of the six extraocular muscles of each eye and precision between the two eyes. Second, the size and clarity of the two images must be compatible; this is known as *sensory fusion.* Only when these two prerequisites have been met can the brain combine what the two eyes see into a single percept.
- *Stereopsis:* Binocular depth perception or three-dimensional vision.

- *Convergence and divergence:* The ability of both eyes to turn inward toward the medial plane and outward from the medial plane.

For a more detailed description of the function of these components, see the textbook by Gentile.[57]

Visual-Cognitive Functions

Interpretation of the visual stimulus is a mental process involving cognition, which gives meaning to the visual stimulus (visual-cognitive process). The visual-cognitive components are visual attention, visual memory, visual discrimination, and visual imagery.

Visual Attention

Visual attention involves the selection of visual input. It also provides an appropriate time frame through which visual information is passed by the eye to the primary visual cortex of the brain, where visual-perceptual processing can occur. Voluntary eye movements of localization, fixation, ocular pursuit, and gaze shift lay the foundation for optimal functioning of visual attention.[71] The following are the four components of visual attention:

- *Alertness:* Reflects the natural state of arousal. *Alerting* is the transition from an awake to the attentive and ready state needed for active learning and adaptive behavior.
- *Selective attention:* The ability to choose relevant visual information while ignoring less relevant information; it is conscious, focused attention.
- *Visual vigilance:* The conscious mental effort to concentrate and persist at a visual task. This skill is exhibited when a child plays diligently with a toy or writes a letter.
- *Divided,* or *shared, attention:* The ability to respond to two or more simultaneous tasks. This skill is exhibited when a child is engaged in one task that is automatic while visually monitoring another task.

Visual Memory

Visual memory involves the integration of visual information with previous experiences. Long-term memory, the permanent storehouse, has expansive capacity. In contrast, short-term memory can hold a limited number of unrelated bits of information for approximately 30 seconds.

Visual Discrimination

Visual discrimination is the ability to detect features of stimuli for recognition, matching, and categorization. *Recognition* is the ability to note key features of a stimulus and relate them to memory; *matching* is the ability to note the similarities among visual stimuli; and *categorization* is the ability mentally to determine a quality or category by which similarities or differences can be noted. These three abilities require the capability both to note similarities and differences among forms and symbols with increasing complexity and to relate these findings to information previously stored in long-term memory.

Visual-perceptual abilities aid the manipulation of a visual stimulus for visual discrimination.[144] Because visual perception has not been consistently defined, resources on visual perception use different terms and categories to define the same visual-perceptual skills. At times this contributes to confusion, because different disciplines may define the same terms differently.

It is also important to note that a distinction exists between object (form) vision (ventral stream) and spatial vision (dorsal stream).[67,84] Object vision is implicated in the visual identification of objects by color, texture, shape, and size (i.e., what things are). Spatial vision, which is concerned with the visual location of objects in space (i.e., where things are), responds to motor information and seems to be integral to egocentric localization during visuomotor tasks.[72] As discussed earlier, these two classes of function are mediated by separate neural systems. The cortical tracts for both object vision and spatial vision are projected to the primary visual cortex, but the object vision pathway goes to the temporal lobe and the spatial vision pathway goes to the inferior parietal lobe. These anatomic divisions have been verified repeatedly. However, researchers have emphasized differences in how these two areas use visual information.[63,64] Visual information about object characteristics permits the formation of long-term perceptual representations that support object identification and visual learning. Spatial vision provides information about the location of object qualities that are needed to guide action, such as adjusting the hand during reach to the size and orientation of an object.

Based on studies done with individuals who had acquired brain damage, these two functions have been shown to be independent.[98,100] That is, disturbances of object recognition can occur without spatial disability, and spatial disability can occur with normal object perception.[46] Following are definitions of the object (form) and spatial-perceptual skills, although they are not entirely separate entities.

Object (Form) Perception

Form discrimination and processing involves multiple visual areas in the brain. It is thought that form perception is accomplished by two processes with two separate systems carrying different aspects of form information.[67] The first system, the abstract visual form system (AVF) is thought to perform abstract processing to recognize types of forms. The AVF system is used when the visual form information should be processed and stored in an abstract, nonspecific manner. For example, when a child is scanning the gym supply cabinet for a soccer ball, he is attempting to find a ball but not a specific ball. The second system, specific visual form (SVF) system, provides specific processing to distinguish different instances of a type of form. The SVF system processes input in a manner that produces specific output representations that distinguish different instances of the same type of form—for example, the child searching for his soccer ball among those of his teammates after practice is over.

- *Form constancy:* The recognition of forms and objects as the same in various environments, positions, and sizes. Form constancy helps a person develop stability and consistency in the visual world. It enables the person to recognize objects despite differences in orientation or detail. Form constancy enables a person to make assumptions regarding the size of an object even though visual stimuli may vary under different circumstances. The visual image of an object in the distance is much smaller than the image of the same object at close range, yet the person knows that the actual sizes are equivalent. For example, a school-aged child can identify the letter *A* whether it is typed, written in manuscript, written in cursive, written in upper or lower case letters, or italicized.
- *Visual closure:* The identification of forms or objects from incomplete presentations. This enables the person quickly to

recognize objects, shapes, and forms by mentally completing the image or by matching it to information previously stored in memory. This allows the person to make assumptions regarding what the object is without having to see the complete presentation. For example, a child working at his or her desk is able to distinguish a pencil from a pen, even when both are partly hidden under some papers.

- *Figure-ground recognition:* The differentiation between foreground or background forms and objects. It is the ability to separate essential data from distracting surrounding information and the ability to attend to one aspect of a visual field while perceiving it in relation to the rest of the field. It is the ability to visually attend to what is important. For example, a child is able visually to find a favorite toy in a box filled with toys, scissors in a cluttered drawer, his or her mother in a crowded room, or a shirtsleeve on a monochromatic shirt.

Spatial Perception

There are two types of spatial relations: categorical spatial relations (above-below, right-left, on-off) and coordinate spatial relations (specify locations in a way that can be used for precise movements).[130]

- *Position in space/visual spatial orientation:* The determination of the spatial relationship of figures and objects to oneself or other forms and objects. This provides the awareness of an object's position in relation to the observer or the perception of the direction in which it is turned. This perceptual ability is important to understanding directional language concepts such as in, out, up, down, in front of, behind, between, left, and right. In addition, position in space perception provides the ability to differentiate among letters and sequences of letters in a word or in a sentence. For example, the child knows how to place letters equal spaces apart and touching the line; he or she is able to recognize letters that extend below the line, such as *p, g, q,* or *y*. Another aspect of spatial perception, now referred to as *object-focused spatial abilities,* focuses on the spatial relations of objects irrespective of the individual.[154] This includes skills evaluated by many formal assessments; however, poor performance on a formal test may or may not be linked to functional behavior.
- *Depth perception:* The determination of the relative distance between objects, figures, or landmarks and the observer and changes in planes of surfaces. This perceptual ability provides an awareness of how far away something is, and it also helps people move in space (e.g., walking down stairs, catching a ball, pouring water into a glass, parking a car). Depth perception is the third dimension beyond the two-dimensional image in the retina.[123] Binocular vision, along with monocular cues such as texture, shading and linear perspective, all contribute to perception of three-dimensional shape and distance. Visual acuity and ocular alignment must also be adequate. The parietal lobe has been associated with depth perception.
- *Topographic orientation:* The determination of the location of objects and settings and the route to the location. *Wayfinding* depends on a cognitive map of the environment. These maps include information about the destination, spatial information, instructions for execution of travel plans, recognition of places, keeping track of where one is while moving about, and anticipation of features. These are important means of monitoring one's movement from place to place.[46] In addition, the images a person sees must be recognized if he or she is to make sense of what is viewed and if the individual is to find his or her way around.[46] For example, the child is able to leave the classroom for a drink of water from the water fountain down the hall and then return to his or her desk.

Visual Imagery

Another important component in visual cognition is visual imagery, or *visualization.* Visual imagery refers to the ability to "picture" people, ideas, and objects in the mind's eye even when the objects are not physically present. Developmentally, the child is first able to picture objects that make certain sounds and those that are familiar by taste or smell. The ability to picture what words say while reading is the next step. For example, the child can imagine the character of a book based on the written description. This level of visual-verbal matching provides the foundation for reading comprehension and spelling.

Motor and Process Skills

Client factors may affect performance skills that in turn may affect activities and occupations. Motor skills of posture, mobility, and coordination may be affected by poor visual skills. For example, in the area of mobility, research has shown the importance of vision in the development of proprioception of the hand prior to the onset of reaching in newborn infants.[33] This can explain why young babies spend much time visually examining their hands. By 5 to 7 months, infants, in preparation for reaching, may use the current sight of the object's orientation, or the memory of it, to orient the hand for grasping; sight of the hand has no effect on hand orientation at this point.[96] If problems occur in visual memory affecting the memory of the hand, the hand may not be properly oriented during reach, and this affects coordination.

Process skills of knowledge, temporal organization, organization of space and objects, and adaptation all can be affected by visual perception. Children who have acquired damage to the white matter around the lateral ventricles or damage to the posterior parietal lobes can find it difficult to use vision to guide their body movements.[47] For example, a floor boundary between carpet and linoleum can be difficult to cross because it looks the same as a step. Black-and-white tiled floors can be frightening to walk across. At a curb, the foot may be lifted to the wrong height, too early, or too late, and walking down stairs without a banister is difficult and dangerous.

Developmental Framework for Intervention

Warren presented a developmental framework based on a bottom-up approach to evaluation and treatment.[157] Using the work of Moore,[62] Warren suggested that with knowledge of where the deficit is located in the visual system, the therapist could design appropriate evaluation and treatment strategies to remediate basic problems and improve perceptual function.[157] To apply this approach, the occupational therapist must have an understanding of the visual system, including both the visual-receptive and visual-cognitive components. Although Warren's model was presented as a developmental

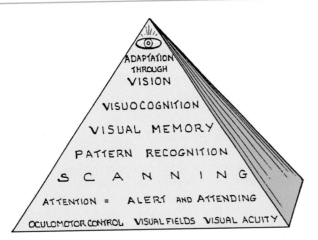

FIGURE 12-2 Hierarchy of visual-perceptual skills development. (From Warren, M. [1993]. A hierarchical model for evaluation and treatment of visual perceptual dysfunction in adult acquired brain injury. I. *American Journal of Occupational Therapy, 47,* 42-54.)

framework for evaluation and treatment of visual-perceptual dysfunction in adults with acquired brain injuries, it is useful as a model for children with visual-perceptual deficits. A hierarchy of visual-perceptual skill development in the central nervous system is presented in Figure 12-2. The definitions of components of each level are provided in the following list and are used in later descriptions of intervention.

1. *Primary visual skills* form the foundation of all visual functions.
- *Oculomotor control* provides efficient eye movements that ensure that the scan path is accomplished.
- *Visual fields* register the complete visual scene.
- *Visual acuity* ensures that the visual information sent to the CNS is accurate.
2. *Visual attention.* The thoroughness of the scan path depends on visual attention.
3. *Scanning.* Pattern recognition depends on organized, thorough scanning of the visual environment. The retina must record all the detail of the scene systematically through the use of a scan path.
4. *Pattern recognition.* The ability to store information in memory requires pattern detection and recognition. This is the identification of the salient features of an object.
- Configural aspects (shape, contour, and general features)
- Specific features of an object (details of color, shading, and texture)
5. *Visual memory.* Mental manipulation of visual information needed for visual cognition requires the ability either to retain the information in memory for immediate recall or to store for later retrieval.
6. *Visual cognition.* This is the ability to mentally manipulate visual information and integrate it with other sensory information to solve problems, formulate plans, and make decisions.

Warren's model provides a framework for assessing vision alone, without consideration of the other sensory systems. When visual-perceptual problems relate to sensory integration (SI) dysfunction, models based on SI theories can guide evaluation and intervention.[20] These models consider organization of multisensory systems and the influence of vision as it integrates with other sensory systems.

Vision can be viewed as a dynamic blending of sensory information in which new visual and motor input are combined with previously stored data and then used to guide a reaction. Research demonstrates an expansive interconnectivity of sensory systems.[143] Studies of brain activity confirm that when an individual is using the visual system, many areas of the brain are activated. Evidence of full brain activity during visualization supports the concept that vision should be viewed in the totality of all sensory systems.

DEVELOPMENTAL SEQUENCE

Visual-Receptive Functions

As with other areas of development, the development of visual-receptive process and abilities takes place according to a prescribed timetable, which begins in the womb. By gestational week 24, gross anatomic structures are in place, and the visual pathway is complete. Between gestational weeks 24 and 40, the visual system, particularly the retina and visual cortex, undergoes extensive maturation, differentiation, and remodeling.[62] As early as the fifth gestational month, eye movements are produced by vestibular influences.[43] At birth the infant has rudimentary visual fixation ability and brief reflexive tracking ability. The visual system at this age is relatively immature compared with other sensory systems, and considerable development occurs over the next 6 months.[62]

Toward the end of the second month, accommodation, convergence, and oculomotor subsystems are established.[15] Stereopsis is evident at about 2 months of age; it does not appear to depend on visual recognition and does not need to be taught.[160] Maximum accommodation is reached at 5 years of age, and the child should be able to sustain this skill effort for protracted periods at a fixed distance.

Controlled tracking skills progress in a developmental pattern from horizontal eye movements to eye movements in vertical, diagonal, and circular directions. By kindergarten a child should be able to move the eyes with smooth control and coordination in all directions. This can be demonstrated by asking the child to follow with the eyes a moving object located 8 to 12 inches from the child's face. If the child moves the head as a unit along with the eyes, this skill is still developing. Visual acuity is best at 18 years of age and tends to decline thereafter.

Visual-Cognitive Functions

Vision enables infants to acquire information from multiple locations at a range of distances and is a means for infants to organize information received from their other senses.[142] By coordinating visual and auditory input, infants accumulate information as they explore places, events, and individuals in the physical and social environments.[137] Some visual-cognitive capacities are present at birth, whereas other higher-level visual-cognitive abilities are not fully developed until adolescence. This development occurs through perceptual learning, the process of extracting information from the environment.

Perceptual learning increases with experience and practice and through stimulation from the environment.

Object (Form) Vision

Long before infants can manipulate objects or move around space, they have well-developed visual-perceptual abilities, including pattern recognition, form constancy, and depth perception. Infants as young as 1 week of age show a differential response to patterns, with complex designs and human faces receiving more attention than simple circles and triangles. The infant learns to attend to relevant aspects of visual stimuli, to make discriminations, and to interpret available cues according to experiences. Babies can organize visual information in at least three ways. Perception of brightness emerges first by 2 months of age. By 4 months, most infants can group objects by shape and proximity.[49]

Visual perception develops as the child matures, with most developmental changes taking place by 9 years of age. However, children vary in the rate at which they acquire perceptual abilities, in their effective use of these capacities, and in the versatility and comfort with which they apply these functions.[89]

The child first learns to recognize an object based on its general appearance and not by specific details. As the child learns to classify objects into categories and types, it becomes apparent that he or she is able to extract the features that make the object part of that category.[108] For example, the child learns to categorize cars as certain types or to classify animals according to their species. Williams estimated the developmental ages when primary visual-perceptual skills develop (Table 12-1).[161]

Bouska and colleagues described three areas in which a child demonstrates increasing ability to discriminate visually.[15] These areas include (1) the ability to recognize and distinguish specific distinctive features (e.g., that *b* and *d* are different because of one feature); (2) the ability to observe invariant relationships in events that occur repeatedly over time (e.g., a favorite toy is the same even when distance makes it appear smaller); and (3) the ability to find a hierarchy of pattern or structure, allowing the processing of the largest unit possible for adaptive use during a particular task (e.g., a map is scanned globally for the shape of a country, but subordinate features are scanned for the route of a river).[59] These skills are important for learning to read and write. Justice and Ezell described emergent literacy as comprising two broad yet highly interrelated domains of knowledge: written language awareness and phonologic awareness.[79] Written language awareness, also referred to as *print awareness*,[135] describes children's knowledge of the forms and functions of printed language (e.g., distinctive features of alphabet letters, storybook conventions, environmental signs).

The child's first perceptions of the world develop primarily from tactile, kinesthetic, and vestibular input. As these three basic senses become integrated with the higher level senses, vision and audition gradually become dominant. Young children or beginning readers tend to prefer learning through their tactile and kinesthetic senses and have lower preferences for visual and auditory learning.[26] At 6 or 7 years of age, most children appear to prefer kinesthetic, tactile, visual, and auditory learning, in that order. They learn easily through their sense of touch and whole-body movement and have difficulty learning through listening activities. The predominant reading style of primary grade children and struggling readers is global, tactile, and kinesthetic.[26] Global reading methods (i.e., recorded stories, shared reading) start with a modeled story, practice words from the story, and teach phonics skills. This differs from analytic reading methods (e.g., phonics) that teach sounds letters make, then practice words containing the sounds taught, and proceed to stories. Tactile learners recall what they touch, are often doodlers, and learn better when they can touch or manipulate objects (such as a reading game). Kinesthetic learners recall what they experience and learn when engaged in physical activity (e.g., acting in plays, floor games, building models).[27]

Research shows that struggling readers prefer and do better in classrooms that allow for movement, have some comfortable seating and varied lighting, and enable students to work with relevant ease in different groupings.[44] Research indicates that when the student's environmental preferences are met, they are more likely to associate reading with pleasure, to read for longer periods, and overall read at higher levels.[44] Generally, boys are less auditory and verbal and remain kinesthetic longer than girls. Around third grade most children become highly visual, and not until fifth grade do many children learn well through their auditory sense. However, it is important to remember that reading style strengths and preferences develop at different times and rates.[26]

In the young child, visual discrimination of forms precedes by years the visual-motor ability to copy forms. Throughout elementary school, the child assimilates more internal detail of figures and develops greater ability to understand, recall, and recreate such configurations. Children begin to use

---

TABLE 12-1   Developmental Ages for Emergence of Visual-Perceptual Skills

Perception	Developmental Age
OBJECT (FORM)	
Figure-ground perception	Improves between 3 and 5 years of age; growth stabilizes at 6 to 7 years of age
Form constancy	Dramatic improvement between 6 and 7 years of age; less improvement from 8 to 9 years of age
SPATIAL	
Position in space	Development complete at 7 to 9 years of age
Spatial relationships	Improves to approximately 10 years of age

Modified from Williams, H. (1983). *Perceptual and motor development.* Englewood Cliffs, NJ: Prentice Hall.

simultaneous and sequential data to develop strategies, and cognitive or learning styles begin to emerge. In addition, children learn best through their dominant sensory input channel. About 40% of school-age children remember visually presented information, whereas only 20% to 30% recall what is heard.[25]

Information processing in the visual-perceptual–motor domain has been identified as one of the major factors that predict readiness for the first grade. There is evidence that the child who enters school with delayed perceptual development may not catch up with his or her peers in academic achievement.[52] Of the children who have difficulty reading in first grade, 88% have difficulty reading at the end of fourth grade.[78] Adequate perceptual discrimination is considered necessary for the development of the literacy skills of reading and writing.[86,136] An important aspect of developing early literacy is termed *alphabetics*. This includes phonemic and phonologic awareness, letter recognition, print awareness, and phonics. Letter recognition/identification, defined as knowing the names of the letters of the alphabet, supports reading acquisition. Measures of the ability to name letters have been shown to be predictors of reading development, especially when letter naming is taught in conjunction with other beginning reading skills. *Print awareness* refers to knowledge or concepts about print, such as the following: (1) print carries a message; (2) there are conventions of print such as directionality (left to right, top to bottom), differences between letters and words, distinctions between upper and lower case, punctuation; and (3) books have some common characteristics (e.g. author, title, front/back). It has been shown that print awareness supports reading acquisition (e.g., decoding). Occupational therapists are not primarily responsible for teaching students to read or write but may address many of the performance skills to support student literacy outcomes.[8]

Children gradually develop the abilities to attend to, integrate, sort, and retrieve increasingly larger chunks of visual data. These stimuli from the environment usually arrive for processing either in a simultaneous array or in a specific serial order.[89] An example of *simultaneous processing* involves observing and later trying to recall what someone wore.

Sequential processing involves the integration of separate elements into groups, where the elements have a specific arrangement in time with each element leads only to one other. Sequential processing enables the child to perceive an ordered series of events.[60] An example of sequential processing is the visual information provided in the written instructions for assembling a plastic model. An effective learner in the classroom needs to be able to evaluate, retain, process, and produce both simultaneous and sequential packages of information or action. In addition, children must learn to analyze and synthesize material containing more detail at a faster rate.

In adolescence, perceptual skills are enhanced by their interrelationship with expanding cognitive skill. Thus the adolescent can imagine, create, and construct complex visual forms. The adolescent is able to manipulate visual information mentally to solve increasingly complex problems, formulate plans, and make decisions. Of the children who are poor readers at the end of third grade, 75% remain poor readers in high school.[131] Teenager rites of passage such as obtaining a driver's license or independent dating may be challenging or impossible for an individual with severe visual-perceptual deficits.

Spatial Vision

In the developmental process of organizing space, the child first acquires a concept of vertical dimensions, followed by a concept of horizontal dimensions. Oblique and diagonal dimensions are more complex, and perception of these spatial coordinates matures later. A 3- to 4-year-old child can discriminate vertical lines from horizontal ones, but children are unable to distinguish oblique lines until about 6 years of age.[37] The ability to discriminate between mirror- or reverse-image numbers and letters, such as *b* and *d*, and *p* and *q*, does not mature in some children until around 7 years of age.[75]

The child develops an understanding of left and right from the internal awareness that his or her body has two sides[140]; this understanding of left and right, called *laterality*, proceeds in stages. A child's awareness of his or her own body is generally established by 6 or 7 years of age. Before 7 years of age, a child is not yet ready to handle spatial concepts on a strictly visual basis. The child must relate them to his or her own body.

Around the eighth year the child begins to project laterality concepts outside himself or herself. The child then develops *directionality*, or the understanding of an external object's position in space in relation to himself or herself. This allows the child to handle spatial phenomena almost exclusively in a visual manner. By sensing a difference between body sides, the child becomes aware that figures and objects also have a right and a left. The child "feels" this visually.

Directionality is thought to be important in the visual discrimination of letters and numbers for both reading and writing. The child first learns these concepts in relation to himself or herself and then transfers them to symbols and words.

Role of Vision in Social Development

The importance of vision in facilitating infants' participation in social interactions has been widely recognized.[99] Facial expressions are an important way to communicate emotions.[76] Infants respond to attentive, social initiations from their parents by visually focusing on their parents' eyes, smiling, and occasionally shifting gaze to scan their parents' faces and the environment. Mutual gaze between parents and infants facilitates emotional attachment. Adults' facial expressions appear to be the major driving force during social interactions with infants younger than 6 months. Infants discriminate between happy and sad facial expressions by 3 months of age. Toward the end of the first year an infant can shift attention from one person to another person, or to an object of mutual interest in joint attention paradigms.[42] Social imitation then shifts from simple reactions to another person's facial expressions to imitations of another person's actions with objects. Toddlers will imitate a peer's action on an object, but only when identical objects are available.

VISUAL-PERCEPTUAL PROBLEMS

Visual-Receptive Functions

The importance of good vision for classroom work cannot be overemphasized. More than 50% of a student's time is spent working at near-point visual tasks such as reading and writing.

Another 20% is spent on tasks that require the student to shift focus from distance to near and near to distance, such as copying from the board. For more than 70% of the day, therefore, tremendous stress is put on the visual system.[115] Many students with visual dysfunction may have difficulty meeting the behavioral demands of sitting still, sustaining attention, and completing their work. Academic instruction in the first years places great demand on the child's visual processing skills, with emphasis on recognition, matching, and recall. In early elementary grades, periods of sustained near work are infrequent, and visual stimuli (letters) are relatively large and widely spaced.

Visual efficiency becomes a more significant need in later elementary grades, middle school, and high school. Letters and text become smaller and more closely spaced and reading requires more comprehension effort for extended periods of time. Students visually attend for sustained periods of near work.[102]

Learning-related vision problems represent deficits in two broad visual system components: visual efficiency and visual information processing.[13] Figure 12-3 presents a sample list of behaviors noted in children with specific visual problems.[102] In addition, individuals with functional vision problems may exhibit[56]:

- Difficulty completing school tasks in a timely manner
- Avoidance of reading work
- Visual fatigue
- Adaptation of the visual system through the development of a refractive error to perform near-centered visual tasks
- Distraction or inattention as a secondary problem, thus decreasing the opportunity for practice and learning

Impairment of oculomotor control can occur through disruption of cranial nerve function or disruption of central neural control. The pattern of oculomotor dysfunction depends on the areas of the brain that have been injured and the nature of the injury.[88] Oculomotor problems can limit the ability to control and direct gaze. In addition, when large amounts of energy must be used on the motor components of vision, little energy may be left for visual-cognitive processing.[72] Warren[157] and Scheiman[125] present detailed descriptions of oculomotor deficits and other deficits seen in visual-receptive components.

At least 20% of students with learning disabilities have been found to have prominent visual information–processing problems. The prevalence of visual efficiency problems in children with learning disabilities is thought to be in the 15% to 20% range.[126] Accommodative disorders have been reported in 60% to 80% of individuals with visual efficiency problems; accommodative insufficiency is the most prevalent type.[102] Convergence insufficiency is the most common convergence anomaly.

Refractive Errors

A child who is nearsighted has blurred distant vision but generally experiences clarity at near point. The child who is farsighted frequently has clear distant and near vision but has to exert extra effort to maintain clear vision at near point. The child with astigmatism experiences blurred vision at distance and near, with the degree of loss of clarity depending on the severity of the astigmatism. Measures of visual acuity alone do not predict how well children interpret visual information.[72] Other determinants include the ability to see objects in low-contrast lighting conditions, the ability of the eye to adapt to different lighting conditions, visual field problems, accommodation, and other oculomotor functions.[72,74]

If accommodation takes longer than previously described, words appear blurry and the child tends to lose his or her place, missing important information and understanding. When accommodation for near objects is poor, presbyopia exists; this individual is described as farsighted.

If the conditions of motor fusion and sensory fusion have not been met, allowing binocular fusion to occur (this process was described previously), single binocular vision is at best difficult and at worst impossible. If one eye overtly turns in, out, up, or down because of muscular imbalance, the condition is known as *strabismus,* sometimes referred to as a *crossed* or *wandering eye.* This can result in double vision or mental suppression of one of the images. This, in turn, can affect the development of visual perception. Some children have surgery to correct an eye turn. Although this intervention can correct the eye cosmetically, it does not always result in binocular vision.

Another type of binocular dysfunction is called *phoria.* Phoria refers to a tendency for one eye to turn slightly in, out, up, or down, but overt misalignment of the two eyes is absent. Phoria requires the child to expend additional mechanical effort to maintain motor fusion of the two eyes, whether focusing near or far. The extra effort frequently detracts from the child's ability to process and interpret the meaning of what he or she sees.

Visual-Cognitive Functions

Attention

The integrity of the attention system is considered to be a prerequisite for higher cognitive functions. To review, visual attention is composed of alertness, selective attention, vigilance, and shared attention. If the child's state of alertness or arousal is impaired, the child may demonstrate behaviors of overattentiveness, underattentiveness, or poor sustained attention.[144] Children who are overattentive may be compelled to respond to visual stimuli around them rather than attend to the task at hand, may be easily distracted by visual stimuli, and may demonstrate continual visual searching behaviors. Children who are underattentive may have difficulty orienting to visual stimuli, may habituate quickly to a visual stimulus, and may fatigue easily. At this level a child may refrain from attending to a familiar stimulus. A child with poor sustained attention may demonstrate a high activity level and may be easily distracted.

Selective attention is the next level of visual attention, and a child with difficulty in this area demonstrates a reduced ability to focus on a visual target. The child may have difficulty screening out unimportant or irrelevant information and may focus on or may be distracted by irrelevant stimuli. A child with difficulty in selective attention is easily confused. The child may focus on unnecessary tasks or information and therefore not obtain the specific information needed for the task. Selective attention is critical for encoding information into memory and successfully executing goal-directed behavior.

A child with reduced vigilance skills shows reduced persistence on a visual task and poor or cursory examination of visual stimuli. The child cannot maintain visual attention. The more

CHECKLIST OF OBSERVABLE CLUES TO CLASSROOM VISION PROBLEMS

1. **Appearance of eyes**
   One eye turns in or out at any time _____
   Reddened eyes or lids _____
   Eyes tear excessively _____
   Encrusted eyelids _____
   Frequent styes on lids _____
2. **Complaints when using eyes at desk**
   Headaches in forehead or temples _____
   Burning or itching after reading or
      desk work _____
   Nausea or dizziness _____
   Print blurs after reading a short time _____
3. **Behavioral signs of visual problems**
   a. **Eye movement abilities (ocular motility)**
      Head turns as reads across pages _____
      Loses place often during reading _____
      Needs finger or marker to keep place _____
      Displays short attention span in
         reading or copying _____
      Too frequently omits words _____
      Repeatedly omits "small" words _____
      Writes uphill or downhill on paper _____
      Rereads or skips lines unknowingly _____
      Orients drawings poorly on page _____
   b. **Eye teaming abilities (binocularity)**
      Complains of seeing double (diplopia) _____
      Repeats letters within words _____
      Omits letters, numbers, or phrases _____
      Misaligns digits in number columns _____
      Squints, closes, or covers one eye _____
      Tilts head at extreme angle while working
         at desk _____
      Consistently shows gross postural
         deviations at all desk activities _____
   c. **Eye-hand coordination abilities**
      Must feel things to assist in any
         interpretation required _____
      Eyes not used to "steer" hand
         movement (extreme lack of
         orientation, placement of words
         or drawings on page) _____
      Writes crookedly, poorly spaced:
         cannot stay on ruled lines _____
      Misaligns both horizontal and vertical
         series of numbers _____
      Uses hand or fingers to keep place
         on the page _____
      Uses other hand as "spacer" to control
         spacing and alignment on page _____
      Repeatedly confuses left-right directions _____
   d. **Visual-form perception (visual compar-
      ison, visual imagery, visualization)** _____
      Mistakes words with same or similar
         beginnings _____
      Fails to recognize same word in next
         sentence _____
      Reverses letters and/or words in
         writing and copying _____
      Confuses likenesses and minor
         differences _____
      Confuses same word in same sentence _____
      Repeatedly confuses similar beginnings
         and endings of words _____
      Fails to visualize what is read either
         silently or orally _____
      Whispers to self for reinforcement
         while reading silently _____
      Returns to "drawing with fingers" to
         decide likes and differences _____
   e. **Refractive status (e.g., nearsightedness,
      farsightedness, focus problems)** _____
      Comprehension reduces as reading
         continued; loses interest too quickly _____
      Mispronounces similar words as
         continues reading _____
      Blinks excessively at desk tasks and/or
         reading; not elsewhere _____
      Holds book too closely; face too close
         to desk surface _____
      Avoids all possible near-centered tasks _____
      Complains of discomfort in tasks that
         demand visual interpretation _____
      Closes or covers one eye when reading
         or doing desk work _____
      Makes errors in copying from chalk-
         board to paper on desk _____
      Makes errors in copying from reference
         book to notebook _____
      Squints to see chalkboard, or requests
         to move nearer _____
      Rubs eyes during or after short periods
         of visual activity _____
      Fatigues easily; blinks to make chalk-
         board clear up after desk task _____

NOTE: Students found to have any of the visual or eye problems on the checklist should be referred to a behavioral optometrist. Referral lists of behavioral optometrists are available from Optometric Extension Program Foundation, 2912 S. Daimler, Santa Ana, CA 92705.

FIGURE 12-3   Checklist of observable clues to classroom vision problems.

complex the visual structure of an object, the lengthier the process of visual analysis and the greater the vigilance skills needed. Impaired sustained attention is associated with error awareness[95] as well as with working memory to hold and manipulate information.[133] A child with deficits in shared attention can focus well only on one task at a time. He or she may be easily confused or distracted if required to share visual attention between two tasks.

Enns and Cameron suggested that visual inattention is the result of an inability to select the features that differentiate objects in a visual array.[48] The child cannot see, recognize, or isolate the salient features and therefore does not know where to focus visual attention. Luria suggested that problems of visual recognition represent a breakdown of the active feature by feature analysis necessary for interpretation of a visual image.[92] The current psychological literature focuses on such constructs as mental resource, automaticity, and stimulus selection.[3] The research focuses on the attention demands that numerous competing stimuli make on individuals with a limited capacity to process those stimuli and on the fact that these exteroceptive stimuli can be processed either with awareness (i.e., effortful processing) or automatically (i.e., effortless processing).

Memory

The child with visual memory deficits has poor or reduced ability to recognize or retrieve visual information and to store visual information in short- or long-term memory. The child may fail to attend adequately, may fail to allow for storage of visual information, or may show a prolonged response time. The child may demonstrate the inability to recognize or match visual stimuli presented previously because he or she has not stored this information in memory, or the child may be unable to retrieve it from memory.[144] The child may have good memory for life experiences but not for factual material and may fail to relate information to prior knowledge. He or she may demonstrate inconsistent recall abilities and poor ability to use mnemonic strategies for storage.

Visual sequential memory problems are seen when the child has difficulty recalling the exact sequence of letters, numbers, symbols, or objects. Visual spatial memory deficits are seen when the child has difficulty recalling the spatial location of a previously seen stimulus and is unable to identify or reproduce it.

Visual Discrimination

The child with poor discrimination abilities may demonstrate impaired ability to recognize, match, and categorize. Ulman proposed that a finite set of visual operations, or *routines,* are performed to extract shape properties and spatial relationships.[152] Usually an individual recognizes an object by orienting to its top or bottom. A child with poor matching skills may demonstrate difficulty matching the same shape presented in a different spatial orientation or may confuse similar shapes. A child with poor matching skills also may have difficulty recognizing form in a complex field.

Object (Form) Vision

Children with form constancy problems may have difficulty recognizing forms and objects when they are presented in different sizes or different orientations in space or when differences in detail exist. This interferes with the child's ability to organize and classify perceptual experiences for meaningful cognitive operations.[106] This may result in difficulty recognizing letters or words in different styles of print or in making the transition from printed to cursive letters.

A child with a visual closure deficit may be unable to identify a form or object if an incomplete presentation is made; the child therefore would always need to see the complete object to identify it. For example, a child would have difficulty reading a sign if the letters were partly occluded by tree branches.

The child with figure-ground problems may not be able to pick out a specific toy from a shelf. He or she also may have difficulty sorting and organizing personal belongings. The child may overattend to details and miss the big picture or may overlook details and miss the important information. Children with figure-ground problems may have difficulty attending to a word on a printed page because they cannot block out other words around it. The child with figure-ground difficulties may not have good visual search strategies. Marr suggested that control of the direction of gaze is a prerequisite for efficiency of visual search.[93] Cohen described the following visual search strategies[34]:

1. The viewer looks for specific visual information and makes crude distinctions between figure and ground by isolating one figure from another.
2. The viewer determines which figures are most meaningful (the process stops here when recognition is immediate).
3. When recognition is not immediate, the viewer makes a hypothesis about the visual information received and directs attention to selected items to test the hypothesis.

Rogow and Rathwill found that good readers more frequently proceeded from the left to the right and from the top down to find "hidden figures" than did poor readers.[117] Good readers were also more flexible in their approach; they rotated the page as needed and were not content until they found as many hidden figures as possible. The good readers also were less distressed by ambiguity, and they understood that pictures could be viewed in different ways.

Spatial Vision

A child with position in space difficulty has trouble discriminating among objects because of their placement in space. These children also have difficulty planning their actions in relation to objects around them and may show delayed gross motor skills. They may show letter reversals in writing or reading past 8 years of age and may show confusion regarding the sequence of letters or numbers in a word or math problem (e.g., was/saw). Writing and spacing letters and words on paper may be a problem. The children may show difficulty understanding directional language such as in, out, on, under, next to, up, down, and in front of. They may show inconsistent directional attack when reading.

Decreased depth perception can affect the child's ability to walk through spaces and to catch a ball. The child may be unable to determine visually when the surface plane has changed and may have difficulty with steps and curbs. Transference of visual-spatial notations across two visual planes can make copying from the blackboard difficult. Faulty interpretation of the spatial relationships can contribute to a problem with sorting and organizing personal belongings. The child may show confusion in right and left.

A child who has diminished topographic orientation may be easily lost and unable to find his or her way from one location to the next. The child may also demonstrate difficulty determining the location of objects and settings and may not recognize the images that help people find their way around the environment.[46] The child may be unable to walk from home to school without getting lost.

Diagnoses with Problems in Visual Perception

When children with disabling conditions have visual problems, the effects of the visual impairments can be tremendous. Numerous studies have found a high frequency of vision problems among individuals with disabilities.[32] Severe refractive errors are common among children with developmental problems,[117] and impaired visual attention can have a pervasive negative influence on the functional behavior of these children. Often considered distractible, these children may be able to locate objects but have difficulty sustaining eye contact or recognizing objects visually.[117]

Retinopathy of prematurity (ROP) is the single most cited cause of blindness in preterm infants. However, the number of infants with ROP has declined in past 25 years because of changes in medical interventions for premature infants.[136] Cortical visual impairment also occurs in preterm infants and is generally associated with severe CNS damage, such as periventricular leukomalacia. Other visual disorders common in preterm children include lenses that are too thick, poor visual acuity, astigmatism, extreme myopia, strabismus, amblyopia, and anisometropia (unequal refraction of the eyes).[5] These children also have difficulty processing visual information. Scores for visual attention, pattern discrimination, visual recognition, memory, and visual-motor integration are lower than those for full-term infants.[29,120,132] Studies of older children suggest that these problems often persist.[117]

Children with developmental disabilities commonly have a coexisting diagnosis of blindness or other visual impairment. These children also may have sensory integrative deficits that further complicate their functional abilities.[119]

Children with cerebral palsy (CP) frequently have been identified as a group with visual-perceptual deficits.[17,21] Children with CP often have a strabismus, oculomotor problems, convergence insufficiencies, or nystagmus. These problems may also limit the ability to control and direct visual gaze.[117]

Early research indicated that the degree of perceptual impairment in individuals with CP was related to the type and severity of the motor impairment.[10] In a comparison study, children with CP scored significantly lower on a motor-free test of visual perception than typical children.[96] These findings supported earlier studies that showed that a group of children with spastic quadriplegia demonstrated the greatest problems in visual perception. Children with left hemiplegia scored significantly lower than control children on motor-free visual tests, but children with right hemiplegia did not.[21]

In children with language delay, poorly developed visual perception may contribute to the language difficulties. For example, language moves from the general to the specific. Young children call every animal with four legs a dog. Eventually they are able to discriminate visually between dogs and lions, and the vocabulary follows the visual-perceptual lead. Next, they can tell Dalmatians from Dachshunds, but they are unable to recognize that both are dogs. Finally, the ability to categorize and generalize emerges somewhere between 7 and 9 years of age. In addition, the child who has visual-spatial perception deficits may show difficulty understanding directional language, such as in, on, under, and next to.

Visual-perceptual problems are found more frequently in individuals who have significantly higher verbal scores than performance scores on intelligence testing. Not all children with learning disabilities have visual-perceptual problems.[70] A recent study suggests that early brain damage can give rise to specific visual-perceptual deficits, independent of, although occurring in association with, selective impairment in nonverbal intelligence.[138]

Children with learning disabilities may have difficulty filtering out irrelevant environmental stimuli and therefore have erratic visual attention skills. Children who have difficulty interpreting and using visual information effectively are described as having visual-perceptual problems because they have not acquired adequate visual-perceptual skills despite having normal vision.[144] Children with developmental coordination disorder (DCD) obtained significantly lower scores compared with typically developing children on a motor-free test of visual perception.[147] Although group differences were statistically significant, some of the children with DCD did not have general visual-perceptual dysfunction.

Dyslexia is best understood as a neurocognitive deficit that is specifically related to reading and spelling processes. Dyslexia can occur for two different reasons. One cause is that the reader has difficulty decoding words (single word identification) and encoding words (spelling).[132] A second reason for dyslexia is that the reader makes a significant number of letter reversals (b – d), letter transpositions in words when reading or writing (sign – sing) or has right-left confusion.[66]

Daniels and Ryley studied the incidence of visual-perceptual and visual-motor deficits in children with psychiatric disorders.[39] In their study, deficits in visual-motor skills occurred far more frequently than deficits in visual-perceptual skills. When visual-perceptual problems occurred, they did so in conjunction with visual-motor skill problems.

Some children with autism have demonstrated poor oculomotor function.[121] Children with autism often do not appear to focus their vision directly on what they are doing.[103] A possible explanation is that they use peripheral vision to the exclusion of focal vision. One study found that children with autism spend the same amount of time inspecting socially oriented pictures, have the same total number of fixations, and have scan path lengths similar to those of typically developing children.[153] These results do not support the generally held notion that children with autism have a specific problem in processing socially loaded visual stimuli. The study authors suggested that the often-reported abnormal use of gaze in everyday life is not related to the nature of the visual stimuli, but that other factors, such as social interaction, may play a role.

Effects of Visual-Perceptual Problems on Performance Skills and Occupations

The effects of visual-perceptual problems may be subtle. However, when the child is asked to perform a visual-perceptual task, he or she may be slow or unable to perform it. Because visual-perceptual dysfunction affects the child's ability to use tools and to relate materials to one another,[4] bilateral manipulative skills are affected to a greater degree than the child's basic prehension patterns indicate. The child with visual-perceptual deficits may show problems with cutting, coloring, constructing with blocks or other construction toys, doing puzzles, using fasteners, and tying shoes. Visual perception deficits also can influence children's areas of occupation, such as activities of daily living (ADLs), education, work, play, leisure, and social participation.

Children with visual-perceptual problems may demonstrate difficulty with ADLs. In grooming, the child may have difficulty obtaining the necessary supplies and using a brush and comb and mirror to comb and style the hair. Applying toothpaste to the toothbrush may be difficult for the child. Using fasteners; donning and doffing clothing, prostheses, and orthoses; tying shoes; and matching clothes may present problems. Skilled use of handwriting, telephones, computers, and communication devices may present difficulty for the child with visual-cognitive problems. Instrumental ADLs, such as home management, may present problems. For example, the child may have trouble sorting and folding clothes. Community mobility may be difficult because the child is unable to locate objects and find his or her way. In play, the child may demonstrate difficulty with playing games and sports, drawing and coloring, cutting with scissors, pasting, constructing, and doing puzzles.

Classroom assignments may present problems for the child with visual-perceptual problems. He or she may have difficulty with educational activities such as reading, spelling, handwriting, and math. The educational problems seen in the school-aged child are considered in some detail next. Visual processing deficits are considered developmental. With maturation and experience the performance of the child with deficits improves, but the rate of maturation of skill continues to lag.

Problems in Reading

The role of phonologic processing deficits in the understanding of reading disability is significant.[146] These deficits are manifested in the failure to use or properly understand phonologic information when processing written or oral language. This is seen in the inadequacy of phonemic awareness, the poor understanding of sound-symbol correspondence rules, and the improper storage and retrieval of phonologic information. Deficits in short- and long-term memory can also affect comprehension.

At least a subgroup of children with reading problems confuses orientation and visual recognition of letters.[161] The characteristics of printed (written) information make reading possible; these include a word's graphic configuration, orthography (order of letters), phonology (sounds represented), and semantics (meaning). The child benefits from these multiple simultaneous cues in reading. If the child has difficulty with one characteristic, he or she can rely on perception of the other characteristics to extract the meaning. In early reading, children first encounter the visual configuration (graphics) and orthographics of a printed word. The child then must break the written word into its component phonemes (phonology), hold them in active working memory, and synthesize and blend the phonemes to form recognizable words (semantics). Visual word recognition seems to involve a subphonemic level of processing.[91] After practice, this step is accomplished and the word then can be dealt with as a gestalt or in its entirety rather than letter by letter and added to the child's growing sight vocabulary. Sight vocabulary consists of words that are instantly recognized as gestalts. As the child's reliance on sight vocabulary increases, decoding takes less time and automaticity

develops, which allows the child to begin to concentrate on comprehension and retention.

Understanding sentences requires adding two more variables, context (word order) and syntax (grammatical construction), to the skills previously discussed.[90] For reading paragraphs, chapters, and texts, it is assumed that decoding is automatic. A hierarchy can be assumed such that any developmental dysfunctions that impair decoding or sentence comprehension impede text reading.

The segmenting of written words in early reading calls for a variety of skills. First, children must be able to recognize individual letter symbols. This requires visual attention, visual memory, and visual discrimination. Two aspects of word reading are important for comprehension: accuracy and speed. The more attentional resources are consumed by lower level process (i.e., word identification), the fewer resources are available for comprehension.

Letter knowledge contributes significantly to reading and should be measured in preschool, kindergarten, and first grade. The prerequisite skills of letter naming and phonemic awareness should be assessed early in kindergarten.

Visual-perceptual attributes are different from the capacity to assimilate visual detail. The child may be diagnosed as having visual-perceptual problems when he or she is limited in attending to or extracting data presented simultaneously. In this instance the child does not have difficulty with the specific perceptual content but with the amount of information that must be simultaneously perceived to understand the whole.

Children with visual discrimination deficits may not be able to recognize symbols and therefore may be slow to master the alphabet and numbers. Their relatively weak grasp of constancy of forms may make visual discrimination an inefficient process. Some children cannot readily discern the differences between visually similar symbols. Confusion between the letters p, q, and g and between a and o, as well as letter reversals, may result, such as the notorious differentiation between b and d. A meta-analysis was conducted using 161 studies to examine the relationship between visual-perceptual skills and reading achievement.[83] The findings suggest that visual perception is an important correlate of reading achievement and should be included in the complex of factors predicting it. Visual discrimination abilities (form perception and spatial perception) are somewhat less important at advanced stages of the learning-to-read process than they are during the initial stages of reading acquisition.[16]

Confusion over the directionality and other spatial characteristics of a word may result in weak registration in visual memory, again possibly causing significant delays in the consolidation of a sight vocabulary. Even frequently encountered words need to be analyzed anew each time they appear. A child with visual-spatial deficits has difficulty with map reading and interpretation of instructional graphics such as charts and diagrams. Graphic representations require the child to integrate, extract the most salient elements from, condense, and organize the large amount of stimuli presented at once. Again, the child may not have difficulty with the perceptual content, but the amount of information to be assimilated simultaneously is more than the child can integrate and remember.[90]

Memory deficits affect reading in a number of ways. Children with visual memory problems may be unable to remember the visual shape of letters and words. Such children may also demonstrate an inability to associate these shapes with letters, sounds, and words.[65] Children with weaknesses of visual-verbal associative memory have difficulty establishing easily retrievable or recognizable sound-symbol associations. They are unable to associate the sound, visual configuration, or meaning of the word with what is seen or heard. Children who have difficulty with active working memory also may have difficulty holding one aspect of the reading process in suspension while pursuing another component. This ability is closely related to perceptual span, or the ability to recall the beginning of the sentence while reading the end of it. The child must take a second look at the beginning of a sentence after reading the end of it.

With severe dysfunction, recognition of words may be impaired,[90] which interferes with the acquisition of sight vocabulary. Problems with visual perception might be suspected in a child who appears to be better at understanding what was read than at actually decoding the words. This child has good language abilities but some trouble processing written words.

According to Raymond and Sorensen, children with dyslexia have been shown to have normal detection but abnormal integration of visual-motion perception.[111] The authors suggest that perhaps a collection of inefficient information-processing mechanisms produces the characteristic symptoms of dyslexia.

Problems in Spelling

Research by Giles and Terrel does not support the hypothesis that proficient spelling is mediated by visual memory.[60] They suggest that spelling skills may depend on be visual recognition or visual imagery ability. Children with impaired processing of simultaneous visual stimuli may have difficulty with spelling. Their inability to visualize words may result from indistinct or distorted initial visual registration. Such children who have strong sound-symbol association may spell the word phonetically (e.g., lite for light) yet incorrectly.

Problems in Handwriting and Visual Motor Integration

Handwriting requires the ability to integrate the visual image of letters or shapes with the appropriate motor response. Handwriting difficulties affect between 10% to 30% of school-age children. Visual-cognitive abilities may affect writing in a variety of situations. Children with problems in attention may have difficulty with correct letter formation, spelling and the mechanics of grammar, punctuation, and capitalization. They also have difficulty formulating a sequential flow of ideas necessary for written communication. For a child to write spontaneously, he or she must be able to revisualize letters and words without visual cues. A child with visual memory problems may have difficulty recalling the shape and formation of letters and numbers. Other problems seen in the child with poor visual memory include mixing small and capital letters in a sentence, writing the same letter many different ways on the same page, and being unable to print the alphabet from memory. In addition, legibility may be poor, and the child may need a model to write.

Visual discrimination problems may also affect the child's handwriting. The child with poor form constancy does not recognize errors in his or her own handwriting. The child may be unable to recognize letters or words in different prints and therefore may have difficulty copying from a different type of print to handwriting. The child may also show poor recognition of letters or numbers in different environments, positions, or sizes. If the child is unable to discriminate a letter, he or she may have difficulty forming it. A child with visual-closure difficulty always needs to see the complete presentation of what he or she is to copy. A child with figure-ground problems may have difficulty copying because he or she is unable to determine what is to be written; the child therefore may omit important segments or may be slower than peers in producing written products.

Visual-spatial problems can affect a child's handwriting in many ways. The child may reverse letters such as *m*, *w*, *b*, *d*, *s*, *c*, and *z* and numbers such as *2, 3, 5, 6, 7,* and *9.* If the child is unable to discriminate left from right, he or she may have difficulty with left–to-right progression in writing words and sentences. The child may overspace or underspace between words and letters and may have trouble keeping within the margins. The most common spatial errors in handwriting involve incorrect and inconsistent spacing between writing units, and variability in orientation of major letter features when the letter is written repeatedly.[155] When a child has a spatial disability, he or she may be unable to relate one part of a letter to another part and may demonstrate poor shaping or closure of individual letters or a lack of uniformity in orientation and letter size.[163] The child may have difficulty placing letters on a line and adapting letter sizes to the space provided on the paper or worksheet. Pilot studies have begun to explore the relationship between visual-cognitive skills and handwriting.[164] Tseng and Cermak found that visual perception shows little relationship to handwriting, whereas kinesthesia, visual-motor integration, and motor planning appear to be more closely related to it.[148] Further research is necessary to better understand the role of visual perception in handwriting.

Failure on visual-motor tests may be caused by underlying visual-cognitive deficits, including visual discrimination, poor fine motor ability, or inability to integrate visual-cognitive and motor processes, or by a combination of these disabilities. Therefore, careful analysis is necessary to determine the underlying problem. Tseng and Murray examined the relationship of perceptual-motor measures to legibility of handwriting in Chinese school-age children.[149] They found visual-motor integration to be the best predictor of handwriting. Weil and Cunningham-Amundson studied the relationship between visual-motor integration skills and the ability to copy letters legibly in kindergarten students.[159] A moderate correlation was found between students' visual-motor skills and their ability to copy letters legibly. The researchers found that as students' scores on the Developmental Test of Visual-Motor Integration (VMI) increased, so did scores on the Scale of Children's Readiness in PrinTing (SCRIPT). Also, students who were able to copy the first nine forms on the VMI were found to perform better on the SCRIPT. Daly, Kelley, and Krauss partly replicated the Weil and Cunningham-Amundson study and found a strong positive relationship between kindergarten students' performance on the VMI and their ability to copy letter forms legibly.[38] They suggest that students are ready for formal handwriting instruction once they have the ability to copy the first nine forms on the VMI.

Extensive research on the relationship between visual-motor integration and handwriting skills has been completed. Studies of handwriting remediation suggest that intervention is effective. There is some evidence that handwriting difficulties do not resolve without intervention.[51]

Problems in Mathematics

Poor visual-perceptual ability is significantly related to poor achievement in mathematics, even when controlling for verbal cognitive ability. Therefore, visual perceptual ability, and particularly visual memory, should be considered to be among the skills significantly related to mathematics achievement.[85] Consequently, visual-perceptual ability, and particularly visual memory skill, should be assessed in children with poor achievement in mathematics. The child with visual-perceptual problems can have difficulty aligning columns for calculation, and answers therefore are incorrect because of alignment problems and not calculation skills. Worksheets with many rows and columns of math problems may be disorienting to children with figure-ground problems. Children with poor visual memory may have difficulty using a calculator. Visual memory difficulties also may present problems when addition and subtraction problems require multiple steps. Geometry, because of its spatial characteristics, is very difficult for the child with visual-spatial perception problems. Recognition, discrimination, and comparison of object form and space are part of the foundation of higher-level mathematic skills. The visual imagery required to match and compare forms and shapes is difficult for students with visual-perceptual problems, which interfere with their ability to learn these underlying skills.

A longitudinal investigation that studied the relationship of sensory integrative development to achievement found that sensory integrative factors, particularly praxis, were strongly related to arithmetic achievement.[102] This relationship was found at younger ages (6 to 8 years), and the strength of the association declined with age (10 to 12 years).

EVALUATION METHODS

Evaluation of visual-perceptual functions requires the therapist to consider the entire process of vision and examine the relationship of visual function to behavior and performance.[129] Visual-receptive and visual-cognitive components may represent different issues in a child's school performance. Problems can and do exist in either area, with differing effects on the learning process. However, visual-receptive components can influence the information obtained for visual-cognitive analysis. Because receptive and cognitive components are important in the visual processing of information, assessment of each child should be conducted using an interdisciplinary approach, recognizing that the interplay of visual-receptive abilities, visual-cognitive skills, and school success is different for each child.

Reports generated by other educational or medical specialists often provide standardized measures of performance. Securing this information often eliminates the need for the occupational therapist to spend time administering additional visual-motor or visual-perceptual tests that yield the same information. This information also can help the occupational therapist select alternative measures that yield different data that could further help in understanding a child's problem. An interview with the teacher or classroom observation should be a major component of the assessment process. For example, information on visual stimulation in the classroom, which could affect the child's attention and focus, should be determined. The therapist might also determine whether most visual work for copying is done at near point or far point. The child's parents also should be interviewed, and they should be included as part of the team in the diagnosis and treatment of the child.

Through the interdisciplinary approach, the occupational therapist's findings can be integrated with those of the reading specialist, psychologist, speech-language pathologist, parent, and classroom teacher. By combining test results and analysis of the child's performance, the team members ascertain the nature of the interaction of the disability with the activity. A vision specialist, such as an ophthalmologist or an optometrist, may be needed to assess visual-receptive dysfunction and to remediate the condition.

Evaluation of Visual-Receptive Functions

Evaluation should begin by focusing on the integrity of the visual-receptive processes, including visual fields, visual acuity, and oculomotor control.[158] In children who have deficits in these foundational skills, insufficient or inaccurate information about the location and features of objects is sent to the CNS, and the quality of their learning through the visual sense is severely affected. Warren suggested that what sometimes appear to be visual-cognitive deficits are actually visual-receptive problems, which may include oculomotor disturbances.[156] Therefore, visual-receptive and visual-cognitive deficits may be misdiagnosed. The occupational therapist should be familiar with visual screening, because evaluation of vision and oculomotor skills assists in the assessment and analysis of their influence on visual perception and functional performance.[144]

Visual screening consists of basic tests administered to determine which children are at risk for inadequate visual functions.[15,72] The purpose of the screening is to determine which children should be referred for a complete diagnostic visual evaluation. Therefore, the purpose of screening the visual-receptive system is to determine how efficient the eyes are in acquiring visual information for further visual-cognitive interpretation. The checklist presented in Figure 12-3 can alert the therapist to visual symptoms commonly found in children who demonstrate poor visual performance.

Perimetry (computerized measurement of visual field by systematically showing lights of differing brightness and size in the peripheral visual field), confrontation, and careful observation of the child as he or she performs daily activities provide useful information about field integrity.[165] For example, missing or misreading the beginning or end of words or numbers may indicate a central field deficit.

The child's refractive status, which is the clinical measurement of the eye, should be determined. A school nurse or vision specialist usually performs this test. The refractive status reflects whether the student is nearsighted (myopic), farsighted (hyperopic), or has astigmatism. Several methods can be used to determine a child's refractive status. One method, the Snellen test, is used to screen children at school or in the physician's office. However, it measures only eyesight (visual acuity) at 20 feet. This figure, expressed commonly as 20/20 for normal vision, has little predictive value for how well a child uses his or her vision. It is estimated that the Snellen Test detects fewer than 5% of visual problems.[129] When a child passes this screening, he or she may be told that the existing vision is fine. However, it is only the eyesight at 20 feet that is fine.

Some schools and clinics use a Telebinocular or similar instrument in vision screening. This device provides information on clarity or visual acuity at both near and far distances, as well as information on depth perception and binocularity (two-eyed coordination). Warren suggested that the Contrast Sensitivity Test is best for measuring acuity.[158] A pediatric version of this test is available (Vistech Consultants, Dayton, Ohio).

The occupational therapist may observe oculomotor dysfunction in the child. The screening test should answer several questions, including the following[73,165]:

1. Do the eyes work together? How well?
2. Where is visual control most efficient and effective? Least efficient and effective?
3. What types of eye movements are quick and accurate? Which are not?
4. Does the child move his head excessively when reading? Skip lines when reading?

Screening tools that can be used by occupational therapists are presented in Table 12-2.

In addition, the child's ocular health should be evaluated. The presence of a disease or other pathologic condition, such as glaucoma, cataracts, or deterioration of the nerves or any part of the eye, must be ruled out. An interview with the family regarding significant visual history helps identify any conditions that may be associated with visual limitations. This information can also be obtained from a review of the child's records and from consultation with other professionals involved in direct care of the child (e.g., teacher or physician).

When visual problems are detected in screening, the child may be referred to a vision specialist such as an optometrist. The specialist can help determine whether the child has a visual problem that might be causing or contributing to school difficulties. The therapist then will be able to understand the effect those deficits have on function and can devise intervention strategies by designing and selecting appropriate activities that are within the child's visual capacity.[15]

Evaluation of Visual-Cognitive Functions

Clinical evaluation and observation may be the occupational therapist's most useful assessment methods. The therapist should observe the child for difficulty selecting, storing, retrieving, or classifying visual information. Observations may include visual search strategies used during visual-perceptual tasks (e.g., outside borders to inside), how the child approaches the task, how the child processes and interprets visual information, the child's flexibility in analyzing visual information, methods used for storage and retrieval of visual information, the amount of stress associated with visual activities, and whether the child fatigues easily during visual tasks. The therapist should analyze the tasks observed carefully to determine what visual skills are needed and to identify the areas in which the child has difficulty.

Tsurumi and Todd have applied task analysis to the nonmotor tests of visual perception.[150] This information greatly assists the therapist in analyzing the results of these tests. Currently, the best method for evaluating visual attention in children is informal observation during occupational performance tasks. Standardized assessments that may be used include the following:

- *Bruininks-Oseretsky Test of Motor Proficiency (2nd Ed.) (BOT-2)*[19]: An individually administered, standardized test for individuals 4 through 21 years of age. The test measures a wide array of motor skills. The eight subtests include fine motor precision, fine motor integration, manual dexterity,

TABLE 12-2 Vision Screening Tests

Test	Authors	Description
Visual Screening	Bouska, Kauffman, & Marcus (1990)[15]	Comprehensive screening test of distance and near vision, convergence near point, horizontal pursuits, distant and near fixations, and stereoscopic visual skills to identify children who should be referred to a qualified vision specialist for a complete diagnostic visual evaluation.
Sensorimotor Performance Analysis	Richter & Montgomery (1991)*	Assessment of visual tracking, visual avoidance, visual processing, and hand-eye coordination during gross and fine motor tasks.
Pediatric Clinical Vision Screening for Occupational Therapists	Scheiman (1991)†	A test that screens accommodation, binocular vision, and ocular motility.
Clinical Observations of Infants	Ciner, Macks, & Schanel-Klitsch (1991)[32]	Description methods for testing vision in early intervention programs.

*Richter, E., & Montgomery, P. (1991). *The sensorimotor performance analysis.* Hugo, MN: PDP Products.
†Scheiman, M. (1991). *Pediatric clinical vision screening for occupational therapists.* Philadelphia: Pennsylvania College of Optometry.

bilateral coordination, balance, running speed and agility, upper-limb coordination, and strength. This test has been the most widely used standardized measure of motor proficiency and has good reliability and validity.

- *Test of Visual Analysis Skills*[122]: An untimed, individually administered, criterion-referenced test for children 5 to 8 years of age. The child is asked to copy simple to complex geometric patterns. The purpose of the assessment is to determine if the child is competent at or in need of remediation for perception of the visual relationships necessary for integrating letter and word shapes. Reliability and validity of this test indicate that the psychometric properties are adequate.

Visual-Spatial Tests

- *Jordan Left-Right Reversal Test, revised*[77]: An untimed, standardized test for children 5 to 12 years of age that can be administered individually or to a group. It is used to detect visual reversals of letters, numbers, and words, and the test manual includes remediation exercises for reversal problems. The test takes about 20 minutes to administer and score and has good test-retest reliability and criterion-related validity.

Visual-Perceptual Tests

- *Test of Visual-Perceptual Skills (Non-Motor), Third Edition (TVPS-R)*[94]: A norm-referenced test for children 4 to 18 years of age that can be administered individually or to a small group. The subtests include visual discrimination, visual memory, visual-spatial relationships, form constancy, visual-sequential memory, visual figure-ground and visual closure. The test uses black and white designs as stimuli for perceptual tasks, and responses are made vocally or by pointing.
- *Developmental Test of Visual Perception, Second Edition (DTVP-2)*[68]: A norm-referenced test for children 4 to 10 years of age that is unbiased relative to race, gender, and handedness. The eight subtests include hand-eye coordination, copying, spatial relationships, position in space, figure-ground competence, visual closure, visual-motor speed, and form constancy. This test has been shown to have strong normative data and good reliability and validity.
- *Componential Assessment of Visual Perception (CAVP)*[113]: A computer-assisted evaluation tool that was designed as a process-based approach to the evaluation of visual-perceptual functioning in children and adults with neurologic disorders. Promising clinical usefulness has been reported in terms of utility, ease of use, format, and appeal.[112]
- *Motor-Free Visual Perception Test, Third Edition (MVPT-3)*[35]: A norm-referenced test that is quick and easy to administer. Scoring requires adding the number of correct choice responses. This test has a high test-retest reliability and internal validity. Also, criterion validity is determined relative to academic performance.
- *Test of Pictures, Forms, Letters, Numbers, Spatial Orientation, and Sequencing Skills*[54]: A norm-referenced

test for children 5 to 9 years of age that can be administered individually or to a group. The test, which has seven subtests, measures the ability to perceive forms, letters, and numbers in the correct direction and to perceive words with letters in the correct sequence.

Visual-Motor Integration Tests

- *Wide Range Assessment of Visual Motor Abilities (WRAVMA)*[1]: A norm-referenced, standardized test for children 3 to 17 years of age. Assesses and compares visual-spatial skills through the matching subtest, fine motor skills through the pegboard subtest and integrated visual-motor skills through the drawing subtest. Each subtest requires 4 to 10 minutes and offers easy administration and sound psychometric properties.
- *The Developmental Test of Visual-Motor Integration, 5th Edition, Revised (VMI)*[6]: This test assesses three subtest areas for individuals 2 to 19 years of age and has strong content, concurrent and construct validity.

These tests can be used to evaluate how the child is processing, organizing, and using visual-cognitive information. Care should be taken in interpreting and reporting test results because it is not always clear what visual-perceptual tests are measuring. Because of the complexity of the tests, it is certain that they tap different kinds and levels of function, including language abilities.

The effectiveness of any treatment method is largely determined by how the child is diagnosed; therefore, careful analysis of test results and observations is important. Burtner et al. provided a critical review of seven norm-referenced, standardized tests of visual-perceptual skills frequently administered by pediatric therapists.[22] Each assessment tool was critically appraised for its purpose, clinical utility, test construction, standardization reliability, and validity. Discussion focused on the usefulness of these assessment tools for describing, evaluating, and predicting visual-perceptual functioning in children.

INTERVENTION

Theoretical Approaches

The theoretical approaches that guide evaluation and treatment of visual-perceptual skills can be categorized as *developmental, neurophysiologic,* or *compensatory.* The developmental model devised by Warren,[157,158] described in a previous section, is based on the concept that higher level skills evolve from integration of lower level skills and are subsequently affected by disruption of lower level skills. Skill levels in the hierarchy function as a single entity and provide a unified structure for visual perception. As pictured in Figure 12-2, oculomotor control, visual field, and acuity form the foundational skills, followed by visual attention, scanning, pattern recognition or detection, memory, and visual cognition. Identification and remediation of deficits in lower level skills permit integration of higher-level skills. Occupational therapists who follow this model need to evaluate lower level skills before proceeding to higher level skills to determine where the deficit is in the visual hierarchy and to design appropriate evaluation and intervention strategies.

The *neurophysiologic* approaches address the maturation of the human nervous system and the link to human performance. These approaches help create environmental accommodations to sensory hypersensitivity and visual distractibility. They also promote organization of movement around a goal, reinforcing the sensory feedback from that movement. Neurophysiologic approaches emphasize the importance of postural stability for oculomotor efficiency. The role of visual perception as part of sensory integration and the way the child perceives his or her environment are discussed in Chapter 11. The neurophysiologic approaches focus on improving visual-receptive and visual-cognitive components to enhance a child's occupational performance.

Learning theories and behavioral approaches emphasize a child's development of visual analysis skills. The therapist provides the child with a systematic method for identifying the pertinent, concrete features of spatially organized patterns, thereby enabling the child to recognize how new information relates to previously acquired knowledge on the basis of similar and different attributes. Because the child learns to generalize to dissimilar tasks, that improvement in visual-perceptual skills leads to increased levels of occupational performance.

In *compensatory approaches*, classroom materials or instructional methods are modified to accommodate the child's limitations. The environment can also be altered or adapted. The therapist may work with the classroom teacher on behalf of the child to provide necessary supports. Adaptation and compensation techniques can include reducing classroom visual distractions, providing visual stimuli to direct attention and guide response, and modifying the input and output of computer programs. In daily living skills, adaptations to increase grooming, dressing, eating, and communication skills can be made. In play situations, toys can be made more accessible, and in work activities, adaptations can be made to promote copying, writing, and organizational skills. Box 12-1 outlines compensatory instruction guidelines.

Perceptual training programs use learning theories to remediate deficits or prerequisite skills and have been implemented in the public schools for more than 2 decades. Occupational therapists generally use activities from these approaches in combination with neurophysiologic and compensatory approaches.

Optometry and occupational therapy have common goals related to the effects of vision on performance.[72,125] When

a visual dysfunction is identified, sometimes only environmental modifications (e.g., changes in lighting, desk height, or surface tilt) are needed to alleviate the problem. In many cases, glasses (lens therapy) are prescribed to reduce the stress of close work or to correct refractive errors. In other cases, optometric vision therapy may be prescribed by an optometrist and carried out collaboratively with an occupational therapist. Through vision therapy, optometrists provide structured visual experiences to enhance basic skills and perception. Vision training is well supported by evidence but should be performed only under supervision of an optometrist. Collaboration between the occupational therapist and the optometrist is supported by case studies and clinical judgment.

Intervention Strategies

For a child of any age, an important treatment strategy is education regarding the problem the child is experiencing.[150] The occupational therapist can help interpret the functional implications of the vision problem for the child and his or her parents, caregivers, and teachers. At times this can be the most helpful intervention for the child. This section presents intervention suggestions according to age groups. However, activities should be analyzed and then selected according to the child's needs rather than according to his or her age group.

These activities illustrate both the developmental and compensatory approaches. Often activities combine approaches. For example, when classroom materials are adapted so that the print is larger and less visual information is presented (compensatory approach), the child might be better able to use visual-perceptual skills, with resulting improvement in those skills (developmental approach). For each age group, the focus of intervention is occupation in natural environments. The aim of occupational therapy intervention is to reduce activity limitations and enhance participation in everyday activities.[145]

Infants

Glass presented a protocol for working with preterm infants in a neonatal intensive care unit (NICU).[62] Dim lighting allows the newborn to spontaneously open his or her eyes. Stimulation of the body senses (e.g., tactile-vestibular stimulation) can influence the development of distance sense (e.g., visual), which matures later.[120,151] On the basis of research of neonatal vision, Glass suggested ways to use the human face as the infant's first source of visual stimulation. The intensity, amplitude, and distance of the stimulus depend on whether the intent is to arouse or quiet the infant. Glass also recommended beginning with softer, simpler forms and three-dimensional objects and varying the stimuli based on whether the intent is to soothe or arouse the infant. Mobiles hung over cribs should be placed approximately 2 feet above the infant and slightly to one side. This allows for selective attention by the infant. In addition, Glass suggested that black and white patterns be reserved for full-term infants who are visually impaired and unable to attend to a face or toy.[62] Once a visual response is elicited with the high-contrast pattern, a shift to a pattern with less contrast should be made. Recent studies suggest that 3- to 5-month-old infants may be attracted to toys that reflect

---

BOX 12-1 Compensatory Instruction Guidelines

1. Limit the amount of new material presented in any single lesson.
2. Present new information in a simple, organized way that highlights what is especially pertinent.
3. Link new information with the information the child already knows.
4. Use all senses.
5. Provide repeated experiences to establish the information securely in long-term memory; practice until the child knows it and does not need to figure it out.
6. Group children with similar learning styles together.

ight or flash light congruently with a sound.[107] At the age of 4½ months, the preference for the familiar precedes the preference for novel as infants examine visual stimuli.[116] This presentation of stimuli is important in the formation of memory representations.

Preschool and Kindergarten

Occupational therapists can help preschool and kindergarten teachers organize the classroom activities to help children develop the readiness skills needed for visual perception. Teachers should understand the increased need for a multisensory approach with young children who are struggling with shape, letter, and number recognition. For example, the child might benefit from tactile input to learn shapes, letters, and numbers. By using letters with textures, the child has additional sensory experiences on which he or she can rely when visual skills are diminished. Children should be encouraged to feel shapes, letters, and words through their hands and bodies. Letters can be formed with clay, sandpaper, beads, or chocolate pudding (Figure 12-4). Studies have shown that the incorporation of visuo-haptic and haptic exploration of letters in reading training programs facilitates 5-year-old children's understanding of the alphabet.[41]

All preschool, kindergarten, and primary classes should include frequent activities that develop body-in-space concepts to improve spatial perception. Even with a range of levels of understanding among young students, group activities, such as Statue, shadow dancing, and Simon Says, can reinforce body-in-space comprehension. Children benefit from watching and imitating one another. The therapist may pair children so that one can model for the other in an obstacle course or other gross motor

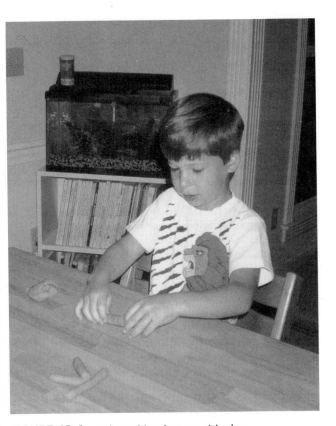

FIGURE 12-4 Kyle making letters with clay.

activity. Appendix 12-A on the Evolve website lists publications describing activities for both classroom teachers and therapists.

Shared storybook reading has been found to provide a particularly useful context within which to promote at-risk preschoolers' emergent literacy knowledge.[80] Further study has shown placing that emphasis on the print concepts by talking about and by pointing to the print increases visual attention to it. Children attended to print significantly more often when being read a storybook with large narrative print, relatively few words per page, and multiple instances of print embedded within the illustrations.[81]

Studies of handwriting suggest that no significant difference in letter writing legibility exists between kindergartners who use paper with lines and those who use paper without lines.[38,159] The study investigators suggest that teachers allow kindergarten children to experiment with various types of writing paper when initially learning proper letter formation.

Elementary School

Therapy should begin at the level of the visual hierarchy where the child is experiencing difficulty. If the child is experiencing difficulty with visual-receptive skills, cooperative efforts between the occupational therapist and the optometrist may be helpful. The school-based occupational therapist's objectives for improving visual-receptive skills (as these appear on student's individualized education program) are to support the child's academic goals and appropriate curricular outcomes.

Organizing the Environment

Visual perception affects a child's view of the entire learning environment. Visually distracting and competing information can be problematic to the child who has not yet fully developed his or her skills. The child may require that the classroom be less "busy" visually to allow him or her to focus on learning. Limiting a distractible child's peripheral vision by using a carrel is often helpful (Figure 12-5). In addition, the level of illumination needs to be monitored, and glare must be controlled.

The child needs a stable postural base that allows his or her eyes to work together. Children often sit at ill-fitting furniture, which can compound their problems. The occupational therapist can help the teacher properly position the child. The therapist can add bolsters to seat backs, put blocks under the child's feet, or provide the child with a slant board if any of these materials will help the child use vision more efficiently or increase productivity. The therapist can also stress the importance of encouraging different positions for visual activity. Figure 12-6 shows such alternative positions as prone, "television position" for sitting, and side-lying for visual-perceptual activities such as reading. Each position should place the child in good alignment and should offer adequate postural support.

Children may benefit from color-coded worksheets to help them attend to what visually goes together. However, children with color vision problems may have difficulty with educational materials that are color coded, particularly when the colors are pastel or muddy. Therefore, it is important to differentiate an actual visual color deficit from a problem either with color naming or with color identification.[32]

Christenson and Rascho proposed strategies to assist the elderly in topographic orientation, and these can be adapted for children.[30] The authors found that use of landmarks and signage can enhance wayfinding skills and topographic orientation. They recommend the use of pictures or signs that are

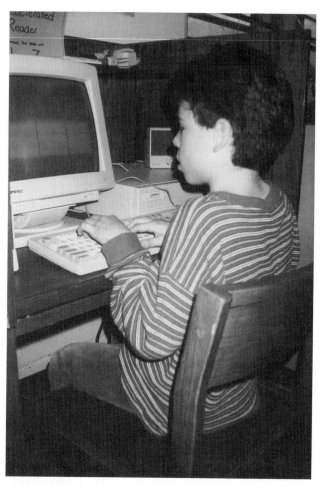

FIGURE 12-5 Todd in a study carrel.

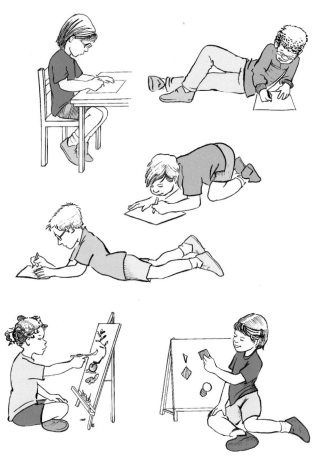

FIGURE 12-6 Alternate positions for visual-perceptual activities.

realistic and simple and that have high color contrast. For example, a simple, graphic depiction of a lunch tray with food could be used for the cafeteria door.

Visual Attention

With a sensory processing approach, general sensory stimulation or inhibition may be provided during or before visually oriented activities to improve visual attending skills. If the child is overaroused, the therapist can diminish sensory input to calm him or her; if the child is underaroused, the therapist selects alerting activities to increase the level of arousal.

For the child with impaired visual attention, the therapist addresses goals using varied activities and time segments that are achievable. The therapist identifies activities that are intrinsically motivating to the child because these help maintain the child's attention. The therapist should plan activities together with the child and use as many novel activities as possible. Most challenging to the therapist is adapting or modifying task activities while maintaining a playful learning environment for the child. For example, the therapist may have many activities focusing on the same visual-perceptual problem, and he or she changes activities frequently, depending on the child's sustained attention to the task. The therapist also gradually increases the amount of sustained attention needed to complete the task. Elimination of extraneous environmental stimuli is helpful at each level of visual attention.

The occupational therapist can be a consultant to the classroom teacher suggesting ways to improve the child's attention to learning in the classroom. For instance, the therapist can provide activities during a classroom session and then leave further suggestions for activities that the teacher can implement during the week. Specific components of attention could be addressed in a hierarchical manner so that intervention tasks gradually place greater demands on attention (e.g., progressing from sustained attention to divided attention).

Visual attention skills are enhanced by activities that are developmentally appropriate and visually and tactilely stimulating. Manual activities such as drawing or manipulating clay encourage the eyes to view the movements involved.[117] In addition, the hand helps educate the eye about object qualities such as weight, volume, and texture and helps direct the eye to the object.[117] Simultaneous hand and eye movements construct internal representations of objects and improve object recognition.

Activities to compensate for limitations in attention include (1) placing a black mat that is larger than the worksheet underneath it to increase high contrast, thereby assisting visual attention to the worksheet; (2) drawing lines to group materials; and (3) reorganizing worksheets.[144] Visual stimuli on a worksheet or in a book can be reduced by covering the entire page except the activity on which the student is working or by using a mask that uncovers one line at a time (Figure 12-7). Reducing competing sensory input in both the auditory and visual modalities can be helpful for some students with poor visual

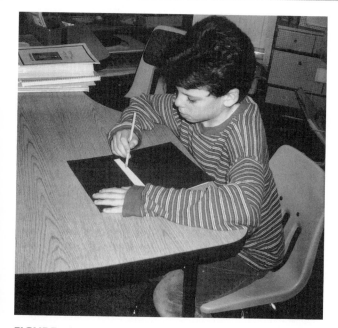

FIGURE 12-7   Todd uses a mask to uncover one line at a time.

attention. For example, headphones can be worn when working on a visual task. Good lighting and use of pastel-colored paper helps reduce glare. Encouraging children to search for high-interest photographs or pictures can help increase visual attention skills.[117] *Where's Waldo?* and similar books are highly motivating and encourage children to develop search strategies and visual attention.

Other suggestions include cueing the child to important visual information by using a finger to point, a marker to underline, or therapist verbalization to help the child maintain visual attention. For example, children tend to look at a picture when it is named. The therapist can use large, colorful pictures combined with rhyming chants to encourage attention to the pictures.[117] Visual work should be presented when the student's energy is highest and not when he or she is fatigued.[117] Strategy training can be used to control distractibility, impulsivity, or a tendency to lose track or to overfocus.[145] Intervention strategies may include the following[50]:

- Attending to the whole situation before attending to parts
- Taking timeouts from a task
- Monitoring the tendency to become distracted
- Searching the whole scene before responding
- Teaching self-instruction
- Devising time-pressure management strategies[50]

Visual Memory

Children with visual memory problems need consistent experiences; the therapist therefore should consult with the parents and teachers so that this consistency can be maintained at home and in the classroom. There is no evidence that repetitive practice of word lists or objects generalizes to other material.[31] Instead, memory strategies may help with encoding or with the retrieval of memory. Grouping information in ways that provide retrieval cues can help a child remember interrelated data.[127] Several strategies may be helpful. *Chunking* is organizing information into smaller units, or chunks. This can be done by cutting up worksheets and presenting one unit or task at a time. *Maintenance rehearsal* (repetition) helps the

child hold information in his or her short-term memory but seems to have no effect on long-term storage. An example of this strategy would be repeating a phone number until the number is dialed. *Elaborative rehearsal* is a strategy by which new information is consciously related to knowledge already stored in long-term memory. By the time a child is 8 years of age, he or she can rehearse more than one item at a time and can rehearse information together as a set to remember. Children can also relate ideas to more than one other idea.

Mnemonic devices are memory-directed tactics that help transform or organize information to enhance its retrievability through use of language cues such as songs, rhymes, and acronyms. Gibson suggested that memory is composed primarily of distinctive features (what makes something different).[58] If the child has good visualization, this can be used as a memory strategy for encoding information. Occupational therapists can help the child determine differences in visual stimuli to promote storage in memory. Playing games such as Concentration, copying a sequence after viewing it for a few seconds, or remembering what was removed from a tray of several items can be enjoyable ways to increase visual memory (Case Study 12-1). The therapist first provides the student with short, simple tasks that he or she can complete quickly and successfully; gradually, as the student accomplishes tasks, the therapist increases their length and complexity.

External strategies and aids can also be used, such as notebooks, hand-held computers, and tape recorders, to name a few. Also, tasks and environments can be rearranged so that they are less demanding on memory.[143] Examples include labeling drawers with the contents inside them, making cue cards with directions for tasks, and posting signs to help the child find his or her classroom. Emotional memory has been shown to be the strongest kind of memory. When students are deeply interested and emotionally involved in what they are reading, they are more likely to comprehend and learn from it.[23]

Visual Discrimination

The therapist must use task analysis to design an intervention program. Remediation should follow an orderly design[15] so that the child can make sense of each performance. By analyzing the continuum of a task, the therapist can grade the activity from simple to complex to allow success while challenging the child's visual abilities.[11] Intervention strategies should aim to help children recognize and attend to the identifying features by teaching them to use their vision to locate objects and then to use object features as well as other cues to form identification hypotheses.[127] Teaching children to scan or search pictures visually instructs the child in the value of looking for and finding meaning. With high-interest materials the therapist can teach the child to look from top to bottom and left to right.[117] Using pictures from magazines, the therapist removes an important part of a picture and asks the student to identify what part is missing. Drawing, painting, and other art and craft activities encourage exploration and manipulation of visual forms. As the child moves from awareness to attention and then to selection, he or she becomes better able to discriminate between the important and unimportant features of the environment.

Occupational therapists can assist teachers in reorganizing the child's worksheets. Color-coding different problems may assist the child in visually attending to the correct section. Worksheets can also be cut up and reorganized to match the

CASE STUDY 12-1   Todd

When Todd was a 9-year-old student in the third grade, most of his day was spent in the regular third grade classroom, where he functioned at grade level in all areas of academics except reading. Todd received daily resource room instruction in this area. This instruction consisted of copying, worksheet completion, and drill and repetition techniques and did not include opportunities for manipulative activities.

An occupational therapy evaluation indicated that Todd's perceptual skills were delayed about 2 years, with weaknesses noted in visual-spatial relations, figure-ground perception, and visual sequential memory. From interviewing the teacher, the therapist learned that Todd was not moving from learning to read to reading to learn. His decoding was not automatic; therefore, he was spending considerable time figuring out what the words were rather than comprehending what he was reading. He also reported that his eyes tired easily while reading. Good eye movements were needed to sustain reading for longer periods. Because of poor spatial abilities, Todd had difficulty discerning differences in visually similar symbols and had difficulty with words that differed only by sequence (*three* and *there*) or spatial orientation

(*dad* and *bad*). The third grade reading books had more print per page and fewer illustrations to give cues. Too many words on the page made it difficult for Todd because of his poor figure-ground abilities. He demonstrated an inability to recall the exact order of words, poor sight vocabulary, and poor spelling caused by poor visual sequential memory.

The therapist referred Todd for optometric evaluation because of his reported visual fatigue during reading tasks. Planning together with Todd, the therapist and the teacher developed strategies to assist him in increasing his visual memory. Initially, short visual memory tasks were used, and gradually the length of tasks was increased. This was done using visual memory games (such as Concentration) and activities on the computer. In addition, visual discrimination tasks were started, beginning with simple forms and moving to forms that were more complex.

In consultation with the teacher, the therapist recommended reducing the amount of print per page and masking what was not immediately needed when this could not be done. Phonics approaches to word recognition were recommended (see Table 12-3), as were using verbal mediation to decode words.

---

child's visual needs. It is important gradually to phase out the restructuring of the worksheets so that the child can eventually use the sheets as they are presented in the workbooks.

When a child has problems copying from the chalkboard, the occupational therapist may recommend that the chalkboard be regularly cleaned in an effort to reduce clutter and provide high contrast for chalk marks. Notations on chalkboards, bulletin boards, or overhead transparencies should be color coded, well spaced, and uncluttered. These practices can reduce figure-ground problems. The therapist may also suggest that the teacher reduce use of the chalkboard by having the children copy from one paper to another with both papers in the same plane. A teacher may be encouraged to try bean bag games in which the targets are placed at approximately the same distance from the child's eyes as the chalkboard so that a student can practice focusing and fixating the eyes near and far in play.

Reducing the amount of print on a page (less print, fewer math problems) and providing mathematical problems on graph paper with numbers in columns in the 1s, 10s, and 100s places help students with figure-ground difficulties. Masking the part of the worksheet not being worked on can help the child focus on one problem at a time. Cooper proposed a theoretic model for the implementation of color contrast to enhance visual ability in the older adult.[36] Principles of color contrast and the ways in which color contrast can be achieved by varying hue, brightness, or color saturation, of an object in relation to its environment are the foundation of the method of intervention. This helps a child identify the relevant information, such as the classroom materials and supplies.

Decoding Problems in Reading

Children who have difficulty distinguishing between similar visual symbols may benefit from a multisensory approach. This includes tracing the shapes and letters, hearing them, saying

them, and then feeling them, allowing a number of routes of processing to help supplement weak visual-perceptual processing. Thus the child sees it, hears it, traces it, and writes it. Eating letters is an activity children love; alphabet cereal, gelatin jigglers, and cookies in the shape of letters can be served for snacks. Children can trace the letters with frosting from tubes onto cookies and with catsup from packets.

For children with word recognition difficulty, the initial emphasis should be on recognition rather than retrieval. The child can be given a choice of visually similar words to complete sentences that have single words missing. In addition, using word families (ball, call, and tall) to increase sight vocabulary enhances word recognition skills. Phonic approaches may also be the best reading instruction method for children with poor word recognition. Textbooks recorded on CDs can be ordered from local and state libraries from the American Printing House for the Blind (1839 Frankfurt Ave., P.O. Box 6085, Frankfurt, KY 40206). The student can hear and read the textbook at the same time, which provides input through two sensory modalities.

If the child has strong verbal skills, verbal mediation (talking through printed words) should be stressed, and the child could be encouraged to describe what he or she sees to retain the information. A strategy that may assist a child who reverses letters in words is to follow along the printed lines with a finger. This technique helps stress reading the letters in the correct sequence. Reading material rich in pictorial content (e.g., comic books), pictures with captions and cartoons, and computer software designed to enhance sight vocabulary can strengthen these associations. Verbal instruction to guide and support the child's nonverbal problem-solving processes and direct verbal training on a spatial task have been shown to be an effective treatment strategy for children with nonverbal learning difficulties.[53]

Several studies support the use of colored filters to improve reading skills.[14,128] Color overlays have been used for children with difficulty reading due to visual fatigue and visual perceptual distortions that are reported as movement of the print (jumping, fading, disappearing, blurring), merging of the print and background, and patterns within the print. Research suggests that they may be a beneficial tool to use when children have reading difficulties. Blaskey et al. investigated the effectiveness of Irlen (colored) filters for improving comfort and reading performance and for determining whether traditional optometric intervention would be effective in relieving the symptoms commonly reported by people seeking help through the use of Irlen filters.[12] Results revealed that subjects in both treatment groups showed improvement in vision functioning. Although the subjects in the Irlen filter group did not show any significant gains in reading rate, work recognition in context, or comprehension, they did report increased comfort in vision when reading.

The What Works Clearinghouse collects, reviews, and reports on studies of education programs, products, practices, and policies in selected topic areas, using a set of standards based on scientifically valid criteria. Programs in early childhood education including print awareness and beginning reading are reviewed. The site can be accessed at http://www.w-w-c.org or http://www.whatworks.ed.gov.

Visualization

The development of visualization techniques, or visual imagery, may be delayed. Like all skills, this proceeds from the concrete to the abstract. Therapists can start by helping students picture something that they can touch or feel. Using a grab bag with toys or objects inside that the child identifies without vision is a good way to do this.

As material becomes less concrete, more visual skills are drawn into play. A student might be asked to visualize something that he or she has done. The occupational therapist can facilitate the child's thinking by reminding him or her to consider various factors, such as color, brightness, size, sounds, temperature, space, movement, smells, and tastes. The hope is that once the child practices verbally, he or she will generalize the visualization process to reading.[7]

Children with poor visualization may have difficulty spelling and may need to learn spelling rules thoroughly. They may also demonstrate reading comprehension problems. In addition, they may have difficulty forming letters because they are unable to visualize them. This would become evident when the child writes from dictation. Sometimes the child can visualize a letter from the sound, but it is reversed or missing parts.

Learning Styles

All students have a preferred learning style.[24,26] When a student is taught through his or her preferred style, the child can learn with less effort and remember better.[44,114] Figure 12-8 shows diagnostic learning styles. All students need to be taught through their strongest senses and then reinforced through their next strongest sense.

Auditory learners recall at least 75% of what is discussed or heard in a normal 40- to 45-minute period. Visual learners remember what they see and can retrieve details and events by concentrating on the things that they have seen. Tactual and kinesthetic learners assimilate best by touching, manipulating, and handling objects. They remember more easily when they write, doodle, draw, or move their fingers. It is best to introduce material to them through art activities, baking, cooking, building, making, interviewing, and acting experiences. If a child has weaknesses in visual processing, it is more

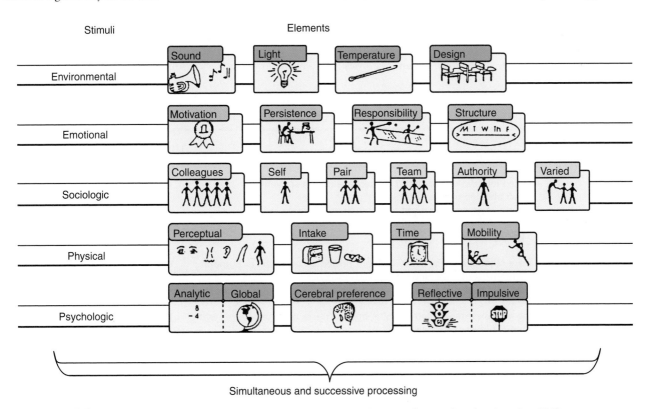

FIGURE 12-8 Diagnostic learning styles. (Courtesy Rita Dunn, EdD, St. John's University, Jamaica, NY.)

BOX 12-2 Suggestions for Tactile and Kinesthetic Learners

- At story time, give the child a prop that relates to the story. The child can act out something that he or she just heard using the prop.
- Provide letter cubes for making words.
- To enable the student to build models and complete projects, provide simple written and recorded directions (the child sees and hears written directions simultaneously, which increases understanding and retention).
- Use games such as bingo, dominoes, or card games to teach or review reading skills. These activities allow movement and peer and adult interaction.
- Use writing activity cards. Paste colorful, high-interest pictures on index cards and add stimulating questions.[26]
- Encourage the child to participate actively while he or she reads. For example, children can write while they read, underline or circle key words, place an asterisk in the margin next to an important section as they read, and inscribe comments when appropriate.
- Use glue letters.
- Use blocks from a Boggle game.
- Play Scrabble.

difficult for him or her to learn through the visual sense. This child may learn more effectively through the kinesthetic and tactile senses. Box 12-2 presents suggestions for kinesthetic learning.

Occupational therapists can greatly assist teachers by helping to determine a child's perceptual strengths and weaknesses so that an appropriate reading program can be matched to the child's preferred perceptual modality. Once the child is in first grade, it is important to determine what reading program the teacher is using. Table 12-3 matches reading methods to perceptual strengths and weaknesses and global and analytic styles.

In addition to perceptual strengths, the therapist must keep in mind the child's preferred manner of approaching new material. For instance, global learners require an overall comprehension first and then can attend to the details. Analytic learners piece details together to form an understanding.

Visual-Motor Integration

To review, the therapist should first focus on the underlying visual-receptive functions and then focus on the visual-cognitive functions. This should proceed in the sequence of visual attention, visual memory, visual discrimination, and specific visual discrimination skills. A multisensory approach to handwriting may be helpful to a child with visual-cognitive problems. Working with the eyes closed can be effective in reducing the influence of increased effort that vision can create and in lessening the visual distractions. Keeping the eyes closed can also improve the awareness of the kinesthetic feedback from letter formation.

The therapist should be aware of which handwriting approach is used in the classroom. The child whose preferred learning style is based on an auditory system can be assisted in learning handwriting through use of a talking pen. Handwriting programs that appear easier for children with visual-cognitive problems include Loops and Other Groups[9] and Handwriting Without Tears.[101] Olsen described strategies to help children correct or avoid reversals. During handwriting lessons, the child should proofread his or her own work and circle the best-formed letters. Chapter 19 has comprehensive information on developing handwriting skills.

Children with visual-spatial problems often choose random starting points, which can confuse the writing task from the onset. Concrete cues must be used to teach abstract handwriting concepts. For example, colored lines on the paper or paper with raised lines can be helpful for the child who has difficulty knowing where to place the letters on the page. In addition, green lines drawn to symbolize *go* on the left side of the paper and red lines to symbolize *stop* on the right side may help a child know which direction to write his or her letters and

TABLE 12-3 Matching Reading Methods to Perceptual Strengths

Reading Method	Description	Reading Style Requirements
Phonics	Isolated letter sounds or letter clusters are taught sequentially and blended to form words.	Auditory and analytic strengths
Linguistic	Patterns of letters are taught and combined to form words.	Auditory and analytic strengths
Orton-Gillingham	Consists of phonics and tactile stimulation in the form of writing and tracing activities.	Auditory and analytic strengths combined with visual weaknesses
Whole word	Before reading a story, new words are presented on flash cards and in sentences, with accompanying pictures.	Visual and global strengths
Language-experience	Students read stories that they have written.	Visual, tactile, and global strengths
Fernald	Language-experience method, plus student traces over new words with index finger of writing hand.	Tactile and global strengths combined with visual weaknesses
Choral reading	Groups read a text in unison.	Visual and global strengths
Recorded book	Students listen two or three times to brief recordings of books, visually track the words, then read the selection aloud.	Visual and global strengths

From Carbo, M. (2007). *Becoming a great teacher of reading: Achieving high rapid reading gains with powerful differentiated strategies.* Thousand Oaks, CA: Corwin Press.

BOX 12-3   Postulates for Change

Reversal error in individual letters and numbers. Occupational therapists can take an active role in helping to reduce letter and number reversal errors by providing the following:
- Activities that offer an opportunity to practice writing individual letters and numbers, focusing on the distinctive features of letter forms with contrasting orientation, such as *b* and *d*
- Activities that afford an opportunity to practice detecting distinctive features of individual letters and numbers, such as tracing, coloring, and pointing
- Demonstration, naming of letters and numbers, and descriptions of the differences between the orientations of individual letter forms that are likely to be reversed

Reversal error in letter order of words and numbers. Occupational therapists can take an active role in reducing reversal errors in letter order of words and numbers by engaging students in the following:
- Activities that provide an opportunity to practice writing words, focusing on the distinctive features of letter forms with contrasting sequences, such as *was* and *saw*
- Activities that provide an opportunity to analyze patterns of words and numbers in relation to one's own body and space
- Activities that encourage the child to start writing at the left position of a line
- Prompts or visual cues at the left side of the paper as a reminder of where to start writing

From Lee, S. (2006). A frame of reference for reversal errors in handwriting: A historical review of visual-perceptual theory. *School System Special Interest Section Quarterly, 13*(1), 1-4.

words. Upright orientation of the writing surface may also lessen directional confusion of letter formation (*up* means up and *down* means down) versus orientation at a desk on a horizontal surface, where *up* means away from oneself and *down* means toward oneself.[127]

Directional cues can be paired with verbal cues for the child who commonly reverses letters and numbers. These cognitive cues rely on visual images for distinguishing letters and include the following:
1. With palms facing the chest and thumbs up, the student makes two fists. The left hand will form a *b* and the right hand will form a *d*.
2. Lower case *b* is like *B*, only without the top loop.
3. To make a lower case *d*, remember that *c* comes first, then add a line to make a *d*.

The therapist can develop cue cards for the student to keep at his or her desk with common reversals. Lee has developed a frame of reference for reversal errors in handwriting based on visual-perceptual theory.[87] See Box 12-3 for the postulates for change as outlined by Lee.

Children with visual-cognitive problems often overspace or underspace words. The correct space should be slightly more than the width of a single lower case letter. When a child has handwriting spacing problems, the occupational therapist may recommend using a decorated tongue depressor or a pencil to space words, or simply have the child use his or her finger as a guide. The child can also imagine a letter in the space to aid in judging the distance.

When students need additional help to stop at lines, templates with windows can be used in teaching handwriting. These templates can be made out of cardboard with three windows; one for one-line letters (*a, c, e, i, m,* and *n*), one for two-line letters (*b, d, k, l,* and *t*), and the third for three-line letters (*f, g, j, p, q, z,* and *y*). It is important to consider that visual memory is used to recognize the letters or words to be written, and motor memory starts the engram for producing the written product. Therefore it may be that motor memory, not visual memory, is the basis for the problem.

Dankert, Davies, and Gavin evaluated whether preschool children with developmental delays who received occupational therapy would demonstrate improvement in visual-motor skills.[40] The children received a minimum of one individual 30-minute session and one group 30-minute session per week for one school year. Their performance was compared with that of two control groups: typically developing peers who received occupational therapy and typically developing peers who did not receive occupational therapy. The results showed that the students with developmental delays demonstrated statistically significant improvement in visual-motor skills and developed skills at a rate faster than expected compared with typically developing peers.

Computers
Many excellent educational computer programs for young children are already on the market. Software programs that are highly motivating for children of all ages are available. Living books on the computer reinforce the written word with the spoken word and assist in developing a sight-word vocabulary.

The computer can be used as a motivational device to help increase the child's attention to the task. It also provides a means to practice skills in an independent manner. Drill and practice software record data on accuracy and the time taken to complete the drills, allowing the therapist to record the child's progress. The therapist can adapt the computer program by changing the background colors to those that enhance the child's visual-perceptual skills. The therapist can also enlarge the written information so that less information is present on the screen. Sands and Buchholz provide a discussion on the use of computers in reading instruction.[124] Appendix 12-A on the Evolve website includes a list of computer software and hardware companies that provide current information on technologic and educational resources available for children with a variety of special needs.

Studies have shown that children's use of computer-based activities resulted in improved performance. For example, using single-subject reversal design study, Cardona, Martinez, and Hinojosa examined five children 3 to 5 years of age who had developmental disabilities to measure the effectiveness of using a computer to increase attention to developmentally appropriate visual analysis activities.[28] The results suggested that each child's attention to task performance improved during the computer-based activities as measured by the number of off-task behaviors. Sitting tolerance and visual attention to the task did not change. All participants seemed to be interested in and motivated to engage in the computer-based activities.

More research is needed to examine a longer intervention phase and the effectiveness of computer-based intervention in natural settings such as a classroom. Authors who have studied the effects of computer games in kindergarten-age children recommend their use in improving visual-perceptual skills.[104] Their findings indicate that, on the basis of required time and motivation level, computer games are more efficient than other educational programs.

Currently a considerable body of literature supports the use of virtual environment technology to train spatial behavior in the real world.[45] Occupational therapists should incorporate this information into their interventions.

SUMMARY

Children with visual-perceptual problems often receive the services of occupational therapists. This chapter described a developmental approach that emphasizes methods of identifying the underlying client strengths and deficits in visual-receptive and visual-cognitive skills. The relationship of these components to various performance skills was described. Using the developmental approach, the occupational therapist helps the child increase his or her visual-perceptual skills by addressing the skill problems that appear to be limiting function. By adapting classroom materials and instruction methods, the therapist also helps the child compensate for visual-perceptual problems. Intervention often includes a combination of developmental and compensatory activities. This holistic approach enables the child with visual-perceptual problems to achieve optimal function and learning.

Little evidence exists in the occupational therapy literature regarding treatment effectiveness for visual-perceptual problems in children. See Table 12-4 for results of visual-perceptual treatment. As a profession, occupational therapy has identified that visual-perceptual problems are within its domain of practice. Further, occupational therapy practitioners, authors, and researchers have defined practice models and intervention activities to remediate visual-perceptual problems. The next step is to systematically test the effectiveness of these intervention programs.

TABLE 12-4 Evidence of Visual-Perceptual and Visual-Motor Treatment

Author(s)*	Study Design	Sample Size	Outcome Intervention	Summary of Results
Krebbs, Eickelberg, Krobath, & Baruch (1989)	1 group nonrandomized	6 students with spina bifida aged 9-12	6 min of active exercise, rest, or figural learning	Significant increase in peripheral vision after active exercise
Aki & Kayrhan (2003)	Random assignment to 2 groups	40 children with low vision	Group 1—Same activities given physiotherapy 3/wk for 3 mo, visual-perceptual training Group 2—Same activities for a home program	Significant increase found in both groups. Significant increase for Group 1 in FCP, PS, and reading performance. Increased academic skills and ADLs
Sovik (1981)	Random assignment to 3 groups	36 3rd graders	6 wks Group 1—classroom instruction plus lab 1×/wk during 6 weeks for 60 min Group 2—classroom instruction Group 3—Control conventional instruction	Experimental groups scored significantly higher than control in accuracy in copying, tracking, and writing and children in Group I scored higher than those in Group 2.
Fox & Lincoln (2008)[53]	A-B-A single case experimental design	2 children aged 8–9 with nonverbal learning disabilities	Nonverbal construction tasks using verbal mediation	Improved in ability to complete nonverbal construction tasks with verbal mediation showed no improvement with practice alone
Ratzon, Efrain, & Bart (2007)	Random into 2 groups, experimental and control. Before and after two tests administered.	52 1st grade students in Israel	12 sessions 1×/wk for 45 min following motor learning theories, multisensory theory, Benbow activities	Intervention group made significant gains both in the total score on the graphomotor test and on fine motor test

TABLE 12-4 Evidence of Visual-Perceptual and Visual-Motor Treatment—Cont'd

Author(s)[*]	Study Design	Sample Size	Outcome Intervention	Summary of Results
Palisano (1989)	6 months	34 children with learning disabilities	Group 1—OT 2/wk in small or large group settings Group 2—consultation from OT through a wkly large group session in the classroom and a 30 min/wk consultation with the teacher to provide a monthly lesson plan of follow-up activities to be performed 3×/wk for 6 mo	Both groups improved on the standardized assessments of gross and fine motor abilities, VMI and V-P skills
Dankert, Davies, & Gavin (2003)[40]	Quasi-experimental two-factor mixed design. Three groups of preschool children of differing disability levels and amounts of therapy received for 8 mo. Assessed pre-, mid-, and post-therapy sessions.	Group 1—12 preschool children with DD Group 2—16 preschool children c/o disabilities Group 3—preschool children without disabilities	Group 1— minimum of OT 1 individual 30-min session/wk and 1 group 30-min sessions/wk for 1 school year Group 2—1 30-min OT group session/wk Group 3—no TV	OT can effectively improve visual motor skills. Children who received OT made significant gains after 8 mos. And they acquired skills at a rate that exceeded typical development.
Lahav, Apter, & Ratzon (2008)	Randomized control trial	169 poor children in regular kindergarten or first grade	12 wks of treatment—45-min sessions Group 1—directive visual-motor intervention (DVMI) Group 2—nondirective supportive intervention (NDSI) Group 3—no treatment	NDSI kindergarten children significantly improved in VMI skill compared with DVMI and no treatment No significant differences among first graders No significant difference among groups in improvement in psychological adjustment or self-esteem Kindergarteners may benefit from the positive and meaningful relationships inherent in NDSI

*Complete source information follows:

Aki, E., & Kayihan, H. (2003). The effect of visual perception training on reading, writing and daily living activities in children with low vision. *Fizyoterapi Rehabilitasyon, 14*(3), 95-99.

Krebbs, P., Eickelberg, W., Krobath, H., & Barvch, I. (1989). Effects of physical exercise on peripheral vision and learning in children with spina bifida manifesta. *Perceptual and Motor Skills, 68,* 167-174.

Lahav, O., Apter, A., & Ratzon, N. (2008). A comparison of the effects of directive visuomotor intervention versus nondirective supportive intervention in kindergarten and elementary school children. *Journal of Neural Transmission, 115*(8), 1231-1239.

Palisano, R. J. (1989). Comparison of two methods of service delivery for students with learning disabilities. *Physical and Occupational Therapy in Pediatrics, 9*(3), 79-100.

Ratzon, N. Z., Efraim, D., & Bart, O. (2007). A short-term graphomotor program for improving writing readiness skills of first-grade students. *American Journal of Occupational Therapy, 61*(4), 399-405.

Sovik, N. (1981). An experimental study of individualized learning/instruction in copying, tracking, and handwriting based on feedback principles. *Perceptual and Motor Skills, 53,* 195-215.

REFERENCES

1. Adams, W., & Sheslow, D. (1995). *Wide range assessment of visual motor abilities manual.* Wilmington, DE: Wide Range, Inc.
2. American Occupational Therapy Association (AOTA). (2008). Occupational therapy practice framework: Domain and process (2nd ed.). *American Journal of Occupational Therapy, 62,* 625–683.
3. Arguin, M., Cavanagh, P., & Joanette, Y. (1994). Visual feature integration with an attention deficit. *Brain and Cognition, 24,* 44–56.
4. Ayres, A. J. (1979). *Sensory Integration and the Child.* Los Angeles: Western Psychological Services.
5. Batshaw, M. L., Pellegrino, L., & Roizen, N. (2007). *Children with handicaps: A medical primer* (6th ed.). Baltimore: Brookes.
6. Beery, K. E., & Beery, N. A. (2004). *Developmental Test of Visual-Motor Integration with supplemental Developmental Tests of Visual Perception and Motor Coordination: Administration, Scoring, and Teaching Manual* (5th ed.). Upper Saddle River, NJ: Pearson.
7. Bell, N. (1991). *Visualizing and verbalizing for language comprehension and thinking.* Paso Robles, CA: Academy of Reading Publishers.
8. Bell, B., & Swinth, Y. (2005). Defining the role of occupational therapy to support literacy development. *School System Special Interest Section Quarterly, 12*(3), 1–4.
9. Benbow, M. (1990). *Loops and other groups.* Tucson, AZ: Therapy Skill Builders.
10. Birch, H. G. (1964). *Brain damage in children: The biological and social aspects.* New York: Williams & Wilkins.
11. Blanksby, B. S. (1992). Visual therapy: A theoretically based intervention program. *Journal of Visual Impairment and Blindness, 86,* 291–294.
12. Blaskey, P., Scheimen, M., Parisi, M., Ciner, E. B., Gallaway, M., & Sleznick R. (1990). The effectiveness of Irlen filters for improving reading performance: A pilot study. *Journal of Learning Disabilities, 23,* 604–612.
13. Borsting, E. (1996). Visual perception and reading. In R. Garzia (Ed.), *Vision and reading.* St. Louis: Mosby.
14. Bouldoukian, J., Wilkins, A. J., & Evans, B. J. W. (2002). Randomised controlled trial of the effect of coloured overlays on the rate of reading of people with specific learning difficulties. *Ophthalmic & Physiological Optics, 22,* 55–60.
15. Bouska, M. J., Kauffman, N. A., & Marcus, S. E. (2006). Disorders of the visual perception system. In D. A. Umphred & R. T. Lazaro (Eds.), *Neurological rehabilitation* (6th ed.). St. Louis: Elsevier.
16. Bowers, P. G., & Ishaik, G. (2003). RAN'S contributions to understanding reading disabilities. In H. L. Swanson, K. R. Harris, & S. Graham (Eds.), *Handbook of learning disabilities* (pp. 140–157). New York: Guilford Press.
17. Breakey, A. S., Wilson, J. J., & Wilson, B. C. (1994). Sensory and perceptual functions in the cerebral palsied. *Journal of Nervous and Mental Diseases, 158,* 70–77.
18. Deleted in proofs.
19. Bruininks, R. H., & Bruininks, R. (2005). *Bruininks-Oseretsky Test of Motor Proficiency* (2nd ed., BOT-2). Upper Saddle River, NJ: Pearson Assessment.
20. Burpee, J. D. (1997). Sensory integration and visual functions. In M. Gentile (Ed.), *Functional visual behavior: A therapist's guide to evaluation and treatment options.* Bethesda, MD: American Occupational Therapy Association.
21. Burtner, P. A., Dukeminier, A., Ben, L., Qualls, C., & Scott, K. (2006). Visual perceptual skills and related school functions in children with hemiplegic cerebral palsy. *New Zealand Journal of Occupational Therapy, 53*(1), 24–29.
22. Burtner, P. A., Wilhite, C., Bordegaray, J., Moedl, D., Roe, R. J., & Savage, A. R. (1997). Critical review of visual perceptual tests frequently administered by pediatric therapists. *Physical and Occupational Therapy in Pediatrics, 17,* 39–61.
23. Caine, R. N., Caine, G., McClintic, C., & Klimek, K. (2005). *12 Brain mind learning principles in action.* Thousand Oaks, CA: Corwin Press.
24. Carbo, M. (1992). *Reading Style Inventory (Revised).* Roslyn, NY: National Reading Styles Institute.
25. Carbo, M. (1997). Reading styles times twenty. *Educational Leadership, 54,* 38–42.
26. Carbo, M. (2007). *Becoming a great teacher of reading: Achieving high rapid reading gains with powerful, differentiated strategies.* Thousand Oaks, CA: Corwin Press and National Association of Elementary School Principals.
27. Carbo, M. (2008). Best practices for achieving high, rapid reading gains. *The Education Digest, 73*(7), 57–61.
28. Cardona, M., Martinez, A. L., & Hinojosa, J. (2000). Effectiveness of using a computer to improve attention to visual analysis activities of five preschool children with disabilities. *Occupational Therapy International, 7,* 42–56.
29. Caron, A., & Caron, R. (1981). Processing of relational information as an index of infant risk. In S. Friedman & M. Sigman (Eds.), *Preterm birth and psychological development.* New York: Academic Press.
30. Christenson, M. A., & Rascho, B. (1989). Environmental cognition and age-related sensory change. *Occupational Therapy Practice, 1,* 28–35.
31. Cicerone, K. D. (2000). Evidence-based cognitive rehabilitation: Recommendations for clinical practice. *Archives of Physical Medicine and Rehabilitation, 81,* 1596–1615.
32. Ciner, E. B., Macks, B., & Schanel-Klitsch, E. (1991). A cooperative demonstration project for early intervention vision services. *Occupational Therapy Practice, 3,* 42–56.
33. Clifton, R. K., Muir, D. W., Ashmead, D. H., & Clarkson, M. G. (1993). Is visually guided reaching in early infancy a myth? *Child Development, 64,* 1099–1110.
34. Cohen, K. M. (1981). The development of strategies of visual search. In D. F. Fisher, R. A. Monty, & J. W. Senders (Eds.), *Eye movements: Cognition and visual perception.* Hillsdale, NJ: Erlbaum.
35. Colarusso, R. P., & Hammill, D. D. (2003). *Motor-Free Visual Perception Test* (3rd ed.). Novata, CA: Academic Therapy Publications.
36. Cooper, B. A. (1985). A model for implementing color contrast in the environment of the elderly, *American Journal of Occupational Therapy, 39,* 253–258.
37. Cratty, B. J. (1970). *Perceptual and motor development in infants and children.* New York: Macmillan.
38. Daly, C. J., Kelley, G. T., & Krauss, A. (2003). Relationship between visual-motor integration and handwriting skills of children in kindergarten: A modified replication study. *American Journal of Occupational Therapy, 57,* 459–462.
39. Daniels, L. E., & Ryley, C. (1991). Visual-perceptual and visual-motor performance in children with psychiatric disorders. *Canadian Journal of Occupational Therapy, 58*(30), 137–141.
40. Dankert, H. L., Davies, P. L., & Gavin, W. J. (2003). Occupational therapy effects on visual-motor skills in preschool children. *American Journal of Occupational Therapy, 57,* 542–549.
41. de Boisferon, A. H., Bara, F., Gentaz, E., & Cole, P. (2007). Preparation of young children to read: Effects of visual-haptic exploration of letters and visual perception of writing motions. *L'Annee Psychologique, 107,* 537–564.
42. D'Entremont, B., Hains, S. M. J., & Muir, D.W. (1997). A demonstration of gaze following in 3-to-6 month olds. *Infant Behavior and Development, 20,* 569–572.
43. DeQuiros, J. B., & Schranger, O. L. (1979). *Neuropsychological fundamentals in learning disabilities.* Novato, CA: Academic Therapy Publications.
44. Dunn, R., Griggs, S. A., Olson, J., Gorman, B., & Beasley, M. (1995). A meta-analytic validation of the Dunn and Dunn

learning styles model. *Journal of Educational Research, 88*, 353–363.

45. Durlach, N., Allen, G., Dorken, R., Garnett, R., Loomis, J., Templeman, J., et al. (2000). Virtual environments and the enhancement of spatial behavior. *Presence: Teleoperators and Virtual Environments, 9*, 593–616.

46. Dutton, G. (2002). Visual problems in children with damage to the brain. *Visual Impairment Research–2002, 4*, 113–121.

47. Dutton, G., Ballantyne, J., Boyd, G., Bradnam, M., Day, R., McCulloch, D., et al. (1996). Cortical visual dysfunction in children: A clinical study. *Eye, 10*, 302–309.

48. Enns, J. T., & Cameron, S. (1987). Selective attention in young children: The relation between visual search, filtering, and priming. *Journal of Experimental Child Psychology, 44*, 38–63.

49. Farran, E. K., & Cole, V. L. (2008). Perceptual grouping and distance estimates in typical and atypical development: Comparing performance across perception, drawing, and construction tasks. *Brain & Cognition, 68*, 157–165.

50. Fasotti, L., Kovacs, F., Eling, P., & Brouwer, W. H. (2000). Time pressure management as a compensatory strategy training after closed head injury. *Neuropsychological Rehabilitation, 10*, 47–65.

51. Feder, K. P., & Maynemer, A. (2007). Handwriting development, competency, and intervention. *Developmental Medicine & Child Neurology, 49*, 312–317.

52. Fegans, L. V., & Merriwether, A. (1990). Visual discrimination of letter-like forms and its relationship to achievement over time in children with learning disabilities. *Journal of Learning Disabilities, 23*, 417–425.

53. Fox, T., & Lincoln, N. (2008). Verbal mediation as a treatment strategy for children with non-verbal learning difficulties. *International Journal of Therapy and Rehabilitation, 15*(7), 315–320.

54. Gardner, M. F. (1992). *Test of Pictures-Forms-Letters-Numbers-Spatial Orientation & Sequencing Skills.* Burlington, CA: Psychological and Educational Publications.

55. Deleted in proofs.

56. Garzia, R. (1994). The relationship between visual efficiency problems and learning. In M. M. Scheiman & M. W. Rouse (Eds.), *Optometric management of learning-related vision problems.* St. Louis: Mosby-Year Book.

57. Gentile, M. (1997). *Functional visual behavior: A therapist's guide to evaluation and treatment options.* Bethesda, MD: American Occupational Therapy Association.

58. Gibson, E. J. (1991). Perceptual learning and the theory of word perception. *Cognitive Psychology, 2*, 351.

59. Gibson, E. J., & Levin, H. (1975). *The psychology of reading.* Cambridge, MA: MIT Press.

60. Giles, D. C., & Terrell, C. D. (1997). Visual sequential memory and spelling ability. *Educational Psychology, 17*, 245–253.

61. Gilfoyle, E., Grady, A., & Moore, J. (1990). *Children adapt* (2nd ed.). Thorofare, NJ: Slack.

62. Glass, P. (1993). Development of visual function in preterm infants: Implications for early intervention. *Infants and Young Children, 6*(1), 11–20.

63. Goodale, M. (2000). Perception and action in the human visual system. In M. S. Gazzaniga (Ed.), *The new cognitive neurosciences* (2nd ed., pp. 365–377). Cambridge, MA: MIT Press.

64. Goodale, M., & Milner, L. S. (1992). Separate visual pathways for perception and action. *Trends in Neuroscience, 15*, 20–25.

65. Greene, L. J. (1987). *Learning disabled and your child: A survival handbook.* New York: Ballantine Books.

66. Griffin, J. R., Christensen, G. N., Wesson, M. D., & Erickson, G. B. (1997). *Optometric management of reading dysfunction.* Boston: Butterworth-Heinemann.

67. Gulyas, B., Heywood, C. A., Popplewell, D. A., Roland, P. E., & Cowey, A. (1994). A visual form discrimination from color or motion cues: Functional anatomy by positron emission tomography. *Proceedings of the National Academy of Science USA, 92*, 9965–9969.

68. Hammill, D. D., Pearson, N. A., & Voress, J. K. (1993). *Developmental Test of Visual Perception* (2nd ed.). Austin, TX: Pro-Ed.

69. Hendry, S. H. C., & Calkins, D. J. (1998). Neuronal chemistry and functional organization in the primate visual system. *Trends in Neurosciences, 21*, 244–349.

70. Hung, S. S., Fisher, A. G., & Cermak, S. A. (1987). The performance of learning-disabled and normal young men on the test of visual-perceptual skills. *American Journal of Occupational Therapy, 41*, 790–797.

71. Hyvarinen, L. (1994). Assessment of visually impaired infants. *Ophthalmology Clinics of North America, 7*, 219–225.

72. Hyvarinen, L. (1995). Considerations in evaluation and treatment of the child with low vision. *American Journal of Occupational Therapy, 49*, 891–897.

73. Hyvarinen, L. (1995). *Vision testing manual.* La Salle, IL: Precision Vision.

74. Hyvarinen, L. (1988). *Vision in children: Normal and abnormal.* Medford, Ontario: Canadian Deaf, Blind and Rubella Association.

75. Ilg, F. L., & Ames, L. B. (1981). *School readiness.* New York: Harper & Row.

76. Izard, C. (1997). Emotions and facial expressions: A perspective from differential emotions therapy. In J. A. Russell & J. M. Fernandez-Dols (Eds.), *The psychology of facial expression.* New York: Cambridge University Press.

77. Jordan, B. A. (1991). *Jordan Left-Right Reversal Test* (3rd ed.). Los Angeles: Western Pscyhological Services.

78. Juel, C. (1988). Learning to read and write: A longitudinal study of 54 children from first through fourth grades. *Journal of Educational Psychology, 80*, 437–447.

79. Justice, L. M., & Ezell, H. K. (2001). Descriptive analysis of written language awareness in children from low income households. *Communication Disorders Quarterly, 22*, 123–134.

80. Justice, L. M., & Ezell, H. K. (2002). Use of storybook reading to increase print awareness in at-risk children. *American Journal of Speech-Language Pathology, 11*, 17–29.

81. Justice, L. M., & Lankford, C. (2002). Preschool children's visual attention to print during storybook reading: Pilot findings. *Communication Disorders Quarterly, 24*(1), 11–21.

82. Kandel, E. R., Schwartz, J. H., & Jessell, T. M. (1991). *Principles of neural science.* New York: Elsevier Science.

83. Kavale, K. (1982). Meta-analysis of the relationship between visual perceptual skills and reading achievement. *Journal of Learning Disabilities, 15*, 42–51.

84. Kosslyn, S., Chabis, C. F., Marsolek, C. J., & Koenig, O. (1992). Categorical versus coordinate spatial relations: Computational analyses and computer simulations. *Journal of Experimental Psychology of Human Perceptual Performance, 18*, 562–577.

85. Kulp, M., Earley, M., Mitchell, G., Timmerman, L., Frasco C., Geiger, M., et al. (2004). Are visual perceptual skills related to mathematics ability in second through sixth grade children? *Focus on Learning Problems in Mathematics, Optometry and Vision Science, 80*, 431–436.

86. Kulp, M. T., & Schmidt, P. P. (1996). Visual predictors of reading performance in kindergarten and first grade children. *Optometry Vision Science, 73*, 255–262.

87. Lee, S. (2006). A frame of reference for reversal errors in handwriting: A historical review of visual-perceptual theory. *School System Special Interest Section Quarterly, 13*(1), 1–4.

88. Leigh, R.J., & Zee, D.S. (1983). *Neurology of eye movements.* Philadelphia: F.A. Davis.

89. Levine, M. (1987). *Developmental variation and learning disorders.* Cambridge, MA: Educators Publishing Service.

90. Levine, M., Hooper, S, Montgomery J., et al. (1993). Learning disabilities: An interactive developmental paradigm. In G. R. Lyon, D. B. Gray, N. A. Krasnegor, & J. F. Kavanagh (Eds.), *Better understanding learning disabilities: New views from research*

and their implications for education and public policy. Cambridge, MA: Educators Publishing Service.

91. Lukatela, G., Eaton, T., Lee, C., & Turvey, M. T. (2001). Does visual word identification involve a sub-phonemic level? *Cognition, 78,* B41–B52.

92. Luria, A. (1966). *Higher cortical functions in man.* New York: Basic Books.

93. Marr, D. (1982). *Vision.* San Francisco: Freeman.

94. Martin, N. (2006). *Test of Visual Perceptual Skills* (3rd ed.). Novato, CA: Academy Publishers.

95. McAvinue, L., O'Keeffe, F., McMackins, D., & Robertson, I. H. (2005). Impaired sustained attention and error awareness in traumatic brain injury: Implications for sight. *Neuropsychological Rehabilitation, 15(5),* 569–587.

96. McCarty, M. E., Clifton, R. K., Ashmead, P. L., Lee, P., & Goubet, N. (2001). How infants use vision for grasping objects. *Child Development, 72,* 973–987.

97. Menken, C., Cermak, S. A., & Fisher, A. G. (1987). Evaluating the visual-perceptual skills of children with cerebral palsy. *American Journal of Occupational Therapy, 41*(10), 646–651.

98. Milner, A. D., & Goodale, M. A. (1993). Visual pathways to perception and action. In T. P. Hicks, S. Molotchnikoff, & T. Ono (Eds.), *The visually responsive neuron: From basic neurophysiology to behavior* (pp. 317–337). New York: Elsevier Science.

99. Muir, D. W., & Nadel, J. (1998). Infant social perception. In A. Slater (Ed.), *Perceptual development: Visual, auditory, and speech perception in infancy* (pp. 247–286). East Sussex, UK: Psychology Press.

100. Necombe, F., & Ratcliff, G. (1989). Disorders of spatial analysis. In E. Boller & J. Grafman (Eds.), *Handbook of neuropsychology* (Vol. 2). New York: Elsevier Science.

101. Olsen, J. Z. (2008). *Handwriting without tears: First grade printing teacher's guide.* Cabin John, MD: Handwriting Without Tears.

102. Optometric Extension Program Foundation. (2006). Santa Ana, CA: The Foundation.

103. Osterling, J., & Dawson, G. (1994). Early recognition of children with autism: A study of first birthday videotapes. *Journal of Autism and Developmental Disorders, 24,* 247–257.

104. Parham, L. D. (1998). The relationship of sensory integrative development to achievement in elementary students: Four-year longitudinal patterns. *Occupational Therapy Journal of Research, 18,* 105–127.

105. Perov, A., & Kozminsky, E. (1989). The effect of computer games practice on the development of visual perception skills in kindergarten children. *Computers in the Schools, 6(3/4),* 113–122.

106. Piaget, J. (1964). *Development and learning.* Ithaca, NY: Cornell University Press.

107. Pizur-Barnekow, K., Kraemer, G. W., & Winters, J. M. (2008). Pilot study investigating infant vagal reactivity and visual behavior during object perception. *American Journal of Occupational Therapy, 62,* 198–205.

108. Quinn, P. C. (1998). Object and spatial categorization in young infants: "What" and "Where" in early visual perception. In A. Slater (Ed.). *Perceptual development: Visual, auditory, and speech perception in infancy.* Psychology Press.

109. Rafal, R. D., & Posner, M. I. (1987). Cognitive theories of attention and the rehabilitation of attentional deficits. In M. J. Meier, A. L. Benton, & L. Diller (Eds.), *Neuropsychological rehabilitation.* New York: Guilford Press.

110. Ratcliff, G. (1987). Perception and complex visual processes. In M. J. Meier, A. L. Benton, & L. Diller (Eds.), *Neuropsychological rehabilitation* (pp. 182–201). New York: Guilford Press.

111. Raymond, J. E., & Sorensen, R. E. (1998). Visual motion perception in children with dyslexia: Normal detection but abnormal integration. *Visual Cognition, 5,* 389–404.

112. Reid, D. T., & Jutai, J. (1994). *The Componential Assessment of Visual Perception manual.* Toronto, Ontario: University of Toronto, Department of Occupational Therapy.

113. Reid, D. T., & Jutai, J. (1997). A pilot study of perceived clinical usefulness of a new computer-based tool for assessment of visual perception in occupational therapy practice. *Occupational Therapy International, 4,* 81–98.

114. Reutzel, D. R., & Smith, J. A. (2004). Accelerating struggling readers' progress: A comparative analysis of expert opinion and current research recommendations. *Reading and Writing Quarterly, 20,* 63–89.

115. Ritty, J. M., Solan, H., & Cool, S. J. (1993). Visual and sensory-motor functioning in the classroom: A preliminary report of ergonomic demands. *Journal of the American Optometric Association, 64*(4), 238–244.

116. Roder, B. J., Bushnell, E. W., & Sasseville, A. M. (2001). Infant preferences for familiarity and novelty during the course of visual processing. *Infancy, 1*(4), 491–507.

117. Rogow, S. M. (1992). Visual perceptual problems of visually impaired children with developmental disabilities. *Re:View, 24*(2), 57–64.

118. Rogow, S. M., & Rathwill, D. (1989). Seeing and knowing: An investigation of visual perception among children with severe visual impairments. *Journal of Vision Rehabilitation, 3*(3), 55–66.

119. Roley, S., & Schneck, C. (2001). Sensory integration and the child with visual impairment and blindness. In S. Smith Roley, E. Blanche, & R. Schaff (Eds.), *Sensory integration and developmental disabilities.* Tucson, AZ: Therapy Skill Builders.

120. Rose, S. A. (1980). Enhancing visual recognition memory in preterm infants. *Developmental Psychology, 16,* 85.

121. Rosenhall, J., Johansson, E., & Gilberg, C. (1988). Oculomotor findings in autistic children. *Journal of Laryngeal Otology, 102,* 435–439.

122. Rosner, J. (1999). *Test of Visual Analysis Skills.* Academic Therapy.

123. Sakata, H., Taira, M., Kusunoki, M., Murata, A., & Tanaka, Y. (1997). The TINS lecture: The parietal association cortex in depth perception and visual control of hand action. *Trends in Neurosciences, 20*(8), 350–357.

124. Sands, S., & Buchholz, E. S. (1997). The underutilization of computers to assist in the remediation of dyslexia. *International Journal of Instructional Media, 24*(2), 153–175.

125. Scheiman, M. (1997). *Understanding and managing vision deficits: A guide for occupational therapists.* Thorofare, NJ: Slack.

126. Scheiman, M., Gallaway, M., & Coulter, R. (1996). Prevalence of vision and ocular disorders in a clinical pediatric population. *Journal of the American Optometric Association, 67,* 193–202.

127. Schneck, C. M. (1998). Intervention for visual perceptual problems. In J. Case-Smith (Ed.), *Occupational therapy: Making a difference in the school system.* Bethesda, MD: American Occupational Therapy Association.

128. Scholber, M., & Mateer, C. (2001). *Cognitive rehabilitation: An integrative neuropsychological approach.* New York: Guilford Press.

129. Scott, L., McWhinnie, H., Taylor, L., Stevenson, M., Irons, P., Lewis, E., et al. (2002). Double-masked placebo-controlled trial of £9, precision spectral filters in children who use coloured overlays. *Ophthalmic & Physiological Optics, 14,* 365–370.

130. Seiderman, A. S., & Marcus, S. E. (1990). *20/20 is not enough: The new world of vision.* New York: Alfred A. Knopf.

131. Sergent, J. (1991). Judgments of relative position and distance on representations of spatial relations. *Journal of Experimental Psychology: Human Perception and Performance, 91,* 762–780.

132. Shaywitz, B. A. (1997). The Yale Center for the study of learning and attention: Longitudinal and neuro-biological studies. *Learning Disabilities: A Multidisciplinary Journal, 8,* 21–30.

133. Shaywitz, S. E. (1998). Dyslexia. *New England Journal of Medicine, 338,* 307–312.

134. Sigman, M., & Parmelee, A. (1974). Visual preferences of four-month-old premature and full-term infants. *Child Development, 45,* 959–965.

135. Snow, C., Burns, M. S., & Griffin, P. (Eds.). (1998). *Preventing reading difficulties in young children*. Washington, DC: National Academy Press.

136. Sortor, J., & Kulp, M. (2003). Are the results of the Beery-Buktenica Developmental Test of Visual-Motor Integration and its subtest related to achievement test scores? *Optometry and Vision Science, 80,* 758–763.

137. Spelke, E. S., & Cortelyou, A. (1981). Perceptual aspects of social knowing: Looking and listening in infancy. In M. E. Lamb & L. R. Sherrod (Eds.), *Infant social cognition: Empirical and theoretical considerations* (pp. 61–83). Hillsdale, NJ: Erlbaum.

138. Stiers, P., De Cock, P., & Vandenbussche, E. (1999). Separating visual perception and non-verbal intelligence in children with early brain injury. *Brain and Development, 21,* 397–406.

139. Stiles, S., & Knox, R. (1996). Medical issues, treatments, and professionals. In M. C. Holbrook (Ed.), *Children with visual impairments: A parent's guide* (pp. 21–48). Bethesda, MD: Woodbine House.

140. Suchoff, I. B. (1987). *Visual-spatial development in the child* (2nd ed.). New York: State University of New York, State College of Optometry.

141. Swinth, Y. L., & Handley-Moore, D. (2004). Supplementary lesson 8: Handwriting, keyboarding, and literacy: What is the role of occupational therapy? In Y. L. Swinth (Ed.), *Occupational therapy in school-based practice: Contemporary issues and trends* (online course). Bethesda, MD: American Occupational Therapy Association.

142. Teplin, S. W. (1995). Visual impairment in infants and young children. *Infants and Young Children, 8,* 18–51.

143. Thelan, D., & Smith, L. B. (1994). *A dynamic systems approach to the development of cognitions and action.* Cambridge, MA: MIT Press.

144. Todd, V. R. (1999). Visual perceptual frame of reference: An information processing approach. In P. Kramer & J. Hinojosa (Eds.), *Frames of reference for pediatric occupational therapy* (2nd ed., pp. 205–256). Baltimore: Williams & Wilkins.

145. Toglia, J. P. (2003). Cognitive-perceptual retraining and rehabilitation. In E. B. Crepeau, E. S. Cohen, & B. A. B. Schell (Eds.), *Willard and Spackman's occupational therapy* (10th ed., pp. 607–629). Philadelphia: Lippincott Williams & Wilkins.

146. Torgesen, J. K., Wagner, R. K., & Rashotte, C. A. (1994). Longitudinal studies of phonological processing and reading. *Journal of Learning Disabilities, 27,* 276–286.

147. Tsai, C., Wilson, P. H., & Wu, S. K. (2008). Role of visual-perceptual skills (non-motor) in children with developmental coordination disorder. *Human Movement Science, 27,* 649–664.

148. Tseng, M. H., & Cermak, S. A. (1993). The influence of ergonomic factors and perceptual-motor abilities on handwriting performance. *American Journal of Occupational Therapy, 47,* 919–926.

149. Tseng, M. H., & Murray, E. A. (1994). Differences in perceptual-motor measures in children with good and poor handwriting. *Occupational Therapy Journal of Research, 14,* 19–36.

150. Tsurumi, K., & Todd, V. (1998). Tests of visual perception: What do they tell us? *School System Special Interest Section Quarterly, 5*(4), 1–4.

151. Turkewitz, G., & Kenny, P. A. (1985). The role of developmental limitations of sensory input on sensory/perceptual organization. *Developmental and Behavioral Pediatrics, 6,* 302.

152. Ulman, S. (1986). Visual routines. In S. Pinker (Ed.), *Visual cognition* (pp. 97–159). Cambridge: MIT Press.

153. Van der Geest, J. N., Kemner, C., Camfferman, G., Verbaten, M. N., & Van Engeland, H. (2002). Looking at images with human figures: Comparison between autistic and normal children. *Journal of Autism and Developmental Disorders, 32*(2), 69–75.

154. Voyer, D., Voyer, S., & Bryden, M. P. (1995). Magnitude of sex differences in spatial abilities: A meta-analysis and consideration of critical variables. *Psychological Bulletin, 117,* 250–270.

155. Wann, J., & Kardirkamanathan, M. (1991). Variability in children's handwriting: Computer diagnosis of writing difficulties. In J. Wann, A. Wing, & N. Sovik (Eds.), *Development of graphic skills: Research, perspectives, and educational implications* (pp. 223–236). Academic Press: London.

156. Warren, M. (1990). Identification of visual scanning deficits in adults after CVA. *American Journal of Occupational Therapy, 44,* 391–399.

157. Warren, M. (1993). A hierarchical model for evaluation and treatment of visual perceptual dysfunction in adult acquired brain injury. I. *American Journal of Occupational Therapy, 47,* 42–54.

158. Warren, M. (1993). A hierarchical model for evaluation and treatment of visual perceptual dysfunction in adult acquired brain injury. II. *American Journal of Occupational Therapy, 47,* 55–66.

159. Weil, M. J., & Cunningham-Amundson, S. J. (1994). Relationship between visuomotor and handwriting skills of children in kindergarten. *American Journal of Occupational Therapy, 48,* 982–988.

160. Westheimer, G., & Levi, D. M. (1987). Depth attraction and repulsion of disparate foveal stimuli. *Vision Research, 27*(8), 1361–1368.

161. Williams, H. (1983). *Perceptual and motor development.* Englewood Cliffs, NJ: Prentice-Hall.

162. Willows, D. M., & Terepocki, M. (1993). The relation of reversal errors to reading disabilities. In D. M. Willows, R. S. Kruk, & E. Corcois (Eds.), *Visual processes in reading and reading disabilities* (pp. 265–286). Hillsdale, NJ: Erlbaum.

163. Ziviani, J. (2006). The development of graphmotor skills. In A. Henderson, & C. Pehoski (Eds.), *Hand function in the child: Foundations for remediation* (pp. 184–193). St. Louis: Mosby.

164. Ziviani, J., Hayes, A., & Chant, D. (1990). Handwriting: A perceptual motor disturbance in children with myelomeningocele. *Occupational Therapy Journal of Research, 10,* 12–26.

165. Zoltan, B. (2007). *Visual processing skills. Vision, perception, & cognition* (4th ed.) Thorofare; NJ: Slack.

Psychosocial Issues Affecting Social Participation

Debora A. Davidson

Temperament
Attachment
Child abuse
Social competence
Stress
Mental health
Mental disorder
Anxiety disorders
Mood disorders
Pervasive
  developmental
  disorders
Attention deficit
  disorder
Disruptive behavior
  disorders
Students with
  emotional
  disturbance

Classroom-based
  psychosocial therapy
Outpatient mental
  health services
Day treatment
  programs
Residential treatment
  centers
Juvenile justice system
Inpatient psychiatric
  hospitals
Activity groups
Social learning and
  behavioral
  approaches

6. Define the roles of occupational therapists who provide services to children and youth with psychosocial disorders, as well as those of other team members.
7. Understand evaluation and intervention processes related to the special needs of children and youth whose occupational performance has been affected by psychosocial problems.

The promotion of the child's social participation within the contexts of family, friendships, classmates, caregivers, and teachers is an essential domain of occupational therapy in all practice settings.[5,50,56,135,181] Achievement of developmental milestones and occupational goals is the result of continuously evolving interactions between aspects of the individual child and the environmental contexts that envelop him or her. Social relationships constitute a critical chunk of that environment; the mutual influences of the individual and his or her social contexts help determine the child's quality of life and participation in those social contexts.

This chapter is organized as follows: It (1) describes dynamic aspects of healthy psychosocial development within the child and the family, (2) outlines common causes of psychosocial problems in children and adolescents and their implications for occupational performance, (3) describes the roles of occupational therapy practitioners and other team members within a variety of intervention settings, and (4) introduces selected evaluation and intervention methods, including intervention goals for common psychosocial needs.

The unifying frame of reference for this chapter is the person-environment-occupation (PEO) model.[106] The PEO model emphasizes the dynamic interaction between the individual and various aspects of the environment and how these interactions influence occupational performance. "Person" factors include qualities of the individual such as gender, age, developmental levels, skills, preferences, and values. "Environment" factors encompass the social, cultural, economic, political, and physical contexts that the child functions within. Person and environment factors are viewed as reciprocally influential and as directly relevant to the child's occupational performance. "Occupations" are the everyday tasks and activities that an individual performs, ranging from very basic actions, such as eating and using the toilet, to highly sophisticated activities, such as

1. Understand the dynamic interaction of emotional, cognitive, neurobehavioral, and environmental factors as they influence aspects of occupational performance through the course of typical development during infancy, childhood, and adolescence.
2. Explain means of promoting the psychosocial wellness of infants, children, and youth within natural contexts.
3. Identify the diagnostic hallmarks and contributing factors of common mental health conditions, and relate these to the occupational performance of children and adolescents.
4. Understand the continuum of services available to children and youth with psychosocial disorders.
5. Explain the variety of service delivery models and frames of reference used by occupational therapists in psychosocial settings.

working a calculus problem, flirting with a classmate, or roller-blading. Appreciating and understanding the elements of the PEO model and their potential for dynamic interaction enable occupational therapists to approach intervention holistically and effectively.

TEMPERAMENT: A "PERSON" FACTOR THAT INFLUENCES AND IS INFLUENCED BY THE ENVIRONMENT

Children vary in their development of interests, habits, talents, and social competence. Standardized pediatric tests reveal variations among children in the rate and sequence of their acquisition of motor, language, and cognitive skills. Curiosity about these differences among children has inspired decades of research. Chess and Thomas were among the first scholars to study children's styles of responding to various experiences and carrying out activities such as sleeping, eating, and exploring objects.[158] Their work developed the concept of *temperament*. Temperament refers to a collection of inborn, relatively stable traits that influence how individuals process and respond to the environment and that contribute to the development of personality and everyday functioning.[154] Chess and Thomas identified nine basic characteristics of temperament, which remain useful today. These are (1) activity level, (2) rhythmicity (i.e., the degree to which the child's patterns of sleeping, eating, and play are predictable), (3) approach to or withdrawal from novel situations, (4) intensity of emotional responses, (5) sensory threshold, (6) mood (general emotional state), (7) adaptability, (8) distractibility, and (9) attention span and persistence.[33] Temperament characteristics are not considered to be inherently good or bad, and they are not under the control of the child or the parents. However, behaviors arising from temperament traits may be more or less adaptive or pleasing, depending on the context. Children whose temperament style approaches extremes on any of the nine parameters may have more difficulty negotiating the social and emotional demands of childhood. The environmental demands and expectations must always be considered, however, when attempting to predict the effects of temperament on occupational performance. Research indicates that the assessment of each child's temperament is influenced by the observer's point of view and that the determination of function or dysfunction has much to do with the situational compatibility with the family and other social environments.[171]

Chess and Thomas were interested in learning about the influence of personality characteristics on the parent-child relationship and the child's development.[35] They applied the concept *goodness of fit* (from statistics) to interpersonal relationships. When the expectations of persons important to the child are compatible with the child's temperament, there is a good fit (Case Study 13-1). When the child's temperament is at odds with parental expectations, mutual distress may result. Although Chess and Thomas focused on parent-child fit, other research has supported the findings in teacher and peer relationships.[90,91]

Chess and Thomas (1983) identified three common patterns of temperament from the nine temperament traits described above. They gave these combinations the labels *easy child*, *difficult child*, and *slow-to-warm-up child* (Figure 13-1). The *easy child* is positive in mood and approach to new stimuli.

> ### CASE STUDY 13-1 Theresa
>
> Theresa is a highly active, inquisitive 8-year-old who likes to move around and interact with others and dislikes sedentary activities. Although her mood is generally happy, Theresa's emotional responses are intense, and she expresses her feelings loudly. Theresa's temperament is a good fit for running with her friends on the playground, and her peers regard her as someone who is exciting and fun to be with. Theresa's temperament is not such a good fit when she attends church services with her family; they often scold and correct Theresa for looking around, moving, and talking.

This child is calm, expressive, malleable, and has a generally low to moderate activity level. Children characterized as easy tend to adapt effectively to changing situations and demands. The *difficult* child is at the opposite end of the temperament spectrum. Characteristics that characterize this style are a negative mood and approach, slow adaptability, a high activity level, and high emotional intensity. Extremes of sensory threshold often occur among children with a difficult temperament pattern. A *slow-to-warm-up* child demonstrates mild-intensity negative reactions to new stimuli in combination with slow adaptation. These children require repeated exposures to new environments before they feel comfortable. Once a slow-to-warm-up child has established a routine, he or she usually functions well, but transitions are often problematic for children of this temperament type. Research has linked various temperament characteristics to parental stress in child-rearing,[34] certain psychiatric disorders in adulthood,[87,129] adolescent substance abuse,[179] and disruptive behavioral disorders.[68] A growing body of research supports the notion that temperament, although inborn, is not unchanging across a child's lifespan. Experiences and environmental circumstances such as the interpersonal styles of the primary caregivers have been assessed as having potentially significant influence on the developing child's temperament style.[17] These findings suggest that therapeutic intervention can be helpful in situations lacking goodness of fit between child and caregiver.

Occupational therapists often see children who are in distress and whose behavior is disruptive or upsetting to the family. Practitioners can help parents, caregivers, teachers, and children to explore and understand their temperaments and learn to predict when behavior may not match environmental demands (e.g., a very active child at the theater, a slow-to-warm-up child beginning a new school year). This perspective may decrease frustration and increase the possibility of organizing environments and activity demands to promote goodness of fit and successful occupational engagement.

ATTACHMENT: A DYNAMIC INTERACTION OF BIOLOGY AND ENVIRONMENT

A child's neuromaturational progress greatly influences social participation. The healthy, full-term infant is biologically prepared to participate in interactions with a nurturing and consistent caregiver, resulting in a loving attachment that is

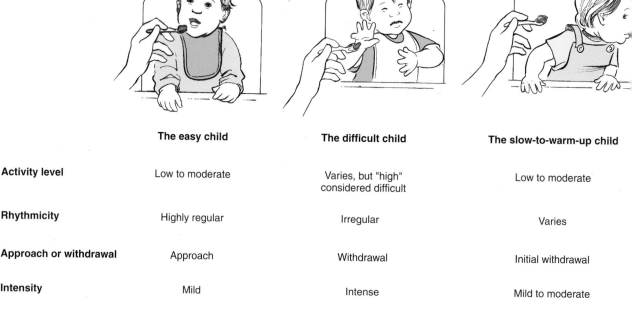

	The easy child	The difficult child	The slow-to-warm-up child
Activity level	Low to moderate	Varies, but "high" considered difficult	Low to moderate
Rhythmicity	Highly regular	Irregular	Varies
Approach or withdrawal	Approach	Withdrawal	Initial withdrawal
Intensity	Mild	Intense	Mild to moderate
Sensory threshold	Moderate	Extreme, high or low	Moderate
Mood	Pleasant	Unpleasant	Varies, but not extreme
Adaptability	Easily adapts	Slow to adapt	Slow to adapt
Distractibility	Varies	Varies	Varies
Attention span and persistence	Varies	Extreme, high or low	Varies

FIGURE 13-1 Temperament types: easy, difficult, and slow-to-warm up child.

essential for healthy development.[11] As the infant nurses, cuddles, gazes with fascination at her mother's face, and responds to comforting, emotions result that will become the foundation of the baby's self-concept and a safe base from which to explore the world.[159] Simultaneously, the mother experiences hormonal and neurochemical effects from interacting with her infant that promote feelings of well-being, protectiveness, and love for her baby.[77] Healthy attachment occurs when the caregiver and infant consistently interrelate in such a way that the infant develops confidence that the needs will be met and that he is safe and cared for.[16,116] Many experts contend that the quality of early attachment influences the capacity to form relationships later in life.[55,73,178] Some researchers are studying the influence of early attachment experience on neurodevelopment itself at the biochemical and cellular levels.[58,101,115] Thompson asserts that the quality of early relationships is "far more significant on early learning than are educational toys, preschool curricula, or Mozart CDs" (p. 11).[159]

Traits and behaviors of the parent and the child interact dynamically within environmental contexts to determine the quality of attachment that develops; each party is simultaneously influencing and influenced by the other and by other features of the environment.[60] Researchers have identified four patterns of attachment behavior between parents and infants: secure, avoidant, resistant or ambivalent, and disorganized/disoriented.[2,...] These are illustrated in Table 13-1.

Parent-child attachment relationships continuously chang in relation to the child's and the parent's stages of develop ment and changing environmental circumstances.[144] As th infant becomes mobile and then develops language and se care skills, the caregiving style of the parent adjusts accor ingly, and the attachment relationship is altered. Attachme patterns may also be influenced by environmental factors su as the loss or addition of family members. Adjustments attachment continue throughout the child's development course, and in the best circumstances the positive reciproc initiated early in infancy will be maintained throughout.

Understanding that patterns of attachment between chi dren and their parents can change implies that attachment a process that can be influenced.[11] This notion is support by research with high-risk infants and mothers who receive intervention to promote healthy attachment through thre home visits focused on teaching mothers how to observe ar respond effectively to their infants' behaviors.[168] The grou of 50 receiving the training developed significantly mo secure attachments than did those in the control group. The

TABLE 13-1 Patterns of Attachment in Infants and Parents

Attachment Style	Characteristic Caregiver Behavior	Characteristic Infant Behavior
Secure	Emotionally available, responsive to infant's emotional and physical needs in a timely, consistent, and effective manner	Seeks proximity to parent, but as mobility develops explores the immediate environment; demonstrates mastery motivation and self-confidence; misses parent on separation, but easily comforted on parent's return
Avoidant	Emotionally unavailable, typically not adequately responsive to infant's communications of need	Avoids parent; emotionally blunted; interacts with objects in the environment rather than with the parent
Resistant or ambivalent	Inconsistently available and responsive to infant's communications of need; caregiving style is determined by parent's moods and is an unpredictable combination of adequate and inadequate responses	Is clingy and preoccupied with the parent; does not actively explore the environment; is difficult to comfort after separation; mood may be angry or passive
Disorganized/ disoriented	Highly anxious or threatening toward the child; does not respond effectively or appropriately to infant's communications; may be abusive or psychotic	Is disorganized or disoriented when interacting with the parent; displays approach-avoidance behaviors including staring and "freezing," clinging, or huddling on the floor

effects from interventions to promote attachment have been found in other studies as well.[40,169]

Many infants, children, and adolescents served by occupational therapists have neurodevelopmental problems. Children who have intrinsic difficulty with receptive and/or expressive communication, sensory processing, or motor performance have a different social experience than do those who are developing typically.[142] Difficulty with feeding, an inability to establish regular patterns of activity and sleep throughout the day and night, resistance to cuddling, and other behaviors common to infants with neurologic dysfunction are incompatible with easy attachment, and may place the process at risk. Environmental factors such as a parent's long hours of work can limit the time available for child-focused interaction, potentially interfering with the attachment process. Likewise, a parent whose behavior is anxious, irritable, emotionally disengaged, or who has difficulty interpreting and responding to the child's communications cannot fully participate in reciprocal interaction. When such behaviors are frequent, attachment is at risk. Occupational therapists can support healthy interaction between caregivers and children by understanding this essential process, educating parents about their child's development and communication style, and helping them to generate solutions for problems that inhibit strong attachment formation. They can help families identify causes of stress in their daily and weekly routines and structure solutions to address them. These could involve prioritizing goals, working together to get tasks completed more efficiently, and making mindful choices about how to use time to improve quality of life and family relationships.

CHILD ABUSE AND NEGLECT: PROBLEMS WITH THE PARENT-CHILD RELATIONSHIP AND ENVIRONMENT

At its most extreme, inadequate attachment formation between a parent and a child can be a factor in the abuse or neglect of the child. This is a common problem for children and families, affecting at least 905,000 American children in 2006.[166]

Nearly 8% of the victims of child abuse or neglect had diagnosed disabilities. The Federal Child Abuse Prevention and Treatment Act (CAPTA), (42 U.S.C.A. §5106g), as amended by the Keeping Children and Families Safe Act of 2003, defines child abuse and neglect as follows:

- Any recent act or failure to act on the part of a parent or caretaker which results in death, serious physical or emotional harm, sexual abuse or exploitation; or
- An act or failure to act which presents an imminent risk of serious harm.

Child abuse has been categorized as neglect, physical abuse, sexual abuse, medical neglect, or "other" maltreatment; the various forms of child abuse may occur in combination.

- *Neglect* is defined as the withholding of nutrition, shelter, clothing, medical care, such that the child's health is endangered. Undersupervision and abandonment are included in this category. This is the most common form of child abuse, accounting for about 64% of reported cases.
- *Physical abuse* affects about 16% of victims. This type of abuse includes punching, shaking, kicking, biting, throwing, burning, and other forms of injurious punishment.
- *Sexual abuse* is estimated to occur at a rate of about 9% and includes any seduction, coercion, or forcing of a child to observe or participate in sexual activity for the sexual gratification of a more powerful individual.
- *Medical neglect* is a failure by the caregiver to provide for the appropriate health care of the child although financially able to do so, or offered financial or other means to do so. This kind of maltreatment affects 2% of the reported cases.
- *"Other"* types of maltreatment constitute 15% of the reported cases. These include emotional abuse, such as the withholding of affection, chronic humiliation, threatening harm to the child or those he or she cares about, and criticism. Abandonment and congenital drug addiction also fall under this reporting category.[166]

Developmental and psychological outcomes that have been associated with childhood abuse include traumatic brain injury, depression, substance abuse, posttraumatic stress disorder, learning disorders, conduct disorders, and personality disorders.[9,22,53,78,83,85,103] These problems can have long-term occupational consequences, including the increased risk of involvement in violent and nonviolent crime and of not completing high school.[104] Most tragically, approximately 1530 children died from the effects of abuse or neglect in 2006.[166] Clearly, such pathology is incompatible with healthy family functioning.

Attachment patterns between parents and children are the result of a dynamic interaction of factors related to the child, the parent, and the environment. Risk factors for child abuse and neglect have been identified in these three arenas (Table 13-2). No single factor is consistently associated with child abuse. The more risk factors present and the more severe each of these is, the higher the risk of abuse and neglect within a family.

A child's level of risk decreases with age, with infants suffering the highest rate of abuse.[166] Disability increases the risk of child maltreatment. The incidence of abuse and neglect may be as high as 3.4 times greater for children with disabilities than for those without.[157] Disabilities that have been associated with an increased risk of maltreatment include behavioral disorders, communication disorders, cognitive disabilities, physical impairments, and craniofacial anomalies.[46,84,157,173,176] Any condition that prolongs a child's dependency or stimulates parental rejection adds to the risk of abuse or neglect. For example, having a "difficult" temperament or being born prematurely increases risk.[59,153] Most of the young clients seen by occupational therapy practitioners have delayed development in one or more areas and are, as a group, at increased risk for abuse and neglect.

Environmental factors interact dynamically with features of the child to affect the levels of risk for abuse and neglect. Certain qualities of the parents (particularly the mother, who is usually the primary caretaker) have been identified as risk factors. These include having a personality that is characterized by immaturity, a history of having been abused, egocentrism, impulsivity, and alcohol or drug abuse.[131,149,184] Characteristics of the larger community may further contribute to environmental risk factors. Poverty has been shown to correlate positively with increased rates of child abuse and neglect.[44,150] Social isolation is a powerful risk factor, placing children in single-parent families at significantly higher risk for abuse than those in two-parent families.[82] Communities with high crime rates present a combination of a cultural acceptance of aggressive behavior, high levels of economic distress, and the social isolation that results when residents are fearful to step out onto the street.

Although poverty and a parent's troubled background may increase the likelihood of child abuse, high levels of social integration and community morale appear to be mediating factors that can reduce its incidence.[61] Successful intervention and prevention programs address family and community needs for safe and enjoyable places to gather and engage in meaningful occupation.[174] A meta-analysis of abuse prevention and family wellness programs indicated that the most effective programs supported parents by using a strengths-based, empowerment approach. Successful programs continued over 6 months and provided at least two sessions per month.[113] Occupational therapists have opportunities to intervene with individuals and families through direct service, program development, consultation, and administrative roles.

Children who are experiencing physical abuse and/or neglect may bear outward signs of this, and therapists should always observe for bruises, cuts, or other injuries, or behaviors that may reflect pain. The appropriateness of the child's clothing for weather conditions and fit should be noted over time. This is not to assess fashionableness but adequacy. The occupational therapist asks the child about his or her eating and sleeping habits and activities through the day when at home, asks about how the adults at home respond to children's misbehavior (e.g., "What kinds of things do you do that get you in trouble sometimes?" "What happens then?") Given gentle encouragement, some children will describe inadequate or unsafe situations. School-based personnel should observe what the child has brought for lunch or how the child responds to food that is offered; a child with too little to eat at home

TABLE 13-2 Risk Factors for Child Abuse

Factors	Examples
Physical and Emotional Abuse	
Parent factors	Youth/immaturity
	Substance abuse
	Low empathy
	Difficulty interpreting child's communications
	Impulsiveness
	Limited coping skills
	Lack of knowledge about child development
	Unrealistic expectations
	Emotionally needy
	History of abuse
	Disappointment in child's gender or appearance
Child factors	Prolonged dependency for developmental or medical reasons
	"Difficult" temperament
	High activity level
	Limited skill at interpreting parent's nonverbal communications
	Appearance is displeasing to the parent
Environmental factors	Social isolation, lack of support
	Culture that condones or encourages aggression/abuse
	Poverty
Child Neglect	
Parent factors	Depression or other mental disorders
	Cognitive limitations
	Substance abuse
	History of extreme deprivation
Child factors	Prolonged dependency for developmental or medical reasons
Environmental factors	Social isolation, lack of support
	Poverty
	Family disorganization

may hoard food or eat more than is typical. Socially, children from abusive homes may behave in a variety of ways that reflect individual temperaments and coping styles. Behaviors may range from being withdrawn and guarded to acting intrusive and demanding. Often children who have been abused are themselves aggressive, but this is not universal.[97] Many abused children are socially immature and emotionally needy. The description of resistant/ambivalent and disorganized/disoriented attachment styles also fits many of these children.

Occupational therapy practitioners are mandated by federal law to report suspected cases of abuse and neglect to state child protective services agencies.[36] Reports of suspected child abuse or neglect may be made by telephone and should be followed with a letter documenting the child's demographic information, specific observations leading to the report, and the practitioner's contact information. Referrals to child protective services are held in confidence, and persons who submit referrals in good faith are protected by law from prosecution. Statutes and information about reporting abuse or neglect for each state are available on the child welfare policy website (http://www.childwelfare.gov/systemwide/laws_policies/state/). Discovery of a practitioner's failure to report suspected cases of abuse or neglect may result in prosecution and/or disciplinary action by the practitioner's licensing board or in the civil courts.

Referrals to child protective services are reviewed and classified according to the situational risk. Families who are evaluated often receive a variety of intervention services, including respite care, parenting education, assistance with housing, day care, home visits, individual and family counseling, substance abuse treatment, and transportation. Fewer than 20% of the children whose families are investigated for abuse and neglect are taken into protective foster care.[166]

ENVIRONMENTAL FACTORS AND SOCIAL PARTICIPATION

Social participation can only be fully experienced when children and families live within supportive environments that provide opportunities for self-expression and connection with others. When these conditions are unmet, even for a limited time, occupational performance suffers. When conditions are less than adequate for prolonged periods, the child's very course of development may be altered, with lifelong effects. Assessing the nature of a child's environment is a critical stage of clinical reasoning when trying to determine the psychosocial contributors to occupational dysfunction.

Environmental factors that relate to psychosocial performance may be roughly divided into those that are relatively brief and those that are more long-term (Box 13-1). Time-limited events include personal and family stressors that are keenly experienced and then resolved over a period of weeks or months. Long-term events or situations are those in which the stressors are pervasive and continue for months or years. These categories are further described in the next sections. Although they are useful for general conceptual purposes, they should be applied with caution. Whether an event or circumstance falls into one category or another is partially dependent on the coping style and circumstances of the individual affected. For example, the death of a grandparent may be an

---

BOX 13-1 Environmental Stress and Its Effects on Children

TIME-LIMITED ENVIRONMENTAL STRESS FACTORS*
Changing schools or child care providers
Illness of an immediate family member
Death of a family member or friend
Temporary financial crisis
Family relocation
Temporary marital distress of parents
Divorce with closure

LONG-TERM ENVIRONMENTAL STRESS FACTORS*
Violence in the home or neighborhood
Chronic illness of a parent
Death of a parent
Chronic poverty
Long-term homelessness
Chronic parental conflict
Societal discrimination/prejudice

*These categorizations are general examples. Whether a stress is experienced in a time-limited or chronic fashion is ultimately dependent on multiple individual and environmental factors.

---

event that a child feels acutely sad about for several weeks and then adjusts to, especially if the relationship was limited by distance or other factors. For a child who is very sensitive, or for whom the grandparent was a primary caregiver, such a loss could result in months of grief. If the child did not know the grandparent at all, the loss may be irrelevant.

Time-Limited Environmental Stress and Its Impact on Occupational Performance

Short-acting environmental conditions such as the death of an extended family member or friend, temporary marital crises, a change of school or day care, or a family relocation, can have significant effects on the child's social participation. A survey of 56 school-based occupational therapists indicated that many of the students with whom they worked experienced such loss and grief in their lives and that their behavior reflected this.[123] Children's reactions to such events often include decreased performance in play or academic activities. The child may act preoccupied, fatigued, or uninterested in usual pastimes. Sometimes children temporarily "lose" their skills in self-care and revert to more dependent, infantile ways.[182] They may become emotionally overreactive and engage in provocative behavior such as fighting or disobeying adults' directives.[125] Occupational therapists can help children and adolescents to cope with times of increased stress through establishing a therapeutic relationship, asking about how the child is feeling and the events that are occurring in their lives, providing opportunities for self-expression through activities, and communicating with the rest of the team to ensure the best possible communication and support throughout the child's day. Educating the child, family, and others who are in contact with the child regarding typical grief reactions and ways to respond to these can also facilitate the child's passage through difficult experiences (Case Study 13-2).

CASE STUDY 13-2   Brooke

Brooke is a 3-year-old girl who has been receiving occupational therapy services for developmental dyspraxia. One month ago Brooke's mother gave birth to Ryan. Initially Brooke responded to this event with positive excitement and continually begged to hold and help care for her brother. However, during the past week she has been talking "baby talk," resisting bedtime, and even wet her pants on two occasions, with no visible embarrassment or remorse. Brooke's parents are understandably concerned, and they are wondering what to do. They tried telling her to "talk like a big girl" and ignored her when she used infantile language. They have been irritable and exasperated at bedtime, as both parents are exhausted from getting up at night with the baby. Now that she has wet her pants, they are fearful that Brooke may have a "major psychological problem." The occupational therapist, who has been working with Brooke and her family for several months, responds, "You all have your hands full, with the changes and demands of a new baby in the family! I can see that everyone is working to capacity to cope, including Brooke. She is showing her stress the way 3-year-olds do. She has regressed in her development in some ways; the way she talks, needing lots of extra support at bedtime, and not using the potty all of the time. The good news is that these behaviors are very normal for preschoolers who are stressed, and they are temporary. As the family finds its new routines, so should Brooke. The challenging news is that Brooke probably really does need extra attention right now, just when time and energy are so stretched. Let's try to think creatively about who might be able to pitch in, to provide Brooke with some extra attention. Perhaps her aunt or grandpa could take her to the zoo or to make cookies? Also, if someone can take over little Ryan's care for short periods, you will be able to give Brooke the special time with you that she so needs. There are some wonderful children's books that explore how it feels to become an older sister or brother; reading one of these with Brooke may give her some emotional relief. Looking at videos or photos of Brooke's infant years and reminiscing with her about what a cute and cared-for baby she was (and what an adorable 3-year-old she is now) may also provide her some reassurance as to her position in the family. Taking a nap cuddled up together might be restorative to both of you. You will know what methods work for her when she requests to repeat them! I think that by meeting some of her extra needs now, you can hasten Brooke's return to her 3-year-old self. What are your thoughts?"

Chronic Environmental Stress and Its Impact on Occupational Performance

Long-term sources of social stress are circumstances and events that do not resolve over the course of weeks or months (see Box 13-1). Examples of these are poverty, social discrimination, and severe family dysfunction that may occur when one or both parents suffer from substance abuse or other mental disorders. These kinds of environmental conditions may have long-term effects on children's development and social participation through the lifespan, especially if combined with other complications such as the child's own neurodevelopmental problems.

More than 17% of children in the United States live in poverty. Of the children aged 18 and younger living in poverty, approximately 24% are black, 21% are Hispanic, 10% are white, and 10% are Asian.[164] Long-term poverty has been associated with a number of serious problems for children and adolescents and for the adults who care for them.[32,42] Having a low income and living in a crime-ridden environment have been shown to correlate with increased risk of having newborns born prematurely or with low birth weight, both of which increase the risk for subsequent developmental and health problems.[120]

The home environments of families with few resources may offer limited access to items that are considered to be "necessities" by a majority of members of the culture, such as books, toys, a telephone, television, or computer. The language opportunities in low-income homes are often different and reduced when compared with those found in middle-class homes (Case Study 13-3).[108] Due to a combination of health and environmental factors, children who live in chronic economic deprivation are at increased risk for having lower cognitive abilities and more behavioral problems.[18,42] Parents who experience the stress of chronically worrying about meeting basic needs for food, shelter, and safety are more prone to discipline their children harshly, have marital conflicts, experience depression, and have substance abuse problems.[15,42,86,121] They may be too overwhelmed, discouraged, or disorganized to become involved in their children's schooling. These conditions place many low-income students at a disadvantage and diminish their future opportunities. Some children who have experienced lifetimes of severe family and community dysfunction reach adolescence feeling hopeless about their futures. Their occupational performance is clearly affected by this as they struggle with society's expectations to further their education in order to prepare for a productive adulthood, while from the discouraged adolescent's perspective this is impossible to achieve.

Case Study 13-3 illustrates how poverty and other chronic stress factors can affect a child's occupational performance, both in terms of the preparation for and availability of opportunities to achieve social participation. Although environmental factors are clearly influential in determining a child's occupational performance, the PEO model reflects a balance of emphasis among its three components.[106] Each individual has capacities and desires that strongly influence occupational expression. The following section provides information regarding the role that mental functioning plays in the enactment and development of children's occupational performance.

MENTAL HEALTH FACTORS AFFECTING SOCIAL PARTICIPATION

Children's developmental progress and occupational performance depend as much on how well their psychosocial needs are being met as they do on the adequacy of the nutrition and

Marcus is a 15-year-old boy who is a ninth-grade student in a large public high school. Marcus's family has struggled with poverty for many generations. He lives in a neighborhood where he has observed drug-related activities, fighting, and adults' sexual behavior on a regular basis. His favorite uncle was killed in a knife fight last year. Marcus's cousin, a rising-star basketball player, was permanently disabled in a shooting. Last week one of his teachers quit her job after being mugged in her classroom. Marcus's mother has a 10th-grade education and four children, whom she is raising independently. She has a day job as a hotel maid and a night job as a cashier in a convenience store. She is chronically exhausted and irritable. She encourages all of her children to work hard in school so they can have a better life than hers. Marcus is also exhausted. He tries to go to school and

to do what he can to help his mother, but he sees no real way out of their current situation. The bills are always greater than the family's resources. In Marcus's environment it seems that no matter how hard people try they never seem to get ahead, and often they do not even survive. The teachers at school seem critical and uncaring, and Marcus is made anxious by their questions and reprimands. Schoolwork is difficult, boring, and unrelated to his real concerns. When he was a child, Marcus wanted to be a professional football player or a doctor when he grew up. Now he is convinced that these were childish, impossible dreams, but he has no new plans with which to replace them. He is on the verge of quitting school and has no job skills. His likelihood of eventually achieving a satisfying career and contributing positively to the community is extremely small.

shelter they receive. In 1999, Dr. David Satcher, Surgeon General of the United States Public Health Service, supervised the publication of the results of a multiagency effort sharing the expertise of hundreds of service providers, researchers, and consumers. The Surgeon General's Report on Mental Health states: "From early childhood until death, mental health is the springboard of thinking and communication skills, learning, emotional growth, resilience, and self-esteem. These are the ingredients of each individual's successful contribution to community and society" (Chapter 1, Introduction & Themes).[167]

A fixed definition of mental health is difficult to formulate; behaviors and beliefs that are construed as "healthy" by one individual in a particular context may be considered to be inappropriate or unhealthy by someone else or in another context. The Surgeon General's definition of mental health suggests cultural variables influence what behaviors are expected and, therefore, how mental health is defined: "Mental health is a state of successful performance of mental function, resulting in productive activities, fulfilling relationships with other people, and the ability to adapt to change and to cope with adversity. Mental health is indispensable to personal well-being, family and interpersonal relationships, and contribution to community or society."[167] For example, American parents of Northern European descent often value independence and achievement. Such parents might be concerned about the behavior of their five-year-old son, who wants his mother to help him with dressing and bathing, even though he can do these things for himself. This behavior might cause them to wonder if their child is immature or "spoiled." Parents from a cultural background that promotes a climate of interdependence, such as that found in Japan, might expect such behavior and find it quite acceptable. It is clear that practitioners must be competent in assuming a multicultural approach in order to effectively evaluate social and emotional behavior.

Children and adolescents' ability to participate socially and academically may be severely impaired by poor mental health. It is estimated that nearly 13% of children have mental or emotional problems, and 32.8% have mental and emotional problems along with other types of functional disorders.[82] It is thought that increasing numbers of children are being diagnosed with mental disorders as a result of combination of

increasingly sensitive diagnostics and contributing social pressures and problems.[37,71,140,184] Effective interventions for these types of conditions typically require a combination of family education, special services at school, various therapies for the child and family, and, often, medication.

Occupational therapists approach their work with a client-centered, occupational performance—rather than a medical or pathology-focused—perspective.[26,106] However, client-centered approaches do not preclude understanding the nature and course of a client's illness or disability. To develop and implement client-centered, contextually appropriate intervention, the child's symptoms, medication effects and side effects, and prognosis must be understood. Additionally, practitioners who recognize the diagnostic hallmarks of mental disorders that occur in childhood and adolescence can play an important role in referring children and adolescents in need of a diagnostic evaluation to specialists such as psychologists or psychiatrists. In many settings the occupational therapist may be the only team member who understands the symptoms and various interventions for mental disorders and their implications for occupational performance in school, child care, and at home. The following section presents an overview of selected mental disorders that can affect children and their implications for occupational performance. It is not unusual for individuals to experience multiple disorders simultaneously, such as depression and anxiety, Asperger's syndrome and depression, or cognitive impairment and attention deficit disorder.[6] A common criterion for all diagnoses of mental disorder is that the individual's daily life and activities are significantly impaired by the symptoms.[6]

SELECTED MENTAL DISORDERS COMMONLY AFFECTING CHILDREN AND ADOLESCENTS

Mood Disorders

Mood disorders involve long-term changes in the child's prevailing emotions. The presence of symptoms may be cyclic, increasing and decreasing periodically, but they may last for months or years if untreated.[6,99] The diagnostic criteria for *major depression* stipulates that symptoms must have reached a level of severity that results in changes in occupational performance or significant distress during daily activities.[6] Depression manifests as persistent or repeated episodes of a combination of irritability, loss of interest in and enjoyment of usual activities, increased or decreased activity level, sadness, periods of crying, decreased energy, inability to concentrate and learn, agitation, sleep and/or appetite disturbance, anxiety, guilt, and/or thoughts of death or suicide. Depression is estimated to occur in 3% of children and 8% of teens.[124] Children and adolescents who have experienced clinical depression are at increased risk to have repeated episodes into adulthood.[6,69,100] The diagnostic evaluation of depression should be made by a psychologist or psychiatrist through structured interviews with the child and parents.[124,146] Ascertaining a diagnosis in children may be complicated because the outward symptoms may appear inconsistently; the child may play and seem happy some of the time. Intervention often includes a combination of medications and psychotherapy or counseling parents.[124,146] Brief hospitalization may be required if there is risk of suicide.

Occupational performance and satisfaction are adversely affected by the symptoms of depression. Difficulty with thinking and the loss of enjoyment and interest reduce the child's motivation to play and decrease ability to attend and learn in school. Children with depression may sleep during the day, even in classes, and often experience aches and pains. They often complain of being tired or bored during previously preferred activities. Activity levels may be decreased or increased, so the child may be chastised for being "lazy" or "out of control," depending on the situation. Unexpected tearfulness or displays of temper place the child in social jeopardy with adults and peers. Changes in appetite may affect social interactions during meals, as the child is scolded for eating too little or too much. There may be resistance to attending family, church, and other social activities. Among the most occupationally debilitating aspects of depression are the child's feelings of incompetence, hopelessness, and helplessness. These emotions, however irrational, are symptoms of depression that can prevent children and adolescents from participating in activities that involve any risk of failure or humiliation: deciding which answer to choose on a test, raising one's hand in class, inviting a peer to play, or joining in a game. Adolescents with depression must add the anxiety and self-doubt of depression to the feelings of self-consciousness typically experienced at this phase of life. Depression increases the risk of alcohol and drug use, as sufferers seek relief from emotions that are overwhelmingly painful.[6,112]

Bipolar disorder, or manic-depressive illness, is increasingly being recognized as a condition that often emerges during childhood or adolescence.[25,72] Individuals with bipolar disorder experience "mania," or periods of extreme overactivity, agitation, irritability, rapid ("pressured") speech, and reduced periods of sleep.[6] Less often, children and adolescents may display elation, giddiness, or grandiosity.[19,88] Episodes of mania are juxtaposed by periods of typical or depressed mood. These mood states may fluctuate quite rapidly, sometimes even presenting as mixed states, or can alternate over a period of weeks or months.[6,25] Sometimes a child's changes in mood may be difficult to distinguish from voluntary behaviors aimed at provoking or controlling others.[88] Mania in children may be misdiagnosed as attention deficit disorder, oppositional defiant disorder, or temporal lobe epilepsy.[72] During manic phases some people have confused and bizarre thinking that may involve feelings of omnipotence, euphoria, and/or hallucinations. Children and adolescents with bipolar disorder are prone to episodes of aggression and despair and may pose a danger to themselves or others.[72] Approximately 10% to 12% of adolescents with recurrent episodes of major depression will develop bipolar disorder.[6] Individuals with bipolar disorder are at increased risk for suicide, especially during transitions from a manic to depressed mood state. A diagnostic evaluation should be completed by a psychologist or psychiatrist specializing in the care of children and adolescents, using structured interviews with the child and parents and direct behavioral observation. Intervention often includes medication, psychotherapy or counseling, and client/family education.[72,88,146]

Children and adolescents who have bipolar disorder may have periods of time when their behavior is noticeably "out of character" or socially inappropriate, or they may seem consistently irritable and active.[19] Behaviors that are commonly experienced during low levels of mania include continuously talking, attention-seeking, disregard for others' feelings or social norms, abruptly changing emotions, and impulsiveness. The child may resist adults' attempts at guidance or correction or correct him and may act "bossy" toward adults. There may be aggressive outbursts toward property, other children, adults, or himself or herself. These behaviors are not compatible with performance as a student and may occur sometimes even if the child is taking medication. It is important that the adults who regularly interact with a child who has recurring symptoms of bipolar disorder know that these behaviors may not always be under the child's control and have plans in place to respond effectively, avoiding behavioral outbursts that are disruptive or dangerous. Occupational therapy should include helping the child adopt regular sleeping habits, learn about the illness, engage in effective stress management strategies, and learn ways to communicate well with others. All team members should participate in monitoring the child's behavior as it relates to medication effects. Some of the most effective medications used to treat bipolar disorder can cause life-threatening side effects if the child becomes dehydrated or the timing of dosage is incorrect.[25]

Anxiety Disorders

Anxiety disorders are characterized by pervasive and persistent (longer than 6 months) feelings of uneasiness, fearfulness, or dread that are not founded on realistic concerns.[6] Estimated to occur in 4% to 13% of children, anxiety is a relatively common problem that is thought to result from a combination of inborn/genetic traits and environmental factors.[25] The diagnosis of an anxiety disorder is made by a psychiatrist or psychologist through observation, interviews with the child and family, and self-report questionnaires.[145] Symptoms of anxiety and depression often occur together, and medications and psychotherapy may be combined to address both kinds of problems.[25,88] Subclinical levels of anxiety may also have a negative impact on children's occupational performance and social participation and should receive attention by occupational therapists and others who work with children in schools and other settings.

Social anxiety disorder is estimated to affect up to 11% of all children and adolescents.[38] Characteristic symptoms include excessive worrying about others' evaluations of oneself or about one's past and future behavior. Those affected exhibit considerable self-consciousness and a high need for reassurance by others.[6,70,107] Children and adolescents who have social anxiety may be unable to participate in many of the activities in which they would like, or are expected, to engage.[13,151] Any time the child feels he is at risk of criticism or embarrassment, he may become overwhelmed by automatic reactions such as a racing heart, blushing, feeling out of breath, and perspiring. Thinking is derailed by emotions of fear or even panic. The anxious child's behavioral reactions to these overwhelming emotions (e.g., crying, resisting an activity, having a tantrum) may draw critical attention from others, further increasing social anxiety. Acute anxiety reactions can occur in an array of daily situations, such as being called on to perform in class, taking a piano lesson, walking into church, or learning to drive a car. Such experiences are subjectively unpleasant and may cause embarrassment due to others' real or imagined reactions. Children and adolescents who have symptoms of social anxiety avoid and miss out on participating in many required and cherished activities.[45]

Obsessive-compulsive disorder (OCD), another subset of the anxiety disorders, is characterized by intrusive thoughts and repetitive behaviors that have little or no functional purpose beyond decreasing tension.[6] OCD has been measured as affecting relatively few children and adolescents (fewer than 1%), but is thought by some experts to be underreported, as its expression is often confined to the home.[63] Symptoms of obsessive-compulsive disorder may occur consistently or episodically, but they tend to be durable over many years, and are exacerbated by stress.[160] OCD typically emerges between the ages of 6 to 15 years in males and 20 to 29 years in females.[6]

Children and adolescents with OCD may spend many hours per day engaging in behaviors such as hand washing, counting objects, arranging objects in a particular way, checking on the status of something (such as whether an appliance is unplugged), or cleaning. These behaviors may be visible to the casual observer or performed surreptitiously. In either case, if the repetitive activity is interrupted or prevented, the affected individual experiences anxiety. Intervention typically includes medication, client and family education, and cognitive behavioral therapy.[25,63] Children and adolescents with neurologic impairments such as learning disabilities, Tourette's syndrome, and autistic spectrum disorders are at increased risk of also having OCD.[63,145]

The daily balance of activity is negatively affected by the amount of time spent on obsessive-compulsive rituals in children and adolescents with this disorder. Tasks that would ordinarily take minutes may require hours as the child restarts the process again and again. Task interruption may occur as he or she stops to readjust unrelated objects or to wash hands repeatedly. Studying, packing a book bag, bathing, using the toilet, and getting dressed are just some examples of activities that could be severely affected by obsessive-compulsive symptoms. The child or adolescent with OCD also suffers socially, because even though he may know that his repetitive actions are irrational and, by others' standards, "weird," he feels compelled to continue doing them. It becomes easier to spend time alone and at home, rather than to cope with others' reactions and misunderstanding. Occupational therapists can support team interventions by helping affected children and adolescents to understand the nature of this neurologically based disorder, teaching stress management skills, and helping them identify and reduce exposure to environmental triggers that stimulate obsessive thoughts.

Attention Deficit Disorder

Attention deficit disorder is characterized by significant difficulty with selective and/or sustained attention to tasks; this central problem may be accompanied by difficulties with overactivity and/or impulsivity. Attention deficit disorders are estimated to affect 8% of children and adolescents, with more boys than girls represented.[6] A diagnosis is made through structured observations in a variety of settings and across time. Intervention often includes a combination of medication, behavior management, client education, support, and environmental adaptation.[185]

Children and adolescents with attention deficit disorder may have difficulty performing tasks in environments that are moderately or highly stimulating, such as the typical classroom or household. When trying to engage in activities, the child may have to work at continuously redirecting her attention from extraneous sounds and sights and back to the targeted task. Reading comprehension and listening skills are often affected. Impulsiveness may result in acting before thinking, leading to errors on schoolwork or inappropriate social behavior. Adolescents with attention deficit disorder may have difficulty following through on commitments due to disorganization and forgetfulness. They are less able to organize their time and materials than most of their peers. They may have difficulty sustaining effort on tasks, quickly become "bored" and leave tasks unfinished.

Occupational therapy for children with attention deficits should address the personal, environmental, and occupational factors. Children and teens can be taught to understand that they have a neurologically based problem. They can then learn ways to manage this through adherence to medication routines and attending and responding to their sensory and emotional states. Framing the child's difficulty as a set of solvable problems, rather than as deliberate misbehavior, can help all parties feel better and behave more productively. Teachers, parents, and clients can learn ways to create and maintain physical environments that minimize auditory and visual distractions during tasks that require concentration and to modify tasks to allow well-timed breaks and opportunities for feedback. All involved parties can learn to structure and support a well-regulated routine of daily activities, with established and balanced patterns of sleeping, eating, work, and play.

Disruptive Behavior Disorders

Oppositional defiant disorder (ODD) is characterized by a well-established pattern of disobedience and hostility toward authority figures that lasts for over 6 months. Children who fit this diagnosis often have excessive displays of temper, are irritable, deliberately refuse to comply with rules and directives, blame others for their actions, and act vindictively.[6] They seek to provoke others by verbally threatening or insulting them. ODD is generally diagnosed by 8 years of age, and rarely after early adolescence; rates of its occurrence range from 2% to 16%.[6]

Conduct disorders are characterized by the many of the same behaviors as those seen in oppositional defiant disorder, but include more intrusive and severe forms of chronic misbehavior such as physical aggression toward property, animals, or people, theft, and/or lying. Environmental factors appear to play a large role in the development of disruptive behavior disorders; there is also evidence of genetic influence and a high rate of co-occurrence with neurologically based problems such as learning disabilities and attention deficit disorder.[38] Many children with a conduct disorder are also diagnosed as having depression and/or attention deficit disorder and may receive medication for these problems.

Disruptive behavior disorders affect up to 10% of children and adolescents and seriously impede participation in family, school, and community activities.[6,38] Conduct disorders place children at risk of harming others, breaking the law, and being placed in restrictive correctional or mental health facilities. Occupational therapists with clients who have disruptive behavior disorders are positioned to join a team effort to help children learn prosocial, adaptive ways to enjoy school, play, and rejuvenation. This begins with establishing a therapeutic alliance that includes well-understood and maintained expectations for positive behavior and reliable and fair consequences for behavioral infractions.[38] Therapy that promotes achievement of recognition and feelings of competence through engaging in valued activities provides children with alternatives to antisocial behavior and motivation to behave in ways that allow participation in the larger community. Teaching the child how to use anger and stress management techniques, social interaction skills, and conflict resolution skills can be part of the occupational therapy plan. Consultation with other team members may include helping teachers and parents identify educational and functional tasks that are motivating, highly structured, and provide the "just right" level of challenge for that particular child or adolescent.

Autism Spectrum Disorders

Autism spectrum disorders, which manifest within the first 3 years of life, are characterized by (1) abnormal ways of relating to people, objects, and events; (2) delayed or missing speech, language, and/or nonverbal communication skills; and (3) restricted, repetitive, and stereotyped patterns of behavior, interests, and/or activities.[6] Children with autism spectrum disorder exhibit a wide range of ability and variation in severity of symptoms. At one extreme, children have functional language and cognitive skills at levels that allow their participation in typical classrooms; children at the other end of the spectrum are functionally nonverbal and require continuous assistance and accommodation. Problems that may co-occur with autistic spectrum disorders include sensory processing dysfunction, cognitive impairment, anxiety, depression, hyperactivity, seizure disorder, fragile X syndrome, and tuberous sclerosis.[127] The diagnosis of autism spectrum disorder has increased over the past 20 years, spurring debate as to whether this marks an actual increase in the incidence of the disorders or an increased sensitivity in diagnosing new cases.[71] The number of special education students classified as having autism spectrum disorder increased by 189,000 between 1994 and 2006.[81] Current estimates indicate that approximately 1 in 150 children have an autism spectrum disorder.[31] This apparent increase has been attributed variously to a broadening of the diagnostic criteria, the advent of assessments that allow earlier diagnosis, and a possible increase in mistaking other language and cognitive disorders for autism.[71,146] Children with autistic spectrum disorders may grow up to achieve full independence and community participation in adulthood or may require assistance throughout their lives. An individual's long-term outcome is determined by a combination of factors, including the severity of the autistic disorder, cognitive ability, and social factors.[39]

Intervention for problems associated with autism spectrum disorders often includes behavioral methods, psychoeducational approaches, communication interventions, social skills training, and a variety of medications to address specific symptoms.[6,127,136,146] (See Chapter 14 for additional information on this topic.) There is a growing body of evidence linking autistic disorders and sensory processing dysfunction.[51,75] Occupational therapy may include sensory integration therapy, life skills training, and social skills training.[10,74,114] Clinical trials have demonstrated positive effects for most of these interventions; however, the evidence is limited (see Case-Smith & Arbesman's review of intervention applied by occupational therapists[29]). As with all interventions, families should be encouraged and supported in making a critical evaluation of the evidence to date before engaging in a particular intervention.[146]

The Occupational Therapist's Role Relative to Psychotropic Medication

All of the mental disorders described above may be treated with medications as a central or adjunctive intervention. Research evidence to date indicates that, just as for adults, a combination of medication and therapy is more effective than either approach alone for anxiety and attention deficit disorders.[64,92,98,136] The use of psychotropic medications among children and adolescents has increased significantly over the past 15 years.[64,132] Approximately 17% to 22% of all students receiving special education services use psychotropic medications; this includes 42% to 52% of students classified as having emotional disturbance.[130]

Many children who receive occupational therapy services take psychotropic or seizure medications. The medical management of such drugs is made challenging by the children's rapid growth and development, as well by as the lack of research to guide decision making.[64,88] Although occupational therapists do not administer medications, they should stay apprised of their clients' medications, and assume responsibility to be informed about the medications' expected effects, possible side effects, and precautions. As a general guideline, therapists should consistently observe their clients for positive changes and possible unwanted drug effects and report these to the prescribing physician and in the client's official record. Brown and colleagues have published a useful array of forms that can be used to systematically document behaviors and symptoms that reflect a child's responses to medication.[25] Any time a child displays an abrupt or marked change in his state of arousal (e.g., acts unusually drowsy or agitated), demonstrates signs of neurologic change (such as previously unobserved motor or cognitive difficulties), or complains of discomfort such as nausea or headaches, the possibility of medication side effects should be considered. If the observed symptoms are severe or of sudden onset, the situation should be treated as a medical emergency requiring the immediate notification of the child's parents and evaluation by a qualified medical practitioner, such as a physician or registered nurse. All such observations and referrals should be documented by the occupational therapy practitioner in a timely manner.

Children and adolescents with psychological and behavioral problems live, work, and play in an array of environments. Their problems and needs may become apparent in a variety of ways, depending on the context. The following section explores the wide range of possible settings in which occupational therapists work with children whose occupational performance is affected by psychosocial dysfunction and how occupational therapy may be practiced in each.

PRACTICE ENVIRONMENTS

This section describes ways in which occupational therapists provide psychosocial intervention in a representative selection of settings and to illustrate how occupational therapists apply holistic, client-centered approaches. A variety of treatment settings are described, representing a continuum from less to more psychiatrically oriented and from less to more intensive and restrictive. The mission, clientele, services, frames of reference, and staffing patterns for each type of facility, as well as traditional or potential roles for occupational therapists in each setting, are outlined. Case studies synthesized from the author's clinical experiences illustrate psychosocial intervention in a variety of traditional and nontraditional settings.

Therapeutic environments may include early childhood intervention programs, public schools, outpatient mental health services, day treatment programs, residential treatment centers, correctional facilities, and inpatient acute care hospitals. Some of these programs are designed specifically to assist children and adolescents who have identified mental health problems; other programs are oriented toward meeting more general developmental, educational, or social needs. Occupational therapists are established practitioners in some of these settings and are pioneers in other settings. In any case, pediatric occupational therapists have the knowledge base, the skills, and the opportunities to provide psychosocial intervention to children and adolescents with mental health and social problems in all service settings.

Early Childhood Intervention Programs

The primary mission of early childhood intervention (ECI) programs is the prevention and amelioration of developmental disabilities in children from birth to 3 years of age. According to the Individuals with Disabilities Act (IDEA), clients include infants and toddlers who are diagnosed as having developmental delay, those who are considered to be at risk for developmental problems, and their families. Although infants and toddlers are referred primarily to early intervention for evaluation and treatment of neurologic and physical conditions, children may be referred when their development is at risk because

of parental mental health problems, such as chemical dependency, domestic violence, parental depression, or other psychiatric disorders. Occasionally the identified infant may have a diagnosed mental disorder, such as failure to thrive or pervasive developmental disorder.[6]

Professionals working in ECI programs are likely to use developmental, neurodevelopmental, rehabilitative, behavioral, interactional, and familial systems as frames of reference (Table 13-3). Occupational therapists, educated to recognize and treat persons with mental illness, contribute significantly to the ECI team's effectiveness with high-risk families. For example, mothers who are experiencing anxiety or depression are often unable to meet their infant's needs for responsive interaction.[41,80,137] Parents who are addicted to drugs are at increased risk of neglecting or abusing their children.[149,184] Occupational therapists can observe clients for signs of problems such as depression and substance abuse and can facilitate clients' access to evaluation and treatment by a qualified care provider. Environmental stressors such as poverty, social isolation, and community violence also need to be evaluated and addressed, since they play a part in a family's ability to meet the needs of infants and children.[44,64,79,174] If the parent of a child with medical complications reports that the family is having difficulty following through with the child's care because of unemployment and marital stress, the ECI team is positioned to refer the parents for financial assistance, work placement, and counseling services. Once these concerns are resolved, parents have more energy available for child care. If there appears to be a danger of child abuse or neglect, the occupational therapist is mandated by law to report these concerns to the state child protection agency. Case Study 13-4 presents an example of family-centered early intervention.

Public School Systems

Students whose special needs are primarily psychosocial are classified by the school system as *emotionally disturbed* (ED). Federal regulations for IDEA define this special education classification as:

> a condition exhibiting one or more of the following characteristics over a long period of time and to a marked degree, which adversely affects educational performance: (A) An inability to learn that cannot be explained by intellectual, sensory, or health factors; (B) An inability to build or maintain satisfactory interpersonal relationships with peers or teachers; (C) Inappropriate types of behavior or feelings under normal circumstances; (D) A general pervasive mood of unhappiness or depression; or (E) A tendency to develop physical symptoms or fears associated with personal or school problems. This category does not include children who demonstrate socially maladjusted behavior (e.g., delinquency, school truancy, conduct disorder) in the absence of the problems previously listed. Other categories in which psychosocial problems and behavioral disorders are often present include pervasive developmental disorders, mental retardation, and traumatic brain injuries [Code of Federal Regulations, Title 34, § 300.7(c)(4)(i)].

Emotional disturbance was the primary disability category for about 1 in 12 special education students in the year 2000 to 2001.[82] The rate of educational diagnoses of emotional

TABLE 13-3 Settings for Psychosocial Treatment of Children and Adolescents

	Early Childhood Intervention Programs	School Systems	Outpatient and Day Treatment Programs	Residential Treatment Centers	Correctional Facilities	Inpatient Hospitals
Frames of reference	Developmental Neurodevelopmental Rehabilitation Behavioral Family systems	Educational Developmental Behavioral	Behavioral Cognitive Developmental Psychodynamic Family systems Neurobehavioral	Behavioral Developmental Milieu	Behavioral Educational	Developmental Neurobehavioral Behavioral Cognitive Psychodynamic Family systems
Clientele	Families of children aged 0–3 yr who are diagnosed with developmental delay or are at risk for delay	Children and adolescents 2–18 yr of age	Children and adolescents 5–18 yr of age and their families	Children and adolescents 5–10 yr of age, sometimes families	Children and adolescents 10–18 yr of age	Children and adolescents 3–18 yr of age
Staffing	Dominant team style: 2 and 3 Special educators Speech-language pathologists Audiologists Occupational therapists Physical therapists Social workers Psychologists Nurses Nutritionists	Dominant team style: 1 and 2 Educators Special educators Speech-language pathologists Occupational therapists Physical therapists Counselors Psychologists Administrators	Dominant team style: 1, 2, and 3 Psychiatrists Psychologists Social workers Nurses Counselors Occupational therapists Art therapists Recreational therapists Music therapists	Dominant team style: 2 and 3 Houseparents Psychologists Social workers Educators	Dominant team style: 1 and 2 Guards Police officers Parole officers Lawyers Psychologists Psychiatrists Social workers Educators Counselors Occupational therapist	Dominant team style: 1 and 2 Psychiatrists Nurses Unit staff Psychologists Social workers Occupational therapists Recreational therapists Music therapists Art therapists

CASE STUDY 13-4 Vanessa

Vanessa, who is 16 years of age, and her 4-month-old daughter, Nicole, live independently in a subsidized housing development in a large city. Nicole was referred to an early childhood intervention (ECI) program by her pediatrician, who was concerned about the possibility of developmental delay related to her low birth weight and probable fetal alcohol syndrome effects. Nicole was evaluated by the center's interdisciplinary team and was found to be a passive baby who rarely interacted with people or the environment, had low muscle tone, and was slow to drink from a bottle. Because of transportation problems, Vanessa decided that she would prefer home-based intervention. The team agreed that the occupational therapist would provide therapeutic and case management services.

The therapist worked with Nicole and Vanessa individually and together. To coordinate care, she established communication with two other agencies that were also providing services to the family: the state's department of children and family services and the public health department. Intervention with Nicole was focused on increasing her arousal level and responsiveness to the environment, developing motor control, and improving her efficiency in eating. Neurodevelopmental, sensory integrative therapy, and feeding techniques were applied to reach these goals. The therapist provided a selection of toys each week and encouraged Vanessa to give Nicole opportunities to move and explore the environment.

Vanessa was initially shy and guarded with the therapist but became increasingly comfortable after several weeks. The therapeutic relationship was forged when the occupational therapist and Vanessa worked together to assemble a colorful mobile for the baby's crib. During that session, Vanessa confided that she was living in fear of Nicole's father, who had beaten Vanessa repeatedly during her pregnancy and was threatening her life if she did not agree to let him move into the apartment.

The occupational therapist assisted Vanessa in contacting a battered women's service organization, which offered support groups, crisis shelter, legal services, and adult education programs. She also helped Vanessa identify family members who might be able to assist with child care and to help with occasional transportation needs. During the course of their relationship, the occupational therapist continued to listen to Vanessa's concerns and encouraged her to pursue the resources that were available to her. She also monitored the home situation for potential violence toward Nicole, in case a referral to child protective services was needed. Additionally, she maintained regular communication with the referring pediatrician, who assisted with monitoring Nicole's health and the family's progress.

Although Vanessa consistently expressed strong feelings of affection and the desire to be a good mother to Nicole, the therapist observed that the mother-infant interactions were often poorly synchronized, resulting in frustration for both.

The occupational therapist taught Vanessa to recognize Nicole's changing states of arousal and to time her attempts to engage the baby in social play when Nicole was calm and alert. Vanessa learned to involve Nicole in developmentally appropriate interactive activities such as "peek-a-boo," gentle tickling, and "so big." She also learned the importance of providing Nicole with a variety of sensory, motor, and language experiences.

After 6 months of therapy, Vanessa was regularly attending educational and support activities sponsored by the women's shelter. She planned to enroll in her school's vocational training program. Nicole had become appropriately active and sociable, and both she and her mother interacted warmly in a manner that bespoke their mutual emotional development and attachment. The therapist in this example helped the family address key psychosocial needs through direct intervention and community referral. The ECI team carried out its mission by providing direct assistance and coordinating the provision of services among various agencies. As with most young families, the psychosocial and physical needs of the infant could only be met fully when those of the primary caregiver were also met.

---

disturbance increases with age and grade level. Most children in need do not receive professional mental health care, so the public schools serve more children with behavioral and emotional disorders than any other agency.[76] Students with mental health problems do not qualify for special education services unless their symptoms significantly disrupt their school performance, so their needs are often underserved at school, as well as in the community and health care systems.[12] Occupational therapists working in the schools have an important responsibility to observe the students with whom they work for signs of emotional distress, as many children with mental health problems also have the learning and attentional disorders that are typically referred for services at school.

The primary mission of public education is academic and social preparation for future education and work roles. Research shows that this goal has been largely unreached for students who have emotional and behavioral problems.[20,27,110,177] Students with moderate to severe behavioral problems are unable to take full advantage of education and experience repeated academic and social failure. More than 50% of students with emotional or behavioral disorders drop out of high school.[165] These students have a significantly increased risk for economic dependency and crime.[20,175] The public schools represent an arena in which occupational therapists have an unrealized opportunity to have a tremendous effect on the lives of children with psychosocial problems.[12,123] See Chapter 24 for further description of school mental health programs.

A variety of school settings serve special education students with ED. Self-contained classroom arrangements allow students whose behavior is frequently disruptive or otherwise inappropriate to receive intensive behavioral intervention while being educated in a small group setting. However, students in such classrooms are segregated from peers and role models and suffer the stigma of being identified as "different." This segregation contradicts the goal of full inclusion of special education students in regular education settings. In a full inclusion model, students attend regular education classrooms with support services that may include a resource room for specific subjects, classroom aides, crisis intervention, and counseling services. Benefits of this approach include regular exposure to a typical school environment, opportunities to interact with typically developing peers, and positive experiences that reinforce learning of social skills. Problems can arise with this approach when the teachers have large numbers of students and little training in preventing or managing disruptive behaviors. Teachers and students then feel inadequate and frustrated.

Many classroom teachers incorporate social skills training programs into their regular curricula. These programs are suitable for all children, and they address areas such as communication and social skills,[66] violence prevention,[23] and drug abuse prevention.[67] Such educational programs can provide an excellent means of developing prosocial thinking and behavior in typically developing children. However, these programs do not provide the intensive guidance required by many children and adolescents who have psychosocial dysfunction affecting performance in these areas.[143]

School-based therapeutic intervention is directed toward enhancing students' academic and future vocational performance with an emphasis on both scholastic and social development. Traditionally the school psychologist, counselor, or social worker assumes responsibility for evaluating psychosocial needs and may work with students in individual or small group sessions. These professionals serve the needs of all students, not just those in special education, and may not have an extensive clinical background in psychopathology.[110] They apply behavioral, cognitive, and developmental approaches (see Table 13-3).

Many leaders in education and occupational therapy believe that the services provided to students with behavioral disorders are inadequate in quantity and quality.* Teachers express despair as they sacrifice creative educational methods to address behavioral crises. Parents of students with behavioral disorders are frustrated by the paucity of services to address their children's particular needs. All parents are concerned about their children's safety and education while they are at school.

Occupational therapy activity groups have been described as effective for elementary students who have social and behavioral difficulties.[50,147,148] Motivating activities such as planning and preparing meals, creating craft projects, producing a newspaper, performing skits and plays, and refinishing furniture help students develop competencies in daily living skills while practicing adaptive responses to interpersonal challenges and developing self-confidence. The goal of this type of approach is to support improved occupational functioning in the classroom and other school settings. Students' behavioral improvements in occupational therapy task groups have been shown to generalize to the classroom and other contexts, thus winning the support of educators and administrators in the school.[1,148] Agrin speculated that the students' future success in less restrictive settings could be predicted by the development of their social skills in the activity groups.[1]

Students who are referred for occupational therapy services to address fine motor, perceptual, or orthopedic problems may also have social and emotional needs that impair academic performance. Case Study 13-5 exemplifies how one student's

multiple needs were addressed. General education teach● are working with increasing numbers of special needs childre● including those who have educational diagnoses of emotion● disturbance. Additionally, their classrooms include childr● who are not enrolled in special education, but who a● troubled and preoccupied with acute and/or chronic life stre● ses such as poverty, community violence, and family turmo● In some schools the majority of students are trying to lea● despite a climate of constant crises in their homes and neig● borhoods. Behavioral disruptions are frequent and educato● feel endangered and unsupported. Occupational therapi● are positioned to provide consultation to teachers who ne● ideas regarding environmental adaptation and group manag● ment and to help determine which students should be referr● for occupational therapy or other related services evaluatior● By educating and supporting teachers, therapists can have● positive influence on the school experiences of hundreds ● children.

The School to Work Opportunities Act (1994) and IDE● (2004) both reflect the high priority placed on preparing stu● dents for gainful employment. Middle and high school studen● who have emotional and behavioral problems are considered b● many to be among the most challenging to transition succes● fully into independent living and satisfying, economically su● taining work.[27,111,175] Although no universally successf● means have been identified, research to date indicates that th● most promising interventions include individualized plannin● that involves the student and parents. The intervention shoul● also include social skills training and support, classroom educa● tion regarding work values and life skills, and actual work expe● rience in positions where the fit between students and jobs● optimal.[110] Age- and situation-appropriate occupations shoul● be emphasized over performance components training, an● environments should be structured to facilitate students' suc● cess.[24,134] Occupational therapists are able to provide any an● all of these interventions, and they can serve educational team● as well as transitional planning specialists.

School-based occupational therapists do not consistentl● emphasize psychosocially oriented intervention.[12,30,123] O● the basis of a review of the special education literature, Schult● concluded that teachers would welcome the kind of assistanc● that occupational therapists can provide in improving students● social skills.[147] School administrators who are concerned abou● occupational therapists meeting the needs of the traditiona● referrals may initially be less encouraging. School-based thera● pists who are committed to providing holistic services need t● educate and persuade colleagues regarding the potential effec● tiveness of occupational therapy approaches to help student● meet central academic goals by developing essential skill● needed for social participation. This may be approached directl● through discussions with key administrators, in-services for tea● chers and related services professionals, program development● and case-by-case demonstration. Occupational therapists shoul● advocate including psychosocial goals in students' individua● education programs. Trends in inclusionary and transitiona● education have created an atmosphere in which occupationa● therapy leadership in comprehensive holistic intervention● approaches are needed and often welcomed. Examples of evi● dence-supported, activity-based interventions used by school● based occupational therapists in their work with students with● emotional disturbances are listed in Box 13-2.

---

*References 12, 30, 56, 110, 119, 148.

CASE STUDY 13-5   Dylan

Dylan was an 8-year-old second grader who was referred for an occupational therapy evaluation because his handwriting was slow and illegible. The teacher completed a Pre-assessment Checklist (see Figure 13-2), indicating that Dylan often exhibited problems with incomplete and careless work, disorganized work habits, and peer relations characterized by teasing and rejection, as well as the handwriting difficulty that precipitated the referral.

Assessments that could be helpful include:

- Classroom, lunchroom, and PE class observations to learn about Dylan's abilities to attend to and follow through on tasks, his social behavior, his fine and gross motor performance, and the physical, sensory, and social environments. These will help to determine personal, environmental, and occupational strengths and limitations.
- A standardized evaluation of handwriting, such as the Evaluation Tool of Children's Handwriting[7] and observation of Dylan's spontaneous writing and drawing in classroom and quiet settings. This will help to evaluate the precise nature of Dylan's handwriting problems and the contextual factors that may help or hinder his performance.
- As information about Dylan's performance and abilities is gathered and understood, the occupational therapist should decide whether further evaluation is needed to plan intervention. Assessments of visual perception (such as the Test of Visual Perceptual Skills), general fine and gross motor skills (such as the Bruininks-Oseretsky Test of Motor Proficiency II), and/or sensory processing (such as the Sensory Profile) may be warranted if additional information about the nature of Dylan's problems is needed.

During the evaluation session Dylan was polite and compliant. His affect was generally sad, and he made frequent self-disparaging comments, such as "I'm not good at this." When motor testing was completed, the occupational therapist asked about Dylan's feelings about school this year and whether he had anyone in his class with whom he played on a regular basis. He reported feeling "okay" about school in general, but said, "I don't have any friends at school. They all say I'm fat and dumb." Dylan's fine motor skills and handwriting were significantly below average. Classroom observation revealed that Dylan was seated near the center of the room, and amidst several active classmates. His attempts to join in their conversations were imitative and immature and generally ignored. His sitting posture was poor, and he looked around the room, rather than at the teacher or his papers. Dylan went largely unnoticed by the teacher, who was busy controlling the large group, and he spent a lot of the session disengaged from the relay race activity. At lunch, Dylan had difficulty opening food packaging and did not finish eating before it was time to leave.

Evaluation Results: Dylan's school performance was enhanced by his capacity for cooperation and good manners. Identified areas for improvement included Dylan's general fine motor skills, handwriting speed and quality, attention to tasks, seated positioning, and social interactions with peers. Long-term goals, negotiated between Dylan and the rest of the educational team, included (1) producing written work that was complete and legible at least 80% of the time, and (2) having at least two friends in his classroom, with whom he could work and play on a regular basis.

Dylan was enrolled in 30 minutes per week of occupational therapy with two other second graders. The group worked on developing writing and cutting skills by making group collages with themes, such as, "I can be a friend by. . ." and "The five best things about me are. . . ." They also drew pictures of what they would like to be doing 20 years in the future and wrote and illustrated collective stories. Group members discussed their ideas and, with guidance and encouragement from the therapist, began to listen to one another, express their ideas, and give and accept positive feedback. The boys shared ideas about how to make friends and cope with teasing and rejection. Dylan and another boy developed a friendship that continued outside of the sessions. The group members voted to name themselves "The Tuesday Club," adding to their sense of belonging. Concurrently, the therapist worked with Dylan's teacher on adaptations that would facilitate improved organization, handwriting performance, and social interactions. Together they designed a chart to reward desirable classroom behaviors and simplified his worksheets to allow smaller units of work and more frequent feedback. Last, the occupational therapist advised the parents regarding recreational opportunities, such as YMCA day camp and Boy Scouts, which would further enhance Dylan's social and motor skills.

After one semester of occupational therapy, Dylan's grades improved significantly. His mother reported that he no longer resisted attending school on most days and Dylan reported satisfaction with his school performance and social life. The teacher was pleased both with Dylan's progress and with her success in using a behavior charting system. At that point the occupational therapist reduced intervention to biweekly monitoring and occasional consultation with the teacher.

The therapist in this example met the concerns of the referring teacher, who could not read the student's writing, and the concerns of the student, who felt isolated and anxious at school. Both problems significantly impaired the student's academic progress and were effectively and efficiently addressed through a combination of direct service and consultation.

Mental Health Services

In the United States, mental health services for children and adolescents have been chronically underfunded, with the result that most young people who have mental disorders do not gain access to expert professional services.[109,163,167,183] In 1992, Congress responded to this problem by authorizing the Comprehensive Community Mental Health Services for Children and their Families Program.[165] This program provides federal funding through demonstration grants to states and communities and is designed to develop and promote effective ways to organize, coordinate, and deliver mental health services and supports for children and adolescents and their families. Private foundations have joined in the effort, resulting in the coordination of multiple agencies within communities working together

---

BOX 13-2 Examples of Activity-Based Intervention for Students with Emotional Disturbances

- Yoga: Yoga has been found to be effective in helping children to reduce stress and improve motor control and attention.[62] Yoga groups can provide opportunities for children with and without special needs to interact and benefit from this popular form of exercise.
- ALERT program: This combination of sensorimotor and cognitive-behavioral activities helps children and teachers to identify the child's level of neurologic arousal and provides tools for the child's self-regulation.[188]
- Social skills groups: A variety of social skills group formats can be helpful in improving children's abilities related to getting along with peers and adults.[180] Occupational therapists can engage children in seated or active play while modeling, teaching, and prompting appropriate social behavior, such as taking turns, making requests, and asking to play.

---

to provide innovative, client-centered, culturally appropriate services. A universal goal of contemporary community-based mental health services for children is to facilitate successful participation within the family, community, and school. Best-practice standards for children with severe and complex needs involve a "wraparound" planning and management process, in which the family and all involved care providers work closely together to ensure well-coordinated, comprehensive intervention.[183] Although few occupational therapists identify mental health settings as their primary site of practice, many practice in settings that participate in the coordinated care of young people with mental health problems.[126] These settings include early intervention services, day care programs, preschools, schools, and hospital-based outpatient clinics. Although most mental health centers and private practices do not include occupational therapists as part of their core team, occupational therapists can participate as valuable ad hoc members of the extended, community-based mental health team and as consultants. Understanding the forms and functions of contemporary mental health systems allows occupational therapists to engage effectively with the professionals working within the system and to join in providing coordinated care from a unique perspective.

Outpatient treatment is the mental health intervention most commonly accessed by children and adolescents.[167] Outpatient mental health services may be provided through freestanding clinics, hospital-based programs, publicly funded community mental health centers, health maintenance organizations, and private practices. Funding sources may include the clients' families, private insurance, Medicaid, federal grants, and state monies.[102,118] An agency's sources of funding influence the types of clientele served and the types of services provided.

Children and adolescents who seek outpatient mental health services often have significant behavioral disturbances that have caused moderate to severe levels of disturbance for family, school, or community members.[102] The primary goals of outpatient mental health services are the diagnosis and management of mental health problems to improve functioning within the community and prevent crises necessitating hospitalization.

The child's initial contact with an outpatient mental health practitioner—typically a social worker, psychologist, psychiatrist, or licensed counselor—consists of an intake interview exploring the nature and severity of the child's and the family's problems. Responses to the interview form the basis for decisions regarding appropriate evaluation and intervention. Possible dispositions include outpatient evaluation at a later date or crisis evaluation with immediate short-term intervention.

Frames of reference used in outpatient programs and practices vary, but they commonly draw from cognitive behavioral, behavioral, family systems, neurobiologic, and psychodynamic theories (see Table 13-3). Treatment approaches are most commonly goal-focused and time-limited and involve the family and school. Clients generally attend one or two 1-hour sessions per week for a specified period. In publicly funded mental health centers, payment for services is based on the individual's income. Third-party payers have varied levels of coverage for mental health care. Therapeutic modalities commonly include play therapy (for young children), talking therapy, expressive art, therapeutic board games, group discussions, family discussions, and parenting education sessions. These programs can be staffed by a combination of psychologists, social workers, psychiatrists, psychiatric nurses, and licensed counselors.[118]

Day treatment programs and therapeutic schools are offered in a variety of settings, including psychiatric hospitals, community mental health facilities, and schools for students with special needs.[141] Such programs provide a therapeutic level of intensity between outpatient intervention and hospitalization and are popular for clinical and economic reasons.[5] Clients typically attend programming from 4 to 6 hours per day, 5 days per week, and are at home during evenings and weekends.[21] Interventions often include a variety of therapies including occupational therapy and specialized academic classes.

Day treatment programs or schools can facilitate a child's transition from the hospital back to the home and community, provide crisis stabilization, allow comprehensive evaluation, or serve as an intensive therapeutic alternative to outpatient or inpatient treatment.[141] Programming often follows a psychoeducational model and may include vocational evaluation and training for adolescents.[128] A psychiatrist or psychologist who specializes in child and adolescent mental health or a special educator typically leads intervention teams. Other team members are listed in Table 13-3 and can include occupational therapists.

Occupational therapy activities in day programs can address academic, sensorimotor, daily living, and psychosocial goals. Crafts, role-playing exercises, cooperative action games, board games, cooking, sensorimotor interventions, and field trips are popular modalities in such occupational therapy programs. Hygiene and grooming, telephone and e-mail etiquette, how to order food in a restaurant, and other such daily living needs can be addressed. Working with the client's parents, child care providers, teachers, job coach, or school-based occupational therapist can facilitate the transition from intensive day treatment programs to the community and public school and enhance the carryover of interventions and goals. The family may also benefit from assistance with locating and securing social and leisure resources. Case Study 13-6 describes how a consultative model of intervention can be used to assist with

CASE STUDY 13-6   Mario

Mario was 17 years of age and had diagnoses of mild mental retardation, anxiety disorder, and impulse control disorder. He had a lifelong history of poor socialization with people outside of his family, separation anxiety, and occasional temper tantrums. He also took medications for a seizure disorder and asthma. Mario was admitted to day treatment after a series of explosive episodes during which he broke furniture and a window.

Mario, his family, and the treatment team decided that Mario would begin a job training program as part of his day treatment. It was determined that the occupational therapist would arrange and implement this. The supervisor at the job training site expressed both interest and a little trepidation at the notion of working with a client who had a history of psychiatric disturbance with aggressive behavior. The occupational therapist's task included helping Mario to develop and use new interpersonal and practical skills needed for success in his training, such as meeting new people, asking questions, maintaining acceptable standards of dress and grooming, and reading a clock. This was accomplished through group and individual sessions at the day treatment program. Another part of the intervention involved preparing the job training site to work effectively with Mario.

To facilitate the transition, the occupational therapist visited the job training site to evaluate its appropriateness for Mario and to establish a working relationship with the staff. The occupational therapist then accompanied Mario to his interview at the job training program. As the job trainer and Mario discussed the program's operations, the therapist made suggestions to increase Mario's chances of success. One suggestion was for Mario to write the program schedule into his pocket calendar and to negotiate with the job trainer times needed for regular psychiatric or medical appointments. Another suggestion was for the job trainer to provide Mario with a written list of basic expectations for participation in the program, such as arriving on time, wearing appropriate clothing, and bringing a sack lunch. Mario's need for a high degree of structure and routine was discussed, and the supervisor provided him with a detailed schedule of activities for the upcoming week. The occupational therapist also facilitated Mario's asking the supervisor questions about issues that she knew he was concerned with, such as what would happen if he made mistakes and what he should do if he was confused or had questions. The occupational therapist also helped Mario answer the job training supervisor's concerns about Mario, such as how they should respond if he were to become agitated. (Mario suggested that he could take a break in the break room if he felt overwhelmed, and the therapist gave the supervisor her cell phone number.) The occupational therapist, Mario, and the job training supervisor left the interview feeling prepared and excited about working together.

Once Mario began the job training program, he experienced periods of intense anxiety and agitation, causing concern to his supervisor and coworkers. The supervisor called the occupational therapist, who visited the job training facility. Through discussion with Mario, the occupational therapist was able to establish that he had become upset when he was given conflicting or inconsistent directives from different supervisors. It was also observed that Mario did not interact with coworkers, even if they greeted him.

The therapist met with Mario and the supervisor to negotiate a plan. It was decided to (1) assign Mario routine tasks that needed to be performed the same way each time, as much as possible; (2) limit Mario's supervision to one person at a time; and (3) encourage Mario to verbalize his feelings of confusion, anxiety, and frustration to his supervisor before he felt overwhelmed. The therapist assisted Mario and his supervisor in writing and signing a behavioral contract that outlined consequences for behavioral outbursts: a 30-minute break after the first outburst and suspension without pay for the remainder of the day if there was a second outburst. Finally, the occupational therapist spent some time in the company lunchroom helping Mario meet and get to know his coworkers. Once Mario and his coworkers were mutually comfortable, he was able to demonstrate his full potential as a reliable and capable worker.

---

the transition of a client from day treatment back to full community involvement. The focus in this example is on educating and problem solving with personnel from another agency.

Residential Treatment Centers

About 3% of children and adolescents receiving state-funded mental health services utilize *residential treatment centers,* facilities providing around-the-clock care.[165] Residential care is highly restrictive and costly and is typically utilized only when other means of intervention have failed. Lengths of stay in residential treatment centers vary from weeks to years and are influenced by funding constraints, the facility's philosophy, and the needs of the client and family.[155] Program philosophies range from highly institutional to more naturalistic and homelike environments, and some facilities provide educational programs on-site. Residential treatment centers vary in size from tens to hundreds of residents. The most common reasons for placement are aggressive behaviors toward self or others, mental disorders with severe and persistent symptoms, lack of family supports, and abuse. More than half of the children admitted into residential care come from other congregate care settings, such as acute care hospitals, juvenile corrections, foster homes, and other residential care centers.[3]

The immediate mission of residential care programs is to provide a safe and therapeutic environment for children and adolescents whose behavioral, emotional, and social problems preclude their safety and competence in the community.[156] The intended outcome of residential care is for children and adolescents to function as full participants within the community and family, foster family, transitional living, or independent living settings. Experts in the area of residential care assert that treatment may include individual, group, and family therapy sessions. To be meaningful, therapeutic intervention must continue in the everyday experiences of children as they interact with child care staff and their peers.[14,52,156]

The effectiveness of intervention is determined by the skills of the therapeutic, educational, and childcare staff in building relationships, managing children's behavior, and structuring leisure and work activities.[48,162]

Staffing reflects each residential care facility's philosophy and target populations. All residential care facilities employ childcare workers who are paraprofessionals with various levels of expertise. Other team members include psychiatrists, psychologists, social workers, nurses, teachers, and "therapeutic activities personnel," who may include occupational therapists.[3] Some residential treatment facilities may contract occupational therapy services that can include consultation to the house staff regarding the residents' developmental needs and limitations, ways to organize and guide household responsibilities to include the residents, and ways to teach residents self-care and community living skills (Case Study 13-7). Other occupational therapists provide services within the residential centers' school programs, addressing goals related to academic and social performance. Frames of reference often used in residential care include cognitive behavioral, behavioral, psychodynamic, and psychoeducational approaches.[89,156] Children who live in even the most deluxe institutional settings do not have access to many occupational experiences that are a part of the daily activities for children in family homes and the community. At this time, occupational therapy is not a mandated service as determined by accreditation standards for residential

---

CASE STUDY 13-7   The Diners' Club

The occupational therapist at a residential care home for children ages 6 to 17 years was approached by one of the special educators with a concern about two of the students: no one among the children or staff wanted to eat near them because they were so messy and rude at mealtimes. "It's like eating with hogs!" she exclaimed. Eating is an activity of daily living that affects individuals' physical, emotional, and social quality of life on a daily basis and is part of the occupational therapist's domain of practice.

The occupational therapist arranged to have lunch in the common dining room in order to observe the students eating. It was apparent that the two identified students were not alone in their problems with eating and that the problems were multileveled. The dining room was large and noisy. Round tables with seating for up to eight people were scattered across the area, with chairs placed on the tabletops until the diners arrived to take them down. The tabletops were scarred and sometimes sticky. As people were seated, it was noted that the staff sat together and children sat together. There was a lot of friendly banter and jostling as everyone gathered their trays of food, silverware, and beverages. The dining room staff knew each child by name and joked with them in a gentle way. During the meal the conversation at the children's tables was mainly procedural, such as "Give me the salt." And "Move down!" The children in question (and many others) ate hurriedly and often used their fingers to lift wet and sticky food. They had numerous spills, for which they were scolded by peers and adults. They took huge bites and talked with their mouths full. Sometimes they played with the food, making disgusting concoctions. The dining room looked like a disaster area when the meal ended. The mealtime did not seem relaxing or pleasant for these children, and they were clearly not ready for public dining.

The occupational therapist met with the clinical director and multidisciplinary staff and proposed a new lunchtime therapy group: the Diners' Club. The group would meet twice weekly at lunchtime with the occupational therapist and a cotherapist, either an occupational therapy student or one of the teachers, and would include up to six children per session. Each session would last 6 weeks, and goals would be individualized. Typical goals would include using utensils as needed and with skill; using a napkin to clean mouth and hands while holding the napkin on the lap until needed; pouring beverages effectively; making polite social conversation; saying "please," "thank you," and "no thank you" as appropriate; and learning to appreciate the enjoyment that a relaxed meal can bring. The team approved the idea with enthusiasm, and many nominations for the first 6-week session were discussed and decided upon. The manager of the dietary service was included in the discussion and offered to support the effort by providing a tablecloth and centerpiece for sessions, which were to take place at a corner table at the back of the dining hall.

Attractively decorated invitations to the Diners' Club were given to the referred students the next week, and they were all very excited. Each of the students met with the occupational therapist to learn more about the group, and all accepted eagerly. Before the first Diners' Club session, each child was observed eating at least one meal and met with the therapist to determine his or her personal goals. Diners' Club lunches began about 20 minutes before the lunch hour, with all participants meeting at the special table, which was always decked out with the tablecloth, flowers, and something special to eat: for example, a bowl of mints, a Jell-O salad to share, or a pitcher of punch. Each place had silverware and a napkin correctly arranged. The group began by greeting each member and making some polite small talk. Then there would be a brief didactic and demonstration on the topic of the day, such as, "What foods require a knife and fork? How should one hold and use a fork?" or, "What should you do if... you drop your spoon? ...you burp loudly? ...you can't stand the food that someone has passed your way in a serving dish?" After discussion, "Club" members and staff filed up to the serving area and picked up trays of food to bring back to the table. Good manners were modeled and reinforced during interactions with the dining hall staff. Then the meal itself was a laboratory in good manners and fine dining. When the meal ended, each member had a brief conversation with the therapists about their progress on their goals that meal.

At the end of the 6-week session, each diner received a certificate of completion. All of the club members had made significant progress toward their goals and expressed satisfaction with their achievement. Staff members were likewise pleased with the children's progress and were noted to comment positively on the students' mealtime behavior between sessions. The facility administrators were so pleased that they offered funding to take the Diners' Club graduates out for a restaurant meal to celebrate and try out their new capabilities!

care facilities. Published literature describing or testing the effectiveness of occupational therapy within residential care facilities for children is minimal. As a member of a small community of practitioners who have provided occupational therapy in residential care for more than 10 years, this author asserts that occupational therapy can have a tremendous impact on the quality of life and effectiveness of residential treatment in preparing children and adolescents for successful transitions to lives in the larger community. Direct intervention with the children and adolescents in residential care can include many of the goals and approaches outlined in the discussion of occupational therapy in day treatment programs. Additionally, occupational therapists can facilitate the resident's participation in community activities such as shopping, playing sports, participating in activity clubs, and attending church. Opportunities for as much family interaction as possible during such activities increase the benefits of such experiences.[93,155]

Juvenile Corrections

The more than 100,000 children and adolescents who are housed by the juvenile justice system share many of the needs of those in residential treatment centers and represent another underserved group with serious psychosocial and occupational needs.[82] Youth who have been incarcerated for committing crimes often have serious emotional disturbances that have not been addressed therapeutically.[8] In a review of the literature on juvenile detention, Goldstrom and colleagues estimated that up to 95% of youth in the juvenile justice system have mental, emotional, or behavioral health problems, 20% of these with severe mental disorders.[65] Those incarcerated are completely removed from the home and community and lack opportunities to gain or maintain skills they need to reintegrate into the community on release. Boredom and hopelessness can contribute to antisocial behavior within the facility, posing a danger to the prisoners and staff. Most correctional institutions for youth provide traditional psychotherapeutic care but not rehabilitation-focused care.[82] Occupational therapists should be involved in the comprehensive psychiatric and functional evaluations of children and adolescents who are either under consideration for psychiatric commitment or who are to be tried as adults. They can provide therapeutic services to address their psychosocial and daily living skills needs and help to educate staff members about the developmental and neurobehavioral issues that this group shares. Youth offenders who are enrolled in diversional programs or who are being treated in state or other psychiatric facilities would be good candidates for occupational therapy.

Inpatient Psychiatric Hospitals

Inpatient psychiatric hospitals provide the most restrictive, intensive, and costly therapeutic intervention.[167] They are used for children and adolescents who pose a serious safety risk to themselves or others, have complicating medical conditions, or require specialized teams for rapid diagnosis and stabilization.[138] Very often individuals are hospitalized when in crisis, such as after a suicide attempt, an assault, or a psychotic episode. Sometimes patients are admitted for comprehensive psychological and medical evaluation of complex chronic

problems. Due to the high cost of inpatient care, lengths of stay are brief, with a range of 2 to 27 days and a median of 4.5 days.[28]

Inpatient psychiatric units may be found in general hospitals, state psychiatric hospitals, and private psychiatric hospitals. Child and adolescent inpatient psychiatric units are usually locked facilities that are directed by a psychiatrist and staffed by nurses and paraprofessionals who are trained in the care and management of severely impaired patients.[47] The treatment team is interdisciplinary and may include psychiatrists, nurses, paraprofessional direct care staff, psychologists, neuropsychologists, and social workers. The professional staff apply a variety of psychosocial theories, with neurobiologic and cognitive behavioral approaches among the most commonly used. Due to brief lengths of stay, occupational therapists are rarely part of the core intervention team in acute care psychiatric units for children and adolescents. An occupational therapist may be brought in to contribute to the developmental, neurodevelopmental, and functional evaluations for severely impaired patients.

The case examples presented throughout this chapter depict a number of ways to intervene with children and adolescents who have psychosocial problems. The following section outlines occupational therapy evaluation and intervention options more specifically and in more detail.

EVALUATION AND INTERVENTION

Evaluation

The evaluation process is foundational to the intervention process and largely determines its success. Evaluating children who exhibit behavioral problems can be challenging, due to the complex nature of the task and the fact that the child may be unable to cooperate with traditional assessment approaches. As much information as possible should be gleaned indirectly from past and current school or medical records. Evaluating therapists can learn a great deal from teacher and parent checklists and naturalistic observations in typical contexts, such as various settings within the school, home, institution, and community.

The evaluation process begins with an occupational profile that includes an occupational history, the client's perceptions of current occupational functioning, the client's concerns about occupational performance, and priorities for intervention.[4] A thorough occupational profile includes information about the person, environment, and occupations. The occupational profile may be obtained through informal interviews or with the assistance of a structured interview such as the Canadian Occupational Therapy Performance Measure.[105] An interview or paper-and-pencil activity may be used to gain an understanding of the child's habits and balance of activity. Some children are better able to express their concerns and hopes for the future in pictures. For them a large piece of paper and some colorful markers or crayons, along with an invitation to "draw a picture of yourself doing something" or "make a picture of some things you want to be doing next month" may give the therapist and the child a way to begin their dialog. The purpose of beginning the evaluation process with an occupational profile is to obtain a sense of the scope and immediacy of issues concerning the client. For occupational therapists working with children, the "client" includes the referring adult, who could be a parent, a teacher, a foster parent, or some other closely involved person. When the child is very young, has limited functional communication, or is being seen in the context of school, the occupational profile should include information from the involved adults. This information will guide decisions about subsequent steps in the evaluation process and help with formulating intervention goals and methods, facilitating their efficiency and quality.

In school settings, a pre-assessment checklist for teachers to complete prior to evaluation can help to define issues of concern and inform teachers about the scope of occupational therapy (Figure 13-2). This tool is designed with items related to written schoolwork listed first, and cast with a positive slant ("Works independently on written assignments"). The last 12 items relate more to cognitive and social performance, and the items are cast from a more problem-oriented perspective ("Has difficulty learning new motor tasks"). Teachers rate the consistency of performance and then may write in specific concerns. The results can help to target areas of strength and possible limitations that require further evaluation.

One of the most valuable assessment methods with children and adolescents who have social participation problems is to observe them interacting with peers or family members during motivating activities such as crafts, board games, or preparing and enjoying food.[133] During such sessions the therapist can see the child in action as she responds to opportunities to initiate interactions, make choices, share opinions, request help, try something new, cope with competition or conflict, and other typical demands of social participation. The activity-focused session can also allow observations of performance areas, such as functional reading, planning and organization, safety awareness, concentration, problem solving, postural control, or small tool use. If the session includes classmates, family members, or others with whom the child relates at home or school, information about the child's social environment is also gathered.

An evaluation of play can provide invaluable, multifaceted information about a child's social, emotional, cognitive, and motor development and addresses a critical area of occupational performance. Assessments for this purpose include structured observational measures, such as the Preschool Play Scale[94-96] or the Test of Playfulness.[152] Florey and Greene outline an activity observation guide to facilitate practitioners' evaluation of play in children aged 6 to 12 years.[57]

The Social Skills Rating System was developed by psychologists to evaluate and classify social behavior in students from kindergarten through 12th grade.[66] There are three versions of the protocols, each for a different grade range. Through a combination of teacher, parent, and student (self-) rating scales, this tool measures perceived performance in the domains of social skills, academic competence, and problem behaviors. The 30 social skills scale items are stated in positive terms (e.g., "Initiates conversation with peers") and include items indicative of cooperation, assertion, responsibility, empathy, and self-control. Respondents are asked to rate the items in terms of frequency and importance. The problem behavior items, answered only by parents and teachers, classify behaviors as externalizing (behaviors that are intrusive or disruptive), internalizing (behaviors reflecting anxiety or sadness), and

hyperactivity. The Social Skills Rating System results are easily translated into intervention and individualized education plan goals and objectives.

The School Function Assessment (SFA) is an observational assessment that assists with the evaluation of school performance of students with disabilities.[43] It is administered as a paper-and-pencil form that can be completed by the occupational therapist, child's teacher, and others who know his school behavior well. It is followed by a structured interview that elaborates on the written responses. More than 100 items on the SFA pertain to social participation in categories of functional communication, memory and understanding, following social conventions, compliance with adult directives and school rules, task behavior/completion, positive interaction, behavior regulation, and safety.

The Occupational Therapy Psychosocial Assessment of Learning (OTPAL) uses a combination of observation and interviewing to evaluate students' psychosocial abilities as they relate to their specific school environment.[161] This assessment is designed for children in elementary school who have been identified as having social participation difficulties.

Standardized assessments of skills, such as measures of the child's fine and gross motor abilities, developmental levels, handwriting, sensory integration, and cognitive-perceptual abilities, should be employed as needed for intervention planning. Some standardized assessments such as the *Miller Function and Participation Scales*[122] include behavioral checklists that provide valuable insight from the parent's or teacher's perspective.

General guidelines for the structured evaluation of students who may resist following directions are:

1. Remember that the main goal is first to form a therapeutic alliance and then to measure the student's best performance on assessment items.
2. Allow extra time for relationship building and breaks during the assessment sessions. Take several brief sessions to complete the battery, if that is needed to ensure a valid measure. Do not be afraid to stop a session early if the child becomes agitated or intractable; crisis prevention is always preferable to crisis intervention.
3. Ask the teacher beforehand for tips about the child's preferences and dislikes. Find out what behavior management techniques work well in the classroom and what interaction styles to avoid. Ask if there is any history of aggressive behavior and, if so, what forms it takes.
4. Be prepared to use rewards to help the child persevere. Favored items include stickers, small candies, and an enjoyed activity at the session's end.
5. Involve the student as a partner in the evaluation process by explaining the nature and purposes of the assessments, interviewing personably, asking for feedback, and making responsive adjustments as often as possible.

Intervention

If it is to be meaningful and effective, intervention with children and adolescents who have social performance problems must include goals that directly address these concerns. These goals should relate directly to the contexts and activities in which the child needs and wants to participate. Examples of such goals are presented next for James, a 10-year-old who wants to participate in the general physical education classes but has

Please rate the student's performance as it compares with that of most of the other children in his or her class	Usually	Sometimes	Never
Works independently on written assignments			
Writing is legible			
Writing is efficient/speed is adequate			
Writing is accurate for copied work			
Writing is accurate for spontaneous work			
Completes all parts of worksheets			
Written work is neat			
Approach to work is logical, organized			
Independently identifies errors in work			
Independently corrects errors in work			
Persists when tasks are challenging			
Seeks help as needed			
Works at a reasonable pace			
Reads at a level close to his/her cognitive level			
Follows instructions and rules			
Cooperates with peers			
Cooperates with teachers			
Expresses emotions appropriately			
Focuses on tasks despite typical distractions			
Stays seated, refrains from excessive fidgeting			
Appears uncoordinated			
Bumps into people or things			
Trips or falls			
Knocks things over			
Holds objects in an unusual manner			
Has trouble cutting with scissors			
Acts before thinking			
Is under- or over-active (circle one)			
Has difficulty learning new motor tasks			
Seeks unusual sensations (smelling, twirling, rubbing)			
Over-reacts to: movement, heights, touch, sounds, smells (circle any that apply)			
Under-reacts to: movement, heights, touch, sounds, smells (circle any that apply)			
Engages in body-rocking			
Scratches, pinches, strikes, or bites self			
Chews or mouths non-food objects			
Disregards or over-reacts to pain (circle one)			
Appears anxious			
Harms or destroys property			
Is verbally aggressive (threatens, curses)			
Is physically aggressive toward peers or adults			

FIGURE 13-2 Pre-Assessment Checklist for Teachers (Revised).

struggled with frequent behavioral "meltdowns" and noncompliance. The intervention team has designed the following goals:

Long-term goal I: James will participate successfully in physical education classes, requiring 0 to 1 verbal correction per class session by (date).

Short-term goal Ia: Given verbal reminders and adult support, James will consistently take turns with peers during a 20- minute ball game by (date).

Short-term goal Ib: James will independently locate his "square" upon entering the gym, and, given occasional verbal cues, will sit or stand on his square as directed by the teacher on 4 of 5 days by (date).

Short-term goal Ic: James will refrain from leaving the gym without permission 100% of the time by (date).

Short-term goal Id: Given opportunities to take brief "breaks" as needed, James' behavior will be age-appropriate and polite during sports and games in physical education classes, on 4 of 5 opportunities by (date).

Contemporary models of occupational therapy emphasize interventions using activities within their natural contexts.[4,106] In order to be optimally therapeutic, activities must

- Be interesting and motivating to the client
- Challenge at least one (preferably more than one) of the skills or abilities targeted for improvement
- Be graded to challenge the child at a level that requires effort and facilitates learning but does not overwhelm
- Provide a sense of fun, rejuvenation, and/or satisfaction

Schultz described such an approach with boys who have been classified with behavior disorders in school, using the model of Occupational Adaptation (Research Note 13-1).[147,148]

In contrast with the environmentally focused approach of Occupational Adaptation, other interventions may be occupation-focused in which the therapists provide highly structured activities. For example, behavioral methods such as point- or token-reward systems may be incorporated into activities-based therapy (Case Study 13-8). This type of operant behaviorism has been well researched and found to be effective in promoting new skills.[139] However, operant behavioral approaches have been criticized by some because they take power away from the naturalistic environmental influences and the child's learning and place it more on the artificial rewards and the therapist.[148,170] Ideally, operant behavioral methods, if used at all, are temporary facilitators for children who have learned to get their needs met through unacceptable behaviors and who can quickly learn adaptive behaviors, given a temporary reward that is then faded as the naturally occurring social rewards become available.

A more socially based behavioral approach is that of *rational intervention (RI)*, a cross-disciplinary decision making system that assists those interacting with children and adolescents with the clinical reasoning needed to make immediate responses that facilitate social participation (Table 13-4).[49] The primary goal of RI is to help children attain and maintain behaviors that are adaptive and appropriate for participation in natural contexts and to create a consistent approach that supports this for all staff members and adult family members who interact with the child. General principles of RI are as follows:

- Every interaction between a child and an adult is a learning session.
- Intervention begins with the adult's consistent enactment of respectfulness and caring toward the child.

RESEARCH NOTE 13-1

Schultz, S. 1992. School-Based Occupational Therapy for Students with Behavioral Disorders. Occupational Therapy in Health Care, 8, 173-196.

ABSTRACT

A 2-year intervention project was implemented to test basic concepts of the theory of Occupational Adaptation with fourth- through sixth-grade boys who received special education services for emotional disturbance. These students had historically been in trouble for behaving badly in school and were expected by many teachers and administrators to act dangerously or out of control. The boys attended small groups, where they participated in craft activities that were motivating and appropriately challenging. The therapist's role was to arrange and maintain an environment that supported the participants' efforts toward learning ways of adapting to new and familiar challenges, social and otherwise. The participants were supported in evaluating their own performance, with minimal and carefully chosen direction from the therapist. If a participant was aggressive toward another person or property, he was instructed to leave that session and allowed to try again the next. As the students progressed, they began to give one another corrective and positive feedback. Once the group achieved sufficient progress during parallel craft activities, the challenge was increased to focus on cooperative group projects, such as the development and creation of a hallway display depicting social studies concepts. Positive changes in the boys' observed social participation were attributed to a combination of improvements in the boys' adaptive capacities and changes in the social environment at school. During her 2 years of intervention with the boys, Schultz observed that the adults and students had developed negative expectations of the students who had emotional disturbances, such that inappropriate and maladaptive behavior was inadvertently encouraged. When the group members behaved appropriately within the school context, expectations and opinions about them began to shift, resulting in improved environmental support for future successes.

IMPLICATIONS FOR PRACTICE:

- By facilitating goodness-of-fit among the client, environment, and activities, the occupational therapy allows the client to demonstrate his or her competence
- When teachers and others are given an opportunity to observe the positive qualities and competencies of children whose prior actions have been alienating, the social environment can change from hostile to supportive.
- Intervention that occurs in the natural environment can result in beneficial long-term effects.
- The main goals of intervention are all persons' immediate safety and the continuous improvement of the child's ability to make decisions that support successful participation in life, at home and in the community.

CASE STUDY 13-8 Max

Max typically shouts and tosses over board games when he fears losing, resulting in broken games and negative interactions. The therapist initially talks with Max about his behavior, and they discuss ways to better cope. Although he can describe alternative ways to handle his distress, Max continues to act inappropriately when playing competitive games. Max is enrolled in small activity group sessions during which the children play board games. The players are intermittently rewarded with praise and small treats for "being patient" and "good sportsmanship." As Max becomes more capable and the natural rewards of enjoying a game with friends become available to him, he requires less structure and fewer artificial rewards in order to maintain his role as a player in the games. Soon he can engage in this type of play as well as other children his age.

TABLE 13-4 Levels of Social Appropriateness and Rational Intervention

Level	Child's Behavior	Rational Interventions
5	Is within an functional range for acceptable performance in the community	Facilitate
4	Approximates that which is acceptable, with minor errors	Facilitate, monitor, or gently correct: Alter the environment Redirect Model Cue Discuss alternatives
3	Not positive, but not disruptive or dangerous (*May be withdrawn, passive, quietly off task*)	Facilitate, monitor, or gently correct: Alter the environment Redirect Model Cue Discuss alternatives
2	Is disruptive but not dangerous (*Noncompliant with rules and directives, making rude sounds or gestures, cursing*)	Gently correct: Alter the environment Redirect Model Cue Discuss alternatives and/ or moderately correct: Timeout
1	May escalate to dangerous level (*Shouting, verbal or physical threats of violence, spitting, pinching, or hitting self, harming expendable property*)	Gently correct: Alter the environment Cue verbally Explain outcomes/ alternatives and/or moderately correct: Time-out
0	Is imminently harmful to self or others (*Striking, kicking, biting, head-banging, cutting, running away, destroying valuable property*)	Strongly correct: Time-out Physically manage Seclusion room Physically restrain

- Opportunities for making choices and decisions are built into daily activities as often as possible. Children should have regular, frequent opportunities to practice skills needed for community living through educational and leisure experiences in the community.
- In order to promote children's opportunities for decision making, adults should impose the least amount of external control needed to maintain safety and promote positive, functional behavior.

When using an RI approach, the therapist initially observes and assesses the child's behavior and then classifies it as belonging in one of three color-coded zones (Case Study 13-9). *Green zone behaviors* are adaptive and would be acceptable in most community and home settings. *Yellow zone behaviors* are mildly to moderately problematic and require monitoring, environmental modification, or cueing to facilitate adaptive social behavior. *Red zone behaviors* present a threat or actuality of danger to the child or others and require direct and immediate verbal or physical management. Therapeutic responses include facilitation, monitoring, gentle correction, moderate correction, and strong correction and may be incorporated into therapy sessions and all social participation contexts (Box 13-3).

SUMMARY

Children and adolescents with emotional, cognitive, and behavioral problems have limited participation in home, school, and community life. Social problems such as poverty, family sociopathic conditions, and cultural violence have been linked with an increased incidence of psychosocial dysfunction in young people.[37,140,184] Such social problems are steadily increasing in our country, while mental health services for young people continue to be inadequate in quantity and quality. Occupational therapists who work with children and adolescents have the knowledge and skills to help improve their clients' occupational functioning by addressing key psychosocial needs. This may be accomplished through individual and group therapy, program development, and consultation. Pediatric occupational therapists in all settings need to be psychosocial practitioners to meet effectively the urgent and growing needs of young people and their families.

CASE STUDY 13-9 Brenda

Brenda is an occupational therapist who works at a therapeutic school for children with behavioral and emotional problems. Today she is helping to care for the children during recess. As Brenda walks around the busy playground area, she encounters many scenes, each of which requires rational intervention.

Scene 1: Three children have acquired a basketball. They are discussing what to play and seem to be making headway toward consensus. This is functional, safe, Level 5 behavior; Brenda leaves them to their game.

Scene 2: A girl keeps running into the midst of a kickball game that is in progress, and the players are shouting angrily at her. It appears to Brenda that the girl wants to play the game but does not have the skills to ask to join. This is Level 4 behavior: generally positive, but not well executed. Brenda gives the child a verbal cue, calling out to her, "Ask Tom if you can be on his team!" She watches to make sure the intervention is successful, then moves on.

Scene 3: Brenda notices a boy who has tied a garden hose into a series of knots. She approaches and asks him to take the knots out of the hose. The boy responds, "Get lost, Bozo!" and keeps making knots in the hose. Although this behavior is inappropriate and rude, it is not dangerous. It is a Level 2, Yellow Zone behavior. Brenda says, "Tying up the hose can damage it. Please take out the knots now. I will help if you like." The boy abruptly stands and swings the hose at Brenda, missing her by several feet. His behavior has digressed to Level 3, in the Red Zone, and could be potentially dangerous. Brenda responds in a calm, firm voice, "Please put the hose down right now, or you will have to go inside for the rest of recess." The boy drops the hose and says, "You're mean! You took away my recess!" Brenda recognizes this as an improvement, and responds supportively, "I'm glad you decided to put down the hose. Let's hurry and fix it, so you'll have more time to play outside."

BOX 13-3 Response Options in Rational Intervention

FACILITATION
- Observe unobtrusively
- Improve the environmental supports (e.g., provide comfortable seating and a quiet work area for children who want to play a board game together)

MONITORING
- Observe visibly, so children are aware of adult presence
- Express encouragement as needed
- Facilitate children's problem solving by asking guiding questions

GENTLE CORRECTION
- Alter the environment as needed (e.g., change the seating arrangement to reduce conflict between participants)

- Remind children of rules, expectations, or new skills that may be used
- Join the activity and model adaptive behavior
- Redirect the child to an alternative activity
- Discuss alternatives to the current behavior

MODERATE CORRECTION
- Give the child a break from the activity through redirection

STRONG CORRECTION
- Formal time-out (the child is seated away from the activity for 1 to 5 minutes, until calm)
- Physical management of the child and removal from the activity and/or the activity area

---

REFERENCES

1. Agrin, A. (1987). Occupational therapy with emotionally disturbed children in a public school. *American Journal of Occupational Therapy*, 7, 105–114.
2. Ainsworth, M. D., Blehar, M. C., Waters, E., & Wall, S. (1978). *Patterns of attachment: A psychological study of the strange situation*. Hillsdale, NJ: Earlbaum.
3. American Association of Children's Residential Treatment Centers. (1999). Outcomes in children's residential treatment centers: A national survey. Washington, DC: AACRC.
4. American Occupational Therapy Association Commission on Practice. (2002). Occupational therapy practice framework: Domain and process. *American Journal of Occupational Therapy*, 56(6), 609–639.
5. American Occupational Therapy Association. (2004). Psychosocial aspects of occupational therapy. *American Journal of Occupational Therapy*, 58(6), 669–672.

6. American Psychiatric Association. (2000). Diagnostic and statistical manual of mental disorders (4th ed., text rev.). Washington, DC: American Psychiatric Association.
7. Amundson, S. (1995). *Evaluation Tool for Children's Handwriting*. Homer, AK: OT Kids.
8. Atkins, D., Pumariega, A., Rogers, K., Montgomery, L., Nybro, C., Jeffers, G., et al (1999). Mental health and incarcerated youth: II. Prevalence and nature of psychopathology. *Journal of Child and Family Studies*, 8(2), 193–204.
9. Bagley, C., & Mallick, K., (2000). Prediction of sexual, emotional and physical maltreatment and mental health outcomes in a longitudinal cohort of 290 adolescent women. *Child Maltreatment*, 5, 218–226.
10. Baker, J. (2003). *Social skills training for children and adolescents with Asperger's syndrome and social-communications problems*. Shawnee Mission, KS: Autism Aspergers Publishing.
11. Barnekow, K., & Kraemer, G. (2005). The psychobiological theory of attachment: A viable frame of reference for early

intervention providers. *Physical and Occupational Therapy in Pediatrics, 25,* 3–15.

12. Beck, A., Barnes, K., Vogel, K., & Grice, K. (2006). The dilemma of psychosocial occupational therapy in public schools: The therapists' perceptions. *Occupational Therapy in Mental Health, 22,* 1–17.

13. Beidel, D. C., Turner, S. M., & Morris, T. L. (1995). A new inventory to assess child social phobia: The Social Phobia and Anxiety Inventory for Children. *Psychological Assessment, 7,* 73–79.

14. Beker, J., & Feuerstein, R., (1991). The modifying environment and other environmental perspectives in group care: A conceptual contrast and integration. *Residential Treatment for Children and Youth, 8*(3), 21–36.

15. Belle, D. (1990). Poverty and women's mental health. *American Psychologist, 45,* 385–389.

16. Belsky, J. (1999). Quantity of nonmaternal care and boys' problem behavior/adjustment at ages 3 and 5: Exploring the mediating role of parenting. *Psychiatry, 62*(1), 1–20.

17. Belsky, J., Fish, M., & Isabella, R. (1991). Continuity and incontinuity in infant negative and positive emotionality: Family antecedent and attachment consequences. *Developmental Psychology, 27,* 421–431.

18. Bendersky, M., & Lewis, M. (1994). Environmental risk, biological risk, and developmental outcome. *Developmental Psychology, 30,* 484–494.

19. Biederman, J. (1997). Is there a childhood form of bipolar disorder? *Harvard Mental Health Letter, 13,* 8.

20. Blackorby, J., & Wagner, M. (1996). Longitudinal post school outcomes of youth with disabilities: Findings from the National Longitudinal Transition Study. *Exceptional Children, 62,* 399–413.

21. Block, B., & Lefkovitz, P. (1992). *Standards and guidelines for partial hospitalization.* Alexandria, VA: American Association for Partial Hospitalization.

22. Boden, J., Horwood, L., & Fergusson, D. (2007). Exposure to childhood sexual and physical abuse and subsequent educational achievement outcomes. *Child Abuse and Neglect, 31,* 1101–1114.

23. Botvin, G., Griffin, K., & Nichols, T. (2006). Preventing youth violence and delinquency through a universal school-based prevention approach. *Prevention Science, 7.* Retrieved May 2009, from http://www.springerlink.com/content/g7437517441m5lll/fulltext.html

24. Brollier, C., Shepherd, J., & Markley, K. (1994). Transition from school to community living. *American Journal of Occupational Therapy, 48,* 346–353.

25. Brown, R., Carpenter, L., & Simerly, E. (2005). *Mental health medications for children: A primer.* New York: Guilford Press.

26. Burke, J. P. (2003). Philosophical basis of human occupation. In P. Kramer, J. Hinojosa, & C.B. Royeen (Eds.), Perspectives in *human occupation: Participation in life* (pp. 32–44). New York: Lippincott Williams & Wilkins.

27. Carson, R. R., Sitlington, P. L., & Frank, A. R. (1995). Young adulthood for individuals with behavioral disorders: What does it hold? *Behavioral Disorders, 20,* 127–135.

28. Case, B., Olfson, M., Marcus, S., & Siegel, C. (2007). Trends in inpatient mental health treatment of children and adolescents in U.S. community hospitals between 1990 and 2000. *Archives of General Psychiatry, 64,* 89–96.

29. Case-Smith, J., & Arbesman, M. (2008). Evidence-based review of interventions for autism used in or of relevance to occupational therapy. *American Journal of Occupational Therapy, 62,* 416–429.

30. Case-Smith, J., & Archer, L. (2008). School-based services for students with emotional disturbance: Findings and recommendations. *OT Practice, 13,* 17–21.

31. Centers for Disease Control and Prevention. (2008).

32. Chafel, J. A., & Hadley, K. G. (2001). Poverty and the well-being of children and families. In C. E. Walker & M. C. Roberts (Eds.), *Handbook of clinical psychology* (pp. 48–71). New York: John Wiley & Sons.

33. Chess, S. (1997). Temperament: Theory and clinical practice. *The Harvard Mental Health Letter, 14*(5), 5–7.

34. Chess, S., & Thomas, A. (1983). Dynamics of individual behavioral development. In M. D. Levine, W. B. Carey, A. C. Crocker, & R. T. Gross (Eds.), *Developmental-behavioral pediatrics* (pp. 158–175). Philadelphia: W.B. Saunders.

35. Chess, S., & Thomas, A. (1987). *Know your child.* New York: Basic Books.

36. Child Welfare Information Gateway. (2008). Home page. Retrieved May 2009, from http://www.childwelfare.gov/

37. Constantino, J. (1993). Parents, mental illness, and primary health care of infants and young children. *Zero to Three, 13*(5), 1–10.

38. Cooley, M. (2007) *Mental health and learning disorders in the regular classroom: How to recognize, understand, and help challenged (and challenging) students succeed.* Minneapolis: Free Spirit Publishing.

39. Coplan, J. (2000). Counseling parents regarding prognosis in autistic spectrum disorder. *Pediatrics, 105.* Retrieved May, 2009, from http://www.pediatrics.org/cgi/content/full/105/5/e65

40. Cornell, T., & Hamrin, V. (2008). Clinical interventions for children with attachment problems. *Journal of Child and Adolescent Psychiatric Nursing, 21,* 35–47.

41. Correia, L., & Linhares, M. (2007). Maternal anxiety in the pre- and postnatal period: A literature review. *Review of Latino-American Enfermagem, 15,* 677–683.

42. Costello, E. J., Compton, S., Keeler, G., & Angold, A. (2003). Relationships between poverty and psychopathology: A natural experiment. *Journal of the American Medical Association, 290,* 2023–2029.

43. Coster, W., Deeney, T., Haltiwanger, J., & Haley, S. (1998). *School function assessment.* San Antonio, TX: Psychological Corporation.

44. Coulton, C., Korbin, J., Su, M., & Chow, J. (1995). Community level factors and child maltreatment rates. *Child Development, 66,* 1262–1276.

45. Crick, N. R., & Ladd, G. W. (1993). Children's perceptions of their peer experiences: Attributions, loneliness, social anxiety and social avoidance. *Developmental Psychology, 29,* 244–254.

46. Cuevas, C., Finkelhor, D., Ormrod, R., & Turner, H. (2009). Psychiatric diagnosis as a risk marker for victimization in a national sample of children. *Journal of Interpersonal Violence, 24*(4), 636–652.

47. Dalton, R., & Forman, M. (1992). *Psychiatric hospitalization of school-age children.* Washington, DC: American Psychiatric Press.

48. Daly, D., Schmidt, M., Spellman, D., Criste, T., Dinges, K., & Teare, J. (1998). The Boys' Town residential treatment center: Treatment implications and preliminary outcomes. *Child and Youth Care Forum, 27*(4), 267–279.

49. Davidson, D. (2001). Measuring the outcome of Rational Intervention: A behavior management approach for children and adolescents in residential care. Unpublished manuscript.

50. Davidson, D., & LaVessar, P. (1998). Facilitating adaptive behaviors in school-aged children with psychosocial problems. In J. Case-Smith (Ed.), *AOTA self-study series: Occupational therapy: Making a difference in school based practice.* Bethesda, MD: American Occupational Therapy Association.

51. Dunn, W. (2002). Sensory processing issues associated with Asperger syndrome: A preliminary investigation. *Focus on Autism and Other Developmental Disabilities, 56,* 97–102.

52. Durrant, M. (1993). *Residential treatment: A cooperative, competency-based approach to therapy and program design.* New York: W.W. Norton.

53. Egeland, B., Sroufe, A., & Erickson, M. (1983). The developmental consequences of different patterns of maltreatment. *Child Abuse and Neglect, 7,* 459–469.

54. Erker, G., Searight, H. R., Amant, E., & White, P. (1993). Residential versus day treatment for children: A long-term follow-up study. *Child Psychiatry and Human Development, 24,* 31–39.

55. Feeny, J. A. (1996). Attachment, caregiving, and marital satisfaction. *Personal Relationships, 3,* 401–416.

56. Florey, L. (1989). Nationally speaking: Treating the whole child: Rhetoric or reality? *American Journal of Occupational Therapy, 43,* 365–368.

57. Florey, L., & Greene, S. (2008). Play in middle childhood. In L. D. Parham, & L. S. Fazio (Eds.) *Play in occupational therapy for children* (2nd ed., pp.279–299). St. Louis: Mosby.

58. Fox, N., & Card, J. (1999). In C. E. Walker, & M. C. Roberts (Eds.), *Handbook of clinical psychology* (3rd ed., pp. 226–245). New York: John Wiley & Sons.

59. Frodi, A. (1981). Contribution of child characteristics to child abuse. *American Journal of Mental Deficiency, 85,* 341–345.

60. Fuertes, M., Lopes Dos Santos, P., Beeghly, M., & Tronick, E. (2006). More than maternal sensitivity shapes attachment: Infant coping and temperament. *Annals of the New York Academy of Sciences, 1094,* 292–296.

61. Gabarino, J., & Kostelny, K. (1992). Child maltreatment as a community problem. *Child Abuse and Neglect, 16,* 455–464.

62. Galantino, M., Galbavy, R., & Quinn, L. (2008). Therapeutic effects of yoga for children: A systematic review of the literature. *Pediatric Physical Therapy, 20,* 66–80.

63. Gilbert, B. O., Greening, L., & Dollinger, S. J. (2001). Neurotic disorders in children: Obsessive-compulsive, somatoform, dissociative, and post-traumatic stress disorders. In C. E. Walker & M. C. Roberts (Eds.), *Handbook of clinical psychology* (3rd ed., pp. 414–431). New York: John Wiley & Sons.

64. Gleason, M., Egger, H., Emslie, G., Greenhill, L., Kowatch, R., Lieberman, et al (2007). Pharmacological treatment for very young children: Contexts and guidelines. *Journal of the American Academy of Child and Adolescent Psychiatry, 46,* 1532–1572.

65. Goldstrom, I., Jaiquan, F., Henderson, M., Male, M. A., & Manderscheid, R. W. (2000). Jail mental health services: A national survey. In R. W. Manderscheid & M .J. Henderson (Eds.), *Mental Health, United States, 1998* (DHHS Publication No.SMA-99-3285, pp. 176–187). Washington, DC: U.S. Government Printing Office.

66. Gresham, F., & Elliot, S. (1993). Social skills intervention guide: Systematic approaches to social skills training. *Special Services in the Schools, 8,* 137–158.

67. Griffin, K. W., Botvin, G. J., & Nichols, T. R. (2006). Effects of a school-based drug abuse prevention program for adolescents on HIV risk behaviors in young adulthood. *Prevention Science, 7,* 103–112.

68. Harden, P. W., & Zoccolillo, M. (1997). Disruptive behavior disorders. *Current Opinions in Pediatrics, 9,* 339–345.

69. Harrington, R., Fudge, H., Rutter, M., Pickles, A., & Hill, J. (1990). Adult outcomes of childhood and adolescent depression I. *Archives of General Psychiatry, 47,* 465–473.

70. Harvard Health Publications. (2004). Children's fears and anxieties. *Harvard Mental Health Letter, 21*(6), 1–4.

71. Harvard Health Publications. (2005). In brief: Is the rate of autism rising? *Harvard Mental Health Letter, 22*(3), 6.

72. Harvard Health Publications. (2007). Bipolar disorder in children: Difficult to diagnose, important to treat. *Harvard Mental Health Letter, 23*(11), 1–4.

73. Hazan, C., & Zeifman, D. (1999). Pair bonds as attachments. In J. Cassidy & P. Shaver (Eds.), *Handbook of attachment: Theory, research, and clinical applications* (pp. 336–354). New York: Guilford Press.

74. Hickman, L., & Orentilicher, M. (2001). Transition from school to adult life for students with autism. In H. Miller-Kuhaneck (Ed.), *Autism: A comprehensive occupational therapy approach* (pp. 237–268). Bethesda, MD: American Occupational Therapy Association.

75. Hilton, C., Graver, K., & LaVessar, P. (2006). Relationship between social competence and sensory processing in children

with high functioning autism spectrum disorders. *Research in Autism Spectrum Disorders, 1,* 164–173.

76. Hoagwood, K., Burnes, B., Kiser, L., Ringeisen, H., & Schoenwald, S. (2001). Evidence-based practices in child and adolescent mental health services. *Psychiatric Services, 52,* 1179–1189.

77. Hofer, M. (1994). Hidden regulators in attachment, separation, and loss. *Monographs for the Society for Research in Child Development, 59,* 192–207, 250-283.

78. Hoffman-Plotkin, D., & Twentyman, C. (1984). A multimodal assessment of behavioral and cognitive deficits in abused and neglected preschoolers. *Child Development, 55,* 794–802.

79. Humphry, R. (1995). Families who live in chronic poverty: Meeting the challenge of family-centered services. *American Journal of Occupational Therapy, 49,* 687–693.

80. Hurley, K., Black, M., Papas, M., & Caufield, L. (2008). Community and international nutrition: Maternal symptoms of stress, depression, and anxiety are related to nonresponsive feeding styles in a statewide sample of WIC participants. *Journal of Nutrition, 138,* 799–805.

81. IDEAdata.org. (2008). Data tables for OSEP state reported data. Retrieved August, 2008, from https://www.ideadata.org/index.html

82. Jans, L., Stoddard, S., & Kraus, L. (2004). *Chartbook on mental health and disability in the United States.* An InfoUse Report. Washington, DC: U.S. Department of Education, National Institute on Disability and Rehabilitation Research.

83. Jasinski, J. L., Williams, L. M., & Siegel, J. (2000). Childhood physical and sexual abuse as a risk factor for heavy drinking among African-American women: A prospective study. *Child Abuse and Neglect, 24,* 1061–1071.

84. Jaudes, P. K., & Diamond, L. J. (1985). The handicapped child and child abuse. *Child Abuse and Neglect, 9,* 341–347.

85. Johnson, R., Kotch, J., Catellier, D., Winsor, J., Dufort, V., Hunter, W., et al. (2002). Adverse behavioral and emotional outcomes from child abuse and witnessed violence. *Child Maltreatment, 7,* 179–186.

86. Jones-Webb, R. J., Snowden, I., Herd, D., Short, B., & Hannan, P. (1997). Alcohol-related problems among black, Hispanic, and white men: The contributions of neighborhood poverty. *Journal of Studies on Alcohol, 58,* 539–545.

87. Kagan, J., & Zentner, M. (1996). Early childhood predictors of adult psychopathology. *Harvard Review of Psychiatry, 3,* 341-350.

88. Katic, A., & Steingard, R. J. (2001). Pharmacotherapy. In C. E. Walker & M. C. Roberts (Eds.), *Handbook of clinical psychology* (3rd ed., pp. 928–951). New York: John Wiley & Sons.

89. Kennedy, P., Kupst, M., Westman, G., Zaar, C., Pines, R., & Schulman, J. (1990). Use of timeout procedures in a child psychiatry inpatient milieu: Combining dynamic and behavioral approaches. *Child Psychiatry and Human Development, 20,* 207–216.

90. Keogh, B. K. (1986). Temperament and schooling: Meaning of "goodness of fit"? *New Directions in Child Development, 31,* 89-108.

91. Keogh, B. K., & Burstein, N. D. (1988). Relationship of temperament to preschoolers' interactions with peers and teachers. *Exceptional Child, 54,* 456–461.

92. Khalid-Khan, S., Santibanez, M., McMicken, C., Rynn, M. (2007). A social anxiety disorder in children and adolescents: Epidemiology, diagnosis, and treatment. *Pediatric Drugs, 9,* 227–237.

93. Knis-Matthews, L., Richard, L., Marquez, L., & Mevawala, N. (2005). Implementation of occupational therapy services for an adolescent residence program. *Occupational Therapy in Mental Health, 21,* 57–72.

94. Knox, S. (1974). A play scale. In M. Reilly (Ed.), *Play as exploratory learning: Studies in curiosity behavior.* Beverly Hills, CA: Sage.

95. Knox, S. (1997). Development and current use of the Knox Preschool Play Scale. In L. D. Parham, & L. S. Fazio (Eds.), *Play*

in occupational therapy for children (1st ed., pp. 35–51). St. Louis: Mosby.

96. Knox, S. (2008). Development and current use of the Revised Knox Preschool Play Scale. In L. D. Parham & L. S. Fazio (Eds.), *Play in occupational therapy for children* (2nd ed., pp. 55–70) St. Louis: Mosby.

97. Kolko, D. J. (2002). Child physical abuse. In J. E. B. Myers, L. Berliner, J. Briere, C.T. Hendrix, C. Jenny, et al. (Eds.), *The APSAC handbook on child maltreatment* (2nd ed.). Thousand Oaks, CA: Sage.

98. Kolko, D., Bukstein, O., & Barron, J. (1999). Methylphenidate and behavior modification in children with ADHD and co-morbid ODD or CD: Main and incremental effects across settings. *Journal of the American Academy of Child and Adolescent Psychiatry, 38,* 578–586.

99. Kovacs, M., Feinberg, T. L., Crouse-Novak, M. A., Paulauskas, S. L., & Finkelstein, R. (1984). Depressive disorders in childhood. I. *Archives of General Psychiatry, 41,* 229–237.

100. Kovacs, M., Feinberg, T. L., Crouse-Novak, M. A., Paulauskas, S. L., & Finkelstein, R. (1984b). Depressive disorders in childhood. II. *Archives of General Psychiatry, 41,* 643–649.

101. Kraemer, G. (1992). A psychobiological theory of attachment. *Behavioral and Brain Sciences, 15,* 493–541.

102. Landolf, B. (2005). Out-patient private practice model. In R. Steele & M. Roberts (Eds.), *Handbook of mental health services for children, adolescents, and families.* New York: Kluwer Academic/Plenum Publishers.

103. Lang, A., Aarons, G., Gearity, J., Laffaye, C., Satz, L., Dresselhaus, T., et al. (2008). Direct links between child maltreatment, posttraumatic stress disorder, and women's health. *Behavioral Medicine, 33,* 125–135.

104. Lansford, J., Miller-Johnson, S., Berlin, L., Dodge, K., Bates, J., & Pettit, G. (2007). Early physical abuse and later violent delinquency: A prospective longitudinal study. *Child Maltreatment, 12,* 233–245.

105. Law, M., Baptiste, S., Carswell, A., McColl, M., Polatajko, H., & Pollack, N. (2005). *The Canadian Occupational Performance Measure* (revised). Ottawa, Ontario: Canadian Association of Occupational Therapy.

106. Law, M., Cooper, B., Strong, S., Stewart, D., Rigby, P., & Letts, L. (1996). The person-environment-occupation model: A transactive approach to occupational performance. *Canadian Journal of Occupational Therapy, 63,* 9–23.

107. Leary, M.R., & Kowalski, R.M. (1995). *Social anxiety.* New York: Guilford Press.

108. Locke, A., Ginsborg, J., & Peers, I. (2003). Development and disadvantage: Implications for the early years and beyond. *International Journal of Language and Communication Disorders, 37,* 3–15.

109. Lourie, I. (2003). A history of community child mental health. In A. Pumariega & N. Winters (Eds.), *Handbook of community-based systems of care: The new child and adolescent community psychiatry.* New York: Jossey-Bass.

110. Maag, J. W., & Katsiyannis, A. (1996). Counseling as a related service for students with emotional or behavioral disorders: Issues and recommendations. *Behavioral Disorders, 21,* 293–305.

111. Maag, J., & Katsiyannis, A. (1998). Challenges facing successful transition for youths with E/BD. *Behavioral Disorders, 23,* 209–221.

112. Macro International, Inc. (1997). *Annual report to congress on the evaluation of the comprehensive community mental health services for children and their families program.* Atlanta, Georgia.

113. MacLeod, J., & Nelson, G. (2000). Programs for the promotion of family wellness and the prevention of child maltreatment: A meta-analytic review. *Child Abuse and Neglect, 24,* 1127–1149.

114. Mailloux, Z., & Roley, S. S. (2001). Sensory integration. In H. Miller-Kuhaneck (Ed.), *Autism: A comprehensive occupational therapy approach.* Bethesda, MD: American Occupational Therapy Association.

115. Main, M. (1995). Attachment: Overview, with implications for clinical work. In S. Goldberg, R. Muir, & J. Kerr (Eds.), *Attachment theory: Social, developmental, and clinical perspectives* (pp. 407–474). Hillsdale, NJ: Analytic Press.

116. Main, M. (1996). Overview of the field of attachment. *Journal of Consulting and Clinical Psychology, 64,* 237–243.

117. Main, M., & Solomon, J. (1990). Procedures for identifying infants as disorganized/disoriented during the Ainsworth Strange Situation. In M. T. Greenberg, D. Cicchetti, & E. M. Cummings (Eds.), *Attachment in the preschool years: Theory, research, and intervention* (pp. 121–160). Chicago: University of Chicago Press.

118. Manderscheid, R. W., & Sonnenschein, M. A. (1992). *Mental health, United States, 1992* (DHSS Publication No. ADM 92-1942). Washington, DC: US Government Printing Office.

119. Martin, K., Lloyd, J., Kauffman, J., & Coyne, M. (1995). Teachers' perceptions of educational placement decisions for pupils with emotional and behavioral disorders. *Behavioral Disorders, 20,* 106–117.

120. Masi, Hawkley, L., Piotrowski, Z., & Pickett, K. (2007). Neighborhood economic disadvantage, violent crime, group density, and pregnancy outcomes in a diverse, urban population. *Social Science in Medicine, 65,* 2440–2457.

121. McLoyd, V. C. (1990). The impact of economic hardship on black families and children: Psychological distress, parenting, and socioemotional development. *Child Development, 61,* 311–346.

122. Miller, L. (2006). *Miller Function and Participation Scales (M-FUN).* New York: Harcourt.

123. Milliken, B., Goodman, G., Bazyk, S., & Flinn, S. (2007). Establishing a case for occupational therapy in meeting the needs of children with grief issues in school-based settings. *Occupational Therapy in Mental Health, 23,* 75–100.

124. Milling, L. S. (2001). Depression in preadolescents. In C. E. Walker & M. C. Roberts (Eds.), *Handbook of clinical psychology* (3rd ed., pp. 373–392). New York: John Wiley & Sons.

125. Moller, B. (2001). A grieving child. *The ASCA School Counselor, 39,* 14–17.

126. National Board for Certification in Occupational Therapy. (2008). *Executive summary for the practice analysis study.* Retrieved September 2008, from http://www.nbcot.org.

127. National Institutes of Mental Health. (2007). Autism spectrum disorders: Pervasive developmental disorders (addendum January 2007). Retrieved August, 2008, from http://www.nimh.nih.gov/health/publications/autism/complete-publication.shtml.

128. Nelson, R., & Condrin, J. (1987). A vocational readiness and independent living skills program for psychiatrically impaired adolescents. *Occupational Therapy in Mental Health, 7,* 105–113.

129. Nigg, J., & Goldsmith, H. (1998). Developmental psychopathology, personality, and temperament: Reflections on recent behavioral genetics research. *Human Biology, 70*(2), 387–412.

130. Office of Special Education and Rehabilitation Services, U.S. Department of Education. (2005). *25th annual report to congress on the implementation of the individuals with disabilities education act.* Retrieved September 20, 2008, from http://www.ed.gov/about/reports/annual/osep/2003/25th-vol-1.pdf.

131. Ogata, S., Silk, K., Goodrich, S., Lohr, N., Westen, D., & Hill, E. (1990). Childhood sexual and physical abuse in adult patients with borderline personality disorder. *American Journal of Psychiatry, 147,* 1008–1013.

132. Olfson, M., Blanco, C., Liu, L., Moreno, C., & Laje, G. (2006). National trends in the outpatient treatment of children and

adolescents with antipsychotic drugs. *Archives of General Psychiatry, 63*, 679–685.

133. Olson, L. (2006). *Activity groups in family-centered treatment: psychiatric occupational therapy approaches for parents and children.* New York: Haworth Press.

134. Orentlicher, M. L., & Olson, L. J. (2004). Transition from school to adult life for students with autism. In H. Miller-Kuhaneck (Ed.), *Autism: A comprehensive occupational therapy approach* (2nd ed.). Bethesda, MD: American Occupational Therapy Association.

135. Peloquin, S. (1993). The patient-therapist relationship: Beliefs that shape care. *American Journal of Occupational Therapy, 47*, 935–942.

136. Pfefferbaum, B. (1997). Posttraumatic stress disorder in children: A review of the past 10 years. *Journal of the American Academy of Child and Adolescent Psychiatry, 36*, 1503–1511.

137. Pickens, J., & Field, T. (1993). Facial expressivity in infants of depressed mothers. *Developmental Psychology, 29*, 986–988.

138. Pottick, K., McAlpine, D., & Andelman, R. (2000). Changing patterns of psychiatric inpatient care for children and adolescents in general hospitals, 1988-1995. *American Journal of Psychiatry, 157*, 1267–1273.

139. Powers, S. W. (2001). Behavior therapy with children. In C. E. Walker & M. C. Roberts (Eds.), *Handbook of clinical psychology* (3rd ed., pp. 4825–4839). New York: John Wiley & Sons, Inc.

140. Prothro-Stith, D. (1991). *Deadly consequences: How violence is destroying our teenage population and a plan to begin solving the problem.* New York: Harper Collins.

141. Pruitt, D., & Kiser, L. (1991). Day treatment: Past, present, and future. In M. Lewis (Ed.), *Child and adolescent psychiatry: A comprehensive textbook.* Baltimore: Williams & Wilkins.

142. Richardson, P. (2002). The school as social context: Social interaction patterns of children with physical disabilities. *American Journal of Occupational Therapy, 56*, 296–304.

143. Robinson, K. & Rapport, L. (2002). Outcomes of a school-based mental health program for youth with serious emotional disorders. *Psychology in the Schools, 3*, 661–676.

144. Rothbart, M. K. (1991). Temperament: A developmental framework. In J. Strelau & A. Angleitner (Eds.), *Explorations in temperament: International perspectives on theory and measurement* (pp. 2235–2260). London: Plenum Press.

145. Rothe, E. M., & Castellanos, D. (2001) Anxiety disorders in children and adolescents. In H. B. Vance, & A. J. Pumariega (Eds.), *Clinical assessment of child and adolescent behavior* (pp. 383–412). New York: John Wiley & Sons.

146. Sabatino, D. A., Webster, B., & Vance, H. B. (2001). Childhood mood disorders: History, characteristics, diagnosis, and treatment. In H. B. Vance & A. J. Pumariega (Eds.), *Clinical assessment of child and adolescent behavior* (pp. 413–449). New York: John Wiley & Sons.

147. Schultz, S. (1992). School-based occupational therapy for students with behavioral disorders. *Occupational Therapy in Health Care, 8*, 173–196.

148. Schultz, S. (2003). AOTA continuing education article: Psychosocial occupational therapy in schools. *OT Practice*, September 2003, CE-1-CE-8.

149. Sidebotham, P., & Golding, J. (2001). Avon longitudinal study of parents and children. *Child Abuse and Neglect, 25*, 1177–1200.

150. Sidebotham, P., & Herson, J. (2006). Child maltreatment in the "children of the nineties": A cohort study of risk factors. *Child Abuse and Neglect, 30*, 497–522.

151. Silverman, W. K., & Ginsberg, G. S. (1998). Anxiety disorders. In T. H. Ollendick & M. Hersen (Eds.), *Handbook of child psychopathology* (3rd ed., pp. 239–268). New York: Plenum Press.

152. Skard, G., & Bundy, A. (2008). Test of Playfulness. In L. D. Parham & L. S. Fazio (Eds.), *Play in occupational therapy for children* (2nd ed., pp. 71–91). St. Louis: Mosby.

153. Spencer, N., Wallace, A., Sundrum, R., Bachus, C., & Logan, S. (2006). Child abuse registration, fetal growth, and preterm birth: A population based study. *Journal of Epidemiology and Community Health, 60*, 337–340.

154. Sperry, L. (2003). *Handbook of diagnosis and treatment of DSM-IV-TR personality disorders* (2nd ed.). New York: Brunner-Routledge.

155. Spreat, S., & Jampol, R. (1997). Residential services for children and adolescents. In R. T. Ammerman & M. Hersen (Eds.), *Intervention in the real world context: Handbook of prevention and treatment with children and adolescents* (pp. 106–133). New York: John Wiley & Sons.

156. Stein, F. (1995). *Residential treatment of adolescents and children: Issues, principles, and techniques.* Chicago: Nelson-Hall Publishers.

157. Sullivan, P. M., & Knutson, J. F. (2000). Maltreatment and disabilities: A population-based epidemiological study. *Child Abuse and Neglect, 24*, 1257–1273.

158. Thomas, A., Chess, S., & Birch, H. (1968). *Temperament and behavior disorders in children.* New York: New York University Press.

159. Thompson, R. (2002). The view from research: The roots of school readiness in social and emotional development. *The Kauffman Early Education Exchange, 1*(1), 8–29.

160. Thomsen, P., & Mikkelsen, H. (1995). Course of OCD in children and adolescents. *Journal of the American Academy of Child and Adolescent Psychiatry, 34*, 1432–1440.

161. Townsend, S., Carey, P., Hollins, N., Helfrich, C., Blondis, M., Hoffman, A., et al (2001). *Occupational therapy psychosocial assessment of learning.* Chicago: Model of Occupational Therapy Products.

162. Trieschman, A., Whittaker, J., & Brendtro, J. (1969). *The other 23 hours: Child-care work with emotionally disturbed children in a therapeutic milieu.* Chicago: Aldine Publishing Company.

163. Tuma, J. (1989). Mental health services for children: The state of the art. *American Psychologist, 44*, 188–199.

164. DeNavas-Walt, C., Proctor, B., & Lee, C. (2006). Income, Poverty, and health insurance coverage in the United States. U.S. Census Bureau.

165. U.S. Department of Health and Human Services. (2004). *Comprehensive community mental health services program for children and their families.* Retrieved September 20, 2008, from http://mentalhealth.samhsa.gov/publications/allpubs/Ca-0013/default.asp.

166. U.S. Department of Health and Human Services, Administration on Children, Youth and Families. (2006). *Child maltreatment 2006.* Washington, DC: U.S. Government Printing Office. Retrieved September 15, 2008, from http://www.acf.hhs.gov/programs/cb/stats_research/index.htm#can

167. U.S. Public Health Service. (1999). *Mental health: A report of the Surgeon General.* Retrieved May, 2009, from http://www.surgeongeneral.gov/library/mentalhealth/home.html

168. van den Boom, D. (1990). Preventive intervention and the quality of mother-infant interaction and infant exploration in irritable infants. In W. Koops, H. J. G. Soppe, J. L. van der Linden, P. C. M. Molenaar & J. J. F. Schroots (Eds.), *Developmental psychology behind the dikes: An outline of developmental psychology research in the Netherlands* (pp. 249–270). Amsterdam: Eburon.

169. van IJzendoorn, M., Juffer, F., & Duyvesteyn, M. (1995). Breaking the intergenerational cycle of insecure attachment: A review of the effects of attachment-based interventions on maternal sensitivity and infant security. *Journal of Child Psychology and Psychiatry, 36*, 225–248.

170. VanderVen, K. (1995). "Point and level systems": Another way to fail children and youth. *Child and Youth Care Forum, 24*, 345–367.

171. Vaughn, B. R., & Bost, K. K. (1999). Attachment and temperament: redundant, independent, or interactive influences on interpersonal adaptation and personality development? In J. Cassidy & P. Shaver (Eds.), *Handbook of attachment: Theory, research, and clinical applications* (pp. 198–225). New York: Guilford Press.

172. Vaughn, S., Kim, A., Sloan, C., Hughes, M., Elbaum, B., & Spridhaur, D. (2003). Social skills interventions for young children with disabilities: A synthesis of group design studies. *Remedial and Special Education, 24,* 2–15.

173. Verdugo, M. A., Bermejo, B. G., & Fuertes, J. (1995). The maltreatment of intellectually handicapped children and adolescents. *Child Abuse and Neglect, 19,* 205–215.

174. Vondra, J. I. (1990). Sociological and ecological factors. In R. T. Ammerman & M. Hersen (Eds.), *Children at risk: An evaluation of factors contributing to child abuse and neglect* (pp. 149–165). New York: Plenum Press.

175. Wagner, M. M. (1995). Outcomes for youths with serious emotional disturbance in secondary school and early adulthood. *Future Child, 5*(2), 90–112.

176. Wald, R. L., & Knutson, J. F. (2000). Childhood disciplinary experiences reported by adults with craniofacial anomalies. *Child Abuse and Neglect, 24,* 1623–1627.

177. Walker, R., & Bunsen, T. (1995). After high school: The status of youth with emotional and behavioral disorders. *Career Development of Exceptional Individuals, 18,* 97–107.

178. Waters, E., & Stroufe, A. (1983). Social competence as a developmental construct. *Developmental Review, 3,* 79–97.

179. Weinberg, N., Rahdert, E., Colliver, J., & Glantz, M. (1998). Adolescent substance abuse: A review of the past 10 years. *Journal of the American Academy of Child and Adolescent Psychiatry, 37*(3), 252–261.

180. Williams, M., & Shellengerger, S. (1996). *How does your engine run? A leader's guide to the ALERT program for self-regulation.* Albequerque, NM: Therapy Works.

181. Williamson, G. (1993). Enhancing the social competence of children with learning disabilities. *Sensory Integration Special Interest Section Newsletter, 16,* 1–2.

182. Willis, C. (2002). The grieving process in children: Strategies for understanding, educating, and reconciling children's perceptions of death. *Early Childhood Education Journal, 29,* 221–226.

183. Winters, N., & Pumariega, A. (2007). Practice parameter on child and adolescent mental health care in community systems of care. *Journal of the American Academy of Child and Adolescent Psychiatry, 46,* 284–299.

184. Wolfner, G., & Gelles, R. (1993). A profile of violence toward children: A national study. *Child Abuse and Neglect, 17,* 197–212.

185. Zametin, A. J., & Ernst, M. (1999). Review article: Problems in the management of attention-deficit-hyperactivity disorder. *New England Journal of Medicine, 340*(1), 40–46.

14

Interventions and Strategies for Challenging Behaviors

Renee Watling

OBJECTIVES

1. Describe reasons for behavior problems.
2. Explain how to prevent challenging behaviors from occurring.
3. Describe interventions for existing challenging behaviors.
4. Identify and describe specific strategies in behavior management.
5. Using case studies, discuss examples of behavioral intervention.

STRATEGIES FOR MANAGING DIFFICULT BEHAVIOR

Children with a variety of disability conditions may display challenging or inappropriate behaviors that interfere with daily life activities (Case Study 14-1). Behavior management strategies designed to prevent and reduce challenging behaviors are an important component of occupational therapy intervention for any child whose behaviors are interfering with occupational performance. This chapter introduces behavior management theories and presents strategies that have proven effective in preventing and reducing challenging or unacceptable behavior in children.

Much of what is known about challenging behavior and the strategies to facilitate behavior change has emerged from the fields of education and psychology. Robust research from these professions provides a wealth of knowledge that occupational therapists can apply to help understand why challenging behavior occurs, how to prevent challenging behavior, and how to intervene when a child exhibits challenging behavior (Table 14-1).

Behavior Happens

Behavior is an expressive act by an individual that can have many different forms and meanings. Whether a certain behavior is appropriate and acceptable is dependent on the context and contextual norms for the given situation. For example, in a public school building it would be inappropriate and unacceptable for a student to run out of a classroom onto the playground when the teacher passes out a work assignment; however, the same behavior would be appropriate and desirable in response to a ringing fire alarm. In turn, it is considered inappropriate and unacceptable for a child to scream and withdraw when his dinner plate loaded with green beans is placed on the table, but screaming and withdrawal are acceptable and possibly even anticipated when a child receives an immunization shot. As dynamic organisms with constantly active neurological, physiological, and physical systems, human beings interact with environments, materials, and other dynamic organisms. With so many variables at play, the possibility of a mismatch between two or more variables is likely. When such a mismatch occurs, undesired or inappropriate behavior may be exhibited.[21]

Inappropriate behavior can take many forms. Passive behaviors such as noncompliance, withdrawal, avoidance, inattention, or lack of response are not overtly disruptive but still interfere with occupational performance and participation. Active behaviors such as direct refusal to engage, opposition, aggression toward people or property, or self-injurious behavior not only interfere with occupational performance and participation but can also be disruptive or harmful. Both passive and active forms of inappropriate behavior can be difficult to manage.

Children exhibit challenging and inappropriate behaviors for many reasons. Some of these are internal and emerge from a lack of skill or ability to perform in a desired manner. Other reasons are related to external factors. Box 14-1 identifies some of the internal and external factors that influence behavior.

Purposes

To effectively manage difficult behavior, it is critical to remember that all behavior serves a purpose. Decades of research has identified three primary purposes of challenging behavior: (1) obtaining a desired object or event, (2) avoiding a situation,

CASE STUDY 14-1	Sam and Eli

Sam is a 2½-year-old boy who lives with his mother, father, and 6-year-old brother. Sam enjoys staying at home to play with his toys or watch movies. He plays by himself for unlimited periods of time. He spends many hours a day driving his cars and trucks back and forth while lying prone and watching the wheels turn. If his brother plays with the cars, Sam screams uncontrollably until the car is returned to him. Another of Sam's favorite activities is playing with balls. He pulls the basket of balls to the top of the stairs where he bounces them off the wall and down the stairs into the family room over and over. If someone else retrieves one of the balls or tries to engage Sam in a ball game, an ear-piercing scream is heard before Sam deteriorates into a kicking, screaming tantrum.

Sam's brother Eli is 6 years old. He attends kindergarten 5 days each week, where he follows the classroom routine, engages with teacher-directed activities, and plays side by side with his peers. At home, Eli plays by himself for up to 30 minutes at a time. He prefers activities such as coloring and playing with dinosaur figurines. His favorite color is blue and his coloring pictures show all shades of the hue. His favorite dinosaur is a Tyrannosaurus rex and Eli can recite a number of known facts about this creature. When a visitor comes to the family home, Eli inundates the person with incessant talk about the T-rex. His eye contact is spontaneous but fleeting. He is easily distracted, looking away from a task to investigate all noise or movement around him. When approached by others, Eli gives a quick "Hi" then directs his gaze to the person's shoulder and begins reciting facts about the T-rex.

Sam eats approximately 10 different foods. His diet is restricted by his own preferences for certain tastes and textures, and also by intolerance for gluten. His mother is careful to prepare foods that are gluten free and that she knows Sam will eat. He is able to use a spoon and fork moderately well but prefers to use his fingers for self-feeding. He refuses all fruits, vegetables, and dairy products. His mother has expressed concern about Sam's nutrition. His behavioral rigidity considerably impacts the family's daily life. He does well on weekdays during the school year while his brother is at school. On school days, Sam accompanies his mother on errands to one familiar place at a time if mother brings favorite toys and a snack. If mother tries to combine two errands into one trip, Sam tantrums and refuses to exit the car. Sam's behavior is much more erratic on weekends and holidays, when the schedule is inconsistent and more people are in the home.

Both Sam and Eli are diagnosed with developmental disabilities.

or (3) escaping from an undesired object, event, or demand.[9] The purpose of a given episode of challenging behavior can be accurately identified only by the person executing the behavior or through careful analysis of those factors that maintain and strengthen the behavior. However, while a challenging behavior is being displayed, the individual likely is not in a state in which he can articulate the purpose of the behavior. This can be problematic for others who are experiencing the effects of the behavior and who want the behavior to stop. Functional behavioral analysis (FBA) is a formal process for evaluating the factors influencing behavior including the antecedents (events occurring before and triggering the behavior) and consequences (events after the behavior that also serve to reinforce the behavior). An FBA can be resource intensive and often is reserved for situations in which extreme or dangerous behaviors are occurring. The formal FBA process is described later in the chapter. For less severe situations, the FBA can be conducted informally by determining mismatches between the person and the context that are in effect when the challenging behavior is being executed.

Being Prepared for Problem Behavior

A variety of general strategies can be implemented to help create a context in which challenging behaviors are less likely to occur and more readily managed if they do occur. The following methods are suggested as general approaches to being prepared for problem behavior. These strategies are recommended as first steps in working to reduce the possibility of problem behavior; as children become more skilled, it is appropriate to adjust the type, structure, frequency, and intensity of supports provided.

Ruling Out Pain or Illness

Children experiencing pain or illness can act out in a variety of ways.[2] Pain-based behaviors can be especially difficult to identify in children who are nonverbal. Behaviors associated with pain or illness may have a sudden onset, be associated with a certain body position, be cyclic, or occur frequently for no apparent external reason. If behaviors appear to be associated with pain, the occupational therapy practitioner should work with others to determine whether the behavior is driven by pain and, if appropriate, should follow through with recommendations to remediate the source of pain.

Establishing Predictability and Consistency

Maintaining a consistent context in relation to schedule, environment, people, and demeanor helps to allay a child's anxiety about what is going to happen next.[8] When anxiety is diminished, the child has more resources available to direct toward self-management and productivity. Children are more successful when expectations, environments, people, and situations are familiar. As much as is possible, the occupational therapy practitioner should work to increase the known and decrease the unknown. Examples of strategies are scheduling activities in a similar order and location from day to day, keeping the physical arrangement and furnishings in the environment consistent, offering the same type of activities, establishing consistent social expectations, and arranging to have the same people interact with the child during the same activities.

Creating a Calm Atmosphere

Keeping the physical environment clean and organized creates a sense of order and predictability. Children know where to find desired items and they know which areas to avoid if there

TABLE 14-1 Selected Single-Subject-Design Studies of Behavior Management Interventions

Authors	Research Design	Research Questions/ Hypothesis	Sample	Measures	Intervention	Findings
Dettmer, Simpson, Myles, & Ganz (2000)	Single subject reversal ABAB	Effectiveness of visual supports to aid transition between activities	2 children with autism ages 5 and 7 yr	Duration of time to transition with and without the visual support	Visual schedule representing sequence of daily activities	Significant decrease in latency to transition and number of adult-delivered instructions when visual supports were used
Foxx & Meindl (2007)	Single subject AB	Intensive behavior management program to treat aggression and create academic challenge	13-yr-old boy with autism and history of progressively aggressive and destructive behaviors	Frequency of behaviors pre- and post-treatment	Functional assessment, token economy, reinforcement, overcorrection, crisis management	Reduction in negative physical and verbal behaviors to near zero levels within 6 mo accompanied by increased time engaged in educational activities
Scattone, Wilczynski, Edwards, & Rabian (2002)	Single subject multiple baseline across participants	Effectiveness of individualized social story at reducing specific disruptive behaviors	3 children with autism ages 7 yr, 7 yr, and 15 yr	Frequency of disruptive behavior pre- and post-intervention	Social stories developed and implemented according to Gray's (1998) guidelines	Each child demonstrated a decrease in the targeted disruptive behavior after implementation of the intervention
Schindler & Horner (2005)	Single subject, concurrent multiple baselines across settings	Effect of functional communication skills training on generalized reduction of problem behavior in multiple settings	3 children with autism ages 4–5 yr	Frequency of problem behavior, use of functional communication skills	Low-effort interventions and functional communication training	Low-effort interventions are more effective at reducing problem behaviors in multiple settings when used after functional communication skills training

Dettmer, S., Simpson, R. L., Myles, B. S., & Ganz, J. B. (2000). The use of visual supports to facilitate transitions of students with autism. *Focus on Autism and Other Developmental Disabilities, 15,* 163-169; Foxx, R. M., & Meindl, J. (2007). The long term successful treatment of the aggressive/destructive behaviors of a preadolescent with autism. *Behavioral Interventions, 22,* 83-97; Scattone, D., Wilczynski, S. M., Edwards, R. P., & Rabian B. (2002). Decreasing disruptive behaviors of children with autism using social stories. *Journal of Autism and Developmental Disorders, 32,* 535-543; and Schindler, H. R., & Horner, R. H. (2005). Generalized reduction of problem behavior of young children with autism: Building trans-situational interventions. *American Journal on Mental Retardation, 110,* 36-47; Gray, C. (1998). Social Stories and comic strip conversations with students with Asperger's syndrome and high functioning autism. In E. Schopler, G. Mesibov & L. Kunce (Eds.), *Asperger syndrome or high functioning autism?* (pp. 167-198). New York: Plenum Press.

BOX 14-1   Factors That Influence Behavior

INTERNAL FACTORS
- Desire for control
- Fatigue
- Illness
- Ineffective communication
- Pain
- Poor emotional regulation
- Poor self-regulation
- Poor sensory processing

EXTERNAL FACTORS
- Task demands greater than skill level
- Change in schedule
- Unfamiliar person
- Unfamiliar place

re items that are off limits. In addition, maintaining a calm demeanor when mishaps occur can help to minimize chaos and preserve a sense of order. Children often react to the stress and anxiety displayed by others with a disorganization of their own behavior. When adults remain calm, a sense of order is maintained and the child is at ease.

Attending to Appropriate Behaviors

It has been said that for every negative comment, a child should hear at least eight positive comments.[11] Adults should consistently reward and reinforce appropriate behaviors by attending to them, complimenting the child on his behavior, and identifying specifically what the child did that was appreciated. Specific feedback can increase the child's awareness of the behaviors that are desired. Although general feedback can help a child build confidence in his ability to produce desired behaviors, specific feedback helps the child know exactly what to do the next time and increases the likelihood that the desired behaviors will occur again.

Using "Do" Statements

Similar to providing specific feedback, using "do" statements tells a child exactly what is desired. Rather than telling a child "Don't pull Susie's hair," the occupational therapy practitioner rephrases the statement to direct the child to do a behavior that is desired: for example, "Use your hands for nice touching." In contrast with the "don't" statement, the "do" statement appeals to the child's desire to please and helps to keep a positive atmosphere. Modeling the instructed behavior while saying the instruction helps to reinforce what is being communicated.

Keeping Perspective

Challenging behavior happens despite preventive measures. As children learn and grow through new stages of development and independence, they continually seek to discover where limits exist, where their capabilities lie, and what they are allowed to do. It is important for the practitioner to be prepared to respond whenever the challenging behavior occurs, so that expectations for appropriate behavior are quickly and effectively re-established.

BEHAVIOR MANAGEMENT APPROACHES

Three primary approaches to managing challenging behavior are presented in this chapter: (1) preventing challenging behavior from occurring, (2) supporting desired behaviors, and (3) intervening when challenging behavior already exists. Strategies associated with each of these approaches are discussed in this section.

Preventing Challenging Behavior

Strategies for preventing challenging behavior are similar to the general strategies for supporting appropriate behavior. However, these strategies can be very effective when a child is known to have a repertoire of challenging behaviors and the goal is to prevent those behaviors from emerging.

Minimizing Aversive Events

Children often demonstrate inappropriate behaviors in response to events that they find aversive (Case Study 14-2).[9] To minimize aversive events, situations and scenarios must be perceived through the child's eyes. In other words, the occupational therapy practitioner should think about what it is that the child finds aversive. Often these are things that adults or other children do not consider problematic. Careful consideration of a particular child's temperament, personality, likes, dislikes, skills, abilities, and sensory processing tendencies can be helpful in identifying those conditions and events that the child finds aversive. When an aversive condition is identified, minimizing the frequency, intensity, or duration of the condition can help to reduce the child's reactive behaviors. If the correct events or conditions are not identified and addressed, no change in the behavior should be expected.

Sharing Control

Children often have very little control over their environments and the situations that surround them throughout the day. By allowing the child to choose activities, determine the order of events, or contribute his ideas about what should happen, the occupational therapy practitioner can instill a sense of value and build self-esteem. The experiences of making acceptable choices, contributing to a collaborative effort, and giving valued input not only help the child to feel important but can foster a sense of commitment to the therapeutic relationship. In turn, this can create the desire to preserve the relationship through effective and appropriate behaviors.

Providing an Environment That Promotes Successful Engagement

Challenging behaviors often occur when a child is bored or unoccupied. Providing an environment that promotes engagement can reduce boredom and thereby reduce occurrences of unacceptable behavior.[10] Environments that promote engagement offer both structured and unstructured activities that are appropriate to the child's level of development, are enjoyed by the child, and allow the child to experience success. Supplies and materials should be readily available to the child in locations that allow independent access. Strict rules about how and where materials are used should be relaxed to allow creativity and ingenuity. A child who is dynamically engaged in productive activity is less likely to engage in inappropriate or unacceptable behaviors.

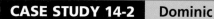

CASE STUDY 14-2   Dominic

Dominic has an extensive collection of train engines that he keeps arranged in a row on his bedroom floor. A new train engine is a treasure to Dominic. He will carry it with him for days after receiving it and carefully determine its placement in his collection at bedtime. His satisfaction with determining each train's placement is celebrated with laughter, clapping, and jumping. If the trains are disrupted, as occurs when the floor is vacuumed, Dominic becomes upset, making guttural vocalizations of increasing intensity while rocking back and forth. When he recovers from being upset, Dominic meticulously works to ensure that each train engine is in the correct order and placement.

The challenging behaviors that Dominic displays when his trains are disrupted can be avoided by giving careful attention to the situation. First, Dominic should be prepared in advance for the need to move the trains. For example, his mother should inform him that she needs to vacuum the floor and allow Dominic the time to carefully move his trains on his own. Second, support and assistance should be offered when the trains are disrupted. For example, Dominic should be informed when the trains become disrupted, and the person responsible should offer to assist Dominic in replacing the trains. The assistance should be provided in a manner meaningful and acceptable to Dominic, whether that is handing the trains to him one at a time, pointing to the place in line where each train should be placed, or simply being near Dominic as he works on replacing each train.

Increasing Communication Effectiveness

Children who do not have an effective means of communication often use behavior to deliver a message. Messages about pleasant experiences or enjoyable activities may be communicated through a smile, hug, or clapping. However, messages about pain, an undesired activity or location, or an unpleasant situation may be communicated through a variety of inappropriate methods such as screaming, hitting, throwing, or destroying property. Being attentive to a child's efforts to communicate is a first step in preventing situations that lead to frustration with communication barriers. Providing a means for the child to express both positive and negative messages effectively and efficiently can reduce inappropriate behaviors associated with lack of functional communication.[6] Working with a speech-language pathologist to identify and implement the most effective and appropriate communication system is highly recommended. Strategies that can be helpful include using physical gestures or sign language and exchanging written symbols or icons. Strategies should be appropriate for the child's ability level and should be portable for easy accessibility in all environments and situations.

In addition to providing an effective means for the child to communicate, it is equally important that the child receives and comprehends messages directed to him. This responsibility often falls to the speaker because many children are not able to express that they do not understand a message. Awareness by the receiver that a message has been communicated but not understood can be very frustrating. When the message is not acted on, the sender becomes frustrated at the lack of response. The receiver is not only at a loss to decipher the message, but may also receive verbal and/or nonverbal communication about the sender's growing frustration. This scenario can result in increased anxiety, which may lead to behavioral outbursts. Using simple language to convey messages, allowing additional time for processing of information, and supplementing verbal information with gestures or visual information can increase the possibility that messages are received and understood by the child, reducing the likelihood of frustration and resulting behavioral reactions.[14]

Clarifying Expectations

When activities or schedules are similar from day to day, assumptions may be made that expectations are known. Children, while sensing the comfort of a familiar environment, schedule, and social structure, do not necessarily attach performance expectations to environments or situations. Uncertainty about what is expected may lead the child to unknowingly act in inappropriate ways or to act out to test the limits. Many children respond best when rules are clearly established and limits are defined. Explicitly communicating expectations about what the child is supposed to do and how he is expected to act can alleviate any misconceptions or misunderstandings and promote the child and therapist having the same expectations.[21]

Supporting Self-Regulation

Many children who demonstrate challenging behavior also have difficulty managing responses to environmental stimuli (see Chapter 11 on sensory integration). Ambient noise, flickering lighting, constant movement of others, inadvertently being bumped, and other unpredictable or intense environmental stimuli can be anxiety-producing for persons who respond intensely to these stimuli. The result can be physiologic over-arousal such that the individual's sympathetic fight-or-flight response occurs. This response can manifest as behaviors such as aggression toward others, violence, self-injurious behaviors, or immediate and intense withdrawal from the situation. For these children, disorganized behavior may be a precursor to problem behavior.

The occupational therapy practitioner should watch for disorganized behavior and help the child to identify when behavior is becoming disordered. This may include informing the child of his disorganized behavior by specifically describing the behavior that was observed, identifying the context in which the behavior occurred, and describing what behavior would have been more appropriate to the context. In addition, the therapist should help the child develop a repertoire of more appropriate responses. Careful attention to and management of stimuli present in the environment can prevent the "fight, flight, or fright" response from occurring, allowing the individual to participate

BOX 14-2 Environmental Modifications to Support Self-Regulation

- Minimize ambient noise by adding carpeting, closing classroom door, turning off appliances, removing fluorescent lighting.
- Reduce visual stimulation by removing decorations from walls, closing curtains on windows, closing classroom door, providing a study carrel.
- Reduce situations that may result in accidental bumping or brushing against the child. Pay attention to stationary activities as well as activities requiring movement.

- Create zones for specific types of activities (e.g., quiet work, messy work, moving bodies).
- Install dimmer switches for lighting.
- Provide a hideout so child can withdraw from over-stimulating conditions.
- Arrange classroom seating to minimize possibility of child's being bumped or jostled.
- Rearrange the schedule to allow moving through the school building or visiting community locations at times when it is not crowded.

in the environment successfully. Box 14-2 identifies some suggested environmental modifications.

Matching Demands to Abilities

When performance demands exceed an individual's abilities, that person can become frustrated, angry, avoidant, or aggressive. Conversely, when performance demands are too low and do not match or challenge an individual's abilities, the person can become bored or uninterested in a task or activity. Either of these situations can result in challenging behavior as the individual expresses frustration with the mismatch between demands and abilities.[10] Creating individualized expectations and designing the just right challenge for each child can help alleviate frustration and create a just-right match between each child's performance demands and performance abilities.

SUPPORT POSITIVE BEHAVIOR

Strategies for supporting positive behaviors can be powerful tools in preventing situations that elicit problem behaviors. Some of the strategies are global and can be particularly useful for group situations in which more than one child requires assistance in managing appropriate behavior.[19] Other strategies are individualized to a particular child. All of the strategies should be implemented consistently and predictably to create a context that supports the child's ability to be successful.

General Strategies

Meeting Sensory Needs

Sensory input is an inherent part of life. Every experience and situation is saturated with sensation. Sensory information is received, interpreted, and managed by the central nervous system through a variety of chemical and electrical mechanisms. The central nervous system produces behavioral and emotional responses to this input. When an individual's processing of sensory information is ineffective or inaccurate, erratic behaviors that are inappropriate to the context or situation can be displayed.[1] These behaviors can take many forms. Often the behaviors can be identified as sensation-seeking or sensation-avoiding.[5] Sensation-seeking behaviors result in increased quantity or intensity of sensory input to the nervous system. In contrast, sensation-avoiding behaviors result in a decreased quantity or intensity of sensory input to the nervous system.

In and of themselves, sensation-seeking and sensation-avoiding behaviors are not inappropriate, but they may occur with inappropriate intensity, at inappropriate times, without regard for safety of others or the environment. By being aware of and taking efforts to meet an individual's sensory needs, such situations can be avoided, allowing the individual to have greater success in interacting with the people, objects, and situations around them. This can be accomplished through a variety of strategies ranging from intense one-on-one intervention to a range of sensory-based strategies that are embedded in the daily routine. An example of addressing challenging behavior by meeting sensory needs is presented in Case Study 14-3. In addition, see Chapter 11 for a discussion of sensory integration dysfunction and strategies to meet sensory needs.

Building New Skills

Children who have deficits in performance areas can become frustrated with the frequent experience of poor performance or lack of success. As mentioned before, frustration can lead to demonstration of undesired behaviors as a way of expressing or dealing with the frustration.[12] Thus, it is important that occupational therapists incorporate efforts to build new skills into their intervention plans. When developing the intervention plan, those skills that appear to pose the greatest barriers to independence in self-care, physical mobility, play, or education are often prioritized. However, it also is important to include development of skills that will enable the child to experience success in the regular daily occupations of social interaction and contextual participation. Box 14-3 identifies skills that are easily overlooked but are important to social participation. These should be incorporated into the occupational therapy intervention plan in an effort to build new skills and reduce frustration and the resulting problem behaviors.[21]

Specific Strategies

Increasing Compliance Through Contingency Methods

Many children resist engaging in tasks that they do not enjoy. Resistance can take many forms including, but not limited, to withdrawal, refusal, avoidance, and aggression. Contingency methods such as offering rewards or using a token economy can help to elicit participation in nonpreferred activities. Contingency methods are based on the principle of allowing access to a desired event contingent upon performance of or

CASE STUDY 14-3   Stephen

Stephen is a 10-year-old boy enrolled in the third grade. His teacher states that Stephen often has difficulty with attention to tasks, following directions, and completing his work. He constantly fidgets with his clothing and does not sit still in his chair. He is frequently sent to the principal's office for disrespecting teachers' authority and having an uncooperative attitude. He often has a scowl on his face and does not greet others or participate in social interactions. His comments are negative and demeaning toward others. He does not receive compliments or praise but deflects these comments by highlighting a rule that was broken or promise not kept. A recent psychological evaluation resulted in a diagnosis of oppositional defiant disorder.

The classroom teacher requested an occupational therapy evaluation to address Stephen's difficulty in performing the handwriting required to complete his schoolwork. In addition to poor development of intrinsic hand musculature, the occupational therapy evaluation identified difficulties in processing visual, auditory, and tactile sensory inputs such

that behavior and fine motor performance were affected. The occupational therapist recommended modifications to Stephen's classroom to address his sensitivity to bright lights, ambient noise, and unexpected touch. The placement of his desk was moved from the center of the classroom to the side, near the teacher's desk; a study carrel was brought into the classroom; and Stephen was allowed to wear sunglasses in class during work time. The occupational therapist collaborated with the classroom teacher to develop an activity plan incorporating regular opportunities for movement and physical effort to help meet Stephen's need for increased proprioceptive input. In addition, she conducted an in-service for the school staff instructing them on the relationship between poor sensory processing and ineffective behavioral regulation, the importance of addressing sensory needs as a first step in helping children to more effectively regulate behavioral responses to others, and the need to intentionally teach and reinforce those behavioral skills that the child needs to develop.

BOX 14-3   Skills That Promote Social Participation

Communicating wants, desires, dislikes
Compliance with requests
Cooperation with adults and peers
Flexibility
Giving an object on request
Independent play:
- Ability to initiate
- Ability to sustain
- Ability to conclude

Making choices
Parallel play
Social play
Variety in play
Sharing
Turn taking
Waiting

---

compliance with something else. For example, during intervention a child who enjoys blowing bubbles would be allowed to play with bubbles only after he completed a therapist-directed task such as pencil-paper work. Contingency approaches are commonly used in everyday life for children—access to outdoor play is not granted until the child puts on his coat; dessert is not served unless the child finishes her dinner. By withholding the desired item or activity until after the child completes the mandatory task, motivation is increased and compliance is gained.

Token Economies

Token economies are similar to withholding strategies, but are more complex. A system in which the child earns tokens for desired behaviors is established and taught. Examples of behaviors that are reinforced are compliance with a rule,

completion of a certain task or part of a task, and keeping hands out of mouth. The tokens can be exchanged for privileges such as 2 minutes of play with a preferred toy, a piece of candy, or the opportunity to play a game on the computer. In essence, certain privileges are withheld from the child until he has sufficient tokens to buy them. The tokens are earned through performance of desired tasks, engagement in prescribed activities, or demonstration of appropriate behavior. In establishing the token economy, the specific behavior for which tokens can be earned should be specified, as should the number of tokens each behavior is worth. For example, a child might earn one token for engaging in seat work for 3 minutes without needing redirection, or earn two tokens for spontaneously sharing art supplies with another child. In addition, the privileges or items that the child can purchase with the tokens and the cost of each should be established at the outset of establishing the token economy.

Token economies can be very simple, involving merely the earning of tokens and purchasing of rewards, or they can be made more complex by incorporating tokens given for undesired behaviors (Case Study 14-4). In this system, the child earns one color of token (often green or white) for desired behaviors and another color (often red) for undesired behaviors. The tokens for desired behavior have purchasing value and those for undesired behavior decrease purchasing value. For example, a child might earn one green token for each 2 minutes that he remains seated during independent work time and one red token each time he moves out of his chair. At the end of a 10-minute work period, the child has four green tokens and two red tokens. Each red token cancels out one green token, leaving the child with two tokens for that period of time.

Positive Reinforcement

Positive reinforcement is a specific strategy that has been established as a powerful behavior change technique. Positive reinforcement is the contingent presentation of a type of

CASE STUDY 14-4 Stephen

In addition to addressing Stephen's sensory needs, the occupational therapist worked with Stephen and his teacher to develop a behavior contract outlining expectations for appropriate interactions with the teacher, school staff, and other children. The contract includes a token economy and specifies the positive behaviors that Stephen is expected to display. He will earn a green token for each desired behavior, a red token for undesired behavior, and specific graduated consequences for not abiding with the contract. Green tokens are earned for specific occurrences of appropriate interactions with others and for maintaining appropriate on-task classroom behavior for a specified duration of time. Red tokens are given to Stephen for occurrences of inappropriate social interactions, off-task behavior, swearing, and noncompliance with the teacher's instructions. Tokens are counted and exchanged at the end of each school day for a choice from the school prize box, 5 minutes of free choice from a specified set of activities, and opportunities for special activities such as ice cream with the principal.

consequence that, when presented immediately after a behavior, increases the probability of that behavior occurring again.[17] In other words, a consequence that strengthens a behavior functions as a positive reinforcer for that behavior. Consider the mother who gives in and hands her child a cookie to stop the crying that began when the mother first denied the child's request for the cookie. Though the mother's purpose in giving the cookie was to stop the crying, the crying resulted in his obtaining a desired object. In other words, from the child's perspective, the crying worked. The likelihood that the child will behave in the same manner in the future (i.e., cry) has been increased by the positive reinforcer (obtaining the cookie). The power of positive reinforcement to effect behavior change has more than 40 years of empirical support[15,16,23-25]; however, occupational therapy practitioners typically are not trained in these techniques.[22] Strategic and effective use of this method could increase desired behaviors and reduce challenging behaviors, thereby supporting client engagement in therapeutic activities.

Alternate Preferred and Nonpreferred Activities

At times, all children need to participate in or complete tasks or activities that they do not enjoy. Attempts to gain the child's compliance in a nonpreferred task can lead to opposition, withdrawal, or outright refusal. If the adult keeps pressing the child to comply, challenging behaviors can escalate. One strategy for gaining compliance is to alternate the nonpreferred activity with one or more preferred activities. This strategy is similar to the contingency approaches in which a desired activity or event is withheld until the child performs a therapist-directed task. To implement this strategy successfully, the nonpreferred activity should seamlessly follow the preferred activity and should be presented in a matter-of-fact manner that does not highlight the child's lack of preference for the activity. By strategically and seamlessly sequencing the nonpreferred activity to come just after a preferred activity, the child is more likely to comply because the activity seems to flow from the one he just completed (Case Study 14-5).

CASE STUDY 14-5 Anastasia

Anastasia is a 5-year-old girl with a diagnosis of developmental delay. She demonstrates many signs of sensory processing dysfunction including sensory-seeking behaviors, distractibility, and high frequency of movement. These behaviors result in nonengagement in tabletop activities. Anastasia's mother has brought her to occupational therapy with concerns about readiness for school, specifically her unwillingness to engage in pencil-paper activities. During the evaluation, Anastasia refused to complete the writing activities on standardized testing of fine motor and visual-motor skills. During observations, Anastasia used a static tripod grasp while drawing on a chalkboard. She was able to approximate continuous circles, but no other shapes. Her attention was fleeting and she did not return to the chalkboard spontaneously or upon request.

Evaluation results identified significant deficits in fine motor and visual motor skills as well as poor processing of vestibular, tactile, and proprioceptive input. The occupational therapist began intervention using a sensory integration approach. As part of therapy sessions, Anastasia participated in obstacle courses in which she was challenged to push, pull, climb, swing, jump, ride a scooterboard around obstacles, and crawl. As Anastasia's distractibility decreased and her willingness to engage in therapist-directed activities increased, the occupational therapist began to incorporate pencil-paper tasks into the obstacle courses. After using a hand-over-hand motion to pull herself up a ramp while riding prone on a scooterboard, then jumping off the ramp platform into a mountain of pillows and crawling through a tunnel, Anastasia sat on a therapy ball and drew straight lines on paper mounted on a slantboard. Anastasia was not allowed to continue the obstacle course until she completed the pencil-paper task. Over time, the occupational therapist gradually increased the complexity of drawing, the duration of the drawing task, and the quality of work expected. As she alternated between the sensory-based activities she needed to become prepared and organized for table work with the table work activities, Anastasia's willingness to engage and her duration of engagement increased, allowing her to develop new skills.

Addressing Transitions

Transition between activities or environments can be particularly problematic times during which challenging behaviors emerge. Some practical strategies can support children during transitions and help to minimize noncompliance or refusals.

In school situations, the classroom schedule often dictates when a transition needs to occur. Adults have strategies such as watching the clock and having awareness of how much time has passed, which helps them anticipate a pending transition. Children do not have the same strategies, and transitions can appear to be arbitrarily imposed.

A transition routine can help to set the stage for a positive transition. Transition routines consist of using the same set of events each time a transition needs to occur. Singing a particular song or using a hand-clapping pattern are simple, distinct events that can be used to signal transitions. Using the same strategies for each transition provides familiarity, establishes context, and communicates expectations, all of which can help children transition successfully.

Timers provide an objective signal that something is about to occur.[7] Because once it is set, a timer operates independently of an adult, the implication that changes are arbitrarily imposed by the adult is reduced. To implement use of a timer, the occupational therapy practitioner shows it to the child and informs him of what will happen (e.g., "The timer will make a beeping sound. When you hear the beeping sound, it will be time to clean up the blocks and come to the table for snack."). The practitioner trains the child in how to turn the timer off. When the timer signals, the practitioner cues the child that the timer is beeping, helps the child turn off the timer, and reminds the child what the sound meant (Case Study 14-6).

Once use of the timer is established, it can be applied in a variety of contexts and situations. Children can learn to operate the timer themselves as a way to self-monitor use of time and compliance with time limits. Alarm clocks can be used in a similar manner as timers to indicate events that occur at a specific time of day such as time to go to the bus stop, time to get ready for bed, or time to leave for an appointment.

Another excellent method of supporting successful transitions is the use of *visual schedules*.[4] These are particularly useful in situations where the schedule remains relatively similar from day to day or week to week. Either picture icons or word cards can be arranged on a schedule board to represent the sequence of activities or events that is going to occur. Children can follow the visual representation of the sequence. Depending on a given child's abilities, he or she can learn to use the visual schedule independently, consulting it when one activity is completed or when a transition is indicated. Some visual schedules merely represent activity sequences with no time allotted. Other schedules are time-based and indicate day of the week, time of day, and the activity that will be occurring. Many visual schedules use removable cards so that the schedule can be modified easily if the schedule changes. Some schedules are posted on poster board mounted to the wall; others are secured in a binder or notebook that is easily transported from one setting to another. The form of the schedule and the amount of support given to the child in using the schedule are individualized to the child's capabilities.

General Support Strategies

Many challenging or inappropriate behaviors can be ameliorated through the use of general positive strategies. Providing extra time for a child to process a verbal instruction or organize an appropriate response to a stimulus can alleviate anxiety and stress and the resulting behavioral reaction. Providing encouragement that communicates belief in the child's ability to succeed can improve self-esteem and a sense of self-worth.[18] Giving explicit instructions in how to approach or complete a task can alleviate fears of failure that may cause a child to withdraw or disengage from an activity. Providing specific feedback about the child's efforts and what could be done differently next time can also build confidence and motivate a child to try again rather than walk away from a task with a feeling of despair. These strategies are examples of therapeutic use of self. The therapist uses the therapist-client interactions strategically to support the client in whatever challenge he or she is experiencing and to communicate belief in the individual's ability to

---

CASE STUDY 14-6 | **Meg**

Meg is a 4-year-old girl with autism. She enjoys playing with alphabet blocks and her toy piano. Meg has extreme difficulty concluding her play to transition to a different activity. When a transition is imposed on her, Meg demonstrates one of two predictable responses: a complete lack of response as if she did not hear the instruction or extreme refusal to transition expressed by screaming and stamping feet. At times, the behavior can escalate into a full-blown tantrum including hitting, kicking, dropping to the floor, and throwing toys.

Meg is enrolled in a preschool classroom for children with developmental disabilities. Transition between activities occurs multiple times each day as the children engage in different play centers, circle time, snack time, and outdoor play.

Meg's difficulties with transitions often disrupt the class. The occupational therapist works with Meg on a weekly basis and introduces a timer to help her learn how to conclude an activity. Within 3 days Meg consistently responds when the timer signals. She alerts to the sound, discontinues her activity, and turns the timer off. Sometimes she returns to her activity and re-engages, but when cued by the teacher or occupational therapist, she is able to transition to the next activity. By the end of 9 school days, Meg reliably alerts to the sound of the timer, discontinues her activity, and consults a visual schedule to determine what she is to do next. She then activates the timer for a preset duration of time and transitions to the activity indicated on her schedule.

achieve his or her desires. Effective therapeutic use of self leads to a partnership between the therapist and the client that is empowering and encouraging.[20] The power of these experiences can help to prevent misbehaviors that are associated with feelings of despair and low self-esteem.

INTERVENE WHEN CHALLENGING BEHAVIORS ALREADY EXIST

The best practice approach to managing challenging and problematic behaviors that already exist combines FBA with a positive behavioral support (PBS) plan.[13] This comprehensive approach is a highly structured, dynamic process that addresses the problem behavior within the natural context. The FBA is a 5-step process consisting of (1) team building and goal setting, (2) functional assessment of the behavior, (3) hypothesis development, (4) development of the comprehensive support plan, and (5) implementation and outcome monitoring of the plan including refining the plan as needed.[3] Occupational therapists may be part of the FBA process because they often have personal knowledge of the client and direct experience with the behavior of focus. Each of the five steps of the FBA process is described briefly in the following paragraphs.

The first step of the FBA process is to gather a team of individuals who will collaborate to work together for the child's best interest. Ideally, the team includes the child's parents or caregivers as recognized experts on the child and as partners in the intervention process. Together with the caregivers, the team works to first identify desired outcomes for the child.[3] Conversation and planning centers around understanding the child as a "whole" person, including the child's capacities and areas needing further development. This process creates a foundation upon which the intervention and support plans are built.

Step two involves the comprehensive functional assessment of the specific behavior. Efforts focus on clearly describing the challenging behavior, the context(s) in which it occurs, the antecedents and consequences that maintain the behavior, and the functions of the behavior. The goal of this step is to understand the purpose of the behavior and when the behavior is most and least likely to occur. Data collection is the best method for understanding the purpose of the behavior and the events that maintain the behavior. Data can be gathered by interviewing people who have direct knowledge of the child and experience with the behavior, observing the child where and when the behavior is most likely to occur, reviewing records in which the behavior has been documented, and gathering information about contextual variables such as health or changes in other environments or activity schedules.

The third step in the FBA process is to develop hypotheses about the behavior including the antecedents (factors that trigger the behavior), consequences (responses to the behavior), and communicative function of the behavior (request something or avoid/escape from something). Hypotheses statements are generated based on the information gathered in step two.

Fourth, a comprehensive behavior support plan is developed. The plan itself has four elements: (1) a functional assessment of behavior provides a foundation for the intervention plan, (2) multiple intervention strategies are used, (3) the plan is applied throughout the day, and (4) the elements of the plan are consistent with the values and resources of the child receiving support and the persons providing support.[13] The collaborative effort of the team to gather data about the behavior and develop hypotheses about the function and reinforcing events surrounding the behavior are used to understand the behavior and the functional purpose it is serving for the child. This understanding is used to develop the intervention component of the plan, which includes strategies aimed at preventing the challenging behavior from occurring and strategies aimed at helping the child develop new skills that effectively and efficiently achieve the same function as the challenging behavior. The new skills are taught to the child as replacement strategies for the challenging and undesired behavior. The plan also includes contingencies for both the challenging and the replacement behaviors. The contingencies for demonstration of the replacement behavior are designed to reinforce and strengthen use of the new behavior, whereas the contingencies for the challenging behavior are designed to discourage its use.

The final step of the PBS process is implementation of the plan and measurement of outcomes. Once the plan is developed, it is tested for goodness of fit with the personal, physical, and social contexts of the child, family, and other service providers to ensure that all persons involved in implementing the plan are equally comfortable using the plan in their respective situations. Ensuring goodness of fit is a critical step in increasing the likelihood that the plan is used. As the plan is implemented, the team evaluates the effectiveness of the plan in producing the desired results: reduction of the challenging behavior and production of the replacement behaviors. The team meets periodically to review plan effectiveness and the child's progress. Modifications and adjustments are made as needed followed by implementation and monitoring of the revised plan (Case Study 14-7).

SUMMARY

Challenging and inappropriate behaviors are demonstrated by children with a wide range of developmental disabilities and can interfere with engagement in occupation, prevent participation in context, and create situations that are potentially harmful. When problem behaviors exist, reducing the problem behavior should be a primary focus of occupational therapy intervention. Effective management of challenging behavior includes not only improving an individual's behavioral competence but also creating contexts that support positive behaviors and intentionally managing consequences. Occupational therapy practitioners have knowledge and skills in task analysis, human behavior, and occupational engagement, enabling them to effectively analyze problem behavior, develop behavioral intervention plans, and implement behavior management strategies.

CASE STUDY 14-7   Jessie

Seven-year-old Jessie was suspended from his second grade classroom because of uncontrollable aggressive outbursts that included yelling at the teacher, refusing to complete schoolwork, overturning desks, and throwing school supplies. The behaviors had been building throughout the fall and culminated with punching the teacher in early December. An FBA was initiated in November and revealed that Jessie's behaviors escalated whenever work demands involved extended writing and during collaborative group work activities. The occupational therapist had observed Jessie's handwriting abilities in October at the request of the classroom teacher. Jessie used a mature tripod grasp, was able to form letters correctly, and had good upper extremity positioning and postural support for handwriting tasks. Jessie was able to perform handwriting activities without difficulty when copying from a sample or when writing personal information such as his name. The occupational therapist observed signs of anxiety when Jessie was asked to write creatively, documenting that he "seemed unable to generate ideas or topics to write about and he became flushed, fidgeted with his pencil, and stated that the assignment was 'stupid'."

During the FBA it was discovered that signs of anxiety often preceded Jessie's behavioral outbursts and that the outbursts were worse later in the day during the creative writing lessons. Jessie also showed signs of anxiety during collaborative work activities. When group work was assigned, Jessie fidgeted with materials in his desk and did not join his group until specifically instructed by the teacher. He did not join in the group discussions or participate in work activities. Rather, he remained at the fringe of the group. If his participation was requested by a peer or instructed by the teacher, Jessie shifted his weight and looked around anxiously, often giving excuses for not working. If pushed to participate, he verbally refused with increased vocal intensity and volume and sometimes shoved a desk or chair. The FBA team hypothesized that the behaviors were a result of poor ability to cope with anxiety and that writing and social situations were anxiety-producing for Jessie.

The FBA team had worked together to develop a plan to better match writing and social demands to Jessie's abilities, provide support during writing assignments, and provide intervention to develop social skills that would support his ability to participate in group learning activities.

In addition to modifications the teacher made to assignments, the occupational therapist provided recommendations for modifying the classroom environment to decrease anxiety-producing situations and add coping supports. She also designed a program aimed to help Jessie develop improved self-regulation of behavior, body scheme, fine motor coordination, and social skills. Some classroom-wide strategies included seated isometric exercises for the entire class at key times during the school day, regularly scheduled dimmed lighting and whispered voice times, and a "cozy corner" for independent use by students. The occupational therapist also worked with Jessie, his teacher, and the school counselor to identify two peers with whom Jessie could work to build his social skills. She provided training sessions with the students, teacher, and counselor including instruction on teamwork, complimenting, turn taking, and collaboration. Data collection forms were used to track Jessie's behavior. A change in the frequency and intensity of Jessie's behavior was seen almost immediately and, within 3 weeks of implementing the program, Jessie's inappropriate behavior had diminished to occasional verbal outbursts with no physical aggression.

REFERENCES

1. Baker, A. E., Lane, A., Angley, M. T., & Young, R. L. (2008). The relationship between sensory processing and behavioural responsiveness in autistic disorder: A pilot study. *Journal of Autism and Developmental Disorders, 38,* 867–875.
2. Bauman, M. (2008). *Autism: Emotion and behavior—is it all in the brain?* Paper presented at R2K: Research 2008 Sensory Integration. Long Beach, CA: Emotions, and Autism.
3. Buschbacher, P. W., & Fox, L. (2003). Understanding and intervening with the challenging behavior of young children with autism spectrum disorder. *Language, Speech, and Hearing Services in Schools, 34,* 217–227.
4. Dettmer, S., Simpson, R. L., Myles, B. S., & Ganz, J. B. (2000). The use of visual supports to facilitate transitions of students with autism. *Focus on Autism and Other Developmental Disabilities, 15,* 163–169.
5. Dunn, W. (1997). The impact of sensory processing abilities on the daily lives of young children and their families: A conceptual model. *Infants and Young Children, 9*(4), 23–35.
6. Durand, V. M., & Carr, E. G. (1992). An analysis of maintenance following functional communication training. *Journal of Applied Behavior Analysis, 25,* 777–794.
7. Ferguson, A., Ashbaugh, R., O'Reilly, S., & McLaughlin, T. F. (2004). Using prompt training and reinforcement to reduce transition times in a transitional kindergarten program for students with severe behavior disorders. *Child and Family Behavior Therapy, 26,* 17–24.
8. Flannery, K. B., & Horner, R. H. (1994). The relationship between predictability and problem behavior for students with severe disabilities. *Journal of Behavioral Education, 4,* 157–176.
9. Foxx, R. M. (1996). Twenty years of applied behavior analysis in treating the most severe problem behavior: Lessons learned. *Behavior Analyst, 19,* 225–235.
10. Foxx, R. M. & Meindl, J. (2007). The long term successful treatment of the aggressive/destructive behaviors of a preadolescent with autism. *Behavioral Interventions, 22,* 83–97.
11. Grazier, P. B. (1995). *Starving for recognition: Understanding recognition and the seven recognition do's and don'ts.* EI Network. Retrieved October 9, 2008, from http://www. teambuildinginc.com/article_recognition.htm

12. Horner, R. H. (2000). Positive behavior supports. *Focus on Autism and Other Developmental Disabilities, 15,* 97–105.

13. Horner, R. H., & Carr, E. G. (1997). Behavioral support for students with severe disabilities: Functional assessment and comprehensive intervention. *The Journal of Special Education, 31,* 84–104.

14. Horner, R., Carr, E., Strain, P., Todd, A., & Reed, H. (2002). Problem behavior interventions for young children. *Journal of Autism and Developmental Disorders, 32,* 423–446.

15. Koegel, R. L., Koegel, L. K., Frea, W. D., & Smith, A. E. (1995). Emerging interventions of children with autism: Longitudinal and lifestyle implications. In R. L. Koegel & L. K. Koegel (Eds.), *Teaching children with autism: Strategies for initiating positive interactions and improving learning opportunities* (pp. 1–16). Baltimore: Paul H. Brookes.

16. Koegel, R. L., O'Dell, M., & Dunlap, G. (1988). Producing speech in nonverbal autistic children by reinforcing attempts. *Journal of Autism and Developmental Disorders, 18,* 525–538.

17. Malott, R. W., Malott, M. E., & Trojan, E. A. (2000). *Elementary principles of behavior* (4th ed.). Upper Saddle River, NJ: Pearson.

18. McMinn, L. G. (2000). *Growing strong daughters.* Grand Rapids, MI: Baker.

19. OSEP Technical Assistance Center on Positive Behavior Supports and Intervention. (2008). *School-wide PBS.* Retrieved on December 23, 2008 from http://www.pbis.org/schoolwide.htm

20. Taylor, R. R. (2008). *The intentional relationship: Occupational therapy and use of self.* Philadelphia: F.A. Davis.

21. Watling, R. (2005). Interventions for common behavior problems in children with disabilities. *OT Practice, 10,* 12–15.

22. Watling, R., & Schwartz, I. S. (2004). The issue is: Understanding and implementing positive reinforcement as an intervention strategy for children with disabilities. *American Journal of Occupational Therapy, 58,* 113–116.

23. Williams, J. A., Koegel, R. L., & Egel, A. L. (1981). Response-reinforcer relationships and improved learning in autistic children. *Journal of Applied Behavior Analysis, 14,* 53–60.

24. Wolf, M., Risley, T., & Mees, H. (1964). Application of operant conditioning procedures to the behaviour problems of an autistic child. *Behavior Research and Therapy, 1,* 305–312.

25. Zannolli, K., & Daggett. (1998). The effects of reinforcement rate on the spontaneous social initiations of socially withdrawn preschoolers. *Journal of Applied Behavior Analysis, 31,* 117–125.

15

Feeding Intervention

Linda M. Schuberth • Lauren M. Amirault • Jane Case-Smith

KEY TERMS

Feeding
Eating
Mealtime
Oral structures
Oral motor
 development
Suck/Swallow/Breathe
 coordination
Swallowing phases

Oral motor swallowing
 evaluation
Videofluoroscopic
 swallow study (VFSS)
Dysphagia
Cleft lip and palate
Non-oral feeding
Nutrition

OBJECTIVES

1. Describe the acquisition of feeding, eating, and swallowing skills as developmental milestones.
2. Describe the anatomic landmarks and four phases of swallowing or deglutition.
3. Outline the cranial nerves involved in feeding and swallowing.
4. Explain the components of a feeding, eating, and swallowing evaluation.
5. Assess feeding difficulties in children within the larger context of the family's cultural, social, and behavioral routines around food and mealtimes.
6. Classify common abnormalities and disorders related to the phases of swallowing.
7. Identify factors that may warrant further evaluation, including a videofluoroscopic swallow study.
8. Describe additional diagnostic and medical testing that may be used in a comprehensive evaluation.
9. Understand the developmental and psychosocial implications for a child whose nutritional intake is altered.
10. Identify medical, developmental, behavioral, and social issues that contribute to feeding, eating, and swallowing problems.
11. Explain the team approach to evaluating and treating the child from a biopsychosocial perspective.
12. Describe intervention strategies for feeding, eating, and swallowing deficits.
13. Define altered food textures and liquid consistencies.

FEEDING: DEFINITION AND OVERVIEW

The process of feeding, eating, and swallowing is critical for health and wellness and plays an integral part in the child's social, emotional, and cultural maturation. At the most basic level, the process of taking in adequate nutrition is essential for normal growth and development.

Throughout childhood, from infancy and all the way through adolescence, dietary requirements are constantly changing. At the same time, a child's development gradually moves from complete dependence toward independent self-feeding. This dynamic process depends on the acquisition of both complex oral motor and fine motor skills. Indeed, mealtimes allow a child to explore new tastes and textures, while at the same time encouraging the development of motor skills through finger feeding and the use of utensils. Equally important, the feeding process is marked by social contact with other children, parents, and family and is thus essential for development of social interaction skills in the child. Children learn to communicate needs and desires through verbal and nonverbal cues. Feeding is one of the earliest instances in a child's life where he or she learns to signal hunger, satiety, and thirst among other needs and desires. Finally, because this complex process is shaped by cultural and social norms, it often lays the foundation for the acquisition of certain customs and rules of sociocultural behavior.

Feeding—sometimes called *self-feeding*—is defined as the process of setting up, arranging, and bringing food from the plate or cup to the mouth. *Eating* is the ability to keep and manipulate food or fluid in the mouth and swallow it. *Swallowing* is a complex act in which food, fluid, medication, or saliva is moved from the mouth through the pharynx and the esophagus, and into the stomach.[4]

Children develop problems with feeding, eating, and swallowing as a result of medical, oral, sensorimotor, and behavioral factors, either alone or in combination.[55] Medical conditions include prematurity, neuromuscular abnormalities, structural anomalies, gastroesophageal diseases, food allergies, and tracheostomy. Children with developmental disabilities may fail to meet basic nutritional needs because of delayed or deficit oral motor and self-feeding skills. Oral motor dysfunction causing poor nutrition is strongly associated with poor growth and adverse health outcomes.[27,63] Clinical findings may include food refusal/selectivity, vomiting, swallowing difficulty, prolonged mealtimes, poor weight gain, and failure to thrive.

Behavioral problems are very common in children with feeding disorders. Food refusal and/or food selectivity can often signal negative interaction between children and their caregivers. However, they may be, and often are, secondary to underlying medical causes such as reflux or food allergy. In fact, both medical and behavioral etiologic factors are often present, making definitive diagnosis difficult.

The Role of the Occupational Therapist

Of all the activities of daily living, none is more life-sustaining than eating. Occupational therapists and occupational therapy assistants have long played an integral role in providing essential services and comprehensive management to children who have problems with one or more aspects of the feeding process. A competent occupational therapist should therefore be familiar with the following:

- Basic anatomy and physiology
- Growth and developmental milestones
- Nutrition
- Medical conditions and their impact on feeding
- Social and emotional factors that can affect feeding

Some occupational therapists work in specialized facilities as part of a multidisciplinary team that often consists of pediatric specialists, including gastroenterologists, developmental pediatricians, allergists, otolaryngologists (also known as ENTs), nurse practitioners, nutritionists, speech–language pathologists, behavioral psychologists, and social workers, all of whom work in tandem to evaluate and manage complex cases. However, many therapists work in school settings or as solo practitioners and are often the first to detect a child's difficulties with feeding. In either instance, the occupational therapist has a well-defined, unique role in the assessment and management of feeding, eating, and swallowing disorders.

THE MEALTIME: AN OVERVIEW

Mealtime is generally a family time that provides physical, cognitive, and emotional nourishment of all members. Meals arrange the day temporally, organizing it into periods and signaling that certain activities end and new ones begin. Mealtimes provide a routine and a structure and offer a time for relaxation, communication, and socialization. At mealtimes, parents and children communicate symbolically and emotionally while at the same time satisfying very basic needs.[22] Many believe that to nourish a child is to nurture a child. Thus, mealtimes are cultural rituals and, as such, an integral part of a family's life, a time for bonding and sharing.

Caregivers and children engage in both shared and individual roles during mealtimes. Usually, the child is expected to remain seated, to attend to the caregiver, to feed himself or herself, to communicate with others at the table, and, generally, to follow the table manners and routines. The caregiver is expected to provide food in quantities sufficient to satisfy hunger, to assist in feeding younger children, to communicate and interact with other family members, and to establish mealtime norms and routines.

A child's mealtime participation changes as he or she goes through the different stages of growth and development, from infancy to adulthood. During infancy, the parents are responsible for feeding or assisting the child. During the preschool and school-age years, the parents' role shifts toward oversight, communication, and discipline. Almost all parents try to create a pleasant and relaxing family atmosphere during meals. This could be challenging and not always easy to achieve if a child has a disability that affects eating performance. The child's temperament, health, and disposition and the parent's health and mood are all important factors contributing to mealtime social interactions.

Contextual Influences on Mealtime

Family composition determines who is present at mealtime. The child may be fed in an isolated setting alone with his mother or may sit with all family members around the dinner table. Large families may have chaotic or noisy mealtimes. Such an environment creates difficulties for a child with hypersensitivities or high sensory arousal. Caregivers may not notice that a child has poor intake when many are present at the dinner table. On the flipside, large families have extra hands to assist in a child's feeding if needed. Sometimes, children who need a quieter environment or who need maximal assistance are fed separately before or after the other family members. Sometimes only one family member can feed the child successfully. When a child has only one feeder, the responsibility for feeding around the clock can, over time, become stressful and exhausting for the feeder.

In some cultures, children are fed by a caregiver throughout the preschool years, whereas in others, infants are encouraged to self-feed despite the ensuing mess. For example, Puerto Rican mothers may continue to feed their children well into their preschool years, whereas Anglo mothers encourage self-feeding much earlier. Puerto Rican mothers who feed their children as toddlers generally emphasize respectful relations and appropriate interpersonal relationships during the meal. In contrast, Anglo mothers who allow self-feeding at 12 months of age tend to emphasize the young child's independence and autonomy.[59] Cultural beliefs also determine the amount and type of food that parents believe their children should eat. For example, southern African American children are often given sweetened tea to supplement their diet, because parents believe that tea enhances the physical and cognitive abilities of a child.[41] The tea, however, may replace other drinks (e.g., milk) that have more vitamins and nutrients.

A family's socioeconomic status also has an impact on mealtime and feeding patterns. Families in poverty may be unable to provide sufficient food or may eat cheaper foods that tend to be high in carbohydrates and fat. A parent's educational level, which is often related to socioeconomic status, can affect a child's diet because an undereducated parent may lack knowledge of basic nutrition. Obesity and hunger coexist in high-poverty areas. Diets of low-income consumers may be high in sugars and fat because they are the cheapest source of nutrition.

According to the results of the annual survey of the U.S. Census Bureau, those at greatest risk of being hungry live in households that are headed by a single woman; that are Hispanic or Black; or with incomes below the poverty line. Overall, households with children have food insecurity at almost double the rate for households without children. According to survey undertaken by the U.S. Department of Agriculture in 2006, 35.5 million persons are food insecure, of which 12.6 million are children.[24] Food insecurity refers to the lack of access to enough food to fully meet basic needs at all times because of a lack of financial resources.[47] UNICEF defines undernutrition as being underweight for age, too short for age (stunted growth), dangerously thin for height (wasted), and deficient in vitamins and minerals.[66]

A single parent may be under greater stress and may not be able to provide structured mealtimes, causing the child to have chaotic mealtime patterns. In the absence of mealtime structure, the child may graze throughout the day whenever hungry, eating whatever is easily available. Adolescent parents may not have access to information on child development and feeding and may feed their young children inappropriate foods or foods with poor nutritional value.

Feeding and mealtime patterns vary from family to family, and factors beyond the ones described above may be at play. Interviewing parents about the degree of flexibility they allow a child who refuses to eat, Humphry and Thigpen-Beck found that older, better-educated parents were more likely to be flexible.[36] Parents who placed emphasis on discipline and obedience were less likely to be flexible with a child's refusal to eat. Clearly, social context can be helpful in understanding a family's feeding strategy and how parents interpret and respond to a child's mealtime behavior.[37]

Personal Influences on Mealtime

A caregiver's personality traits and other individual factors can also shape mealtime and affect a child's ability to feed. When the caregiver does not enjoy feeding a child or approaches it as a chore, the task can lose much of its meaning, changing the mealtime experience for both the adult and the child. For example, some caregivers are anxious about feeding and tend to be controlling when the child is a poor eater. The caregiver may have preconceived ideas about how much the child should eat and force food on the child or become disappointed with the child's intake. A controlling parent may find that the child desires control of what he or she eats, and a battle of the wills may result.

Personal/individual factors that influence mealtime include the child's health, eating skills, and communication/interaction skills. Children with feeding/eating problems can require extra time, special food preparation, adaptive equipment, and a structured protocol for the caregiver. This chapter discusses some health problems and delayed or deficient oral motor skills that can affect feeding. Occupational therapists are often called on to provide intervention in such circumstances.

DEVELOPMENTAL SEQUENCE OF MEALTIME PARTICIPATION

Progression of Mealtime Participation

In the first 6 months of life, parents feed their infant in their arms. Feeding is a time for bonding, characterized by close holding and warmth, eye contact, and nonverbal communication between the parents (or other primary caregivers) and the child. A typical interaction between child and parent may be the parent's stroking and touching the infant, who responds by grasping the mother's breast or hair or the father's shirt or fingers. Although the parent determines what the infant eats, it is the infant who typically sets the pace, duration, and end of a meal. When this interaction is less than smooth, the parent may compensate by trying to exercise more control. Positive early mealtime experiences solidify the bond between parent and child and strengthen the relationship between them.

An infant becomes more independent between 7 and 24 months. For example, a 7-month-old infant can usually finger feed. By 18 months, the child is typically attempting to use a spoon and a cup. As independence grows, so do the chaos and messiness of mealtimes. Although the parent continues to select the foods for the child, the child can now choose whether to eat or refuse the food. During this time, the toddler gets a greater variety of foods. The child moves out of the parents' arms and into a high chair or a booster seat. The toddler studies his or her foods and truly enjoys making a mess. Most toddlers explore the sensory qualities of foods, such as texture, with their hands and tongues. Parents encourage their child's efforts at self-feeding and allow him or her to try different foods, while ensuring they limit those difficult to chew and/or digest. Eating, however, continues to be time for communication, by now both verbal and nonverbal. Parents begin to describe the child's foods and thus provide a source for new vocabulary. In fact, words denoting food are often among the first words acquired by many toddlers.

Once the child is about 2 years old and is feeding relatively independently, he or she usually becomes a full participant in family mealtime. The child sits at the table, where she or he can observe and mimic the actions and behaviors of fellow meal participants. By preschool, children begin to eat some or all of the foods that other family members are eating. Family members become models for appropriate feeding behaviors and instruct the child in the basics of self-feeding. For most preschool children, mealtimes are enjoyable social times, marked by a sense of togetherness and an altogether positive, relaxing environment. Disability, however, can have a negative effect on mealtimes and hinder or slow the progression and accomplishment of these outcomes. Too much pressure on preschoolers to eat more, eat neatly, or eat certain foods may create anxiety about eating and may be harmful in the long run by making eating a less than enjoyable physical, sensory, and social activity.

Development of Oral Structures

Intact oral structures and cranial nerves are prerequisites for normal eating and drinking. Various aspects of oral motor development emerge as the child begins to control jaw, tongue, cheek, and lip movement. The anatomic structures of the mouth and throat change significantly during the first 12 months. The growth and development of the oral structures allow for increasingly mature feeding patterns. Table 15-1 lists the oral structures involved in feeding.

The newborn has a small oral cavity filled with fat pads inside the cheeks and the tongue. The small and tight oral cavity allows the child to grasp and easily compress the nipple during breast-feeding and to achieve automatic suction. The negative pressure caused by the sucking movements of the jaw extracts liquid from the nipple.[44] Thus, a full-term healthy newborn can suck easily and successfully from a breast or bottle nipple.

TABLE 15-1 Functions of Oral Structures in Feeding

Structure	Parts	Function during Feeding
Oral cavity	Hard and soft palate, tongue, fat pads of cheeks, upper and lower jaws, and teeth	Contains the food during drinking and chewing and provides for initial mastication before swallowing
Pharynx	Base of tongue, buccinator, oropharynx, tendons, and hyoid bone	Funnels food into the esophagus and allows food and air to share space; the pharynx is a space common to both functions
Larynx	Epiglottis and false and true vocal folds	Valve to the trachea that closes during swallowing
Trachea	Tube below the larynx supported by cartilaginous rings	Allows air to flow into bronchi and lungs
Esophagus	Thin and muscular esophagus	Carries food from the pharynx, through the diaphragm, and into the stomach; it is collapsed at rest and distends as food passes through it

Modified from Wolf, L. S., & Glass, R. P. (1992). *Feeding and swallowing disorders in infancy: Assessment and management.* Tucson, AZ: Therapy Skill Builders.

The structures in an infant's throat are also in close proximity to one another. The epiglottis and soft palate are in direct approximation. As a result, the liquid from the nipple safely passes from the base of the tongue to the esophagus. During swallowing, the larynx elevates and the epiglottis falls over it to protect the trachea. Therefore, aspiration is less likely before 4 months of age, and the infant can safely feed in a reclined position.

As the infant grows, the neck elongates, and the configuration of the oral and throat structures changes. The oral cavity becomes larger and more open, the tongue becomes thinner and more muscular, and the cheeks lose much of their fatty padding. With the increase in oral cavity space, the tongue, lips, and cheeks provide greater control of liquid and food within the mouth. New sucking patterns develop enabling the infant to handle liquid without the structural advantages of early infancy. These include up-and-down movements of the tongue to extract liquid from the nipple. The increasing oral space also provides room to advance food texture and to move the tongue in the rotary pattern required during chewing.[69]

As the infant approaches 12 months of age, the hyoid, epiglottis, and larynx descend, creating space between these structures and the base of the tongue. The hyoid and larynx become more mobile during swallowing, elevating with each swallow. The greater complexity of the suck-swallow-breathe sequence leads to greater coordination among these structures. The elongated pharynx increases the risk of aspiration during feeding in reclined position as the pull of gravity accelerates the flow of liquid into the entrance of the esophagus. Figure 15-1 shows the structures of the mouth and pharynx of the infant.

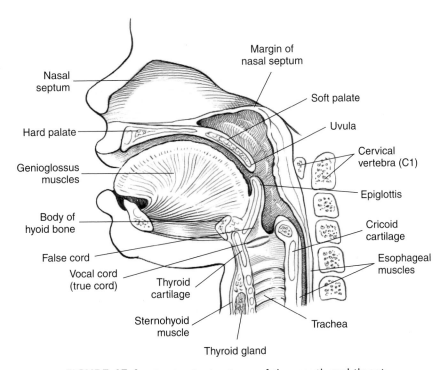

FIGURE 15-1 Anatomic structures of the mouth and throat.

Phases of Swallowing

There are four defined phases of swallowing. The *oral preparatory* phase is under voluntary control and the area of oral motor/feeding intervention. Oral manipulation using the jaw, lips, tongue, teeth, cheeks, and palate results in the formation of a bolus. The amount of time varies depending on the texture of food/liquid. The trigeminal (V), facial, (VII), glossopharyngeal (IX), and hypoglossal (XII) cranial nerves are listed in Box 15-1.

The second phase is the *oral* phase, also under voluntary control. This phase begins when the tongue elevates against the alveolar ridge moving the bolus posteriorly and ends with the onset of the pharyngeal swallow lasting for 1 to 3 seconds. The third phase is the *pharyngeal* phase, also lasting 1 to 3 seconds, which starts with the trigger of the swallow at the anterior faucial arches. The hyoid and larynx move upward and anteriorly, and the epiglottis retroflexes to protect the opening of the airway. It ends with the opening/relaxation of the cricopharyngeal sphincter. The *final* phase is the esophageal, which, along with the pharyngeal phase, is not under voluntary control. It starts with the contraction of the cricopharyngeus muscle and ends with relaxation of the lower esophageal sphincter, allowing food to enter the stomach. The duration is 8 to 10 seconds.

ORAL MOTOR DEVELOPMENT ASSOCIATED WITH EATING SKILLS

Sucking, drinking, biting, and chewing are closely linked to the child's overall motor development. Oral patterns evolve along with the child's changing nutritional needs, growing desire for self-feeding, and increasingly greater ability to communicate.[7] Table 15-2 summarizes the sequence of eating skills development.

Coordination of Sucking, Swallowing, and Breathing

The sucking reflex is present in the fetus and is the predominant method of feeding during the first 8 to 10 months of life. Sucking can be either nonnutritive or nutritive, and each one is different. Nonnutritive sucking, the goal of which is not to feed but rather to calm, occurs when a child is sucking on a pacifier. It is marked by rapid, rhythmic movements, occurring at a speed of about two sucks per second. By contrast, the nutritive pattern occurs when a child is sucking on a source of nutrition, such a bottle nipple. It is rhythmic, but its rhythm

is marked by alternating bursts with pauses, which allows the infant to breathe and rest between sucking bursts.

Premature infants of 33 weeks' gestational age or less are typically fed by nonoral methods such as an intravenous line or a nasogastric tube. The reason for this is that infants younger than 33 weeks, although capable of rhythmic nonnutritive sucking, have insufficient strength and endurance for nipple feeding. A 35-week-old healthy premature baby typically has sufficiently strong jaw and tongue movements to be fed orally, at least part of the time.

Two important factors that determine the ability to feed are sucking rhythm and type of suction (i.e., negative pressure for expression of liquid) that the infant achieves and sustains over time.[21] Both compression and suction are required for the expression of liquid.[69]

To achieve suction and compression, the infant seals his or her lips around the nipple and simultaneously moves the tongue back and forth and up and down. By 36 weeks of gestational age, most premature infants can take all food by mouth and are able to suck nearly as well as a full-term infant.

The full-term infant (37 to 42 weeks' gestation) has strong oral reflexes that enable him or her to take in liquid nutrition without difficulty. Exposed to tactile stimulation near the mouth (such as gentle touching of the lips), the hungry infant reacts by turning the head (rooting reflex), which permits him or her to latch onto any potential source of nutrition. The infant also exhibits gag and cough reflexes to prevent liquid from entering the airway.

The amount of liquid consumed during a meal is determined by three factors: rate or speed of sucking, force of suction or compression, and length of feeding time. Thus, infants who suck faster and pull more forcefully on the nipple and take in more fluid may finish eating in less time than those who suck more slowly or weakly. The sucking pattern of the full-term infant is rhythmic, sustained, and efficient. Sucking speed and force begin to decrease with satiety. Each infant has a unique sucking pattern that may vary from feeding to feeding depending on factors such as fatigue and hunger. Most infants complete an oral feeding in 20 to 25 minutes.

An infant's first sucking pattern is called *suckling*.[44] During suckling, the tongue moves back and forth, and the jaw opens and closes, following the movement of the tongue.[70] Typically, the tongue extends to, but not beyond, the border of the lips. Suckling is the predominant sucking pattern during the first 4 months of life. At 1 month of age, a hungry infant usually performs one suck per swallow. However, as the infant becomes satiated, he or she decreases the force of suction, taking in less and less liquid with each sucking motion. The rate slows down to about two to three sucks per swallow. Slight liquid loss and air intake may occur with suckling and are primarily observed in the second and third months, after the infant's physiological flexion has disappeared but before the infant has acquired mature oral motor control.

At 4 months of age, the tongue begins to move up and down, the hallmark movement of true sucking. The wide jaw excursions of the young infant are reduced, less liquid is lost, and nipple suction force increases. By 4 months of age, the infant is capable of taking in 20 or more sucks from the breast or bottle before pausing. Swallowing occurs intermittently (after four to five sucks) and without pausing. Breathing slows during sucking and occurs within and between sucking sequences. Occasionally, the infant

TABLE 15-2   Developmental Sequence of Eating Skills

Age	Type of Food	Sucking/Drinking Skills	Swallowing	Biting and Chewing
1 mo	Liquids only	Uses a suckling or sucking pattern	Tongue moves in extension–retraction to swallow	Does not bite or chew
3 mo	Liquids or puréed	Uses a suckling or sucking pattern Tongue moves in extension/retraction	Uses a primitive suckle–swallow pattern Sequences 20 or more sucks from bottle/breast	Rarely exhibited; may demonstrate reflexive biting
5 mo	Eats puréed foods Formula or breast milk remain primary sources of nutrition	Continues to use sucking pattern Tongue moves up and down One sip at a time taken from cup	Choking on breast or bottle is rare Takes puréed food well	Uses a primitive phasic bite-and-release pattern Biting is not yet controlled or sustained Jaw moves up and down in munching and biting
6 mo	Liquids and puréed foods	No longer loses liquids during sucking Uses a suckling or sucking pattern for cup drinking Tongue moves up and down on bottle but in extension–retraction with cup Has difficulty drinking from a cup and loses liquids	Swallows thicker puréed foods and some lumpy foods Uses long sequences of sucking, swallowing, and breathing with breast or bottle May cough or choke when using a cup	The up-and-down jaw movements are more variable and less automatic Uses diagonal rotary movement when moving the tongue to the side Some tongue lateralization when food is placed to the side Lips help to hold the food in place for chewing
9 mo	Soft foods, mashed table foods	Strong sucking pattern, no liquid loss	Uses long sequences of sucking during cup drinking Takes one to three sucks before stopping to swallow or breathe	Munches with diagonal movements as food is transferred from center to sides Voluntary biting on food and objects Lips are active with jaw during chewing Uses lateral movements to transfer food from the center to sides of mouth
12 mo	Easily chewed foods including meats, coarsely chopped foods	Most of liquid is now from a cup Uses a sucking pattern (up-and-down tongue movement) May lose liquid when using a cup	Swallows liquids and semisolid foods with tongue-tip elevation At times exhibits tongue protrusion Lips are closed during swallow	Controlled, sustained bite with soft cookie Begins rotary chewing movements Lips are active during chewing Easily transfers food from the center to both sides
18 mo	Coarsely chopped table foods, including most meats and raw vegetables	Mature sucking patterns Jaw is stable when drinking from the cup	Uses tongue-tip elevation with swallowing Swallows solid foods with easy lip closure No loss of food	Uses a controlled sustained bite on a hard cookie Chews with lips closed Demonstrates rotary chewing
24 mo	All table foods, all foods except those with skins, very tough meats, or foods that break into large pieces	Adult-like sucking patterns: up-and-down tongue movements	No liquid loss Swallows solid foods with easy lip closure Tongue-tip elevation used for swallowing	During chewing, can transfer food from both sides of the mouth Lips are closed during chewing Uses circular rotary movements when transferring food across the midline from one side to the other

Ages are approximate and may vary among infants.
Adapted from Glass, R., & Wolf, L. (1998). Feeding and oral motor skills. In J. Case-Smith (Ed.), *Pediatric occupational therapy and early intervention*. Boston: Butterworth Heinemann; Morris, S. E., & Klein, M. (2000). *Prefeeding skills* (2nd ed.). San Antonio, TX: Therapy Skill Builders.

may cough or choke when he or she momentarily loses coordination of sucking, swallowing, and breathing.

The 6-month-old infant demonstrates strong up-and-down tongue movement with minimal jaw excursion during sucking. Jaw stability increases and allows for better control of tongue movement. The lip seal is tighter, and liquid loss no longer occurs. In fact, 6 months is the age when many caregivers in the United States introduce the cup, usually a sipper cup with a spout. When first presented with a cup, the infant will try to use a suckling pattern so the jaw continues to move up and down, and the tongue moves back and forth in the mouth. The wide jaw excursions can result in some liquid loss. An infant's early attempts at cup feeding may be accompanied by some coughing.

At 9 months of age, the infant continues to feed from the bottle nipple using strong sucking patterns. When drinking from a cup, the jaw is not consistently stable on the rim of the cup, which makes drinking from a cup somewhat messy at that age. The infant stops to swallow or breathe after one to three sucks from the cup.

At 12 months of age, many infants make a full transition from bottle to cup for drinking during mealtime but may continue to bottle-feed at other times. Jaw stability, and consequently cup support, continues to be somewhat of a challenge. The infant may try to overcompensate by protruding his or her tongue slightly beneath the cup for additional support. At this age, elevation of the tongue tip during swallowing occurs for the first time. He or she bites on the rim of the cup to make the jaw more stable and obtain greater control of the cup. By 12 months of age, sequences of three suck-swallows occur during cup drinking.[44]

By 15 to 18 months of age, the infant has excellent coordination of sucking, swallowing, and breathing. When drinking from a cup, the infant's swallowing follows sucking without pauses. Coughing or choking rarely occurs.

At 24 months of age, the child can efficiently drink from a cup. He or she uses both up-and-down tongue movements and tongue tip elevation. Internal jaw stabilization develops, and the jaw appears still. The jaw becomes stable enough to support the rim of the cup, and biting on it is no longer necessary. The child swallows with easy lip closure and does not lose liquids from the cup. Lengthy suck-swallow sequences occur.

As the infant gains more control of jaw, tongue, and lip movement, he or she also learns to coordinate and arrange oral movements into rhythmic patterns of sucking, swallowing, and breathing.[16] The intricate synchronization among the oral structures is perhaps more important to the feeding process than the development of control of any one oral structure by itself.

Biting and Chewing

An infant's first biting or chewing movements are reflexive. At 4 to 5 months of age, the infant uses a rhythmic, stereotypic, phasic bite-and-release pattern on almost any substance placed in the mouth (e.g., a soft cookie, a cracker, or a toy). The jaw moves up and down rather than sideways and diagonally. When the phasic bite-and-release pattern occurs rhythmically and repeatedly, it is called *munching*. A munching pattern is characterized by vertical jaw movement and a back-and-forth tongue movement. The ability to move the tongue and jaw sideways is not yet developed at this age.

The munching pattern allows the infant to successfully eat pureed or soft foods that dissolve quickly.[65]

By 7 to 8 months of age, the infant begins to exhibit variations in this up-and-down munching pattern. He or she begins to use some diagonal jaw movement when the texture of the food requires the jaw to move both horizontally and vertically. The infant continues to use the phasic bite-and-release pattern when he or she bites on a cookie; thus, the jaw closes abruptly on the cookie and the infant sucks on it. The jaw holds the cookie, but the infant cannot yet successfully bite through it. A piece is broken off while the jaw remains closed on the cookie. When the infant receives food on a spoon, the upper lip actively cleans it from the spoon. The lips become more active during sucking and maintaining the food within the mouth.

By 9 months of age, the infant handles pureed and soft foods well. He or she continues to use a munching pattern, but the up-and-down jaw movements are now interspersed with diagonal movements. The infant transfers the food from the center of the mouth to the side using lateral tongue movements. The same lateral movements keep the food on the side during munching, making that process effective in mastication of soft or mashed table food. The lips are active during chewing, so they make contact as the jaw moves up and down.

Rotary chewing movements develop at approximately 12 months of age and are made possible by the increasing stability, control, and mobility of the jaw, evidenced by the child's sustained, well-graded bite on soft cookies. The tongue is actively involved in chewing by moving food from the center of the mouth to the sides, licking food from the lips, and demonstrating tip elevation on occasion. The infant is able to retrieve food on the lower lip by drawing it inward into the mouth.

At 18 months of age, the infant exhibits well-coordinated rotary chewing. He or she is able to chew soft meat and various table foods. The child can control and sustain bites and can bite off a piece of a hard cookie or a pretzel. The tongue becomes increasingly mobile and efficiently moves food within the mouth.

At 24 months of age, the child can eat most meats and raw vegetables.[65] The child can grade and sustain the bite and can easily bite on hard foods. The circular jaw movements that characterize mature chewing are present at this age. The tongue transfers food from one side of the mouth to the other using a rolling movement and moves skillfully to clear the lips and gums. Lip closure during chewing prevents loss of food.

Self-Feeding

The caregiver can introduce new challenges to the feeding process even before the child shows full mastery in a certain area of performance. Table 15-3 outlines the developmental sequence of self-feeding. The ages are approximate and overlapping.

Children are often eager to feed themselves. As early as 6 months of age, the infant may bring his or her hands up to the bottle and try to hold it. The caregiver should not prop the bottle because the infant lacks the motor skills necessary to remove the bottle if choking occurs. Also, the infant typically lacks the cognitive understanding that a dropped bottle can be retrieved and put back into the mouth. Infants older than 8 months of age actively hold the bottle, but caregivers should monitor their self-feeding to ensure adequate intake,

TABLE 15-3   Developmental Continuum in Self-Feeding

Age (mo)	Eating and Feeding Performance	Concurrent Changes in Performance Components		
		Sensorimotor	**Cognition**	**Psychosocial**
5–7	Takes cereal or puréed baby food from spoon	Has good head stability and emerging sitting abilities; reaches and grasps toys; explores and tolerates various textures (e.g., fingers, rattles); puts objects in mouth	Attends to effect produced by actions, such as hitting or shaking	Plays with caregiver during meals and engages in interactive routines
6–8	Attempts to hold bottle but may not retrieve it if it falls; needs to be monitored for safety reasons		Object permanence is emerging and infant anticipates spoon or bottle	Is easily distracted by stimuli (especially siblings) in the environment
6–9	Holds and tries to eat cracker but sucks on it more than bites it; consumes soft foods that dissolve in the mouth; grabs at spoon but bangs it or sucks on either end of it	Good sitting stability emerges; able to use hands to manipulate smaller parts of rattle; guided reach and palmar grasp applied to hand-to-mouth actions with objects	Uses familiar actions initially with haphazard variations; seeks novelty and is anxious to explore objects (may grab at food on adult's plate)	Recognizes people once regarded as strangers; emerging sense of self
9–13	Finger feeds self a portion of meals consisting of soft table foods (e.g., macaroni, peas, dry cereal) and objects if fed by an adult	Uses various grasps on objects of different sizes; able to isolate radial fingers on smaller objects	Has increased organization and sequencing of schemas to do desired activity; may have difficulty attending to events outside visual space (e.g., position of spoon close to mouth)	Prefers to act on objects than to be passive observer
12–14	Dips spoon in food, brings spoonful of food to mouth, but spills food by inverting spoon before it goes into mouth	Begins to place and release objects; likely to use pronated grasp on objects like crayon or spoon	Recognizes that objects have function and uses tools appropriately; relates objects together, shifting attention among them	Has interest in watching family routines
15–18	Scoops food with spoon and brings it to mouth	Shoulder and wrist stability demonstrate precise movements	Experiments to learn rules of how objects work; actively solves problems by creating new action solutions	Internalizes standards imposed by others for how to play with objects
24–30	Demonstrates interest in using fork; may stab at food such as pieces of canned fruit; proficient at spoon use and eats cereal with milk or rice with gravy with utensil	Tolerates various food textures in mouth; adjusts movements to be efficient (e.g., forearm supinated to scoop and lift spoon)	Expresses wants verbally; demonstrates imitation of short sequence of occupation (e.g., putting food on plate and eating it)	Has increasing desire to copy peers; looks to adults to see if they appreciate success in an occupation; interested in household routines

because infants are easily distracted once they satisfy their initial hunger.

Typically, finger feeding develops quickly and naturally by about 8 months of age when the infant receives soft cookies or crackers to hold. At this age, infants exhibit a radial digital grasp, which positions the cookie for entry into the mouth. From 9 to 13 months of age, the infant develops several important abilities, including better control of sitting posture, improved sitting balance, refined pincer grasp with controlled release, and refined isolated forearm and wrist movements, all of which greatly improve self-feeding skills. By 12 months of age, finger feeding is generally a preferred and enjoyed activity and occurs simultaneously with certain psychosocial changes that signal the infant's increased desire for independence, often manifested by refusal to be fed. The selection of finger foods should match the child's oral–motor skills (e.g., cooked vegetables are easily grasped and mashed with the tongue and gums).

Infants younger than 1 year of age will grasp, wave, and bang spoons during feeding. Around 12 months of age, the infant demonstrates an understanding of the spoon's function by poking at a bowl of food with a spoon and bringing it to the mouth. Because visual monitoring of the spoon's position is poor and the infant has difficulty sequencing scooping movements or adjusting the forearm and wrist, the food often slips from the spoon before it reaches the mouth. Attending to the whole activity and recognizing when the spoon is empty, which requires sufficient cognitive changes to use feedback, is necessary before the infant starts to control the wrist and forearm sufficiently for spoon-feeding. Infants will frequently insist on self-feeding even though independence means less success at satisfying hunger.

Full spoon-feeding proficiency emerges between 15 and 18 months of age when the infant begins to bring a spoon with sticky food, such as yogurt, into the mouth with minimal spillage. The infant holds the spoon in a pronated gross grasp and uses primarily shoulder movement to bring it to the mouth. By 24 months of age, the child spoon-feeds without spillage, balancing the spoon to hold a variety of foods. He or she holds the spoon in the radial fingers with the forearm supinated and is able to obtain the food and efficiently place the spoon into the mouth. Between 30 and 36 months of age, the child may begin to prefer a fork for stabbing foods and may learn to eat foods that are more difficult to balance on a spoon (e.g., cold cereal and rice with gravy).

Drinking

Infants as young as 6 months may demonstrate interest in drinking from a cup, but cup-drinking skills do not emerge fully until 12 months of age. At that time, the infant is better able to correctly position the cup to the mouth and to tip it at a degree that makes spillage less likely. There are several types of cups that can facilitate an infant's acquisition of cup-drinking skills. The first type used by the infant is a cup with a lid and a spout. It may have handles or it may be a small cup that the infant can hold in one hand. Placing only a little liquid in the cup initially decreases spillage and allows the child to control the flow. At 24 months of age, the child may begin to use a small 4- to 6-ounce cup without a lid, but spillage is inevitable at this juncture.

The ability to drink from a straw emerges at about 2 years of age, but it may become a skill even earlier if the caregiver exposes the child to straw drinking at a younger age. Use of a straw requires good lip seal and strong suction to bring the liquid into the mouth (Figure 15-2). In addition to the oral motor skills required to draw the liquid into the mouth, cognitive skills are needed to figure out how to use the straw. The infant often bites or blows on the straw before learning how to suck through it. This framework of typical development should help the therapist identify problems and establish realistic intervention goals and expected outcomes.[16]

EVALUATION

Feeding Problems: An Overview

The process of analyzing and identifying problematic areas should always start by asking parents and caregivers questions about feeding, eating, and swallowing. In addition, the therapist should elicit information about the child's medical history

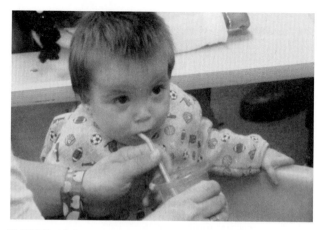

FIGURE 15-2 Using a straw to drink requires lip pursing and active lip seal. (Courtesy Jayne Shepherd.)

and evaluate the child for clinical signs of underlying disorders (Box 15-2).

Any evaluation for possible feeding problems should start by assessing mealtime participation, as well as by gathering information and impressions of the feeding situation from the caregivers. The child's developmental status and health history are also important in identifying feeding problems, as well as for making decisions about further evaluation and subsequent intervention. Usually, such information can be easily obtained from the child's medical records, from written and oral interviews with the parents and caregivers, and by mere observation. Such data often give the occupational therapy practitioner a general picture and may point to the feeding problem and, sometimes, to its underlying cause. The therapist obtains information about current feeding practices by asking the parents to describe feeding over the course of a typical day. This open-ended inquiry, as opposed to multiple-choice questions, allows the parents to bring forward their concerns. After these initial impressions, the therapist can ask more targeted questions, focusing on certain areas of interest, and obtain even more comprehensive information.

A discussion of the feeding problem from the parents' perspective is critical because it helps identify their primary concerns. For example, are the parents most concerned about weight gain or is it the length of time required for feeding that poses a problem? Does the child seem to lose most of the food consumed during feeding (e.g., through vomiting or reflux)? Is the child's behavior during feeding causing distress for the entire family during mealtime? Although the parents' expressed concerns become the focus of the subsequent intervention, the therapist should always consider other concerns expressed by professionals (such as doctors or other health care personnel) in developing a feeding plan, especially when these concerns differ from those expressed by the parents.

The parents also provide the team with information about the child's developmental and feeding histories. Obtaining this information helps the therapist identify the root of the feeding problem (e.g., if longstanding sensory or behavioral issues have affected feeding). Inquiring about the feeding history helps the therapist get a sense of any possible frustration and the parents' ability to cope with the child's feeding issues. The techniques used by parents may be helpful in identifying

BOX 15-2   Feeding History and Caregiver Concerns

1. Caregiver's primary concerns about feeding
   - Limited or inadequate consumption of food
   - Difficulty sucking or drinking
   - Problems with biting, chewing, or managing age-appropriate textures
   - Coughing, choking, or congestion during feeding
   - Refusal to try new foods, textures, or utensils
2. Pertinent medical history
   - Birth history
   - Major illnesses
   - Surgeries or hospitalizations
3. Diagnostic testing and results
   - Videofluoroscopic swallow study
   - Testing for gastroesophageal reflux
   - Food allergy work-up
4. Current nutritional status
   - Weight-for-age
   - Height-for-age
   - Body mass index (weight-for-height percentile)
5. Developmental and neuromotor status
   - Muscle tone
   - Cognitive development
   - Language skills
   - Gross and fine motor skills
   - Adaptive skills
6. Developmental feeding history
   - Breast- or bottle-feeding
   - Age at introduction of infant cereal or baby foods
   - Transition to solid food textures
   - Cup or straw-drinking experience
7. Current feeding methods and schedules
   - Food textures and amounts
   - Utensils, cups, and/or bottles
   - Positioning and location
   - Length of meals
   - Dependent or independent
   - Strategies used during meals
8. Child's behavior reactions during meals
   - Indication of hunger
   - Interest and enthusiasm for eating
   - Behavioral response to different feeders
   - Frequency of crying, gagging, or refusal
   - Events that lead to termination of the meal

Modified from Schuberth, L., Flanagan, J., & Cramer, T. (2008). Occupational therapy assessment and intervention. In P. J. Accardo (Ed.), *Capute & Accardo's neurodevelopmental disabilities in infancy and childhood* (3rd ed., pp. 97-107), Baltimore: Paul H. Brookes.

appropriate intervention strategies. Parents whose children have received therapy services in the past probably have important information to share regarding interventions that worked and those that did not. The interview can also help the therapist determine which parent or caregiver would do best in implementing recommendations, initiating a referral to an oral motor or feeding program, and discussing information about the child's progress in developing eating/feeding skills.

Recorded developmental histories are important because they supplement the parents' report and offer additional insights for the therapist. The written reports of other occupational and physical therapists, speech-language pathologists, early childhood specialists, and teachers provide fundamental knowledge about the child. For example, a child with a sustained hospitalization may not have had enough opportunities to progress, or an early history of restricted upper extremity movement may lead to restricted oral play, influencing sensory systems and, by extension, the ability to eat. Understanding the child's developmental course and rate of change in other occupational performance areas such as object play and social interactions is important for the therapist to set realistic goals, prioritize objectives, and choose appropriate intervention strategies.

Although these issues are discussed separately, feeding problems are seldom attributable to a single cause and usually are the result of delays or impairments in multiple areas. For example, children with severe sensory problems generally have oral motor skill delays, and children with swallowing disorders often have motor deficits.

Neuromotor Evaluation

The occupational therapist then completes a "hands-on" evaluation of generalized muscle tone, neuromuscular status, and general developmental level. Observation of movement initiation and transition patterns allows the occupational therapist to observe whether abnormal tone could be affecting feeding, eating, and/or swallowing. Muscle tone abnormalities interfere with the ability to maintain upright posture and head/neck alignment. They may also lead to difficulty grading or sustaining oral motor patterns, uncoordinated breathing, drooling, decreased oral exploration, and limited self-feeding. The use of adapted seating systems during the evaluation helps determine the optimal position for feeding. For many children, the upright position is the most effective and provides airway protection. For others some degree of recline may allow for better head control and retention of food.

Examination of Oral Structures and Oral Motor Patterns

The oral sensorimotor examination is the third part of the evaluation. The initial step is observation of symmetry, size, and range of motion of oral structures, including the jaw and larynx proceeding intraorally to the gums, dentition, hard and soft palate, and tongue. A thorough examination of the tongue is critical because the tongue serves many functions in feeding/eating and swallowing. At rest, the tongue should have a well-defined shape, with a nicely rounded tip and a central groove, and be seated inside on the bottom of the oral cavity. Increased oral tone may cause the tongue to be retracted, humped, or have tip elevation and may often be the primary cause of feeding difficulties. Children with food refusal and normal oral tone sometimes use these tongue positions as a defensive posture. In contrast, hypotonia may cause the tongue to be flat, lack a midline groove, and extend beyond the lips.

Eating and Feeding Performance

The final aspect of the comprehensive clinical assessment is the observation of the actual feeding/eating and swallowing process to assess level of performance and to analyze how motor, sensory, cognitive, and communication skills contribute to performance. It is important that the observation mimic those conditions as closely as possible under which the child normally eats and uses foods the child would typically eat. Parents or caregivers can either bring a meal from home or help the therapist select the menu. The therapist places the child in his or her typical feeding position, provides familiar utensils, and asks a parent or caregiver to feed the child the initial portion of the meal.

Observing the parent–child interaction gives the therapist clues about factors that may affect the child's food intake. During this time, the therapist reflects on the potential meaning of the occupation of eating to the child and his or her interest in participating. Observing the parent–child interaction also provides insights into the everyday context of feeding to help formulate recommendations. The following are signs to watch for:

- Does the parent talk to the child?
- Does the child send clear cues regarding readiness to eat, satiation, or preferences to foods?
- Does the parent respond to the child's nonverbal cues?

The therapist also needs to use a variety of textures while observing the child eating if this is age appropriate. When possible, the therapist precedes a trial of different textures with relaxed play with the child so that he or she becomes comfortable. Nonintrusive play can also help to establish rapport.

To observe the child's sensory responses, the therapist should use various textures and attempt placement of food in different parts of the mouth. When the child exhibits aversive responses to food inside the mouth, the parent is asked if the responses are typical or exaggerated because of discomfort with an unfamiliar feeder.

Videofluoroscopic Swallow Study (VFSS)

To further analyze the child's feeding and eating issues, the therapist may need to return to the child's medical record for additional information. Does the child have a medical condition that leads to feeding problems or poor weight gain? Instances of pneumonia and frequent and prolonged upper respiratory infection may indicate a swallowing problem. To confirm or rule out swallowing problems, a videofluoroscopic swallow study may be needed.

The modified barium swallow study is the radiographic procedure of choice for assessing the oral, pharyngeal, and upper esophageal anatomy, and the physiology of the stages of swallowing. It is particularly useful in identifying aspiration or the risk of aspiration and in tailoring treatment for infants and children with feeding disorders. The test can also be helpful in detecting problems related to head and neck positioning, bolus characteristics, rate and sequence of presentation, and food/liquid consistencies. The results of the test can be helpful in identifying compensatory techniques to minimize the risk of aspiration and maximize eating efficiency.[9] The therapist selects the types of food textures based on the child's current diet and feeding goals and mixes them with liquid or paste barium.[58] It is important to remember that the VFSS only shows a brief sample of swallowing, and positioning, amount, and order of food/liquid bolus presentation is up to the occupational therapist or speech pathologist conducting the study.[8]

VFSS is used to analyze the swallow mechanism and is particularly important for children who aspirate or are at high risk for aspiration because of severe motor problems.[29] Factors that suggest swallowing problems include gagging, coughing, choking, nasopharyngeal reflux, increased congestion, wet vocal quality, and the occurrence of respiratory infections and/or pneumonia.[46] Aspiration may be silent, so a thorough history and feeding observation are critical. The therapist should distinguish aspiration from penetration. Penetration describes the flow of food or liquid underneath the epiglottis into the laryngeal vestibule but not into the airway. It does not pass through the vocal folds. Aspiration refers to food entering the airway before, during, or after a swallow. Because the recording shows the food traveling through the mouth and pharynx, the therapist receives real-time, detailed information about the swallowing problem.[60,69] The results of the VFSS indicate the safety and appropriateness of oral feeding and guide the therapist's recommendations.[71] These may include modified positions and textures for the parents to use during feeding that appear to result in optimal swallowing patterns without aspiration. Although the VFSS gives the therapist important information and insight about the swallowing problem, it may not always be representative of the child's typical feeding in a more natural environment.

Medical Conditions Affecting Eating

Feeding problems may be associated with specific medical diagnoses. Children with cerebral palsy may be either hypotonic or hypertonic. Facial hypotonia often results in an open-mouth resting posture, drooling, and decreased sensory awareness. Children with hypertonia often present with a strong tongue thrust or bite reflex.[54] Congenital oral–facial anomalies such as cleft lip and palate and micrognathia may be associated with Pierre-Robin malformation sequence or may be part of Stickler syndrome.[69] Children with Down syndrome often have a small oral cavity, hypotonia, and macroglossia, all of which can contribute to feeding difficulties. Other structural abnormalities that could impact feeding are tracheoesophageal fistula and esophageal atresia, as well as gastrointestinal problems such as gastroesophageal reflux and dysmotility.

Complicated pulmonary and feeding issues are well documented in the premature infant.[34,67] The Neonatal Oral-Motor Assessment Scale (NOMAS)[50] is the visual observation method most commonly used to assess the nonnutritive sucking and the nutritive sucking skills of infants up to approximately 8 weeks postterm.[20]

Behavioral difficulties often manifest as food refusal or food selectivity but are often associated with some medical problem such as pain from reflux or an allergic reaction and are often maintained over time by behavioral factors.[15] Food refusal can also be associated with poor dentition or sensitive gums. Caregivers sometimes neglect oral hygiene in children with oral motor dysfunction, oral hypersensitivity, or in those demonstrating food refusal.

Gastroesophageal reflux (GER) is an increasingly common problem in the general population and may be an underlying cause of swallowing dysfunction in children. GER occurs when the lower esophageal sphincter does not close properly or opens spontaneously, and stomach contents move upward (acid reflux) into the esophagus. During the first year of life, mild GER is common, resulting in occasional spitting up or vomiting, but it is transient and is generally not considered a medical problem. True gastroesophageal reflux disease (GERD) results from more prolonged reflux that causes clinical signs and symptoms including regurgitation, nausea, chest pain, coughing, and other respiratory problems. During feeding, infants or young children with GERD may be unusually irritable, arch their backs, and refuse food completely, which leads to poor weight gain.[45]

The presence and extent of GERD can be confirmed by an esophageal pH probe. The probe is inserted into the esophagus through the nose to monitor abnormal acid levels, usually over a 24-hour period. Radiology studies including barium swallow or upper GI series can detect anatomic abnormalities such as hiatal hernia and assess peristalsis in the esophagus. If the GERD causes aspiration, the x-ray film may show lung changes. An upper endoscopy with esophageal biopsy (also referred to as an esophagogastroduodenoscopy [EGD]) can diagnose inflammatory conditions such as reflux esophagitis or eosinophilic esophagitis, commonly associated with allergies. Fiberoptic endoscopic evaluation of swallowing with sensory testing (FEESST) is a relatively new tool that allows direct visualization of the larynx and pharynx to observe penetration, aspiration, spillage, and residual material.[45] Gastroesophageal scintigraphy or "milk scan" assesses the severity of GERD using a noninvasive nuclear medicine scanning technique that involves the ingestion and tracking of radiolabeled milk as it moves through the esophagus and stomach.[53]

Contextual Factors

Evaluation of the context (environment) in which feeding occurs is essential to the development of intervention plans. In some cases, feeding problems are based primarily on contextual issues, including physical, social, temporal, and cultural. Box 15-3 lists some of the contextual factors that should be considered in assessing feeding.

Understanding the contextual factors that influence mealtimes and feeding performance helps determine the basis for the problem and possible solutions. Certain contextual factors can be changed easily (e.g., a child can be positioned in a chair that is more upright and has straps that maintain good alignment); however, cultural beliefs and family routines are less amenable to change and should be accommodated in the intervention plan. Contextual factors may determine the success of the intervention (i.e., which recommended strategies the family will implement). For example, if the caregivers do not value or prioritize the child's independence in feeding, they are unlikely to follow through with suggestions to increase feeding independence.

The assessment findings are discussed and interpreted by team members, including the family, to develop a cohesive intervention plan. Any intervention for feeding problems should be holistic, meaning that it considers the whole child, involves the family, and involves collaboration with professionals from other disciplines as needed.[60,64]

INTERVENTION: GLOBAL CONSIDERATIONS

Problems with feeding, eating, and swallowing are caused by multiple underlying factors. If feeding problems persist as the child grows older, new problems or skill impairments may appear that further complicate the intervention needs. For example, children with dysphagia who require nonoral feeding for an extended period of time may experience subsequent developmental delays in self-feeding skills because of lack of experience. Occupational therapists can provide direct intervention for children with feeding, eating, and swallowing disorders to improve functional participation in mealtimes. Throughout the intervention process, therapists must consider medical and nutritional problems that often coexist with the child's feeding disorder and collaborate with physicians and nutritionists to create an optimal intervention plan.

Feeding activities occur multiple times throughout the day within a variety of natural environments, and occupational therapists must work closely with families and other caregivers to ensure carryover within daily routines. Children with oral feeding difficulties often require one-on-one attention or increased caregiver time and effort throughout each day. Mealtimes may

---

BOX 15-3 Guiding Questions to Evaluate the Contexts for Feeding

PHYSICAL
- Is seating and positioning adequate? supportive? Does it provide stability?
- Are head, neck, shoulders, and pelvis well aligned?
- Is space adequate for eating activities?
- Are noise and activity levels conducive to eating?

SOCIAL
- Who feeds the child?
- Who is present during the meal?
- What is the nature of the social interaction among family members during the meal?

- What communication/interaction occurs between caregiver and child during feeding?

TEMPORAL
- Is sufficient time allotted and available for a relaxing meal?
- How often is the child fed?
- How long does feeding take?

CULTURAL
- How do cultural beliefs and values influence mealtime?
- What foods does the family eat?

be quite stressful for parents, especially when the child's oral feeding difficulties create ongoing problems with nutrition and growth. Whenever possible, typical family mealtime routines should be preserved within the intervention program. Therapists should consider the caregivers' time investment and provide realistic recommendations that do not significantly increase the burden of care within the family system. Parents of children with feeding, eating, and swallowing disorders may benefit from peer support groups, which have been shown to strengthen caregivers' abilities to cope with stressful problems on a day-to-day basis.[17]

Occupational therapists use a holistic approach when developing a treatment plan for children with feeding, eating, and swallowing disorders. Consideration is given to many different overlapping areas described within the Occupational Therapy Practice Framework, including child factors, performance skills, activity demands, contexts, and family patterns.[5] A comprehensive intervention plan may include environmental adaptations, positioning recommendations, sensory development activities, behavioral strategies, neuromuscular handling techniques, food texture modifications, adaptive equipment, or suggestions to improve independence in self-feeding.

Safety and Health

Basic safety guidelines should be followed when providing occupational therapy treatment. Children who demonstrate clinical signs of aspiration may require additional assessment with videofluoroscopy to determine appropriate feeding goals. Therapists must also consider the child's nutritional status and prioritize treatment goals to maximize a child's ability to meet basic nutritional needs. Some interventions may require implementation outside of regular meal sessions, so as not to disrupt the child's ability to meet oral intake requirements.

The Occupational Safety and Health Administration mandates the use of gloves during therapy activities when there is potential for contact with mucous membranes within the mouth.[48] Another critical factor when working with different food textures is the understanding that certain foods carry a high choking risk and require modifications or close supervision with young children, especially round slices of hot dogs, small hard candies, nuts, popcorn, raw carrots, fruits with seeds, and chewing gum.

INTERVENTION STRATEGIES

Environmental Adaptations

Occupational therapists often recommend changes to the mealtime environment to promote success with oral feeding. Environmental adaptations may be recommended to change the structure of the child's daily mealtime routines. Specifically, therapists may provide intervention recommendations for scheduling and location of meals, length of meal periods, sensory stimulation within the environment, or changes to the order of mealtime activities.

Children often benefit from regularly scheduled meals at consistent times or locations from day to day. When parents allow children to snack or consume liquids throughout the day, there may be little opportunity for children to become hungry during mealtimes, when more nutritious foods are presented. Consistently scheduled meals and snacks allow the child to experience periods of time without eating, which may promote hunger cues and more interest in eating.[44] Children should also have a consistent location for meals, such as sitting in a high chair or at a specific table. Wandering around while eating or having meals in different locations every day may be distracting for young children and does not help to establish positive mealtime behaviors.[39]

Some children may require shorter meal lengths. Children with neuromuscular impairments may eat slowly and have long meal periods because of oral motor or self-feeding difficulties. Parents of children with poor growth may prolong mealtimes to try to encourage more food intake. When mealtimes are longer than 30 to 40 minutes on a regular basis, the demands on the child and the caregiver become extremely high. Children who become fatigued during prolonged meals may expend increased energy to sustain the feeding, outweighing any benefits from additional oral intake.[29] Children with delayed gastric emptying or gastroesophageal reflux may benefit from smaller, more frequent meals throughout the day.[44] Larger meals may create more discomfort or episodes of vomiting in children with gastrointestinal disorders.

The amount of sensory stimulation and number of distractions within the environment may also impact a child's oral feeding skills. Many children show improved oral feeding when environmental distractions are limited. Limiting the sensory stimuli within the environment may be beneficial for children who are concentrating on independent self-feeding, children who are hypersensitive to environmental stimuli, and infants with disorganized suck-swallow-breathe coordination. A calming sensory environment can be created with dim lights, reduced noise, soft or rhythmic music, and limited interruptions. Alternatively, some children may eat better when environmental distractions are present during mealtimes. Active toddlers may consume more food or have improved ability to remain seated at a meal when they are allowed access to a favorite toy or television show. The use of distraction may also help some children with defensive behaviors, to reduce the child's focus on the discomfort of the oral feeding activity.[50]

Occupational therapists may also consider the order of presenting foods and liquids during meal sessions. Some children have more success when challenging oral feeding activities are presented at the beginning of the meal, when the child is feeling hungry and their muscles are less fatigued. When the challenging task creates disruption or distress and impacts the child's oral intake for the remainder of the meal, therapists may consider implementing a new intervention outside of meals or during a smaller snack session.

Positioning Adaptations

Oral motor and feeding activities require skilled movement and coordination of many small muscle groups. Children with postural instability and neuromuscular impairments have difficulty with oral motor control if they do not have adequate positioning support. Positioning changes may have an immediate impact on some difficult oral motor problems such as tonic bite and tongue thrust movement patterns. When a therapist is making positioning adaptations, proximal support (i.e., support at the trunk and neck) influences distal movement and control. For this reason, therapists should consider positioning throughout the child's whole body. Positioning of the feet, legs, and pelvis influences the child's trunk stability. Stability, muscle tone, and activity in the trunk muscles affect the child's ability to move or stabilize the head and neck. The position and muscle activation of the child's head and neck influence jaw movements. Finally, good jaw stability and freedom of movement influence the child's tongue and lip control.[44] Providing external postural stability, excellent alignment, and comfort during oral feeding activities optimizes a child's oral motor skills and oral intake.

In general, positioning adaptations provide stability in the trunk and support the child in a midline orientation with the head and neck aligned in neutral or slight flexion during oral feeding. The child's age, size, neuromuscular status, and self-feeding skills must be considered, as well as the caregiver's position and comfort. Lastly, positioning adaptations should promote social interaction and communication during mealtimes.

Infants may be supported in a variety of positions during oral feeding. Side-lying within the caregiver's arms is a common position during breast-feeding. This position may also be recommended for children who have difficulty coordinating sucking, swallowing, and breathing, because the impact of gravity does not immediately draw the liquid into the pharyngeal space. It may be difficult for the caregiver to hold a child in a side-lying position for prolonged periods, especially with older children or infants with hypotonia. Infants may also be supported in supine position within the caregiver's arms or on a caregiver's thighs facing the caregiver (Figure 15-3). The supine position provides excellent alignment and midline orientation for infants who take formula from a bottle. An infant seat, car seat, or a Tumble Forms Feeder Chair (Figure 15-4) may be adapted with small rolls to provide head and trunk support or slight shoulder protraction to help an infant hold his or her own bottle. Both of these positioning options allow the feeder to have two hands free, creating opportunities to provide oral motor support or implement handling techniques.

For older infants and toddlers who are engaging in spoon-feeding activities, additional positioning options are available. A regular high chair may provide adequate trunk support and can be easily adapted with small towel rolls for additional foot support or lateral support. The height of a standard high chair

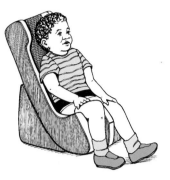

FIGURE 15-4   Tumble Forms Feeder Chair offers support and an adjustable feeding angle.

also allows caregivers to sit comfortably at a table, promoting social interaction between the child and the family.

Older children with neuromuscular impairments may require a wheelchair or a Rifton chair (Figure 15-5) to provide optimal support during oral feeding. A variety of options and accessories are available for customization of these positioning devices. Within a seated position, the child should have supported feet and neutral pelvic alignment. Lateral trunk or arm supports, a pelvic strap, or a tray may help to provide more stability for the trunk. Wheelchairs may also be

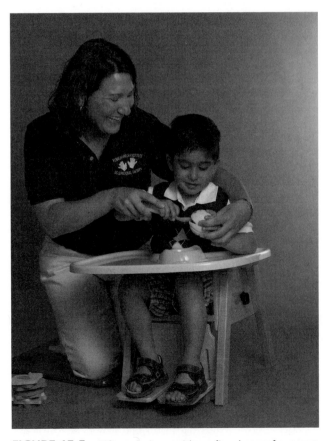

FIGURE 15-5   Rifton chair provides a firm base of support to trunk and feet during self-feeding. (Courtesy Kennedy Krieger Institute.)

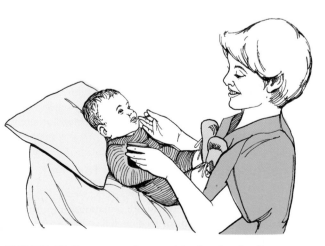

FIGURE 15-3   Face-to-face positioning for feeding.

customized with a padded vest strap or humeral wings to help promote a forward position of the shoulders and arms for added stability.

Research has been conducted to evaluate the use of adaptive seating in children with neuromuscular impairments and developmental delays. Results from this research indicate that children demonstrated improved head control, reaching, grasping, sitting posture, and visual tracking when using positioning devices, as well as decreased dependence on caregivers during activities of daily living.[35] Hulme and colleagues reported that optimal positioning included vertical head and trunk position, hip flexion greater than 90 degrees, knee flexion at 90 degrees, and feet supported on a flat surface.[35]

Therapists may need to work with families to determine whether positioning equipment will fit comfortably within the home and to evaluate caregiver perceptions about adaptive equipment. Reilly and Skuse studied positioning during mealtimes within the home for children with cerebral palsy.[52] They found that positioning problems were common among children with cerebral palsy; however, only 50% of parents who received adaptive positioning devices used the equipment regularly. Occupational therapists must evaluate each child and caregiver individually to determine the best options for positioning during oral feeding, provide education about the benefits of proper positioning, and suggest alternatives to adaptive equipment when necessary.

Interventions for Sensory Problems

Abnormal sensory processing, such as hypersensitivity to food tastes, textures, or smells, can create significant problems with oral feeding. Children with oral hypersensitivity often react negatively to touch near or within the mouth. They may turn away from feeding or tooth-brushing activities, restrict food variety, gag frequently, or have difficulty transitioning to age-appropriate food textures. Children diagnosed with generalized tactile defensiveness have a significantly higher incidence of oral hypersensitivity and oral feeding difficulties compared with typical peers.[62] Oral hypersensitivity is also common in children who have received extensive medical interventions. Medical interventions such as intubation, orogastric or nasogastric tube feeding, or frequent oral suctioning may have caused ongoing distress or gagging, affecting the development of the sensory systems. Early feeding problems experienced in infancy, such as gastroesophageal reflux or swallowing difficulties, may have created negative associations between food consumption and discomfort.[61] The child's sensory system becomes overprotective, and hypersensitivities may continue long after the noxious stimuli or swallowing impairments are eliminated. Children with developmental and neurologic conditions, including diagnoses such as autism, pervasive developmental disorders, cerebral palsy, traumatic brain injury, genetic conditions, and generalized sensory integration dysfunction may also exhibit oral hypersensitivity.

In most young children, oral exploration and gradual adaptation are natural processes assisted by oral feeding and associated comfort and caregiver bonding. Children who experience prolonged periods of nonoral feeding may demonstrate signs of oral hypersensitivity.[64] When the child's oral sensory system is not challenged to explore tastes and textures of objects and foods during critical periods of development, the child may have difficulty adjusting to new oral stimuli at a later developmental stage.[61]

Occupational therapists create opportunities for gradual oral sensory exploration through play and positive experiences to reduce oral hypersensitivity. Children may tolerate greater sensory input if the activity is under the child's control and provided in the context of a motivating, developmentally appropriate activity.[14] Therapists provide access to textured objects, teethers, or vibrating toys, and playfully encourage the child to explore them with his or her hands, face, and mouth. Therapists may also engage the child in songs or games to encourage self-directed touch to the face, or play dress-up with hats, scarves, or sunglasses.

Children with oral hypersensitivity may benefit from generalized sensory deep pressure or calming strategies such as slow, linear rocking before oral stimulation. Infants may be encouraged to soothe themselves with hand-to-mouth activities or a pacifier.

Children may gradually improve acceptance of therapist-directed touch with firm pressure that is first applied distally on the body, such as on the arms or shoulders, before moving to touch near the face. A variety of tools can be used to provide stimulation within the mouth, including a gloved finger, a warm washcloth, a Nuk brush, a Pro-Prefer (nonridged) device, an infant or child toothbrush, or a teething ring. Applying firm pressure to the child's gums or palate may help to reduce oral hypersensitivity. Older children with more mature oral motor skills may enjoy whistles, oral sound-making games, bubbles, and blow toys to improve oral sensory processing.

During feeding activities, the occupational therapist introduces new flavors and textures gradually. A lollipop or teething ring can be dipped into a new flavor of food. Children may advance their oral feeding skills when slight changes are made to their current preferred foods. The therapist can gradually thicken a food, combine strained baby foods with pureed table foods for stronger flavors, or change food temperatures to expand the child's sensory experiences. The therapist or parent should provide consistent praise and encouragement for the child's oral exploration and feeding attempts.

Some children with sensory integration dysfunction have low sensory registration and may demonstrate poor oral sensory awareness. These children may frequently seek oral sensory stimulation by mouthing their hands, toys, or clothing. They may have decreased awareness of drooling or try to overstuff their mouths when eating. Occupational therapists may establish a treatment program to provide enhanced oral sensory input intermittently throughout the day. Oral activities with a Nuk brush, cold washcloth, or vibrating device can be used to provide oral sensory stimulation.[39] During mealtimes, foods with strong flavors and cold temperatures may help the child take appropriately sized bites of food. Children who consistently overstuff their mouths when eating may require foods that are cut into pieces, verbal cues, or supervision for safety.

Neuromuscular Interventions for Oral Motor Impairments

A wide range of children demonstrate oral motor impairments that affect the development of feeding skills. Oral motor problems are seen frequently in children with global neuromuscular impairments resulting from cerebral palsy, traumatic brain injury, prematurity, or genetic conditions such as trisomy 21. Children without neuromuscular impairments may also demonstrate oral motor problems when they are delayed in transitioning from a bottle to a cup or from puréed foods to textured foods. Inexperience with normal feeding activities may contribute to oral motor weakness and coordination difficulties. Oral hypersensitivity may cause a child to retract his tongue back within the mouth to avoid stimulation, contributing to maladaptive oral movement patterns. Occupational therapists include oral motor activities within a comprehensive intervention plan to promote strength and coordination for the development of functional oral feeding skills.

Whenever possible, oral motor activities should include foods or flavors to incorporate taste receptors and facilitate the integration of both sensory and motor skills for a functional response. Hypersensitive children may tolerate nonnutritive activities initially, before they are able to accept the additional sensory input that food flavors provide.

Jaw weakness is often seen in children with oral feeding difficulties. This may contribute to an open-mouth posture at rest, drooling, food loss during feeding, difficulty with chewing a variety of age-appropriate foods, or poor stabilization when drinking from a cup. Jaw weakness and instability may also affect lip closure for spoon feeding and control during swallowing. Occupational therapists may facilitate jaw strength with a variety of nonnutritive or nutritive activities. Nonnutritive strengthening activities may include sustained biting or repetitive chewing on a resistive device or flexible tubing (Figure 15-6) before the introduction of food textures. Nutritive jaw strengthening activities may include biting or chewing on fruits or vegetables encased in a mesh pouch or progressive resistive activities with a variety of solid or chewy foods placed over the molar surfaces.[56]

Children with neuromuscular impairments may have strong patterns of abnormal oral movement. A tonic bite may be seen, in which a child bites down forcefully in response to a stimulus and has subsequent difficulty opening or relaxing the jaw. Poor trunk and head control and positioning in an extension pattern may contribute to a tonic bite. Assisting the child into flexion of the neck with good trunk and shoulder support helps to reduce this pattern. A strong tongue thrust movement pattern may also be present, where the tongue forcefully protrudes beyond the border of the lips during oral feeding activities. A well-supported and slightly flexed position reduces the severity of this abnormal movement pattern. Children with tongue thrust may also benefit from oral motor activities to facilitate tongue lateralization and placement of the spoon or food bolus to the sides of the mouth rather than at midline.[11]

Children may demonstrate immature forward-backward tongue movements during feeding, poor dissociation of the tongue from the jaw, and poor tongue lateralization to control textured food over the molar surfaces. Occupational therapists may engage the child in activities to facilitate tongue movements such as encouraging the child to make silly faces in a mirror or to lick lollipops or favorite flavors at the corners of the mouth or within the cheeks. Stimulating the sides of the tongue and inside the cheeks with a Nuk brush or oral motor tool may encourage tongue lateralization. Elevation of the tongue tip can be facilitated when touching the tip of the tongue with an oral motor device and providing slight pressure on the anterior hard palate just behind the front teeth.[11,33]

Problems affecting the lips and cheeks include abnormal tightness or weakness. Children may demonstrate lip or cheek retraction, making it difficult for the child to assume or sustain lip closure. Good lip closure and lip seal are needed to assist the child with oral food control and prevent anterior spillage during feeding. It is also very difficult to swallow with retracted lips and cheeks because the lips seal the oral cavity to create pressure to propel the food bolus into the pharyngeal cavity. Slow perioral and intraoral cheek stretches can help promote lip closure before initiating functional activities with spoon-feeding or whistles.

Evidence reporting the efficacy of oral motor intervention is extremely limited. Research Note 15-1 describes one study evaluating oral motor intervention in children with cerebral palsy. However, numerous authors suggest that oral motor therapy is an important component of a global treatment approach for children with feeding problems.[6,18,42]

Adaptive Equipment

A variety of adaptive equipment is available for feeding activities, including adaptive spoons, forks, cups, and straws. Adaptive equipment may promote improvement in oral motor control, increase independence in self-feeding, or compensate for a motor or sensory impairment.

Occupational therapists should consider the properties of the spoon or fork used in feeding activities. A spoon with a shallow bowl may help a child with decreased lip closure. A spoon with bumps or ridges on the bottom of the bowl or a chilled metal spoon may provide additional sensory input for a child with decreased sensory registration. A rubber-coated or dense plastic spoon may be used as an alternative to a metal spoon for a child who bites down on the utensil. Utensils with shorter handles or larger grip diameters may help a child to self-feed more independently.[39]

A child first learning to drink from a straw may do well with a shorter or smaller straw, such as one that typically comes with a juice box. These straws require less oral suction and deliver a

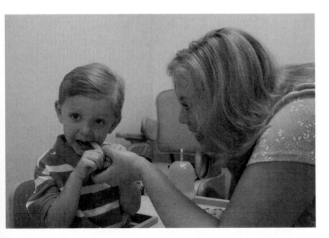

FIGURE 15-6   Using a resistive device to improve oral motor skills for advanced food textures. (Courtesy of Kennedy Krieger Institute.)

RESEARCH NOTE 15-1

Gisel, E. G. (1994). Oral-motor skills following sensorimotor intervention in the moderately eating-impaired child with cerebral palsy. Dysphagia, 9, 180-192.

ABSTRACT

This study looked at the efficacy of oral sensorimotor treatment in children with cerebral palsy. Outcomes were reported for nutrition anthropometrics, such as weight and skin fold parameters. Additional outcomes were reported for functional oral feeding activities, including spoon feeding, biting, chewing, cup-drinking, straw-drinking, swallowing, and drooling. Twenty-seven American toddlers and school-aged children with cerebral palsy completed the 20-week study. Comparisons were made among treatment groups: protocols comprised 20 weeks of oral sensorimotor treatment, 20 weeks of chewing-only treatment, and 10 weeks of no treatment followed by 10 weeks of treatment. During the treatment phase, oral motor therapy or chewing was completed daily for 5 to 7 minutes prior to snack or lunch. Oral motor treatment interventions were described in detail, and included activities to stimulate tongue lateralization, lip closure, and chewing skills. The results showed a positive treatment effect at the end of the 20-week period for all three treatment groups, with improvements noted in the areas of spoon-feeding, chewing, and biting skills. Each group showed improvements in different functional oral feeding skills, however, improvements were noted in the third group only after treatment was initiated in the second 10-week period. Improvements in nutrition anthropometrics, cup-drinking skills, and videofluoroscopic swallowing results were not significant for any of the three treatment groups.

IMPLICATIONS FOR PRACTICE

Oral motor and chewing interventions may be effective to improve some oral feeding activities; however, the research evidence continues to be limited. Occupational therapists should carefully, objectively, and regularly evaluate whether progress is being demonstrated in their patients. Therapists may also supplement oral motor therapy with a variety of interventions, including food texture modifications, sensory-based activities, postural and respiratory activities, positioning adaptations, and behavioral techniques as part of a comprehensive treatment plan to improve feeding skills in this population.

smaller liquid bolus. Children who require thickened liquids or those with decreased lip closure may benefit from the use of a relatively short straw with a larger diameter. Therapists may also consider using a straw with a specialized one-way valve. When liquid is pulled into a valved straw, it does not fall back into the cup if the child loses suction. A cup with a handle on it may help a child with poor fine motor skills to drink more independently. U-shaped cut-out cups help to maintain a neutral head position when drinking liquid. Clear cut-out cups also allow the therapist or caregiver to easily see liquid entering the child's mouth when physical assistance is provided for drinking activities.

Modifications to Food and Liquid Properties

Different consistencies of liquid require different oral motor and oral sensory demands (Box 15-4). Thin liquids presented from an open cup are the most difficult to control within the mouth. Thick, lumpy, or pasty foods such as oatmeal require more oral motor strength and sensory tolerance when compared with smoother and thinner puréed foods. Occupational therapists may recommend changes to food or liquid properties to compensate for a variety of swallowing, oral motor, and oral sensory deficits.

Thickened liquid is easier to control with the lips and tongue, moves more slowly within the mouth, and allows the child more time to organize a bolus for effective swallowing without early spillage into the pharyngeal cavity. Children with dysphagia may not be able to coordinate swallowing with thin liquids, and aspiration and penetration events are more common with thin liquids when evaluated with videofluoroscopic swallow studies.[13,26,43] Thickened liquids may also be used to compensate for oral motor difficulties when a child is first learning to drink from an open cup, even when the child has pharyngeal competence with thin liquids from a bottle or sip cup. When a therapist recommends thickened liquids, the child's liquid intake and hydration status must be closely monitored to ensure the child is meeting daily fluid requirements.

A variety of foods and supplements can be used to thicken liquids. Simply Thick is one type of commercial gel thickener; it is tasteless and does not add any texture to the liquid, even after the liquid has been sitting out for some time. Other commercial thickeners include powder thickeners such as Diafoods Thick-It and Thick-It 2, and Resource Thicken-Up. Puréed or baby food fruits and vegetables may be used to create blenderized smoothies. Dried infant cereals or mashed potato flakes may be added to thicken formula or milk. Yogurt or pudding may be added to create blenderized milkshakes. Each thickener has different sensory, nutrition, and thickening properties, all of which should be considered in a therapist's recommendations.

There are also multiple different textures and sensory properties of foods that may be considered within an intervention plan. Foods with a smooth, even, cohesive consistency, such as yogurt and strained fruits or vegetables, are easier to manage when a child has oral sensory and oral motor impairments. Foods that are dense, crunchy, sticky, or uneven in consistency are more difficult to manage. Table 15-4 provides examples of food progressions based on texture and consistency.

BOX 15-4 Liquid Consistencies Categorized from Thinnest to Thickest

- **Thin:** The consistency of water or juice. Many formulas and milk products have a slightly higher viscosity than that of clear liquids; however, they are still considered thin liquids. Soup broth and foods that melt are also considered thin liquids.
- **Nectar:** The consistency of tomato juice, including many natural fruit nectars (such as apricot nectar or pear nectar) and some store-bought yogurt smoothies.
- **Honey:** The consistency of honey, which slowly drips off a spoon

TABLE 15-4 Food Progression Based on Texture and Consistency

	Puréed	Junior, Coarse Puréed	Wet-Ground, Mashed	Soft, Dissolvable	Chopped, Soft Solid	Full Diet
Meats and meat substitutes	Strained meats or proteins; foods are blenderized to a smooth, even consistency	Commercial junior foods; soft meats finely ground in a food grinder with added liquids; scrambled eggs that are mashed; hummus	Ground meats with gravy; scrambled soft eggs; mashed tofu	Ground meats; regular scrambled eggs; tofu	Small pieces of soft meats; hard-cooked eggs, deli-sliced turkey or ham	Cut-up meats; stew; almonds or nuts
Dairy products	Thinned pudding; plain yogurt; strained cottage cheese	Fork-mashed cottage cheese; tapioca pudding; thickened cream soups	Cottage cheese	Yogurt with soft fruits; American cheese slices	Cheddar or Swiss cheese	All dairy products
Breads and cereals	Infant cereals thinned with milk	Thicker infant cereals; Cream of Wheat	Cooked cereals such as oatmeal	Breads, muffins, crackers, cereal (without milk), pancakes; well-cooked pasta or rice	Dry cereals with milk; sandwiches with smooth filling cut into small pieces; firmer pasta or rice	Sandwiches with various fillings
Fruits and vegetables	Strained fruits and vegetables	Junior fruits; junior vegetables; regular unstrained applesauce; mashed potatoes or yams	Fork-mashed, soft canned fruits without skins; soft ripe mashed fresh fruits; fork-mashed, well-cooked vegetables	Canned fruits (peaches, pears) or soft ripe fruits cut into small pieces (peeled); well-cooked vegetables	Canned fruits of increased texture (fruit cocktail); regular bite-sized pieces of cooked vegetables cut into small pieces	Raw fruits; dried fruits; raw vegetables with fibers or skins (corn, celery, peppers); vegetable soups, mixed salads

---

BOX 15-5 Levels of Food Texture for Dysphagia Management

Level 1: Puréed—Puréed foods that are homogeneous, cohesive, or pudding-like.
Level 2: Mechanically Altered—Cohesive, moist, semisolid foods that may require some chewing. Ground or minced meats and fork-mashed soft fruits and vegetables are included in this diet level. Most bread products, crackers, and dry foods are excluded.
Level 3: Advanced—Soft–solid foods that require more chewing ability, such as crackers, breads, cooked vegetables, soft fruits, and meats. Excludes some fruits with skins, hard or crunchy vegetables, tough meats such as beef or pork steak, and foods that are very sticky or dry.
Level 4: Regular—No food restrictions.

Data from American Dietetic Association: National Dysphagia Diet Task Force. (2002). *National dysphagia diet: Standardization for optimal care.* Chicago: American Dietetic Assoc.

The National Dysphagia Diet provides standardized terminology when describing food texture modifications in dysphagia management.[3] Although pediatric therapists often use additional descriptors for food textures, such as "junior" or "ground," some institutions have begun using the terminology from the National Dysphagia Diet (Box 15-5).

When presenting foods and liquids, therapists may alter the size of the bite or sip of liquid. When first beginning to advance with a new skill for the child, therapists may present a food or liquid in a small, consistent bolus size. For example, offering one teaspoon of liquid (5 mL) from a small cut-out cup may help a therapist to clearly evaluate the child's oral motor and swallowing skills when compared with unmeasured free access sips. Similarly, offering a smaller food bolus when trying a new taste or texture may promote greater success for the child.

Consideration should be given to other sensory properties of foods, such as taste or temperature. Cold foods or foods with strong flavors, including tangy, salty, or sour foods, may be beneficial for children with decreased oral sensory awareness. Bland, room-temperature, or slightly warm foods may increase intake in hypersensitive children.

Behavioral Interventions

Food refusal often begins with the presence of underlying medical or skill problems. Children with gastroesophageal reflux, constipation, or food allergies may feel uncomfortable when eating and develop food refusal behaviors as a result.[61] Children who gag with textured foods or refuse cup-drinking may not have adequate sensory or motor skills to manage these feeding activities. However, a child's refusal behaviors and oral aversion may persist long after the initial medical, sensory, or skill problems have been adequately managed. Inconsistencies may be seen in which the child accepts cup-drinking in the preschool setting but refuses to drink from a cup at home. Behavioral "power struggles" may develop during mealtimes. In many cases, occupational therapists may need to include behavioral treatment strategies within the comprehensive intervention program to promote successful advancement of oral feeding.

Separate from underlying medical or skill problems, many typical children refuse new foods when they are first introduced as toddlers. Evidence has been reported that it takes multiple presentations of a food before a child feels comfortable with it and before a true food preference can be determined.[12,40] Some caregivers will try a new food once or twice and then give up. Children with autism or food refusal behaviors may become more selective over time, gradually eliminating foods from their diet. Therapists should encourage parents to offer small amounts of a new food across multiple meal sessions to allow the child sufficient time to adapt to the new taste or texture.

A child's refusal to eat may contribute to caregiver stress, and mealtimes may become a battleground, with increasing levels of negative or stressful interactions.[31] Therapists try to create new positive interactions and child associations around feeding activities and mealtimes. Therapists and caregivers should have a relaxed, confident, and caring demeanor during oral feeding and therapy activities. Offering choices and turn taking during an activity may help a child have a sense of control and increase willingness to participate during mealtimes. For example, a caregiver may offer a choice of two different foods or the therapist may allow the child to choose which activity is performed first.

When implementing behavior management strategies, it is important to determine an appropriate form of praise or reinforcement for the child's positive behaviors. The occupational therapist can provide clear expectations and break the activity down into small, achievable steps. When the expectations are small and achievable, the child has the opportunity to experience praise and positive reinforcement for participation and success. Consistent success with an activity should be attained before the demand is increased.[23] If the demands are increased rapidly or if the activity is continued indefinitely until the child's refusal behaviors intensify, he or she may quickly learn to refuse more strongly to escape the activity the next time it is presented. When behavioral strategies are implemented with gradual progression of new skills, positive reinforcement, and clear expectations, the child learns to trust the therapist or caregiver, and the negative behaviors may quickly decrease in frequency and intensity.

It is not unusual for children with feeding disorders to experience negative behaviors when trying new oral feeding activities. Negative behaviors may include crying, pushing the spoon or cup away, or spitting the food out. Children may also occasionally cough, gag, or perhaps even vomit when trying new oral feeding activities. When parents or therapists react strongly to these events and immediately end the activity, the child may begin to gag, cough, or cry more frequently at the onset of the meal as a way to quickly escape the demand. Multiple research studies have supported the use of differential attention during mealtimes, where positive reinforcement is combined with ignoring or redirection of inappropriate behaviors to improve oral intake.[10,38,51] Another study showed that positive reinforcement and regular exposure to nonpreferred foods significantly improved oral consumption and self-feeding skills.[68] Occupational therapists may suggest the use of a visual schedule or timer set in advance to help the child clearly understand when the activity is finished, rather than having the parent end the meal when the child's behavior has escalated. This clear end to the activity may also help the child transition from the difficult or new task back to their usual routine of feeding.

nterventions to Improve Self-Feeding

Children experience delays in self-feeding skills because of physical or neuromuscular deficits, cognitive or visual impairments, ensory processing difficulties, behavioral refusal, or poor motiation to eat. Each of these underlying causes creates different hallenges for the intervention plan. Children will have the most uccess when they have begun to demonstrate an interest in self-eeding and an interest in exploring food more independently. Within each intervention plan, the therapist's goal is to facilitate he child's success and gradually decrease the amount of physical ssistance or adaptive equipment required in self-feeding.

For children with physical or neuromuscular deficits, it is articularly important to create a balance between the effort of elf-feeding, oral motor, and swallowing safety, the overall ength of the meal, and the child's nutritional needs. Therapists nay implement self-feeding activities for only a portion of the neal, or during a smaller snack session, to allow practice and kill development opportunities. Adaptive positioning or adapive feeding equipment can be used to facilitate grasp patterns r hand-to-mouth movements. When providing positioning ecommendations, therapists attempt to support correct posural alignment and stability to allow the child greater control f the arm in space while bringing the spoon to the mouth. Adaptive positioning to support self-feeding activities may nclude a chair that provides good postural support and allows ccess to a stable tray or table for increased arm stability. A raised tray or table surface may provide more trunk and shoul-ler stability while decreasing the distance the child needs to nove the spoon or fork from the bowl to the mouth. Stabilizing he elbow on the table or tray can also help reduce the physical lemand of self-feeding, prolonging the child's endurance.

Dycem or a nonskid placemat may help to prevent move-nent of the dish or bowl to compensate for uncoordinated rm movements. Children may have improved independence vhen self-feeding with foods that stick to the spoon or with scoop-dish that has raised edges. Some dishes also have a suc-ion cup on the bottom to help secure them to the table.

A utensil with a built-up handle that is not weighted may help to compensate for a weak grasp pattern. Children with everely impaired grasping skills may benefit from a utensil that as straps to secure it to the hand in a stable position. Toddlers vho are first learning to self-feed may benefit from a utensil hat has a shorter handle. A curved handle may help to com-ensate for limited forearm or wrist coordination.

There are also a variety of adaptations that can be made to help children drink liquids more independently. Cups with a vide base or cups with lids may help reduce spillage when the child is placing the cup on a table. Some children may benefit from a long straw placed within a cup that is secure in a cup-holder, reducing the need to lift or move the cup with the hands.

Children with cognitive or behavioral problems may benefit from backward chaining of self-feeding, with gradually decreas-ing levels of assistance provided. During the first step of this backward chain, children may be required only to move the spoon with their hand for the last few inches before it reaches the mouth. The therapist can scoop the food onto the spoon or provide hand-over-hand assistance for the remainder of the task. Klein and Delaney suggest a utility hand-hold for providing physical assistance during spoon feeding, whereby

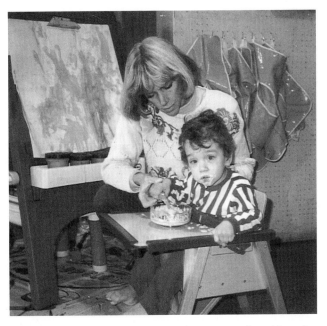

FIGURE 15-7 The therapist supports and guides the child's hand during self-feeding using the thumb on hand dorsum and finger in his palm.

the caregiver uses the middle or index finger to hold the spoon within the child's hand, and places the thumb on the back of the child's wrist (Figure 15-7).[39] Using this technique, the ther-apist can apply varying amounts of pressure in the palm to facil-itate grasp, while also assisting with appropriate wrist movements needed for self-feeding. The occupational therapist praises and encourages the child for each step of his or her prog-ress toward independent self-feeding.

When encouraging self-feeding in children with visual impairments, therapists may recommend consistent orienta-tion of food and drink on the placemat. For example, placing the cup in the 2 o'clock position next to the plate or placing different foods in consistent locations within the dish may improve the child's awareness of the mealtime environment for improved independence.

Children with sensory defensiveness may be less willing to explore food with their hands to finger feed independently. Therapy activities to reduce generalized hypersensitivity out-side of mealtimes are indicated to prepare the child for self-feeding. During mealtimes, therapists may try a variety of spoons, such as those with a small diameter or smooth handle, to improve a child's tolerance. Some children may be more willing to try self-feeding when they are simply provided with a napkin or moist cloth to reduce their discomfort if the feed-ing activity becomes messy.

INTERVENTION: SPECIFIC REFERRAL PROBLEMS AND MEDICAL DIAGNOSES

Dysphagia

When aspiration or pharyngeal dysphagia affects a child's abil-ity to eat safely, occupational therapists may recommend food or liquid consistency adaptations, such as thickened liquids for children who aspirate with thin liquids. When thickened liquids are recommended, collaboration with physicians and nutritionists is required to help ensure the child's nutrition and hydration needs are met. Some children who are prescribed thickened liquids have poor acceptance of the new liquid and reduce their oral intake. Therapists may consider a variety of liquid thickeners to benefit the child to help improve compliance. More recent research suggests there may also be alternatives to thickeners, such as carbonated liquids, to reduce aspiration or penetration (Research Note 15-2). Comprehensive caregiver training is needed to ensure understanding of clinical signs of aspiration, methods for modifying liquids, and safety precautions during oral feeding.

Positioning is also very important for children who have dysphagia. Supportive positioning can have a major impact on the child's oral motor and swallowing skills. A chin-tuck position may be recommended when the child has delayed swallow initiation. During a videofluoroscopic swallow study, a delay is typically seen as pooling of food or liquid in the pharyngeal space located close to the opening of the larynx.

RESEARCH NOTE 15-2

Bulow, M., Olsson, R., & Ekberg, O. (2003). Videoradiographic analysis of how carbonated thin liquids and thickened liquids affect the physiology of swallowing in subjects with aspiration on thin liquids. Acta Radiologica, 44, 366-372.

ABSTRACT
The purpose of this study was to evaluate how carbonated thin liquids affected swallowing physiology during videofluoroscopic assessments. Participants were evaluated with a variety of liquid consistencies during a videofluoroscopic swallow study. Forty adults who demonstrated aspiration with thin liquids were then included in this study and received additional assessment with carbonated thin liquids. Of the 40 participants, 36 had a diagnosed neurologic impairment. Data were analyzed to compare carbonated liquids with thin liquids and thickened liquids in the frequency of aspiration/penetration, pharyngeal transit time, and pharyngeal retention during swallowing. The results indicated that carbonated liquids significantly reduced aspiration/penetration events and demonstrated faster pharyngeal transit time when compared with both thin liquids and thickened liquids. Carbonated liquids also demonstrated significantly decreased pharyngeal retention when compared with thickened liquids. When thickened liquids were compared with thin liquids, significantly fewer penetration and aspiration events were noted with the thickened liquids.

IMPLICATIONS FOR PRACTICE
The use of both thickened liquids and carbonated thin liquids by individuals who demonstrate aspiration or penetration with thin liquids is supported by this descriptive study. Although this study has not yet been duplicated with a pediatric population, the results suggest that carbonated liquids may reduce aspiration in children known to aspirate thin liquids. Carbonated liquids may be an alternative to thickened liquids.

When the child is positioned with a slight chin tuck, the laryngeal opening may become smaller, reducing the risk of aspiration or penetration. Occasionally, a chin-tuck position may be contraindicated for young infants who have laryngomalacia or tracheomalacia (softening of the cartilage within the larynx or trachea), because their soft tissues may be more prone to collapse.[57] Garon also reported problems associated with the chin-tuck position in dysphagic adults with abnormal epiglottic movement patterns after a neurologic insult.[28] Occupational therapists need to make individualized positioning recommendations based on a comprehensive assessment and provide follow-up services to evaluate the outcomes of positioning changes on oral feeding skills.

Adaptations to the mealtime structure may be made to compensate for dysphagia. Occupational therapists may recommend reducing the meal length to compensate for weakness or muscle fatigue. Some children with poor oral control require multiple swallows to clear one bite of food. If a child is unable to complete a subsequent swallow in response to a verbal prompt, an empty spoon offered in the same way as a bite of food may stimulate oral movements to prompt a second swallow. Therapists may also provide recommendations for the pace of oral feeding to allow the child sufficient time to swallow and to promote safety. More difficult foods, liquids, or self-feeding activities may need to be limited or presented within the first few minutes of a meal session when the child is less fatigued. Children may also benefit from a smaller food or liquid bolus achieved through the use of a controlled-flow cup, small, measured sips, or a smaller spoon.

Occupational therapists may consider implementing oral motor activities with cold stimulation or thermal gustatory stimulation to the anterior faucial arches located in the back of the mouth to facilitate a reflexive swallow response.[2] Cold stimulation may also be provided with a frozen lemon-glycerin swab, a cotton swab dipped in water and frozen, or small amounts of lemon sherbet on a Nuk brush or other oral device. Offering chilled foods or liquids may also help to create a more efficient swallow.[57]

Research studies have been completed with adult and pediatric clients evaluating the use of neuromuscular electrical stimulation (NMES) in the treatment of dysphagia. In some cases, NMES resulted in significant improvements in swallow function when other traditional interventions had failed.[19,25] VitalStim therapy has been approved by the U.S. Food and Drug Administration as a safe treatment modality. The neuromuscular electrical stimulation is provided to strengthen or reeducate muscles on the face and anterior neck to promote swallowing and reduce dysphagia. VitalStim therapy may be administered only by therapists who obtain specialty training and certification.

Food Refusal or Selectivity

Some children referred to occupational therapists are highly selective or "picky" eaters. Initial recommendations may include consultation with physicians to consider gastroesophageal reflux disease, food allergies, digestive problems, or structural abnormalities. Occupational therapists may also work to address underlying skill deficits or swallowing safety concerns, which may contribute to food refusal behaviors. When management of medical or skill problems has been optimized, children may continue to demonstrate ongoing food refusal or food selectivity behaviors.

Children with food refusal or selectivity often benefit from environmental adaptations, including mealtime structure for consistent feeding times, reducing grazing, or excessive liquid consumption outside of meals, consistent eating locations, and consistent length of meals. These environmental strategies will promote hunger cues, limit access to less nutritious foods, and create structure within the meal to establish positive eating patterns.

Occupational therapists may also consider interventions to reduce oral hypersensitivity and improve oral sensory exploration skills. Children with food selectivity frequently react to the sensory properties of new foods. Interventions to reduce oral hypersensitivity and generalized defensiveness outside of meal sessions may help the child to prepare for the new feeding challenges.

Finally, therapists may recommend or implement behavioral treatment strategies within a comprehensive intervention program to reduce food refusal and food selectivity. Behavioral strategies may include positive reinforcement when a child explores, tastes, or swallows a nonpreferred food and adapting the activity demand to gradually build on small, achievable steps.

Delayed Transition to Textured Foods

Children who are unable to transition to age-appropriate food textures frequently have a combination of oral sensory and oral motor problems, and some may also demonstrate behavioral refusal. Occupational therapists may implement nonnutritive oral motor activities to reduce hypersensitivity and improve oral motor coordination. Jaw strengthening and repetitive chewing activities without the demand for swallowing may assist the child to build oral motor skills. Increased tolerance for food textures is typically addressed by placing crumbs on a piece of chewy tubing or slowly adding rice flakes to a puréed food. Children who consume baby foods should begin to transition to puréed table foods to adjust to stronger flavors and a wider variety of oral sensations. Children may practice chewing foods encased within a mesh feeding bag to experience repetitive chewing with less risk for gagging or choking. Therapists may provide praise or behavioral reinforcement for the child's participation in challenging new activities. When a child is able to take a few small bites of textured food safely outside of primary meal sessions, therapists may begin to integrate these new skills slowly within meals, such as during the first 5 to 10 bites. Rapidly increasing the demands within the meal session before the child has adequate motor or sensory skills may affect oral intake or nutritional status and create stressful child–caregiver interactions. Box 15-6 is helpful in recognizing the foods that may be indicated and contraindicated in children with immature oral motor skills.

Delayed Transition from Bottle to Cup

There are a variety of reasons why a child may have difficulty transitioning from breast or bottle-feeding to drinking from a cup. Efficient cup-drinking requires more mature oral motor movements. Difficulty transitioning from the bottle to the cup can be caused by poor jaw stability, oral control, or

---

BOX 15-6 Foods Indicated and Contraindicated for Children with Immature Oral-Motor Skills

PROPERTIES OF INDICATED FOODS
Even consistency
Increased density and volume
Thick (liquids)
Uniform texture
Stays together (will not break up in the mouth)
Easy to remove and suck

PROPERTIES OF CONTRAINDICATED FOODS
Multiple textures and consistencies (tacos, vegetable soup, stews, and salads)
Sticky (peanut butter)
Greasy (fried foods)
Tough (red meat, processed meats, and diced fruit)
Fibrous and stringy (celery, citrus fruits, and raw vegetables)
Skins (raw fruits and peanuts)
Spicy (pepper and horseradish)
Seeds and nuts (plain or in breads and cakes)
Thin (liquids such as water, broth, coffee, tea, and apple juice)
Quickly liquefying (Jell-O, ice cream, and watermelon)
Foods that break up in the mouth (some cookies and flaky pastries)
Hard/crunchy (carrots)

---

pharyngeal coordination to manage a more unpredictable liquid bolus. Children with a history of failure-to-thrive may have prolonged dependence on bottle or breast feeding as the most reliable method to meet their nutritional or hydration needs. When a child is orally hypersensitive, he or she may dislike the intermittent touch of the cup on the outside of the lips or spillage that often occurs during early cup-drinking activities.[39] Hypersensitive children may also seek the calming, organizing sensory input that comes from sucking during bottle or breast feeding.

To help children prepare for cup-drinking activities, therapists may initially work on jaw stability, lip closure, tongue movements, and oral sensitivity through positioning, handling, and oral motor activities. Cups with nonspill valves within the lid require stronger lip closure and oral suction abilities and may be more difficult to use for children with neuromuscular impairments. A spouted cup may initially make it easier for a child to suck the liquid or form a bolus within the mouth. Spouted cups may also provide similar sensory input to bottle-feeding for children with sensory defensiveness. When drinking from a cup with a spout, the child may need to tilt the head back, which may create additional difficulties if the child has extensor posturing, poor head control, or pharyngeal swallowing problems. Use of a cut-out cup may help to reduce head and neck extension and allows the therapist to easily observe the flow of liquid and the child's mouth movements during drinking activities.

With free-flowing liquid from an open cup or nonvalved spouted cup, children should be positioned in a more upright position to encourage bolus formation within the mouth, without the impact of gravity creating an uncontrolled flow into the pharyngeal space. Children may also benefit from thickened

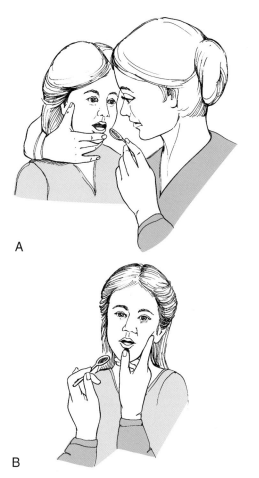

A

B

FIGURE 15-8 Jaw control and oral support. **A,** From the side. **B,** From the front.

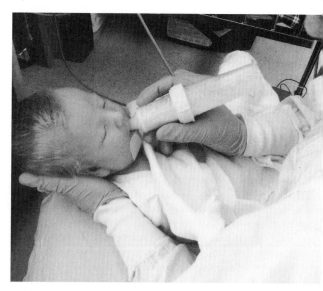

FIGURE 15-9 Infant using Habermann feeder. (Courtesy Jayne Shepherd.)

liquids when first learning to drink from a cup to compensate for decreased oral control or pharyngeal swallowing skills. External jaw support can be provided by the therapist, where the therapist's index finger is underneath the lower mandibular bone, and the thumb is placed on the anterior chin. Providing jaw support while sitting beside the child with the arm around the back of the child's neck may allow the therapist to provide additional stability for the child to maintain adequate head alignment (Figure 15-8). Children often bite on the rim or spout of the cup to gain additional jaw stability. They also may push the cup into the corners of their lips or rest their tongue on the rim of the cup for additional sensory input.[39] These patterns should decrease over time as the child becomes more skilled in managing liquids from a cup.

Cleft Lip and Palate

A cleft lip or palate is a separation of parts of the mouth usually joined together at midline during the early weeks of fetal development. A cleft lip is separation of the upper lip and often the upper dental ridge. A cleft palate is a separation of the hard or soft palate and may occur with or without a cleft lip. Because of the lack of closure between the oral and nasal cavities, young infants have difficulty creating suction to express liquid from a nipple.[30] After surgical repair of the cleft, older children may have difficulty with active lip movement, oral defensiveness, or nasopharyngeal reflux during oral feeding.

Occupational therapists typically recommend compensatory positioning, equipment, and strategies for oral feeding before surgical repair of the cleft. A variety of nipples are available to compensate for oral structural problems. The Habermann nipple was developed specifically for infants with cleft palate to deliver flow without requiring suction (Figure 15-9). It has a one-way valve that allows the infant to express fluid through compression alone, without requiring suction.[30] This nipple allows the infant to independently control milk flow. Long nipples may help deposit liquid toward the back of the infant's mouth beyond the cleft to decrease liquid flow into the nasal passageway. Additional considerations for choosing appropriate nipples for infants with cleft palate are provided in Table 15-5. Some children with an open cleft may require a special bottle that can be squeezed by the parent to deposit formula into the infant's mouth. Children with an open cleft may have more success when positioned upright or in the side-lying position during oral feeding. They also may require frequent breaks to allow for burping during oral feeding.

After surgical repair of a cleft, occupational therapists may perform scar massage, initiate activities to reduce oral hypersensitivity, and reassess the oral feeding method. Some children may have ongoing problems with nasopharyngeal reflux during oral feeding, where food or liquid enters the nasal cavity. Therapists may evaluate which food or liquid textures are more problematic for the child, suggest alternating bites of food with sips of liquid, or recommend a specific bolus size to reduce the functional impairment.

Other Structural Anomalies

Other structural anomalies include micrognathia and macroglossia. *Micrognathia* is defined as a small, recessed jaw. *Macroglossia* is a term used when the tongue is disproportionately large in comparison with the size of the mouth or jaw. Therapists need to consider the impact of the size and position of

TABLE 15-5   Nipple Characteristics Related to Use with Children Who Have Oral Structural Defects

Nipple Type	Characteristics
Long, thin nipples	Work well when the tongue is recessed; can bring the tongue forward
Single nipple hole	Results in a steady liquid stream, which can be easier to handle than bursts of liquid
Wide nipple	Can be compressed for liquid expression for the child with a cleft palate
Broad-based nipple	Can help the infant with a cleft lip gain suction
Nipple with cross-cut hole	Can create an uneven liquid flow or a burst of fluid that is difficult for the infant to control
Nipple with enlarged hole	Should be used with great care; when the caregiver enlarges the hole, it is difficult to predict what type of liquid flow will result
Soft, pliable nipple	Appropriate for infants with cleft palates who are unable to achieve suction
Nuk nipple	Has the hole on top of the nipple and should not be used with children with cleft palates; this nipple may be functional if its position on the tongue is reversed

oral structures on respiration and oral movement patterns during feeding. Therapists may use different nipples, utensils, or positioning adaptations to help compensate for these structural differences. For example, infants with micrognathia may benefit from prone positioning to help draw the tongue into a more forward position, allowing improved respiration and nipple compression during bottle-feeding.

Structural anomalies of the esophagus include esophageal strictures, tracheoesophageal fistula, and esophageal atresia. With tracheoesophageal fistula or esophageal atresia, the structural abnormalities are repaired surgically. Children with structural anomalies of the esophagus are at increased risk for functional problems with feeding, eating, and swallowing associated with poor esophageal motility. Esophageal motility describes how quickly foods and liquids move through the esophagus and empty into the stomach. Liquids and smooth, runny foods empty into the stomach more quickly than thick, fibrous, or more solid foods. Children who have a history of esophageal structural anomalies may have problems advancing to higher food textures as a result of decreased esophageal motility. Occupational therapists may recommend adapting food textures to maximize oral intake, alternating bites of food with sips of liquid to help clear the esophagus, slowing the pace of feeding, or encouraging a subsequent dry swallow after each bite of food to help compensate for delayed esophageal motility.

Transition from Nonoral Feeding to Oral Feeding

Nonoral feeding with a gastrostomy, nasogastric tube, or other method is indicated when a child is unable to meet his or her nutrition or hydration needs by mouth. Nonoral feeding methods may be used when the child has dysphagia; complex heart, respiratory, or other medical conditions; or gastrointestinal problems. Other children require nonoral feeding methods simply because they are unable to consume enough food or liquid by mouth to demonstrate adequate growth and hydration. Inadequate nutrition or hydration can severely limit a child's motor development, cognitive development, and health.[29] The placement of a gastrostomy tube or the use of other nonoral feeding methods can be a temporary measure to promote the child's nutritional status and growth.[64]

When children receive nonoral feeding, they are at risk for developing oral motor and oral sensory impairments because of limited oral feeding experiences. Nasogastric and orogastric tubes may also create sensory distress for the child during the placement of the tube. When these tubes are needed over a long period of time, they are typically re-inserted or replaced every month, causing further sensory distress to the child. Occupational therapists may provide an intervention program to provide ongoing oral exploration activities and social engagement during nonoral feeding. The goal is to create positive social and oral exploration experiences on a daily basis and ultimately link these pleasurable experiences with the satiation of hunger.

If there is a history of aspiration dysphagia or if oral feeding is not medically safe, the child may suck on a pacifier or engage in mouth play with teethers, spoons, and toys during nonoral feeding. Therapists and caregivers can engage in games that include touch and exploration around the face and mouth. Children may also benefit from games that encourage them to make different sounds with their mouth, give kisses, or blow whistles or bubbles. Whenever possible, therapists should encourage families to include their child in mealtime routines, such as sitting with the family at the table during tube feedings and oral play activities.

When the child is medically cleared to have nutritive stimulation, therapists and caregivers can provide flavors or tastes of foods by dipping a finger, pacifier, spoon, or toy into juice, formula, or puréed foods. Children who receive nonoral feeding may have limited opportunities to experience typical feelings of hunger. This is especially true when children require nonoral feedings on a continuous schedule across many hours during the day. Children who are able to tolerate more compressed bolus feedings may have more opportunities to experience hunger, which may increase the child's motivation to consume some foods by mouth. As the child is beginning to advance oral intake skills, therapists need to collaborate with physicians or nutritionists, who can determine appropriate schedule changes and reductions in nonoral nutrition.

Children who have tracheostomies often require nonoral feeding methods. The risk and complications of aspiration are significantly increased in a child with a tracheostomy because of the fragility of the respiratory system.[1] This may be related to the changes in pressure created by the new opening in the laryngeal cavity or poor laryngeal mobility. Children with a tracheostomy may be ready for nutritive stimulation when they are able to manage their own saliva without frequent suctioning and can tolerate a Passy Muir valve or cap, which may help to create more normalized pharyngeal swallowing coordination.[32] Occupational therapists must collaborate with physicians and complete comprehensive assessments of swallowing before initiating nutritive oral feeding activities in children with tracheostomies. Before receiving medical clearance for oral feeding, children with tracheostomies will benefit from oral exploration and desensitization activities when oral feeding is not possible.

When children are medically cleared and have sufficient oral motor and swallowing skills to consume larger amounts of food by mouth, they may continue to demonstrate strong oral aversions, hypersensitivity, or refusal to engage in oral feeding activities. Transitioning from nonoral to oral feeding is a gradual process and may require a variety of oral sensory, skill development, and behavioral intervention activities over a period of time.

SUMMARY

The causes of pediatric feeding, eating, and swallowing disorders are diverse and complex. Occupational therapists must consider the whole child during the assessment and intervention process, including multiple overlapping child factors and performance skills, activity demands and contexts, and family patterns (Case Study 15-1). This chapter has provided a foundation of knowledge for the occupational therapist to improve a child's safety during oral feeding, promote acceptance of age-appropriate foods or liquids, and advance functional independence during mealtimes. The assessment and treatment of pediatric feeding disorders require interdisciplinary collaboration between the occupational therapist and other members of the child's treatment team. As with most occupational therapy

---

CASE STUDY 15-1   Marco

Marco was a 4½-year-old boy referred for an evaluation of feeding, eating, and swallowing. His problems with oral feeding began early in infancy. He had difficulty latching on during breast feeding attempts and did not have adequate weight gain; therefore, he was introduced to bottle feeding at 1 month of age. He coughed and sputtered during bottle-feeding in infancy, often at the end of the feeding. Marco was very particular about the type of nipple used with his bottle and did not take his bottle whenever a different nipple was attempted. Baby foods were first introduced at 6 months of age. With baby foods, Marco gagged, refused to open his mouth, and turned away after the first few bites. His parents stopped trying baby foods for a few weeks, and then they would try again. Marco demonstrated similar responses with every attempt. Marco's parents later insisted that Marco sit at the dinner table at the start of family meals, where he was encouraged to try some new foods. He would occasionally lick a potato chip or a pretzel during these meals. If Marco persisted in his refusal, his parents would allow him to leave the table after a few minutes.

As a toddler, Marco continued to be dependent on formula from a bottle, and he continued to have difficulty growing and gaining weight. At the advice of the primary care physician, Marco's mother stopped bottle-feeding and attempted to transition to cup-drinking when Marco was 4 years old. Marco then refused to eat or drink anything for 3 days, he was admitted to the hospital for correction of dehydration, and he started nasogastric tube feedings. After 3 weeks of nasogastric feeding, a gastrostomy tube was placed.

Marco lived in a rural community and had limited access to medical and therapy services. Marco had never had a modified barium swallow study. He had no history of pneumonia; however, he had occasional unexplained low-grade fevers, which the parents attributed to teething. Marco received a private speech–language evaluation approximately 2 months before the occupational therapy feeding evaluation, and concerns were reported with receptive language, expressive language, and articulation. Marco was scheduled to enroll in a preschool class in the fall.

EVALUATION FINDINGS

At the time of the evaluation, Marco received 100% of his nutrition from PediaSure via his gastrostomy tube on a continuous schedule over 16 hours. He was unable to tolerate an increase in his tube-feeding, with leakage around the gastrostomy tube site and discomfort noted.

Marco grimaced during the oral motor assessment; however, he was able to participate with encouragement, clear expectations, and praise. He gagged when stimulation was provided on his tongue or palate and demonstrated retraction in his cheeks and tongue. He did not like stimulation on the outer surfaces of his molars or within his cheeks. Marco used a weak, nonrhythmical munching pattern and required multiple verbal and physical jaw prompts during a nonnutritive chewing activity. He had a positive tongue lateralization response during therapist facilitation and a closed-mouth posture at rest, with no evidence of drooling. Oral–facial muscle tone appeared to be within normal limits. During a baseline feeding observation, Marco licked a pretzel and drank 1 sip of water from an open cup after receiving maximum encouragement from his mother. Marco was ambulatory, alert, sociable, and able to communicate basic needs. During observations of play, he did not want to explore "squishy balls" with his hands during the evaluation, and he pulled away during a scissors activity when the paper began to touch the back of his hand.

INTERVENTION

Before the start of intervention, Marco was referred for an evaluation by a gastroenterologist. An endoscopy was completed, which showed significant esophagitis and gastroesophageal reflux disease, but no evidence of allergies. Marco began antireflux medication. Marco was not referred for a videofluoroscopic swallow study because of the severity of his refusal to consume food or liquid by mouth. Marco was monitored throughout his treatment program for clinical signs of dysphagia.

Because Marco's family lived in a rural area with limited availability of treatment services, he was referred for an intensive day-treatment program to improve his oral feeding skills. He received interdisciplinary treatment consisting of

CASE STUDY 15-1   Marco—cont'd

occupational therapy, behavioral psychology, and speech–language treatment. He also received consultations with a nutritionist, gastroenterologist, and social worker. Occupational therapy services were provided 3 to 4 times per week for 30-minute sessions, for a total of 5 weeks. Occupational therapy sessions integrated sensory, motor, and behavioral treatment techniques to improve Marco's ability to consume a variety of foods, manage liquids from a cup, and improve self-feeding skills. Specific occupational therapy activities included the following:

- Sensory: Marco demonstrated oral hypersensitivity, with symptoms of generalized tactile defensiveness. During treatment, Marco engaged in play-based sensory activities with finger paint, craft activities, "squishy balls," Play Doh, clay, rice, and water play. Oral sensory preparatory activities included slow deep-pressure touch beginning on the arms and shoulders before progressing to the outer cheeks and lips. During oral motor and feeding activities, the occupational therapist provided a napkin to compensate for Marco's poor tolerance for messiness when spills happened.

- Behavior: Marco often refused to try new feeding and oral motor activities The occupational therapist implemented behavioral strategies to offer choices when possible and set clear, consistent expectations. Enthusiastic praise and other reinforcements (e.g., a favorite toy or game) were provided after participation in oral feeding and difficult activities. A timer was used for transitions. Activities were graded to provide a gradual increase in demands that were consistent with Marco's oral motor and oral sensory skill level. Toward the end of the treatment program, external toy reinforcements were gradually decreased to encourage self-motivated participation.

- Oral Motor: Marco had oral motor impairments limiting his ability to manage a variety of foods. He demonstrated jaw weakness and tightness or retraction in his cheeks, lips, and tongue. Initially during meal sessions, Marco was offered puréed foods to maximize his oral intake and compensate for his oral motor and oral sensory difficulties. During occupational therapy sessions (e.g.,

outside of mealtimes), Marco quickly improved his tolerance for oral motor activities when they were combined with behavior management and sensory processing techniques. The occupational therapist was able to complete cheek and lip stretches to improve management of food in the buccal cavity during chewing. After these stretches, Marco was encouraged to activate these muscles by exploring a variety of whistles. Intraoral activities were provided with a Nuk brush, vibration, toothette sponge, flavor sprays, lollipops, and a regular toothbrush. Marco also participated in jaw-strengthening activities. Expectations were increased gradually when Marco's oral motor skills were adequate to manage more textured foods. Initially, Marco would mash small amounts of cracker crumbs placed in his mouth for mashing. He then began biting and munching small pieces of dissolvable solid foods, and then progressed to a wider variety of soft solids, such as cooked vegetables and canned fruits. Marco's cup-drinking skills were also advanced gradually, with small single sips at first, leading up to consecutive sips and swallows from an open cup.

DISCHARGE STATUS

At the time of discharge from the feeding program, Marco was consuming 100% of his nutrition needs by mouth, eating a wide variety of foods, and self-feeding almost all of his food independently. He continued to be anxious whenever a new food was introduced, and would need some physical prompts and behavioral strategies to "try it out" before he would attempt to eat the food independently. He demonstrated significantly improved jaw strength, oral motor coordination, and oral sensory responses. He was able to take ½-inch pieces of soft–solid foods during snack sessions. He continued to be somewhat slow with his chewing, so he was on a fork-mashed texture in meal sessions. Marco was referred for weekly speech and occupational therapy services after discharge for continued work on higher food textures and language. Marco's mother was also provided with a comprehensive program to continue his oral feeding development at home.

---

interventions, inclusion of primary caregivers within all stages of the assessment and treatment program is extremely important to the child's ultimate success within natural environments.

REFERENCES

1. Abraham, S. S., & Wolf, E. L. (2000). Swallowing physiology of toddlers with long-term tracheostomies: A preliminary study. *Dysphagia*, 15, 206–212.
2. Ali, G. N., Laundl, T. M., Wallace, K. L., deCarle, D. J., & Cooke, I. J. (1996). Influence of cold stimulation on the normal pharyngeal swallow response. *Dysphagia*, 11, 2–8.
3. American Dietetic Association: National Dysphagia Diet Task Force. (2002). *National dysphagia diet: Standardization for optimal care*. Chicago: American Dietetic Association.
4. American Occupational Therapy Association. (2006). *Specialized knowledge and skills in feeding, eating, and swallowing for occupational therapy practice*. Bethesda, MD: American Occupational Therapy Association, Inc.
5. American Occupational Therapy Association. (2008). Occupational therapy practice framework: Domain and process, second edition. *The American Journal of Occupational Therapy*, 62(6), 609–639.
6. Arvedson, J. C. (1998). Management of pediatric dysphagia. *Otolaryngologic Clinics of North America*, 31, 453–476.
7. Arvedson, J. C. (2006). *Swallowing and feeding in infants and young children*. GI Motility Online. Retrieved May 27, 2007, from http://www.nature.com/gimo/contents/pt1/full/gimo17.html
8. Ardveson, J. C., & Brodsky, L. (2002). Instrumental evaluation of swallowing. In J. C. Arvedson & L. Brodsky (Eds.), *Pediatric swallowing and feeding: Assessment and management* (2nd ed., pp. 356). Albany: Singular/Thomson Learning.

9. Arvedson, J. C., & Lefton-Greif, M. A. (1998). *Pediatric video-fluoroscopic swallow studies: A professional manual with caregiver guidelines.* San Antonio: Communication Skill Builders.

10. Babbitt, R. L., Hoch, T. A., Coe, D. A., Cataldo, M. F., Kelly, K. J., Stackhouse, C., et al. (1994). Behavioral assessment and treatment of pediatric feeding disorders. *Journal of Developmental and Behavioral Pediatrics, 15,* 278–291.

11. Beckman, D. (2000). Oral motor assessment and intervention. Paper presented at the Oral Motor Assessment and Intervention I conference, Charlotte, NC.

12. Birch, L. L., & Marlin, D. W. (1982). I don't like it; I never tried it: Effects of exposure on two-year-old children's food preferences. *Appetite, 3,* 353–360.

13. Bulow, M., Olsson, R., & Ekberg, O. (2003). Videoradiographic analysis of how carbonated thin liquids and thickened liquids affect the physiology of swallowing in subjects with aspiration on thin liquids. *Acta Radiologica, 44,* 366–372.

14. Bundy, A. C., & Koomar, J. A. (2002). Orchestrating intervention: The art of practice. In A. C. Bundy, S. J. Lane, & E. A. Murray (Eds.), *Sensory integration: Theory and practice* (2nd ed.). Philadelphia: F.A. Davis.

15. Byars, K., Burklow, K. A., Ferguson, K., O'Flaherty, T., Santoro, K., & Kaul, A. (2003). A multicomponent behavioral program for oral aversion in children dependent on gastrostomy tube feedings. *Journal of Pediatric Gastroenterology and Nutrition, 37,* 473–480.

16. Carruth, B. R., & Skinner, J. D. (2002). Feeding behaviors and other motor development in healthy children (2-24 months). *Journal of the American College of Nutrition, 21*(2), 88–96.

17. Chamberlin, J., Henry, M. M., Roberts, J. D., Sapsford, A. L., & Courtney, S. E. (1991). An infant and toddler feeding group program. *The American Journal of Occupational Therapy, 45,* 907–911.

18. Christensen, J. R. (1989). Developmental approach to pediatric neurogenic dysphagia. *Dysphagia, 3,* 131–134.

19. Christiaanse, M., Glynn, J., & Bradshaw, J. (2003). *Experience with transcutaneous electrical stimulation: A new treatment option for the management of pediatric dysphagia.* Winston-Salem, NC: Wake Forest School of Medicine, University Health Sciences.

20. da Costa, S. P., & van der Schans, C. P. (2008). The reliability of the Neonatal Oral-Motor Scale. *Acta Paediatrica, 97,* 21–26.

21. Daniels, H., Devlieger, H., Casaer, P., & Eggermont, E. (1986). Nutritive and non-nutritive sucking in preterm infants. *Journal of Developmental Physiology, 8,* 117–121.

22. DeVault, M. L. (1991). *Feeding the family: The social organization of caring as gendered work.* Chicago: Chicago Press.

23. Fischer, E., & Silverman, A. (2007). Behavioral conceptualization, assessment, and treatment of pediatric feeding disorders. *Seminars in Speech and Language, 26,* 223–231.

24. Food Research Action Center. (2006). *Hunger in the U.S.* Retrieved September 2008 from http://www.frac.org.

25. Freed, M. L., Freed, L., Chatburn, R. L., & Christian, M. (2001). Electrical stimulation for swallowing disorders caused by stroke. *Respiratory Care, 46,* 466–474.

26. Friedman, B., & Frazier, J. B. (2000). Deep laryngeal penetration as a predictor of aspiration. *Dysphagia, 15,* 153–158.

27. Fung, E. B., Samson-Fang, L., Stallings, V. A., Conaway, M., Liptak, G., & Henderson, R. C. (2002). Feeding dysfunction is associated with poor growth and health status in children with cerebral palsy. *Journal of the American Dietetic Association, 102,* 361–368.

28. Garon, B. (2003). Swallow dysfunction: New research evidence. Paper presented at Keep Pace Seminars conference, Baltimore.

29. Gisel, E. G., Applegate-Ferrante, T., Benson, J. E., & Bosma, J. F. (1995). Effect of oral sensorimotor treatment on measures of growth, eating efficiency and aspiration in the dysphagic child with cerebral palsy. *Developmental Medicine and Child Neurology, 37,* 528–543.

30. Glass, R. P., & Wolf, L. S. (1999). Feeding management of infants with cleft lip and palate and micrognathia. *Infants and Young Children, 12,* 70–81.

31. Greer, A. J., Gulotta, C. S., Masler, E. A., & Laud, R. B. (2008). Caregiver stress and outcomes of children with pediatric feeding disorders treated in an intensive interdisciplinary program. *Journal of Pediatric Psychology, 33,* 612–620.

32. Gross, R. D., Mahlmann, J., & Grayhack, J. P. (2003). Physiologic effects of open and closed tracheostomy tubes on the pharyngeal swallow. The Annals of Otology, Rhinology, and Laryngology, 112, 143–152.

33. Hanson, J. (2004). *Lip prints: Home program for oral-motor skills.* Austin, TX: Pro-Ed.

34. Hawdon, J. M., Beauregard, N., & Kennedy, G. (2000). Identification of neonates at risk of developing feeding problems in infancy. *Developmental Medicine and Child Neurology, 42,* 235–239.

35. Hulme, J. B., Gallacher, K., Walsh, J., Niesen, S., & Waldron, D. (1987). Behavioral and postural changes observed with the use of adaptive seating by clients with multiple handicaps. *Physical Therapy, 67,* 1060–1067.

36. Humphry, R., & Thigpen, B. (1997). Caregiver role: Ideas about feeding infants and toddlers. *Occupational Therapy Journal of Research, 17,* 237–263.

37. Humphry, R., & Thigpen-Beck, B. (1998). Parenting values and attitudes: Views of therapists and parents. *The American Journal of Occupational Therapy, 52,* 835–843.

38. Kerwin, M. E. (1999). Empirically supported treatments in pediatric psychology: Severe feeding problems. *Journal of Pediatric Psychology, 24,* 193–214.

39. Klein, M. D., & Delaney, T. A. (1994). *Feeding and nutrition for the child with special needs.* Tucson, AZ: Therapy Skill Builders.

40. Koivisto Hursti, U. K. (1999). Factors influencing children's food choice. *Annals of Medicine, 31*(Suppl. 1), 26–32.

41. Lee, E. J., Murry, V. M., Brody, G., & Parker, V. (2002). Maternal resources, parenting, and dietary patterns among rural African American children in single-parent families. *Public Health Nursing, 19,* 104–111.

42. Logemann, J. A. (1998). *Evaluation and treatment of swallowing disorders* (2nd ed.). Austin, TX: Pro-Ed.

43. Miller, C. K., & Willging, J. P. (2003). Advances in the evaluation and management of pediatric dysphagia. *Current Opinion in Otolaryngology & Head and Neck Surgery, 11,* 442–446.

44. Morris, S. E., & Klein, M. D. (2000). *Pre-feeding skills* (2nd ed.) Tucson, AZ: Therapy Skill Builders.

45. National Digestive Disease Information Clearinghouse. *Heartburn, Gastroesophageal Reflux (GER), and Gastroesophageal Reflux Disease (GERD).* Retrieved May 2008 from http://digestive.niddk.nih.gov/ddiseases/pubs/gerd/.

46. Newman, L. A., Keckley, C., Petersen, M. C., & Hamner, A. (2001). Swallowing function and medical diagnoses in infants suspected of dysphagia. *Pediatrics, 108*(6), E106.

47. Nord, M., Andrews, M., & Carlson, S. (2006). *Household food security in the United States.* Economic research report No. (ERR. 49). United States Department of Agriculture. Retrieved May 2008 from http://www.ers.usda.gov/Publications/ERR49/.

48. Occupational Safety and Health Administration. (1991). *Federal Register, 56*(235).

49. Palmer, M. M. (1993). Identification and management of the transitional suck pattern in premature infants. *Journal of Perinatal and Neonatal Nursing, 7,* 66–75.

50. Palmer, M. M., & Heyman, M. B. (1993). Assessment and treatment of sensory- versus motor-based feeding problems in very young children. *Infants and Young Children, 6,* 67–73.

51. Piazza, C. C., Patel, M. R., Gulotta, C. S., Sevin, B. M., & Layer, S. A. (2003). On the relative contributions of positive reinforcement and escape extinction in the treatment of food refusal. *Journal of Applied Behavior Analysis, 36,* 309–324.

2. Reilly, S., & Skuse, D. (1992). Characteristics and management of feeding problems of young children with cerebral palsy. *Developmental Medicine and Child Neurology, 34*, 379–388.

3. Rogers, B., Arvedson, J., Buck, G., Smart, P., & Msall, M. (1994). Characteristics of dysphagia in children with cerebral palsy. *Dysphagia, 9*, 69–73.

4. Rogers, B., & Senn, K. (2008). Pediatric Dysphagia. In P. J. Accardo (Ed.), *Capute & Accardo's neurodevelopmental disabilities in infancy and childhood* (3rd ed., pp. 145–167). Baltimore: Paul H. Brookes.

5. Rommel, N., DeMeyer, A. M., Feenstra, L., & Veereman-Wauters, G. (2003). The complexity of feeding problems in 700 infants and young children presenting to a tertiary care institution. *Journal of Pediatric Gastroenterology and Nutrition, 37*, 75–84.

6. Rosenfeld-Johnson, S. (2005). *Assessment and treatment of the jaw.* Tucson: Talk Tools Innovative Therapists International.

7. Ruark McMurtrey, J. (2007). Best practices for behavioral management of pediatric dysphagia. *Pediatric Feeding and Dysphagia Newsletter, 7*(3), 1–5. Salt Lake City, UT: Hiro Publishing.

8. Schuberth, L. M. (1994). The role of occupational therapy in diagnoses and management. In D. N. Tuchman & R. Walter (Eds.), *Disorders of feeding and swallowing in infants and children* (pp. 115–1300). San Diego, CA: Singular Publishing Group.

9. Schulze, P. A., Harwood, R. L., & Schoelmerich, A. (2001). Feeding practices and expectations among middle-class Anglo and Puerto-Rican mothers of 12-month-old infants. *Journal of Cross-Cultural Psychology, 32*, 397–406.

10. Schwarz, S. M. (2003). Feeding disorders in children with developmental disabilities. *Infants and Young Children, 15*, 29–41.

11. Skuse, D. (1993). Identification and management of problem eaters. *Archives of Disease in Childhood, 69*, 604–608.

62. Smith, A. M., Roux, S., Naidoo, N. T., & Venter, D. J. (2005). Food choice of tactile defensive children. *Nutrition, 21*, 14–19.

63. Sullivan, P. B., Juszezak, E., Lambert, B. R., Rose, M., Ford-Adams, M. E., & Johnson, A. (2002). Impact of feeding problems on nutritional intake and growth: Oxford feeding study II. *Developmental Medicine and Child Neurology, 44*, 461–467.

64. Tarbell, M. C., & Allaire, J. H. (2002). Children with feeding tube dependency: Treating the whole child. *Infants and Young Children, 15*, 29–41.

65. Toomey, K. (2002). Feeding strategies for older infants and toddlers. *Pediatric Basics: The Journal of Pediatric Nutrition and Development, 100*, 2–11.

66. UNICEF—Progress for Children. (2006). *Nutrition, survival, and development.* Retrieved May 2008 from http://www.unicef.org/progressforchildren/2006n4/undernutritiondefinition.html.

67. Vergara, E. R., & Bigsby, R. (2004). *Developmental and therapeutic interventions in the NICU.* Baltimore: Brookes.

68. Werle, M. A., Murphy, T. B., & Budd, K. S. (1993). Treating chronic food refusal in young children: home-based parent training. *Journal of Applied Behavior Analysis, 26*, 421–433.

69. Wolf, L. S., & Glass, R. P. (1992). *Feeding and swallowing disorders in infancy: Assessment and management.* Tucson, AZ: Therapy Skill Builders.

70. Yokochi, K. (1997). Oral motor patterns during feeding in severely physically disabled children. *Brain & Development, 19*, 552–555.

71. Zerilli, K. S. & Stefans, V. A., & DiPietro, M. A. (1990). Protocol for the use of videofluoroscopy in pediatric swallowing dysfunction. *The American Journal of Occupational Therapy, 44*, 441–446.

CHAPTER 16

Activities of Daily Living

Jayne Shepherd

OBJECTIVES

1. Describe the effects of context on a child's performance and parental expectations for activities of daily living (ADLs).
2. Identify the body structures and functions, performance skills, performance patterns, and activity demands that may affect a child's ADL performance.
3. Identify evaluation procedures and methods in ADLs that target child and family preferences for intervention.
4. Describe intervention strategies and approaches, both general and specific.
5. Describe the selection and modification of equipment, techniques, and environments for certain ADL occupations.

Activities of daily living (ADLs) encompass some of the most important occupations children learn as they mature. Self-care or ADLs include learning how to take care of one's body, such as toilet hygiene, bowel and bladder management, bathing and showering, personal hygiene and grooming, eating and feeding, dressing, and functional mobility.[1] Other ADLs tasks include caring for a personal device and learning to express sexual needs.[1] As the child matures, he or she learns to perform ADLs in socially appropriate ways so that he or she can engage in the other occupations within the family unit and the community such as education, play, leisure, rest and sleep, social participation, instrumental activities of daily living (IADLs), and work. Often when a child is young, he or she performs ADLs as co-occupations of caregivers and children, especially when the child has a disability. Parents often establish the routines for bathing, dressing, feeding, and delegate more complex ADLs to others.[1,80,127,149]

This chapter discusses the dynamic interaction of child factors, contexts, activity demands, and performance skills and patterns that allows a child to engage in ADL occupations in a variety of environments. Evaluation methods, intervention approaches, and strategies for improving outcomes in ADL activities are reviewed. Typical development, limitations, and modifications for toileting, dressing, bathing, grooming, and performing other related ADL tasks are described (feeding is discussed in Chapter 15). Examples of adaptations to physical and social environments are provided, with consideration given to cultural, temporal, virtual, and personal influences.

IMPORTANCE OF DEVELOPING ADL OCCUPATIONS

The foundations for mastering ADLs begin in infancy and are refined throughout the various stages of development. As unique individuals living in certain contexts, children learn these activities at varying rates and have occasional regression and unpredictable behaviors. Cultural values, parental expectations, social routines, and the physical environment influence when children begin to bathe, dress, groom, or toilet themselves. Overall, society and families assume that children develop increasing levels of competence and self-reliance to meet their own ADL needs. Growth and maturity allow the child to participate in various roles and environments with decreasing levels of adult supervision for ADLs.

When a child is born with or acquires a disability, parental and child expectations for ADL and daily living independence are modified. Occupational therapists are instrumental in helping parents and children learn how to modify activity demands and routines so that children perform ADL tasks within their everyday environments. Active participation in ADLs has several benefits for the child, including maintaining and improving bodily functions and health (e.g., strength, endurance, range of motion [ROM], coordination, memory, sequencing, concept formation, body image, cleanliness in hygiene) and problem solving while mastering tasks that are meaningful and purposeful to the child. This task mastery leads to increased self-esteem, self-reliance, and self-determination and gives the child a sense of autonomy. When children dress themselves, they may choose their own clothing, participate in dress-up during playtime, put on a coat when going outside, change clothes for gym class, or dress in a uniform to work at a estaurant. As the child learns new ADL tasks, he or she develops a sense of accomplishment and pride in his or her abilities. This increasing independence also gives parents, teachers, and other caregivers more time and energy for other tasks[53] while the child contributes to the family unit.

As a child learns new ADL tasks, routines or patterns of observable behaviors develop. These repetitive routines (e.g., morning routine for getting ready for school, bedtime routines) are embedded within the family culture and environment.[40,128] Therapists ask parents about daily routines and customs at home or school that may influence a child's ADL performance. Some examples of questions to consider asking are "When are children expected to be toilet trained or independent in brushing their teeth? How is your child expected to get from room to room in your house or within school? Can you please describe your morning routine?"

Routines help satisfy or promote the completion of ADL tasks to meet role expectations within home, school, community, and work environments. They are culturally based and often are a combination of what is expected but also what is practical.[50] Each family, teacher, employer, or community organization may follow a unique routine for self-care tasks. For example, the family may require a toilet break anytime they are going somewhere, and teachers may allow students to use the toilet at fixed times during the day. Sometimes routines become damaging and hinder performance of ADL.[1,40,128] For example, a child with autism or obsessive-compulsive disorder may be quite rigid about how he performs his grooming tasks and is inflexible when Aunt Lou visits and the placement of items in the bathroom changes.[149] He also may routinely wash his hands after he touches any object. These patterns of behavior now interfere, instead of support, ADL performance. Families may have routines or no routines that affect ADL performance (e.g., when they eat, when bathing occurs, how often laundry is done, or how children are expected to manage personal items such as glasses, retainers). As a child matures, he becomes more responsible for developing and maintaining routines that become habits to prevent further illness and maintain health and well-being. Checking skin conditions, maintaining cleanliness during toileting or bathing, preventing cavities through tooth brushing, and maintaining personal care devices such as orthotics or catheters are a few of the healthy living routines that help the child meet role expectations for community living.

FACTORS AFFECTING PERFORMANCE

Child factors, the performance environment, contextual aspects, and the specific demands of the self-care activity, as well as the child's performance skills, affect the child's ability to participate successfully in ADL occupations. ADLs are performed in a context of interwoven internal and external conditions, some from within the child (bodily functions and body structures related to the disability; personal and cultural contexts) and others around the child (social and physical environments; virtual, cultural, and temporal contexts).[1] During ADL occupations, the context influences the activity demands, which vary in object use, space and social demands, sequencing and timing, required actions, bodily functions, and the body structures involved. As therapists consider these

factors, they determine the knowledge and performance skills (goal-directed actions) and patterns the child needs to learn self-care.

Child Factors and Performance Skills

Occupational therapy intervention to increase ADL function considers what the child and family value and the context in which tasks occur. The levels of independence, safety, and adequacy of occupational performance of the child and family determine the child's ADL occupations in various contexts.

Specific child factors (body structures and functions), performance skills, and performance patterns will affect ADL performance. For example, children with tactile hypersensitivity may cry during dressing and refuse to dress despite having the motor and cognitive skills to do so. Children with visual impairments may need to use their sense of touch when brushing their hair.[102] A child with cerebral palsy may not have the postural control to sit up during dressing but may have the sensory perceptual skills (e.g., right-left discrimination and figure-ground) to dress in a side-lying position. A child with attention-deficit disorder may have all the motor and sensory perceptual skills to complete a self-care task, but his or her cognitive organization, sequencing, and memory may interfere with adequate, safe performance.[139]

Interest level, self-confidence, and motivation are strong forces that help children attain levels of performance that are either above or below expectations. Children with intellectual disabilities, traumatic brain injury, or multiple disabilities have trouble in coordination, initiative, attention span, sequencing, memory, safety, and ability to learn and generalize activities across environments. However, with instruction and opportunity, ADLs sometimes become the tasks these children perform most competently.[79,111]

The child's disability or health status may affect his or her ability to perform ADL tasks and may also affect caregiver–child interaction during ADL tasks. The child's capacity for learning and ability to complete difficult tasks safely are considered. Pain, fatigue, the amount of time the child needs to complete the task, and the child's satisfaction with his or her performance influence the choice of ADL occupations.[69] In a study by Kadlec, Coster, Tickle-Degnen, and Beeghly,[76] caregiver–child responsiveness was videotaped for three groups of 30-month-old children and their caregivers. Groups included children born full term, children born at a very low birth weight with no white matter disorders, and children born at very low birth weight with white matter disorders. During feeding and dressing activities, mothers of the very-low-birth-weight children tended to adjust to their child's motor and cognitive needs by giving more directive and positive emotional and social assistance during ADLs than parents of children who were born full term. Similarly, in both high- and low-risk groups of children, Landry, Miller-Loncar, and Smith found high responsiveness of caregivers when involved in daily activities.[91] Information from these studies may help therapists consider how caregivers actively support ADL participation by modifying the social and physical environment or by changing the demands of the ADLs.[76,79] The first-hand knowledge of parents and caregivers about strategies that "work" with their child and within their family routines is essential to consider in planning ADL intervention.[5,50,128,129]

Children who are acutely ill or who have multiple disabilities that require numerous procedures throughout the day (e.g., tube feeding, tracheotomy care, bowel and bladder care) may not have the time or energy to work on ADL tasks. For example, Jenna, a 10-year-old child with a C6 spinal cord injury and quadriplegia, can dress herself independently within a 45-minute period, but she and her family prefer that someone else dress her so that she has more energy for school tasks. Children with multiple disabilities may physically be unable to do all or any part of ADL tasks, but they can partially participate or direct others on how to care for them (Case Study 16-1). When children are hospitalized for long periods, they often need to have some control over their participation in self-care routines. Figure 16-1 shows how doing a small part of self-care routines is possible and meaningful for children in the hospital with acute illnesses.

Performance Environments and Contexts

The initiation and completion of ADL tasks are influenced by the context of the tasks, including interwoven conditions both internal and external to the child (e.g., personal, cultural, temporal, and virtual contexts) and around the child (physical and social environments). Children in early and middle childhood often perform ADLs in different settings. The four primary settings that children experience are home, school, community, and work. Once the occupational therapist understands the contexts in which occupation occurs, intervention strategies congruent with the demands of the activity are chosen or aspects of the environment that are barriers to the child's performance of ADL tasks are modified. Although this section has divided the contexts into various areas, all of the areas are interrelated.

Personal and Temporal Contexts: Family Life Cycle and Developmental Stage

Age, gender, education, and socioeconomic status define the personal context for ADL occupations.[1] In assessing dressing, awareness of the personal context is critical in choosing age- and gender-appropriate clothing that is within the family's budget. The time of day or year; the life stage of the child or other family members; and the duration, sequence, or past history of the activity are included in the temporal context.[1]

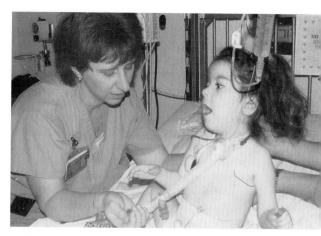

FIGURE 16-1 Partial participation. This child partially participates in hair combing and picks out her barrettes while therapists support her in her hospital bed.

Consider Cory, who is learning to tie his shoes. A routine method is established so he does the task the same way every time he tries it (e.g., first pull both laces tight, then make an X). Cory practices it every time he tries to tie his shoes but becomes frustrated easily. If mom and dad work, practicing shoe tying before going to school can work if they all get up 15 minutes earlier in the morning and Cory doesn't become frustrated with the time constraints. When the season changes, Cory must not only tie his shoes, but also don boots and extra clothes (e.g., mittens and snow pants). With these additional time constraints, his parents may decide to practice shoe tying at a different time of the day.

Children typically master ADLs in a sequence, achieving specific tasks as overall competency increases. The sequence of ADL development helps therapists and families form realistic expectations for children at different ages and helps determine the appropriate timing for teaching these occupations. By considering the child's age, therapists determine when it is time to stop working on specific preparatory or therapeutic activities. For example, 6-year-old Tilly has received occupational therapy for 5 years to enhance eating by trying to increase lip closure and to develop a more efficient suck-swallow pattern. If she has not learned this over the past 5 years, what are her chances of learning it this year? It may be time for the therapist to work on self-feeding strategies or on an IADL activity, such as operating an appliance with a switch for meal preparation.

Families vary in their ability and availability to assist and encourage the child to perform ADLs. This ability often depends on where the family and child are in the family life cycle, the personal factors or characteristics of the child, and the family's ability to spend time and be flexible in everyday routines.[5,146,149] When their child is an infant, parents often seek instruction on feeding, dressing, and bathing. By 3 years of age, the child's self-feeding, dressing, and toileting skills may become issues for parents if the child has a disability. For example, if Mary is the last of seven children, increased ADL independence in feeding or dressing may be less important because her older siblings love to feed and dress Mary. As Mary transitions into a daycare setting or another sibling is born, learning basic ADL skills may become a priority.

> ### CASE STUDY 16-1   Karina
>
> Four-year-old Karina is hospitalized every 2 months because of respiratory complications related to a muscular disorder. Like most 4-year-old girls, Karina has an opinion about and preference for how her hair is styled, and she likes to wear barrettes, ribbons, jewelry, and pretend makeup. Karina has a tracheotomy, poor endurance, limited strength, and limited postural control to sit independently. Although sitting independently in bed to groom herself is limited by these client factors, with partial participation, Karina is still part of the activity. She can sit up and bend forward with physical support from the therapists, reach and choose her barrettes, and comb her hair with assistance.

When the child enters elementary school, typically by 6 years of age, functional mobility in the school environment, dressing (especially outerwear), toileting, socialization with peers, grooming (e.g., washing the hands and face), and functional communication (e.g., writing, drawing, and expressing needs) become increasingly important. As older siblings become more aware of and sensitive to the child's disability, they may ignore their brother or sister in community settings or be more motivated by the therapist to help the child learn ADL tasks.

During adolescence (13 to 21 years), parents and child can begin to have different concerns and goals for therapy. Both may be concerned about the adolescent's independence in ADL; however, adolescents may have more concerns about fitting in with a social group.[101] When children who require maximum physical assistance in ADLs approach adulthood, they may become a great concern to parents. For the first time, parents may not have the physical strength to handle the daily care needs of their child or may voice concerns about the child's safety if someone else provides the caretaking.

Increasing independence in ADL tasks during adolescence often determines whether a child will fit in with peers, obtain a job, or go to college outside the school and family environment. The child takes on increased responsibility for managing ADL routines, caring for personal devices, and perfecting grooming skills (e.g., shaving, hair styling, skin care, braces). During this stage, families further investigate current community resources as they think about future living arrangements, vocational opportunities, and the availability of other recreational activities for their child.[146] Additional IADL tasks are introduced to promote independence during this stage, including caring for clothing, preparing meals, shopping, managing money, and maintaining a household.[65] Parent issues may focus on the child's ability to express sexual needs, to be safe in many environments, and to respond appropriately to emergencies.

Social Environment

The social environment, family, other caregivers, and peers provide encouragement and support ADL independence. They also shape expectations regarding the child's ADL occupations. In large families, different members may be assigned to perform or to help with specific ADL tasks for a child with a disability; in other families, the parent may be the sole person responsible for the daily living needs of the child. Family expectations, roles, and routines for managing daily living needs also influence the child's development of ADL and performance patterns.[146] For example, parents living on a farm may expect their child to get up at dawn, put on overalls and boots, do chores such as feeding the animals, receive home schooling, and help sell eggs to augment the family income.

When planning treatment, the therapist considers personal characteristics of family members, such as temperament, coping abilities, flexibility, and health status (see Chapter 5).[146] For example, the mother may place her older child in the "mothering" role if she is depressed and unable to get out of bed and begin the morning routine. Parents with intellectual disabilities or mental health problems may need to see a therapist modeling a behavior to learn how to cue and structure a task for their children.[38,146] Parents with physical problems may need instructions and practice in using specific techniques and assistive devices safely.

An analysis of social routines helps determine when and how ADLs are taught. Routines may differ significantly across home, school, community, and recreational environments. The variation in routine may confuse or disorganize children with intellectual disabilities, autism, or attention-deficit disorders, but may be motivating to children without attention, sensory, or cognitive problems. School-based and early intervention therapists need to be aware of the social routines so that they can choose appropriate times to teach tasks. When tasks are taught or practiced at times and places where they occur naturally, they more quickly become part of the child's behavior repertoire.[15] For example, school-based therapists may meet children at the bus to work on functional mobility and may be present as the child removes his or her coat to work on dressing. When tasks are embedded throughout all environments, children have multiple opportunities to practice activities and learn how to use the natural cues in the environment to modify their behavior. Social interactions and networks of peer buddies are extremely powerful in motivating children[71] and helping them succeed in self-care. Judie Schoonover, an occupational therapist and assistive technology specialist in Virginia, describes creative routines to practice ADL tasks within the school routine:

> Rehearsing routines such as dressing and undressing for toileting with students with limited cognition is not meaningful when practiced separate from their daily routines. They do not understand why they are undressing, then pulling their pants right up without using the toilet! Instead, I have asked their mothers to send snacks to school in something that snaps, unbuttons, or zips. Guess what? Undoing fasteners to get a snack out is far more engaging, and doesn't require weekly OT sessions in the therapy room.
>
> Another strategy I've used for a child working on an IEP goal of shoe tying or buttoning (but who doesn't wear buttons or tie shoes!) is to talk with her teacher about incorporating tying a bow as part of her behavior plan. Whenever the child accomplishes a task in class, she buttons a button on an incentive chart or ties a bow on a special dowel rather than put[ting] a sticker on a chart (p. 10).[62]

Cultural Context

As therapists work with children and families in an array of service provision models, they must be aware of their own and others' cultural beliefs, customs, activity patterns, and expectations for performance in ADLs.[97] An occupational therapist may become involved with a family because someone else believes that services are needed, and the family may not welcome the therapist's personal questions about the child's and family's self-maintenance occupations and routines. Cultural expectations of the family, caregivers, and social group as a whole may determine behavior standards. Family beliefs, values, and attitudes about childrearing, autonomy, and self-reliance influence how parents perceive ADLs. In Anglo-European cultures, parents usually are concerned about children meeting developmental milestones,[64] while other cultures (e.g., Hispanic) may be more relaxed about milestone attainment.[155] Children may not be taught to button their coat, tie shoes, or cut food until a later age because parents may value this role as part of their caregiving and affection for the child.[22]

Social role expectations and routines are influenced by culture. In a study by Horn, Brenner, Rao, and Cheng, African American parents expected toilet training routines to begin at an earlier age (18 months) than did Caucasian parents of a higher income level (25 months).[70] Many Anglo-European parents encourage children to become independent and self-reliant.[64] In contrast, many Hispanic families[155] and Asian families[22] may encourage dependency or interdependency in the family. Routines for dressing, feeding, bathing, going to bed, and carrying out household tasks vary among cultural groups. For example, bathing may occur less than once a day in some cultures, and hairstyles and head garments may be worn for different occasions depending on the child's cultural group.

Culture also influences the type and availability of tools, equipment, and materials a child uses to perform ADLs. Customs and beliefs may determine how parents dress their children, what they feed them, what utensils are used for self-feeding, how they prepare food, what type of adaptations are acceptable to them, and how they meet health care needs. For example, by custom, Muslim or non-Muslim families from the Middle East may eat only with the right hand because their left is used for toileting.[96] Economic conditions, geographic location, and opportunities for education and employment can help determine the types of resources and supports that are available to families. Economics influence ADL tasks in many ways: shoes may be old and the wrong size, indoor plumbing may be nonexistent, or nannies may be expected to dress, groom, or feed a young child with disabilities.

Physical Environment

Barriers in the physical environment, including terrain and furniture and other objects, may hinder the child's ability to improve performance of ADLs. Inaccessible buildings and rooms crowded with furniture limit how children in wheelchairs move throughout the environment. On the other hand, a large, open space may be too much room to allow a preschooler to contain his or her excitement and complete ADL tasks. Differences in surfaces also affect mobility; for example, rugs can make using a walker or wheelchair more difficult. Other physical characteristics that the therapist assesses relate to the type of furniture, objects, or assistive devices in the environment and whether they are usable and accessible. What is usable in one environment (e.g., a particular type of toilet at home) may not be usable in other environments, such as a hospital or job site. Sensory aspects of the physical environment often influence performance (e.g., the type of lighting, noise level, temperature, visual stimulation, and tactile or vestibular input of tasks). In particular, children with autism or attention deficit–hyperactivity disorder (ADHD) are often overly sensitive to and distracted by the sensory aspects of an environment.

The objects used to perform ADL tasks may help or hinder ADL performance. Clothing items (e.g., clothes with snaps, hook-and-loop shoes), grooming items (e.g., toothbrushes or toothpaste dispensers of various sizes and designs), or bathing items (e.g., type of soap, bathing mitt, feel of towel) may either motivate or distract the child. ADL objects or assistive devices need to be accepted and "fit" the child and family's preferences and meet the demands of the social, cultural, and physical environment.

Virtual Context

In today's world, the virtual context is considered for ADL evaluation and intervention. Options for teaching ADLs include videos, computers, televisions, personal digital assistants (PDA), or digital memo devices. "Talking books", visual schedules and stories using digital pictures, computer-generated checklists, or CDs may be used as cues to improve dressing, toileting, hand washing, and other ADL skills.[78,133] Recent research has demonstrated the effectiveness of using videos of others (video modeling [VSM]) or videos of the child himself performing a task (video self-modeling).[8,99] These videos may be played on an MP3 player, a PDA, or a computer and uploaded to a website for use at other times.

Older children and adolescents may use the Internet to learn more about fashion and style and to communicate with friends and others with similar disabilities or interests through email, blogs, or forums. Numerous checklists, assessments, and schedulers, and a wealth of information about ADLs can be found online. Parents, teachers, children, and therapists collaborate in the use of these resources to enhance performance. The Evolve website lists Internet resources for ADLs.

Assistive technology may help children with disabilities access the Internet, communicate, or set up reminders to perform ADL occupations (see Chapter 20). Mentors and support groups for individuals learning how to care for their own needs and live in the community are also available. An exceptional website is Blackboards and Band-Aids (http://www.faculty.fairfield.edu/fleitas), which was developed by a nurse to offer a forum for children and adolescents with chronic health care needs to discuss their day-to-day issues. Here children talk about themselves, allowing other professionals, families, siblings, and friends to understand their dilemmas and celebrations while living with a health care problem. Children post reflections about their disease and how they participate in different social situations. They also post poetry, art, and other information.

Activity Demands

The activity demands in certain contexts facilitate or impede the quality of ADL performance. A task analysis helps the therapist understand the complexity and various aspects of the activity. This evaluation involves analyzing the objects used, space and social demands, sequencing and timing, and required actions and skills.[1] Activity demands vary in the clinic, home, school, and community. For example, when an adolescent with a traumatic brain injury is learning to style her hair, the adolescent's performance skills may vary significantly in the occupational therapy clinic from those observed in her hospital or home bathroom. The child's unfamiliarity with the setup of the sink or bathroom may disrupt the flow of motor skills, and the spatial arrangements, lighting, and surface availability may cause process skill problems. For the activity, specific steps are followed and sequenced according to time requirements. (Verbal instruction in sequencing will support performance of ADL tasks—for example, "first you comb the knots out of your hair, then you part the hair and comb it. After a minute of brushing the hair, use the curling iron"). If the adolescent is doing this with friends, the demand on performance skills increases as the number of tasks or steps and the social demand to share supplies and to converse increase. In summary, grading ADL performance involves considering adaptations to the environment, the type of activity or interactions required, and the sequence of the activity. Occupations are viewed according to the environments in which they occur, the demands of the activity, and the child's abilities.

EVALUATION OF ADLs

Families and their children play key roles in determining which evaluation procedures are used. By working collaboratively with families, therapists learn about the child, the various environments in which ADLs occur, the demands of the activities, and the expectations and concerns of the family. When children get older and are able to communicate, the therapist includes them in determining what areas of ADLs are important to them. The parents and the child often become more vested in the results if the therapist gives them a chance to select or refuse evaluations and to choose where and when the evaluation is completed.[54] This approach also gives therapists a better understanding of the contexts in which the child performs occupations and of current performance patterns that may be valued by the family.

Evaluation Methods

Evaluation of ADL begins with an analysis of occupational performance, which may involve collecting data from numerous sources. Interviews, inventories, and structured and naturalistic observations are evaluation methods typically used to measure ADL performance in occupational therapy. The therapist uses these methods alone or in combination to analyze occupational performance (abilities and limitations), develop collaborative goals with children and their families, plan intervention strategies, and/or measure outcomes of treatment. The choice of instrument depends on the reason for the evaluation. Table 16-1 lists some instruments that assess children's ADL performance for different purposes. Each instrument can be rated by interviewing the caregiver or can be completed as an inventory. Each instrument (except the Vineland Adaptive

TABLE 16-1 Instruments for Assessing ADL Performance in Children and Adolescents

Instrument and Publisher	Age Range	Description
ABS-S: 2 AAMR Adaptive Behavior Scale-School (ABS-2) (2nd ed.) (Lambert, Nihira, & Leland, 1993) Pro-Ed 8700 Shoal Creek Blvd Austin, TX 78757-6897 http://www.proedinc.com	3–8.11 yr	• ABS is a standardized, criterion-referenced measure for adaptive behaviors in nine domains related to IADL: independent functioning, physical development, economic activity, language development, numbers and time, prevocational/vocational activity, self-direction, responsibility, and socialization. • Maladaptive behaviors are measured in seven behavior domains. • ABS is useful for children with intellectual disabilities, autism, and behavior disorders.
AMPS Assessment of Motor and Process Skills (6th ed.) (Fisher, 2006a, 2006b) AMPS Project International PO Box 42 Hampton Falls, NH 03844 http://www.ampsintl.com	3 yr–adult	• AMPS is a criterion-referenced test for ADL tasks that assesses the underlying motor and process performance skills used to perform the task. • Clients choose 2 or 3 ADL tasks they want to do (the test has 83 possible tasks, graded easy to hard). • Examiners need to be trained in a course, observe and rate at least 10 clients, and then have their scores calibrated according to rater severity through AMPS International before using the assessment. • AMPS is useful for individuals ages 3 yr or older and with most disabilities. • Test's reliability and validity have been established, and normative data for typical individuals are available.
BDI Battelle Developmental Inventory (Newborg, 2005) Riverside Publishing 425 Spring Lake Drive Itasca, IL 60143-2079 http://www.riverpub.com/contact/index.html	6 mo–8 yr	• ADL domain includes grooming, toilet hygiene, dressing, and eating. • The evaluator can use an in-depth assessment or a screening format.

Continued

TABLE 16-1 Instruments for Assessing ADL Performance in Children and Adolescents—Cont'd

Instrument and Publisher	Age Range	Description
CCITSN Carolina Curriculum for Infants and Toddlers with Special Needs (3rd ed.) (Johnson-Martin, Attermeier, & Hacker, 2004)	0–2 yr	Both CCITSN & CCPSN: • Include self-care as one of the five domains measured (self-care skills assessed in the CCITSN are eating, dressing, and grooming; the CCPSN assesses these three plus toileting). • Include sequences in responsibility, self-concept, and interpersonal skills.
CCPSN Carolina Curriculum for Preschoolers with Special Needs (2nd ed.) (Johnson-Martin, Hacker, & Attermeier, 2004) Brookes Publishing P.O. Box 10624 Baltimore, MD 21285 http://www.brookespublishing.com	2–5 yr	• Provide an assessment log for collecting information. • Give teaching suggestions for routines and modifications. • Can be used with children with visual, motor, and hearing impairments. • Have been field tested in more than 32 locations. • Have high reliability and validity.
COACH Choosing Options and Accommodations for Children (2nd ed.) (Giangreco, Cloninger, & Iverson, 1998) Brookes Publishing P.O. Box 10624 Baltimore, MD 21285 http://www.brookespublishing.com	3–21 yr	• COACH is a curriculum-referenced, transdisciplinary team assessment and curriculum with four domains: personal management, community, home, and vocational. • The instrument is used as a team planning tool in the domains and does not assess specific skills. • Tasks are scored and given a potential priority and rank by each evaluator. • COACH is intended for children with moderate, severe, or profound disabilities but has been used with children with mild disabilities.
FIM Functional Independence Measure FIMware user guide and self-guided training manual, Version 5.20 (1997, 1999) Buffalo, NY 14214: State University of New York at Buffalo. http://www.udsmr.org/	8 yr–adult	• FIM is a functional outcome measure for clients with physical disabilities. • Scores predict the intensity and extent of the assistance needed. • Six domains are assessed: self-care, mobility, locomotion, sphincter control, communication, and social cognition; there are 18 subdomains. • FIM uses a 7-point ordinal scale to measure the level of independence. • The test is norm-referenced and part of the Uniform Data System for Medical Rehabilitation.
HELP Hawaii Early Learning Profile-Revised (Furuno, O'Reilly, Hosaka, Zeisloft, & Allman, 2004) *Inside HELP: An Administration Manual* (Parks, 1999) VORT P.O. Box 11132 Palo Alto, CA 94306 http://www.vort.com	Birth–3 yr	• HELP is a curriculum-referenced assessment. • Self-care is one of six domains that cover 622 skills. • The instrument includes an inventory of developmental skills, an activity guide, and other materials intended for parents with disabilities. • Psychometric testing is not included.
PEDI Pediatric Evaluation of Disability Inventory (Haley, Coster, Ludlow, Haltiwanger, & Andrellos, 1992) Psychological Corporation Therapy Skill Builders 555 Academic Court San Antonio, TX 78204-2498 http://marketplace.psychcorp.com/; http://www.bu.edu/cre/pedi/about-pedi.html	6 mo–7 yr (and older if skills below those of a 7-year-old)	• PEDI is a normative, judgment-based outcome measurement (i.e., caregiver interview and/or observation). • Three domains are measured: self-care, mobility, and social function. • Some of the self-care skills assessed are drinking, utensil use, dressing, brushing the hair, and washing the face. • Functional skills (197 tasks), caregiver assistance (20 tasks), and modifications of adaptive equipment are rated.
SFA School Function Assessment (Coster, Deeney, Haltiwanger, & Haley, 1998)	5–12 yr	• SFA is a criterion-referenced assessment. • The test measures student function in the school setting according to participation in regular class,

TABLE 16-1   Instruments for Assessing ADL Performance in Children and Adolescents—Cont'd

Instrument and Publisher	Age Range	Description
Psychological Corporation Therapy Skill Builders 555 Academic Court San Antonio, TX 78204-2498 http://marketplace.psychcorp.com/		special education class, playground/recess, transportation, bathroom/toileting, transitions, and mealtime/snack time. • Task supports and activity performance are rated. • SFA produces a functional profile compared with that of peers. • The test has high reliability and strong validity.
VINELAND Vineland Adaptive Behavior Scales (Sparrow, Balla, & Cicchetti, 2005) American Guidance Service Circle Pines, MN 55014 http://www.agsnet.com	Birth–18.11 mos. (and low-functioning adults)	• The instrument is a norm-referenced evaluation. • Social competency is assessed, with behavioral observations in daily living skills (personal, domestic, community), communication, socialization, and motor domains. • An optional maladaptive behavior domain is provided for children 5 yr or older. • Three versions are available: interview/survey form; interview/expanded form; and classroom/teacher form (3–12.11 mo); online scoring is available. • The scales are appropriate for students with or without disabilities. • The instrument is reliable and valid for children with intellectual disabilities (Balboni, Pedrabissi, Moltoni, et al., 2001).
WeeFIM Functional Independence Measure for Children (Hamilton & Granger, 2000) WeeFIM II system clinical guide: Version 5.01. (1998, 2000), Buffalo, NY 14214: University at Buffalo.	6 mos.–6 yrs.	• WeeFIM is a functional outcome evaluation for children with physical disabilities. • The instrument determines the amount of caregiver assistance needed. • Three domains are assessed: (1) self-care (eating, grooming, bathing, dressing [upper body and lower body], toileting, bladder management, and bowel management); (2) mobility; and (3) cognitive skills for a total of 18 items. • This instrument is a direct adaptation of the Functional Independence Measure (FIM) for adults. • WeeFIM has high interrater reliability and stability.

Behavior Scales) can also be completed through observation of the child's performance.

For ADL independence, the child must not only complete the task but also obtain and use the supplies the task requires. The therapist generally rates performance according to the child's ability to set up and complete a task and may assess performance by grading the child's level of independence. Table 16-2 presents one example of how the therapist may rate a child's independence in bathing. The therapist may use a system for grading the child's level of independence with any of the methods or purposes discussed next.

An occupational analysis is done both during evaluation procedures and after they have been completed. Rogers, Holm, and Stone suggested that therapists collect four types of data when evaluating ADL performance: (1) precise identification of limitations in the task, (2) causes of limitations, (3) capacity for change, and (4) possible interventions needed.[122] For example, when a child puts on socks, the therapist identifies that pulling the sock up over the ankle is difficult because of problems with upper extremity weakness and the tightness of the sock. Because the child has a neuromuscular disease with

progressive weakness, the capacity to get stronger is absent; therefore, changes in the activity demands or compensatory techniques (e.g., loose-fitting socks or a sock aid) will be needed to enable the child to complete this activity independently. These data help therapists identify appropriate strategies and outcomes in intervention.

Interviews may be informal and unstructured. For example, the therapist may ask the interviewee (e.g., parent, child, teacher, or other significant caregiver) about the child's goals and dreams, abilities, performance patterns (habits, routines, and roles), and characteristics of the environment in which the ADL task occurs. Sometimes simply asking the child, "What do you want to be able to do?" gives the therapist a place to start for further evaluation. The therapist may use interviewing techniques and inventory methods together to obtain useful information about how the child performs in different contexts.

Therapists also commonly use two types of observation. With *structured observation*, the therapist gives the child a task to do and then rates the child's performance in completing it. Structured observation of ADL performance provides

TABLE 16-2   Rating of Self-Care Skill Independence during Task Analysis

Level of Independence	Definition	Bathing Example
Independent	Child does 100% of the task, including setup.	Child gets out needed supplies and equipment and bathes, rinses, and dries himself or herself without assistance.
Independent with setup	After another person sets up the task; child does 100% of the task.	Caregiver places bathtub seat in tub and organizes bath supplies; child bathes, rinses, and dries himself or herself without assistance.
Supervision	Child performs task by himself or herself but cannot be safely left alone; he or she may need verbal cueing or physical prompts for 1%–24% of task.	Child bathes, rinses, and dries himself or herself without assistance but needs monitoring when getting into and out of tub and when washing lower extremities because of poor balance and judgment.
Minimal assistance or skillful	Child does 51%–75% of task independently but needs physical assistance or other cueing for at least 25% of task.	Child bathes and rinses body parts independently but needs physical assistance getting into and out of tub; he or she is cued to monitor water temperature and to dry body parts.
Moderate assistance (26%-50% partial participation)	Child does 26%–50% of task independently but needs physical assistance or other cueing for at least 50% of task.	Child adjusts water temperature and washes and rinses face, torso, and upper extremities independently; he or she needs physical assistance getting into and out of tub and for washing and rinsing lower extremities and back.
Maximal assistance (1%-25% partial participation)	Child does 1%–25% of task independently but needs physical assistance or other cueing for 75% of task.	Child independently washes, rinses, and dries face but needs verbal cues to wash torso; he or she needs physical assistance getting into and out of tub and for washing other body parts.
Dependent	Child is unable to do any part of the task.	Caregiver physically picks up child, places him or her in tub, and washes, rinses, and dries child's body parts; child does not lift body parts to be washed or dried.

Modified from Trombly, C. A., & Quintana, L. A. (1989). Activities of daily living. In C. A. Trombly (Ed.), *Occupational therapy for physical dysfunction* (3rd ed., p. 387). Baltimore: Williams & Wilkins.

information about how well the child performs the task in a structured situation; however, it does not determine whether the child will begin the task at the appropriate time or perform the task in different contexts (e.g., whether the child will dress himself or herself when left alone).

With *naturalistic* or *ecologic observation,* the therapist gathers information in the typical or natural setting in which the activity occurs. Usually the therapist completes a task analysis to identify the activity demands. This includes looking at the steps of the activity, the sequence of these steps, and how the child adapts to the demands of the environment. In a naturalistic task analysis, the therapist evaluates the child's ability to do the task itself and the physical, social, and cultural characteristics of the environment. For example, when observing a child's ability to use the toilet at school, the therapist notes accessibility barriers and the sensory characteristics of the environment. How the child adapts to these factors, the typical classroom routines and expectations for toileting, and any cultural aspects of the toileting process (e.g., type of clothing the child is wearing; which hand is acceptable for wiping) are also noted. After identifying these contexts and the steps and sequence needed to complete the task, the therapist chooses appropriate intervention strategies according to the demands of the activity in the school context. Environmental observation is time consuming, but it provides an abundance of

information when used in a team effort.[119] In addition to evaluating the performance skills and patterns used, the therapist identifies the level of assistance and the number of modifications needed to improve the child's independence.

Ecologic or environmentally referenced assessments are appropriate for all children and are particularly useful for children with moderate to severe disabilities who have difficulty generalizing tasks from one environment to another.[111,153] A *top-down approach* considers the contexts in which the child performs valued occupations in addition to what the child can or cannot perform.[16,25,68] With this approach, the therapist:

- Asks the parent and child what they want or need to do
- Identifies the environments or context in which the task occurs, the steps of the task, and the child's capabilities
- Compares the demands of the task with the child's actual performance skills while completing the task
- Identifies and prioritizes the discrepancies to develop an intervention plan

Team Evaluations

Curriculum-referenced or curriculum-guided assessments are often used by interdisciplinary teams in settings such as early intervention or school system practice. Self-care is often an area of assessment. The Carolina Curriculum for Infants and

Toddlers with Special Needs (CCITSN),[73] the Carolina Curriculum for Preschoolers with Special Needs (CCPSN),[74] and the Hawaii Early Learning Profile[49] are typical curriculum-referenced assessments used in early intervention. Others are listed in Table 16-1.

Giangreco et al. developed a useful transdisciplinary, curriculum-based assessment and guide, Choosing Options and Accommodations for Children (COACH).[54] Therapists use COACH to identify areas of concern (not specific skills) for school-aged children with moderate to severe disabilities and to help plan inclusive educational goals with a family prioritization interview and environmental observations. The team identifies priorities, outcomes, and needed supports for specific environments and across environments in the areas of communication, socialization, personal management, leisure and recreation, and applied academics. Team members plan goals together, write interdisciplinary goals, and then decide which services the child needs. The team may decide that an occupational therapist is needed only as a consultant if the special education teacher is able to address the ADL task adequately.

Measurement of Outcomes

Health care and educational systems are demanding evidence-based practice and cost-effectiveness for therapy intervention. Within the past decade, professionals in the fields of rehabilitation and occupational therapy have developed universal assessments to measure the outcomes of therapy designed to enhance ADL skills (see Table 16-1). Outcomes may include improved occupational performance, adaptation, role competence, health and wellness, satisfaction, prevention, or self-determination/self-advocacy.[1] In addition to providing a means to evaluate children individually, the collection of aggregated ADL assessment results or outcome measures can help justify program expansion or changes in intervention strategies.

In rehabilitation, four primary assessments, which are valid and reliable, are used to measure occupational performance and adaptation to ADL tasks in children and adolescents. The Functional Independence Measure (FIM) is a universal assessment tool developed for adults but also used for children as young as 8 years old.[48] The FIM assesses the severity of a disability and outcome progress after rehabilitation. For children 7 years of age or younger, therapists use the Functional Independence Measure-II for Children (WeeFIM-II).[61,145] The Pediatric Evaluation of Disabilities Inventory (PEDI)[59] is used for children from birth to 7 years of age and has a computer version for scoring.[27] Numerous studies have used these assessment tools to demonstrate positive outcomes in ADL performance for children with brain injuries and other physical disabilities.[6,7,34,86,88] However, the question arises whether a change in an assessment score really means that the child has made significant functional gains in self-care. Haley, Watkins, and Dumas found that occupational therapists, physical therapists, and speech therapists who were blinded to PEDI scores rated the magnitude of functional change in those scores as meaningful when an 11% change had occurred.[60] In a study by Ziviani et al.,[154] the WeeFIM and the PEDI appeared to measure the same construct of self-care, yet Kothari, Haley, Gill-Body, and Dumas suggest the PEDI was better suited to

measure outcomes in children with brain injury.[88] The choice of which assessment to use depends on the characteristics of the child and the context for intervention.

The Assessment of Motor and Process Skills (AMPS) assesses ADL and IADL performance skills in various environments, both familiar (home or school) and unfamiliar (occupational therapy clinic).[43,44] It has been used with children more than 3 years of age from different cultural backgrounds and with an array of disabilities. The AMPS has been used widely in outcome studies, mostly with adolescents and adults; however, it is also appropriate for children.[43,55,113,114,130] In the AMPS, the therapist assesses the dynamic interaction of process and motor skills while the child attempts to meet the demands of the activity in a certain environment. The therapist has a choice of 83 ADL/IADL tasks and gives the child or adolescent a list of approximately 5 to 6 familiar tasks, from which the child chooses 2 to complete. Because the AMPS has a task–challenge hierarchy from very easy to much harder than average, many of the activities are appropriate for children (e.g., putting on socks and shoes, brushing the teeth, folding laundry, setting a table, upper and lower body dressing, making a sandwich, vacuuming, baking brownies, or cooking an omelet). While the child performs the chosen task according to the instructions given, the therapist rates the 16 ADL motor and 20 ADL process skills. The AMPS tasks use a top-down approach that gives a comprehensive view of how efficiently, safely, and independently the child is functioning in performance contexts.[16,43,44] These results help the therapist predict what other ADL the child may or may not be able to perform. The AMPS has potential for evaluating progress over time after clients have been taught adaptive patterns, organizational strategies, and environmental modifications. In a study that compared children with attention deficit–hyperactivity disorder with typical children, Prudhomme-White and Mulligan found the AMPS to be sensitive in identifying deficits in motor and process skills, which may help therapists identify intervention needs (e.g., coordination, calibration, sequencing, memory).[116] A limitation of the AMPS is that the rater must be trained in a 5-day course; then after observing and rating clients, his or her scoring is calibrated according to rater severity. This training and calibration must occur before the assessment is given.

School therapists may not find the PEDI, WeeFIM-II, or FIM to be a useful outcome assessment of school performance. As discussed in Chapter 24, the School Function Assessment (SFA) evaluates the child's participation in six different environments—transportation, transitions, classroom, cafeteria, bathroom, and playground.[26] This assessment gives the therapist a profile of valuable information about self-care performance and role performance in the school environment, which the therapist uses to develop individualized education program (IEP) outcomes. For the School AMPS, the therapist observes the child in the natural school environment while the child does typical school tasks.[46] Currently, the assessment includes 20 possible school tasks in five categories: pen/pencil writing tasks, drawing and coloring tasks, cutting and pasting tasks, computer writing tasks, and manipulative tasks.[41,45,47,56,108] The School AMPS helps therapists assess motor and process skills during typical school graphic communication and communication device tasks. Because modifications to ADL tasks often involve assistive technology (AT), it is important that the therapist consider the emerging outcome AT assessments in this area related to satisfaction and performance (see Chapter 20).

The Canadian Occupational Performance Measure (COPM) assesses a client's perception of his or her ADL skills, productivity, and leisure occupations over time and is useful for assessment and reassessment.[93] The COPM provides an interview framework for children and families to identify how they are performing in everyday occupations and environments and how satisfied they are with their performance. Personal care, functional mobility, and community management are the areas covered in ADL performance, and a structured scoring system is used. The child identifies his or her most important concern and rates his or her performance and satisfaction with that task; this helps the child prioritize intervention goals.[93,101] This self-assessment piece makes the COPM more appropriate for children older than 8 years of age.[93]

The Child Occupation Self Assessment (COSA) is a self-rating tool that a child uses to describe his or her competence ("How well I do the task?") and the importance or value of doing a task ("How important is this to me?") in school, home, and community settings.[81] Observations of ADL and IADL tasks, as well as managing emotions and cognitive tasks, are part of this assessment. There are two versions available: a checklist with visual symbols and a card sort version. For example, one item is "Keep my body clean." The child then rates how well he or she does the task and how important it is to him or her. This tool has good content, structural, and external validity when used with children 6 to 17 years of age but should be used with caution in assessing younger children and children with intellectual disabilities.[89] This tool helps therapists target intervention, which may or may not include self-care tasks.

Another method to measure outcomes in ADL performance is using goal attainment scaling (GAS). GAS was originally developed for adult clients in mental health settings[84] and is currently used by pediatric occupational therapists.[30,83,92,98,104,107] This method allows the child, family, and therapist to set goals and criteria for success. Kiresuk, Smith, and Cardillo recommend using a 5-point scale.[84] To document progress, baseline behavior is scaled and described as 0 or performance expected, +1 for better than expected performance, and +2 for much better than expected performance. To describe a lack of progress or a decrease in capabilities, behavior is scored −1 for less than expected performance or −2 for much less than expected performance.[100] It is suggested that GAS is appropriate for children with moderate to severe disabilities or for children who make small gains in performance such as those in sensory integration treatment.[98] It is an appropriate outcome measurement tool if standardized testing is not available or if outcomes are variable.[84,100] Before intervention, outcome measures are defined after talking with the child and family to find out what type of change would be meaningful. Data are collected over time and then goals are modified for incremental differences. Mailloux and colleagues suggest that GAS may be used across clinical sites for research outcomes.[98] Research Note 16-1 describes a review of the literature on GAS in pediatric rehabilitation[139] and gives suggestions for using GAS.

RESEARCH NOTE 16-1

Steenbeek, D., Ketelaar, M., Galama, K., & Gorter, J.W. (2007). Goal attainment scaling in paediatric rehabilitation: A critical review of the literature. Developmental Medicine in Child Neurology, 49(7), 550-556.

ABSTRACT

In this article, a literature review of goal attainment scaling (GAS) was completed. Three studies in pediatric rehabilitation were reviewed to assess the psychometric properties of GAS. The authors concluded that additional research is needed because only one study investigated interrater reliability (found to be good) and only one study investigated content validity (found to be acceptable). Low concurrent validity was found in one study and no construct validity or content reliability was reported. In six additional studies reviewed by the authors, the use of GAS demonstrated "good sensitivity to change." The authors concluded that GAS is a promising, responsive method to use in pediatric rehabilitation to evaluate individual goals and progress. However, the authors suggest additional research is needed related to the reliability of this method when used with children of different ages and types of disabilities and by therapists of different disciplines.

IMPLICATIONS FOR PRACTICE

- GAS is a sensitive, practical, easy way to measure small individual changes in ADL occupations using occupational therapy intervention.
- Goals are formulated by parents and children first and then clearly defined on a scale. Goals chosen should represent desired functional changes for performing future ADL tasks. Are they valid goals?
- Training on GAS is necessary to ensure goals are objective and discrete, measurable, relevant, and realistic, and use equal intervals for performance on the scale.
- If multiple raters are going to use GAS for measuring progress, interrater reliability should be checked by having the raters watch a video of children doing the task and then having them rate performance.

INTERVENTION STRATEGIES AND APPROACHES

When planning intervention procedures, the therapist considers the child's characteristics and performance skills and patterns in relation to the context and demands of the activity. Therapists need to be sensitive to parents' and other caregivers' needs and concerns. It is helpful to listen to and reassure these individuals while engaging them in observations and problem solving. When planning treatment for children with performance problems in ADLs, the therapist must ask himself or herself the following questions[14,136]:

- What ADL are *useful* and *meaningful* in current and future contexts?
- What are the *preferences* of the child and/or the family?
- Are the activities *age appropriate* (i.e., used by peers without disabilities)?
- Is it *realistic* to expect the child to perform or master this task?

- What *alternative methods* can the child use to perform tasks (e.g., including the use of activity modifications or assistive technology)?
- Does learning this task *improve the child's health, safety, and social participation*?
- Do *cultural issues* influence how tasks are taught?
- Can the task be assessed, taught, and *practiced in a variety of environments*?

Therapists use various approaches to improve ADL skills in children, including (1) promoting or creating; (2) establishing, restoring, and maintaining performance; (3) modifying or adapting the task, method, and/or environment; and (4) preventing problems/educating others.[1] Therapists often use a combination of these approaches and various theoretic orientations to help children participate in ADL occupations. Table 16-3 gives examples of these approaches and possible theoretical orientations for the therapist to use when teaching a child to button his or her shirt. These approaches are discussed throughout each area of ADL tasks in later sections of the chapter.

Promoting or Creating Supports

Therapists often create supports within the environment that offer all children the opportunity to engage in ADL occupations that are age-appropriate and not related to a disability

TABLE 16-3 Approaches to Improving the Performance of Activities of Daily Living

Approach	Appropriate Frame of Reference	Problem: Buttoning Buttons without the Use of the Right Hand
Create or promote	Person-environment-occupation (PEO) Developmental	Suggest opportunities to help all students learn skills needed for buttoning. • Use activities such as dress-up clothes, smocks, lunch bags with buttons or snaps • Provide calendars or number lines with a button or snap activity • Provide a variety of fine motor activities for center time
Establish, restore, and maintain	Developmental Motor control Biomechanical Neurodevelopmental treatment Sensory integration PEO	Use specific activities to establish hand use and prehension patterns for buttoning. • Use coins in a piggy bank; board games with small, thin game pieces; and craft activities (e.g., friendship bracelets, mosaics) to work on hand strength and coordination before beginning with buttons. • Provide tasks to develop, improve, or restore body functions (e.g., ROM of hand; weight bearing to decrease tone; increase sensory input by playing with foam or PlayDoh); use dexterity activities to improve motor skills (coordinate, manipulate, flow, calibrate, grip). • Maintain performance patterns by using a dressing routine or other tasks that provide practice opportunities for buttoning on a regular basis (e.g., have a calendar on which the day of the week has to be buttoned to the calendar); maintain dexterity and strength through a daily exercise routine.
Modify/adapt	PEO Human occupation Rehabilitation Biomechanical Sensory integration Neurodevelopmental treatment	Revise current activity demands or the context to compensate for body function and body structure limitations that affect performance skills and performance patterns. • Adapt the task method: Child uses one-handed buttoning technique, uses a pullover shirt so that buttoning is not an issue, or uses an extra-large shirt with buttons already buttoned; he or she wears the button shirt over a pullover shirt like an open jacket. Cueing performance may include verbal, gestural, physical, or visual prompts. • Adapt the object or use assistive technology: Buttons are replaced with other buttons that have long shanks or that match the child's tactile preference; child uses a buttonhook, elastic sewn-on buttons, or pressure-sensitive tape; child and devices are positioned for stability during activity (e.g., child sits in a chair with arms to button a shirt.) • Adapt the task environment: Child practices buttoning in the bedroom, away from distracting toys or siblings; parent, sibling, or peer is asked to button the shirt; shirt with buttons is used because it is culturally important to a teenager not to wear a pullover shirt.
Prevention/education	Human occupation Developmental Rehabilitation Biomechanical Sensory integration Coping	Educate and prevent failure at buttoning. • Therapist models and teaches the child and the parent how to use the above approaches and lets them practice the approach while he or she watches. • Therapist provides home ideas for developing opportunities to practice games or tasks and gives written/pictorial, verbal, or video instructions. • Therapist consults with daycare provider or teacher to ensure carryover of the method used. • Therapist helps child anticipate possible problems when purchasing clothing with different fasteners and how to ask for help if needed.

Modified from American Occupational Therapy Association (AOTA). (2008). Occupational therapy practice framework: Domain and process. *American Journal of Occupational Therapy, 62*, 625-683; and Dunn, W., Brown, C., & McGuigan, A. (1994). Ecology of human performance: A framework for considering the effect of context. *American Journal of Occupational Therapy, 48*(7), 595-607.

status.[1] This approach offers team or system supports for schools without focusing on the child with a disability.[62] When using this approach, therapists design a program in which school or community groups participate. Possible activities include creating a module or center activity requiring zipping, snapping, and/or buttoning; developing a box of fine motor/self-care activities to distribute to all kindergarten classrooms in the district; giving an in-service presentation to the church or school about self-care development; or participating as a building committee member to make recommendations about universal design for the new bathrooms or gyms being built. When working with families, therapists may promote opportunities for everyone to participate in using a morning checklist for self-care routines. Perhaps a visual picture board will help all the children in the family to understand what tasks are needed for a morning routine.

Establishing, Restoring, and Maintaining Performance

The therapist may attempt to establish ADL performance and patterns using a developmental approach or, if this is not possible, may try to restore or remediate the child's abilities that interfere with performance. To establish ADL patterns, the therapist establishes the child's developmental and chronologic age and plans treatment according to a typical developmental sequence. In this approach, the therapist examines underlying body structures and functions (e.g., strength, tactile discrimination), selects age-appropriate tasks and habits to target in intervention, and gives parents some expectations for skill development.[67] For children with hemiplegia, constraint-induced therapy may establish or restore movement and use of the weaker upper extremity while the other extremity is casted.[114]

In interventions to establish or restore performance, therapists identify gaps in skills and intervene to teach or remediate the underlying problem that is interfering with a child's ADL performance. This approach focuses on the child's deficits in body function and structure to perform ADL activities. Therapists often use biomechanical, motor control, cognitive orientation, neurodevelopmental therapy (NDT), sensory integration, or behavioral approaches to restore performance skills. For preschoolers with moderate fine motor delays, some ways to increase self-care skills are to provide play and targeted fine motor and praxis interventions, which require in-hand manipulation, grasp strength, and eye-hand coordination.[19] Using an NDT approach, the therapist begins with preparatory handling techniques to inhibit the tone before dressing a child with spastic cerebral palsy and tight extensors. In this instance, the therapist places the child in a supine position and slowly rolls the child's hips from one side to the other to reduce the tone, increase ROM, and encourage trunk rotation. After preparation improves the child's task performance, the therapist facilitates movement patterns by stabilizing the pelvis while the child pulls up his or her pants. When using this approach, therapists provide parents and children with suggestions on how to practice these movement patterns in various tasks.

In a motor learning approach, a child may learn how to put on shoes through practicing the whole task in a variety of activities (e.g., dress up, relay races, morning dressing routine) or environments (e.g., home, school, therapy session, gym class). During practice, the child receives specific feedback (e.g., "pull the back of the shoe up when pushing the heel down in the shoe"). Jarus and Ratzon found that mental practice increased acquisition of new bimanual motor skills for children faster than just physical practice.[72] This technique may also help children acquire ADL skills (e.g., mental rehearsal of putting the shoe on the foot).

Mobility Opportunities Via Education (M.O.V.E.) is a structured interdisciplinary program that helps establish and restore sitting, standing, and walking skills for children with severe motor limitations.[11] The M.O.V.E. team plans and provides motor intervention using a motor control or task-oriented approach. Primary goals are eating, toileting, and motor skills; progress is monitored and goals are updated through systematic data collection.[11,144,151] Child-centered goal setting helps the team target functional outcomes (e.g., to stand to pull up pants at the toilet). Activities are used to develop ADL skills for the context in which they are used. Teams are trained together, and it is often difficult to distinguish between therapists and teachers. This approach is used with persons in any age group with moderate to severe motor limitations and is appropriate for children with and without intellectual impairments. Many case studies and testimonials on the M.O.V.E. web site (http://www.move-international.org/) and a few research studies support the effectiveness of this program.[11,151]

Occupational therapists also use behavioral approaches to establish and restore ADL skills. They may use backward or forward chaining to teach the tasks. In *backward chaining*, the therapist performs most of the task, and the child performs the last step of a sequence to receive positive reinforcement for completing the task. Practice continues, with the therapist performing fewer steps and the child completing additional steps. This method is particularly helpful for children with a low frustration tolerance or poor self-esteem because it gives immediate success. In forward chaining, the child begins with the first step of the task sequence, then the second step, and continues learning steps of the task in a sequential order until he or she performs all steps in the task. *Forward chaining* is helpful for children who have difficulty with sequencing and generalizing activities. The therapist gives varying numbers of cues, or prompts, before or during an activity. Therapist or person cues and environment or task cues may occur naturally or artificially in an environment. Therapists use verbal, gestural, or physical cues or a combination of all three.[12,137] Environmental or task cues may include picture sequences or checklists, color coding, positioning, or modifying the sensory properties of the environment or materials used in a task. Figure 16-2 shows an example of a visual picture sequence for hand washing. Reese and Snell described a hierarchical approach to presenting artificial cues from least intrusive (verbal cues), to more intrusive (verbal and gestural cues), to most intrusive (verbal and physical cues).[118] For example, they described this hierarchy of physical cues: (1) shadowing the child's movements, (2) using two fingers to guide the child, and (3) using a hand-over-hand approach to guide movement. The therapist or the parent uses the fewest cues necessary and fades cues to promote independence. Figure 16-3 presents examples of these different types of cues, which can be

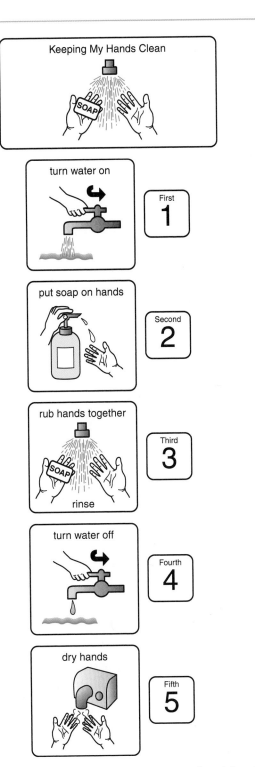

Keeping My Hands Clean

turn water on — First **1**

put soap on hands — Second **2**

rub hands together — Third **3**

rinse

turn water off — Fourth **4**

dry hands — Fifth **5**

FIGURE 16-2 This simple picture sequence gives Adam the needed cues to wash his hands independently. (Courtesy Judith Schoonover, Loudoun County Public Schools, Virginia; Picture Communication Symbols from Mayer-Johnson, Inc, Solana Beach, CA.)

Once self-care routines and patterns are developed, it is important to maintain them and any of the environmental supports that promote continued ADL success. Repetition and the development of habits and routines are essential organizers, particularly for children who take a long time to learn new skills, have poor memory, or thrive on routine or practice. Schedules for toileting or dressing, visual prompts displayed on the wall, a set place for items when grooming, and a checklist for how to clean a splint or contacts are all examples of contextual supports. Health maintenance activities (e.g., self-catheterization, wheelchair push-ups, ROM exercises, taking medication regularly, and eating nutritious meals) support task performance in all occupations, including ADLs such as maintaining a bowel and bladder routine, transferring to the toilet, and dressing.

Adapting the Task or Environment

When adapting or modifying an activity (i.e., using a compensatory approach), the therapist uses alternative physical techniques, substitute movement patterns, or other adaptive performance patterns to enable the child to complete a task. Adaptation strategies may include modification of the task or task method, use of assistive technology, or modification of the environment. Therapists often use a combination of these strategies to improve a child's performance, considering the performance context. Table 16-4 provides examples of typical adaptation approaches used with different functional problems in ADLs.

Therapists practice adaptation or compensatory strategies in various contexts and modify them until they become functional. For example, a child with a bilateral upper extremity amputation may use several compensatory strategies for ADL tasks. As an adapted method, the child may use the feet or mouth to write or dress, or may learn new movement patterns to operate a prosthetic arm (assistive device) for manipulating objects. Adapting the social environment by using a personal assistant or peer in the home or school environment is another adaptation strategy. Modification of the bedroom setup for easier accessibility and placement of clothes in lower drawers that are reachable from a wheelchair are other possibilities.

Adapting or Modifying Task Methods

The therapist often modifies tasks by using grading techniques. *Grading* is the adaptation of a task or portions of a task to fit the child's capabilities. By using a task analysis, the therapist rates subtasks of the activity and varies them according to their degree of ease or difficulty for the child. The therapist may modify the activity demands to compensate for limited capacities and performance skills. He or she may grade the tasks according to specific qualities (e.g., simple to complex). Grading a task may include gradually increasing the number of steps for which the child is responsible, fading the amount of personal assistance or cueing the child receives, or reducing the strength needed or length of time the child takes to complete an activity.

Each ADL involves a series of steps that are performed together in a specific sequence. Through task analysis, the therapist gains an understanding of the sequence of steps involved in each ADL task. When a child cannot complete a

used as a child performs various self-care occupations. Research Note 16-2 presents a review of studies that used different cues for persons with severe and profound disabilities and gives practical suggestions to consider.[90]

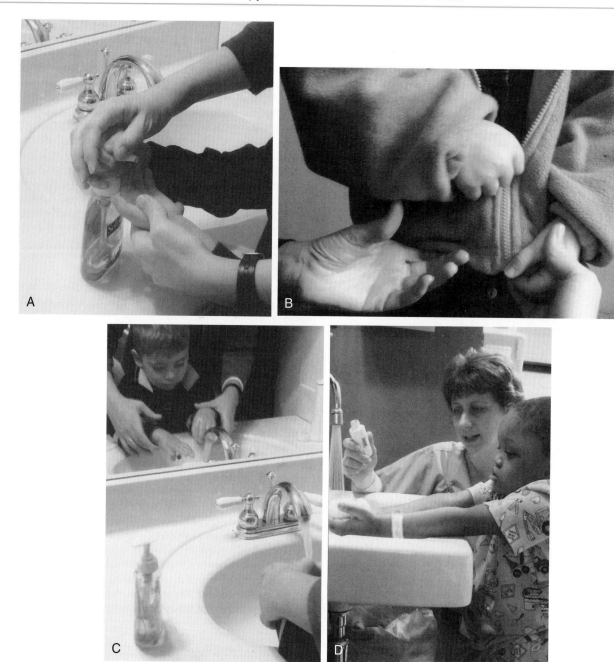

FIGURE 16-3 Hierarchy of cues, from most intrusive to least intrusive. **A,** A hand-over-hand approach is used for squirting soap onto the child's hands. **B,** Two fingers are used to guide zipping of the child's coat. **C,** The therapist shadows her hand over the top of the child's hands to cue hand movements for hand washing. **D,** The therapist verbally cues the child on how to wash the hands.

task independently or when completion of the task requires too much of the child's energy, therapists may suggest *personal assistance*, which the child directs.[135] The therapist uses *partial participation* when a child cannot complete a task independently. The child performs some steps of the task, and a caregiver completes the remaining steps. This helps the child become part of the activity and use his or her current abilities. Partial participation is often used when children are first learning a task or when their abilities are severely limited.[39,58]

Adapting the Task Object or Using Assistive Technology

Several assistive devices are available through equipment vendors, catalogs, and specialty department stores. These devices are changing constantly, and they vary in complexity, price, and quality. Assistive devices are commercially available or are custom-made by the therapist, skilled orthotists, or rehabilitation engineers. By using local and national databases, publications, and Internet searches on product comparison, therapists

RESEARCH NOTE 16-2

Lancioni, G. E. & O'Reilly, M. F. (2001). Self-management of instruction cues for occupation: Review of studies with people with severe and profound developmental disabilities. Research in Developmental Disabilities, 22, 41-65.

ABSTRACT

Learning and maintaining occupations is often difficult for children with severe and profound developmental disabilities. The authors of this paper reviewed studies about this population for the last 15 to 20 years and identified five main strategies of instructional cues: (1) cards with picture cues, (2) computer-aided and stored picture cues, (3) cards with object cues attached, (4) audio recording equipment that stores verbal cues, and (5) self-verbalization of what is being done. The effectiveness of these strategies and the practicality of using the different types of instructional cues were discussed.

IMPLICATIONS FOR PRACTICE

- When choosing cues to facilitate ADL performance, therapists need to consider their effectiveness and practicality.
- It is important not to infer that all children with moderate to severe disabilities will respond the same way to different prompts or that only one type of prompt is appropriate.
- Ask the child and the caregivers their preferences for the type of cue given for completing the task. Attitudes can sabotage the effectiveness of cue use.
- After learning one cue for one step, try to use one cue to do two steps of the self-care task. This will help decrease dependency on the cues, and help lead to using one or two cues for a multistep ADL task.
- Try taking data to see what cueing system works best. For example, does the child remember the steps for dressing with picture card cues or cues stored in a recording device or a PDA or a combination of cues?
- For complex tasks consider using other types of cues such as videos, video monitoring, video self-monitoring, or verbal cues. Take baseline data and data during the intervention to see if performance is improving.

keep informed of the availability of new assistive devices to find equipment for unique or specific problems.

The choice of an assistive device is a cooperative decision made by the child, the parents, therapists, and others who work with the child.[24] Together, these individuals systematically evaluate what the child needs to do, his or her performance contexts, the child's abilities and limitations, and the capabilities of the device itself. They choose the device that has the best "environmental fit." When the device arrives, student, family, and staff are taught to use it to eliminate unnecessary trials or frustrations. At this time, attitudes about the device are addressed (e.g., "This is too difficult to learn.") by providing support and education. Adolescents who are striving to identify with their peers tend to reject devices that call

attention to their disabilities. Children are easily frustrated if use of the device requires skills that exceed their coordination abilities or attention span.

To be worthwhile, an assistive device should meet the following requirements:

- *Assist in the task* the child is trying to complete without being cumbersome
- Be *acceptable* to the child and family and in the contextual environments in which it will be used (e.g., in terms of appearance, functions, upkeep, storage, and amount of time to set up or learn how to use the device)
- Be *practical and flexible* for the environments in which it will be used (e.g., have acceptable dimensions, portability, positioning, and be usable with other assistive devices)
- Be *durable* and easy to clean
- Be *expandable* (i.e., able to meet the child's needs now and when the child has grown and has more sophisticated abilities)
- Be *safe* for the child to use (e.g., physical, behavioral, or cognitive child factors such as drooling, throwing, or difficulty with sequencing do not interfere with use of the device)
- Have a *system of maintenance or replacement* with continued use
- *Meet the cost constraints* of the family or purchasing agency

Overall, the child should complete tasks at a higher level of efficiency using the device than he or she could without it. Trial use of a device is highly recommended; this helps determine the feasibility of its use and demonstrates its value to the child and primary caregivers. Caregiver roles are lightened by using assistive devices and modifications.[112]

Recently, computers and cognitive prosthetic devices have come into use to give children the visual and/or auditory prompts needed to initiate, sequence, sustain, and terminate ADL and work activities.[31,52,57] For example, a "talking book" from Microsoft's PowerPoint helps a child learn how to tie a shoe, how to dress himself or herself, and how to set a table if the technology is nearby. As shown in Figure 16-4, for tying shoelaces, the child or adolescent uses the talking book as a visual and auditory prompt on his or her computer or PDA. Other cognitive prosthetic devices that aid ADL tasks include portable memory aids (e.g., checklists, voice-activated tape recorders), medication alarm pill boxes, watches with specialized features (alarms, schedules, talking), alarm organizers, pagers, sound-activated key rings, and simple switches that program up to three steps.

Adapting the Physical Environment

In all of the approaches discussed, the therapist uses the interaction among the child, the environment, and the contexts to improve performance. Physical environments are adapted by changing the nonhuman characteristics of the environment. This may include simple modifications to the lighting, floor surface, amount and type of furniture or objects, and the overall traffic pattern of the room or building. Sometimes, modifications for architectural and other physical barriers or sensory characteristics are recommended. To facilitate wheelchair access, ramps are installed or furniture may be moved. For example, the family places the computer on a more usable work surface in a more accessible location so that the child who is wheelchair dependent uses it for doing homework or

TABLE 16-4 Typical Adaptation Principles Used with Children and Adolescents with Disabilities

Behavior/Disability	Adaptation Principles
Low vision or hearing (or both)	Use intact or residual senses Amplify sensory characteristics of objects (e.g., color, size, tactile and auditory features) Give cues consistently to determine whether activity is beginning or ending Use tactile, verbal, visual, or object cues (e.g., put hand on washcloth or say, "It's time to wash your face") Use gestures (e.g., point to arm that is put in sleeve first) Decrease auditory and visual distractions
Dislike of being touched (tactile defensive)	Prepare child for touch by giving deep pressure and organized, rhythmic touch Give choices for tactile preferences (e.g., clothes, washcloths, brushes) Let child perform touching on himself or herself (e.g., use toothbrush or wash face or body) Allow child to wear snug clothing (e.g., turtleneck) or loose clothing in accordance with his or her preference
Inability to find clothes or to understand top, front, or bottom	Amplify characteristics Reduce distracters (e.g., place only one utensil on countertop for cooking activity) Use visual or gestural cues (e.g., mark medial border of shoes with "happy faces" to keep shoes on correct feet) Use systematic scanning when searching for objects (e.g., clothes in closet)
Inability to sit up or maintain balance	Provide support externally (e.g., use positioning device) Change position of child (e.g., have child sit to put on shoes or dress in side-lying position) Change position of activity (e.g., keep grooming items together in a bucket on top of the sink)
Limited reach	Reduce amount of reach needed Change position of activity Lengthen handles (e.g., use long-handled bath sponge or reacher)
Difficulty grasping objects	Build up handles of objects (e.g., brushes and spoons) Substitute assistive devices so that grasping is not necessary (e.g., use universal cuffs or straps) Stabilize objects with other body parts (e.g., in teeth or between legs)
Weakness with little endurance	Eliminate gravity (e.g., prop elbow, or dress in side-lying position) Use lightweight objects Use power equipment
Difficulty controlling movement	Provide stable base of support (e.g., sit on floor with wide base) Eliminate need for fine control (e.g., use an enlarged zipper pull) Use weighted devices to give proprioceptive feedback (e.g., weighted toothbrushes and cups)
Poor memory; inability to remember sequences or directions	Establish and practice set routines and sequences Use partial participation, grading techniques, and backward and forward chaining Use visual cues (e.g., pictures, labels, checklists, color coding) Substitute assistive technology (e.g., alarm on watch or timers) Use verbal cues (e.g., "First, then second," jingles, rhymes, songs) Use real-life materials in the setting in which the occupation occurs
Tendency to become easily frustrated; outbursts	Identify purpose of "problem behavior" (e.g., escape, avoid, attention, obtain, transition, or stimulate) by analyzing antecedents and consequences Limit exposure to context associated with misbehavior Use preferred tasks and give choices Reinforce, coach, and expand appropriate alternate behaviors Avoid personal assistance and coaching (use partial participation) Use grading, prompting, fading prompts, and generalization

Developed from Geyer, L. A., Kurtz, L. A., & Byram, L. E. (1998). Prompting function in daily living skills. In J. P. Dormans & L. Peliegrino (Eds.), *Caring for children with cerebral palsy: A team approach* (pp. 323-346). Baltimore: Brookes; and Koegel, L. K., Koegel, R. L., Kellegrew, D., & Mullen, K. (1996). Parent education for prevention and reduction of severe problem behaviors. In L. K. Koege, R. L. Koegel, & G. Dunlap (Eds.), *Positive behavioral support: Including people with difficult behavior in the community* (pp. 3-30). Baltimore: Brookes.

communicating with a brother or sister at college. For some children, therapists minimize sensory stimuli and eliminate visual and auditory distractions. Other children may require increased environmental stimulation (e.g., color or music) to cue their performance. Table 16-5 presents adaptation examples of the physical environment.

Work Surface

The work surface supports the child, materials, tools, and assistive devices in an activity. The boundaries of the workspace help children keep within usable or safe environments. For example, a cutout surface on a table or a lip on a wheelchair tray or sink countertop can serve as a boundary. The therapist adds

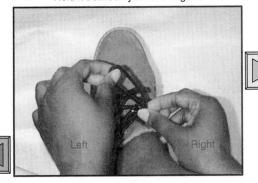

Use your right hand to make a loop
close to the knot.
Hold it between your two fingers.

FIGURE 16-4   Sample talking book. This frame from *Talking Shoes* was created with Microsoft PowerPoint.   (Courtesy Laura Pal and Kelly Showalter, Virginia Commonwealth University, Richmond.)

various textures, colors, and pictures to the work surface area to give sensory cues about boundaries or to structure the task. Even with these modifications, some children (e.g., those with weakness in one side of the body) need assistance in stabilizing objects. Table 16-6 presents suggestions for stabilizing

objects when they are placed on the work surface or held by the child.

Characteristics of the work surface that are amenable to adaptation include height, angle of incline (Figure 16-5), size, distance from the body, distance from other work areas, and general accessibility. Changes in these characteristics enhance the child's function in various ways, including improving arm support, increasing the visual orientation of a task, adapting seat height for easier transfers, and optimizing table height for wheelchair access.

Positioning

Therapists consider the position of the child and the position of the materials or activity when planning intervention. When possible, the therapist uses the most typical position for a given activity with the fewest restrictions or adaptations to stabilize the body for function.[10,42] Children who have problems with posture and movement often lack sufficient control to assume or maintain stable postures during activity performance and thus benefit from adaptive positioning. Adaptive positioning may include using different positions (e.g., sitting instead of standing), low-technology devices (e.g., lapboards, pillows, towel rolls), or high-technology devices (e.g., customized cushions, wheelchairs, or orthotics). If an adaptive device or orthotic is used, the therapist needs to systematically consider whether the device assists or hinders ADL performance. Chafetz et al. found that some

TABLE 16-5   Environmental Adaptations for the Home When Accessibility Is Limited

Architectural Barrier	Structural Changes	Possible Assistive Devices	Task Modifications
Entrances and exits	Hand rails Hand stairs Ramp Built-up terrain to door height Stair lift In-home elevator Increased door width (33 to 36 inches minimum) Step-back hinges Door rehinged to open in or out Pocket or folding door Electric door openers	Straps or loop door handle Lever handles Portable doorknob Built-up key holders Combination locks Environmental control unit	Use different entrance Remove inside doors Use curtains for privacy Use hip or wheelchair to open doors
Bathroom	Increased door width (33 to 36 inches minimum); French doors or accordion door Enlarged room Sink mounted low Open space under cabinet Showers with built-in seat Placement of tub faucets changed Ramped shower stall Toilet bidet installed Linen closet shelves with no door	Safety rails Seat reducer Raised commode seat Step placed in front of commode Wheelchair commode Insulated pipes Single-lever faucets Tub seats Wheelchair shower chair Hydraulic lifts Toilet paper tongs Toilet paper mounting Angled mirror Wall-mounted hairdryer with switch Suction-cupped bucket to hold supplies	Freestanding commode in secluded area Urinal Bed bath Sponge bath Liquid soap Soap on a string Shampoo pump Dry shampoo

Continued

TABLE 16-5 Environmental Adaptations for the Home When Accessibility Is Limited—Cont'd

Architectural Barrier	Structural Changes	Possible Assistive Devices	Task Modifications
Bedroom	Downstairs bedroom Enlarged space Enlarged closet doors Low closet pole Closet storage system with shelves Built-in bookshelves at low and medium heights Cut holes in work surfaces for holding objects and electrical cords Built-in dressers or dressers bolted to the wall Special glides for wall drawers	Leg extenders Bed rails Firm mattress Straps or rope ladders Mounted shoe rack Environmental control units or switches for TV, radio, and light access Enlarged drawer handles or loop added Positioning devices Adaptive chairs	Place bed on floor Keep most-used clothes in accessible drawers Use shelves instead of dresser drawers for clothes Store toys in shoe bag
Kitchen	Enlarged space Lowered countertops Lowered cabinets No cabinets under sink Built-in range top Sliding drawers and organizers in cabinets Wall-mounted, side-by-side oven Dishwasher mounted higher or has front opening Front-opening washing machine		Keep most-used items in low cupboards or on accessible surfaces Hang bowls and pans on wall instead of storing in cabinets Eat on wheelchair lap tray instead of table Keep water in insulated pump bottle on table Use a stool for washing dishes

TABLE 16-6 Stabilization Materials and Application Procedures

Material	Application Procedures
Tape	Applies quickly but often is a temporary solution; includes masking, electrical, and duct tapes (duct tape is sturdy and has holding power).
Nonslip pressure-sensitive matting	Fits under objects or around them and can be glued to objects; friction between materials minimizes slipping and sliding of objects; available in rolls or pads.
Suction cup holders	Hold lightweight materials, maintaining suction between object and work surface; single-faced suction cups can be applied permanently to objects (e.g., with nails, screws, or glue); double-faced suction cups can be moved from object to object.
C-clamps	Secure flat objects to lap trays, table edges, and other surfaces.
Tacking putty	Sticks posters onto walls; holds lightweight objects on surfaces such as tables, lap trays, angle boards, and walls.
Pressure-sensitive hook-and-loop tape (Velcro)	Sewn to cloth or glued to the base of objects and work surfaces; soft loop tape is used on areas that will contact the child's skin or clothing.
Wing nuts and bolts	Secure objects to a table surface or lapboard when holes are drilled through the object and holding surface; sturdy and more permanent.
Magnets	Affix to an object; stabilize objects on metallic surfaces such as refrigerator doors, metal tables, and magnetic message boards.
L-brackets	Hold objects in an upright plane; holes are drilled in both the work surface and the object to correspond with the L-bracket holes; objects are secured with nuts and bolts.
Soldering clamps	Hold small items for intricate work (e.g., mending a shirt, sewing on a button, or putting on a bracelet); mounted to freestanding base; bases are weighted, suction cupped, or held to the surface with a C-clamp.
Elastic or webbing	Attach to or around objects or positioning devices to hold them down; they also secure flat objects straps onto a work surface; straps are secured by tying, pressure-sensitive hook-and-loop tape, D-rings and buckles, grommets, or screws.

children wearing a thoracolumbosacral orthosis had better posture but actually performed less efficiently with dressing when wearing the orthosis.[21]

Alternative body positions are extremely helpful to children with disabilities. These changes help compensate for physical limitations in body functions such as strength, joint movement, control, or endurance and provide relief to skin areas and bony prominences. The therapist considers positions that maximize independent task performance. Key points for stability that enable the child to use available voluntary movement

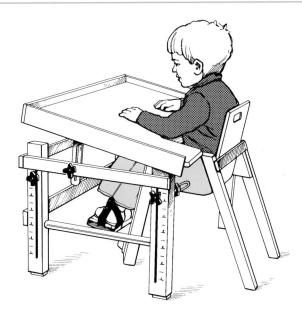

FIGURE 16-5   Commercially available chair with positioning components and a desk with an adjustable height and an adjustable inclined work surface.

are the pelvis and trunk, head, and extremities.[9,42] The following questions guide decision making about positioning:

- Is the child aligned properly? Are the hips, shoulders, and head in good alignment (Figure 16-6)?
- What positions or devices increase trunk stability (e.g., using a hard seat insert or lateral or orthotic supports, using a surface to support the feet, or widening the sitting base by abducting the legs)?
- Is support adequate to maintain upright posture with head in the midline?
- Can the child use his or her hands and visually focus on the task? Sitting and sometimes standing are the most appropriate positions for the child to perform ADL tasks. In addition

to postural alignment, the therapist recommends positions that provide the child with (1) good orientation of his or her body to the work surface and the materials being used; (2) good body and visual orientation to the therapist (if instruction is being given); and (3) the ability to independently get to the place where the ADL occurs, maintain the necessary position, and leave. The therapist modifies chair heights so that the child's feet are touching the floor to support postural stability and facilitate transfers. If the therapist raises the seat height, a footrest is also provided. The therapist shortens or lengthens chair legs with blocks or leg extenders.

Kangas advocates a "task-ready position" for children with moderate to severe motor disabilities.[77] Instead of positioning the child's hips, knees, and ankles at 90-degree angles, Kangas positions them so that they are ready to move. In the task-ready position, the pelvis is secure, the trunk and head are slightly forward so that the shoulders are in front of the pelvis, the arms and hands are in front of the body, and the feet are flat on the floor or behind the knees. The therapist removes or loosens as many restraints or chair adaptations as safely possible so that the child has maximal potential for movement. Such movement, even when subtle, provides visual, vestibular, proprioceptive, and kinesthetic feedback. A carved or molded seat and a seat belt across the thighs give additional sensory feedback and are used for positioning the pelvis and for safety.

Prevention/Education

Problem Solving: Cognitive Approach

Anticipatory Problem Solving

Children learn and perform ADL tasks in a variety of environments, not just in the clinic or the typical place where the task occurs. Anticipatory problem solving is a preventive approach that prepares children and their families for those unexpected events that may occur during self-care occupations.[124] Typically, parents do this with young children during toilet training. They anticipate the child will have accidents in the

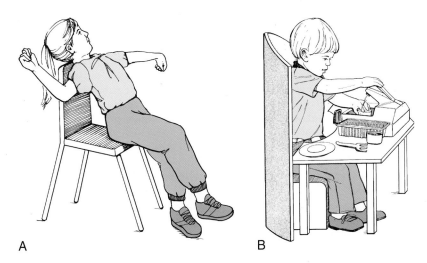

FIGURE 16-6   Sitting postures. **A,** Incorrect sitting resulting from a massive extension pattern and an asymmetrical tonic reflex posture. **B,** Correct sitting posture. Weight is equally distributed on the sitting base, and the feet and elbows are supported.

beginning and bring two changes of clothes in case this does occur. In a study by Bedell, Cohn, and Dumas, parents used anticipatory problem solving to help prevent meltdowns for their children with brain injuries.[5] By thinking ahead (e.g., remembering not to have the child dressed in overalls on gym day; having children wear splints on the weekend and not during the week), parents ensure that their children can actively participate in school activities.

Children and youth also need to be part of anticipatory problem solving. By anticipating problems and generating solutions ahead of time, children can often reduce the anxiety they experience when trying a new task or entering a new environment.[124] Using contextual cues,[17] such as noticing the floor is wet in the bathroom, and practicing different scenarios may be helpful. Schultz-Krohn suggests asking the following questions[124]:

1. *What is the task to be completed and where will it occur?*
2. *What are the objects needed to complete the task?*
   a. *Are these objects available and ready to be used?*
   b. *If the objects are not available (e.g., misplaced, broken, or being used by someone else), what else could be used and who and how will the child ask for help?*
3. *What safety risks or hazards are within the environment or related to the objects being used by this student or other students? How can these risks be avoided?*

Planning a natural teaching incident to occur during an activity (sabotage)[140] gives the child, caregivers, teachers, and therapists a good idea of how well the child can adapt and possibly use the anticipatory problem-solving solutions generated (Case Study 16-2). Giving the child an opportunity to choose a different way to complete or adapt a task promotes self-determination.

Cognitive Orientation Approach

In a similar model, occupational therapy researchers have developed a model of intervention called the Cognitive Orientation to (daily) Occupational Performance (CO-OP).[115] Researchers have studied the application of the CO-OP model in occupational therapy intervention on children with brain injuries, developmental coordination disorders (DCDs), or autism. These studies have demonstrated improvement in skills using the CO-OP.[115,120,121] In this model, children learn verbal problem-solving approaches and cognitive strategies to apply when they incur performance challenges. Talking about the task first, then practicing it, and then practicing and talking about the task (dual tasking) are the three main steps used in the CO-OP model. Research Note 16-3 describes a small study that used the CO-OP approach with boys with DCD.

Coaching and Education

Child and caregiver collaborative education is essential in all therapy for children. By collaborating with others, the therapist helps prevent injuries and possible failure in occupational performance. This collaboration helps children perform ADLs in their environments and helps caregivers and children learn safety information, specific techniques, and coping strategies. When providing information, occupational therapy practitioners consider the learning capacity, preferences, and environmental contexts of children and their families, as well as the demands of the activity.[69]

Because a young child or a child with moderate developmental delays may not be ready to assume ADLs and health maintenance tasks independently, parents, caregivers, and occasionally siblings are responsible for learning appropriate methods and adaptations to perform ADLs. Instructional methods depend on individual preferences, family life cycle needs, and the physical, learning, and psychosocial capacities of children, families, and caregivers.

Hanft, Rush, and Shelden suggest using a coaching approach with children, parents, caregivers, and teachers based on an understanding of their knowledge, skills, and desired outcomes.[63] This requires asking the right questions and having all parties reflect on their progress. Questions that are reflective, comparative, and interpretive are used

---

> ## CASE STUDY 16-2 Nadia
>
> Nadia was injured in a car accident and is now using a wheelchair for functional mobility in middle school while her femur and tibia fractures mend. Before Nadia's injury, she was identified as having a learning disability with problems with spatial relations. Using the anticipatory problem-solving questions from Schultz-Krohn,[125] the outlined questions were answered during therapy. Mom is transporting Nadia to and from school and her tasks to complete are to move safely around the school environment in the halls, classroom, band room, school nurse office, restroom, and cafeteria. She needs a wheelchair, lap tray, and/or book bag, a map of the school, and a way to keep her schoolwork organized. If these objects do not work or are unavailable, the therapist and Nadia generated the following solutions: If a wheelchair does not fit within a small classroom space, she could use her crutches for short distances or a rolling computer chair and ask someone else to push her closer to the table. The occupational therapist, teacher, and mother discuss how to transfer from the wheelchair to a rolling chair or separate bench,
>
> and Nadia practices these transfers ahead of time in case she needs to make these transfers. In addition, the occupational therapist and Nadia discuss her seating arrangements in each class and decide a change in desk placement is needed. If a lap tray is not available, she asks others to carry her cafeteria tray or classroom materials. A divided book bag, which should help with organization, is placed on the back of her wheelchair. A side pocket on the armrest is used for pencils, money, and personal grooming items. Because of Nadia's poor spatial relations, time is taken to review and practice how to use the wheelchair without running into walls or other people. A safe distance from people is established and she asks her teachers to be excused 5 minutes before classes end so she is not in the crowded hallways. Wheelchair maintenance and safety also are discussed, as well as deciding who may assist with the wheelchair. To enhance Nadia's anticipatory problem solving, the therapist may sabotage her mobility performance and provide a natural teaching incident by removing the lap tray or moving classroom chairs to impede her pathway.

RESEARCH NOTE 16-3

Rodger, S., & Liu, S. (2008). Cognitive orientation to (daily) occupational performance: Changes in strategy and session time use over the course of intervention. OTJR: Occupation, Participation and Health, 28*(4), 168-179.*

ABSTRACT

In this study, the authors used the Cognitive Orientation to (daily) Occupational Performance (CO-OP) intervention to help improve the motor performance of four 6- to 9-year-old boys with developmental coordination disorder (DCD) in daily occupations. Ten treatment sessions were videotaped for each subject, and a computer analysis examined the cognitive strategies and changes in strategies used during the sessions. "Session time use referred to the duration of Talking About Task (describing the task or plans that will be executed), Practicing Task (actually doing the task or activity), and Dual Tasking (both talking and doing) coded during video segments observations" (p. 168). The authors examined the use of cognitive strategies within the subjects and across all four subjects during the 10 individual sessions. Each subject had varied results and no patterns of cognitive strategy use were evident. The authors concluded that each child has a unique way of interacting with a task and the environment, and this emphasized the need for client-centered intervention that is individualized, which is the purpose of the CO-OP model.

IMPLICATIONS FOR PRACTICE

- ADL instruction must be individualized for children and is dependent on the interaction of the child factors, interests, and performance skills with the demands of the task and the characteristics of the environment.
- When planning ADL intervention such as washing the face for a child with DCD, consider using some of these CO-OP strategies:
  1. Talking about the task: Determine what face cleanser and cloth to use; where, when, and how it will be used; and what safety precautions are needed for face washing (e.g., water too hot, soap in eyes).
  2. Practicing the task: Grade set-up of the activity by therapist doing it first; practice first with a washcloth with no soap, then practice with a soap; try it in an isolated environment without distractions, try it within therapy sessions, then try it at home.
  3. Dual tasking: While face washing, discuss how he is or is not following safety precautions, what is working such as the pressure he is using or the pattern he is using to wash the entire face.

throughout the coaching process. Questions to reflect (e.g., what, who, when, where), compare (how), and interpret (e.g., why did this work? what other issues may arise?) give the therapist needed information to help coach the child and family. Hanft et al. suggest observing, listening, responding, and planning collaboratively with all parties involved in the task.[63] Observing the child where the task naturally occurs is essential. Observing the child and the caregiver and then the child and the therapist and using self-observation via videotape of all or any of the parties helps everyone reflect and know how the child completes the ADL task. Therapists need to listen respectfully and objectively to all parties to understand preferences, concerns, and areas of need when working together. Responding to concerns, giving feedback, and collaboratively deciding how to proceed with a task helps all parties. Finally, coaching requires careful planning: What strategies will they try this week? How will the occupational therapist modify the routine if this does not work? How will the teacher and the therapist give each other feedback?

Therapists present child or caregiver education in various ways by using coaching or other educational methods. They often demonstrate, or model, how to do the task (e.g., tub transfers) when instructing. In addition, the therapist may use visual aids, written instructions, audiotapes, videotapes, and checklists. The method chosen often depends on the comfort level and preferences of the parents and therapists and the contextual demands. In a study by Feldman, videotaped instructions were used to teach parents with limited cognition about child care (including dressing skills) and child safety.[38] The information was learned and retained for longer than 65 months.

Children require multiple opportunities to practice new tasks, and families may need help assessing routines and identifying when children can practice ADL occupations.[87] In a study by Kellegrew, parents used self-monitoring forms to record the number of opportunities their child had to perform an ADL task and the amount of assistance they gave the child during the task.[79] The parents did not receive specific instructional methods; rather, broad concepts were conveyed—for example, that ADL tasks were important, that their children were ready and able to learn, and that their children required many opportunities to practice the tasks. Families were creative in finding ways and opportunities to help their children practice tasks, and skills increased only when children were given multiple opportunities to engage in ADLs. These results suggest that it is important for therapists to assess a child's opportunities to practice tasks when collaboratively developing home ideas for families and their children.

An educational approach provides parents and children the chance to make informed choices about the services, methods, assistive technology, and environmental adaptations they will use.[4] Grading, forward and backward chaining, partial participation, and modeling help train caregivers.[147] Unfortunately, some programs may not place adequate emphasis on educating and informing parents.[82] In this chapter, anticipatory problem solving or CO-OP, as well as coaching and educating caregivers and children, is assumed to be integral to intervention approaches for helping children develop ADL skills.

SPECIFIC INTERVENTION TECHNIQUES FOR SELECTED ADL TASKS

Specific intervention strategies for toilet hygiene and bowel and bladder management, dressing, bathing, and showering, personal hygiene and grooming, and sexual activity are described in this section. Interrelationships among child factors, contexts, and activity demands are considered. Combinations of approaches and strategies that help children become as independent as possible in ADL occupations are presented. As with all occupational therapy, the therapeutic use of purposeful and meaningful activities, consultation, and education are methods used to help others learn ADL occupations.

Toilet Hygiene and Bowel and Bladder Management

Typical Developmental Sequence

Independent toileting is an important self-maintenance milestone, and its achievement varies widely among children. It carries considerable sociologic and cultural significance. Self-sufficiency is often a prerequisite for participation in day care centers, school programs, recreational and community opportunities, and secondary school vocational programs. Like other ADL tasks, toileting is a complex task requiring a thorough analysis of the demands of the activity and the ways the context and the child's capabilities influence performance skills and patterns. To begin to learn this task, a child must be physically and psychologically ready. In addition, parents or caregivers need to be ready to devote the time and effort to toilet training the child. A communication system between caregivers and the child is essential: What cue, word, or gesture is used to say it is time to urinate or defecate? What is expected before, during, and after the toileting task? Is there consistency in how caregivers in different environments help the child manage the task?

At birth, a newborn voids reflexively and involuntarily. As the child matures, the spinal tract is myelinated to a level that allows for bowel and bladder control at the lumbar and sacral areas, and the child learns to control sphincter reflexes for volitional holding of urine and feces. Children are often physiologically ready for toileting if they have a pattern of urine and feces elimination.

Bowel control precedes bladder control, and studies indicate that girls are trained an average of 2½ months earlier than boys.[125] Independence in toileting requires that the child be able to get on and off the toilet, manage fasteners and clothing, clean after toileting, and wash and dry hands efficiently without supervision. Children progress in a developmental sequence, according to each child's unique maturational pattern. The typical developmental sequence for toileting is presented in Table 16-7.

Typical Factors That Interfere with Toileting Independence

Children with spinal cord injury, spina bifida, or other conditions that produce full or partial paralysis require special management for bowel and bladder activities. Loss of control over these bodily functions and smells that result can cause embarrassment and reduce self-esteem. School-age children are characteristically modest about their bodies, and adolescents are struggling with identity issues and the need to be like their peers.

The type of bladder problem depends on the level and type of neurologic impairment. When the lesion is in the lumbar region or below, the reflex arc is no longer intact and the bladder is flaccid (lower motor neuron bladder). When the lesion is above the level of bladder innervation, the result is an automatic bladder (upper motor neuron bladder). The child undertakes training programs to develop an automatic response for

Approximate Age (yr)	Toileting Skill
1	Indicates discomfort when wet or soiled
	Has regular bowel movements
1½	Sits on toilet when placed there and supervised (less than 5 minutes)
2	Urinates regularly
	Shows interest in potty training
	Stays dry for 2 hours or more
	Flushes toilet by self
2½	Achieves regulated toileting with occasional daytime accidents (32.5 to 35 mo)
	Rarely has bowel accidents
	Tells someone that he or she needs to go to the bathroom (31.9 to 34.7 mo)
	May need reminders to go to the bathroom
	May need help with getting on the toilet
	Wakes up dry at night
	Washes hands independently (29 to 31 mo)
	Wipes urine independently (32 mo)
3	Goes to the bathroom independently; seats himself or herself on toilet (33 to 39 mo)
	May need help with wiping
	May need help with fasteners or difficult clothing
4-5	Independent in toileting (e.g., tearing toilet paper, flushing, wiping effectively, washing hands, managing clothing)

TABLE 16-7 Typical Developmental Sequence for Toileting

Modified from Coley, I. (1978). *Pediatric assessment of self care assessment* (p. 145, 149). St. Louis, Mosby; and Orelove, F., & Sobsey, D. (1996). Self-care skills. In F. Orelove & D. Sobsey (Eds.), *Educating children with multiple disabilities* (2nd ed., p. 342). Baltimore: Brookes; Schum, T. R., Kolb, T. M., McAuliffe, T. L., Simms, M. D., Underhill, R. L., & Lewis, M. (2002). Sequential acquisition of toilet-training skills: A descriptive study of gender and age differences in normal children. *Pediatrics, 109*(3), e48.

the upper motor neuron bladder. In children with a flaccid bladder training will be ineffective because the bladder has insufficient tone and requires assistance in emptying.

The therapist works with physicians and nurses to determine bladder training and management programs after medical testing and collaborative discussions with children and their parents. Four main methods used to manage urine are (1) condom catheterization (for males); (2) indwelling catheters; (3) intermittent catheterization (every 4 to 6 hours); and (4) ileal conduits. Parents are asked to restrict the child's fluid intake before program sessions to prevent bladder distention. When girls have partial control of bladder function, they wear disposable diapers or incontinence pads.

A basic principle for success in bowel reeducation is to have a regular, consistent evacuation of the bowel. Bowel program timing is a matter of choice, but a consistent schedule is needed. In some cases, the child receives suppositories and a warm drink before evacuation. This stimulates contraction and relaxation of muscle fibers in the walls of the intestine, moving the contents onward. Other techniques include digital stimulation, massage around the anal sphincter, and manual pressure using the Credé method on the abdomen. Occasionally, removal of the stool by hand or by a colostomy is recommended. As with an ileostomy, colostomy collection bags are emptied and cleansed on a regular basis and the child learns to do this independently as soon as possible.

Children with congenital or acquired neurologic disorders often undergo catheterizations or bowel programs. Compared with the toileting practices of their peers, these additional bowel and bladder tasks require more time; higher cognitive functions to plan, organize, and remember to perform the procedure; and established routines.[143] In addition, children may have difficulty in any of the following areas: maintaining a stable yet practical position; hand dexterity (praxis and speed); perceptual awareness; strength, range of motion, and stability; and accuracy in emptying collection devices. Memory, safety, and sensory awareness are needed for many of these procedures. Although nurses are often the professionals who teach bowel and bladder control methods, the occupational therapist may help establish the hand skills necessary, adapt the context by providing assistive devices or adapted methods, or establish a routine that becomes habitual and easy for the child and helps prevent future infections or embarrassment. Levan, an occupational therapist, describes a "penis paddle" made to assist a young man with self-catheterization.[95] By collaborating with the school nurse, the device was incorporated into the self-catheterization routine.

Closely associated with bowel and bladder care is perineal skin care. The skin is cleansed thoroughly to protect the tissue against the effects of contact with waste matter and to eliminate odor. All children with decreased sensation are susceptible to *decubitus ulcers*, pressure sores that develop rapidly when blood vessels are compressed (e.g., around a bony prominence such as the ischial tuberosity). Daily inspection of the buttocks with a long-handled mirror is needed.

Children with Limited Motor Skills and Bodily Functions

Diapering becomes a difficult task when infants or children have strong extensor and adduction (muscle and movement function) patterns in their legs. Therapists teach the mother restorative or remedial methods to decrease extensor patterns before diapering and to incorporate these methods into the diapering routine. For example, the mother may first place a pillow under the child's hips, flex the hips, and slowly rock the hips back and forth before she helps the child abduct the legs for diapering.

Toileting independence may be delayed in children of all ages with limitations in strength, endurance, range of motion, postural stability, and manipulation or dexterity. With an unstable sitting posture, the child has difficulty relaxing and maintaining a position for pressing down and emptying the bowels. With weakness and limited range of motion, the child may be unable to manage fastenings because of hand weakness or may have problems sitting down or getting up from the toilet seat because of hip-knee contractions or quadriceps weakness.

Cleansing after a bowel movement is difficult if the child cannot supinate the hand, flex the wrist, or internally rotate and extend the arm. An anterior approach may work. The therapist must caution girls against contamination from feces, which cause vaginitis. If possible, girls should wipe the anus from the rear. Solutions to cleansing problems are difficult and often discouraging. These children may require remediation strategies to improve body capacities (e.g., active ROM) or adaptation strategies (e.g., wiping tongs or use of a bidet) to perform the toileting task.

Children with Intellectual Limitations

Children with intellectual disabilities take longer to learn toileting, but they often become independent.[111] Problems with awareness, initiation, sequencing, memory, and dexterity in managing their clothes are typical. As with all children, physiologic readiness for toileting is a prerequisite for training programs. The therapist uses task analysis to determine which steps of the process are problems, and he or she then determines what cues and prompts are needed to achieve the child's best performance. The therapist also evaluates which methods work as successful reinforcement.[137]

According to a large longitudinal study by Joinson et al., school-age children with developmental delay, difficult temperament, and mothers with depression/anxiety are at risk for problems with bowel and bladder control during the day.[75] Therapists need to consider if any of these factors are interfering with toilet training and if additional time, procedures, suggestions, or referrals are needed. Some parents of children with developmental delay may use the Azrin and Foxx[3] training method for toileting. This program is behaviorally based and requires the child to be at least 20 months of age and able to complete prerequisites (e.g., sit independently, imitate, stay dry a couple of hours.). Caregivers spend 4 to 6 hours training in the bathroom with their child while giving positive reinforcement and overcorrection for errors. Sensors in the underwear also may be used to alert the child for wetness. There are a few studies reporting the success of the Azrin and Foxx method, but studies are limited that compare the effectiveness of different toilet training methods for children with disabilities.[85] The Evolve website gives additional resources on toileting.

Adaptation Strategies for Improving Toileting Independence

Adaptation strategies include remodeling or restructuring the environment, selecting assistive devices or different types of clothing, or devising alternative methods to enhance independence. Adaptations to provide privacy are particularly important for the older child and adolescent. The therapist also addresses caregiver needs as the child becomes heavier and more difficult to assist with toileting.

Characteristics of physical and social environments at home or school influence how a child manages toileting hygiene. Helping children determine where to perform the procedure and how to manage it in their home, school, and recreational environments is often a challenge. Social routines and expectations are also important variables for the therapist to consider when making recommendations for managing toileting. These expectations depend on the child's age and abilities and how the family perceives the child's ability to manage this aspect of his or her ADLs.

Social Environment and Temporal Context

Of all ADL tasks, toileting requires the most sensitive approach on the part of those who work with the child on a self-maintenance program. Children may purposely restrict their fluid intake at school to avoid the need for elimination. Unfortunately, limited fluid intake promotes infections, which increases the difficulty of regulating the bowel and bladder. Families, teachers, nurses, and paraprofessionals work with therapists to evaluate the social environment and find the best place, time, and routine for the child. When self-catheterization is done in the school or community environment, the child can ensure privacy by using the health room or a private bathroom stall, or perform this ADL at a time when children are usually not taking bathroom breaks. Carrying catheterization supplies in a fanny pack or a small nylon (nontransparent) bag also protects the child's privacy.

Therapists help children who lack bowel and bladder control to develop routines and health habits that eliminate possible odors. By focusing on performance patterns, the therapist reinforces and incorporates regular cleaning and changing of appliances (collection bags for ileal conduits and colostomies) and urine collection bags into daily schedules. A good fluid intake also is recommended to prevent odors and bacterial growth.

Children with autism often have a difficult time with toileting practices. Maria Wheeler offers a practical guide to toilet training for children with autism and related disorders.[150] Her discussion of support strategies such as modeling, Social Stories, and her numerous examples of common problems and solutions associated with training individuals with autism are excellent. She uses the social context and many visual prompts to structure the steps for toileting. In a small study of preschoolers with autism, video modeling with operant conditioning was more successful in establishing toileting than operant conditioning by itself.[78] Table 16-8 provides suggestions for adapting toileting for students.

Physical Environment

The bathroom often is the most inaccessible room in the house, yet it is essential that every family member have access to it. The floor space may be insufficient to allow the child to turn a wheelchair for a toilet transfer. The location and height of the sink, faucets, towels, soap, and toilet paper may make them inaccessible to young children. Sensory aspects of the objects in the environment may hinder performance. Children with hypersensitivity may have difficulty tolerating bathroom odors (e.g., air freshener, perfumed toilet paper or soap) or tactile sensations (e.g., a towel or a rug by the toilet). Therefore, the bathroom's space, equipment, and objects may need to be adapted or modified.

Toileting Adaptations

Numerous adaptations are available to assist the child in positioning and maintaining cleanliness after toileting. Urinals, catheters, leg bag clamps, long-handled mirrors, positioning devices to provide postural stability or to hold the legs open, and universal cuffs with a catheter or digital stimulator attached are some examples of assistive devices that therapists

---

TABLE 16-8 Analysis and Interventions for Toileting

Area	Analysis	Intervention Ideas
Required (task analysis)	Recognizes signal to go to the bathroom (visual or sensation) Goes to bathroom and closes door Pulls clothes down (only as much as needed) Sits or stands at toilet Urinates or defecates (or words child uses) Gets toilet paper Wipes, then throws toilet paper in toilet Flushes once Pulls clothes up Washes and dries hands Throws away trash Leaves bathroom	Have visual routine on wall (objects, pictures, or action words). Make tasks smaller or larger, depending on child's abilities (e.g., separate washing and drying of the hands). Add task if child is omitting it or is having trouble (e.g., if child is smearing feces, use "WIPE" as one of the steps). Child uses too much toilet paper: (1) Remove toilet paper roll and use Kleenex, or pull off correct amount to be used and hand it to child, or (2) place a tape mark on the wall of how much paper to roll out. Child does not sit: Use timer and instruct child to stay "seated" until timer rings; use potty that is close to the floor.
Client factors (body functions and structures)	Sensations (bladder fullness, voluntary control, emptying bladder, wet or dry, toilet paper texture, noise of flushing) Physiologic readiness Strength, coordination, and endurance to manage clothing and fasteners Balance to stand or sit on toilet Emotional readiness: fears of flushing or disease, need for privacy, attitude toward toileting	Use habit training if no pattern is evident: Go at the same times every day. Have child dress in easy-to-manipulate clothing. Use preparatory activities at other times to build strength and coordination for fasteners. Support child's body (e.g., grab bars, foot support, ring reducer, or potty chair on floor). Change toilet papers or use different material, such as wet wipes or cloth.

TABLE 16-8 Analysis and Interventions for Toileting—Cont'd

Area	Analysis	Intervention Ideas
Environment/contexts (cultural, social, physical, personal, temporal)	*Cultural*: Family and societal expectations of toileting; words used; whether child uses a public bathroom and sits on the toilet seat; institutional practices (e.g., co-toileting in preschool, language used) *Social*: Acceptance of use of a diaper; how child indicates need to toilet (e.g., pee-pee, gestures), others in bathroom, flushing, gender-specific public bathroom rules *Physical*: Size, temperature, sounds; set-up; way to flush, height of toilet, adaptations (toilet seat or potty chair; grab bars or safety frame around toilet); faucets and other fixtures *Personal*: Chronologic age, grade in school, gender *Temporal*: Previous experiences, fears of flushing or disease, need for privacy, attitude toward toileting	Spell out expectations in the beginning. Dedicate a bathroom to toilet training, if possible. Play soft music or toilet song on a tape player. Public bathrooms: Boys need cueing for bathroom behavior and may need a Social Story: leave a space between yourself and someone else at a urinal; keep your pants up over your buttocks while urinating at a urinal; don't talk or look others in the eye while at the urinal; be quick and leave when you are finished; only you will touch your body while in the bathroom (unless catheterization training). If child dawdles in bathroom, have him or her go with a peer buddy or go at a less busy time. If child is fearful, have him or her open door for escape, then flush.
Performance skills (sensory-perceptual, motor-praxis, cognitive, emotional regulation, communication/social)	Posture, mobility, coordination, strength, and effort needed *Cognitive*: initiate, sequence, and terminate How child communicates need to go to bathroom (e.g., physically or by speaking)	Provide way to indicate a need to go: Picture cues of entire sequence Object cues or transitional object Social Story Timer Spoken cues Positioning body on toilet Sensitivity to smells and sounds Physical, gestural cues Ear plugs, timing not after another person used the toilet
Performance patterns (habits, routines, roles)	Recognizes typical routines in the family for eating and drinking Recognizes typical times and patterns when child urinates or defecates Uses habit training to go at a certain time of the day, every day Cleans up accidents by himself or herself without harsh reprimanding Behavior challenge may be provoked by changes in routines.	Limit or increase liquids. Use wet/dry chart to determine typical times for toileting. Use visual schedule for toileting steps (including wiping) and times, as well as times for drinking fluids. Use same routine and rituals for toileting (e.g., particular times or when waking, before trips, after meals). Urge family, school, and day care center all to follow the same routine and collect data.
Activity demands (objects, spatial, social, sequencing, timing)	Placement of potty chair or toilet seat; height of toilet, flushing mechanism, toilet paper dispenser Space in bathroom, arrangement of items Door shut or closed; whether child announces it's time to go Steps to toileting, flushing after going potty; when to close door, get toilet paper or paper towel Public bathroom social expectations	Change layout of objects or accessibility of environment. Include "Shut door" as part of toileting sequence. Discuss public bathroom expectations; have social story available to talk about them. Public bathroom (boys): Use private stall first, then move to urinal.

Compiled from Wheeler, M. (1998). *Toilet training for individuals with autism and related disorders.* Arlington, TX: Future Horizons.

may provide. For children with good postural control but limited ROM or grasp, simple, inexpensive aids include various types of toilet paper tongs and toilet paper–holding devices.

A combined bidet and toilet offers a means of total independence. Several models are available that attach to a standard toilet bowl. A self-contained mechanism spray washes the perineal area with thermostatically controlled warm water and dries it with a flow of warm air. The child operates the controls with the hand or foot (Figure 16-7). Various special cushions designed to prevent tissue trauma are available commercially.

The type of clothing worn during toileting often hinders the child's independence or the caregiver's ability to promote

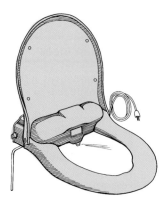

FIGURE 16-7 Electrically powered bidet makes it possible to clean the perineal area independently, without using hands or paper.

independence. Tight stretch garments are often recommended to help with postural control, but these garments may result in problems with toileting independence or incontinence.[109] For children who wear diapers, a full-length crotch opening with a zipper or a hook-and-loop (e.g., Velcro) closure makes changes easier. When children are first learning toilet training, the use of elastic-waisted diapers that pull up gives them the opportunity to practice this part of the toileting sequence while protecting clothing from accidents. As children mature, they may be responsible for changing their own diapers or caring for their appliances and equipment. Girls may wear wrap-around or full skirts because these are easy to put on and adjust for diaper changes or toileting. The child reaches and drains leg bags with greater ease when the pants have zippers or hook-and-loop closures along the seams. Flies with long zippers or hook-and-loop closures make it easier for boys to urinate or catheterize themselves when in wheelchairs.

Adaptations for Unstable Posture

When children sit on the toilet, they need postural security. When toilet seats are low enough that the feet rest firmly on the floor, the abdominal muscles that aid in defecation effectively fulfill their function. Reducer rings are used for small children to decrease the size of the toilet seat opening and thus improve sitting support. A step in front of the toilet helps small children get onto it. Safety rails that attach to the toilet or wall can assist with balance and allow free use of the child's hands. For the child who has outgrown small training potties, freestanding commodes may be useful when wheelchair access to the bathroom is impossible. A toilet chair that rolls into place over the toilet is another option. Commodes that feature such modifications as adjustable legs; safety bars; angled legs for stability; and padded, upholstered, and adjustable backrests and headrests are often helpful to caregivers. Commodes are also available with seat-reducer rings, seat belts, and adjustable footrests.

Menstrual Hygiene

In adolescence, girls need to learn how to care for menstrual needs. As puberty begins, hormones increase and moodiness, emotional turmoil, irregular bleeding, menstrual cramps, and poor hygiene may emerge.[117] For girls with intellectual disabilities, understanding the changes in their body and learning new hygiene skills may be difficult. Depending on the child's disability, puberty may occur between 9 and 16 years of age,

and avoiding abuse and reproductive concerns require consideration. These topics are discussed in this chapter's section on sexual activity.

Puberty is often a difficult time for parents, and they may approach their child's physician for menstrual suppression medication and contraception.[117] Options for gynecological care are important to discuss with parents and the youth. A pelvic or breast examination is part of maintaining health and is needed to detect possible health problems. A physician who is familiar, patient, and sensitive to the adolescent with disabilities is needed. The California Department of Developmental Services has developed a manual for physicians about how to conduct a gynecological exam for women with disabilities, and it is a helpful resource for parents.[134]

Menstrual management is part of toileting hygiene, and many skills, routines and habits, and adaptations may be recommended for the young adolescent with a disability and her caregivers. Similar to girls with normal development, young girls with disabilities need to be prepared, before menarche, for the changes that will occur to their body. They need reassurance that bleeding and sometimes cramps are part of growing up and are normal. Parents and therapists may work with the young adolescent to understand changes in the body and moods, as well as the methods (e.g., wearing pads or tampons) and hygiene habits necessary for managing menstruation.

Teaching Methods for Girls with Limitations in Cognition

For girls with autism, Wrobel suggests using stories and visual cues to help girls learn about menstruation and advising them to inform their teacher or parent when bleeding occurs.[152] Techniques suggested are using photo-sequencing cards, red food coloring placed on a sanitary pad, repetitive practice of how to place the pad in the panties, wearing the pad for a few days at a time before the onset of menarche, and instruction in proper wrapping and disposal of the pad. Wrobel warns that if practice begins with a certain type of pad or panties, it may be difficult to change to something else. In her book, specific stories, pictures, and examples are given related to the hygiene of menstruation, changing pads at school, getting cramps, and keeping menstruation private. These same techniques and ideas are applicable for girls with intellectual disabilities. Besides visual and physical cues, adaptations such as using PDAs or other types of reminders can help the adolescent girl manage her menstrual care. Alarms on watches, PDA timers, or cues are used to help the adolescent change her pad every 3 to 4 hours or remind her that her period may begin this week. Using anticipatory problem solving or the CO-OP method, parents and caregivers can ensure that the adolescent has extra supplies or clothing to manage any mishaps.

Occupational therapists may recommend to parents that they explain menstruation using an anatomically correct doll to simulate menstrual care. Individuals with intellectual disabilities have difficulty generalizing, and this method is not as effective as practicing the actual task during menses.[37] Using dolls may be more appropriate for younger girls when first learning about body parts and sexuality.

Teaching Methods for Physical Limitations

For girls with significant physical and/or cognitive disabilities, therapists can train caregivers to help with menstrual care ADLs.[58] When deficits in managing bodily functions impede independent menstrual care, the M.O.V.E. program[11] may assist in restoring the range of motion, postural control, or coordination needed to participate in this hygienic task. Adaptive devices for menstrual care are similar to aids used for toilet hygiene. Long-handled mirrors, positioning devices to provide postural stability (e.g., grab bars, toilet safety frames) or to hold the legs open, toilet paper tongs, and universal cuffs with a tampon inserter attached are some examples of assistive devices that therapists may provide. If a bidet is available, this may also help with cleanliness during menstruation. To manage sanitary pads, trial and error with materials of different sizes and types (e.g., adhesive strips of the bottom or on wings, underwear with elastic straps for the pad) is needed. Some girls may opt to use a diaper, especially if they are already wearing one. The social and physical environments and temporal context are considered. Where is the menstrual care performed? What is acceptable to the adolescent within this context (e.g., materials, adaptive equipment, positioning, amount of assistance from others)? How do the physical environment and daily habits and routines help or hinder menstrual care?

In Australia, occupational therapists are involved with the Health and Well-Being Network and provide intervention strategies to address menstrual needs of adolescents and women with disabilities.[18] Together with other team members they created a booklet and kit to help families and professionals explore attitudes, practical strategies, and other options for managing menstrual care.[33]

Dressing

Typical Development

For a typical child, achieving independence in dressing usually takes 4 years of practice. Characteristically, learning to undress comes before learning to dress. Caregivers introduce self-dressing in a natural way, at bedtime, by allowing the child to complete the final step in pulling off a garment. Similarly, when the child becomes more goal-directed and motivated to be independent, he or she is ready to try the more difficult tasks of learning to put on clothing. Often the caregiver uses backward chaining by putting the garment on the child and allowing the child to complete the action. Gradually the child performs more of the task and the caregiver performs less. A parent-friendly book that assists caregivers in using backward chaining and collecting data is authored by Turner, Lammi, Friesen, and Phelan.[147] Table 16-9 presents the typical development of dressing.

Dressing requires children to use a variety of performance skills and patterns to meet the unique demands of the activity. They need to know where their bodies are in space and how body parts relate while they use visual and the kinesthetic systems to guide arm and leg movements. The visual and somatosensory systems enable the child to understand form and space and how clothing conforms to and fits on the body. Dynamic postural stability is important as the child reaches, bends, and shifts his or her center of gravity while getting dressed. If the child avoids crossing the midline and performs dressing tasks on the right side of the body with the right hand and those on the left with the left hand, he or she most likely will have difficulty with tasks that require both hands to work together, such as fastening clothing and tying shoelaces. How the child coordinates the two sides of the body, manipulates the

TABLE 16-9   Typical Developmental Sequence for Dressing

Age (yr)	Self-Dressing Skills
1	Cooperates with dressing (holds out arms and legs)
	Pulls off shoes, removes socks
	Pushes arms through sleeves and legs through pants
2	Removes unfastened coat
	Removes shoes if laces are untied
	Helps pull down pants
	Finds armholes in pullover shirt
2½	Removes pull-down pants with elastic waist
	Assists in pulling on socks
	Puts on front-button coat or shirt
	Unbuttons large buttons
3	Puts on pullover shirt with minimal assistance
	Puts on shoes without fasteners (may be on wrong foot)
	Puts on socks (may be with heel on top)
	Independently pulls down pants
	Zips and unzips jacket once on track
	Needs assistance to remove pullover shirt
	Buttons large front buttons
3½	Finds front of clothing
	Snaps or hooks front fastener
	Unzips zipper on jacket, separating zipper
	Puts on mittens
	Buttons series of three or four buttons
	Unbuckles shoe or belt
	Dresses with supervision (needs help with front and back)
4	Removes pullover garment independently
	Buckles shoes or belt
	Zips jacket zipper
	Puts on socks correctly
	Puts on shoes, needs assistance in tying laces
	Laces shoes
	Consistently identifies the front and back of garments
4½	Puts belt in loops
5	Ties and unties knots
	Dresses unsupervised
6	Closes back zipper
	Ties bows
	Buttons back buttons
	Snaps back snaps

Modified from Klein, M.D. (1983). *Pre-dressing skills.* Tucson, AZ: Communication Skill Builders.

clothing, grips fasteners, and calibrates the amount of strength and effort determines how the activity is completed. Cognitive skills such as choosing the appropriate clothing, temporally organizing and remembering the steps of the task, and adapting to contextual changes (e.g., new materials, noise in the environment, placement of clothing) also affect dressing outcomes.

Typical Problems and Intervention Strategies

Limitations in Cognitive and Sensory Perceptual Skills

Children who have underlying cognitive and perceptual deficits may also have problems in processing performance skills. They may demonstrate problems with choosing, using, and handling clothing. These may include difficulty distinguishing right and left sides of the body, putting a shoe on the correct foot, turning the heel of a sock, or differentiating the front of clothing from the back or identifying the correct leg or sleeve. Applying concepts such as above, in front of, or behind may be difficult for these children. Temporal organization, especially initiating, continuing, sequencing, terminating, and organizing the dressing task, is often problematic for children with intellectual disabilities or autism. The pacing may be too slow or too fast, and they may be unable to remember instructions or use environmental cues to find their clothing or to notice or benefit from their mistakes. Instead, they may continue to use the same unsuccessful action to put on the clothing or use fasteners. The therapist helps the child use a compensatory approach for this by modifying the demands of dressing in various environments. Artificial cues such as color coding or labeling dressers or bins with pictures or words help children locate objects for dressing within the bedroom environment. Picture charts and checklists help the child remember the sequence of steps in a task and provide a routine for completing it.

Behaviorally, the child may become frustrated with the complexity of certain dressing tasks. Language deficits may restrict the child's ability to express personal preferences or frustrations. Sometimes children refuse to dress because they have no choice in what they are going to wear or the style they prefer. Given control or choice in dressing, children often become more engaged in the task and motivated to do it themselves.

Frustration may increase when the child is faced with tasks that require fine manipulations if coordination is limited or if the child has sensory modulation problems. Often, a behavioral approach can help the child acquire independence. After making a baseline assessment, the therapist carefully analyzes the demands of each dressing task. Once the therapist determines the limitations and strengths in performance skills and patterns, he or she uses partial participation and backward and forward chaining methods. Environmental and task adaptations include visual charts or pictures, Social Stories, checklists, and clothing that is easy to manipulate (e.g., slightly larger clothing, stretchy materials, pullover shirts, and loafers). Simultaneous prompting in the dressing activity itself helps children learn the task.[131] Figure 16-8 presents an example of a visual story used for a child who has sensory deficits and who dislikes changes in routines or dressing for outside play. The repetition of positive statements makes the child more ready to follow the routine in the story and initiate the task.

Video modeling (VM) and video self-modeling (VSM) are well-researched techniques used by a variety of professionals to teach children with disabilities social tasks and ADLs.[8,99] This research suggests that children may learn a task more quickly by watching themselves model a task on video than by watching a therapist or caregiver modeling the task for the child.[13,99] In the VM technique a child learns a specific dressing skill by watching a video of someone putting on a coat. In a VSM technique, by contrast, videos are edited so a child watches himself correctly put on the coat. For children with intellectual limitations, dressing was learned more quickly when the speed of the VSM was slower.[13] Research evidence across disciplines supports the use of VM and VSM for children with autism, with VSM being more effective in improving performance.[8,99] Research Note 16-4 cites a review of these techniques and provides suggestions for using VM and VSM collaboratively with teams. Additional research is needed to document the effectiveness of these methods in assisting children with different intellectual or emotional disabilities.

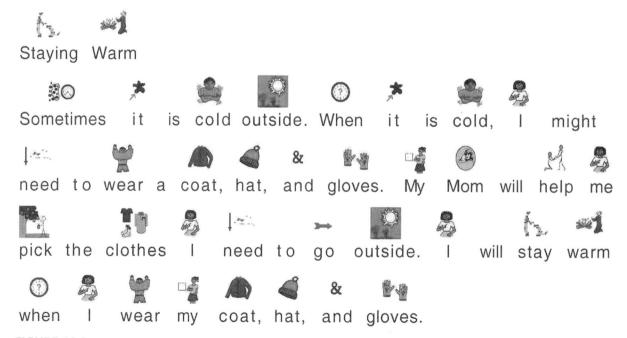

FIGURE 16-8 This example of a story is used before Mimi goes out for recess, to help her rehearse what she is going to do and help her understand why. (Courtesy Rebecca E. Argabrite Grove, Loudoun County Public Schools, Virginia; story created with Pix Writer by Slater Software, Guffey, CO.)

RESEARCH NOTE 16-4

Bellini, S. & Akullian, J. (2007). A meta-analysis of video modeling and video self-modeling interventions for children and adolescents with autism. Exceptional Children, 73(3), 264-287.

ABSTRACT

A meta-analysis of 23 studies (single subject design) of children with autism spectrum disorder (ASD) was completed by the authors. Video modeling (VM) and video self-modeling (VSM) effectiveness were reviewed. The authors used the "percentage of non-overlapping data points (PND)" to determine the effects of intervention, maintenance, and generalization effects. The results of the meta-analysis suggest that video modeling and VSM meet evidence-based practice criteria as strategies to address behavioral functioning, social communication sills, and functional skills. Functional skills in two studies included ADL skills. In addition, results found that when VM and VSM are used to teach skills to persons with autism spectrum disorders, these skills are maintained and are often used across settings.

IMPLICATIONS FOR PRACTICE

- Video modeling or video self-modeling for teaching ADL skills may increase the success of the intervention (PND = 89%), maintain that effect (PND = 100%), and generalize (PND = 97%) across settings for students with autism spectrum disorder.
- Showing a short video (2 to 3 minutes) of another child doing the task (e.g., putting on a shirt) prior to working on the task itself may quicken learning the task sequence.
- In VSM, the child watches himself perform the ADL task correctly, which may help the child be more attentive and interested in the task. Specific computer software merges the various clips of the child performing the task correctly. It may take multiple videotaped sessions to get a usable video.
- Videos of ADL skills placed on a home or school computer, television or a PDA, may help incorporate this intervention strategy into home or school routines to increase the rate of improvement.

Physical or Motor Limitations

Children with various conditions find dressing difficult because of the coordination and the range and strength required for pulling clothes on and off and connecting fasteners. Children with DCD can have difficulty completing dressing (and managing toileting and utensil use) because of slowness, disorganization, frustration, and a history of depending on others to do the task.[106] Dunford, Missiuna, Street, and Sibert found that children with DCD (5 to 10 years of age) reported concerns about their self-care skills even though therapists and parents did not identify these concerns.[35] Children with arthritis who have pain with finger movement frequently require assistance during a flare-up of their disease. Their ability to move their arms freely or reach certain areas of the body is limited. Children with the use of only one hand find it difficult to zip trousers, tie shoelaces, and button shirts or blouses. Establishing or restoring the child's strength or coordination may help, but in most cases the child learns adaptive techniques, often through his or her own experimentation or use of assistive technology. Children with cerebral palsy often have difficulty balancing and controlling arm and leg movement when donning and removing clothing. Limited dexterity may also interfere with dressing. Therapists suggest methods to modify the demands of the activity; such as supportive positioning or the use of adaptive aids such as buttonhooks, rings on zippers, one-handed shoe fasteners, or hook-and-loop closures. Because clothing manufacturers recognize the value of universal design, many of these adaptations are available commercially.[126] Table 16-3 gives other examples of how to improve fastening abilities.

Adaptive Methods for Dressing Children with Motor Limitations

Although it is common to dress an infant while he or she is lying in the supine position, this position frequently increases extensor tone in infants with neurologic impairment. For this reason, some therapists advocate placing the infant prone across the knees, with the infant's hips flexed and abducted, thereby inhibiting leg extensor and adduction tone. When the infant gains head and trunk control, the caregiver dresses him or her in a sitting position with the child's back resting against and supported by the caregiver's trunk. In this position, the infant has an opportunity to observe his or her own body during dressing.

When dressing an infant with increased extensor tone, the caregiver carefully bends the infant's hips and knees before putting on shoes and socks (Figure 16-9) and brings the infant's shoulders forward before putting his or her arm through a sleeve. Flexing the child's hip and knee decreases postural tone and makes dressing easier. When a child achieves sitting balance, a good way to proceed with dressing is to place the child on the floor and later on a low stool, continuing to provide support where needed from the back. Orientation to the child's body parts should remain a focus in the social interaction. The caregiver helps the child understand how the body relates to the clothes and to the various

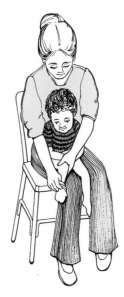

FIGURE 16-9 When dressing a child who is hypertonic, the caregiver should carefully flex the hip and knee before putting on socks and shoes.

positions (e.g., "The arm goes through the sleeve" and "The head goes through the hole at the top of the shirt").

When the child is older and heavier, there may be no alternative but to dress the child while he or she is in the side-lying or supine position. Placing a hard pillow under the child's head, thus slightly raising his or her shoulders, makes it easier for the caregiver to bring the child's arms forward and to bend his or her hips and knees. If it is possible to maintain the child in a side-lying position, this posture may make it easier for the caregiver to manage the child's arms and legs and for the child to assist in the dressing task (Figure 16-10).

Adaptive Methods for Self-Dressing

The child who has hand coordination but poor balance may be able to take advantage of the function that he or she possesses when in a side-lying position, with the effect of gravity lessened. For the child who sits but is unstable, a corner of two adjoining walls or a corner seat on the floor may provide enough postural support for independent dressing. Sitting balance is more precarious as the child reaches when donning overhead garments or pants and shoes; therefore, the child needs additional external support. Sitting in chairs with arms or sitting on the floor against a wall may improve performance.

The occupational therapist helps improve the child's dressing by offering the parent and the child various problem-solving strategies from which the child and parents may choose. Once the method is chosen, anticipatory problem solving is used to help prepare the child for unexpected events within the environment. Table 16-10 offers choices in problem solving that are used for putting on and taking off different garments. Clothing selections, assistive technology, and adaptations to the task are methods for improving a child's performance in self-dressing.

Increased attention to the needs of individuals with disabilities has been shown over the past decade, with some adaptive clothing becoming available through catalog supply companies. These companies generally offer attractive, fashionable clothing that meets functional requirements yet conforms in appearance to the child's peer group standards and fashion trends. Modifications should be inconspicuous, and the appearance of the clothing should not single out the wearer. When possible, clothing should conceal physical disabilities or at least should not attract attention to them. Clothing should contribute to the wearer's sense of well-being. Functionally, the design of the clothing should enable the wearer

to take care of personal needs, help maintain proper body temperature, and provide freedom of movement.

Most clothing is made for individuals in a standing position. For those who spend long hours in a wheelchair, the sitting position causes pulling and straining on some areas of the garment and a surplus of fabric in others. The caregiver makes alterations to provide more comfort in sitting (e.g., pants that are cut higher in the back and lower in the front and cut larger to give additional room in the hips and thighs).[126] A longer inseam also allows the proper hem height for pants when sitting (rests on top of shoe). Pockets in the back may cause shearing or skin breakdown with prolonged sitting. Instead, pockets are placed on the top of the thigh or on the side of the calf for easy access. Front and side seams are sewn with hook-and-loop fasteners or zippers and wrist loops to assist in donning. Pullover tops with raglan and gusset sleeves allow more room when maneuvering a wheelchair. If the shirt is cut longer in the back and shorter in the front, it is easier to keep a neat appearance. Rain or winter capes are comfortable in a wheelchair. They are cut longer in the front to cover the child's legs and feet and shorter in the back so that they do not rub against the wheel of the chair.[126]

For children who wear orthoses for spinal support, front openings that extend from the neck to the lower abdomen make self-dressing easier, whereas back openings are easier when others dress the child.[94,126] Caregivers should use larger clothing that fits over orthoses but should avoid loose sleeves for children who push wheelchairs because the sleeve may become caught in the spokes of the wheel. The child who wears an ankle–foot orthosis may need to have clothing reinforced to protect against rubbing. This is done by sewing fabric patches inside the garment where friction and stress occur and by adapting the pants with side seams and hook-and-loop closures so that the pants go over the orthosis more easily.

When children require gastrostomy feedings, tracheotomy care, catheterization, or diapering, they need clothing that allows easy access. Caregivers may sew moisture-resistant fabric into the seat of pants, on collars, on attaching bibs, and on sleeve cuffs (if the child bites clothing).[142] Jumpsuits or shirts with hook-and-loop closures at the gastrostomy site, neckline, or shoulder, crotch, or pant leg allow caregivers to perform medical procedures without removing the child's clothing.[94,126,142] Refer to the Evolve website for Internet resources on dressing methods, clothing, and other suggestions.

Bathing or Showering

Typical Development

A child's interest in bathing begins before 2 years of age, when he or she begins to wash while in the tub. By 4 years of age, children wash and dry themselves with supervision. It is not until 8 years of age that children independently prepare the bath and shower water (e.g., the appropriate depth and temperature) and independently wash and dry themselves.

Good grooming habits are important for all children but take on added significance for children with disabilities. At an early age, the caregiver needs to encourage and help the child with a disability to achieve cleanliness to maintain his or her health. Bathing should be a pleasurable activity. For the parent of a child who lacks postural stability, bathing becomes a tedious task that requires constant attention and alertness.

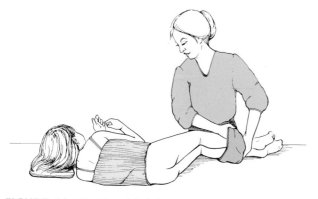

FIGURE 16-10   The side-lying position may reduce stiffness and make dressing easier.

TABLE 16-10   Adaptation Strategies for Dressing with Different Types of Garments

Garment	Design Features of Clothing or Assistive Technology Adaptations for Easier Dressing	Adaptations to Task Method
Pull-up garments	Large size Stretchy material Loops sewn into waistband Elastic waistbands, but not too tight Pressure-sensitive tape Zipper pulls Dressing sticks	Sit on chair Lie on floor Lie on side and roll side to side to pull up pants Use chair or grab-bar to stabilize oneself while pulling up pants Put weak or affected extremity in first
Pullover garments	Large, easy opening for head Flexible rib knit fabric Large armholes and sleeve openings; raglan sleeves Elastic cuffs and waistbands	Lay garment on lap, floor, or table, front side down; put arms in and flip over head Use a template to position garment as above Pull garment over head, then put arms in first Put weak or affected extremity in second
Front-opening garments	Loose style Fullness in back of garment On shirt or jacket, collar of different color from main garment Short-sleeve garments first, proceeding to long-sleeve garments Raglan sleeves Garment with no closures or one or two buttons (e.g., sweater, jacket)	Lay garment on lap, floor, or table, with neck of garment toward child; put in arms, duck head, extend arms, and flip garment over head; shrug shoulders and use arms to help garment fall into place Put weak or affected arm in first, pull up to shoulder; follow collar, then put in other arm Use a template for placement of garment
Buttons	Flat, large buttons Buttons contrast in color with garment Buttons with shanks (easier to grasp) Buttons sewn on loosely Buttons sewn on one side; hook-and-loop tape on both sides to close shirt or pants Front buttons first, proceeding to side and back buttons	Use pullover styles instead of buttons Button all but the first two or three buttons and put shirt on like a pullover Begin buttoning with bottom button (easier to see and align) Use a buttonhook Use elastic thread to sew on sleeve buttons; put on sleeve without buttoning Use backward chaining
Zippers	Nylon zippers (easier than metal) Zipper tabs or rings Zipper pulls Hook-and-loop tape instead of zipper while pulling up zipper tab with other hand Longer zippers (more space for donning and doffing clothes) Front zippers first, proceeding to side and back zippers	Sit to gain stability Stand to keep jacket zipper flat Hold zipper taut with one hand at bottom of zipper For side zipper, lean against wall to hold bottom of zipper
Socks	Soft, stretchy socks Large size Tube sock (no set place for heel) Ankle socks first, proceeding to calf or over-the-calf Loops sewn into socks Sock aide or donner	Sit on stable surface (e.g., chair, floor) Lie on back and prop foot on opposite knee Fold or roll sock before putting it over the toes and pulling up Use backward chaining
Shoes	Long-opening shoes (many eyes) with loose laces Broad shoe (not tight) Slip-on shoes Hook-and-loop tab closures Elastic laces already tied Elastic curly laces that do not need tying Tabs at heels for pulling shoes on Long-handled shoehorns	Sit on stable surface (e.g., chair, floor) Prop up foot on stool or chair Lie on back and prop foot on opposite knee Flex legs and point toes downward Use gravity to help push heel into shoe (e.g., child pushes down on a hard surface)

The work involved multiplies as the child grows and becomes larger and heavier.

Cultural expectations and social routines for bathing vary, and the therapist should consider them when assessing a child's independence. The therapist must respect family preferences on how often a person bathes and with whom (e.g., parent and child bathing together).

Establishing or Restoring Performance

Therapists often use bathing therapeutically to improve body capacities that interfere with independence. A warm bath may calm a child who is distressed and may decrease tonicity and increase ROM and independent movement.[20] When a child has hypersensitivity, water play, rubbing with a washcloth, and deep pressure or rubbing while drying the child may help reduce the child's sensitivity to touch. For children who have difficulty interacting with others or the environment, bath play may motivate the child to explore objects, engage in pretend play, and interact with a sibling or parent.[20]

For children with motor limitations, the therapist may prepare the child to participate more fully in self-bathing. The therapist may use activities to improve range of motion, bilateral coordination, grasp, postural control, and motor planning before teaching bathing. Activities or games (e.g., Simon Says) that require a child to reach above or behind or down to the toes may give children the body awareness and necessary movement for self-bathing. While the child is in the tub, many bath toys (e.g., pour, squeeze or wind-up toys, soap crayons, floating boats) are useful to increase ROM, coordination, play skills, and interactions with others. Body paints are useful in cueing and motivating the child to "wash the part with the paint or X on it."

Adapting the Task or Environment

The caregiver's positioning and handling are prime considerations in adapting bathing of children. Children with cerebral palsy may lose their balance when startled. Keeping the child's head and arms forward when lifting and lowering him or her into the tub prevents a reaction of full extension. The caregiver should use slow, gentle movements with the child and provide simple verbal cues about the steps of bathing. Draining the tub and wrapping the child in a towel before lifting him or her from the tub makes the child feel more secure.

Parents often need suggestions for bathing a child who is hypersensitive to touch or temperature. This child may avoid bathing at all costs and is at risk of getting hurt while in the tub. Understanding the child's sensory needs and using adaptive techniques may help bathing become a positive experience for both parent and child. Preparatory activities that give the child deep pressure before bathing are sometimes helpful, especially deep pressure to the head before shampooing. The child may prefer washing the back and extremities first, and then the stomach and face, using rhythmic, organized, deep strokes. Some parents and children find a hand-held shower with an eye guard hat useful for removing soapsuds (especially during hair washing) and avoiding getting soap in the eyes. Adjusting the water flow or temperature of the hand-held shower and allowing the child to operate it gives the child more control over the direction of the water pressure on his or her body. Sometimes, with children who have tactile sensitivity, using a cup with water is a more relaxing way to rinse off than a shower spray. Wrapping the child in a tight towel after bathing and holding the child with deep pressure also helps.

Adaptive positioning or special equipment may give support that helps the child feel safe and secure. Bath hammocks fully hold the body and enable the parent to wash the child thoroughly (Figure 16-11, *A*). A light, inconspicuous bath support offers design features well adapted to the needs of children with motor deficits (Figure 16-11, *B*). The front half of the support ring swings open for easy entry and then locks securely, holding the child at the chest to give trunk stability. Various kinds of bath seats and shower benches (Figure 16-11, *C*) are available to the older child for help in bathtub seating and transfers. For the child with severe motor limitations who is lying supine in the tub in shallow water, a horseshoe-shaped inflatable bath collar (Figure 16-11, *D*) supports the neck and keeps the child's head above water. A bath stretcher is constructed like a cot and fits inside the bathtub at rim or midtub level to minimize the caregiver's bending while transferring and bathing the child. As discussed earlier, sometimes home modifications such as rolling shower stalls or built-in bath benches are better solutions to increase independence and/or to protect the caregiver's back.

Prevention/Education for Bathing Safety

Parent and child education about bathing safety helps prevent injury. Constant monitoring until the child demonstrates safety in the tub is necessary. Sometimes parents do not teach independence in bathing because they worry that the child may injure himself or herself if they are not there. Following a safe routine for bathing, teaching the child what he or she is and is not allowed to do in the tub or shower, and grading the amount of assistance and monitoring helps develop independence. Nonslip bath mats beside the tub and in the tub are essential for safety. Grab bars and their placement require careful thought and planning in each individual case. A rubber cover for the bathtub faucet prevents injury if the child touches it or slips and hits his or her head. Faucets need to be marked for temperature, and children can be directed to begin running their own bathwater by first putting on the cold water, then slowly adding hot water.

Through coaching and/or educational materials, parents are taught to use good body mechanics during bathing to prevent back injury. To lessen strain, it is best for the adult to sit on a stool beside the tub or to kneel on a cushion. Lifting is done with the knees bent and the back straight, with the legs used for power. As children get older and heavier, a Hoyer lift or an easily accessed shower stall arrangement may be necessary. Parents may need assistance in planning renovations that will assist the child in being independent and/or assist them for the future growth of the child.

Personal Hygiene and Grooming

Skill Development

By 2 years of age, children imitate their parents when brushing their teeth. Supervision of tooth brushing continues until about 6 years of age. Tooth brushing is especially difficult for the child with oral sensitivity. The child should use his or her preferred brushing methods until tolerance improves and he or she accomplishes more thorough cleaning. A small, soft brush is easier to move around in the mouth, especially if the child has a tongue thrust or gag reflex. When the child's gums are tender, the caregiver may substitute a soft, sponge-tipped Toothette for a brush. For the child who brushes independently, an electric toothbrush or oral irrigation device (e.g., Water-Pik) allows more thorough cleaning. This is a good solution for children with limited dexterity, although for children with weakness, an electric toothbrush may be too heavy to manage.

If a child has problems with a weak grasp, the caregiver can enlarge the toothbrush handle with sponge rubber or add a hook-and-loop strap. One-handed flossing tools are available

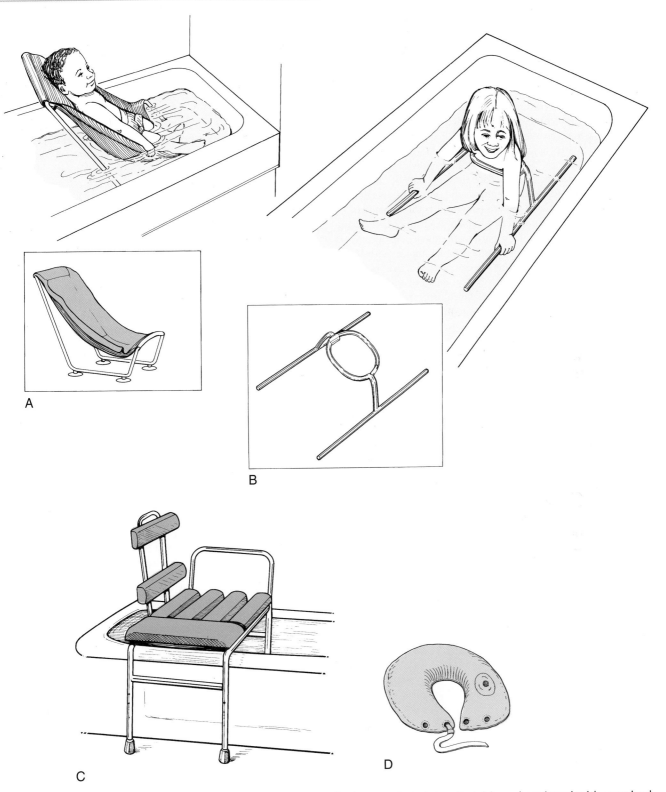

FIGURE 16-11   Adapted seating equipment for bathing. **A,** The hammock chair is adjustable and equipped with oversized suction feet. It fully supports the child who has no sitting balance and poor head control. **B,** Trunk support ring is lightweight and compact and fits all bathtubs. **C,** A shower bench aids seating and transfers. **D,** An inflatable bath collar can be used when the child is in either the supine or the prone position.

in large and small sizes and are adapted by increasing the width or length of the handle. A hand-over-hand technique helps a child learn how to direct the toothbrush in the mouth and to reach all teeth (Figure 16-12). As the child starts doing the movement, gestures or only verbal prompts may be needed. As always, a routine sequence for tooth brushing, gradual fading of cues, and visual pictures about the process assist the child with underlying memory or performance skill problems.

Face washing, hand washing, and hair care are typical grooming activities taught to preschoolers and young children. The child's culture, family values, and individual interests strongly influence the timing of the development of grooming independence. Adolescence begins at the onset of puberty and is a period of remarkable growth toward physical, sexual, emotional, and social maturity. The physiologic changes that occur at puberty are attributable in part to the increased output of hormones by the pituitary gland. For example, body hair grows, and the sebaceous glands become more active, producing oily secretions. With these physical changes and different social expectations (depending on the culture), new self-maintenance tasks emerge, including skin care, hair styling, hair removal, and the application of cosmetics.

In their book, *Caring for Myself*,[51] Gast and Krug give verbal and visual sequences for brushing teeth, getting a haircut, hand washing, bathing, and going to the doctor. The book offers practical prompts, optional considerations for working with sensory issues, and ways to generalize skills and embed self-care activities within a routine. Templates for Social Stories, which are modifiable for different children, are available for parents and therapists.

Intervention

Grooming is an aspect of ADLs that is highly influenced by cultural values. The therapist must respect the child and family's preferences in hairstyle, cosmetics, and routines. The family and child or adolescent need to take the lead in identifying their concerns and priorities in this area. Problem solving follows the principles and approaches identified in the first sections of this chapter. Case Study 16-3 is an example of an adolescent who desires independence in grooming.

Sexual Activity

While the therapist is working with children on ADL tasks such as bathing or personal hygiene, sexuality questions may arise. Although society often still views persons with disabilities as asexual beings,[105] children and adolescents of all disabilities are sexual beings. Sexual activities need to be discussed to prevent social exploitation, abuse, sexually transmitted diseases, and pregnancy. Children with developmental disabilities are more prone to the risk of exploitation because often (1) they must depend on others for basic needs; (2) they frequently have multiple caregivers; (3) their connection with authority figures is one of learned helplessness or nondiscriminatory compliance; and (4) they have difficulty with social, reasoning, judgment, and problem-solving skills.[110,141] Children with communication disorders are at high risk for exploitation, and specific phrases or comments may need to be programmed into their augmentative communication device to protect them from exploitation.[23]

For therapists working with children on very personal daily living activities, it is important to help children differentiate between necessary touch (e.g., diaper changing, catheter instruction, menstrual care, hygiene) and intimate touch. Hinsburger suggested that therapists and parents always do the following[66]:

- Ask permission before touching
- Describe what they are doing and why
- Facilitate participation when performing necessary touch activities
- Communicate with the child about what was done and why and about any feelings after intimate touch

Parents may be receptive to discussing their child's sexuality, or they may feel unprepared to address these issues. If parents and professionals begin talking about sexuality education in early childhood (e.g., body, gender, touching, privacy,

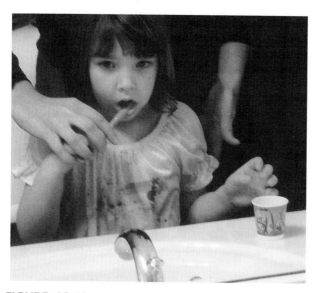

FIGURE 16-12 A hand-over-hand approach works well for Lydia, who is sensitive to tooth brushing, as she is participating in the activity and directing which part of the teeth she wants to brush first.

CASE STUDY 16-3 | **Josie**

Josie demonstrates incoordination, poor memory, and limited judgment, but she wants to be independent in her grooming. Josie has worked on improving her coordination so that she can brush her own hair or manipulate the grooming materials, but adaptation strategies are essential to increase her independence in grooming. The occupational therapist recommends that Josie use a brush with a built-up handle, rest her elbow on the table while brushing her hair to stabilize her ataxic movements, use a checklist and visual model, and ask a peer to help style her hair. Josie and her parents are educated about ways to incorporate grooming tasks into everyday routines by placing visual and natural cues in the environment. such as keeping the deodorant on the dresser. Leaving facial cleansing equipment out on the sink gives Josie a visual cue to use it before applying makeup.

expressing affection, and boundaries), the need to approach complex subjects such as refusal behavior, dating, birth control, and sexuality rights will not be as difficult a transition. Melberg-Schwier and Hingsburger have written an excellent book to guide parents as they embark on this topic.[103] If the child is under 18 years of age, therapists must obtain parental permission to discuss sexuality issues. Therapists need to consider the contextual aspects of the child's family and social groups and determine whether it is appropriate to discuss sexuality and who should discuss it (receiver and informant). Therapists who decide to enter a discourse on sexuality must consider their own knowledge, beliefs, and attitudes so that they give children and their families the correct information in a nonjudgmental way. Occupational therapists may refer the child to someone who is more knowledgeable about sexuality and more comfortable discussing it. Responsible therapists are careful to separate their personal values with regard to sexuality from those of the client and family. The Evolve website gives a number of online resources for talking about sexuality with children with disabilities.

Children and adolescents with cognitive problems related to intellectual disabilities or a traumatic brain injury often need guidelines for expressing their sexuality appropriately in various contexts.[28,29] Appropriate touch from others, dress and hygiene, masturbation, touching of others, and appropriate interactions with the opposite gender are areas in which education is required to prevent abuse and prosecution from the courts for sexual misconduct. Adolescent girls and boys need preparation for the changes that will occur in their bodies at puberty. Body changes, personal care, privacy, masturbation, and emotional changes are areas to address. Menstrual care for girls and wet dreams and erections for boys need discussion before and when they occur.

As children are transitioning into adolescence, questions about how a specific disability (e.g., spina bifida, spinal cord injury) affects sexual abilities and activities often emerge.[123] Older adolescents with chronic health conditions need specific answers and ideas for expressing sexuality in a healthy way.[132] An adolescent may question the physical and psychosocial aspects of sexuality and his or her ability to conceive. Information about contraceptive use and techniques for avoiding intercourse are essential for the adolescent to avoid unwanted pregnancies. As adolescents with disabilities consider conceiving and bearing children in the future, it may be helpful to talk to other parents with disabilities or become aware of online support groups and resources. Table 16-11 presents the information children need about sexual activity across the age span.

Annon developed the PLISSIT model to teach people with disabilities about sexuality.[2] This model is based on four phases of information-giving: (1) permission to ask about sexuality; (2) limited information given; (3) specific suggestions; and (4) intensive therapy (usually provided by a trained counselor or psychologist who understands sexuality in individuals with disabilities). This model teaches staff about sexuality issues and informs clients about who is willing to discuss sexuality with them. In some settings, staff members wear a button saying, "I'm askable" to designate comfort in talking about sexuality.[32] While practicing bed mobility, dressing, personal hygiene, positioning, and communication/interaction skills, the adolescent often asks sexuality questions.

Depending on the situation and the therapy setting, therapists address these questions in the context in which the questions are asked. For example, while practicing bed mobility, 17-year-old Belinda, who recently suffered a spinal cord injury, asks, "How can I ever have sex with a guy? Can I have a baby?" With prior parental permission, this may be an opportune time to discuss contraceptives, positioning, use of intact senses, control of distracting environmental stimuli, and the medical need to empty her bladder before sexual activity. Referral to her physician or to a gynecologist who is knowledgeable about women with disabilities is appropriate, as is referral to her psychologist or counselor. If the parents approve, therapists give additional information in a written, oral, or video format and provide the adolescent with the opportunity to talk to older adolescents or adults who have similar disabilities. Sexuality education needs a team approach, and therapists may work with physicians, nurses, or pharmacists to discuss the use of certain medicines and how they affect sexual function.[36] Memory aids for medicine schedules or contraceptive use may also be helpful. If the therapist is uncomfortable talking about sexual activity, the client should be told this and referred to someone who has the comfort level and knowledge to answer questions.

Care of Personal Devices

With maturity, children learn to take care of their personal devices such as hearing aids, glasses, contact lenses, orthotics, prosthetics, catheters, and/or a variety of pieces of assistive technology used for toileting, grooming, feeding, and dressing. As the child learns how to use these devices, it is essential that he or she know how to clean and maintain them. How many glasses are lost or broken because they are not put back in a case or splints melted by being left in a car? By encouraging children to take responsibility for these devices, perhaps many of these "mishaps" could be avoided.

Performance Patterns

Routines and habits for maintaining items helps children care for their assistive devices. In collaboration with the child, parent, or teacher, therapists can help establish a routine for daily or weekly maintenance of items. Embedding this routine at a naturally occurring time helps the child remember to do the task. For example, the child cleans her catheter when she gets home from school; before bed, she places it back in the fanny pack for the next day. This is often an opportune time to discuss health maintenance activities and routines. Table 16-12 gives an example of health care maintenance for typically developing children and children with spina bifida. Case Study 16-4 shows how developing a routine can help a child care for an assistive device.

Directing Others

Not all children have the motor and praxis skills to clean their glasses, to wash their adaptive utensils, or fill a wheelchair cushion with air. Asking someone else to do the task or to put equipment away and directing others on how to care for an adaptive aid are possibilities. The child may say, "My wheelchair is riding rough. Would you mind checking the tire pressure?" or "My splint strap is broken." Educating children about their adaptive devices gives them a feeling of

TABLE 16-11 Typical Sexuality Concepts Discussed with Children and Adolescents with Disabilities

Age (yr)	Typical Behaviors or Concepts to Learn
Birth–2	Touches genitals for sensory pleasure
	Experiences affection and touch
3–5	Shows interest in genitals of the opposite sex
	Learns proper names of genitals (social demands)
	Plays "Show me" games with other children
	Understands that others should not touch his or her genitals
	Learns that some behaviors are acceptable in public, others are to be done in private (e.g., masturbation, undressing)
	Begins to learn privacy rights (e.g., close doors, knock and wait to enter, close blinds)
	Begins to learn rules for touch and affection boundaries and authority figures
6–8	Knows differences between boys and girls
	Names body parts correctly
	Learns basic elements and language of reproduction and pregnancy
	Learns about relationships (e.g., friends, mutual respect) and decision making
	Thinks about social responsibility
	Understands appropriate and inappropriate social and sexual behaviors
	Understands necessary (e.g., personal hygiene) and intimate touch
	Avoids and reports sexual exploitation (understands necessary touch and intimate touch)
9–11	Shows interest in social relationships
	Discusses body image
	Discusses sexuality within family
	Understands personal boundaries
	Knows how to use refusal skills
	Understands body changes that will occur during puberty (and any impact on his or her disease or disability)
	Knows about reproduction and pregnancy
	Learns about sexually transmitted diseases and the need to abstain from sexual intercourse
	Avoids or reports sexual abuse (understands necessary touch and intimate touch)
12–18	Is sensitive and private about body
	Compares body with others' and may be critical
	Asks questions about changes occurring (physical and emotional)
	Shows more interest in caring for body (e.g., hair, face, exercise)
	Discusses sexuality and sexual identity with friends
	Uses preventive health care routinely (e.g., breast, gynecologic, and testicular examinations)
	Begins dating and learning about communication and love
	Uses values to guide actions in intimacy
	Expresses sexuality through dress, body movement, or intercourse
	Understands reproduction, pregnancy, and birth control
	Knows how to use contraceptives and prevent diseases (safe sex)
	Asks for or is given genetic counseling
	Identifies and uses community sexual health services

Compiled from Couwenhoven, T. (2001). Sexuality education: Building a foundation of healthy attitudes. *Disability Solutions, 4*(6), 1-8. Available at: http://www.disabilitysolutions.org/4-6.htm; Lawrence, K. E., & Niemeyer, S. (1994). Behavior management and psychosocial issues: Sexuality issues. In K. E. Lawrence & S. Niemeyer (Eds.), *Caregiver education guide for children with developmental disabilities: Aspen Reference Group* (pp. 236-245). Frederick, MD: Aspen; and National Information Center for Children and Youth with Disabilities (NICHCY). (1992). Sexuality education for children and youth with disabilities. *NICHCY News Digest, 1*(3), 1-6.

responsibility for the device and may help to prevent breakdown or nonuse of the device. This also incorporates the skills needed for self-determination in the future.

SUMMARY

This chapter presented a wide range of options for enhancing ADL skills in children and adolescents with disabilities. Typical developmental sequences and special methods for evaluating ADLs were presented. The environmental context in which ADLs occur, the child's capacities, and the demands of the task, as well as parent and child preferences, were discussed in the planning of evaluation and intervention. Performance skills during an activity and performance patterns were noted as influences on the outcomes of intervention. Intervention strategies were illustrated, including task adaptation, assistive technology, environmental modification, and research related to video modeling, prompting, and using a cognitive approach to teaching ADL tasks. The importance of positioning and orienting the child to the work surface was stressed. As technology changes and outcome data become available, occupational therapists must continue to remain knowledgeable about current research, methods, and equipment that promote independent ADL functioning in children with disabilities.

TABLE 16-12   Health Care Maintenance for Typically Developing Children and Children with Spina Bifida

Age (yr)	Health Care Maintenance with Typical Development*	Additional Health Maintenance Issues for Child with Spina Bifida
5–9	Follows safety rules at home and school Informs others of emergencies Uses basic first aid techniques for minor injuries Tells other when he or she is sick Cares for health care items with reminders (e.g., glasses, toothbrush) Routinely washes hands; takes a bath and washes hair with reminders Assists in getting medicine ready	Does pressure reliefs and checks for skin breakdown (e.g., legs, buttocks, and feet) with reminders Tells others when he or she is injured or feels sick (e.g., headache, pain, swelling, or change in bowel and bladder patterns) Cares for personal adaptive devices (e.g., crutches, wheelchair, or catheters) with reminders Performs self-catheterization at home and school Carries a list of current medicines and doctors' names
10–14	Recognizes when he or she is getting sick or needs to see a doctor Knows emergency procedures (e.g., phone numbers, who to call, what to do) Cares for health care items (e.g., glasses, braces, retainers, facial scrubs) Uses first aid procedures Eats nutritious meals with supervision Exercises with supervision Takes medicine with supervision Avoids cigarettes, drugs, and sexual abuse	Recognizes when he or she is injured or feels sick (e.g., headache, pain, swelling, or change in bowel and bladder pattern) Knows dosage of medications Knows names of doctors (e.g., primary care, urologist, neurologist, or orthopedist) Cares for personal adaptive devices (e.g., wheelchair, walker, braces) or instructs others in how to maintain devices Performs self-catheterization in community environments Prevents further health care problems (e.g., drinks to avoid bladder infection, exercises [push-ups]; avoids latex; maintains good hygiene, eating, and exercise practices)
15–18	Recognizes when a change in medicine or health intervention is needed Makes appointment to see doctors Eats nutritious meals Exercises regularly Cares for personal hygiene and follows good health habits Uses first aid procedures for major and minor injuries Takes medicine when needed Uses birth control as needed	Takes medications independently and knows side effects Knows how to access therapy, doctors, and other health care services Knows how to obtain and pay for medical supplies Prevents secondary disabilities (e.g., manages weight, follows routine medical care, skin care, and equipment maintenance)

Modified from Ford, A., Schnorr, R., Meyer, L., Davern, L., Black, J., & Dempsey, P. (1989). *The Syracuse community-reference curriculum guide* (pp. 324-327). Baltimore: Brookes; Peterson, P. M., Rauen, K. K., Brown, J., & Cole, J. (1994). Spina bifida: The transition into adulthood begins in infancy. *Rehabilitation Nursing*, *19*(4), 229-238.
*Adherence to protocols for medicines, personal devices, health routines, and so on.

CASE STUDY 16-4   Feddah

Feddah is 9 years old and has worn hearing aids for 2 years, after having viral meningitis. Until last month, her parents cared for the hearing aids until Feddah "wanted to do it herself." Because her parents are encouraging Feddah to be self-determined, they thought this was a good idea. Unfortunately, last week, Feddah had a very severe ear infection that the doctor attributed to improper cleaning of her hearing aids. Mom happened to mention this problem to the occupational therapist, who was seeing Feddah to increase her written production and dexterity in manipulating objects. The therapist collaborated with Mom, the audiologist, and Feddah to develop a routine and a visual schedule to clean her hearing aids. Feddah's hearing aid case is left on the dresser as a naturally occurring cue to remind her to remove, clean, and put away the hearing

aids each night. By using anticipatory problem solving,[125] the therapist and Feddah discussed the task and where the wipes and hearing aid case should be kept. They also discussed how to clean the hearing aids when wipes were not available and how she would handle the care of her hearing aids when on a sleepover. Feddah anticipated that her friend's little sister may try to play with her hearing aids and that she had better ask her friend's mother to help her find a safe place for her hearing aid box. If she forgot her hearing aid box, she would ask for a Baggie to store the aids. Figure 16-13 gives an example of a task analysis and data collection sheet for tracking Feddah's routine and success in caring for her own hearing aids. By means of this tracking sheet, the therapist could see if Feddah's performance was improving.

Continued

Name: ___Feddah___ Week of: ___May 21st___
Activity: ___Cleaning hearing aid___ Environment: ___Home in bedroom___
Verbal cue: ___"Time to go to bed and take out your hearing aids"___
Physical set up: ___Feddah is at her dresser that is waist high.___
Visual cues: ___Tissues, wipes, hearing aid box is out on dresser top as a visual reminder to do this every night.___

Steps	Task Analysis	Dates					Comments
		5/21	5/22	5/23	5/24	5/25	
1	Turn off hearing aid	√-	√=	√	√	√	
2	Remove hearing aid from ear before bathing or bed.	√	√	√	√	√	Consistent!
3	Wipe ear mold surfaces with a tissue	A (V)	A(V)	√	√	√	
4	Disinfect the ear mold surface with a disinfectant towelette (non-alcohol based)	A(P)	A(P)	A(V)	√-	√-	Rubs hearing aid too vigorously.
5	Check batteries to hearing aid	0	0	A(V)	A (V)	√-	Added a visual picture to remember this.
6	Place hearing aid back in hearing aid box for storage	A (V)	√-	√-	√-	√	
7	Keep in a safe and cool place	√	√	√	√	√	
Total Steps Completed This Day	Target √ = Did it	2	2	4	4	5	Making progress this week!! She is really learning the task.
	√- = Did most of it	1	2	1	2	2	
	A = Did with verbal (V) or physical prompt (P)	1 P 2 V	1 P 1 V	2 V	1 V	0	
	0 = Didn't do it	1	1	0	0	0	

FIGURE 16-13 Sample task analysis and data collection sheet for hearing aid maintenance.

REFERENCES

1. American Occupational Therapy Association. (2008). Occupational therapy practice framework: Domain and process. (2nd ed.). *American Journal of Occupational Therapy, 62*, 625–683.
2. Annon, J. (1976). The PLISSIT model: A proposed conceptual scheme for the behavioral treatment of sexual problems. *Journal of Sex Education and Therapy*, 1–15.
3. Azrin, N. H., & Foxx, R. M. (1974). *Toilet training in less than a day.* New York: Simon & Schuster.
4. Bayzak, S. (1989). Changes in attitude beliefs regarding parent participation in home programs. *American Journal of Occupational Therapy, 43*, 723–728.
5. Bedell, G. M., Cohn, E. S., & Dumas, H. M. (2005). Exploring parents' use of strategies to promote social participation of school-age children with acquired brain injuries. *American Journal of Occupational Therapy, 59*, 273–284.

6. Bedell, G. M., Haley, S. M., Coster, W. J., & Smith, K. W. (2002). Developing a responsive measure of change for paediatric brain injury inpatient rehabilitation. *Brain Injury, 16,* 659–671.

7. Bedell, G. M., Haley, S. M., Coster, W. J., & Smith, K. W. (2002). Participation readiness at discharge from inpatient rehabilitation in children and adolescents with acquired brain injury. *Pediatric Rehabilitation, 5,* 107–116.

8. Bellini, S. & Akullian, J. (2007). A meta-analysis of video modeling and video self-modeling interventions for children and adolescents with autism. *Exceptional Children, 73,* 264–287.

9. Bergen, A. F., & Colangelo, C. (1985). *Positioning the client with CNS deficits: The wheelchair and other adapted equipment* (2nd ed.). Valhalla, NY: Valhalla Rehabilitation Publications.

10. Bergen, A. F., Presperin, J., & Tallman, T. (1990). *Positioning for function: Wheelchairs and other assistive devices.* Valhalla, NY: Valhalla Rehabilitation Publications.

11. Bidabe, D. L., Barnes, S. B., & Whinnery, K. W. (2001). M.O.V.E.: Raising expectations for individuals with severe disabilities. *Physical Disabilities: Education and Related Services, 19*(2), 31–48.

12. Biederman, G. B., Fairhall, J. L., Raven, K. A., & Davey, V. A. (1998). Verbal prompting, hand-over-hand instruction, and passive observation in teaching children with developmental disabilities. *Exceptional Children, 64,* 503–511.

13. Biederman, G. B., Stepaniuk, S., Davey, V. A., Raven, K., & Ahn, D. (1999). Observational learning in children with Down syndrome and developmental delays: The effect of presentation speed in videotaped modeling. *Down Syndrome Research and Practice, 6*(1), 12–18.

14. Brollier, C., Shepherd, J., & Markley, K. (1994). Transition from school to community living. *American Journal of Occupational Therapy, 48,* 346–353.

15. Brown, L., Schwarz, P., Udvari-Solner, A., Kampschroer, E., Johnson, F., Jorgensen, J., et al. (1991). How much time should students with severe intellectual disabilities spend in regular education classrooms and elsewhere? *Journal of the Association for Persons with Severe Handicaps, 16,* 39–47.

16. Bryze, K., & Curtin, C. (1993). A top-down approach: Relationships to research and occupational performance. *Developmental Disabilities Special Interest Section Newsletter, 2,* 2–4.

17. Candler, C., & Meeuwsen, H. (2002). Implicit learning in children with and without developmental coordination disorder. *American Journal of Occupational Therapy, 56,* 429–435.

18. Carlson, G. (2002). Supporting the health and well-being of people with intellectual disability and high support needs through networking and resource development. *Australian Occupational Therapy Journal, 49,* 37–43.

19. Case-Smith, J. (1996). Fine motor outcomes in preschool children who receive occupational therapy services. *American Journal of Occupational Therapy, 50,* 52–61.

20. Case-Smith, J. (2000). ADL strategies for children with developmental deficits. In C. Christiansen (Ed.), *Ways of living: ADL strategies for special needs* (pp. 83–121). Bethesda, MD: American Occupational Therapy Association.

21. Chafetz, R. S., Mulcahey, M. J., Betz, R. R., Anderson, C., Vogel, L. C., Gaughan, J. P., et al. (2007). Impact of prophylactic thoracolumbosacral orthosis bracing on functional activities and activities of daily living in the pediatric spinal cord injury population. *Journal of Spinal Cord Medicine, 30*(Suppl. 1), S178–S183.

22. Chan, S., & Lee, E. (2004). Families with Asian roots. In E. W. Lynch & M. J. Hanson *Developing cross-cultural competence: A guide for working with children and their families,* (3rd ed., pp. 251–354). Baltimore: Brookes.

23. Collier, B., McGhie-Richmond, D., Odette, F., & Pyne, J. (2006). Reducing the risk of sexual abuse for people who use augmentative and alternative communication. *Augmentative and Alternative Communication, 22,* 62–75.

24. Copley, J., & Ziviani, J. (2004). Barriers to use assistive technology for children with multiple disabilities. *Occupational Therapy International, 11,* 229–243.

25. Coster, W. J. (1998). Occupation-centered assessment of children. *American Journal of Occupational Therapy, 52,* 337–344.

26. Coster, W., Deeney, T. A., Haltiwanger, J. T., & Haley, S. M. (1998). *School Function Assessment: User's manual.* San Antonio, TX: Therapy Skill Builders.

27. Coster, W. J., Haley, S. M., Ni, P., Dumas, H. M., & Fragala-Pinkham, M. A. (2008). Assessing self-care and social function using a computer adaptive testing version of the Pediatric Evaluation of Disability Inventory. *Archives of Physical Medicine and Rehabilitation, 89,* 622–629.

28. Couwenhoven, T. (2001). Sexuality education: Building a foundation of healthy attitudes. *Disability Solutions, 4*(6), 1–8. Web site: http://www.disabilitysolutions.org/4-6.htm

29. Couwenhoven, T. (2007). *Teaching children with Down Syndrome about their bodies boundaries, and sexuality.* Bethesda, MD: Woodbine Books.

30. Cusick, A., McIntyre, S., Novak, I., Lannin, N., & Lowe, K. (2006). A comparison of goal attainment scaling and the Canadian Occupational Performance Measure for paediatric rehabilitation research. *Pediatric Rehabilitation, 9,* 149–157.

31. Davies, D. K., Stock, S. E., & Wehmeyer, M. L. (2002). Enhancing independent task performance for individuals with mental retardation through use of a handheld self-directed visual and audio prompting system. *Education and Training in Mental Retardation & Developmental Disabilities, 37,* 209–218.

32. Dawe, N. J., & Shepherd, J. T. (1985). Occupational therapy in the sexuality program of a rehabilitation hospital. *American Occupational Therapy Association Physical Disabilities Special Interest Section Newsletter, 8,* 1–2.

33. Disability Office of South Australia. (2008). *Managing menstrual care: A resource guide about managing menstruation for women with intellectual disabilities.* Adelaide, SA: Government of South Australia: Department for Families and Communities. Retrieved December 1, 2008, from http://www.dfc.sa.gov.au/pub/tabid//185/itemid/634/School-age-and-youth-820-years-with-a-disabilit.aspx

34. Dumas, H. M., Haley, S. M., Fragala, M. A., & Steva, B. J. (2001). Self-care recovery of children with brain injury: Descriptive analysis using the Pediatric Evaluation of Disability Inventory (PEDI) functional classification levels. *Physical and Occupational Therapy in Pediatrics, 21,* 7–27.

35. Dunford, C., Missiuna, C., Street, E., & Sibert, J. (2005). Children's perceptions of the impact of developmental coordination disorder on activities of daily living. *British Journal of Occupational Therapy, 68,* 207–214.

36. Dunn, K. L. (1997). Sexuality education and the team approach. In M. L. Sipski & C. J. Alexander (Eds.), *Sexuality education function in people with disability and chronic illness: A professional's guide* (pp. 381–402). Baltimore, MD: Aspen.

37. Epps, S., Stern, R. J., & Horner, R. H. (1990). Comparison of simulation training on self and using a doll for teaching generalized menstrual care to women with severe mental retardation. *Research in Developmental Disabilities, 11,* 37–66.

38. Feldman, M. A. (1999). Teaching child-care and safety skills to parents with intellectual disabilities through self-learning. *Journal of Intellectual and Developmental Disability, 24*(1), 27–44.

39. Ferguson, D. L., & Baumgart, D. (1991). Partial participation revisited. *Journal of the Association for Persons with Severe Handicaps, 16,* 218–227.

40. Fiese, B. H., Tomcho, T. J., Douglas, M., Josephs, K., Poltrock, S., & Baker, T. (2002). A review of 50 years of research on

naturally occurring family routines and rituals: Cause for celebration? *Journal of Family Psychology, 16,* 381–390.

41. Fingerhut, P., Madill, H., Darrah, J., Hodge, M., & Warren, S. (2002). Classroom-based assessment: Validation for the School AMPS. *American Journal of Occupational Therapy, 56,* 210–213.

42. Finnie, N. (1997). *Handling the young child with cerebral palsy at home* (3rd ed.). Woburn, MA: Butterworth-Heinemann.

43. Fisher, A. G. (2006a). *Assessment of Motor and Process Skills: Vol. 1. Development, standardization, and administration manual* (6th ed.). Fort Collins, CO: Three Star Press.

44. Fisher, A. G. (2006b). *Assessment of Motor and Process Skills: Vol. 2. User manual* (6th ed.). Fort Collins, CO: Three Star Press.

45. Fisher, A. G., Bryze, K., & Atchison, B. T. (2000). Naturalistic assessment of functional performance in school settings: Reliability and validity of the School AMPS scales. *Journal of Outcome Measurement, 4,* 504–522.

46. Fisher, A. G., Bryze, K., Hume, V., & Griswold, L. A. (2005). *School AMPS: School Version of the Assessment of Motor and Process Skills* (2nd ed.). Ft. Collins, CO: Three Star Press.

47. Fisher, A. G., & Duran, G. A. (2004). Schoolwork task performance of students at risk for delays. *Scandinavian Journal of Occupational Therapy, 11,* 1–8.

48. Uniform Data System for Medical Rehabilitation. (1998, 2000). *Functional Independence Measure FIMware User Guide and Self-Guided Training Manual, Version 5.20. WeeFIM System^{SM} Clinical Guide: Version 5.01.* Buffalo: State University of New York.

49. Furuno, S., O'Reilly, K., Hosaka, C. M., Zeisloft, B., & Allman, T. (2004). *Hawaii Early Learning Profile* (2nd ed.). Palo Alto, CA: Vort.

50. Gallimore, R., & Lopez, E. M. (2002). Everyday routines, human agency, and ecocultural context: Construction and maintenance of individual habits. *Occupational Therapy Journal of Research, 22,* 70S–77S.

51. Gast, C., & Krug, J. (2008). *Caring for myself.* Philadelphia: Jessica Kingsley.

52. Gentry, L. O. (2003). *Cognitive prosthetics: 21st century tools for the rehabilitation of thinking skills* [online course]. Retrieved September 2, 2003, from http://www.cerebreon.com/courses/cp/

53. Gevir, D., Goldstand, S., Weintraub, N., & Parush, S. (2006). A comparison of time use between mothers of children with and without disabilities. *Occupation, Participation and Health, 26,* 117–127.

54. Giangreco, M., Cloninger, C., & Iverson, V. (1997). *Choosing options and accommodations for children (COACH)* (2nd ed.). Baltimore: Brookes.

55. Gol, D., & Jarus, T. (2005). Effect of social skills training group on everyday activities of children with attention-deficit-hyperactivity disorder. *Developmental Medicine and Child Neurology, 47,* 539–545.

56. Granberg, M., Rydberg, A., & Fisher, A. G. (2008). Activities in daily living and schoolwork task performance in children with complex congenital heart disease. *Acta Pædiatrica, 97,* 1270–1274.

57. Gray, C. (2000). *The new social story book: Illustrated edition.* Arlington, TX: Future Horizons.

58. Griffin, J., Carlson, G., Taylor, M. & Wilson, J. (1996). An introduction to menstrual management for women who have an intellectual disability and high support needs. *International Journal of Disability, Development and Education, 41,* 103–116.

59. Haley, S. M., Coster, W. J., Ludlow, L. H., Haltiwanger, J., & Andrellos, P. (1992). *Administration manual for the Pediatric Evaluation of Disability Inventory.* San Antonio, TX: Psychological Corporation.

60. Haley, S. M., Watkins, M. P., & Dumas, H. M. (2003). Establishing minimal clinically important differences for scores on the pediatric evaluation of disability inventory for inpatient rehabilitation. *Physical Therapy, 83,* 888–898.

61. Hamilton, B. B., & Granger, C. U. (2000). *Functional Independence Measure for Children (WeeFIM-II).* Buffalo, NY: Research Foundation of the State University of New York.

62. Hanft, B., & Shepherd, J. (2008). 2..4…6…8…How do you collaborate? In *Collaborating for student success: A guide for school-based occupational therapy* (pp. 1–34). Bethesda: AOTA.

63. Hanft, B. E., Rush, D. D., & Sheldon, M. L. (2004). *Coaching families and colleagues in early childhood.* Baltimore, MD: Paul H. Brookes.

64. Hanson, M. (2004). Families with Anglo-European roots. In E. W. Lynch , & M. J. Hanson (Eds.), *Developing cross-cultural competence* (3rd ed., pp. 93–126). Baltimore: Brookes.

65. Healy, H., & Rigby, P. (1999). Promoting independence for teens and young adults with physical disabilities. *Canadian Journal of Occupational Therapy, 66,* 240–248.

66. Hingsburger, D. (1993). *I openers: Parents ask questions about sexuality and children with developmental disabilities.* Vancouver, BC: Family Support Institute Press.

67. Hinojosa, J., & Kramer, P. (1999). Developmental perspective: Fundamentals of developmental therapy. In P. Kramer, & J. Hinojosa (Eds.), *Frames of reference for pediatric occupational therapy* (2nd ed.). Baltimore: Lippincott Williams & Wilkins.

68. Hinojosa, J., Kramer, P., & Crist, P. (2005). *Evaluation: Obtaining & interpreting data* (2nd ed.). Rockville, MD: American Occupational Therapy Association.

69. Holm, M. B., Rogers, J. C., & James, A. B. (2003). Interventions for daily living. In E. B. Crepeau , E. Cohn , & B. Schell (Eds.), *Willard and Spackman's occupational therapy* (10th ed., pp. 491–554). Philadelphia: J.B. Lippincott.

70. Horn, I. B., Brenner, R., Rao, M., & Cheng, T. L. (2006). Beliefs about the appropriate age for initiating toilet training: Are there racial and socioeconomic differences? *Journal of Pediatrics, 149,* 151–152.

71. Hughes, C., & Carter, E. W. (2000). *The transition handbook: Strategies high school teachers use that work!.* Baltimore: Brookes.

72. Jarus, T., & Ratzon, N. Z. (2000). Can you imagine? The effect of mental practice on the acquisition and retention of a motor skill as a function of age. *Occupational Therapy Journal of Research, 20,* 163–178.

73. Johnson-Martin, N., Attermeier, S. M., & Hacker, B. (2004). *The Carolina curriculum for infants and toddlers with special needs* (3rd ed.). Baltimore: Brookes.

74. Johnson-Martin, N., Hacker, B., & Attermeier, S. M. (2004). *The Carolina curriculum for preschoolers with special needs* (2nd ed.). Baltimore: Brookes.

75. Joinson, C., Herson, J., von Gontard, A., Butler, U., Golding, J., & Edmond, A. (2008). Early childhood risk factors associated with daytime wetting and soiling in school-age children. *Journal of Pediatric Psychology, 33,* 739–750.

76. Kadlec, M. B., Coster, W., Tickle-Degnen, L., & Beeghly, M. (2005). Qualities of caregiver-child interaction during daily activities of children born very low birth weight with and without white matter disorder. *American Journal of Occupational Therapy, 59,* 57–66.

77. Kangas, K. (1998). *Using your head: Access and integration of independent mobility and communication "head first".* Presentation at TechKnowledgy '98 Conference, Children's Hospital, Richmond, VA, October 28, 1998.

78. Keen, D., Brannigan, K. L., & Cuskelly, M. (2007). Toilet training for children with autism: The effects of video modeling. *Journal of Development and Physical Disabilities, 19,* 291–303.

79. Kellegrew, D. (1998). Creating opportunities for occupation: An intervention to promote the ADL independence of young children with special needs. *American Journal of Occupational Therapy, 52,* 457–465.

80. Kellegrew, D. H. (2000). Constructing daily routines: A qualitative examination of mothers with young children with disabilities. *American Journal of Occupational Therapy, 54,* 252–259.

81. Keller, J., Kafkes, A., Baso, S., Federico, J., & Kielhofner, G. (2005). *Child Occupational Self Assessment (COSA; Version 2.1)*. Chicago: MOHO Clearinghouse.

82. King, G. A., Law, M., King, S., & Rosenbaum, P. (1998). Parents' and service providers' perceptions of the family-centeredness of children's rehabilitation services. *Physical and Occupational Therapy*, 18, 21–40.

83. King, G. A., McDougall, J., Palisano, R. J., Gritzan, J., & Tucker, M. A. (1999). Goal attainment scaling: Is use in evaluating pediatric therapy programs. *Physical and Occupational Therapy Pediatrics*, 15, 31–52.

84. Kiresuk, T. J., Smith, A., & Cardillo, J. E. (1994). *Goal attainment scaling: Applications, theory and measurement*. Hillsdale, NJ: Lawrence Erlbaum.

85. Klassen, T. P., Kiddoo, D., Lang, M. E., Friesan, C., Russell, K., Spooner, C., et al. (2006). The effectiveness of different methods of toilet training for bladder and bowel control. Technology Assessment No/Technology Assessment No. 147 (prepared by the University of Alberta Evidence-Based Practice Center, under contract number 290-02-0023). AHRQ Publication No. 07-E003. Rockville, MD: Agency for Healthcare Research and Quality.

86. Knox, V., & Usen, Y. (2000). Clinical review of the Pediatric Evaluation of Disability Inventory. *British Journal of Occupational Therapy*, 63, 29–32.

87. Koegel, L. K., Koegel, R. L., Kellegrew, D., & Mullen, K. (1996). Parent education for prevention and reduction of severe problem behaviors. In L. K. Koegel, R. L. Koegel, & G. Dunlap (Eds.), *Positive behavioral support: Including people with difficult behavior in the community* (pp. 3–30). Baltimore: Brookes.

88. Kothari, D. H., Haley, S. M., Gill-Body, K. M., & Dumas, H. M. (2003). Measuring functional change in children with acquired brain injury (ABI): Comparison of generic and ABI-specific scale using the Pediatric Evaluation of Disability Inventory (PEDI). *Physical Therapy*, 83, 776–785.

89. Kramer, J. (2008). Validity evidence for the Child Occupational Self Assessment. *The Model of Human Occupation Evidence Brief*. Retrieved November 30, 2008, from http://www.moho.uic.edu/images/KramerDissertationBrief.pdf

90. Lancioni, G. E., & O'Reilly, M. F. (2001). Self-management of instruction cues for occupation: Review of studies with people with severe and profound developmental disabilities. *Research in Developmental Disabilities*, 22, 41–65.

91. Landry, S. H., Miller-Loncar, C. L., & Smith, K. E. (2002). Individual differences in the development of social communication competency in very low birthweight children. In D. L. Molfese & V. J. Molfese (Eds.), *Developmental variations in learning: Applications to social, executive function, language, and reading skills*. Mahwah, NJ: Lawrence Erlbaum.

92. Lannin, N. (2003). Goal attainment scaling allows program evaluation of a home-based occupational therapy program. *Occupational Therapy in Health Care*, 17, 43–54.

93. Law, M., Baptiste, S., Carswell, A., McColl, M. A., Polotajiko, H., & Pollock, N. (2005). *Canadian Occupational Performance Measure* (3rd ed.). Toronto: Canadian Association of Occupational Therapists.

94. Lawrence, K. E., & Niemeyer, S. (Eds.). (1994). *Home care issues/activities of daily living: Caregiver education guide for children with developmental disabilities* (pp. 4:31–4:46). Gaithersburg, MD: Aspen.

95. Levan, P. (2008). A male toileting aide: The penis paddle. *Journal of Occupational Therapy, Schools & Early Intervention*, 1, 68–69.

96. Lynch, E. (2004). Developing cross cultural competence. In E. Lynch & M. Hanson (Eds.), *Developing cross-cultural competence* (3rd ed., pp. 41–78). Baltimore: Brookes.

97. Lynch, E., & Hanson, M. (2004). *Developing cross-cultural competence* (3rd ed.). Baltimore: Brookes.

98. Mailloux, Z., May-Benson, T. A., Summers, C. A., Miller, L. J., Brett-Green, B., Burke, J. P., et al. (2007). The Issue Is—Goal attainment scaling as a measure of meaningful outcomes for children with sensory integration disorders. *American Journal of Occupational Therapy*, 61, 254–259.

99. McCoy, K. & Hermansen, E. (2007). Video modeling for individuals with autism: A review of model types and effects. *Education and Treatment of Children*, 30, 183–213.

100. McDougall, J., & King, G. (2007). *Goal attainment scaling manual: Description, utility and applications in pediatric therapy* (2nd ed.). Ontario, London: Thames Children's Centre. Retrieved December 1, 2008, from http://www.tvcc.on.ca/images/stories/All_PDFs/OurServices/Research/gasmanual2007.pdf

101. McGavin, H. (1998). Planning rehabilitation: A comparison of issues for parents and adolescents. *Physical and Occupational Therapy*, 18, 69–82.

102. McInnes, J. M., & Treffry, J. A. (1993). *Deaf-blind infants and children: A developmental guide*. Toronto: University of Toronto Press.

103. Melberg-Schwier, K. M., & Hingsburger, D. (2000). *Sexuality: Your sons and daughters with intellectual disabilities*. Baltimore: Brookes.

104. Miller, L. J., Schoen, S. A., James, K., & Schaaf, R. C. (2007). Lessons learned: A pilot study of occupational therapy effectiveness for children with sensory modulation disorder. *American Journal of Occupational Therapy*, 61, 161–169.

105. Milligan, M. S., & Neufeldt, A. H. (2001). The myth of asexuality: A survey of social and empirical evidence. *Sexuality & Disability*, 19, 91–109.

106. Missiuna, C., Moll, S., Law, M., King, S. l., & King, G. (2006). Mysteries and mazes: Parents' experiences of children with developmental coordination disorder. *Canadian Journal of Occupational Therapy*, 73, 7–17.

107. Mitchell, T., & Cusick, A. (1998). Evaluation of a client-centered pediatric rehabilitation programme using goal attainment scaling. *Australian Occupational Therapy Journal*, 45, 7–17.

108. Munkholm, M., & Fisher, A. G. (2008). Differences in school-work performance between typically developing students and students with mild disabilities. *OTJR: Occupation, Participation and Health*, 38, 121–132.

109. Nicholson, J. H., Morton, R. E., Attfield, S., & Rennie, D. (2001). Assessment of upper-limb function and movement in children with cerebral palsy wearing lycra garments. *Developmental medicine and child neurology*, 43, 384–391.

110. O'Neill, P. (2002). *Abuse and neglect of children with disabilities: A collaborative response*. Richmond, VA: Virginia Institute for Developmental Disabilities, Virginia Commonwealth University.

111. Orelove, F., & Sobsey, D. (1996). ADL skills. In F. Orelove & D. Sobsey (Eds.), *Educating children with multiple disabilities* (3rd ed., pp. 333–375). Baltimore: Brookes.

112. Ostensjo, S., Carlberg, E. B., & Vollestad, N. K. (2005). The use and impact of assistive devices and other environmental modifications on everyday activities and care in young children with cerebral palsy. *Disability and Rehabilitation*, 27, 849–861.

113. Payne, S., & Howell, C. (2005). An evaluation of the clinical use of the Assessment of Motor and Process Skills with children. *British Journal of Occupational Therapy*, 68, 277–280.

114. Pierce, S. R., Daly, K., Gallagher, K. G., Gershoff, A. M., & Schaumburg, S. W. (2002). Constraint-induced therapy for a child with hemiplegic cerebral palsy: A case report. *Archives of Physical Medicine and Rehabilitation*, 83, 1462–1463.

115. Polatajko, H. J., Mandich, A. D., Miller, L. T. & Macnab, J. J. (2001). Cognitive orientation to daily occupational performance (CO-OP): Part II-The evidence. *Physical and Occupational Therapy in Pediatrics*, 20, 83–106.

116. Prudhomme-White, B., & Mulligan, S. E. (2005). Behavioral and physiologic response measures of occupational task

performance: A preliminary comparison between typical children and children with attention disorder. *American Journal of Occupational Therapy, 59,* 426–436.

117. Quint, E. H. (2003). The conservative management of abnormal bleeding in teenagers with developmental disabilities. *Journal of Pediatric and Adolescent Gynecology, 16,* 54–56.

118. Reese, G. M., & Snell, M. E. (1991). Putting on and removing coats and jackets: The acquisition and maintenance of skills by children with severe multiple disabilities. *Education and Training in Mental Retardation, 26,* 398–410.

119. Rempfer, M., Hildenbrand, W., Parker, K., & Brown, C. (2003). An interdisciplinary approach to environmental intervention: Ecology of human performance. In L. Letts, P. Rigby, & D. Stewart (Eds.), *Using environments to enable occupational performance* (pp. 119–136). Thorofare, NJ: Slack.

120. Rodger, S., & Liu, S. (2008). Cognitive orientation to (daily) occupational performance: Changes in strategy and session time use over the course of intervention. *OTJR: Occupation, Participation and Health, 28,* 168–179.

121. Roger, S., Springfield, E., & Polatajko, H. J. (2007). Cognitive Orientation for daily Occupational Performance approach for children with Asperger's syndrome: A case report. *Physical and Occupational Therapy in Pediatrics, 27,* 7–22.

122. Rogers, J. C., Holm, M. B., & Stone, R. G. (1997). Assessment of daily living activities: The home care advantage. *American Journal of Occupational Therapy, 51,* 410–422.

123. Sawin, K., Buran, C. F., Brei, T. J., & Fastenau, P. S. (2002). Sexuality issues in adolescents with a chronic neurological condition. *Journal of Perinatal Education, 11,* 22–34.

124. Schultz-Krohn, W. (2004). Session 10: Addressing ADLs and IADLs within the school-based practice. In Y. Swinth (Ed.), *Occupational therapy in school-based practice: Contemporary issues and trends.* Bethesda, MD: American Occupational Therapy Association Online Course.

125. Schum, T. R., Kolb, T. M., McAuliffe, T. L., Simms, M. D., Underhill, R. L., & Lewis, M. (2002). Sequential acquisition of toilet-training skills: A descriptive study of gender and age differences in normal children. *Pediatrics, 109,* e48. Available at: www.pediatrics.org/cgi/content/full/109/3/e48

126. Schwarz, S. P. (2000). *Attainment's dressing tips and clothing resources for making life easier.* Verona, WI: Attainment.

127. Segal, R. (2000). Adaptive strategies of mothers with children with attention deficit hyperactivity disorder: Enfolding and unfolding occupations. *American Journal of Occupational Therapy, 54,* 300–306.

128. Segal, R. (2004). Family routines and rituals: A context for occupational therapy interventions. *American Journal of Occupational Therapy, 58,* 499–508.

129. Segal, R., & Frank, G. (1998). The extraordinary construction of ordinary experience: Scheduling daily life in families with children with attention deficit hyperactivity disorder. *Scandinavian Journal of Occupational Therapy, 5,* 141–147.

130. Sellers, S. W., Fisher, A. G., & Duran, L. (2001). Validity of the Assessment of Motor and Process Skills with students who are visually impaired. *Journal of Visual Impairment and Blindness, 95,* 164–167.

131. Sewell, T. J., Collins, B. C., Hemmeter, M. L., & Schuster, J. W. (1998). Using simultaneous prompting within an activity-based format to teach dressing skills to preschoolers with developmental delays. *Journal of Early Intervention, 21,* 132–142.

132. Shapland, C. (1999). Sexuality issues for youth with disabilities and chronic health conditions. In *Healthy and ready to work because everyone deserves a future: An occasional policy brief of the Institute for Child Health Policy* (pp. 1–24). Gainesville, FL: University of Florida, Retrieved August 1, 2003, from http://hctransitions.ichp.edu/policypapers/SexualityIssues.pdf

133. Shipley-Benamou, R., Lutzker, J. R., & Taubman, M. (2002). Teaching daily living skills to children with autism through instructional video modeling. *Journal of Positive Behavior Interventions, 4,* 165–175.

134. Simpson, E., & Lankasky, K. (2001). *Table manners and beyond: The gynecological exam for women with developmental disabilities and other functional limitations.* Retrieved October 21, 2008, from http://www.bhawd.org/sitefiles/TblMrs/cover.html

135. Smith, R., Benge, M., & Hall, M. (2000). Using assistive technologies to enable self-care and daily living. In C. Christiansen (Ed.), *Ways of living: ADL strategies for special needs* (2nd ed., pp. 57–81). Bethesda, MD: American Occupational Therapy Association.

136. Snell, M. E., & Brown, F. (2000). Development and implementation of educational programs. In M. E. Snell & F. Brown (Eds.), *Instruction of students with severe disabilities* (5th ed., pp. 115–165). Upper Saddle River, NJ: Prentice-Hall.

137. Snell, M. E., & Vogtle, L. K. (2000). Methods for teaching self-care skills. In C. Christiansen (Ed.), *Ways of living: ADL strategies for special needs* (2nd ed., pp. 57–81). Bethesda, MD: American Occupational Therapy Association.

138. Steenbeek, D., Ketelaar, M., Galama, K., & Gorter, J. W. (2007). Goal attainment scaling in paediatric rehabilitation: a critical review of the literature. *Developmental Medicine and Child Neurology, 49,* 550–556.

139. Stein, M. A., Szumowski, E., Blondis, T., & Roizen, N. J. (1995). Adaptive skills dysfunction in ADD and ADHD children. *Journal of Child Psychology & Psychiatry, 36,* 663–670.

140. Stowitchek, J. J., Laitinen, R., & Prather, T. (1999). Embedding early self-determination opportunities in curriculum for youth with developmental disabilities using natural teaching incidents. *Journal of Vocational Special Needs Education, 21,* 15–26.

141. Sullivan, P. M., & Knutson, J. F. (2000). Maltreatment and disabilities: A population-based epidemiological study. *Child Abuse and Neglect, 4,* 1257–1273.

142. Sweeney, J. (1989). *Clothing for children with severe disabilities: A guide to adaptive garments for use in the institutional setting.* Alexandria, VA: Special Clothes.

143. Tarazi, R. A., Mahone, E. M., & Zabel, T. A. (2007). Self-care independence in children with neurological disorders: An interactional model of adaptive demands and executive dysfunction. *Rehabilitation Psychology, 52,* 196–205.

144. Thomson, G. (2005). *Children with severe disabilities and the MOVE curriculum: Foundations of a task oriented therapy approach.* Elka Park, NY: East River Press.

145. Tsuji, T., Liu, M., Toikawa, H., Hanayama, K., Sonoda, S., & Chino, N. (1999). ADL structure for nondisabled Japanese children based on the Functional Independence Measure for Children (WeeFIM). *American Journal of Physical Medicine & Rehabilitation, 78,* 208–212.

146. Turnbull, A. P., Turnbull, H. R., Erwin, E. J., & Soodak, L. C. (2004). *Families, professionals, and exceptionality: Positive outcomes through partnerships and trust* (5th ed.). Columbus, OH: Merrill/Prentice Hall.

147. Turner, L., Lammi, B., Friesen, K., & Phelan, N. (2001). *Your child's dressing skills workbook.* Ontario, Canada: CanChild Centre for Childhood Disability Research. Retrieved August 9, 2009, from http://www.canchild.ca/Portals/0/education_materials/pdf/chaining.pdf

148. *WeeFIM II^SM system clinical guide: Version 5.01.* (1998, 2000). Buffalo, NY: University at Buffalo.

149. Werner DeGrace, B. (2004). Families, children with autism and everyday occupations. *American Journal of Occupational Therapy, 58,* 543–550.

150. Wheeler, M. (1998). *Toilet training for individuals with autism and related disorders.* Arlington, TX: Future Horizons.

151. Whinnery, K. W., & Whinnery, S. B. (2007). MOVE systematic programming for early motor intervention. *Infants and Young Children, 20,* 102–108.

152. Wroble, M. J. (2003). *Taking care of myself: A hygiene, puberty and personal curriculum for young people with autism.* Arlington, TX: Future Horizons.

153. York-Barr, J., Rainforth, B., & Locke, P. (1996). Developing instructional adaptations. In F. P. Orelove & D. Sobsey (Eds.), *Educating children with multiple disabilities* (3rd ed., pp. 119–159). Baltimore: Brookes.

154. Ziviani, J., Ottenbacher, K. J., Shephard, K., Foreman, S., Astbury, W., & Ireland, P. (2001). Concurrent validity of the Functional Independence Measure for Children (WeeFIM) and the Pediatric Evaluation of Disabilities Inventory in children with developmental disabilities and acquired brain injuries. *Physical and Occupational Therapy in Pediatrics, 21,* 91–101.

155. Zuniga, M. E. (2004). Families with Latino roots. In E. W. Lynch & M. J. Hanson (Eds.), *Developing cross-cultural competence* (3rd ed., pp. 209–250), Baltimore: Brookes.

SUGGESTED READINGS

Baker, B., & Brightman, A. (2003). *Steps to independence: Teaching everyday skills to children with special needs* (5th ed.). Baltimore: Brookes.

Coucouvanis, J. A. (2007). *The potty journey: Guide to toilet training children with special needs, including autism and related disorders.* Shawnee Mission, KS: Autism Asperger Publishing.

Ducharme, S. H., & Gil, K. M. (1997). *Sexuality after spinal cord injury: Answers to your questions.* York, PA: Brookes, The Maple Press Distribution Center.

Lehman, J., Klaw, R., & Peebles, G. (2003). *From goals to data and back again: Adding backbone to developmental intervention for children with autism.* Philadelphia: Jessica Kingsley.

Mayer, T. K. (2007). *One-handed in a two-handed world* (3rd ed.). Boston: Prince Gallison Press.

Schwier, K. M., & Hingsburger, D. (2000). *Sexuality: Your sons and daughters with intellectual disabilities.* Baltimore: Brookes.

Instrumental Activities of Daily Living and Community Participation

Kathryn M. Loukas • M. Louise Dunn[1]

KEY TERMS

Instrumental activities of daily living
Community participation
Self-determination
Family chores
Life habits
Mentoring roles
Social skills training

OBJECTIVES

1. Define instrumental activities of daily living (IADLs) and community participation for children and youths.
2. Describe how participation in IADLs and community participation contributes to occupational development for children and youths.
3. Describe development of IADLs and community participation.
4. Describe occupational performance by developmental age ranges and disability.
5. Describe personal and environmental influences.
6. Identify and apply professional reasoning, evaluation procedures, and intervention approaches for IADLs and community integration.
7. Describe, apply, and integrate evidence-based and occupation-centered intervention approaches to enhance IADL and community participation for children and youth.
8. Evaluate and synthesize information about the development of IADLs and community participation for children/youth through analysis of case studies.

INTRODUCTION

Peter is a 12-year-old boy who has autism. His parents are worried about how he will take care of himself. They are unsure about his role in the home and how much to ask of him. At school, the occupational therapist had taken a sensory motor approach to Peter's occupational therapy, yet she now sees the need for more skills in independent living for Peter. The education team wonders how much to include Peter in life skills and vocational programming.

Mary is a 16-year-old girl who was in a serious car accident that left her with left-sided hemiplegia and cognitive challenges secondary to a brain injury. She is now struggling with activities she used to find routine. She is unsafe in the kitchen, she has difficulty handling money, and her poor social skills make it difficult to make friends. Mary and her family are concerned about her future and wonder how she can regain the skills she needs for community living.

John is an 8-year-old boy with attention deficit disorder. His parents find it extremely challenging to involve him in household tasks, so they organize and manage his belongings and space. He has extreme difficulty paying attention in sedentary activities. John needs structure and guidance to participate in any community-based activity. John is interested in boy scouts and soccer, but his family has not allowed him to participate because of his behavior.

Instrumental activities of daily living (IADLs) are the more complex aspects of daily living that children and youth develop as they reach adolescence and begin to participate in the community with more autonomy. These activities include care of others, care of pets, child rearing, use of a communication device, community mobility, financial management, health management and maintenance, home management, meal preparation and clean-up, shopping, and safety procedures and emergency responses (American Occupational Therapy Association, 2008). Occupational therapists are experts in IADLs, task analysis, and independent living.

Children initially acquire more skill with IADLs when they reach adolescence and begin to participate in the community with more autonomy. They continue to develop competence in these activities through adolescence into young adulthood. IADLs and community participation include activities that promote self-determination, self-sufficiency, health, and social participation for children/youth of all abilities. IADL competence could be categorized as part of the

[1]We acknowledge the original work of Jayne Shepherd, MS, OTR/L, as a framework for this chapter. We thank Bevin Journey, MSOT, OTR/L, for background research that laid the groundwork for the intervention section of this chapter, as well as the University of New England graduate student research team of Tracy Floyd, Betsy Davis, Amanda Milose, and Erin Shugrue. We also gratefully acknowledge the editorial input of Helene Lohman, OTD, OTR/L and Nancy Davis, OTD, OTR/L of the Creighton University Post-Professional Doctoral program.

"magnificent mundane"[11] and is noted more by its absence than its presence. The magnificent mundane refers to the everyday presence of these tasks and reflects the tacit manner in which children/youth learn and understand their roles in these occupations. As preparation for independent living in the community, IADLs may include home management (e.g., clothing care, cleaning, and household maintenance), shopping and money management, meal preparation and cleanup, community mobility, health maintenance (e.g., taking medications, exercise and nutrition), care of pets and care of others, and safety procedures and emergency responses.[1]

An integral relationship exists between IADLs and community participation. For example, shopping is an IADL task that requires interaction with others in the community. Methods for learning to participate in the community may be tacit, such as learning through observation and assisting with shopping, or more explicit, such as finding and enrolling in community activities. Community participation includes social, play, and leisure activities with peers in the community and neighborhood and structured activities within the neighborhood and community.[6,43]

Recent studies contribute to our understanding of the diverse and complex challenges involved in preparing youth for independent/community living. Youth and adults with physical disabilities reported that they lacked opportunities to direct their health care services by making their own appointments and asking questions of medical and health personnel.[25,32] Adults with physical disabilities reported dependence in shopping, home cleaning, laundry, and use of public transportation.[3] Youth in foster care may lack knowledge and experience with independent living, especially safety and home and health maintenance.[46,49] Children and youth with traumatic brain injury (TBI) often lack opportunities to engage in household tasks and community activities such as shopping and recreational activities.[7]

This chapter provides an overview of the development of IADL skills and community participation, and a description of models that guide practices to promote competence in IADLs and full participation in community living. It further explains how emotional well-being, health, peer relations, and life satisfaction are associated with competence and independence in IADL and community living skills. Evaluation and intervention are discussed and illustrated using case examples.

OCCUPATIONAL DEVELOPMENT OF IADL AND COMMUNITY PARTICIPATION

Successful independent/community living is measured by outcomes related to employment, residing in the community, and community participation. IADLs are embedded in community living.

A large longitudinal study demonstrated that 2 years after leaving school, youth with special needs were more likely to be unemployed, live with their parents, and lack engagement in community activities with peers than youth without disabilities.[9] In a second longitudinal study, youth with special needs showed increased employment and engagement in community activities; however, their involvement lagged behind that of their peers without disabilities.[80] Youth with special needs continued to lag behind nondisabled peers in residing with others or alone in the community.

Self-determination has been identified as a factor that promotes independent community living. Defined as "a combination of skills, knowledge, attitudes, and behaviors that enable a person to engage in goal-directed, self-regulated, autonomous behavior,"[20] self-determination encompasses many of the behaviors and attitudes often referred to as *life skills* that are both innate and learned.[44] These skills include managing personal care and health needs, taking care of one's belongings and space, managing home repairs, arranging transportation, and living interdependently with others. Opportunities to develop problem-solving skills, understand one's own strengths and limitations, and make choices are critical to developing these skills. In fact, youth with mild intellectual and/or learning disabilities who have higher self-determination had greater employment rates, earned higher wages, and had more community involvement at 1 and 3 years out of school than similar youth with low self-determination.[82,83]

Late Adolescence (16 to 18 Years)

By late adolescence, youth are more autonomous and show greater breadth in their IADLs and community participation. Many spend most of their time outside the home, driving or taking public transportation, working a part-time job or volunteering, shopping, managing money, and maintaining a healthful regimen (e.g., taking responsibility for medications, exhibiting awareness of healthful behavior with partners).[25,46,66,72] At this age, many youth prepare hot and cold meals, help with cleanup, and manage their laundry. Box 17-1 provides guidelines about IADLs and community participation expectations for older adolescents.

Physical skill levels may limit opportunities to engage in IADLs tasks and community participation for many youth with physical disabilities; but with adaptations and accommodations, many become competent. Behavioral concerns such as lack of confidence, dependency, or weak social skills may also influence task performance of youth with physical disabilities, especially in community activities.[45]

Youth with acquired brain injury, especially when the brain injury was incurred at a young age, often have cognitive, behavioral, and or social impairments that influence their IADLs and community participation. They often require greater assistance with memory, problem solving, and self-management to initiate and complete tasks, sustain focus on tasks, and interact with others when completing work than they do with mobility.[19] Youth who experience an acquired brain injury are likely to need special coaching and assistance to manage the social demands of using public transportation on their own when they need to attend and interact with others.

Youth with autism spectrum disorder (ASD) may do well with household tasks such as making a snack, yet they have difficulty with tasks that require more interaction such as shopping. These youth are likely to have greater difficulty with tasks that involve relating to others, as would be needed to manage health care needs. Engaging in structured and unstructured leisure activities such as team sports or volunteer activities and going to the mall are challenging for youth with ASD.[33] Finally, acquiring initiative to do IADL tasks and engage in community activities may be difficult for many youth with disabilities.

BOX 17-1 Instrumental Activities of Daily Living and Community Participation: Older Adolescent (16 to 21 Years)

MEAL PREPARATION AND CLEAN-UP
- Plans and prepares simple hot and cold meals
- Puts dishes in dishwasher/puts dishes away
- Safely operates stove, oven, toaster, blender, microwave, and dishwasher

COMMUNITY MOBILITY
- Can obtain driver's license
- Uses public transportation on own

HEALTH MANAGEMENT AND MAINTENANCE
- Transfer to adult health care provider
- Responsible for managing medications
- Attends part of medical appointments alone
- Keeps record of medical history

HOUSEHOLD MAINTENANCE AND MANAGEMENT
- Looks into housing choices
- Attendant services and supported living options
- Does home repairs (e.g., replaces light bulb, replaces fuses)

CLOTHING MANAGEMENT
- Launders own clothes
- Mends clothes as needed

USE OF COMMUNICATION DEVICES
- Keeps in touch with friends by phone, texting, and computer (webcam, e-mail)

SHOPPING AND MONEY MANAGEMENT
- Practices budgeting and banking skills
- Purchases

SAFETY AND EMERGENCY RESPONSE
- Knows how to use fire extinguisher
- Knows what to do in case of fire or emergency

COMMUNITY PARTICIPATION
- Makes plans with peers for informal leisure and recreation activities
- Engages in community programs for youth/adults that match leisure or athletic interests
- Works part time and/or volunteers in community

PERFORMANCE SKILLS
- Motor and sensory skills well developed or adaptations and accommodations identified
- Emphasis more on psychological, social, and cognitive skills
- Takes more responsibility for own routines

Data from Dunn, Coster, Orsmond, & Cohn. (2009). Household task participation of children with and without attentional problems. *Physical and Occupational Therapy in Pediatrics, 29*(3), 234-251; Bloorview Life Skills Institute. (2007). Growing up ready timetable & checklists. Retrieved 6/03/2009 from http://www.bloorview.ca/resourcecentre/familyresources/ growingupready.php; Nollan, K. A., Wolf, M., Ansell, D., Burns, J. Barr, L., Copeland, L., et al. (2000). Ready or not: Assessing youth's preparedness for independent living. *Child Welfare, 79*(2), 159-618; Rodger, S. (2006). I can do it: Developing, promoting, and managing children's self-care needs. In S. Rodger & J. Ziviani (Eds.), *Occupational therapy with children* (pp. 200-221). Oxford, UK: Blackwell Publishing.

Early Adolescence (12 to 15 Years)

For young adolescents, teachers and parents emphasize not only learning from academics and vocational exploration but also home and health management, shopping and meal preparation, and community participation.[25,66,72] School programs attempt to establish not only adolescents' independence but also their ability to work interdependently with others. Young adolescents have increased responsibility for caring for others, managing their laundry, preparing simple, hot meals, and preparing snacks.[46,66,72] Technology, such as the microwave, cell phones, e-mail, and instant messaging/texting, increases young adolescents' opportunities for communication and community participation. Box 17-2 provides guidelines about IADL and community participation expectations for young adolescents.

Youth with disabilities often need additional practice and opportunities to promote autonomy with IADLs and community participation.[7,18] Young adolescents with physical disabilities may not direct others or seek assistance as needed with these IADL and community tasks. Some may be reluctant to express their lack of knowledge about how to prepare a meal and just wait until someone does it for them. In addition, cognitive/behavioral and social skill deficits may impede their autonomy in these areas.[45] Lack of assertiveness may impede their willingness to engage in leisure and recreational activities.

Similar deficits at varying levels also impede participation and performance of youth with TBI, ASD, and learning and intellectual disabilities. Communication deficits and rigidity may make it difficult for young adolescents with TBI and

ASD to do volunteer work or arrange rides to structured recreational activities. Lack of safety awareness and difficulty understanding the needs of others may make taking care of younger siblings or others difficult for young adolescents with TBI and ASD. Their insistence on sameness and lack of flexibility may make negotiating with others difficult, a skill needed in many recreational activities such as group hikes.

Middle Childhood (6 to 11 Years)

In middle childhood (6 to 11 years), formal learning opportunities related to IADL and community participation are limited unless children have significant intellectual disabilities. Children in the middle years prepare for future independent/community living through their engagement in everyday family, afterschool and community, and school activities.[42,54] These occupations give children opportunities to make choices, solve problems, and identify interests and skills that help them develop self-determination, social skills, and performance competency.[59,74,81]

In middle childhood many children engage in family and household routines; however, diversity in what they do and with whom is common. Parents report that they expect their children to take care of their space and materials, help with cleanup after meals, prepare simple cold meals, help with putting away groceries, and care for siblings with supervision.[16] As they engage in these tasks, children develop communication, cognitive, and social interaction skills (e.g., problem solving

BOX 17-2 Instrumental Activities of Daily Living and Community Participation: Younger Adolescent (12 to 15 Years)

MEAL PREPARATION AND CLEAN-UP
- Plans and prepares simple hot and cold meals
- Puts dishes in dishwasher/puts dishes away

COMMUNITY MOBILITY
- Starts to find way around local community
- Arranges rides to friends' houses
- Arranges rides to structured leisure and recreational activities
- Uses public transportation without assistance

HEALTH MANAGEMENT AND MAINTENANCE
- Begins to look for adult health care providers
- Attends some medical appointments alone
- Assists with making medical and dental appointments
- Takes more responsibility for managing medications

HOUSEHOLD MAINTENANCE AND MANAGEMENT
- Participates in discussions with parents about where he or she might live as an adult
- Cleans own space and shared (family) space
- May look after or babysit others or younger sibling
- Vacuums, dusts family space
- Puts away own laundry

USE OF COMMUNICATION DEVICES
- Uses phone, pens, and computers to send and receive information

SHOPPING AND MONEY MANAGEMENT
- May use bank card to deposit or withdraw money
- Purchases items with bank card or money
- May receive allowance, earn money from part-time work
- May purchase own goods at store

SAFETY AND EMERGENCY RESPONSE
- May take course in basic first aid
- Educates self about what to do in case of fire or emergency
- Responsible for personal safety when crossing street, obeying traffic and road signs

COMMUNITY PARTICIPATION
- Engages in informal and structured leisure and recreation with peers
- Keeps in touch with friends by phone, e-mail
- May volunteer in community

PERFORMANCE SKILLS AND PATTERNS
- Motor and sensory skills developed or adaptations and accommodations identified
- Emphasis more on psychological, social, and cognitive skills
- Has developed routines for daily activities, yet may need prompting

Data from Dunn, Coster, Orsmond, & Cohn. (2008). Household task participation of children with and without attentional problems. *Physical and Occupational Therapy in Pediatrics, 29*(3), 234-251; Growing up ready timetable and checklists. Retrieved June 3, 2009 from http://www.bloorview.ca/resourcecentre/familyresources/growingupready.php; Nollan, K. A., Wolf, M., Ansell, D., Burns, J. Barr, L., Copeland, L., et al. (2000). Ready or not: Assessing youth's preparedness for independent living. *Child Welfare, 79*(2), 159-618; Rodger, S. (2006). I can do it: Developing, promoting, and managing children's self-care needs. In S. Rodger & J. Ziviani (Eds.), *Occupational therapy with children* (pp. 200-221). Oxford, UK: Blackwell Publishing.

on encountering difficulty). Community activities include formal structured activities such as sports or music lessons, as well as informal unstructured activities such as riding bikes. Box 17-3 provides guidelines about IADL and community participation expectations for children of middle childhood age.

Physical, cognitive, and social functioning deficits may make it difficult for children with disabilities to develop the skills necessary to participate in these activities. For children with either physical and/or cognitive/behavioral disabilities, generalization of learning to different settings may require specific cognitive and behavioral strategies.[62,64] Children with cognitive/behavioral disabilities such as attention deficit–hyperactivity disorder (ADHD) may clean up after preparing food in a community setting yet not carry over this learning to their home life.[30] Children with ADHD may use social skills during art activities at school yet have difficulty sharing materials and taking turns in afterschool creative art activities. Children with physical disabilities may participate in recreational activities by observing rather than doing.[65] Some may not assist with IADLs such as setting or clearing the table because of the time it takes them to do these tasks or because their physical impairments limit their participation.

Children with TBI may not engage in family routines such as preparing simple cold meals and picking up shared areas because of their high need for coaching. Those with memory impairments will need continual practice and repetition to

organize their belongings for school and non–school-related activities. Their attention deficits may impede their safety when crossing the street. Depending on severity, children with ASD may need assistance to focus and find items on the shelf at the supermarket. They may have tantrums and meltdowns at the supermarket or mall because of overstimulation by sounds, sights, and smells.

Preschool (3 to 5 Years)

In preschool, participation in home day care and community activities frequently occurs with supervision from caregivers or parents. Therefore, family involvement is essential to development of IADL and community participation.[34,68,71]

Availability of free play allows children the opportunity to identify interests, make choices, and learn how to share and take turns. In the Head Start program, much emphasis is placed on promoting self-determination by assisting children to identify when they need help and guiding them to solve problems on their own.[24,71] Furthermore, children with and without disabilities are involved in many naturally occurring learning opportunities through community activities such as shopping, going to neighborhood playgrounds, attending library story hours, taking walks in the neighborhood, or participating in events at community centers.[17] In the home, preschool children assist with many household tasks such as

BOX 17-3 Instrumental Activities of Daily Living and Community Participation: Middle Childhood (6 to 11 Years)

MEAL PREPARATION AND CLEAN-UP
- With supervision, puts dishes in dishwasher/puts dishes away
- Gets own snacks
- Sets and clears table

COMMUNITY MOBILITY
- Rides bicycle, uses rollerblades, scooter around neighborhood
- Makes arrangements with parent for rides to friends' houses, video store, etc.
- Uses public transportation with supervision

HEALTH MANAGEMENT AND MAINTENANCE
- Participates in medication routines (as needed)
- Assists with naming medical concerns (e.g., allergies, asthma, seizures)

HOUSEHOLD MAINTENANCE AND MANAGEMENT
- Puts away own materials, vacuums and dusts own room
- Puts away groceries, helps with recycling
- Organizes materials for school and afterschool events

USE OF COMMUNICATION DEVICES
- Keeps in touch with friends by phone, e-mail
- Answers phone, takes messages

SHOPPING AND MONEY MANAGEMENT
- May have a savings account
- Shops with parent or caregiver
- Finds items on shelves at supermarket

SAFETY AND EMERGENCY RESPONSE
- Can name places to find help or be safe
- Aware of safety with food, fire, and strangers

COMMUNITY PARTICIPATION
- With assistance, gets together with peers for leisure activities, hobbies, movies
- May participate in afterschool programs, community center activities
- Visits with friends or relatives in neighborhood

PERFORMANCE SKILLS AND PATTERNS
- Motor planning and sensory–motor skills continue to develop and are further refined, may be problem areas
- Starting to follow routines for daily activities but requires prompting

Data from Dunn, Coster, Orsmond, & Cohn. (2008). Household task participation of children with and without attentional problems. *Physical and Occupational Therapy in Pediatrics, 29*(3), 234-251; Growing up ready timetable and checklists. Retrieved June 3, 2009 from http://www.bloorview.ca/resourcecentre/familyresources/growingupready.php; Nollan, K. A., Wolf, M., Ansell, D., Burns, J. Barr, L., Copeland, L., et al. (2000). Ready or not: Assessing youth's preparedness for independent living. *Child Welfare, 79*(2), 159-618; Rodger, S. (2006). I can do it: Developing, promoting, and managing children's self-care needs. In S. Rodger & J. Ziviani (Eds.) *Occupational therapy with children* (pp. 200-221). Oxford, UK: Blackwell Publishing.

putting away their own toys, making their beds, putting away their clothes, helping to set the table, and preparing cold snacks.[66] In many families, greater emphasis is on beginning to take care of oneself and one's belongings than on taking responsibility for others.

Little information exists about IADL participation for preschool children with disabilities. For children with physical disabilities, opportunities to perform tasks such as picking up one's toys, making choices about snacks, or pointing to items at the supermarket may provide ways to develop routines and be part of the family. Children with TBI may need coaching and positive supports to promote their ability to pick up their toys and make choices about snacks or community activities.

In summary, age and functional abilities contribute to the extent of children's and youth's participation and performance of IADL and community activities. IADL and community participation are both the means and ends for development of motor and process performance skills.

PERSONAL AND ENVIRONMENTAL INFLUENCES ON IADLS AND COMMUNITY PARTICIPATION

Multiple interrelated internal and external factors influence children's and youth's engagement in IADLs and community activities. The occupational therapist should address personal and environmental factors that may support or limit the child's or youth's participation in IADLs and community activities.

Personal Influences

Factors that are within children and youth include their *interests, preferences*, and *motivation* to engage in activities. Engagement in IADL and community activities requires interest and motivation. Initially, motivation may be promoted with external support; however, to continue to engage in tasks and use skills, children and youth must internalize reasons to do so.[63] Internalization of reasons for performing IADL tasks may relate to increased responsibility and opportunities to do favorite activities or to earn money.[10,31]

Environmental Influences

Factors external to the child comprise five environmental or contextual areas: (1) the natural and built environment (physical context); (2) support and relationships (social context); (3) attitudes, values, and beliefs (cultural context); (4) assistive technology; and (5) service systems and policies.[1,85] These factors can either support or limit children's and youth's participation IADL and community activities.

The natural and built environment (physical context) includes the sensory and physical qualities of the setting (e.g., noise, lighting, temperature, terrain, crowding), building design, and accessibility to materials.[45] Within the home, access to different areas and materials supports participation of children and youth in family activities. In the community, buildings that have accessible entrances and activities on a flat terrain support inclusion of children and youth with physical imitations. Examples of barriers are homes without access to all areas and community centers with activities on multiple levels that lack ramps or elevators. Crowding (e.g., group size) and sensory aspects of the environment are potential barriers for children and youth with physical, sensory, cognitive, and intellectual disabilities.[35,52,60] For children and youth with ADHD, ASD, and intellectual disability, the noise from people talking and the movement of people in a crowd may contribute to behavioral outbursts, anxiety, and aggression, thus decreasing their participation. Noise, visual stimulation, and crowding limit participation because these factors interfere with balance, mobility, and communication for children and youth with physical disabilities.[52]

Support and relationships (social context) are particularly salient factors that influence participation of children and youth in IADL and community activities. At home, support is crucial for participation with family members in everyday activities. Families provide children with opportunities and encouragement to learn household tasks such as mealtime preparation and care of common spaces. Modeling of task performance and discussion of tacit planning processes make learning and understanding these tasks more tangible to children and youth. For example, at home children can observe not only their parents but also their siblings. In addition, children may be mentors to their siblings and guides for their parents. As children mature, they may take on the role of caring for their siblings when parents are out of the home. In the community, children may begin by attending structured afterschool activities such as sports or recreation groups (Figure 17-1), or they may meet with peers to socialize at the mall. As they approach older adolescence, they may also take on roles as mentors at recreational centers or scouting events.

The social environment for IADL participation may vary by setting (e.g., school, home, community, or work). At home, children might observe parents and siblings doing household tasks and attempt to model their actions. Short-term outcomes from participating in mealtime preparation and household tasks include promoting a sense of family and demonstrating positive health and social behaviors.[16,53] Long-term outcomes include preparation for adult roles. Lack of support and diminished opportunities for participation in these mundane tasks can impede development of community living skills (e.g., such as the example of youth in foster homes[46]).

Cultural values and beliefs significantly influence opportunities for IADL and community participation. At home family beliefs about routines and perspectives on time allocation influence children's and youth's engagement in activities at home and in the community.[21,26,78] For example, parents of Asian background tend to value academics and place much less emphasis on IADL activities and autonomy for their children.[87] In contrast, Latino and Navajo families tend to focus on interdependency and promote engagement in household and IADL tasks.[69]

The value of interdependency versus autonomy may influence a family's willingness to support the independence of a child or youth with a disability. Families from African American and Hispanic backgrounds are more likely to plan to have their children with developmental disabilities live with them when the children reach adulthood.[5] These beliefs may also influence the opportunities to engage in IADL tasks and community activities for children and youth with disabilities.

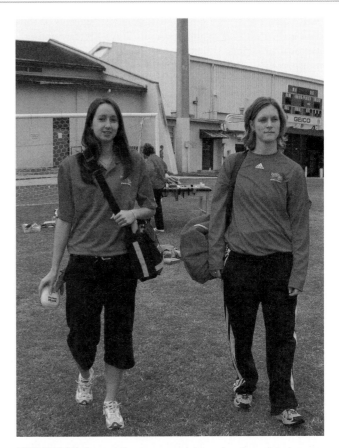

FIGURE 17-1 Adolescents participate in afterschool sports and recreation programs. (From Cummings, N. H., Stanley-Green, S., & Higgs, P. [2009]. *Perspectives in athletic training.* St. Louis: Mosby.)

Parents of children with disabilities, particularly those from lower socioeconomic levels, were less likely to involve their children in household tasks and in interacting with others in the community.[87] Values for engaging in interdependent activities also influence participation in household tasks. For example, parents of children with ADHD tend to emphasize household tasks that involve managing one's own belongings with less focus on shared tasks such as helping at mealtimes.[16]

Community programs that include children and youth of all abilities are supports for community participation.[52] Social stigma, bullying, and marginalization are barriers for children and youth with disabilities.[45,52]

Assistive technology, computers, online resources, and augmentative communication devices are supports used commonly with children and youth who have disabilities to promote their participation in IADL and community activities. Technology and online resources afford opportunities for children and youth of all abilities to connect with others. Information about community activities, employment, shopping, banking, meal planning, public transportation, and health are available online. A growing number of support groups for children and youth with many differing disabilities have set up websites that provide peer mentoring for learning how to live in the community and care for their own needs.

Examples of *service systems* that promote inclusion of children and youth with disabilities are inclusive aftercare and recreational programs, programs with adaptive equipment, and transportation. *Policies*, rules, and standards that govern these services ensure that they are accessible and enable optimal participation of persons with disabilities.[45,85] For children and youth with disabilities, lack of transportation or length of time required to transition to programs can be a barrier to participation in community activities.[35] Another barrier is the lack of policies and funding to cover costs of additional supports that may be needed for inclusion of children and youth with disabilities in out-of-school activities.[35,60]

EVALUATION OF IADL AND COMMUNITY PARTICIPATION

Children, youth, and their families or caregivers play key roles in the evaluation process. These individuals provide relevant information about the settings and contextual features where the children or youth engage in IADL and community activities. Providing youth with greater opportunities to engage in the evaluation process increases their autonomy and prepares them for decision making and management of their health, IADL, and community participation needs. Providing children, youth, and caregivers with opportunities to select or refuse assessments and choose where and when the evaluation is completed increases their investment in collaboration around intervention planning.[27] Evaluation of IADL and community participation may include combinations of the following methods: observation, interview, inventory/questionnaire, performance measures, interest checklists, and chart review. The evaluation may be part of a school-based triennial evaluation required under IDEA and/or transition plan at the request of a pediatrician or health care practitioner, at the parent's request, as part of a medical model assessment, or as part of community models such as foster care. Evaluations may be conducted individually with the child/youth and caregiver, as a team evaluation, or as part of a program evaluation. Table 17-1 provides a listing of available measures, including information about whether assessments measure skills, tasks, and/or environmental factors.

Team Evaluations

Team or arena evaluations often arise when youth meet for transitional planning in schools or when children and youth return to school after hospitalization secondary to medical concerns such as traumatic brain or spinal cord injury. Information from multiple perspectives is helpful for a realistic appraisal of the child or youth's performance in a variety of settings.

Team evaluations also may apply to medical or psychiatric facilities. Medical and rehabilitation facilities may examine IADLs and community participation related to returning home and returning to school. Recently, additional emphasis has been placed on community participation because of research showing concerns in this area for children and youth with acquired or traumatic brain injury and physical disabilities.[8,45] Team members often include, but are not limited to, children and youth, caregivers, occupational and physical therapists, speech therapists, nurses, and physiatrists.

Team evaluations may also be part of community system services. Youth in foster care are monitored and evaluated for independent living skills that include IADLs and community participation.[46,54] This is also true of many at-risk children and adolescents who are in the juvenile system or are homeless. Many are eligible for independent living programs run through welfare agencies.[46] Team members often include, but are not limited to, social workers, foster parents, children and youth in foster care, pediatricians, and occupational therapists. At present, this is an emerging practice area for occupational therapists.[4]

Measurement of Outcomes

Occupational scientists and therapists along with professionals in rehabilitation and health have developed assessments to measure outcomes of IADLs and community participation (see Table 16-1). With the new International Classification of Functioning, Disability, and Health for Children and Youth, outcomes may address participation patterns, activity performance, quality of life, client satisfaction, and contextual supports and barriers.[85]

Assessments for IADLs and community participation are relatively few; most are inventories that are completed by a caregiver. The Vineland Adaptive Behavior Scales II (VABS) is a standardized measure commonly used to measure domestic (IADL) and community skills.[73] This measure provides information about the individual and can be used to assess changes over time. The VABS has often been used with children and youth who have intellectual disabilities and with children with ADHD. The Assessment of Motor and Process Skills (AMPS) is standardized and appears to be sensitive to the progress that children make.[22,23] Studies demonstrated that the AMPS can identify differences in IADLs for children with and without ADHD[30] and for children with hemiplegic cerebral palsy.[79]

Several new participation assessments have recently become available (see Table 17-1). The Children and Adolescent Scale of Participation (CASP)[8] and the Life Habits Questionnaire (LIFE-H)[55] measure participation at home, school, and in the community. These measures produce change scores that can be used to examine outcomes from individual intervention or programmatic outcomes. These measures do not provide information about age ranges but do provide information about the difficulty continuum of the participation items based on Rasch analyses. Measures may be completed by caregiver or teacher and by the child or youth for comparison of perspectives.

The CASP has been used to obtain information about program outcomes for children with TBI.[8] The CASP has 20 items that measure participation for children and youth at home, school, and in the community. Some examples of CASP activities are family chores, responsibility, and expectations at home; social activities with friends in the neighborhood or the community; and shopping.[8] Parents or caregivers compare their child's participation to that of typical children of the same age using a 4-point scale ranging from "age expected" to "unable." This information has been helpful in identifying ongoing intervention concerns after discharge of children with TBI to integrate back into their homes, schools, and communities.

The LIFE-H obtains information about social participation for 5- to 13-year-old children and youth with physical

Text continued on page 529

TABLE 17-1 Instruments for Assessing IADLs and Community Participation for Children and Youth

Instrument and Publisher	Area Assessed	Interview/Inventory	Observation	Age Range	Description
Ansell-Casey Life Skills Inventory (Nollan et al., 2000) Online assessment available at http://www. casselifeskills.org	Person Task	X		8–18 yr	Assessment of life skills, developed for children and youth in foster care, that is completed online and then automatically scored. Categories for life skills include home and money management, health, safety and emergency, transportation. Three age ranges for scale. Criterion-referenced. Good reliability and validity.
ABS-S: 2 AAMR—Adaptive Behavior Scale—School (2nd ed.) (Lambert, Nihira, & Lelan, 1993) Pro-Ed 8700 Shoal Creek Boulevard Austin, TX 78757-6897 http://www.proedinc.com	Person Task	X	X	3–8.11 yr	ABS-S: 2 is a standardized, criterion-referenced measure for adaptive behaviors in nine domains related to instrumental activities of daily living (IADLs): independent functioning, physical development, economic activity, language development, numbers and time, prevocational/vocational activity, self-direction, responsibility, and socialization. ABS is useful for children with intellectual disabilities (ID), autism, and behavior disorders. Administration—Easy to follow instructions. Takes about 1 hour to administer.
AMPS Assessment of Motor and Process Skills (5th ed.) (Fisher, 2003a, 2003b) AMPS Project International P.O. Box 42 Hampton Falls, NH 03844 http://www.ampsintl.com	Person Task	X	X	3 yr–adult	AMPS is a criterion-referenced test for activities of daily living (ADL) and IADL tasks that assess the underlying motor and process performance skills used to perform the task. Examiner training—formal training procedure through course attendance, observation and rating of 10 clients with calibration of scoring through AMPS International required before using AMPS. Established reliability and validity with normative data for typical individuals.
ASK Activity Scale for Kids (Young et al., 2000) Nancy Young, Ph.D. nancyyoung@sickkids.on.ca ASK manual (1996) The Hospital for Sick Children Toronto, Ontario	Person Task	X	X	5–15 yr	Measures performance (what child does) and capacity (what child is capable of doing) for personal care, dressing, eating, locomotion, stairs, play, transfers and standing skills. Excellent reliability and validity. Child and/or parent report. Takes about 30 minutes first time, 10 minutes for repeat tests.
CASP Child and Adolescent Scale of Participation (Bedell, 2004)	Person Environment Task	X		5–12 yr Adolescent data in process	Summed scores allow comparison of individuals across time. Newly developed measure of participation at home, school, and in community.

Continued

TABLE 17-1 Instruments for Assessing IADLs and Community Participation for Children and Youth—Cont'd

Instrument and Publisher	Area Assessed	Interview/ Inventory	Observation	Age Range	Description
Contact author for CASP and for scoring guidelines Gary Bedell, Ph.D., OT gary.bedell@tufts.edu					Consists of four sections that assess Home Participation, School Participation, Community Participation, and Home and Community Living Activities. Parent and caregiver/teacher report measure with youth report and Spanish version under development. Has excellent psychometric properties. Takes ~20 to 30 minutes to complete measure. Scoring: summary scores allow comparison of individuals across time.
CASE Child and Adolescent Scale of Environment (Bedell, 2004) Contact author for CASE and for scoring guidelines Gary Bedell, Ph.D., OT gary.bedell@tufts.edu	Environment Task	X		5–12 yr Adolescent data in process	Newly developed parent report measure that taps all participation indices of ICF. Has excellent reliability and content validity. For individual, program, and population-based assessment Useful for gathering information about environmental supports/problems in following areas: school (support, assistance, services, equipment, attitudes); home/community (including transportation and government policies); physical design of school, home and community; family stress and problems with finances. Takes ~10 to 15 minutes to complete measure. Scoring: summary scores allow comparisons across time.
CHORES Children Helping Out: Responsibilities, Expectations and Supports (Dunn, 2004) Contact author for CHORES and scoring guidelines Louise Dunn, ScD, OTR/L louise.dunn@hsc.utah.edu	Person Environment Task	X		Grade 1–8 ~ 6–14 yr	Parent report measure that examines children's participation in household tasks. Has excellent internal consistency and test-retest reliability for school-aged children (Dunn, 2004) and youth (Dunn, in preparation). Takes ~15 to 20 minutes to complete measure Scoring: summary scores allow comparison of individuals across time. Additional open-ended questions about parents' perspectives on importance and satisfaction with their children's' household task participation.
COACH Choosing Options and Accommodations for Children (2nd ed.) (Giangreco, Cloninger, & Iverson, 1998) Brookes Publishing P. O. Box 10624 Baltimore, MD 21285 http://www. brookespublishing.com	Person Task	X	X	3–21 yr	COACH is a curriculum-referenced transdisciplinary team assessment and curriculum with four domains: personal management, community, home, and vocational. Used as a team planning tool, does not assess specific skills. Intended for children with moderate, severe, or profound disabilities but has been used with children with mild disabilities.

Measure	Components		Age	Description
COPM Canadian Occupational Performance Measure (4th ed.) (Law et al., 2005) Available through: Canadian Association of Occupational Therapists (CAOT) CTTC Building, Suite 3400 1125 Colonel By Drive Ottawa, Ontario K1S 5R1 Canada http://www.caot.ca	Person Task Environment	X	~8 yr through adult	Child, youth, and parent report measure of occupational performance for client-selected self-care, productivity, and leisure concerns. Semistructured interview format with two rating scales: performance and satisfaction with occupational performance. Takes ~30 to 40 minutes to complete. Scoring: summary scores allow comparison of individuals across time. Website provides information about COPM, FAQ and other resources.
COSA Child Occupational Self Assessment (Keller et al., 2005) Available through MOHO Clearinghouse http://www.moho.uic.edu/assessments	Person Task	X		Child and youth self-report measure of occupational competence and importance of activities at school, home, and in the community. Takes ~20 minutes to complete, longer when assistance is needed. Rasch analysis provides information about difficulty levels of items. Scoring information based on individual performance. Provides information for goals and for outcomes.
LIFE-H Life Habits Questionnaire (Noreau et al., 2007) Contact Luc Noreau, PhD for LIFE-H and scoring guidelines Luc.Noreau@rea.ulaval.ca	Person Environment Task	X	5–18 yr	Parent and youth report measure based on ICF participation. Excellent reliability and validity. Examines six categories of participation: interpersonal relationships, communication, personal care, mobility education, and recreation. Examines daily activities (e.g., personal care, mobility, nutrition) and social roles (e.g., recreation, responsibility). Takes ~15 to 20 minutes to complete. Youth may complete as part of interview. Summary scores permit individual comparison over time.
OCAIRS Occupational Circumstances Assessment Interview and Rating Scale (Forsyth et al., 2005) Available through MOHO Clearinghouse http://www.moho.uic.edu/assessments	Person Task Environment	X	Adolescent–adult	Descriptive interview format for gathering data about extent and nature of an individual's occupational participation. Takes ~20 minutes to complete. Summary scores provide information about participation in different settings.
SIB–R Scales of Independent Behavior Revised (Bruininks, Woodcock, Weatherman, & Hill, 1996) http://www.riverpub.com/products/sibr/bruininks.html	Person Task	X	Infancy–80+ yr	Norm-referenced measure of adaptive and maladaptive behaviors Comprised of 14 subscales grouped into 4 clusters: motor skills, social interaction and communication skills, personal living skills, and community living skills. Administration—45 to 60 minutes for full test; 15 to 20 minutes for short form

Continued

TABLE 17-1 Instruments for Assessing IADLs and Community Participation for Children and Youth—Cont'd

Instrument and Publisher	Area Assessed	Interview/ Inventory	Observation	Age Range	Description
TDRWQ **Transition Daily Rewards and Worries Questionnaire** (Glidden & Jobe, 2007) Contact Laraine Glidden for TDRWQ and scoring guidelines lmglidden@smcm.edu	Person Environment	X			Parent report inventory that measures daily rewards and concerns of parents as their adolescents transition to adulthood Good internal consistency (.74 to .85) and adequate test-retest reliability (via confirmatory factor analysis; correlations for four factors ranged from .56 to .68) Assesses positive and negative aspects of adolescent's transition to adulthood by examining four areas: future/adult life, socialization, community resources, and family relations Summary scores permit individual comparison over time
VABS II Vineland Adaptive Behavior Scales II (Sparrow, Balla, & Cicchetti, 2005) American Guidance Service Circle Pines, MN 55014 http://www.agsnet.com)	Person Environment Task	X		Birth–18.11 yrs.	The VABS II is a norm-referenced assessment. Measures daily living skills (personal, domestic, and community). Within these areas, examines communication, socialization and motor domains. Maladaptive behavior domain is available for children 5 yr and older Three versions are available: Interview/survey; interview/ expanded form; and classroom/teacher form (3-12.11 yr) Scales appropriate for students with or without disabilities Reliability and validity established for children with intellectual disabilities (Balboni, Pedrabissi, Molton, et al., 2001)

Data from Bedell, G. M. (2004). Developing a follow-up survey focused on participation of children and youth with acquired brain injuries after discharge from inpatient rehabilitation. *NeuroRehabilitation, 19,* 191-205; Bruininks, R. H., Woodcock, R. W., Weatherman, R. F., & Hill, B. K. (1996). *Scales of independent behavior—revised (SIB-R).* Rolling Meadows, IL: Riverside Publishing; Dunn, L. (2004). Validation of the CHORES: A measure of children's participation in household tasks. *Scandinavian Journal of Occupational Therapy, 11,* 179-190; Fisher, A. G. (2003a). *Assessment of motor and process skills: Vol. 1. Development, standardization, and administration manual* (5th ed.). Fort Collins, CO. Three Star Press; Fisher, A. G. (2003b). *Assessment of motor and process skills: Vol. 2. User manual* (5th ed.). Fort Collins, CO. Three Star Press; Forsyth, K., Deshpande, S., Kielhofner et al. (2005). *The Occupational Circumstances Assessment Interview and Rating Scale (OCAIRS) Version 4.0.* Chicago: MOHO Clearinghouse; Giangreco, M., Clonger, C., & Iverson, V. (1997). *Choosing options and accommodations for children (COACH)* (2nd ed.). Baltimore: Brookes; Glidden, L. M. & Jobe, B. M. (2007). Measuring parental daily rewards and worries in the transition to adulthood. *American Journal on Mental Retardation, 112*(4), 275-278; Keller, J., Kafkes, A; Basu, S., Federico, J., & Kielhofner, G. (2005). *Child Occupational Self Assessment (COSA), version 2.1.* Chicago, IL: MOHO Clearinghouse; Lambert, N. M., Nihira, K., & Leland, H. (1993). *AAMR Adaptive Behavior Scale-School-2.* Austin, TX: Pro-Ed; Law, M., Baptiste, S., Carswell, A., McColl, M. A., Polatajko, H. & Pollock, N. (2005). *The Canadian Occupational Performance Measure.* Ottawa, Canada: CAOT publications ACE; Nollan, K. A., Wolf, M., Ansell, D., Burns, J. Barr, L., Copeland, L., et al. (2000). Ready or not: Assessing youth's preparedness for independent living. *Child Welfare, 79*(2), 159-618; Noreau, L., Lepage, C., Boissiere, L., Picard, R., Fougeyrollas, P., Mathieu, J., et al. (2007). Measuring participation in children with disabilities using the Assessment of Life Habits. *Developmental Medicine & Child Neurology, 49,* 666-671; Sparrow, S., Balla, D., & Cicchetti, D. (2005). *Vineland Adaptive Behavior Scales II.* Circle Pines, MN: American Guidance Services; Young, N. L., Williams, J. I., Yoshida, K. K., & Wright, J. G. (2000). Measurement properties of the Activities Scale for Kids. *Journal of Clinical Epidemiology, 53,* 125-137.

disabilities, TBI, or developmental disabilities.[55] Life habits refer to participation in valued everyday activities such as nutrition, fitness, communication, personal care, and valued social roles such as responsibility and community life. Ratings, on a 10-point scale, measure level of participation difficulty, assistance required (compared with that expected for typically developing peers), and satisfaction.

Preparation for independent and interdependent living often is addressed during adolescence; however, research supports monitoring and assessing these performance areas before adolescence. Because children and youth with disabilities often require additional support to learn and perform these mundane tasks,

assessment and planning before adolescence are needed. The Children Helping Out: Responsibilities, Expectations, and Supports (CHORES) program was developed for these purposes and provides information about participation in household tasks and some aspects of IADLs.[15] In CHORES household tasks include domestic tasks as well as caring for others. Household tasks are organized into two groups: self-care tasks and family-care tasks.[84] Self-care refers to household tasks for which the outcomes primarily affect the individual such as picking up one's clothing or making a cold meal for oneself. Family care refers to household tasks for which the outcomes primarily affect others such as caring for pets and preparing meals (Figure 17-2).

Household Tasks (SC = Self-Care) (FC = Family-Care)	On own initiative (7)	When asked (6)	With supervision (5)	Some assistance (4)	Lot of assistance (3)	Child cannot (2)	Not expected (1)
Puts away own clothes (SC) ☐ Yes ☐ No							
Makes self a cold meal (SC) ☐ Yes ☐ No							
Puts own laundry in hamper (SC) ☐ Yes ☐ No							
Sweeps or vacuums own room (SC) ☐ Yes ☐ No							
Feeds pet (FC) ☐ Yes ☐ No							
Sets or clears the table (FC) ☐ Yes ☐ No							
Takes out garbage/recycling (FC) ☐ Yes ☐ No							
Cares for younger sibling (FC) ☐ Yes ☐ No							

Note: If parent answers "yes," child does item; check off assistance level rating. If parent answers "no," child does not do task; indicate if it is because child cannot or is not expected to do task.

FIGURE 17-2   Examples of CHORES items and ratings for the Children Helping Out: Responsibilities, Expectations, and Supports (CHORES) Program.

Scoring on CHORES provides a way to measure change for individuals across time. Changes are measured by comparing the number of tasks performed and the assistance required to perform household tasks. Two open-ended items provide information about the importance of household task participation to parents and parents' satisfaction with their children's household task participation. Refer to Figure 17-2 for examples of items and rating scales for CHORES.

CHORES provides a way to gather information from parents that can contribute to development of interventions that address goals and concerns related to household task performance, as well as to being part of the family. This information can promote discussions about expectations and opportunities and preparation for independent living for children and youth of all abilities.

Information relative to the perspectives and beliefs of children, youth, and caregivers on participation in the community and in IADLs is essential to client-centered and evidence-based practice. The Canadian Occupational Performance Measure (COPM) is often used for this purpose.

A new outcome-based measure, the Children's Occupational Self Assessment (COSA), measures children's perspectives on their competence and the importance of participation in activities in their homes, schools, and communities.[38] Children rate their competence and importance of activities using a four-point pictorial scale of faces and stars. Examples of IADL items are getting chores done and using money to buy things for themselves.

The Transition Daily Rewards and Worries Questionnaire (TDRWQ) provides a way to measure caregivers' beliefs and concerns for their adolescents who are transitioning to the adult world.[29] The TDRWQ is a 28-item measure with four subscales: positive future orientation, community resources, financial independence, and family relations. Parents or caregivers rate items on a five-point scale from *strongly disagree* to *strongly agree*. Examples are perception of adolescents' adjustment to living out of the home and perception about schools' preparation of adolescents for independent living. This measure affords a way to promote discussion and to develop goals and interventions to address preparation of adolescents for independent and interdependent living.

INTERVENTION PLANNING AND IMPLEMENTATION

Inclusion of the families or caregivers of children with disabilities is essential to promote and reinforce positive self-esteem in everyday life, and to promote self-determination skills for positive social experiences.[28,48,76,82,86] Psychosocial skills and community participation–based interventions should be facilitated long before meeting for transition planning.

As children begin their transition to adult roles, the focus of occupational therapy should move toward independent or interdependent living.[13] As Orentlicher and Michaels note, the therapist's goal at this stage is to enable the adolescent to achieve full status as an adult:

Disability is a natural part of human experiences and it does not diminish the right of the individual to live independently, enjoy self-determination, make choices, contribute to society, pursue meaningful careers, and enjoy full inclusion and integration in the economic, political, cultural and educational mainstream of American society (p. 2).[56]

Transition planning is concerned with the continuing process of moving from a supported home environment to a role of living in the adult community. Adolescents with disabilities or those who are at risk may require more planning, intervention, and support than a typical student.[36,37,51,56,57]

Occupational therapists often provide services in the school setting to children who experience self-care or functional mobility deficits, rendering a prime opportunity for therapists to implement needed skills for independent living. Because independent living involves participation in activities at home and in the community, expansion of services to home and the community is an area that needs further development. Occupational therapists understand and appreciate the important link between occupations and identity.[12,40] Desired outcomes for adolescents with lifelong disabilities include safe, independent or interdependent engagement in occupation in the natural occurring contexts of IADLs in the home or community[1] and the formation of a strong, positive disability identity (Case Study 17-1).[39]

INTERVENTION MODELS AND STRATEGIES

Client-Centered Intervention

Occupational therapy practitioners and the interdisciplinary team often use a psychosocial approach to enhance the child's or youth's sense of control and his/her independence. Empowering an adolescent toward self-determination can facilitate independence.[25,76,82,86] One way this can be accomplished during therapy is to include the child/youth in intervention planning and decisions by making choices and problem solving. Collaborative decision making with the youth and family can foster an intentional relationship that leads to increased occupational performance.[77] This strategy can be replicated in any area of the child or adolescent's program. Health care and education professionals are recognizing the need to prepare youth for monitoring and taking care of their daily needs such as medications, making appointments, and assessing accessibility in the community. Increasing independence in all areas of life through adaptations such as work simplification can also help an adolescent feel more competent and able. Decision making and increasing independence are key to feelings of competence and control that can create "strands of coherence" (p. 236)[61] as the adolescent becomes an adult.

Adaptation/Compensation

An approach frequently used to include people with disabilities in IADLs and community participation is through adaptation/compensation of the environment, task, or person. See Table 17-2 for specific ideas for adaptive success for common physical, cognitive, and psychosocial challenges.

Contextualism

Humphry and Wakeford understand "development of everyday activities as embedded in and inseparable from societal effort to offer occupational opportunities and social processes that are

Kayla is a 12-year-old girl who is spirited and full of life. She is a child with athetoid cerebral palsy that affects her movement in all areas of motor performance, yet her process skills are intact. She is small and thin for her age and has some significant postural control difficulties and fine motor challenges. Occupational therapy services were primarily sensorimotor based with some neurodevelopmental treatment during her primary school years. She attended a therapy swim group and had many areas of adaptation/compensation for eating and feeding, self-care, writing, physical education, music, and art-based activities. She was fully included in school classes with modifications and the assistance of an educational technician.

As Kayla entered middle school, she was less tolerant of occupational therapy in the inclusive setting. She no longer wanted to use her adaptations for eating and feeding in the cafeteria and often did not wear her ankle foot orthotics. Once happy and fun-loving, she became sullen, was rude to her educator technician, was abrupt with other children, and would often sit and cry. Her longtime occupational therapist, having seen her since kindergarten, felt compelled to change directions with Kayla. The occupational therapist explored a more holistic model and used the Model of Human Occupation (MOHO)[39] to frame a revised intervention plan.

VOLITION SYSTEM

Kayla had become discouraged after being the only child with significant physical disabilities in her school for 6 years. She felt different from others. She was frustrated and angry about not being able to perform activities independently. She was self-conscious about her physical differences and did not want to stand out in any way.

HABITUATION

Kayla had developed habits of being somewhat dependent on others. As she entered adolescence, she psychologically wanted to be more independent and break away, but physically could not. Having aid kept her feeling dependent and not in control of her life and social activities. She also began having more difficulty keeping up with her peers academically.

PERFORMANCE CAPACITY

Kayla was beginning to have the "lived body" experience and to develop a "disability identity,"[39] but she had no one to talk to about this emerging identity. She understood the need for adaptations but did not want them to stand out. She was torn between wanting to perform well at school and not wanting to have things done "differently."

EVALUATION

In the assessment interview, the occupational therapist helped Kayla vent her frustrations and talk about her current and future roles. It became apparent that she was concerned about her future and doubted her own capacities. In an educational team meeting, more comprehensive occupational therapy services were put in place to improve Kayla's independence, IADL skills, and psychosocial functioning. Goals were written to improve life skills and community participation.

INTERVENTION STRATEGIES

Independence and self-sufficiency to increase her sense of control: Kayla was asked if she would like to train her new teacher and aide about her use of equipment and her writing, dressing, eating, and reading adaptations. She practiced with her occupational therapist during a summer session, and then she presented her needs to her new teachers the day before school began. This increased her sense of control and improved her compliance with her adaptations. In addition, her family was committed to improving her independence and began involving Kayla in family chores. Chores selected by Kayla and her family included setting the table, dusting, vacuuming, and pet care. Kayla also worked with the occupational therapist to gain the skills to make her own lunch and to use the stove, oven, and dishwasher. This improved meaning and responsibility in her family role identity. In addition, the occupational therapist consulted with the family in assisting Kayla with the fine motor use of her cell phone. These skills increased to the point where Kayla began using her cell phone for programming numbers and emergency contacts. She also learned how to monitor her minutes and keep the phone costs within the billing plan. The use of the cell phone created new access to socialization outside of school and she became more involved in afterschool events.

Discounting and empowering: One issue that had emerged was that Kayla did not want to wear her ankle-foot orthotics (AFOs) and would come to school in mid–high-heeled shoes. This caused her to lose her balance and slip, to the point of its being dangerous. Through community events, the occupational therapists were able to help Kayla realize it was much safer to be comfortable and stable. The therapist was able to persuade Kayla to try some sports activities for people with disabilities. Kayla tried Special Olympics, and she excelled in horseback riding and swimming. School sports were discounted, and adapted sports were highlighted. This improved her community participation as well as her ADL and IADL skills as she traveled. The outcome was positive and reinforcing once she started winning medals. The school supported her by congratulating her over the intercom and displaying her ribbons and medals in a school trophy case.

Developing a disability identity[39]: Kayla's occupational therapist was able to arrange for her to visit Jim, an occupational therapist colleague who had cerebral palsy. Kayla, her mother, and the occupational therapist visited Jim at his outpatient clinic. Kayla watched him work doing hand therapy and conversed easily with him and his client. Jim talked about his wife and two children and how he really learned about independence by going to an Easter Seals camp when he was about her age. He talked about choosing hand therapy because he felt that he could not perform mobility-based occupational therapy. He talked about being a better

Continued

CASE STUDY 17-1   Kayla—cont'd

INTERVENTION STRATEGIES—CONT'D

therapist because clients respected his own disability experience. Kayla and Jim continued to e-mail each other after that visit. Kayla confided to the occupational therapist that she asked him about things she would not discuss with others. Kayla also tried a monthly group for young women with physical disabilities. She found that group "too old and too disabled" and chose not to return. The role modeling motivated Kayla to work on her IADL skills as she envisioned a more independent future.

Sexuality and body image: Kayla's physical development during adolescence provided opportunities for the occupational therapist and Kayla to problem-solve the logistical problems and wonderful opportunities of becoming a woman. Her mother helped her find fashionable clothing that was functional for her to put on independently. She decided to cut her hair stylishly short, because it was difficult to take care of her long hair. The occupational therapy assistant was male and they developed a nice relationship as he appropriately complimented her on her looks and teased her about boys. The occupational therapist consulted with Kayla's mother about talking about sexuality. These natural, dynamic, and developmental techniques supported her IADL skills of self-care and independent living.

Exclusive and inclusive programming: As mentioned earlier, Kayla attended the Special Olympics two to three times a year and went to Easter Seals Camp in the summer for 2 weeks. This was a huge move in the development of independence and disability identity. The occupational therapist also made sure that she continued to participate in school-based activities and she was involved in the school play. Academic support was added that included more small-group learning. In the small groups, Kayla was granted the time with assignments to effectively use her adapted computer and keep work output at a reasonable pace. With more support and a more reasonable pace, Kayla's frustration decreased and her school success increased. She improved in her written communication and numerical abilities when engaged in community activities where these skills were necessary.

Developing a future vision: The local college added a group home–based dormitory that helped college students with

disabilities. Kayla, her occupational therapist, and her family discussed an article about the dorm, and Kayla was very interested; in fact, her aunt was attending that college. Kayla understood that she might always need assistance but could live an interdependent life. She became more tolerant of her education technician's assistance and they developed good communication about how and when to assist. She began to take more initiative in her ADLs and IADLs in the home environment. In collaboration with the occupational therapist, she organized her bedroom, began a filing system that was large and open to accommodate her fine motor needs, and began online banking with her adapted computer.

Community mobility: Occupational therapy practitioners arranged for Kayla, her family, and team members to attend a wheelchair clinic, and she was prescribed a scooter for community mobility. She also had a technology consultation to ensure that her academic technological support was as strong as it could be. These were important steps in establishing her capacity to participate in the community. Kayla again began to thrive.

Outcomes: Individual education program goal areas of community participation, improved independence, and disability identity increased 100% as measured by the educational team. After occupational therapy consultation, the aide in the classroom, although still needed for adaptive assignments and programming, took a less central role and covered the needs of children other than Kayla. Through interviewing and self-assessment, Kayla listed the most significant strategies to her success as her time at summer camp, Special Olympics, and establishment of the mentorship with the occupational therapist with cerebral palsy. She indicated that she felt more in control of her life and more positive about the future. Kayla's family also reported positive outcomes from the comprehensive intervention plan that addressed IADLs and community participation, noting that their perception of Kayla's future had shifted toward more independence. Kayla's IADL skills in home management, telephone/cell phone use, money management, food preparation, shopping, social interaction, and community mobility had improved along with her confidence, self-determination, and positive disability identity.

---

part of participation in everyday activities" (p. 261).[34] The contextual approach suggests that occupational therapy practitioners facilitate IADL and community participation by creating accessible contexts for performance. They advocate for the creation of niches or small communities that foster development of roles, patterns, and skills. The use of therapy techniques in the context of real experiences and natural environments is more valuable and essential to the generalization and transfer of these skills. Emphasis on the natural physical and social contexts can enhance children's development by giving them observation, imitation, and practice opportunities (Case Study 17-2). Approaches that build on natural contexts are described next.

Reverse Inclusion

Instead of including one child with a disability into a program designed for the skill level of typical children, reverse inclusion brings typical children into a program designed for children with special needs. This has been an effective technique to improve age-appropriate behaviors and social skills targeted in the goals and objectives of youth with disability.[70] In reverse inclusion, typical peers are brought into occupational therapy groups, special recreation, adapted physical education, and other avenues. Benefits have been documented both for typical peers serving as role models and for youth with disability.[70]

TABLE 17-2 Adapted Instrumental Activities of Daily Living

Common Client-Based Challenges	Adaptive Strategies	Application
PHYSICAL CHALLENGES		
Decreased range of motion	Position for limited motion Change the task Provide assistance or interdependence	Write a check Provide stable seating and position hand on inclined tabletop Use online banking Have joint checking account
Decreased strength, endurance, and/or functional mobility	Use work simplification/energy conservation techniques Consider time management to work in small chunks of time Use modern energy-saving devices Plan out tasks to maximize energy	Shop Use a scooter or cart Determine best time of day and shop in small increments of time Use a reacher or other device Pay using debit card Plan with list and determine most efficient route in store
Decreased hand function	Build up utensils or use adapted equipment Use universal cuff or other grip substitute Buy pre-cut or prepared items or energy-saving devices	Prepare a meal Use proper equipment Slide items if necessary Use scissors or devices for opening prepared foods Buy items that are pre-prepared
COGNITIVE CHALLENGES		
Safety awareness	Develop strict rules and reinforce them Use of equipment such as wire gloves when cutting in the kitchen Use of a "buddy system" Have a safety plan	Use the bus system Follow directions Travel with a friend Learn bus etiquette including making sure the bus is stopped before entering Alert the driver to safety needs Have an emergency phone
Difficulty with judgment and decision making	Provide an outline or structure to planning Role-play outcomes of decisions Decrease impulsivity through use of strategies such as counting before acting Budget money	Go on an outing Plan the outing Budget money needs Role-play possible social scenarios, including a sexual advance from a stranger (use the Circles Program—described in text discussion of sexuality and body image) Identify possible scenarios for decision making
Decreased overall cognitive ability	Simplify tasks Simplify instructions or use pictures Repeat needed information Present information in small steps—have the client practice	Cook Choose prepared foods Simplify directions by using pictures Keep kitchen organized with pictures on cabinets Work in small groups with small steps to the task—reinforce needed concepts
PSYCHOSOCIAL CHALLENGES		
Difficulty engaging in social communication	Use scripted language Role play	Go to a movie Script and practice asking for a ticket and stating the name of the show Work with asking for popcorn and managing the conversation and money
Behavioral outbursts	Structured routine Positive behavioral supports Reinforcement system for positive behavior	Money management Review finances at a prescribed weekly time

Continued

TABLE 17-2 Adapted Instrumental Activities of Daily Living—Cont'd

Common Client-Based Challenges	Adaptive Strategies	Application
	Relaxation techniques	Set up a reinforcement system to review finances without outburst
		Use breathing techniques for relaxation
Anxiety	Preparation ahead of time	Personal grooming
	Role play	Shave (face; legs), put on deodorant/make-up
	Relaxation techniques	Set up a routine
	Sensory diet (if applicable)	Provide tactile brushing before shaving
		Use guided imagery during grooming
Overly friendly or flirtatious behavior	Use Circles Program to learn proper boundaries	Go to a dance
	Reinforcement for positive behavior	Review Circles Program
	Role-play appropriate behavior	Plan clothing
	Monitor clothing	Social stories to reinforce safe and appropriate behavior
		Sexual education at client's level

Adapted from Kieckhefer, G. M. (2002). *Foundations for successful transition: Shared management as one critical component.* Keynote presentation at the Hospital for Sick Children, Toronto, Canada.

CASE STUDY 17-2   Brenda

Brenda is an experienced school-based occupational therapist. Her practice has evolved to include a group of children with disabilities in the middle and high schools. Brenda has a large caseload and has provided services to these middle school students for many years. She knows the children very well and has a positive relationship with the families. After many transition plans for her middle school students, Brenda is thinking more from the contextual approach and has decided to write goals that target IADL skills, independent or interdependent living, and community participation including prevocational skills.

In collaboration with the speech therapist, Brenda designed a program for a life skills group. This group began with kitchen tasks, where students planned, implemented, and worked together. She implemented safety rules and supervision and targeted the unique needs of each of the four students involved. Brenda designed the kitchen program to meet each student's client factor needs. Randy, a boy with muscular dystrophy, needed adaptations for his physical disabilities; Amanda, a girl with autism, required scripting to communicate with others; Troy, a youth with mental retardation and associated behavioral problems, was assisted by use of a behavioral report card; and Susan, a girl with intellectual disability, followed recipes through a picture-based cookbook. The cooking group required planning and supervision to meet the individual needs of each student as the various IADL skills (e.g., planning a meal; shopping; safe use of cutting utensils; following a recipe; use of the stove, oven, and dishwasher; and safe handling and storage of food) were developed by each youth.

In addition, working as a team, communication, social skills, hygiene, table manners, and polite eating were enhanced in the kitchen group participants.

The kitchen group that planned, shopped, prepared, and sold lunches to the school community worked so well that Brenda and the team of students decided to add a greenhouse to the middle school. The group learned about working and caring for plants. They traveled to a greenhouse and performed prevocational activities with a local farmer. They chose the plant varieties and followed directions to help the plants grow in their own greenhouse. This evolved into a school and community sale in which the students gained the IADL skills of pricing items, budgeting, and managing money. The greenhouse program also assisted with communication skills. The students took great pride in their accomplishments. With input from the students, school team, and parent volunteers, Brenda now plans to add a cottage industry of making greeting cards with photographs and stamping. The students find great meaning in these activities, and their IADL skills have improved significantly. In addition, the school community has embraced these endeavors, and the students have improved their self-esteem and future visions of success.

Therapy becomes identity building when therapists provide environments that help persons explore possible selves and achieve success in tasks that are instrumental to identities they strive to achieve, and when it enables them to validate the identities that they have worked hard to achieve in the past (p. 55).[12]

Supported Inclusion

Young people with disability can be supported in natural environments through the use of assistants, peer partners, and educated classmates. To promote participation supported inclusion usually requires adapted coursework and activities that are consistent with the physical and cognitive abilities of the client.

Family Activities

Occupational therapy practitioners can consult with families regarding ways to include young people with disabilities in family leisure and household activities. This facilitates skills and helps the youth to develop a family role through productive participation in home management and caring for others.[15] Use of the landline telephone and cell phone, health management, money management and access skills, safe interaction with strangers, and use of public transportation systems are IADL skills that often are learned in the home. Families may need the assistance of occupational therapy services to recognize the need for the youth to achieve these milestones and to adapt these skills to the level of the youth.

Community Participation

Occupational therapy practitioners should advocate for increased community participation for children and youth through shopping, attending school or community events, recreational activities, and/or other avenues of involvement. They can consult with the family and teachers on strategies to facilitate the child's use of the telephone, money management, and accessing public transportation. The practitioner can challenge the youth's physical, cognitive, and social skills through incremental, planned activities in the school and community.

Many IADL and community participation skills are dynamic, complex, and multistep activities, such as cooking, doing laundry, shopping, childcare, and accessing transportation. These tasks are further developed when they are applied in a context that holds meaning for the client. Therefore, finding a task that is meaningful and social and serves a purpose of importance to society will enhance performance. This can be done through cottage industries, whereby the adolescents create and sell merchandise, establish a work-based role, or plan and implement an outing, party, or celebration.

Client-Centered Ecological/Experiential

Emergent literature supports self-determination through development of self-image, independent living skills, problem-solving, and active involvement of youth.[76] These researchers advocate for inclusive services that are strength based, widely accessible, and give adolescents opportunities to succeed. Examples of this type of programming are the Community Capacity-Building project, which provided a forum that brought together clients, families, and community stakeholders to increase communication and opportunities,[86] and an occupational therapy program that created a "Life Skills Institute" as a comprehensive framework to support youth with disabilities and their families transition into adult services.[25]

Self-determination can be facilitated through improvement of life skills, social skills, and academics.[76] Facilitating positive changes to the client's physical appearance through use of make-up, jewelry, or fashionable clothing can also promote IADL skills and self-empowerment. Involvement in school-based, recreational, and/or Special Olympics sports or athletics can improve skills, participation, and socialization.[47] Enhancing and facilitating positive peer relationships and roles using psychosocial approaches is a necessary part of any IADL intervention plan. Davidson and Fitzgerald advocate for a client-centered approach that includes beginning realistic career exploration early and addressing all areas of adult independence.[14]

Discounting and empowering are complementary strategies to address empowerment needs in aspects of the client's life. Discounting, or reframing, is a technique that redefines a disability in terms of what a person can do versus what he cannot do.[28,41,50] For example, Evans, McDougall, and Baldwin found that participation of youth with disabilities in many community-based activities without regard to performance fostered development of relationships and social behaviors.[18] These workers found that community participation correlated with employment and self-determination. Reframing can be applied to other areas that may be difficult for a child or adolescent to succeed in (e.g., sports and other physical activities). Placing less importance on one area may close the gap between values and perceived competence, a key element to self-esteem and self-identity.

Focus on Ability and Success

For clients who have spent years listening to their areas of deficit, emphasizing their assets and abilities is essential as they become adolescents. Changing the context from one in which the adolescent client always struggles to one in which he or she can succeed is key to this strategy.[34] For instance, cooking may be an area in which clients with cerebral palsy or other physical impairment have difficulty. Beginning an IADL session with a safe and physically simple task such as dusting may lead to greater success. The adolescent can be encouraged to compare himself or herself to other adolescents with similar disabilities, instead of with typically developing peers. The Special Olympics camps for children with special needs or support groups are places in which adolescents can experience more success and less competition. Inclusion within the community is positive, but it is also important to establish esteem and disability identity with like peers in adolescence.[39]

Incorporation of Sexuality and Body Image

Adolescents are developing physically and psychologically, and occupational therapists support these positive moves toward adulthood. Noticing and appreciating the growth, changes, new interests, moves toward independence, and physical attractiveness can help build self-esteem in children and adolescents. Comments about growth and positive changes can be incorporated into personal care, because both male and female clients may have new personal hygiene needs as well as the desire to dress and groom themselves differently.

It is important to understand that adolescents with disabilities experience the same hormonal changes as in typical adolescents and perhaps have more questions about what these changes may bring. Families often struggle as their child with a disability becomes a sexual being. The occupational therapist has a key role in addressing this area of occupational performance and these typical aspects of adolescent development.[64] One way to accomplish this is to establish clear boundaries for this population, recognized to be vulnerable to sexual abuse.[64] The "Circles Program" facilitates the establishment of physical boundaries for adolescents with developmental disabilities.[75] By teaching safe relationships, appropriate personal space, and sexuality to adolescents with developmental challenges, it is a concrete way of showing clients with intellectual disability how close to let people into their personal space. The concepts of personal space are taught with actual circles around the client: the closest circle indicates the space of closeness with family, the middle circle at forearm length indicates friends, and a wider circle of a full arm's length is taught for keeping personal space between the youth and acquaintances and strangers.[75]

Mentoring and Role-Modeling a Positive Future

Many youth with disabilities do not know what their future might hold. Addressing possible avenues for prevocational and vocational programming, as well as independent living, enables these clients to see a hopeful and positive future. Inclusion has caused many children to be separated from role models with similar disabling conditions. Whenever possible, youth with disabilities need exposure to role models of adults with disability working and thriving in the community. Visiting work sites and group homes can help youth with disabilities and their families form a positive future vision.[25,86]

The use of mentors or positive role models for IADL and community participation skill development is an intervention strategy that can be effectively used to help the youth with disability gain perspective and increase positive self-regard.[2] The adolescent client may also serve as a mentor for others by assisting in a younger classroom, tutoring students in simple reading or math subjects, or bringing cookies to elders in the community. An adolescent can be encouraged to mentor a younger child with a similar disability. A mentoring program that pairs a successful adult from the community with an adolescent with a similar disability can also help to increase the adolescent's confidence.[2] Peer and cross-age tutoring in reading or other academic tasks can assist with positive role identity and improve behavior in youth with disability.[2]

Inclusive Programming for Youth with Disabilities

With the emphasis and importance placed on inclusion, we must seek to have other avenues to provide children and adolescents with experiences with other people with similar abilities. Individualized and person-centered programming such as Special Olympics, specialized summer camp experiences, handicapped ski programs, adaptive sports, support groups, and other avenues should be explored to help the adolescent client develop a disability identity.[39,76] Bedell and colleagues emphasize the importance of creating opportunities for learning daily tasks and social skills for school-aged children with brain injuries.[7] These authors advocate for involvement of parents in creating opportunities in the community to teach skills for regulation of cognitive and behavioral function within the context of daily life occupations.[7]

Social Skills Training

Bedell and colleagues suggest that, in the context of daily life, adolescents with acquired brain injuries are more impaired by social behavior and cognitive issues than by movement-related impairment.[7] Bedell also stresses the importance of close friends and extracurricular activities as a hallmark of resilient children.[6] Support for psychosocial development has been identified as critical to success for adolescents with physical and cognitive/behavioral disabilities.[58,76]

The main purpose of social skills training is to increase communication and participation in the community. Limitations in the youth's ability to socially participate (e.g., communication skills, problem solving, recognizing feelings) can be identified, addressed, and improved. Social skills training can be done one on one through practicing case scenarios or in an inclusion setting with the entire class to address peer relationships. These are IADL and community processes and can be included in these milieus.

Support Groups

Groups that consist of like participants—those of a similar age and disability—can be a useful strategy. Creating community connections for support is an important transition component to adulthood for youth with disabilities.[86] Creation of networks that include parents, teachers, therapists, and community agencies can facilitate and support the process of transition to adulthood for clients with disability.[86] If this cannot be accomplished logistically, virtual support groups and websites can be helpful, so long as the adolescent is monitored while online.

SUMMARY

Occupational therapy practice encompasses the complex process of IADLs and community participation in the lives of children, youth, and their family/support systems. Through the occupational therapy process of assessment, evaluation, intervention, and outcomes analysis, the occupational therapy practitioner uses critical thinking to facilitate IADL skills and community participation into practice. Occupational development is unique to each individual and should be used as a foundation to address the roles, interests, level of independence/interdependence, and quest for meaningful and productive living in clients across settings. As the child/youth develops maturity and skills, the role of parents, professionals, and the youth themselves also evolves. See Table 17-3 for the developmental role continuum.

TABLE 17-3 The Developmental Role Continuum

Stages	Occupational Therapy Practitioner or Other Professional	Parent/Family	Young Person
Late adolescence	Resource for future planning and implementation of adult roles, routines, and community participation	Consultant to youth; supports and guides decisions. Ensures a safety net.	The youth leads and supervises the program through self-determination.
Early adolescence	Consultant for school success, community participation, vocational programming, empowering client, advocacy, transition and family planning	Supervises and monitors program, advocates for the child/youth. Implements IADL and community programming.	Active involvement in direction, plan, and method of programming. Input is given and received. Independence and advocacy are facilitated.
Middle childhood	School- or community-based intervention for education and life skills	Manages and monitors education program. Begins chores and roles in the home.	Participates in program and intervention planning.
Early childhood	Direct intervention and support to child and family	Provides care and makes decisions.	Receives care and follows directions.

REFERENCES

1. American Occupational Therapy Association. (2008). Occupational therapy practice framework: Domain and process. (2nd ed.). *The American Journal of Occupational Therapy, 62,* 609–639.
2. Anderson, L. B. (2007). A special kind of tutor. Professional development and classroom activities for teachers. *Teaching prek-8, 37*(5). Retrieved June 13, 2008, from http://www.teachingk-8.com
3. Andrén, E., & Grimby, G. (2004). Activity limitations in personal, domestic and vocational tasks: A study of adults with inborn and early acquired mobility disorders. *Disability and Rehabilitation, 26,* 262–271.
4. Aviles, A., & Helfrich, C. (2004). Life skill service needs: Perspectives of homeless youth. *Journal of Youth and Adolescence, 33,* 331–338.
5. Barnhart, R. C. (2001). Aging adult children with developmental disabilities and their families: Challenges for occupational therapists and physical therapists. *Physical and Occupational Therapy in Pediatrics, 21*(4), 69–81.
6. Bedell, G. M. (2004). Developing a follow-up survey focused on participation of children and youth with acquired brain injuries after discharge from inpatient rehabilitation. *NeuroRehabilitation, 19,* 191–205.
7. Bedell, G. M., Cohn, E. S., & Dumas, H. M. (2005). Exploring parents' use of strategies to promote social participation of school-aged children with acquired brain injury. *American Journal of Occupational Therapy, 59,* 273–284.
8. Bedell, G. M., & Dumas, H. M. (2004). Social participation of children and youth with acquired brain injuries discharged from inpatient rehabilitation: A follow-up study. *Brain Injury, 18,* 65–82.
9. Blackorby, J., & Wagner, M. (1996). Longitudinal postschool outcomes of youth with disabilities: Findings from the National Longitudinal Study of Youth. *Exceptional Children, 62,* 399–413.
10. Bowes, J. M., Flanagan, C., & Taylor, A. J. (2001). Adolescents' ideas about individual and social responsibility in relation to children's household work: Some international comparisons. *International Journal of Behavioral Development, 25,* 60–68.
11. Chandler, B. E., Schoonover, J., Clark, G. F., & Jackson, L. L. (2008). The magnificent mundane. *School System Special Interest Section Quarterly, 15*(1), 1–4.

12. Christiansen, C. H. (1999). Defining lives: Occupation as identity: An essay on competence, coherence and creation of meaning. *The American Journal of Occupational Therapy, 53,* 547–558.
13. Conaboy, K. S., Davis, N. M., Myers, C., Nochajski, S., Sage, J., Schefkind, S., et al. (2008). *FAQ: Occupational therapy's role in transition services and planning.* Bethesda, MD: American Occupational Therapy Association.
14. Davidson, D. A., & Fitzgerald, L. (2001). Transition planning for students. *OT Practice, September 17.* Bethesda, MD: American Occupational Therapy Association.
15. Dunn, L. (2004). Validation of the CHORES: A measure of children's participation in household tasks. *Scandinavian Journal of Occupational Therapy, 11,* 179–190.
16. Dunn, L., Coster, W. J., Orsmond, G. I., & Cohn, E. S. (2009). Household task participation of children with and without attentional problems in household tasks. *Physical and Occupational Therapy in Pediatrics, 29,* 258–273.
17. Dunst, C. J., Bruder, M. B., Trivette, C. M., & Hamby, D. W. (2005). Young children's natural learning environments contrasting approaches to early childhood intervention indicate differential learning opportunities. *Psychological Reports, 96,* 231–234.
18. Evans, J., McDougall, J. & Baldwin, P. (2006). An evaluation of the "Youth En Route" program. *Physical & Occupational Therapy in Pediatrics, 26*(4), 63–87.
19. Feeney, T., Ylvisaker, M. (2006). Context-sensitive cognitive-behavioural supports for young children with TBI: a replication study. *Brain Injury, 20,* 629–645.
20. Field, S., Martin, J., Miller, R., Ward, M., & Wehmeyer, M. L. (1998). *A practical guide for teaching self-determination.* Reston, VA: Council for Exceptional Children.
21. Fiese, B. H., Tomcho, T. J., Douglas, M., Josephs, K., Poltrock, S., & Baker, T. (2002). A review of 50 years of naturally occurring family routines and rituals: Cause for celebration? *Journal of Family Psychology, 16,* 381–390.
22. Fisher, A. G. (2003). *Assessment of motor and process skills: Vol. 1. Development, standardization, and administration manual* (5th ed.). Fort Collins, CO: Three Star Press.
23. Fisher, A. G. (2003). *Assessment of motor and process skills: Vol. 2. User manual* (5th ed.). Fort Collins, CO: Three Star Press.
24. Forness, S. R., Serna, L. A., Nielsen, E., Lambros, K., Hale, M. J., & Kavale, K. A. (2000). A model for early detection and primary

prevention of emotional or behavioral disorders. *Education & Treatment of Children, 23*(3), 325–345.

25. Gall, C., Kingsnorth, S., & Healy, H. (2006). Growing up ready: A shared management approach. *Physical & Occupational Therapy in Pediatrics, 26*(4), 47–62.

26. Gallimore, R., Goldenberg, C. N., & Weisner, T. (1993). The social construction and subjective reality of activity settings: Implications for community psychology. *American Journal of Community Psychology, 21,* 537–559.

27. Giangreco, M., Clonger, C., & Iverson, V. (1997). *Choosing options and accommodations for children (COACH)* (2nd ed.). Baltimore: Brookes.

28. Gill, C. J., Kewman, D. G., & Brannon, R. W. (2003). Transforming psychological practice and society: Policies that reflect the new paradigm. *American Psychologist, 58,* 305–332.

29. Glidden, L. M., & Jobe, B. M. (2007). Measuring parental daily rewards and worries in the transition to adulthood. *American Journal on Mental Retardation, 112,* 275–278.

30. Gol, D., & Jarus, T. (2005). Effect of a social skills training group on everyday activities for children with attention-deficit-hyperactivity disorder. *Developmental Medicine & Child Neurology, 47,* 539–545.

31. Goodnow, J. J. & Delaney, S. (1989). Children's household work. Task differences, styles of assignment, and links to family relationships. *Journal of Applied Development Psychology, 10,* 209–226.

32. Healy, H., & Rigby, P. (1999). Promoting independence for teens and young adults with physical disabilities. *Canadian Journal of Occupational Therapy, 66,* 240–249.

33. Hillier, A., Fish, T., Cloppert, P., & Beversdorf, D. Q. (2007). Outcomes of a social and vocational skills support group for adolescents and young adults on the autism spectrum. *Focus on Autism and Other Developmental Disabilities, 22,* 107–115.

34. Humphry, R., & Wakeford, L. (2006). An occupation-centered discussion of development and implications for practice. *American Journal of Occupational Therapy, 60,* 258–267.

35. Jinnah, H. A., & Stoneman, Z. (2008). Parents' experiences in seeking child care for school age children with disabilities—where does the system break down? *Children and Youth Services Review, 30,* 967–977.

36. Johnson, D. R. (2007). Challenges of secondary education and transition services for youth with disabilities. Impact: The Institute of Community Integration. Retrieved September 9, 2007, from http://iciumnedu/products/impact/163/overs.html

37. Johnson, D. R., Stodden, R. A., Emanuel, E. J., Luecking, R., & Mack, M. (2002). Current challenges facing secondary education and transition services: What research tells us. *Exceptional Children, 68,* 519–531.

38. Keller, J., Kafkes, A.; Basu, S., Federico, J., & Kielhofner, G. (2005). *Child Occupational Self Assessment (COSA), version 2.1.* Chicago: MOHO Clearinghouse.

39. Kielhofner, G. (2005). Rethinking disability and what to do about it: Disability studies and its implications for occupational therapy. *The American Journal of Occupational Therapy, 59,* 487–496.

40. Kielhofner, G. (2008). *Model of human occupation: Theory and application* (4th ed.). Philadelphia: Lippincott Williams & Wilkins.

41. Kinavey, C. (2006). Explanatory models of self-understanding in adolescents born with spina bifida. *Qualitative Health Research, 16,* 1091–1107.

42. King, G., Law, M., Hanna, S., King, S., Hurley, P., Rosenbaum, P., et al. (2006). Predictors of the leisure and recreation participation of children with physical disabilities: A structural equation modeling analysis. *Children's Health Care, 35*(3), 209–234.

43. King, G., Law, M., King, S., Rosenbaum, P., Kertoy, M., & Young, N. (2003). A conceptual model of the factors affecting the recreation and leisure participation of children with disabilities. *Physical and Occupational Therapy in Pediatrics, 23*(1), 63–90.

44. Kingsnorth, S., Healy, H., & Macarthur, C. (2007). Preparing for adulthood: A systematic review of life skill programs for youth with physical disabilities. *Journal of Adolescent Health, 41,* 323–332.

45. Law, M., Petrenchik, T., King, G., & Hurley, P. (2007). Perceived environmental barriers to recreational, community, and school participation for children and youth with physical disabilities. *Archives of Physical Medicine & Rehabilitation, 88,* 1636–1642.

46. Lemon, K., Hines, A. M., & Merdinger, J. (2005). From foster care to young adulthood: The role of independent transition programs in supporting successful transitions. *Children and Youth Services Review, 27,* 251–270.

47. Loukas, K. M., & Cote, T. (2005). Sports as occupation. *OT Practice, March 21.* Bethesda, MD: American Occupational Therapy Association.

48. Magill, J., & Hurlbut, N. L. (1986). The self-esteem of adolescents with cerebral palsy. *The American Journal of Occupational Therapy, 40,* 402–407.

49. Massinga, R., & Pecora, P. J. (2004). Providing better opportunities for older children in the welfare system [Electronic version]. *Future of Children, 14*(1), 150–173.

50. Mayberry, W. (1990). Self-esteem in children: Considerations for measurement and intervention. *The American Journal of Occupational Therapy, 44,* 729–734.

51. Michaels, C. A., & Orentlicher, M. L. (2004). The role of occupational therapy in providing person centered transition services: Implications for school based practice. *Occupational Therapy International, 11*(4), 209–228.

52. Mihaylov, S. I., Jarvis, S. N., Colver, A. F., & Beresford, B. (2004). Identification and description of factors that influence participation of children with cerebral palsy. *Developmental Medicine and Child Neurology, 46,* 299–304.

53. Moore, K. A., Chalk, R., Scarpa, J., & Vandivere, S. (2002). Family strengths: Often overlooked, but real. *Child Trends Research Brief,* 1–8.

54. Nollan, K. A., Wolf, M., Ansell, D., Burns, J.Barr, L., Copeland, L., et al. (2000). Ready or not: Assessing youth's preparedness for independent living. *Child Welfare, 79*(2), 159–176.

55. Noreau, L., Lepage, C., Boissiere, L., Picard, R., Fougeyrollas, P., Mathieu, J., et al. (2007). Measuring participation in children with disabilities using the Assessment of Life Habits. *Developmental Medicine & Child Neurology, 49,* 666–671.

56. Orentlicher, M. L., & Michaels, C. A. (2000). Some thoughts of the role of occupational therapy in the transition from school to adult life: Part I. *Developmental Disabilities Special Interest Section Quarterly, 7*(2), 1–4.

57. Orentlicher, M. L., & Michaels, C. A. (2000). Some thoughts of the role of occupational therapy in the transition from school to adult life: Part II. *Developmental Disabilities Special Interest Section Quarterly, 7*(3), 1–4.

58. Orsmond, G. I., Krauss, M. M., & Seltzer, K. K. (2004). Peer relationships and social and recreational activities among adolescents and adults with autism. *Journal of Autism and Developmental Disorders, 34,* 245–256.

59. Palmer, S., & Wehmeyer, M. (2003). Promoting self-determination in early elementary school. *Remedial and Special Education, 24,* 115–126.

60. Parish, S. L., & Cloud, J. M. (2006). Child care for low-income school-age children: Disability and family structure effects in a national sample. *Children and Youth Services Review, 28,* 927–940.

61. Peloquin, S. M. (2006). Occupations: Strands of coherence in a life. *The American Journal of Occupational Therapy, 60,* 236–239.

62. Polatajko, H. J., & Mandich, A. (2005). Cognitive orientation to daily occupational performance with children with developmental coordination disorder. In N. Katz (Ed.), *Cognition and occupation*

across the life span (2nd ed., pp. 237–260). Bethesda, MD: American Occupational Therapy Association Press.

63. Poulsen, A. A., Rodger, S., & Ziviani, J. M. (2006). Understanding children's motivation from a self-determination perspective: Implications for practice. *Australian Occupational Therapy Journal, 53*(2), 78–86.

64. Preston, L., & Lewin, J. E. (2006). Understanding issues of sexuality and privacy for individuals with developmental disabilities. *OT Practice, 11*(22), CE1–CE8, Bethesda, MD: American Occupational Therapy Association.

65. Richardson, P. (2003). From roots to wings: Social participation for children with physical disabilities. *Developmental Disabilities Special Interest Section Quarterly, 26*(1), 1–4.

66. Rodger, S. (2006). I can do it: Developing, promoting, and managing children's self-care needs. In S. Rodger & J. Ziviani (Eds.), *Occupational therapy with children* (pp. 200–221). Oxford, UK: Blackwell Publishing.

67. Rodger, S., Ireland, S., & Vun, M. (2008). Can Cognitive Orientation to daily Occupational Performance (CO-OP) help children with Asperger's syndrome to master social and organizational goals? *British Journal of Occupational Therapy, 71*(1), 23–32.

68. Rogoff, B. (2003). *The cultural nature of human development.* Oxford, UK: Oxford University Press.

69. Savage, S. L., & Gauvain, M. (1998). Parental beliefs and children's everyday planning in European-American and Latino families. *Journal of Applied Developmental Psychology, 19,* 319–340.

70. Schoger, K. D. (2006). Reverse inclusion: Providing peer social interactions opportunities to students placed in self-contained special education classrooms. *TEACHING Exceptional Children Plus, 2*(6), Article 3. Retrieved September 8, 20008 from http://escholarship.bc.edu/education/tecplus/vol2/iss6/art3

71. Shogren, K. A., & Turnbull, A. P. (2006). Promoting self-determination in young children with disabilities: The critical role of families. *Infants & Young Children, 19,* 338–352.

72. Simons, D. (2005). Adolescent development. In A. Cronin & M. B. Mandich (Eds.), *Human development & performance* (pp. 216–246). Clifton Park, NY: Thomson Delmar Learing.

73. Sparrow, S., Balla, D., & Cicchetti, D. (2005). *Vineland Adaptive Behavior Scales II.* Circle Pines, MN: American Guidance Services.

74. Spence, S. H. (2003). Social skills training with children and young people: Theory, evidence and practice. *Child & Adolescent Mental Health, 8,* 84–96.

75. Stanfield, J. (2007). *James Stanfield catalogue: Special education, school to life transitions, conflict resolution and violence prevention.* Santa Barbara, CA: James Stanfield.

76. Stewart, D., Stavness, C., King, G., Antle, B., & Law, M. (2006). A critical appraisal of literature reviews about the transition to adulthood for youth with disabilities. *Physical & Occupational Therapy in Pediatrics, 26,* (4), 5–24.

77. Taylor, R. R. (2008). *The intentional relationship: Occupational therapy and use of self.* Philadelphia: F.A. Davis.

78. Turnbull, & Turnbull. (2001). Self-determination for individuals with significant cognitive disabilities and their families. *Journal of the Association for Persons with Severe Handicaps, 26,* 56–62.

79. Van Zelst, B., Miller, M., Russo, R., Murchland, S., & Crotty, M. (2006). Activities of daily living in children with hemiplegic cerebral palsy: a cross-sectional evaluation using the Assessment of Motor and Process Skills. *Developmental Medicine & Child Neurology, 48,* 723–727.

80. Wagner, M., Cameto, R., & Newman, L. (2003). *Youth with disabilities: A changing population. A report of findings from the National Longitudinal Transition Study (NLTS) and the National Longitudinal Transitions Study-2 (NLTS2).* Menlo Park, CA: SRI International.

81. Wehmeyer, M. L., Sands, D. J., & Doll, B. (1997). The development of self-determination and implications for educational interventions with students with disabilities. *International Journal of Disability, Development, and Education, 44,* 305–328.

82. Wehmeyer, M. L., & Palmer, S. B. (2003). Adult outcomes for students with cognitive disabilities three years after high school: The impact of self-determination. *Education and Training in Developmental Disabilities, 38,* 131–144.

83. Wehmeyer, M. L., & Schwartz, M. (1997). Self-determination and positive adult outcomes: A follow-up study of youth with mental retardation or learning disabilities. *Exceptional Children, 63,* 245–255.

84. White, L. K., & Brinkerhoff, D. B. (1981). Children's work in the family: Its significance and meaning. *Journal of Marriage and the Family, 43,* 789–798.

85. World Health Organization. (2007). *International classification of functioning: Child and Youth Version (ICF-CY).* Geneva: Author.

86. Wynn, K., Stewart, D., Law, M., Burke-Gaffney, J., & Moning, T. (2006). Creating connections: A community capacity-building project with parent and youth with disabilities in transition to adulthood. *Physical & Occupational Therapy in Pediatrics, 26*(4), 89–103.

87. Zhang, D. (2005). Parent practices in facilitating self-determination skills: The influences of culture, socioeconomic status, and children's special education status. *Research & Practice for Persons with Severe Disabilities, 30*(3), 154–162.

18 Play

Susan H. Knox

Play forms
Play functions
Play meanings
Playfulness
Play assessments
Constraints to play

Play as a treatment
   modality
Play as an intervention
   goal
Adaptations
Parent education

1. Describe the importance and relationship of play to occupational therapy.
2. Describe play theories in terms of form, function, meaning, and context.
3. Describe play assessments and determine their usefulness for assessment and treatment planning.
4. Describe environmental and individual qualities that facilitate or constrain play.
5. Describe how play is used in intervention.
6. Describe how occupational therapists can become advocates for play in our society.

Play . . . is the way the child learns what no one can teach him. It is the way he explores and orients himself to the actual world of space and time, of things, animals, structures, and people. Through play he learns to live in our symbolic world of meanings and values, of progressive striving for deferred goals, at the same time exploring and experimenting and learning in his own individualized way. Through play the child practices and rehearses endlessly the complicated and subtle patterns of human living and communication, which he must master if he is to become a participating adult in our social life (pp. v-vi).[45]

All children play, and it is through play that they learn about themselves and the world around them. Watching children play is like looking through a window into their very being. Play has been identified as one of the primary occupations in which people engage, according to the American Occupational Therapy Association (AOTA) Practice Framework.[3] As defined by Parham and Fazio, play is "any spontaneous or organized activity that provides enjoyment, entertainment, amusement or diversion" (p. 448) and is "an attitude or mode of experience that involves intrinsic motivation, emphasis on process rather than

product and internal rather than external control; an 'as-if' or pretend element; takes place in a safe, unthreatening environment with social sanctions" (p. 448).[87]

There are two sides of play: the science of play, in which play is a critical aspect of human development that deserves serious study, and the art of play, in which the therapist and the child are players, where there is joy, pleasure, and freedom. Occupational therapists need knowledge and skill in both aspects. This chapter describes play as the child's occupation from a historical perspective, discusses why play is important to occupational therapists, describes methods of assessing play, and discusses play in intervention.

PLAY THEORIES

Clark et al. defined occupations as "the chunks of culturally and personally meaningful activity in which humans engage" (p. 310).[31] People create or orchestrate their daily experiences through planning and participating in occupations.[114] Occupational therapy generally considers work, self-care, leisure, play, and rest to be the major occupations of people. Occupations can be explained through the substrates of form, function, meaning, and context.[31]

Play can be viewed through these substrates of occupation:
- As an activity having certain characteristics (i.e., its form, including motor skill requirements and products)
- As a developmental phenomenon contributing to a child's development and enculturation (i.e., its function, including purposes, processes, and experiences)
- As an experience or a state of mind (i.e., its meaning, including what motivates or satisfies the individual).

Play, like any other activity, takes place within context, which denotes the individual's environments and the personal, physical, and social elements of each environment.

Form

Many play theorists describe play as categories of activities in which children engage.[14,28,33,40] These include such activities as games, building and construction, social play, pretend, sensorimotor play, and symbolic or dramatic play. Children's play activities change over time and reflect their development.[14,83]

Sensorimotor and exploratory play predominate in infancy (Figure 18-1) as infants develop mastery over their own bodies and learn the effect of their actions upon objects and people in the environment.[90,100] Sensorimotor play peaks in the second year of life and then declines. Children continue to use sensory

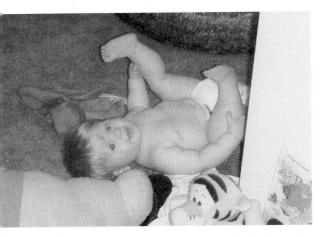

FIGURE 18-1   A first type of sensory motor-exploratory play is the infant's exploration of his or her own body. (Courtesy Dianne Koontz Lowman.)

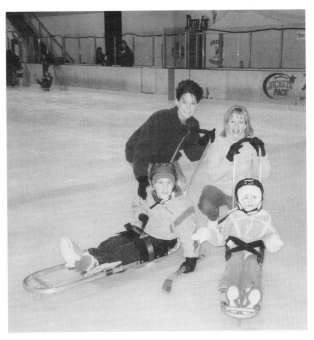

FIGURE 18-2   Play today is often highly structured; for example, this play date takes place at the ice-skating rink. (Courtesy Jill McQuaid.)

motor play when they learn new motor skills. Exploratory play begins in infancy, and by the end of the first year, infants actively explore their surroundings, demonstrate a beginning understanding of cause and effect, and are interested in how things work. In the second year, play centers on combining objects and learning their meaning. Children begin to classify objects and develop purpose in their actions. Exploratory play gradually declines through the preschool years, but it reappears when the child is learning new skills.[14]

Constructive play has identifiable outcomes and predominates during the preschool years as practice. Constructive play remains high during middle childhood and adolescence but becomes more abstract. It may develop into arts and crafts. Symbolic play and pretense develop at the end of the first year and through the second, peaking at around 5 years of age and evolving into dramatic and sociodramatic play. During middle childhood, symbolic play and fantasy play are seen in mental games, secret clubs, and daydreaming, and in language play such as riddles or secret codes.[14] Television, computer games, and movies are also ways of indulging in fantasy play.

Social play begins very early with interaction between the infant and mother, and by age 3, children are able to engage in complex social games. Children use role play to learn about social systems and cultural norms. Garvey described four types of roles seen in group play: (1) functional roles, such as pretending to be a doctor; (2) relational roles, such as pretending to be mother and baby; (3) character roles, such as those from television and movies; and (4) roles with no specific identity.[46] Social play combined with motor play develops into rough-and-tumble play.[14] Games with rules teach children to take turns and to initiate, maintain, and end social interactions.[59] This type of play predominates during the school-age years.[14,44] Social play and games with rules are particularly influenced by the culture. The physical environments available for play, peer groups, and the types of play encouraged by parents have changed as our society has become more urbanized.[83] Currently, time, places, and types of play are more planned and structured, such as with organized sports and "play dates" (Figure 18-2).[66]

Adolescents are concerned with autonomy and being socialized into adult roles. This is a period of transition as obligations, time available for play, changes and refinements of interests, family, and peer pressures all affect teen activity.[83] In a study by Csikszentmihalyi and Larson, the most frequent single activity of adolescents was socializing.[37] Second was television and third was sports, games, hobbies, reading, and music.

Another way to look at the forms of play is through their characteristics. Scholars of play have not identified a single characteristic common to all kinds of play but have suggested many qualities or characteristics of play that differentiate play from non-play. These characteristics include intrinsic motivation, suspension of reality, internal locus of control, and being spontaneous, fun, flexible, totally absorbing, vitalizing, an end in and of itself, non-literal, and challenging.[33,40,55,71,84,96] According to Rubin et al., play is characterized by the following traits: it (1) expresses intrinsic motivation and self-direction; (2) focuses on means rather than ends; (3) is organism-centered rather than object-centered; (4) is noninstrumental or symbolic; (5) shows freedom from externally imposed rules; and (6) reveals active engagement in the activity.[100] Takata defined the following principles of play: (1) it is a complex set of behaviors characterized by "fun"; (2) it involves sensory, neuromuscular, or mental processes; (3) it involves repetition of experience, exploration, experimentation, and imitation; (4) it proceeds within its own time and space boundaries; (5) it functions as an agent for integrating the internal and external worlds; and (6) it follows a sequential developmental progression.[109]

Function

Another way of looking at play is in relation to function, or how play influences adaptation. Play functions include processes, experiences, and purposes. Historically, play has been described as the way a child develops the skills necessary for life,[49,100] as a way of working off surplus energy,[102] or for recreation and relaxation.[100] Modern or contemporary theories emphasize the value of play in contributing to the child's development or to enculturation. They include using play to achieve optimal arousal[15,40] and develop ego function[41] and cognitive skills.[21,90,112] Sociocultural explanations include the development of social abilities,[88,106] role development,[96] and play's contribution to culture.[55,103] Johnson et al. identified three ways to consider play and development: (1) play reflects development; (2) play reinforces development; and (3) play is an instrument for developmental change.[59]

Miller and Kuhaneck conducted interviews on the perceptions of play experiences and play preferences in 10 children between the ages of 7 and 11.[78] The children described "fun" as the core category explaining their choices of play activities. The authors developed a dynamic model for play choice describing the interplay of four characteristics—child, activity, relational, and contextual—that affected the perception of fun.

Meaning

Play meaning refers to the quality of the experience or to a person's state of mind. The attitude a person assumes during play is usually termed playfulness. Liebermann felt that each person has an internal disposition to play that could be described along five dimensions: physical spontaneity, cognitive spontaneity, social spontaneity, manifest joy, and sense of humor.[72] Barnett[8,9] and Barnett and Kleiber[10,11] further related playfulness to the development of cognitive abilities. In the occupational therapy literature, Bundy defined the qualities of playfulness as a person's intrinsic motivation, internal control, and the ability to suspend reality.[23,24] These three elements are best regarded as a continuum, and "it is the sum contribution of these three elements that tips the balance toward play or nonplay, playfulness or nonplayfulness" (p. 219).[24] In addition to these three elements, children give and receive social cues to denote that they are playing.

Knox, in a qualitative study of preschool children's play, identified actions and behaviors that characterized playful children.[64] The playful children showed flexibility and spontaneity in their play and in social interactions, curiosity, imagination, creativity, joy, the ability to take charge of situations, the ability to build on and change the flow of play, and total absorption. Non-playful children were less flexible and had difficulty with transitions or changes, expressed negative or immature affect or speech, often withdrew either physically or emotionally from play sequences, did not have control over situations, and tended to prefer adults or younger children for play.

Blanche explored persons' motivations to engage in meaningful play and identified six motivations: (1) restoring a sense of well-being through quiet activity; (2) exposing oneself to novelty; (3) seeking short-term diversion through light-hearted spontaneous activity; (4) increasing the intensity of involvement in physically and/or mentally stimulating activity; (5) enjoying the ability to master an activity; and (6) creating novelty.[16] She suggested that these motivations can act as potential guides to treatment.

Context

Play also obtains meaning through context. Children's activities can never be isolated from the environment within which they are playing, nor from familial, social, and cultural

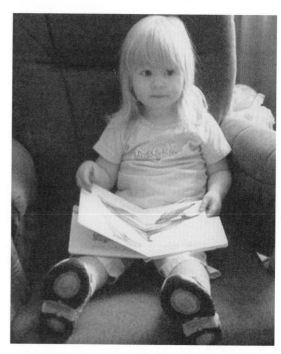

FIGURE 18-3 "Reading" books is an early play activity even before the child is able to actually read. (Courtesy Dianne Koontz Lowman.)

influences. The presence or absence of other persons, animals, the physical setting, and the availability of toys and other objects upon which to interact all have a profound effect on children's play (Figure 18-3). Play context includes cultural and societal expectations of play. Yerxa et al. stated, "The environment provides physical, psychological, social, cultural, and spiritual demands and resources" (p. 7).[114]

A number of authors have studied the effects of the environment, quality of care, and types of interactions between caregivers and children on play behavior.[11,14,54,58] They found that higher socioeconomic status correlated with greater levels of imaginary play, that permissive home environments encouraged creativity, and that high program quality improved children's social interaction and level of play. The variety of materials and opportunities for children to explore and interact with and their ability to control their activities were associated with improved quality of play. In addition, caregivers and peers who were emotionally and verbally responsive helped to improve the child's quality of play. Cultural and ecologic factors also influence the way children play.[59,100] The cultural factors include child-rearing and parental influences, peer experiences, the physical environment, the schools, and the media (Figure 18-4).[12,104] Ecologic influences on play include the effects of stimulus novelty on play, object and material influences, play space density, and indoor versus outdoor play space.

All environments offer affordances for and constraints to an individual's behavior. Knox[63] and Michelman[77] described factors in the environment that either promote or inhibit play. Factors that promote play include the availability of objects and persons, freedom from stress, provision of novelty, and opportunities to make choices. Factors that may inhibit play include external constraints, self-consciousness, too much novelty or challenge, limited choices, and over-competition.

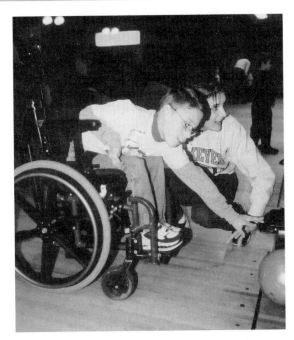

FIGURE 18-4   Mom's enthusiasm and encouragement add to the playfulness experienced in bowling. (Courtesy Jill McQuaid.)

Contextual components that appear to promote play include (1) familiar peers, toys, and other materials; (2) freedom of choice; (3) adults who are nonintrusive or directive; (4) safe and comfortable atmosphere; and (5) scheduling that avoids times of fatigue, hunger, or stress.[100] These elements appear to facilitate playfulness (i.e., the expression of internal motivation and internal control to explore or pretend).

PLAY IN OCCUPATIONAL THERAPY

Play has always been a part of the pediatric occupational therapist's repertoire, although its importance has altered over the years. Adolph Meyer wrote of work, play, rest, and sleep as being the four rhythms that shaped human organization.[76] In one of the earliest articles on play in the occupational therapy literature, Alessandrini referred to play as a "serious undertaking, not to be confused with diversion or idle use of time. Play is not folly. It is purposeful activity, the result of mental and emotional experiences" (p. 9).[1] Richmond spoke of play as the vehicle for communication and growth of the child.[97] Play in the early years of occupational therapy was used for a variety of purposes such as diversion, development of skills, or remediation.

Mary Reilly was instrumental in bringing play into the forefront of occupational therapy in the late 1960s. She described play along a continuum that she called occupational behavior.[96] Through play, children learn skills and develop interests that later affect choices and success in work and leisure. Play is the arena for the development of sensory integration, physical abilities, cognitive and language skills, and interpersonal relationships. In their play, children practice adult and cultural roles and learn to become productive members of society.[14,71,96] Reilly felt that play is a multidimensional system

to adapt to the environment and that the exploratory drive of curiosity underlies play behavior. This drive has three hierarchical stages: exploration, competency, and achievement. Exploratory behavior is seen most in early childhood and is fueled by intrinsic motivation. Competency is fueled by *effectance motivation*, a term defined by White as an inborn urge toward competence.[113] This stage is characterized by experimentation and practice to achieve mastery. Achievement is linked to goal expectancies and is fueled by a desire to achieve excellence. Using this frame of reference, other scholars studying under Reilly expanded the concepts of play. Florey offered a developmental framework of play and explored the concept of intrinsic motivation as being central to play.[43] Takata developed a taxonomy of play and described play epochs based on Piagetian stages,[108,110] and Knox examined play in relation to development for the purposes of evaluation.[63] Robinson described how play is used for the child to learn rules and roles.[98]

In researching the relationship between play and sensory integration, Clifford and Bundy found that children with sensory integration dysfunction differed in play scores on the Preschool Play Scale but that many of their play skills were within normal expectations.[32] This led Bundy to conclude that there were other foundations for play than sensory integration or physical capabilities, and this led to her studies on playfulness.[23-25,105]

Occupational science developed in the late 1980s as an academic discipline to study the nature of occupation and how it influences health. Because play is the primary occupation of children, a number of researchers have studied various aspects of play. Primeau studied parent-child routines and how play is orchestrated into daily routines.[93] She proposed that parents use two types of play strategies: segregation and inclusion. In the segregated strategy, play times were separate from other daily routines, whereas in the inclusion strategy, play was incorporated into other daily routines. Parents use play routines to support their children's learning. Pierce studied object play in infants.[91,92] She described three types of object rules learned by children: (1) object property rules (that is, the child's internal representation of the properties of objects); (2) object action rules (the repertoire of actions on the objects); and (3) object affect rules (those factors affecting object choice and keeping play enjoyable).

Knox expanded the concept of playfulness to study the play styles of preschool children.[66] Four dimensions of play style were identified using grounded theory methods: preferences, attitudes, approach, and social reciprocity. Within these dimensions, elements of style were determined. Preferences included setting, toys, types of play, roles, and playmates. Attitudes included mood, consistency, and humor. Approach included direction, focus, and spontaneity. Social reciprocity included social orientation, responsivity, and flexibility. The children were described in terms of their unique play style and the elements of style were analyzed across the children. Knox found that play style differed among all the children and the way they approached play episodes was dependent on their play style.

PLAY ASSESSMENT

Even though play is considered the child's major occupation, and most occupational therapists would agree that it is important to the child, few therapists routinely evaluate it.[34,36,70]

Couch found that 62% of pediatric occupational therapists who responded to her questionnaire stated that they evaluated play, but less than 20% used criterion-referenced play assessments. Play was usually evaluated through clinical observations or as a part of developmental tests.[34]

Play assessments are usually of four types: (1) those that assess skills in a particular area through play; (2) those that assess developmental competencies; (3) those that assess the way a child plays, including playfulness and play style; and (4) narratives.

Skills

Most of the play assessments described in the literature are designed to evaluate a particular skill area, such as cognition or social interaction. These assessments use structured play settings, materials, and activities or play observations. The assessments described here include those most often cited in the occupational therapy literature. Rosenblatt[99] and Hulme and Lunzer[56] assessed play in relation to language and reasoning. The Piagetian stages of cognitive development have formed the basis of a number of play assessments.[101,106] The classic assessment of the social aspects of play was developed by Parten. She assessed social participation in play of preschool children by examining two dimensions: degree of participation and degree of leadership.[88] Degree of participation included the social interaction during play and was rated as unoccupied, solitary, onlooker, parallel, associative, and organized supplementary play. Degree of leadership included how much the child depended on or directed others in play.

Development

A few assessments rate the developmental skills of the child through play. Linder developed a transdisciplinary play-based assessment that assesses the child in cognitive, social-emotional, language, physical, and motor development through naturalistic play.[73]

Two assessments developed by occupational therapists explore play in its developmental aspects: the Play History[108-110] and the Knox Preschool Play Scale.[19,62,63,65,67] Takata described play developmentally within time and space and felt that play reflected the interaction between the individual and the external environment. The Play History is a semi-structured interview and play observation, yielding information on the child's daily activity schedule. She identified two elements of play: form and content. Form parallels changes in development and includes the choice of play materials, amount and nature of playfulness, and organization in play. Content reflects life's situations and is the expression of the child's immediate needs, impulses, and physical and emotional state. Takata developed a taxonomy of play epochs based on the Piagetian stages to analyze the interview and play observation. Behaviors are classified as evident, not evident, encouraged, and not encouraged. As a result of the analysis, a play prescription can be developed. Behnke and Fetokovich conducted reliability and validity studies on the Play History and found it to be a reliable and valid instrument for assessing children's play behavior.[13] Bryze discussed the play history as a guide to using narrative in assessment of past and present play behavior.[22]

The Knox Preschool Play Scale is an observational assessment designed to describe developmental skills as seen during play for children through 6 years of age.[62,63,65,67] This assessment was revised by Bledsoe and Shepherd[19] and more recently by Knox.[65] The scale describes play in terms of 6-month increments through age 3 and yearly increments through age 6. Four dimensions are examined: space management, material management, pretense/symbolic, and participation. Space management is the manner in which the child learns to manage his or her body and the space around it. Material management is the way in which the child manages his or her material surroundings. The pretense/symbolic dimension is the way in which the child learns about the world through imitation and the development of the ability to understand and separate reality from make-believe. Participation is the amount and manner of social interaction. Children are observed indoors and outdoors and rated on all four dimensions (Case Study 18-1.). Bledsoe and Shepherd examined reliability and validity on the first revision with typically developing children.[19] Harrison and Kielhofner did the same with children with disabilities.[50] Both studies found the scale to be highly reliable and valid. Many studies have been conducted using the Knox Preschool Play Scale, and these have been summarized by Knox.[65,67]

CASE STUDY 18-1   Ellen

Ellen is a 1-year, 3-month-old girl who was referred for home-based occupational therapy for developmental delay. She was born 1 month premature. She has a history of feeding problems with reflux after meals and when she is upset. At the time she was referred, the reflux had partially resolved with small frequent feedings and alternate positioning; however, her mother was reluctant to let her be upset, because she was afraid Ellen would vomit. Ellen is an only child and she lives with her parents in a single-family home.

Ellen's mother was interviewed using the Play History to provide information about her environment, daily schedule, and play experiences and interactions. She was also evaluated with the Knox Preschool Play Scale to provide information about developmental skills as observed in free and facilitated play. Ellen's mother's primary concerns were her reflux, her developmental skills, and her own lack of knowledge about how to play with Ellen. Other mothers seemed to know what to do with their children, and she did not. Her preferred play with Ellen was to read her books.

The information gathered on the Play History is analyzed in terms of what is evidenced or not evidenced in the home environment and what is encouraged or discouraged by her parents. The child's play is compared with the appropriate "epoch" for her age. Ellen's play status worksheet is depicted in Box 18-1.

BOX 18-1 Play Status Worksheet

EXPECTED DESCRIPTION

Epoch: Sensorimotor

Emphasis: Toys, objects for sensory experiences; cause and effect; container play; trial and error; gross motor—stand, sit, walk, pull, climb, pick up; fine motor—bang, carry, open/close, put in and take out, push, pull, relate two objects; people—parents, familiar adults; imitation—of simple actions; setting—home, yard

EVIDENCE

Moderate variety of toys; blocks, nesting and stacking toys, books, stuffed toys, "busy boxes," balls

Freedom around the house for ambulation and exploration; generally plays in the bedroom, family room, and kitchen

Generally likes to play in the same room as mother

Outside grassy area available but not used much

Long attention span for toys

NO EVIDENCE

Mother feels that she doesn't have the imagination or know-how to alter activities to meet Ellen's needs

Little domestic play or imitative play

Hypersensitive to grass and other textures, certain sounds, music

Mother's major concerns have been with Ellen's physical growth, nourishment, and vomiting; as a result she rarely lets Ellen cry or do things that might frustrate her

ENCOURAGED

Mother encourages looking at books while she reads to Ellen

Watches *Sesame Street*

Water play in tub with father; wading pool

Rough-housing with father

Container play, stacking, ball play

Warm, loving relationship with both parents

DISCOURAGED

Little guiding of play or active participation in play on part of mother

Little verbalizing during play by mother; doesn't encourage Ellen's verbalizations

Concrete steps (3) leading out of house to patio; Ellen isn't allowed to creep up or down them yet

---

The information on the Knox Preschool Play Scale is described in terms of four dimensions: space management, material management, pretense/symbolic, and participation. Ellen's play age in each of the dimensions is described in Box 18-2.

Physical or neurologic conditions were not interfering with her development, and it was felt that her delayed skills were primarily a result of lack of experience or stimulation. Her feeding problems were resolving. Her home environment was conducive to play in terms of space, objects, and people. The parent-child relationships were warm and loving, and her mother was eager to learn new ways to stimulate Ellen's play.

BOX 18-2 Knox Preschool Play Scale

SPACE MANAGEMENT: 6- TO 12-MONTH LEVEL

Ellen crawls, pulls to stance, and cruises. She sits with good balance and easily shifts weight in sitting. She plays in either sitting or supported stance against the coffee table. She is beginning to stand unsupported but flops down when balance is challenged. She walks with support from an adult.

MATERIAL MANAGEMENT: 12 TO 18 MONTHS

Ellen puts toys into and takes them out of containers. She pulls and pushes, opens and shuts, bangs, stacks, and puts simple toys together. She puts together familiar single-shape puzzles.

PRETENSE/SYMBOLIC: 12-MONTH LEVEL

Ellen imitates simple actions and novel movements. She is beginning to imitate schemas such as putting a spoon to the doll's face.

PARTICIPATION: 12 MONTHS

Ellen seeks attention from adults and seems to need the attention to prolong her play. She imitates, shows toys, and shares toys. Her expressive language is minimal.

Ellen's weaknesses included the following: she was behind in all areas of development; she showed some mild hypersensitivity to tactile and auditory sensory stimuli; her mother lacked expertise and knowledge in facilitating development and was apprehensive about Ellen's reflux, and she rarely allowed Ellen to challenge herself or become upset. Ellen's mother had few social and emotional supports.

The following goals were established for treatment: (1) improve developmental skills through play; (2) improve play and playfulness; (3) enable Ellen's mother to play with her, incorporate play into their daily routines, and scaffold play to encourage new skills and abilities; and (4) increase Ellen's mother's knowledge of developmentally appropriate play.

The intervention plan included weekly sessions with Ellen and her mother to teach them both play skills and playfulness. Her mother was also encouraged to seek out other resources in the community such as Mommy and Me classes and gym classes. She was also encouraged to set up play dates with other mothers. Ellen's father was included whenever he was available.

Both Ellen and her mother made striking gains with therapy. Ellen's development improved and she became very playful with both her mother and the therapist. Her mother became an active participant in the therapy sessions and became involved in community activities. Individual therapy was terminated when Ellen and her mother enrolled in an early intervention program. A few months later, the therapist visited Ellen and her mother and was pleased with her progress. Ellen was speaking a few words, and she showed the therapist some of the toys and games she played with her mother. Ellen's mother also seemed much happier and appeared to enjoy her daughter more. The experiences they described were typical, playful, and rewarding for both of them.

In this case, play was the primary goal as well as the therapeutic medium used. It illustrates how effective an occupation-based approach can be.

Experience

The third way therapists assess play is to analyze the child's experience or state of mind when playing (i.e., playfulness and play style). Barnett devised a rating scale based on Liebermann's playfulness concepts.[8,9] Children were rated on items representing the five playfulness traits: physical spontaneity, manifest joy, sense of humor, social spontaneity, and cognitive spontaneity.

Bundy developed the Test of Playfulness (ToP), designed to assess the individual's degree of playfulness.[24,25] The scale contains 68 items representing four elements of playfulness: intrinsic motivation, internal control, ability to suspend reality, and framing. The child is rated on scales of extent, intensity, and skill. The ToP can be scored from direct observations or videotapes of children engaged in free play. Bundy and her associates have also developed an assessment of the environment's capacity to support playfulness, the Test of Environmental Supportiveness (TOES).[105]

The previous assessments are based on behavioral observation and parent interviews. Because play is unique to the individual, it is important to obtain the child's own perspective of his or her play, and this is usually done through self-report. Henry developed the Pediatric Interest Profiles, three age-appropriate profiles of play and leisure interests and participation for children from 6 to 9 years of age, from 9 to 12 years, and from 12 to 21 years.[51] The profiles assess what activities the child is doing, the child's feelings about the activity, how skilled they perceive themselves, and with whom they play. They can be used in evaluation in three ways: (1) to conduct a play interview, (2) to identify children and adolescents who may be at risk for play-related problems, and (3) to set play-related goals and identify play or leisure activities to use in intervention.

Advantages and Disadvantages of Evaluating Play

Observing children at play is like looking through a window into their lives. An analysis of children's play is helpful in assessing their physical and cognitive abilities, social participation, imagination, independence, coping mechanisms, and environment.[14,20,46] An evaluation of play and of the child's abilities as seen through play provides important information regarding the child's occupational performance as well as performance skills and patterns.

Play is most often evaluated in routine, self-chosen, familiar activities in naturalistic settings, providing the therapist with a picture of everyday competencies. Play assessments based on identifying what the child can do in play enable the therapist to focus on the child's abilities rather than disabilities.

Some of the disadvantages of play assessments have been summarized by Knox,[66] and Bundy.[24] Because play is an interaction between the child and the environment, the human and physical factors in the environment can substantially influence the child's play.[66] Play assessments that are designed to take place in standardized settings with standardized toys significantly alter and may inhibit the child's play. In addition, although play specifies its own purpose, observed behaviors may have different meanings and serve different purposes for different people. It is difficult for an observer to assess the meaning of play to the participant.

Another limitation is in the amount of time available for observation of the child. The therapist must determine whether the sample of behavior is sufficient, typical, and representative of true play. Knox found that over a prolonged time, a child's play could be vastly different at different times.[66] Also, children engaged in play episodes for prolonged periods (up to 1 hour in some cases). To capture a variety of play behaviors, a therapist needs to observe a child multiple times and in a variety of settings.

Interpreting Play Assessments

Assessment of play should be a part of every occupational therapy evaluation to develop a complete picture of an individual's competence in his or her occupational performance and to plan adequate intervention that focuses on helping that individual participate in meaningful and self-satisfying occupations. Such assessments provide the therapist with a picture of how the individual uses play in his or her daily life. An analysis of play also provides the therapist with a picture of the child's skills in motor, cognitive, and social areas (Figure 18-5). This is especially helpful in assessing a child who does not respond well to standardized developmental testing.

Some of the newer assessments of affect, playfulness, or play style indicate how the individual approaches and gives meaning to the gamut of activities during the day. These instruments hold much promise in helping to determine how an individual balances his or her daily occupations in a meaningful way.

Evaluation in occupational therapy leads to intervention planning. Intervention should capitalize on abilities of the individual to remediate the deficits. Knowledge of the individual's skills, interests, and play style assists in this planning and guides treatment. Bundy offered a number of considerations in observing an individual's play that are useful in developing treatment goals. These include the following[24]:

- In what activities does the child become totally absorbed?
- What does the child get from these activities?

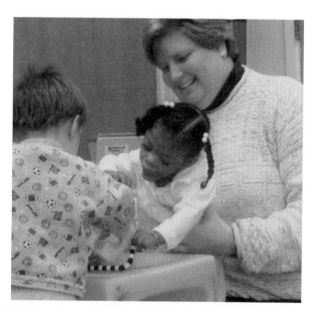

FIGURE 18-5 The occupational therapist assesses motor, cognitive, and social skills during a play activity. (Courtesy Jayne Shepherd.)

Does the child engage routinely in activities in which he or she feels free to vary the process and outcome in whatever way he or she sees fit?

Does the child have the capacity, permission, and support to do what he or she chooses to do?

Is the child capable of giving and interpreting messages that convey "this is play; this is how you should interact with me now"?

CONSTRAINTS TO PLAY

As discussed earlier, play is always influenced by the environment. The effects of the environment on play can be seen in children who have experienced neglect or long hospitalizations. Extreme examples of constraints to play have been seen in some of the reports of children in Romanian orphanages.[29,38] These children showed severe sensory problems, extreme delay in developmental skills, and difficulties in interacting with others. Other characteristics of the play of deprived children included self-stimulation, limited repertoire of activities, decreased social play, and either increased or decreased fantasy play.

When children are hospitalized, they often experience stress of separation, fear of illness, painful procedures, enforced confinement, and disruption of routines.[60] Some of the effects on play behavior include regression to earlier stages of development; decreased endurance and movement; decreased attention span, initiative, and curiosity; decreased resourcefulness and creativity; qualitative decrease in playfulness; decreased affect; and increased anxiety.[61]

Knox, in her study of play styles of preschool children, discussed the importance of the environment on children's play.[66] She found that when children's play styles matched the expectations of the environment, play flourished. When there was a mismatch between play style and the environment, play was stifled.

Effects of Disability on Play Behavior

The play of children with varying disabilities has been described often in the literature.[60,80] However, problems arise in attempts to generalize across or within disabilities. Children are individuals and respond uniquely in different situations, whether or not they have a disability. Descriptions of the play of children with disabilities must be interpreted cautiously.[60] Although it is helpful to examine some of the problems that certain conditions may impose on the child, in actual practice, each child must be considered individually. Bundy stated that although a child's play may not be typical, it was more important for "children to be good at what they want to do" (p. 218).[24]

Some diseases and conditions limit physical interaction with the environment, with toys and other objects, and, to some extent, with people. The child with a physical impairment may display limited movement, strength, and pain when performing daily activities. Social contacts with family and peers may be disrupted by hospitalizations. The play characteristics of children with physical limitations may include fear of movement, decreased active play, and preferences for sedentary activities. The child may also have problems with manipulating toys and show decreased exploration (Figure 18-6). Opportunities for social play are often decreased because of hospitalizations or routines that do not allow for social interaction.[59]

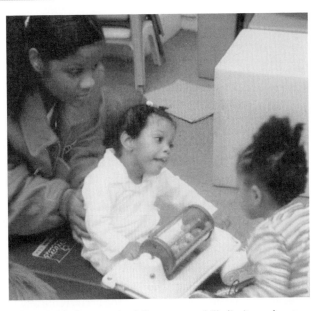

FIGURE 18-6 Impaired fine-motor skills limit exploratory play of this infant with cerebral palsy. Toys that activate to imprecise (full arm) movements are a good choice in play activities. (Courtesy Jayne Shepherd.)

Children with cognitive impairment often show delayed or uneven skills, difficulty in structuring their own behavior, or lack of sustained attention. These characteristics may be manifested in play in preferences for structured play materials, limited or inflexible play repertoires, decreased curiosity, destructive or inappropriate use of objects, decreased imagination, decreased symbolic play, decreased social interaction, decreased language, and increased observer play.[60,80] These children may need more structure and external cues to develop their play skills.

A number of studies have examined the effects of sensory impairment on play, particularly of children with visual or hearing impairments. Kaplan-Sanoff et al.[60] and Mogford[80] noted that children with visual impairment have delays in developing an integrated perception of the world caused by lack of vision and delayed motor exploration of surroundings and objects. The play characteristics of these children are difficulty in constructive play, delays in developing complex play routines with others, and decreased imitative and role play.

The child with a hearing impairment is believed to have problems with decreased inner language, decreased social interactions, and decreased understanding of abstract concepts. These are manifested in play in that imagination becomes more restrictive with age and increased time is spent in noninteractive construction play. Children with hearing impairments demonstrate decreased symbolic play and increased solitary play.[60,80]

Children who have difficulty interpreting and integrating sensory input often have a limited or distorted perception of themselves and of their world, decreased ability to plan and execute motor and cognitive tasks, and poor organization of behavior. Play characteristics of these children include either excessive movement or avoidance of movement, decreased exploration, decreased gross motor or manipulative play, increased observation or solitary play, increased sedentary

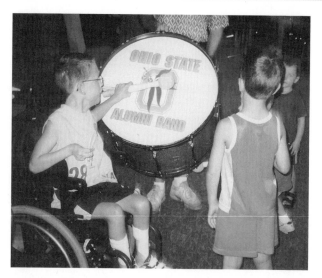

FIGURE 18-7   Matthew, who has cerebral palsy, participates in the pregame rally by playing the drum. (Courtesy Jill McQuaid.)

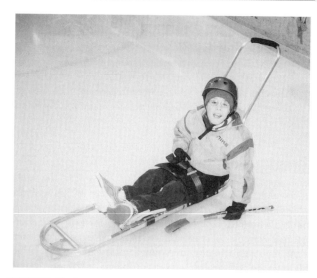

FIGURE 18-8   Matthew takes to the ice using an adapted sled. (Courtesy Jill McQuaid.)

play, a restricted repertoire of play, resistance to change, distractibility, or destructiveness.[5,6,23,80]

Children with autism often have severe sensory integrative problems, as well as social and language deficits. Their play is characterized by a lack of inner and expressive language, stereotyped movements or types of play, decreased imitation and imagination, lack of variety in play repertoires, motor planning problems, decreased play organization, decreased manipulation of toys, decreased construction and combining of objects, and decreased social play.[7,107] Children with autism appear to have a fundamental deficit in play greater than what would be expected in examining specific skills.

Children with cerebral palsy show difficulties in many areas (Figure 18-7). They may show limited and abnormal movement, sometimes have decreased cognitive abilities, have sensory impairments, and often lack opportunities for social play.[42] In play, cognitive abilities are the most decisive factor in limiting play, and children with good cognitive abilities can make adaptations to their physical limitations. Other problems include decreased physical interaction with environment and less interactive play time.[17,18]

Most of the studies of the play of children with disabilities stress the obstacles that the disabling conditions place on the children. Mogford summarized the problems that different disabling conditions have on children's play by stating that all children with disabilities have one thing in common—that their ability to explore, interact with, and master their environment is impaired, depriving them of a normal childhood experience.[80] The occupational therapy practitioner needs to explore supports for play. With adaptations, a child can overcome great obstacles to engage in a favorite activity (Figure 18-8).

PLAY IN INTERVENTION

What differentiates free play from therapeutic play? Free play is intrinsically motivated, fun, and is performed for its own sake rather than having a purpose. The child directs the play.

However, in therapy, goals and objectives are established by the therapist and the parents, who usually direct the play. When external constraints are placed on play, it is perceived as work and no longer contains playful elements. How then can play be used successfully in treatment? Rast stated:

> Play offers a practical vehicle to enlist a child's attention, to practice specific motor and functional skills, and to promote sensory processing, perceptual abilities, and cognitive development. It also serves to support social, emotional, and language development. In the therapeutic setting, play often becomes a tool used to work towards a goal, despite the fact that the goal-oriented, externally controlled aspects of the therapy situation conflict with the essence of play itself (p. 30).[95]

For play to be used successfully in intervention, the child should feel that he or she is choosing or directing the play episode. This is particularly important when the goal is to increase competence in play development. Play and leisure activities are important methods for promoting a child's performance and skills because they have meaning to the individual.

In a study by Couch, Deitz, and Kanny investigating how pediatric occupational therapists use play in intervention, 91% of the therapists rated play as very important.[35] For 95% of the respondents, play was used primarily to elicit motor, sensory, or psychosocial outcomes; only 2% used play as an outcome by itself. The therapists also primarily used adult-directed play versus child-directed play.

The way play is used in intervention is influenced by a number of factors: the therapist's frame of reference, the institution's emphasis on improving performance components and skills, and the family's values and concerns for the physical aspects of the child's disability. Goals and objectives are established in accordance with how the child's disability affects his or her daily occupations and on analysis of occupational performance.[3] Play and leisure activities are used in occupational therapy in three ways: (1) as intervention modalities (to improve specific skills); (2) as an intervention goal (to improve play occupations); and (3) to facilitate playfulness.

Play as a Modality

Three frames of reference that use play as an intervention modality are the developmental, functional, and sensory integrative approaches. Play is most often used when a specific skill needs to be taught or when a specific goal needs to be met. Goals and objectives are established depending on how the disability affects the role performance of the child. Playful activities are used in a more structured or defined sense as a means to achieve the desired goal.

In the developmental frame of reference, play activities are used to develop physical, cognitive, emotional, or social abilities. The play materials are used to entice the child, such as when a toy is used to encourage a child to crawl or when a busy box is used to teach cause-and-effect concepts. Difficulty preserving the qualities of play may arise when therapy goals or techniques require a more structured "hands-on" approach, such as when using a neurodevelopmental treatment technique. Use of play as a modality requires skill and imagination on the part of the therapist to combine approaches successfully and creatively. Anderson, Hinojosa, and Strauch[4] and Blanche[17] provided helpful suggestions for incorporating play into neurophysiologic treatment approaches. Munier, Myers, and Pierce discuss using object play to enhance motivation, address the development of motor skills, facilitate process skills, develop environmental negotiation, facilitate temporal awareness, promote social skills, and support engagement in occupation.[82] Florey and Greene offer strategies for treating children with behavior and emotional problems.[44] Baranak et al.[7] and Spitzer[107] present play engagement strategies for children with autism. These strategies included respecting the child's sensory processing capacities, scaffolding play, using imitation and modeling, and expanding play routines. They also offer suggestions for optimizing attention and organization and augmenting communication.

In the functional frame of reference, play is also used to meet a therapeutic end by adapting the activity, environment, or in therapeutic handling of the child while he or she is engaged in the activity. For example, a child's favorite toy may be positioned in such a way to improve the child's range of motion or adapted to increase the child's strength. In this sense, play is often used as a motivator for action. However, therapists need to be careful in how much they handle or direct the child's play. Germain and Dwyer studied play levels of children with cerebral palsy under two conditions: (1) handled, where the therapist facilitated postural responses while the child played; and (2) unhandled, where the child was engaged in free play.[47] In the handled condition, the children's level of play was lower because the children depended more on the therapist for direction and showed less self-directed play. This study showed the need for balance between giving the child enough support or assistance and giving too much.

In sensory integration, play is valued as the arena through which sensory integration develops.[5,6] To play successfully, children must have adequate sensory integration and be able to make adequate adaptive responses to environmental demands. In therapy, the therapist sets up and manipulates the environment (setting, objects, people) so that the child can choose among activities that potentially offer the "just right" challenge. During treatment, the therapist constantly adjusts the environment, child, or activity to bring about successful adaptation. Bundy provided an excellent description of the role of play within a sensory integrative framework. She concluded:

> Play is a powerful tool for treatment. For many individuals, the most important byproduct of occupational therapy may be the improved ability to play. If it is carefully planned and conducted, therapy using the principles of sensory integration may be very helpful in facilitating the development of play. Likewise, play as a part of a well orchestrated treatment plan, can result in improvements in sensory integration (p. 67).[23]

Mack, Lindquist, and Parham synthesized the commonalities of play from the occupational behavior and sensory integrative viewpoints. They stated:

> In practice, both approaches deem the therapist responsible for structuring adaptive behavior from the child. Thus, the potency of the environment's influence on development is confirmed by both. But from neither perspective does therapy rely solely on environmental manipulation. The child's initiative and active involvement are critical to the therapeutic process. From both perspectives, the intrinsic motivation or self direction of the child is primary in guiding therapy, for importance is placed on the child's inner drive toward mastery. Play, then, is the process through which therapeutic goals are achieved (p. 367).[75]

Play as an Intervention Goal

Burke stated, "An occupation-based view of play is built on basic notions concerning the importance of an occupation to an individual" (p. 201).[27] The use of play as an intervention goal has been described within the occupational science and sensory integration frames of reference, and most recently in the AOTA Practice Framework.[3] In occupational behavior and science, play is viewed as an occupation, determined by the individual and his or her interaction with the environment. The improvement of play skills and playfulness enables competent interaction with the world. Parham stated that enhancement of play itself may be effective in promoting health and well-being.[86]

In an interesting study of the effects of peer play level on preschool children who had delayed play skills, Tanta, Deitz, White, and Billingsley showed that when children were paired with peers who had higher developmental play skills, they showed more initiation and response to initiation than when playing with children with lower play skills.[111] This study suggested that using peers as role models is helpful in developing social play skills.

In Primeau's study of play patterns in families, she suggested that parents modify the environment, incorporate play into the family's routine, and provide verbal suggestions to improve and increase the child's play.[93] Knox emphasized the importance of considering children's play styles in choosing or setting up play environments.[66]

Facilitating Playfulness

The third way play is used therapeutically is to facilitate playfulness in the child. As was stated in the section on assessment of play and leisure, often what individuals play with and how they play may not be as important as the affective quality of their play. Some children with significant or multiple disabilities manage to get great joy and benefit out of play. On the other hand, therapists often see children who are not playful and do not derive pleasure out of even the simplest play interaction. Facilitating playfulness in the child can be an important goal of therapy. Morrison and Metzger stated:

> The more playful child may generalize this flexible approach into environmental interaction beyond play and into other aspects of his or her life. For the child with a condition that impedes his or her ability to interact with the social or physical environment, a flexible (playful) approach may enable the child to succeed more frequently in these difficult situations (p. 540).[81]

Parham suggested strategies that a therapist can use to create a playful atmosphere.[85] The therapist should express a playful attitude through speech, body language, and facial expressions (Figure 18-9). Also, novelty and imaginary play should be used to facilitate playful participation on the part of the child. Bundy stated that the therapist must know how to play to be able to model play for the child.[23] To develop playfulness, the child must develop intrinsic motivation, internal control, ability to suspend reality, and ability to give and read cues.

Facilitating playful interactions is important for any age child with or without a disability. Holloway suggested strategies to encourage playfulness in parents and children within a neonatal intensive care unit.[53] Helping parents learn to read their infant's cues and adapt to the infant's behavioral tempo helps to develop mutually positive experiences that form the basis for playful processes as the infant matures.

Whether the goals of therapy are to use play a medium, to develop play skills, or to develop playfulness, planning intervention must always take into account the interaction among the therapist, the child, and the equipment and play objects in the environment. The therapist needs to create a playful atmosphere and attitude for the child to respond playfully. Six abilities important to facilitating play in a child appear to be that the adult can (1) apply theories of play, (2) analyze activities, (3) let go and let the child lead, (4) empathize, (5) demonstrate spontaneity, and (6) display creativity.[68] Knox, Ecker, and Fitzsimmons developed a program to help therapists and parents follow the child's lead and develop the spontaneity and creativity necessary to weave play and therapy together.[68]

Knowing what is motivating and pleasurable to the child is essential to accomplish goals through play episodes. Knox and Mailloux stated, "When the therapist can make the match between an activity that is highly conducive to achieving a goal and is at the same time attractive to the child as a play experience, then the achievement of goals through play is most likely to occur" (p. 198).[69]

Adaptations

Critical to creating a play atmosphere for children is considering the environment and the objects within it. To foster play, environmental spaces, toys, and equipment should have some flexibility in usage. In an intriguing study, Bundy et al. examined changes in playfulness in a group of typically developing children, ages 5 to 7 years, after new materials (e.g., cardboard boxes, bicycle tires, hay bales, plastic barrels, wood, foam) were introduced to the playground.[26] They found that scores on the Test of Playfulness rose significantly after the intervention and the teachers felt that the children's play had become more active, creative, and social as a result.

In addition, toys and play equipment may need to be adapted for the child to access them optimally. Adaptation of toys and the environment is an important role of the occupational therapist, particularly for the severely involved child. Play spaces should offer a variety of experiences and allow for creativity, illusion, change, and chance. Children need to be able to control the space, i.e., have objects, toys, and people to move and change and freedom to move.[30] The therapist must know the properties of toys as well as how to adapt them appropriately. Switches, adaptive keyboards, or provisions for sensory impairment may be necessary for the child to benefit from and be more independent in play. Play can be enhanced through a variety of augmentative devices ranging from very simple adaptations to complex electronic devices.[39]

Parent Education and Training

Working with parents in relation to play is vitally important if there is to be carryover of the skills and abilities learned in therapy into the child's everyday life. Parents of children with disabilities often attempt to structure therapy into the child's routines. Children with physical disabilities may be involved in therapeutic regimens throughout the day and consequently are deprived of play opportunities. Four barriers to free play

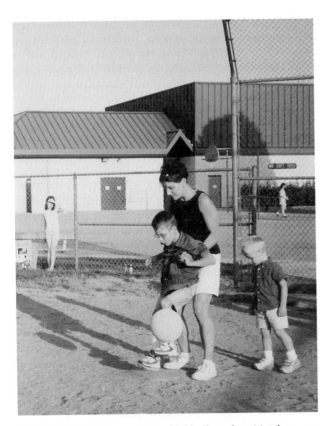

FIGURE 18-9 Mom adapts kickball so that Matthew can play with his brother. (Courtesy Jill McQuaid.)

are (1) limitations imposed by caregivers, (2) physical and personal limitations of the child, (3) environmental barriers, and (4) social barriers.[79] Interventions that support the child's free play and include recommendations about playthings help support the importance of play in overall development.

A goal of therapy is parent education—that is, helping parents understand the importance of play for their child and helping them to interact with their child playfully. Often the parents need help in knowing how to create a balance between doing things for their child and allowing the child to form and carry out his or her own intentions. The therapist may need to model play behavior for the parent, encourage the parent to enter into and contribute to play sequences without directing or controlling them, and help the parent organize or adapt the play environment to meet the needs of the child. By actively involving the parents or caregivers, the therapist helps them appreciate their child's strengths, learn the fun of playing with their child, and develop play skills that will serve them well.

Hinojosa and Kramer stressed the importance of helping families to incorporate play into their lifestyles in order to strengthen interaction with their children and provide typical childhood experiences.[52] They offered a framework for analyzing and understanding family play and provide suggestions to facilitate the inclusion of all members of the family in playful activities.

Societal Concerns

In the last few years, play for all children has diminished. Since 1980, the amount of unscheduled time in the day of an average school-aged child has dropped by 15%.[74] Because of changing family lifestyles, challenges in education, technology, and safety concerns, children today have little time and space for free play. Singer et al. examined the role of play and experiential learning in 16 nations divided into developed countries, newly industrial countries, and developing countries.[104] They gathered information from mothers of 2400 children. They found similarities in all nations, with mothers describing the lack of free play and experiential learning opportunities. A major portion of children's free time was spent watching television.

Other studies have shown many barriers to play. One is over-structuring and over-scheduling of the child's day.[48,66,74,89] Children's afterschool hours are filled with classes, planned activities, and homework. Another barrier is an over-emphasis on early academic achievement. Schools are increasingly moving to eliminate the "playful" parts of school, including recess, gym, sports, and art programs.[48,89] Some states have eliminated recess altogether because it is not considered academic. Academics are being stressed earlier and earlier in our educational systems and parents often feel that, for play to be worthwhile, the adults need to "teach" things during play. A third barrier to play results from parents' concerns for the safety of their children in a culture they perceive as increasingly violent. Outdoor play has decreased markedly and parents schedule "play dates" or planned play experiences. Places for play have decreased also. Many metropolitan areas are severely lacking in park space,[74] and many school playgrounds are often asphalt pads with no playground equipment.

Children are taking part in more organized sports and activities. Although organized activities can be fun and playful, the amount of time and energy children have for less structured free play is reduced. Structured sports do not promote the creativity that is part of play.

The decreases in unstructured, physical play have had a dramatic effect on children. The rise in childhood obesity, as well as in the health problems that accompany obesity, is a major problem facing parents. The over-reliance on television and computers has changed the type of play that children choose and leads to more passivity and reliance on others for entertainment. The increased media exposure has also exposed children to violent themes and content, often without the benefit of parental supervision.

Many organizations including the American Academy of Pediatrics (Ginsburg, 2007),[48] the Association for Childhood Education International, and the American Association for the Child's Right to Play[2] (Isenberg & Quisenberry, 2002)[51] have issued declarations promoting the importance of and need for active play for children.

Occupational therapy practitioners are in a unique position to act as advocates for play, not only for their clients but also for children in general. In 2008, AOTA published a societal statement on play including the following recommendations:

> Occupational therapy practitioners support, enhance, and defend children's right to play as individuals and as members of their families, peer groups, and communities by promoting recognition of play's crucial role in children's development, health, and well-being; establishing and restoring children's skills needed to engage in play; adapting play materials, objects, and environments to facilitate optimal play experiences; and advocating for safe, inclusive play environments that are accessible to all (p. 707).[94]

REFERENCES

1. Alessandrini, N. (1949). Play—a child's world. *American Journal of Occupational Therapy, 3*, 9–12.
2. American Association for the Child's Right to Play. (2007). *IPA declaration of a child's right to play.* Retrieved April 3, 2009, from http//www.ipausa.org/declare/htm.
3. American Occupational Therapy Association. (2008). Occupational therapy practice framework: Domain and process. *American Journal of Occupational Therapy, 62*, 625–683.
4. Anderson, J., Hinojosa, J., & Strauch, C. (1987). Integrating play in neurodevelopmental treatment. *American Journal of Occupational Therapy, 41*, 421–426.
5. Ayres, A. J. (1972). *Sensory integration and learning disorders.* Los Angeles: Western Psychological Services.
6. Ayres, A. J. (1979). *Sensory integration and the child.* Los Angeles: Western Psychological Services.
7. Baranek, G., Reinhartsen, D., & Wannamaker, S. (2001). Play: Engaging young children with autism. In R. Huebner (Ed.), *Autism: A sensorimotor approach to management* (pp. 313–351). Gaithersburg, MD: Aspen.
8. Barnett, L. (1990). Playfulness: Definition, design, and measurement. Play and Culture, 4, 319–336.
9. Barnett, L. (1991). The playful child: Measurement of a disposition to play. *Play and Culture, 4*, 51–74.
10. Barnett, L., & Kleiber, D. (1982). Concomitants of playfulness in early childhood: Cognitive abilities and gender. *The Journal of Genetic Psychology, 141*, 115–127.
11. Barnett, L., & Kleiber, D. (1984). Playfulness and the early play environment. *The Journal of Genetic Psychology, 144*, 153–164.

12. Bazyk, S., Stalnaker, D., Llerena, M., Ekelman, B., & Bazyk, J. (2003). Play in Mayan children. *American Journal of Occupational Therapy, 57,* 273–283.

13. Behnke, C., & Fetokovich, M. (1984). Examining the reliability and validity of the play history. *American Journal of Occupational Therapy, 38,* 94–100.

14. Bergen, D. (1988). *Play as a medium for learning and development.* Portsmouth, NH: Heinemann.

15. Berlyne, D. (1966). Curiosity and exploration. *Science, 15,* 25–32.

16. Blanche, E. (2002). Play and process: adult play embedded in the daily routine. In J. Roopnarire (Ed.), *Conceptual, social-cognitive, and contextual issues in the field of play.* Westport, CT: Ablex Publishing.

17. Blanche, E. (2008). Play in children with cerebral palsy: Doing with—not doing to. In L. D. Parham, & L. Fazio (Eds.), *Play in occupational therapy for children* (2nd ed., pp. 375–394). St. Louis: Elsevier.

18. Blanche, E., & Knox, S. (2008). Learning to play: Promoting skills and quality of life in individuals with cerebral palsy. In A. Eliasson, & P. Burtner (Eds.), *Improving hand function in children with cerebral palsy: Theory, evidence, and intervention* (pp. 357–370). London: Mac Keith Press.

19. Bledsoe, N., & Shepherd, J. (1982). A study of reliability and validity of a preschool play scale. *American Journal of Occupational Therapy, 36,* 783–788.

20. Brown, C., & Gottfried, A. (Eds.). (1985). *Play interactions.* Skillman, NJ: Johnson & Johnson Baby Products.

21. Bruner, J. (1972). Nature and uses of immaturity. *American Psychologist, 27,* 687–708.

22. Bryze, K. (2008). Narrative contributions to the play history. In L. D. Parham & L. Fazio (Eds.), *Play in occupational therapy for children* (2nd ed., pp. 43–54). St. Louis: Elsevier.

23. Bundy, A. (1991). Play theory and sensory integration. In A. G. Fisher, E. A. Murray, & A. C. Bundy (Eds.), *Sensory integration: Therapy and practice* (pp. 46–68). Philadelphia: F. A. Davis.

24. Bundy, A. (1993). Assessment of play and leisure: Delineation of the problem. *American Journal of Occupational Therapy, 47,* 217–222.

25. Bundy, A. (1997). Play and playfulness: What to look for. In L. D. Parham, & L. Fazio (Eds.), *Play in occupational therapy for children* (pp. 52–66). St. Louis: Mosby.

26. Bundy, A., Luckett, T., Naughton, G., Tranter, P., Wyver, S., Ragen, J., et al. (2008). Playful interaction: Occupational therapy for all children on the school playground. *American Journal of Occupational Therapy, 62,* 522–527.

27. Burke, J. (1993). Play: The life role of the infant and young child. In J. Case-Smith (Ed.), *Pediatric occupational therapy and early intervention* (pp. 198–224). Boston: Andover Medical Publishers.

28. Caillois, R. (1958). *Man, play, and games.* New York: The Free Press of Glencoe.

29. Cermak, S. (1996). *Ayres memorial lecture, presented at the Sensory International Annual Symposium.* San Diego, CA.

30. Chandler, B. (1997). Where do you want to play? Play environments; an occupational therapy perspective. In B. Chandler (Ed.), *The essence of play* (pp. 159–174). Bethesda, MD: American Occupational Therapy Association.

31. Clark, F., Parham, D., Carlson, M., Frank, G., Jackson, J., Pierce, D., et al. (1991). Occupational science: Academic innovation in the service of occupational therapy's future. *American Journal of Occupational Therapy, 45,* 300–310.

32. Clifford, J., & Bundy, A. (1989). Play preference and play performance in normal boys and boys with sensory integrative dysfunction. *Occupational Therapy Journal of Research, 9,* 202–217.

33. Cohen, D. (1987). *The development of play.* New York: New York University Press.

34. Couch, K. (1996). *The role of play in pediatric occupational therapy.* Unpublished master's thesis. Seattle, WA: University of Washington.

35. Couch, K., Deitz, J. C., & Kanny, E. M. (1998). The role of play in pediatric occupational therapy. *American Journal of Occupational Therapy, 52,* 111–117.

36. Crowe, T. (1989). Pediatric assessments: A survey of their use by occupational therapists in northwestern school systems. *Occupational Therapy Journal of Research, 9,* 273–286.

37. Csikszentmihalyi, M., & Larson, R. (1984). *Being adolescent.* New York: Basic Books.

38. Daunhauer, L., & Cermak, S. (2008). Play occupations and the experience of deprivation. In L. D. Parham, & L. Fazio (Eds.), *Play in occupational therapy for children* (2nd ed., pp. 251–262). St. Louis: Elsevier.

39. Deitz, J., & Swinth, Y. (2008). Accessing play through assistive technology. In L. D. Parham, & L. Fazio (Eds.), *Play in occupational therapy for children* (2nd ed., pp. 395–412). St. Louis: Elsevier.

40. Ellis, M. J. (1973). *Why people play.* Englewood Cliffs, NJ: Prentice Hall.

41. Erikson, E. (1963). *Childhood and society.* New York: Norton.

42. Finnie, N. (1975). *Handling the young cerebral palsied child at home* (2nd ed.). New York: E.P. Dutton & Company.

43. Florey, L. (1971). An approach to play and play development. *American Journal of Occupational Therapy, 25,* 275–280.

44. Florey, L., & Greene, S. (2008). Play in middle childhood. In L. D. Parham & L. Fazio (Eds.), *Play in occupational therapy for children* (2nd ed., pp. 279–300). St. Louis: Elsevier.

45. Franz, L. (1963). Introduction. In R. Hartley, & R. Goldenson (Eds.), *The complete book of children's play* (pp. v–vi). New York: The Cornwall Press.

46. Garvey, C. (1977a). *Play.* London: Fontana/Open Books.

47. Germain, A., & Dwyre, M. (1988). Unpublished paper presented at the annual conference of the American Occupational Therapy Association, Phoenix, AZ.

48. Ginsburg, K. (2007). The importance of play in promoting healthy child development and maintaining strong parent-child bonds. *Pediatrics, 119,* 182–191.

49. Groos, K. (1976). The play of animals: Play and instinct, and the play of man: Teasing and love play. In J. Bruner, A. Jolly, & K. Sylva (Eds.), *Play: Its role in development and evolution* (pp. 65–83). New York: Basic Books.

50. Harrison, H., & Kielhofner, G. (1986). Examining reliability and validity of the preschool play scale with handicapped children. *American Journal of Occupational Therapy, 40,* 167–173.

51. Henry, A. (2008). Assessment of play in children an adolescents. In L. D. Parham, & L. Fazio (Eds.), *Play in occupational therapy for children* (2nd ed., pp. 71–94). St. Louis: Elsevier.

52. Hinojosa, J., & Kramer, P. (2008). Integrating children with disabilities into family play. In L. D. Parham & L. Fazio (Eds.), *Play in occupational therapy for children* (2nd ed., pp. 321–334). St. Louis: Elsevier.

53. Holloway, E. (2008). Fostering parent-infant playfulness in the neonatal intensive care unit. In L. D. Parham, & L. Fazio (Eds.), *Play in occupational therapy for children* (2nd ed., pp. 335–350). St. Louis: Elsevier.

54. Howes, C., & Stewart, P. (1987). Child's play with adults, toys, and peers: An examination of family and child care influences. *Developmental Psychology, 23,* 423–430.

55. Huizinga, J. (1950). *Homo ludens.* Boston: The Beacon Press.

56. Hulme, I., & Lunzer, E. A. (1966). Play, language and reasoning in subnormal children. *Journal of Child Psychology and Psychiatry, 7,* 107.

57. Isendberg, I., & Quisenberry, N. (2002). Play: Essential for all chilren. A position paper of the Association for Childhood Education International. Retrieved April 2009 from http://www.acei.org/playpaper.htm

58. Jacobs, E., & White, D. (1994). The relationship of child-care quality and play to social behavior in the kindergarten. In H. Goelman & E. Jacobs (Eds.), *Children's play in child care settings* (pp. 85–101). New York: State University of New York Press.

59. Johnson, J., Christie, J., & Yawkey, T. (1999). *Play and early childhood development.* New York: Longman.

60. Kaplan-Sanoff, M., Brewster, A., Stillwell, J., & Bergen, D. (1988). The relationship of play to physical/motor development and to children with special needs. In D. Bergen (Ed.), *Play as a medium for learning and development* (pp. 137–162). Portsmouth, NH: Heinemann.

61. Kielhofner, G., Barris, R., Bauer, D., Shoestock, B., & Walker, L. (1983). A comparison of play behavior in nonhospitalized and hospitalized children. *American Journal of Occupational Therapy, 37,* 305–312.

62. Knox, S. (1968). *Observation and assessment of the everyday play behavior of the mentally retarded child.* Unpublished master's thesis. Los Angeles: University of Southern California.

63. Knox, S. (1974). A play scale. In M. Reilly (Ed.), *Play as exploratory learning* (pp. 247–266). Beverly Hills, CA: Sage.

64. Knox, S. (1996). Play and playfulness in preschool children. In R. Zemke & F. Clark (Eds.), *Occupational science: The evolving discipline* (pp. 81–88). Philadelphia: F.A. Davis.

65. Knox, S. (1997). Development and current use of the Knox Preschool Play Scale. In L. D. Parham & L. Fazio (Eds.), *Play in occupational therapy for children* (pp. 35–51). St. Louis: Mosby.

66. Knox, S. (1999). *Play and playfulness of preschool children.* Unpublished doctoral dissertation. Los Angeles: University of Southern California.

67. Knox, S. (2008). Development and current use of the Revised Knox Preschool Play Scale. In L. D. Parham & L. Fazio (Eds.), *Play in occupational therapy for children* (2nd ed., pp. 55–70). St. Louis: Elsevier.

68. Knox, S., Ecker, C., & Fitzsimmons, L. (2004). *Play outside of the logical.* Paper presented at the Association for the Study of Play Conference, Atlanta, GA.

69. Knox, S., & Mailloux, Z. (1997). Play as treatment and treatment through play. In B. Chandler (Ed.), *The essence of play* (pp. 175–204). Bethesda, MD: American Occupational Therapy Association.

70. Lawlor, M., & Henderson, A. (1989). A descriptive study of the clinical practice patterns of occupational therapists working with infants and young children. *American Journal of Occupational Therapy, 43,* 755–764.

71. Levy, J. (1978). *Play behavior.* Malabar, FL: Robert E. Kruger.

72. Liebermann, J. (1977). *Playfulness: Its relationship to imagination and creativity.* New York: Academic Press.

73. Linder, T. (1993). *Transdisciplinary play-based assessment.* Baltimore: Paul H. Brookes.

74. Louv, R. (2005). *Last child in the woods.* Chapel Hill, NC: Algonquin Books.

75. Mack, W., Lindquist, J., & Parham, D. (1982). A synthesis of occupational behavior and sensory integrative concepts in theory and practice, part 1: Theoretical foundations. *American Journal of Occupational Therapy, 36,* 365–374.

76. Meyer, A. (1922). The philosophy of occupational therapy. *Archives of Occupational Therapy, 1,* 1–10.

77. Michelman, S. (1974). Play and the deficit child. In M. Reilly (Ed.), *Play as exploratory learning* (pp. 157–208). Beverly Hills, CA: Sage.

78. Miller, E., & Kuhaneck, H. (2008). Children's perceptions of play experiences and play preferences: A qualitative study. *American Journal of Occupational Therapy, 62,* 407–415.

79. Missiuna, C., & Pollock, N. (1991). Play deprivation in children with physical disabilities: The role of the occupational therapist in preventing secondary disability. *American Journal of Occupational Therapy, 45,* 882–888.

80. Mogford, K. (1977). The play of handicapped children. In B. Tizard & D. Harvey (Eds.), *Biology of play* (pp. 170–184). Philadelphia: J.B. Lippincott.

81. Morrison, C., & Metzger, P. (2001). Play. In J. Case-Smith (Ed.), *Occupational therapy for children* (4th ed., pp. 528–544). St. Louis: Mosby.

82. Munier, V., Myers, C., & Pierce, D. (2008). Power of object play for infants and toddlers. In L. D. Parham, & L. Fazio (Eds.), *Play in occupational therapy for children* (2nd ed., pp. 219–250). St. Louis: Elsevier.

83. Neulinger, J. (1981). *The psychology of leisure* (2nd ed.). Springfield, IL: Charles C. Thomas.

84. Neumann, E. (1971). *The elements of play.* New York: MSS Information.

85. Parham, D. (1992). Strategies for maintaining a playful atmosphere during therapy. *Sensory Integration Special Interest Section Newsletter, American Occupational Therapy Association, 15,* 2–3.

86. Parham, D. (2008). Play and occupational therapy. In L. D. Parham & L. Fazio (Eds.), *Play in occupational therapy for children* (2nd ed., pp. 3–40). St. Louis: Elsevier.

87. Parham, L. D., & Fazio, L. S. (2008). *Play in occupational therapy with children* (2nd ed.). St. Louis: Elsevier.

88. Parten, M. (1933). Social play among pre-school children. *Journal of Abnormal and Social Psychology, 28,* 136–147.

89. Pellegrini, A. (2008). The recess debate. *American Journal of Play, 1,* 181–191.

90. Piaget, J. (1952). *Play, dreams and imitation in childhood.* London: William Heinemann, Ltd.

91. Pierce, D. (1991). Early object rule acquisition. *American Journal of Occupational Therapy, 45,* 438–449.

92. Pierce, D. (1997). The power of object play. In L. D. Parham & L. Fazio (Eds.), *Play in occupational therapy for children* (pp. 86–111). St. Louis: Mosby.

93. Primeau, L. (1995). *Orchestration of work and play within families.* Unpublished dissertation. Los Angeles: University of Southern California.

94. Primeau, L. (2008). AOTA's societal statement on play. *American Journal of Occupational Therapy, 62,* 707–708.

95. Rast, M. (1986). *Play and therapy, play or therapy. Play: A skill for life.* Rockville, MD: American Occupational Therapy Association.

96. Reilly, M. (1974). *Play as exploratory learning.* Beverly Hills, CA: Sage.

97. Richmond. (1960). Behavior, occupation and treatment of children. *American Journal of Occupational Therapy, 4,* 183–187.

98. Robinson, A. (1977). Play: The arena for acquisition of rules for competent behavior. *The American Journal of Occupational Therapy, 31,* 248–253.

99. Rosenblatt, D. (1977). Developmental trends in infant play. In B. Tizard & D. Harvey (Eds.), *Biology of play* (pp. 33–44). Philadelphia: J.B. Lippincott.

100. Rubin, K., Fein, G., & Vandenberg, B. (1983). Play. In P. Mussin (Ed.), *Handbook of child psychology* (Vol. IV, pp. 694–774). New York: John Wiley & Sons.

101. Rubin, K., Maioni, T. L., & Hornung, M. (1976). Free play behaviors in middle and lower-class preschoolers: Parten and Piaget revisited. *Child Development, 47,* 414–419.

102. Schiller, C. (1957). *Innate motor activity as a basis of learning, instinctive behavior.* New York: International Universities Press.

103. Schwartzman, H. (1978). *Socializing play: Functional analysis, transformations: The anthropology of children's play.* New York: Plenum Press.

104. Singer, D., Singer, J., D'Agostino, H., & DeLong, R. (2009). Children's pastimes and play in sixteen nations: Is free play declining? *American Journal of Play, 1,* 283–312.

105. Skard, G., & Bundy, A. (2008). Test of playfulness. In L. D. Parham & L. Fazio (Eds.), *Play in occupational therapy for children* (2nd ed., pp. 71–94). St. Louis: Elsevier.

106. Smilanski, S. (1968). *The effects of sociodramatic play on disadvantaged preschool children.* New York: John Wiley & Sons.

107. Spitzer, S. (2008). Play in children with autism: Structure and experience. In L. D. Parham & L. Fazio (Eds.), *Play in occupational therapy for children* (2nd ed., pp. 351–374). St Louis: Elsevier.

108. Takata, N. (1969). The play history. *American Journal of Occupational Therapy, 23,* 314–318.

109. Takata, N. (1971). The play milieu—a preliminary appraisal. *American Journal of Occupational Therapy, 25,* 281–284.

110. Takata, N. (1974). Play as a prescription. In M. Reilly (Ed.), *Play as exploratory learning* (pp. 209–246). Beverly Hills, CA: Sage.

111. Tanta, K., Dietz, J., White, O., & Billingsley, F. (2005). The effects of peer-play level on initiations and responses of preschool children with delayed play skills. *American Journal of Occupational Therapy, 59,* 437–445.

112. Vygotsky, L. (1966). Play and its role in the mental development of the child. *Soviet Psychology, 12,* 62–76.

113. White, R. (1959). Motivation reconsidered: The concept of competence. *Psychological Review, 66,* 297–333.

114. Yerxa, E., Clark, F., Frank, G., Jackson, J., Parham, D., Pierce, D., et al. (1989). An introduction to occupational science, a foundation for occupational therapy in the 21st century. *Occupational Therapy in Health Care, 6,* 1–17.

19

Prewriting and Handwriting Skills

Colleen M. Schneck • Susan J. Amundson

OBJECTIVES

1. Describe the role of the occupational therapist in the evaluation and intervention of children with handwriting difficulties.

2. Identify the factors contributing to handwriting readiness for young children.

3. Examine four aspects of functional written communication: the writing tasks in the classroom, legibility, speed, and ergonomic factors.

4. Discuss the performance skills, client factors, performance patterns, and context that influence the student's participation in the writing process.

5. Describe how handwriting fits into the educational writing process.

6. Develop remedial and compensatory strategies to improve a student's performance of written communication, focusing on the actual occupation and the occupational context.

7. Examine the relationship of various pediatric occupational therapy models of practice and handwriting intervention programs.

8. Appreciate the need for gaining more evidence about the effects of occupational therapy intervention on children's handwriting.

Occupational therapy practitioners view the occupations of children to be activities of daily living, education, work, play, and social participation. In the area of education, school-aged children's occupations encompass academic skills such as literacy (including reading and writing), calculation, and problem-solving, as well as nonacademic or functional tasks. Functional tasks may include navigating around classroom furniture and classmates, sharing school supplies with a peer, placing a notebook into a locker, constructing a papier-mâché planet, cutting with scissors, and writing words on paper—all of which support a student's academic performance in the classroom. These academic skills and functional tasks are expected to evolve and strengthen throughout a student's school years.[73]

Handwriting is a critical skill for elementary-aged students to acquire. Writing is a tool for communication; it provides a means to project thoughts, feelings, and ideas.[27] Writing is required when children and adolescents compose stories, complete written examinations, copy numbers for calculations, and write messages to friends and family members. Although computers allow students to type letters and reports, society continues to rely on handwriting to complete forms, write personal notes and messages, and maintain records. Handwriting is more than a motor skill; it requires connecting the letter name with a letterform and recalling a clear visual picture of the letterform from memory, as well as being able to execute the motor pattern required to produce the form.[37] Writing is a complex process requiring the synthesis and integration of memory retrieval, organization, problem solving, language and reading ability, ideation, and graphomotor function.[27] The functional skill of handwriting supports the academic task of writing and allows students to convey written information legibly and efficiently while accomplishing written school assignments in a timely manner.[20,45]

Handwriting consumes much of a student's school day. McHale and Cermak examined the amount of time allocated to fine motor activities and the type of fine motor activities that school-aged children were expected to perform in the classroom.[80] In their study of six classes consisting of two classrooms each from grades two, four, and six in middle-income public schools, they found that 31% to 60% of the children's school day consisted of fine motor activities. Most of these fine motor activities (85%) were paper-and-pencil tasks, indicating that students may possibly spend up to one quarter to one half of their classroom time engaged in paper-and-pencil tasks.

When children are having difficulty with handwriting, problems with written assignments follow. Students with neurologic impairments, learning problems, attention deficits, and developmental disabilities often expend enormous time and effort learning to write legibly.[6,17] Consequences of handwriting difficulties at school may include the following: (1) teachers may assign lower marks for the writing quality of papers and tests with poorer legibility but not poorer content,[26,28,48,100] (2) students' slow handwriting speed may limit compositional fluency and quality,[46,64,111] (3) students may take longer to finish assignments than their peers,[44] (4) students may have problems with taking notes in class and reading them later,[44] (5) students may fail to learn other higher-order writing processes such as planning and grammar, and (6) writing avoidance may develop, contributing later to arrested writing development.[19]

Berninger et al. explain that it is critical for children to learn to write automatically to accomplish the extensive written composition required of them in later elementary grades.[21] Handwriting instruction is important to ensure that children learn the "building blocks of written discourse automatically so that they can focus on other important aspects of writing, such as choosing and spelling words, constructing sentences, and organizing the discourse of composing written texts" (p. 4).[21]

Teachers often request that occupational therapists evaluate a student's handwriting when it interferes with performance of written assignments. In fact, poor handwriting is one of the most common reasons for referring school-aged children to occupational therapy.[25,85,92] Of school occupational therapy referrals, 80% to 85% are for fine motor and handwriting concerns that affect educational performance.

The role of the occupational therapist is to view the student's performance, in this case handwriting, by focusing on the interaction of the student, the school environment, and the demands of school occupations.[3,95] During the evaluation and intervention processes, the practitioner stays focused on (1) the occupation of handwriting, determining which domains of handwriting (e.g., near-point copying or dictation) and which components (e.g., spacing or letter formation) are problematic for the student; (2) the school context (e.g., the curriculum or physical classroom arrangement related to the child's performance; (3) the student's personal context (e.g., cultural, temporal, spiritual, and physical aspects); and (4) student experiences that are interfering with handwriting production.

THE WRITING PROCESS

The No Child Left Behind Act of 2001(NCLB) increased the emphasis on literacy and the contributions of school professionals to developing literacy skills in children. Literacy begins with the basic ability to read and write (functional literacy), which is required in everyday life, and proceeds to advanced literacy, which includes reflecting on knowledge of significant ideas, events, and values of a society.[57]

Preliteracy Writing Development of Young Children

Handwriting is a complex skill that develops over years of practice. Many children begin to draw and scribble on paper shortly after they are able to grasp a writing tool. As young children mature, they write intentionally meaningful messages, first with pictures and then with scribbles, letter-like forms, and strings of letters.[79] The development of a child's writing process in the early elementary grades includes not only mastering the mechanical and perceptual processes of graphics but also the acquisition of language and the learning of spelling and phonology.[104] Typically, children's writing and reading skills develop in parallel processes with one another.[79] Consequently, if a young child is unable to recognize letterforms and understand that these letterforms represent written language, occupational therapists and educators cannot expect the child to write.

As children develop, their scribbling and pictures evolve into the handwriting (i.e., language symbols) specific to their culture. Tan-Lin examined the sequential stages of letter acquisition of 110 children between the ages of 3 and 5 years.[103] Children were observed copying numbers, letters, a few words, and a sentence on three separate occasions over a period of 4 months. She found that the children progressed through the following sequential stages of prewriting and handwriting: (1) controlled scribbles; (2) discrete lines, dots, or symbols; (3) straight-line or circular uppercase letters; (4) uppercase letters; and (5) lowercase letters, numerals, and words. Table 19-1 details the development of prewriting and handwriting in children in the United States. Age levels of handwriting progression listed are only approximations, because variation in skill development is to be expected among young children.

Writing Development of School-Aged Children

Most children learn to write letters in kindergarten, but do not develop fluency until the third or fourth grade, and they do not demonstrate adult speed in writing until the ninth grade.[46] Handwriting requires the integration of both lower-level perceptual–motor processes and higher-level cognitive processes.[50] Correlational studies have found that handwriting skill is strongly linked to eye–hand coordination[4,24,109] and is moderately associated with dexterity.[29] A number of correlational studies found that visual-motor integration is the strongest predictor of handwriting legibility.[110,115] The perceptual-motor processes of handwriting includes visual perception (e.g. when copying from a model), auditory processing (e.g., when words are dictated), and visual motor integration (e.g. when combining the components to write). The cognitive processes involved include executive planning and use of working memory. Handwriting also requires specific language processes,[111] including the ability to hear a word and identify what letters form that word (i.e., turning spoken language into written language).

TABLE 19-1   Development of Prewriting and Handwriting in Young Children

Performance Task	Age Level
Scribbles on paper	10–12 mo
Imitates horizontal, vertical, and circular marks on paper	2 yr
Copies a vertical line, horizontal line, and circle	3 yr
Copies a cross, right oblique line, square, left diagonal line, left oblique cross, some letters and numerals, and may be able to write own name	4–5 yr
Copies a triangle, prints own name, copies most lowercase and uppercase letters	5–6 yr

Bayley, N. (2005). *Bayley scales on infant development* (rev. ed.). San Antonio, TX: Psychological Corporation; Beery, K. E., & Beery, N. (2005). *The Development Test of Visual-Motor Integration.* Cleveland: Modern Curriculum Press; Tan-Lin, A. S. (1981). An investigation into the developmental course of preschool/kindergarten aged children's handwriting behavior. *Dissertation Abstracts International, 42,* 4287A; Weil, M., & Amundson, S. J. (1994). Relationship between visual motor and handwriting skills of children in kindergarten. *American Journal of Occupational Therapy, 48,* 982–988.

When young children first learn to write their letters, they use their vision to guide their hand movements. Although adults rely more on kinesthetic input when writing,[15] children learn the skills by visually analyzing form and space, then linking the image of a letterform to a motor plan. With practice in visually guiding their hand movement, children develop a kinesthetic memory of letterforms. At this point in their learning, writing becomes automatic and minimal cortical processing is required to form letters.[7,15] In primary grades, when students are learning handwriting by copying letters, visual–motor coordination and motor dexterity are critical skills.[111] In older students, who are required to produce substantial amounts of writing, cognitive processes become more important (e.g., planning and linguistic skills). The association between lower level (perceptual–motor) handwriting skills and higher-level (memory and cognition) skills was documented by Graham, who found that difficulties with handwriting can interfere with the execution of the composing processes.[43]

Graham et al. found that handwriting fluency is a predictor of compositional fluency and quality.[45] Once a student has achieved automatic writing, he or she can focus on other aspects of writing (e.g., spelling, grammar, planning, organizing information for writing tasks) and therefore improve composition quality. Because handwriting requires perceptual–motor processes and cognitive processes, students with illegible handwriting may have deficits in either area.

Handwriting Readiness

Some controversy exists as to when children are ready for formal handwriting instruction. Differing rates of maturity, environmental experiences, and interest levels are all factors that can influence children's early attempts and success in copying letters. Some children may exhibit handwriting readiness at 4 years of age, whereas others may not be ready until they are 6 years old.[68,71] A number of authors[4,34,68,118] have stressed the importance of the mastery of handwriting readiness skills before handwriting instruction is initiated. These authors contend that children who are taught handwriting before they are ready may become discouraged and develop poor writing habits that may be difficult to correct later.

Donaghue[34] and Lamme[68] identified six prerequisite skills of children necessary before handwriting instruction begins. These are (1) small muscle development; (2) eye–hand coordination; (3) the ability to hold utensils or writing tools; (4) the ability to form basic strokes smoothly, such as circles and lines; (5) letter perception, including the ability to recognize forms, notice likenesses and differences, infer the movements necessary for the production of form, and give accurate verbal descriptions of what was seen; and (6) orientation to printed language, which involves right–left discrimination and visual analysis to determine when a group of letters forms a word.

The readiness factors needed for handwriting require the integrity of a number of sensorimotor systems. Letter formation requires the integration of the visual, motor, sensory, and perceptual systems. Performance components associated with handwriting include kinesthesia, motor planning, eye–hand coordination, visual–motor integration, and in-hand manipulation. Kinesthesia provides the ongoing error information and references for subsequent repetitions.[71] In addition, it provides information about directionality during letter formation. Good kinesthetic information enhances speed, reduces the need to visually monitor the hand during writing, and influences the amount of pressure applied to the writing implement. Sufficient fine motor coordination is also needed to form letters accurately.[4]

Benbow described six developmental classifications that underlie skilled use of the hands that contribute to greater adeptness in operating a pencil: (1) upper extremity support, (2) wrist and hand development, (3) visual control, (4) bilateral integration, (5) spatial analysis, and (6) kinesthesia.[15] Other authors define readiness for handwriting on the basis of a child's ability to copy geometric forms. Beery[13] and Benbow, Hanft, and Marsh[16] suggested that instruction in handwriting be postponed until after the child is able to master the first nine figures in the Developmental Test of Visual–Motor Integration (VMI).[13] The nine figures are a vertical line, a horizontal line, a circle, a cross, a right oblique line, a square, a left oblique line, an oblique cross, and a triangle.

A study by Weil and Amundson examined 59 kindergarten children who were developing typically (ages 54 to 64 months) and assessed their abilities to copy letterforms as well as the geometric designs on the VMI.[113] The findings indicated that children who were able to copy the first nine forms of the VMI correctly copied significantly more letters than those who were not able to copy the first nine forms, thus providing support for the opinions of Beery[13] and Benbow et al.[16] Weil and Amundson also found that kindergarten children, on average, correctly copied 78% of the letters presented, despite not having received formal handwriting instruction.[113] Based on these results, the authors concluded that most typically developing kindergarten children should be ready for actual handwriting instruction in the latter half of the kindergarten school year.

To develop children's handwriting readiness skills, the occupational therapy practitioner may incorporate activities into therapy sessions or the classroom. Selected activities should be aimed at improving fine motor control and isolated finger movements, promoting prewriting skills, enhancing right–left discrimination, and improving orientation to printed language.[12,15,16,68,84,118]

Some children with significant cognitive or physical impairments may not acquire many of the prerequisite components needed for writing, and they are most successful in written communication using a computer with word processing and word prediction software programs. Other children, despite lacking the prerequisite components for handwriting, may be able to learn to write their name with practice. The occupational therapy practitioner must determine when it is appropriate for the young child to work on prerequisite handwriting skills, the functional skill of handwriting, or both. Activities commonly used with young children to facilitate certain movements, experiences, and perception for handwriting development are listed in Table 19-2. Movements and tasks to encourage handwriting development should be used in the context of what is meaningful and purposeful to the child.

Pencil Grip Progression

The development of pencil grip in young children follows a predictable course for typically developing children but may vary among cultures.[107] Children commonly begin by holding the pencil with a primitive grip—characterized by holding the writing tool with the whole hand or extended fingers,

TABLE 19-2 Activities to Promote Handwriting Readiness

Areas of Handwriting Readiness	Selected Readiness Activities
Improving fine motor control and the isolated finger movements	Roll one-quarter- to one-eighth–inch balls of clay or Silly Putty between the tips of thumb and the index and middle fingers. Pick up small objects (e.g., Cheerios or raisins) with a tweezers. Pinch and seal a Ziploc bag using the thumb opposing each finger. Twist open a small tube of toothpaste with the thumb and index and middle fingers. Move a key from the palm to the fingertips of one hand.
Promoting graphic skills	Draw lines and copy shapes using shaving cream, sand trays, or finger paints. Draw lines and shapes to complete a picture story on blackboards. Form and color pictures of people, houses, trees, cars, or animals. Complete simple dot-to-dot pictures and mazes.
Enhancing right-left discrimination	Perform the "hokey-pokey" dance. Maneuver through obstacles and focusing on the concept of turning right or left. Connect dots at the chalkboard with left-to-right strokes.
Improving orientation to printed language	Label children's drawings based on the child's description. Encourage book-making with child's favorite topics (e.g., special places, favorite foods). Label common objects in the classroom.

pronating the forearm, and using the shoulder to move the pencil. Later, a transitional pencil grip is seen with the pencil being held with flexed fingers. Initially, the forearm is pronated (thumb side downward); later, the forearm is usually supinated. In the mature pencil grip, the pencil is stabilized by the distal phalanges of the thumb and index, middle, and possibly ring fingers, the wrist is slightly extended yet dynamic, and the supinated forearm rests on the table.[38,94,98,107]

Traditionally, teachers and occupational therapy practitioners have stressed the importance of a dynamic tripod pencil grasp.[94,109] In this grip the writing utensil rests against the distal phalanx of the radial side of the middle finger while the pads of the thumb and index finger control it (Figure 19-1).[94] Recent studies[18,31,67,97,98,107,120] have found that a variety of pencil grasp patterns exist among typical adults and children. Frequently observed mature pencil grips, besides the dynamic tripod grasp, include the lateral tripod, the dynamic quadrupod, and the lateral quadrupod. Schneck and Henderson reported in their study of 320 typically developing children that by the age of 6.5 to 7 years, 95% had adopted a mature pencil grasp, either the dynamic tripod (72.5%) or the lateral tripod (22.5%).[98] Outside of the United States, Tseng noted that the lateral tripod grip (42.9%) occurred almost as frequently as the dynamic tripod (44.1%) for typically developing Taiwanese children 5.5 to 6.4 years of age.[107]

In older elementary children, the dynamic quadrupod and lateral quadrupod grips have been identified as functional and mature pencil grasps.[31,67] Thus, the lateral tripod, the dynamic quadrupod, and the lateral quadrupod grips may all be considered acceptable alternatives to the traditionally preferred dynamic tripod grip (see Figure 19-1).

HANDWRITING EVALUATION

When a child with poor handwriting has been referred to occupational therapy, the methods to gather evaluation information must be carefully selected and sequenced. An individual

evaluation is needed because each child with handwriting dysfunction varies from every other child with handwriting problems. A comprehensive evaluation of a child's handwriting includes: (1) the occupational profile; and (2) the analysis of occupational performance.

Initially, the student's performance in the context of classroom standards should be the focus (before moving toward standardized testing). Assembling data and information from various sources gives the occupational therapist an integrated picture of the child's written communication. It also allows the therapist to examine the child's ability to perform other functional school tasks, such as handling school supplies and tools, managing outdoor clothing and fasteners, and organizing school materials. Although poor handwriting is a common referring concern in the classroom, poor performance of other school tasks may have gone unnoticed and should also receive attention from the occupational therapist and educational team.

Occupational Profile

The Occupational Profile describes the student's occupational therapy history, experiences, patterns of daily living, interests, values, and needs. It is designed to gain an understanding of the client's perspective and background.[82] The information for the occupational profile can be gathered by interviewing the child, parent(s), teacher, and other team members. Interviewing the child's parents, educator, and other team members also serves as a mechanism for building rapport.

Interviews

Interviewing the child helps the therapist to understand what is important and meaningful to the child. This information helps the therapist gain an understanding of the child's perspective and background. Because teachers observe their students' daily performance in class, they can share information about the student's abilities and achievements and how the student responds to instruction. A sampling of questions to

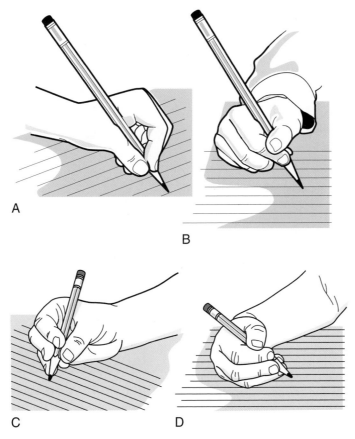

FIGURE 19-1 Mature pencil grips in elementary school children. *A,* Dynamic tripod; *B,* lateral tripod; *C,* dynamic quadrupod; and *D,* lateral quadrupod.

acilitate discussion between the teacher and the occupational therapist is listed in Box 19-1. The educator provides a background picture of the student's capabilities, behavior, and struggles at school.

Cornhill and Case-Smith found that students with poor handwriting, as identified by teacher reports, scored significantly lower on three assessments of sensory motor performance components (eye–hand coordination, visual–motor integration, and in-hand manipulation) than students with good handwriting.[29] In addition, the authors found that scores on assessments of these performance skills could be used to predict scores in the handwriting performance. Teachers report that they evaluate students' handwriting by comparing it with that of classroom peers (37%) or comparing it with student handwriting in a book (35%).[52]

Parents are also a valuable resource for occupational therapists; they provide a different perspective on the child and the child's handwriting abilities. Not only can parents relate the child's developmental, medical, and familial background to the educational team, but they can share invaluable information about the child's interests, social competence, and attitudes toward learning and school.

Parents are considered educational team members, and they provide important perspectives that give the occupational therapist a comprehensive view of the child at home and at school. To facilitate discussion about the child and his or her writing, parents might be asked questions such as the following: (1) Do parents expect the child to complete school assignments or written work at home? (2) What is the child's response

---

BOX 19-1 Questions to Facilitate Discussion among Educational Team Members

1. What are the student's educational strengths and concerns?
2. What is his or her handwriting performance compared with that of peers?
3. What handwriting method (D'Nealian, Zaner-Blöser, Palmer, italics) is being used and what is the student's history with this method?
4. What are the learning standards or curriculum of his or her grade?
5. What seems to be causing the poor handwriting?

6. When does he or she do his or her best written work?
7. When does the performance break down?
8. What strategies for improvement have been tried? Have they worked?
9. Is a student portfolio available on the student's writing development and progress?
10. Are there other daily tasks (e.g., using scissors, getting along with peers, keeping organized) that raise concern for the teacher?

to written homework? (3) How does the child perform his or her written assignments at home and at school? (4) What other writing tasks are expected of the child at home (e.g., corresponding with relatives, recording telephone messages)?

Analysis of Occupational Performance

A comprehensive evaluation of a child's handwriting includes (1) examining written work samples; (2) further discussing the child's performance with the teacher, parent, and other team members; (3) reviewing the child's educational and clinical records; (4) directly observing the child when he or she is writing in the natural setting (i.e., school, home); (5) evaluating the child's actual performance of handwriting; and (6) assessing any performance skills suspected to be interfering with handwriting.

Work Samples

As part of the evaluation process, the occupational therapist accesses the child's handwritten class work or homework. Written work samples may include spelling lessons, mathematical problems, or a story. Ideally, these samples should represent a typical handwriting performance of the child. When reviewing the child's written product, a comparison of the writing samples of the child's peers is also warranted to clarify the classroom standards and teacher expectations. Informal evaluation of the work samples for alignment, size, letter formation, legibility, and slant may indicate the need for further evaluation.

File Review

Relevant information regarding past academic performance, special testing, or receipt of special services can be found in the referred child's educational cumulative file. Medical or clinical reports related to the child's education may also be located in the child's regular or special education files. The child's parents may share academic records and reports with clinic- and hospital-based occupational therapists. This documentation may trigger further conversations among the child's parents and team members.

Direct Observation

Observing the student during a writing activity in the classroom is an essential step in the evaluation process (Figure 19-2). Skilled observation by the examiner usually occurs in the child's classroom and focuses on task performance, attention to task, problem solving, and behavior of the child.[55] Practitioners also note the student's organizational abilities, movement through the classroom, interactions with the teacher and peers, transitions between activities, and overall performance of other school tasks. School contextual features (e.g., the classroom arrangement, lighting, noise level, instructional media), as well as the actual instruction from school personnel, should all be considered in relationship to the student's performance. In addition to a structured protocol for direct observation, the occupational therapist may ask the following:

1. Which writing tasks (for example, copying sentences from the chalkboard or composing a story) are most problematic for the child?

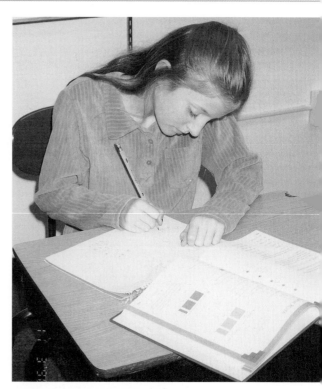

FIGURE 19-2 A girl completes a written assignment at her desk.

2. What behaviors are manifested when the child is required to write? For example, does the child chew on the eraser of the pencil or blow the pencil across the desktop to avoid writing?
3. Can the child engage independently in the task of writing, or does she or he need physical and verbal cues from the teacher or educational assistant?
4. Is the child easily distracted by visual and auditory stimuli during writing, such as a delivery truck driving by the school window?
5. Where does the child sit in the classroom?
6. What curriculum is being followed?
7. Where is the teacher located when he or she gives assignment directions?
8. How does the observed difficulty interfere with the child's learning?

MEASURING HANDWRITING PERFORMANCE

In evaluating the actual task of children's handwriting, the following areas need to be examined: (1) domains of handwriting, (2) legibility components, (3) writing speed, and (4) ergonomic factors. Whether the student writes in manuscript (print), cursive (joined script), or both, these four aspects will help the educational team and parents uncover problematic areas of handwriting and establish a baseline of handwriting function. With accurate and relevant handwriting assessment data, the occupational therapist, the child's parents, and the educational or clinical team will also be able to target specific goals and objectives for the development of written communication.

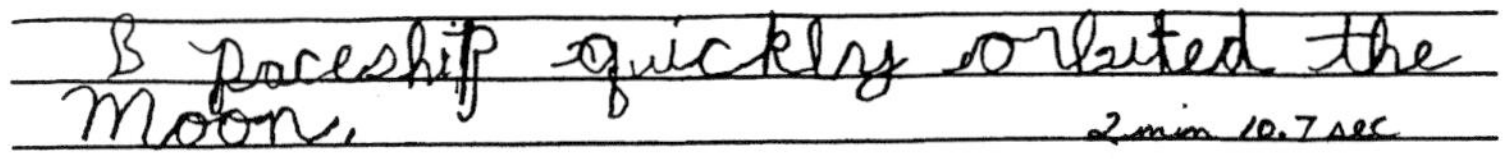

FIGURE 19-3 Cursive handwriting sample exemplifies improper letterforms and disproportionate letter size.

Domains of Handwriting

Evaluating the various domains of handwriting allows the occupational therapist to determine which tasks the child may be having difficulty with and address those tasks in the intervention plan. Handwriting tasks demanded of students, and helpful for intervention planning, include the following:

- Writing the alphabet in both uppercase and lowercase letters along with numbers requires the child to remember the motor engram, form each individual letter and numeral, sequence letters and numbers, and use consistent letter cases.
- Copying is the capacity to reproduce numerals, letters, and words from a similar script model, either manuscript to manuscript or cursive to cursive.
- *Near-point copying* is producing letters or words from a nearby model, commonly on the same page or on the same horizontal writing surface, as when an elementary pupil copies the meaning of a word from a nearby dictionary.
- Copying from a distant vertical display model to the writing surface is termed *far-point copying,* demonstrated by early elementary students writing the words "Happy Valentine's Day" on construction paper cards from the teacher's modeled words on the class chalkboard.
- More advanced than copying, manuscript-to-cursive transition requires a mastery of letterforms in both manuscript and cursive as the child must transcribe manuscript letters and words to cursive letters and words.
- Writing dictated words, names, addresses, and telephone numbers is a skill children will need at school and at home. A higher-level handwriting task combining integration of auditory directions and a motoric response is dictation.
- Composition is the generation of a sentence or paragraph by the child demonstrated by writing a poem, a story, or a note to a friend. The composing process uses the cognitive functions of planning, sentence generation, and revision[56]; thus, this writing task involves complex integration of linguistic, cognitive, organizational, and sensorimotor skills.

Legibility

Legibility is often assessed in terms of its components—letter formation, alignment, spacing, size, and slant.[1,7,47,60,120] However, the bottom line of legibility is readability. Of primary importance is whether what was written by the child can be read by the child, parent, or teacher. In a handwriting evaluation, the components of both legibility and readability need to be assessed.

The influence of legibility components on readability is significant.[47,61] In *letter formation,* Alston identified five features affecting legibility: (1) improper letterforms, (2) poor leading in and leading out of letters, (3) inadequate rounding of letters, (4) incomplete closures of letters, and (5) incorrect letter ascenders and descenders.[1] *Alignment,* or baseline orientation, refers to the placement of text on and within the writing guidelines. *Spacing* includes the dispersion of letters within words and words within sentences[70] and text organization on the entire sheet of paper. Another component of legibility, *size,* refers to the letter relative to the writing guidelines and to the other letters. Finally, the uniformity or consistency of the *slant* or the angle of the text should be observed. Figure 19-3 illustrates errors of letter formation and size in a child's cursive writing.

Although a child's writing sample may still be readable even though a legibility component (e.g., poor sizing) interferes with its appearance, some legibility components have a stronger impact on readability than others. Graham et al. found that the letter formation, spacing, and neatness of 61 fourth-grade students with learning disabilities all significantly correlated with legibility.[47] Typically, legibility is determined by counting the number of readable written letters or words and dividing it by the total number of written letters or words in a writing sample. Figure 19-4 provides the formula to determine word legibility percentage. As reflected in the figure, eight words were written in the child's writing sample; however, only four of them were legible, resulting in 50% word legibility.

Frequently, occupational therapy practitioners and educators want to determine what legibility percentage is appropriate for students at specific grade levels. Likewise, occupational therapists are interested in the "cut-off" legibility percentages for poor and good handwriting. The validity of readability and legibility percentages has been reported in three studies with small samples.

The first study conducted by Talbert-Johnson, Salva, Sweeney, and Cooper asked 15 upper elementary, middle school, and high school students with special needs to copy a short passage in cursive writing.[102] Through a sorting process, easy-to-read handwriting samples scored between 95% and 100% letter legibility, with a mean of 99%. Conversely, difficult-to-read handwriting measured at 60% to 90% letter legibility, with a mean of 78%. In the second study, Reisman found that 51 second grade students receiving handwriting intervention in occupational therapy averaged a 76% legibility rate on a pilot version of the Minnesota Handwriting Test.[92] In a third example, Graham, Berninger, Weintraub, and Shafer, in their study of 900 children who were developing typically in grades one through nine, found that handwriting legibility showed little improvement in the first four elementary grades.[46] Legibility gains were made in the upper elementary grades and maintained through junior high school.

Koziatek and Powell investigated four writing tasks from the Evaluation Tool of Children's Handwriting-Cursive

Word legibility percentage =

$$\frac{\text{Total number of readable words}}{\text{Total number of written words}} = \frac{4}{8} = 50\%$$

FIGURE 19-4 Word legibility percentages are calculated using a simple mathematical formula.

(ETCH-C) with 101 fourth-grade students.[66] They found that the ETCH-C letter and word legibility scores were able to classify and predict children's handwriting grades on report cards. The 75% word legibility level of the ETCH-C could discriminate between satisfactory (C or better grades) and unsatisfactory cursive handwriting.

Although each of the aforementioned studies examining legibility rates used different measures, implications for occupational therapy practice suggest that the range of 75% to 78% appears to discriminate between satisfactory and unsatisfactory handwriting legibility. This range of legibility percentages, however, is not the benchmark for which children warrant occupational therapy services. A student's handwriting may be at the 75% legibility level and still be unreadable. With recommended compensatory strategies from the occupational therapy practitioner, this same child might boost his or her handwriting to a readable level. Thus, no ongoing occupational therapy services may be needed. Determining appropriate educational and therapeutic services for children involves an entire team, including the child's parents, and, of course, should never depend solely on test scores. Thus, the occupational therapist must carefully and comprehensively assess the nature of the child's poor handwriting and give recommendations based on this process.

Writing Speed

A child's rate of writing, or the number of letters written per minute, and its legibility are the two cornerstones of functional handwriting.[7] Students may take longer to complete written assignments, have difficulty taking notes in class,[44] lose their train of ideas for writing,[78] and become frustrated when their handwriting speed is slower than that of their peers. Writing speed typically decreases when the amount of written work or complexity of the writing task increases.[95,114] Upper elementary and older students need not only an adequate writing speed but also the ability to adjust their speed from a hurried, rough draft to a neat, well-paced final one.[114]

Differences in methodologies, subjects, and data collection in relevant studies have resulted in a varied baseline of writing speeds for typically developing children.[108,120] These studies show that children's handwriting speeds develop gradually, becoming faster in each succeeding grade.[46,53,90,91,120,121] However, the studies' findings also suggest that the increase in speed may not be linear but marked by various spurts and plateaus. Handwriting speed per grade level has been found to be highly variable when different study designs and writing conditions are used.

Because of the wide range of handwriting speeds, children's writing rates need to be considered individually within the context of their classroom. Teacher expectations and classroom standards may influence children's writing speeds. Thus, it is appropriate to compare a student's writing speed performance with the rates of classroom peers. In general, handwriting speed is problematic when a student is unable to complete written school assignments in a timely manner. When a student's written expression abilities (e.g., language, spelling) exceed handwriting rate, alternative forms (e.g., keyboarding, word prediction programs) should be considered.

Ergonomic Factors

Writing posture, upper extremity stability and mobility, and pencil grip are ergonomic factors that must be analyzed as the child writes. Sitting posture in the classroom should be observed. Does the child rest his or her head on the forearm or desktop when writing? Is the child falling out of or slumping in his or her chair? Does the child stand beside the desk or kneel in the chair? Are the desktop and the chair at suitable heights?

Stability and mobility of the upper extremities (i.e., the ability to keep the shoulder girdle, elbow, and wrist stable) allow the dexterous hand to manipulate the writing instrument. Does the child write with whole-arm movements? What are the positions of the trunk and writing arm? Does the non-preferred hand stabilize the paper? Does the child apply excessive pressure to the writing tool?

An ergonomic focus for most occupational therapy practitioners is whether a child is holding the pencil properly, or using an atypical pencil grasp. Ziviani reported that different grasp variations are expected.[119] Poor writers tend to demonstrate a greater variety of atypical grasp patterns than legible writers. Mature pencil grips for children now include the dynamic tripod, the lateral tripod, the dynamic quadrupod, and the lateral quadrupod.[31,67,98,107] Unconventional pencil grips do not necessarily affect the speed or the legibility of the child's handwriting.[31,109]

HANDWRITING ASSESSMENTS

Formal or standardized tests are important for assessing the performance of children, as they provide objective measures and quantitative scores, aid in monitoring a child's progress, help professionals communicate more clearly, and advance the field through research. Numerous standardized handwriting instruments are available commercially. Assessment tools commonly used by occupational therapists in the United States include the Children's Handwriting Evaluation Scale,[91] the Children's Handwriting Evaluation Scale—Manuscript,[90] the Denver Handwriting Analysis,[9] the Minnesota Handwriting Test,[93] the Evaluation Tool of Children's Handwriting,[7] the Test of Handwriting Skills,[42] and The Print Tool.[86]

Each of these assessment tools possesses various features regarding domains of handwriting tested (e.g., far-point copying, dictation), age or grade of child (e.g., first and second grades), script examined (e.g., cursive), scoring procedures of the writing performance (e.g., legibility of manuscript), and scores obtained (e.g., percentiles). Typically, tests measure handwriting legibility and speed of handwriting. Scoring procedures for legibility use rating techniques ranging from global and subjective to detailed and specific.[108] Appendix 19-A provides publication information regarding handwriting assessments available to occupational therapists.

For tool selection, the occupational therapist should keep in mind the characteristics of each assessment as well as the strengths and limitations of the tests regarding normative data, reliability, validity, and other psychometric properties (see Chapter 8). Critiques and lengthier descriptions of andwriting assessments by several authors[6,30,92,108] should be reviewed in selecting the most appropriate test. A shortcoming of most handwriting instruments is the low reliability for measuring legibility owing to the subjective nature of judging handwriting legibility.[33] The assessment chosen should match the areas of concern regarding the child's handwriting and should allow for effective intervention planning among the occupational therapist, the child's parents, and other team members.

Factors Restricting Handwriting Performance

To understand more fully which element may be interfering with a child's ability to produce text, the occupational therapist must consider a child's *performance skills, client factors, performance patterns,* and *contextual elements.*[5] As occupational therapists build their clinical reasoning skills, they are able to observe a child struggling to write or view a child's distorted, unreadable handwriting and identify factors that might be interfering with the child's written communication. The example in Case Study 19-1 indicates how various factors may restrict a child's handwriting performance. This example illustrates the complex interactions that occupational therapists must be able to analyze to determine what factors influence a child's ability to engage in an occupation such as handwriting.

Like Natasha, children with poor handwriting typically have a web of factors that restrict their handwriting performance. The occupational therapist must unravel each factor from the others to understand its influence as well as its interaction with other performance factors. For example, Natasha's client factors (i.e., short attention span, impulsiveness) and cultural context (i.e., English as a second language) interact with one another to restrict her handwriting performance. Natasha's short attention span diminishes not only her ability to learn handwriting but also her ability to learn new concepts, including her second language, English. If she is unable to understand the language symbols, words, and syntax of the English language, she will have difficulty reading English. Furthermore, because reading and writing are parallel learning processes, Natasha's handwriting will be impeded. Natasha's handwriting is more likely to improve once effective compensatory and remedial techniques are in place to improve her attention span and her knowledge and use of the English language.

EDUCATOR'S PERSPECTIVE

Writing Process

State standards for written language and literacy, as well as the district curriculum, should be used to guide evaluation and intervention. When educators speak of the writing or composing process, they view it as a goal-directed activity using the cognitive functions of planning, sentence generation, and revision.[56] The actual text production occurs in sentence generation; thus, the child who needs to pay considerable attention to the mechanical requirements of writing may interrupt higher order writing processes, such as planning or content generation. Hence, most educators view the mechanical requirements of handwriting as an integral subset of the writing process. Two factors that teachers indicated most frequently as important for handwriting to be acceptable were (1) correct letter formation and (2) directionality and proper spacing.[52]

Handwriting Instruction Methods and Curricula

During the past decade, an educational debate has focused on teaching handwriting systematically through commercially prepared or teacher-developed programs, or learning it through a "whole-language" approach. The whole-language philosophy purports that both the substance (meaning) of writing and the form (mechanics) of writing are critical for learning to write.[44] Thus, when using the whole-language method as children are learning and mastering handwriting, the teacher gives advice and assigns practice on an individual, as-needed basis. For example, if an educator sees a first-grader struggling to form the letter *m* while writing a story about monsters, he or she may instruct the child regarding the correct letter formation of *m* and encourage extra practice of the letter during the story composition period. Conversely, in a traditional handwriting instruction approach, students are introduced to letter formations and practice them outside of the context of writing. For children with learning disabilities and mild neurologic impairments, regular practice in forming letters is essential in the early stages of handwriting development, yet handwriting should have a meaningful context. Thus, a combination of systematic handwriting instruction

---

> ### CASE STUDY 19-1   Natasha
>
> Natasha, a 9-year-old girl with a traumatic brain injury, has an illegible script marked by overlapping letters, poor use of writing lines, and many dark erasures. When evaluating Natasha's writing performance in her classroom, the occupational therapist observes that her performance skills, particularly her fine motor coordination, are limited. In-hand manipulation skills are poor as Natasha struggles to turn her pencil from the writing position to the erasing position, manage her worksheet, and use her eraser for correcting errors. When she is engaging in classroom activities, the occupational therapist sees that Natasha has a short attention span and impulsiveness. Natasha has difficulty sustaining her attention to desktop work and the teacher's verbal instructions. Furthermore, when the occupational therapist examines a story that Natasha wrote earlier during the day, it is apparent that she has not incorporated the habit of writing her text on the lines of the paper. Because she does not adopt this performance pattern, Natasha's text bumps above and below the writing baseline on her paper, resulting in an unreadable story. Finally, the occupational therapist is told by a classroom paraprofessional that Natasha uses English as a second language due to her recent emigration to the United States. Consequently, the occupational therapy practitioner recognizes that her cultural context may be affecting her overall performance in the classroom.

TABLE 19-3 Evidence on Classroom Instruction

Author	Methods	Evidence
Alston (1995)	Studied British students attending 14 schools that used a systematic handwriting program and 2 schools that used a less systematic approach Correlational	Students taught with systematic and nonsystematic handwriting approaches are equally likely to have handwriting problems
Graham & Harris (1994)	Systematic review	Handwriting best learned by letter formation naturally and in concert with other language skills
Rubin & Henderson (1982)	Questionnaire to all teachers of children 10 yr old in London, U.K. Descriptive	4 of 5 teach handwriting Majority of handwriting lessons were structured for the whole class, supplemented by incidental instruction 68% use workbooks 61% taught handwriting 20–60 min. per week
Stein (1990)	Questionnaire to 274 special education teachers in Michigan (34% return rate) Descriptive	70% handwriting mainly taught by regular teachers, special education provides support
Zaner-Blöser (1993)	Surveyed 4970 K–6 teachers in the U.S. Descriptive	4 of 5 schools require teaching of handwriting 75% use commercial handwriting program Typically spent 30–60 min. per week teaching handwriting 67% thought more emphasis should be placed on handwriting 70% thought handwriting is not as good as it should be 36% received handwriting instruction training in undergraduate degree 50% thought handwriting should be incorporated into language arts

Alston, J. (1995). Assessing writing speeds and output: Some current norms and issues. *Handwriting Review,* 102–106; Graham, S., & Harris, K. R. (1994). The effects of whole language on writing: A review. *Educational Psychology, 2,* 187–192; Rubin, N., & Henderson, S. E. (1982). Two sides of the same coin: Variations in teaching methods and failure to learn to write. *Special Education: Forward Trends, 9,* 17–24; Stein, R. A. (1990). *Teacher-recommended methods and materials for teaching penmanship and spelling to the learning disabled.* ERIC Document Reproduction Service (ED 334 735), Michigan; Zaner-Blöser. (1993). *The Zaner-Blöser Handwriting Survey: Preliminary tabulations.* Zaner-Blöser: Columbus, OH.

and whole-language methods may be most beneficial to this group of children.[44]

In the United States, traditional handwriting instruction programs vary from school district to school district and occasionally from school to school and grade to grade. It is not uncommon for occupational therapy practitioners to receive a referral for a child with poor handwriting who has never had handwriting instruction! See Table 19-3 for evidence on classroom instruction.

The most common instruction methods include Palmer, Zaner-Blöser, italics, and D'Nealian.[4,36,105] See Appendix 19-B for a list of handwriting methods used in schools. Unlike the United States, a few countries, such as the United Kingdom, New Zealand, and Australia,[2,4,62,121] have adopted national curricula for handwriting to improve the standards of handwriting assessment and instruction within their school systems (see Appendix 19-C on the Evolve website for handwriting curricula). Early childhood handwriting curricula should include at least six skill areas: (1) small muscle development, (2) eye–hand coordination, (3) holding a writing tool, (4) basic strokes, (5) letter perception, and (6) orientation to printed language. See Table 19-4 for research on handwriting programs.

Manuscript and Cursive Styles

A generally accepted sequence for handwriting instruction is manuscript writing for use in grades one and two, with children transitioning to cursive writing at the end of grade two

or the beginning of grade three.[12,17,51] The need for manuscript writing may continue throughout life, when students label maps and posters, adolescents complete job or college applications, and adults complete federal income tax forms. By middle school, many students have blended both manuscript and cursive to form their own style of handwriting. To date, no research has decisively indicated the superiority of one script style over the other.

Both manuscript and cursive possess complementary features, and these should be considered when the occupational therapist, child, child's parent, and educational team are collaboratively deciding which style might best serve the child.

Manuscript is endorsed for the following reasons:

1. Manuscript letterforms are simpler and hence are easier to learn.
2. It closely resembles the print of textbooks and school manuals.
3. It is needed throughout adult life for documents and applications.
4. Beginning manuscript writing is more readable than cursive.
5. Ball and stick strokes of manuscript letter formations may be more developmentally appropriate than cursive letters for young children.
6. Manuscript letters are easier to discriminate visually than cursive ones.[11,17,49,51]
7. The traditional vertical alphabet is more developmentally appropriate, easier to read, and easier to write for young children, as well as easier for educators to teach, than the slanted alphabet.

TABLE 19-4 Handwriting Programs Research

Author(s)	Age/Grade and No. of Children	Program(s)/Frameworks used	Time	Measures	Effectiveness
Berninger, Vaughan, Abbott, Rogan, Brooks, Reed, & Graham (1997)	144 first graders	Handwriting styles used: D'Nealian or standard ball & stick Treatment Groups: 1) motor imitation 2) visual cue 3) memory retrieval 4) visual cue + memory retrieval 5) copy 6) control group Rosner's Auditory Analysis Program	Twice a week in 20-min. sessions for 24 lessons	Timed measures of handwriting; 6 finger function tasks; 3 timed handwriting tasks; 3 other tasks; Writing Fluency subtest of the Woodcock-Johnson Psycho-educational Battery—Revised; Vocabulary subtest of the Wechsler Intelligence Scale for Children—3rd edition; Word Attack subtest of the revised Woodcock Reading Mastery Test	Combining numbered arrows and memory retrieval was most effective treatment for improving handwriting and compositional fluency.
Case-Smith (2002)	Second-, third-, and fourth-grade students aged 7-10 yr 29 received occupational therapy intervention, 9 did not	Therapists reported using handwriting practice or activities designed specifically to improve handwriting. They reported using eclectic approaches (ideas from various published curricula and programs) and individualized the intervention emphasis according to individual student needs.	Mean duration of sessions—32.2 min. Mean number of sessions—16.4 (slightly more than twice per month) for 7 mo (school year)	3 subtests of the Developmental Test of Visual Perception (DTVP); Bruininks-Oseretsky Test of Motor Proficiency (BOTMP); translation and rotation were measured using the nine-hole peg test; Evaluation Tool of Children's Handwriting (ETCH); School Function Assessment (SFA)	Students in the intervention group showed significant increases in in-hand manipulation and position in space scores, and improved more in letter legibility scores. Speed and numeral legibility did not demonstrate positive intervention effects.
Graham & Harris (2006)	30 first-grade students (15 were chosen for program)	CASL First Grade Handwriting/Spelling Program—described in article	48 20-min. lessons divided into 8 units, with 6 lessons in each unit	Not specified	Students who participated in program made greater gains in spelling, handwriting legibility and fluency, sentence writing, and vocabulary diversity in their compositions immediately after instruction.
Keller (2001)	Third- and fourth-grade boys	Handwriting Without Tears; use of many sensory integration activities including the program, How Does Your Engine Run?	Twice a week for 30-min. sessions (reported as not being long enough)	Not specified	Students improved cursive writing skills and social skills. They learned which sensory activities helped them to focus and self-regulate. Students felt more confident in handwriting abilities.

Continued

TABLE 19-4 Handwriting Programs Research—Cont'd

Author(s)	Age/Grade and No. of Children	Program(s)/Frameworks used	Time	Measures	Effectiveness
Marr & Dimeo (2006)	26 students ages 6.2–11.9 Grades 1-6	Handwriting Without Tears	1 hr per day for 2 wk	Evaluation Tool of Children's Handwriting; Likert ratings provided by parents pretest, posttest, and 3 mo posttest	Significant changes in legibility of writing the uppercase and lowercase alphabets. Improvements in two subtests of ETCH and in parent ratings.
McGarrigle & Nelson (2006)	16 first-grade students (13 completed end-program testing)	Interventions developed by third-year occupational therapy students. Frameworks used—sensorimotor, biomechanical, teaching—learning principles, and principles of practice when working with indigenous children.	80-min sessions once a week for 6 wk	Beery-Buktenica Developmental Test of Visual-Motor Integration (VMI); Conners' Abbreviated Symptom Questionnaire (ASQ); nonstandardized handwriting measure; non-standardized scissor skills measure	Significant improvements in their sitting posture, pencil grasp, pencil pressure, and paper stabilization/positioning. Students improved their tracing and copying accuracy, and letter inclusion, legibility, and formation when writing their name and letters of the alphabet. Improved in aspects of handwriting, scissor skills, and behavior.
Peterson & Nelson (2003)	59 first-graders (30 selected for intervention group) Students' mean age: 7.1 yr	D'Nealian handwriting; frameworks- biomechanical, sensorimotor, and teaching-learning principles	30-min sessions, twice a week, for 10 wk	Minnesota Handwriting Test	Intervention group demonstrated a significant increase in scores on the posttest of the Minnesota Handwriting Test when compared with scores of the control group.
Ratzon, Efraim, & Bart (2007)	52 first-grade students (24 participants in intervention group)	Graphomotor intervention program developed by Efraim (2002). Activities and tools based on Benbow's[14] recommendations. Frameworks— motor learning, multisensory, and research that found associations between dexterity skills and normal development of visual-motor proficiency	12 sessions, once a week, for 45 min	Beery-Buktenica Developmental Test of Visual-Motor Integration (VMI); Developmental Test of Visual Perception (DTVP-2); Motor Development Scale of the Bruininks-Oseretsky Test of Motor Proficiency	Students in intervention group made significant gains in the total score on the graphomotor test (DTVP-2) and on the fine motor test (Bruininks-Oseretsky Motor Development Scale)

Berninger, V., Vaughan, K. B., Abbott, R. D., Abbott, S. P., Rogan, L. W., Brooks, A., et al. (1997). Treatment of handwriting problems in beginning writers: Transfer from handwriting to composition. *Journal of Education Psychology, 89,* 652–666; Case-Smith, J. (2002). Effectiveness of school-based occupational therapy intervention on handwriting. *American Journal of Occupational Therapy, 56,* 17–25; Graham, S., & Harris, K. R. (2006). Preventing writing difficulties: Providing additional handwriting and spelling instruction to at-risk children in first grade. *TEACHING Exceptional Children, 38,* 64–66; Keller, M. (2001). Handwriting club: Using sensory integration strategies to improve handwriting. *Intervention in School and Clinic, 37,* 9–12; Marr, D., & Dimeo, S. B. (2006). Outcomes associated with a summer handwriting course for elementary students. *American Journal of Occupational Therapy, 60,* 10–15; McGarrigle, J., & Nelson, A. (2006). Evaluating a school skills programme for Australian Indigenous children: A pilot study. *Occupational Therapy International, 13,* 1–20; Peterson, C. Q., & Nelson, D. L. (2003). Effect of an occupational intervention on children with economic disadvantages. *American Journal of Occupational Therapy, 57,* 152–160; Ratzon, N. Z., Efraim, D., & Bart, O. (2007). A short-term graphomotor program for improving writing readiness skills of first-grade students. *American Journal of Occupational Therapy, 61,* 399–405.

Advocates of cursive writing point out the following:

1. Cursive movement patterns allow for faster and more automatic writing.
2. Reversal of individual letters and transpositions of words are more difficult than in manuscript.
3. One continuous, connected line enables child to form words as units.
4. Cursive allows the poor printer a new type of written format, which may be motivating at the child's present maturity level.[10,17,49,51]
5. The brain is not developed for the fine visual–motor distinctions necessary for manuscript.[63]

HANDWRITING INTERVENTION

Planning

In school settings, if the referred child's educational team decides that functional written communication is a priority for the child's educational program, the occupational therapist may be instrumental in directing and guiding this aspect of the program. Typically, the team uses either a remedial or a compensatory intervention approach, or both, to improve the child's written communication. Compensatory strategies improve a student's participation in school with accommodations, adaptations, and modifications for certain tasks, routines, and settings,[8,65,101] whereas remedial approaches improve or establish a student's functional skills in a specific area.

When the team focuses on the occupation of written communication, generally both remedial and compensatory techniques are concurrently used. For example, Hunter, a second-grader, has manuscript handwriting that is unreadable, about 60% of his written letters are not legible, and his writing speed is at the bottom of his class. Although he participates in an intensive multisensory handwriting remediation program, he needs accommodations and strategies that help him achieve functional written communication in the classroom. Consequently, his teacher decided to adjust the time required to complete assignments, allow him to use oral reporting for certain class assignments, or require a lower volume of work to be accomplished than that of his peers. The teacher and the occupational therapist select specific techniques to assist him with legibility, such as spacing between words, sizing letters, and placing text on lines. Readiness activities that are easy to incorporate into the classroom can be embedded in his daily routine.

Initially, the child, the child's parents, and the educational team need to achieve consensus regarding the type of script (e.g., cursive) and the method of handwriting instruction (e.g., Zaner-Blöser) that seems most advantageous for the child to use. Specific intervention techniques and the type, frequency, and duration of service delivery are selected.

When a child's handwriting is very illegible and slow, team members may occasionally decide to incorporate assistive technology, such as a computer or portable word processor. Both the student and the team, particularly the occupational therapy practitioner, must work hard to find a technologic system that allows the student proficiency in text generation.[101] As in handwriting, computer use requires adequate attention, motor control, sensory processing, visual functioning, and self-regulation from the student. Hence, the computer is not a magical tool but one that allows the child to acquire keyboarding and word processing skills through planning, routine instruction, and practice. Two studies of upper elementary students with learning disabilities indicated that handwriting was a quicker mode of generating text than was keyboarding after several months of practice.[74,76] Word processing with word prediction improved the legibility and spelling of written assignments for two of three children with learning disabilities in a single-subject design study.[54] In this age of technology, it is important for all students to develop keyboarding skills for computer use in the classroom, workplace, and home. However, survival handwriting skills will continue to be needed throughout student and adult life. Table 19-5 lists the assistive technology features and the potential benefits of word processing for the student who struggles with handwriting. See Table 19-6 for a description of studies using computer-assisted handwriting instruction programs.

Models of Practice to Guide Collaborative Service Delivery

Models of practice and strategies used by occupational therapists may be unfamiliar to children, educators, parents, and other school personnel. Therefore, the occupational therapist must be able to (1) clearly articulate intervention techniques, activity modifications, and classroom accommodations being used; (2) collaborate with the teacher and others to provide service in the least restrictive environment; (3) implement therapeutic strategies for improving written communication; (4) train others to work with children with handwriting problems; and (5) closely monitor the progress of the child and change aspects of the program to continue improvement.

The overall focus of the educational program is the improvement of student performance in a particular area (e.g., written communication). Occupational therapy models of practice that guide services to improve handwriting include (1) neurodevelopmental, (2) acquisitional, (3) sensorimotor, (4) biomechanical, and (5) psychosocial. Surveys of occupational therapists in the United States[117] and Canada[40] indicate that the most frequently applied theoretical approaches to children's handwriting intervention are multisensory (92%, United States) and sensorimotor (90%, Canada). However, occupational therapists most often combine various theoretical approaches for handwriting intervention,[40] and this use of multiple approaches is advocated in the pediatric occupational therapy literature.[6,24,89]

When considering any intervention plan for handwriting, practitioners should consider the far-reaching parameters of each model of practice along with the overlap and the interplay among them. The occupational therapist must be skillful in the use of one or several models of practice concurrently and in teaching others to implement strategies originating from these models of practice. By remaining focused on the child's occupational outcome related to handwriting and applying various models of practice in the child's educational program, the occupational therapy practitioner can provide appropriate opportunities for the child to learn and master the skill of written communication.

Neurodevelopmental

The *neurodevelopmental theoretical approach* is based on neurologic principles and normal development, focusing on an individual's ability to execute efficient postural responses and

TABLE 19-5 Assistive Technology That Supports Handwriting Skills

AT to Support Writing Skills	Description
Text to speech	Speaks as the student types letters, words, and sentences. Speaks if text is selected and text-to-speech is then activated. May highlight word and/or sentence as it speaks. Voice (e.g., male/female) can be selected as well as speed of speech.
Electronic spell check	Spell check after production of writing. In-line spell check with visual supports. In-line spell check with visual and auditory cues. Phonetic spell check. Talking spelling suggestions for misspelled words.
Picture-supported text	Pictures appear as the students type words. Pictures can be sized and location can often be selected (above or below text). Some programs will allow a choice of picture libraries used with the text including GIFs (animated pictures). Picture supported text often has text-to-speech feature.
Abbreviated expansion	Freestanding or embedded software that allows users to create their own shortened abbreviations for commonly used words or phrases. The abbreviation is often expanded by using a modifier key after the abbreviation is typed into the document. The purpose of abbreviation expansion is to reduce the number of keystrokes needed to create a typed document.
Word prediction	Software-embedded word prediction. Independent word prediction. Frequency-weighting word prediction. Grammatically based word prediction (use of syntactic rules). Phonetic word prediction. Content-specific word prediction (e.g., custom dictionaries, extraction of text from digital reading materials). Adjustable number of word prediction choices displayed. Auditory preview of words predicted before selection. In-line vs. stationary word prediction. Picture-supported word prediction.
Electronic word and sentence banks	When selected, pictures, words, or sentences contained in a cell/button can be placed in a word processing document. Cells/buttons can be combined together to create a grid/toolbar. Cells/buttons/toolbars/grids can be linked so they can be dynamically displayed onscreen at different times. Cells/buttons/toolbars/grids can be scanned so that switch users can have alternate access for writing activities. Some programs will allow "drag and drop" features of words within the word processor so that cells/buttons/grids/toolbars are not needed.
Voice recognition software	The user speaks into a microphone and the words are converted by the computer into text. Users must "train" and "correct" the system for their unique speaking style. Training and correction can be time consuming, but has improved in the last 5 years. Users need to be able to remember specific commands to direct the computer. Environmental noise can be an issue for reliable detection of text. It is a hands-free text entry system.

movement patterns.[60] This model of practice provides an ideal orientation for addressing problems of children who have inadequate neurodevelopmental organization evidenced by poor postural control, automatic reactions, or limb control.[34] Decreased, increased, or fluctuating muscle tone, inadequate righting and equilibrium responses, and poor proximal stability may interfere with successful performance in fine motor activities such as handwriting.

Postural and arm preparation activities are an important component of a comprehensive handwriting program for children with mild neuromuscular impairments and sensory processing problems. For these children, preparing their bodies and hands for handwriting becomes the preliminary ingredient of handwriting intervention. Selecting preparatory activities to address each child's specific deficits and carefully analyzing his

or her response to these activities are both critical in the preparatory phase of the handwriting intervention program. Postural and arm activities can prepare children's bodies to write by (1) modulating muscle tone, (2) promoting proximal joint stability, and (3) improving hand function.

Postural preparation to modulate muscle tone may involve activities to increase, decrease, or balance muscle tone. Traditional activities to increase tone include jumping while sitting on a "hippity-hop" ball and jumping on a mini-trampoline. In the classroom, activities to build tone and strength might include students placing their hands on the sides of their chairs and bouncing in place for a "popcorn ride." They may hold that position with arms extended for a chair pushup. They may perform heavy work such as an arm pushup in a school chair (Figure 19-5).

TABLE 19-6   Computer-Assisted Handwriting Instruction

Author	Methods	Treatment	Evidence
Roberts & Samuels (1993)	36 Canadian students (with and without learning disabilities), grades 4–6 were assigned to 3 groups	Control group: traditional handwriting instruction; Group 1: conventional instruction through a computer; Group 3: computer-based handwriting exercises	Conventional handwriting group improved in five areas (parent's rating, teacher's rating, letter formation, letter size, and alignment). Computer-conventional group improved only in parent ratings and letter closures. The computer exercises group—improved only in teacher rating and the actual computer exercises (this indicates that they were practicing only the exercises and not handwriting).
Sovik (1981)	36 9-year-olds assigned to one of three conditions	Control group: conventional instruction; Group 1: individualized handwriting instruction; Group 2: individualized and computer lab instruction	The computer lab group was better at copying, tracking, and accuracy. Individual instruction group was better at copying than the control group.
Slovik (1984)	12 third graders with poor handwriting randomly assigned to control and experimental groups	Conventional instruction and computer lab instruction vs. conventional instruction only; effects on handwriting	Computer training did not improve speed of writing compared with the control group. Computer training improved the accuracy of writing of the student in the experimental group.

Roberts, G. I., & Samuels, M. T. (1993). Handwriting remediation: A comparison of computer-based and traditional approaches. *Journal of Educational Research, 87,* 118–125; Sovik, N. (1981). An experimental study of individualized learning instruction in copying, tracking, and handwriting based on feedback principles. *Motor Perceptual Motor Skills, 53,* 195–215; Sovik, N. (1984). The effects of a remedial tracking program on the writing performance of dysgraphic children. *Scandinavian Journal of Educational Research, 28,* 129–147.

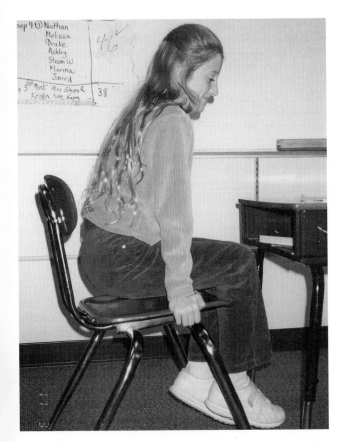

FIGURE 19-5   A girl demonstrates an arm pushup in her school chair.

For children whose muscle tone or activity level needs to be reduced, conventional slow rocking may be achieved by sitting astride a large bolster and moving from side to side to the rhythm of a child's poem recited aloud. In the classroom before writing, a child's postural tone may be decreased by rocking in a rocking chair to the beat of slow, rhythmic instrumental or vocal music from a headset, by snuggling into a beanbag chair, or by participating in a relaxing visual imagery exercise.

Children with poor handwriting frequently exhibit poor proximal stability and strength. To encourage co-contraction through the neck, shoulders, elbows, and wrists, young children may benefit from practicing animal walks, such as the crab walk, the bear walk, the inchworm creep, and the mule kick. Older children may prefer calisthenics, such as doing pushups on the floor or against the wall, performing resistive exercises with elastic tubing or Thera-Band, cooperatively pulling up a partner from a seated position on the floor, or practicing yoga poses that require weight bearing on the upper extremities. Figure 19-6 shows two children engaging in a yoga pose (London Bridge pose) to get ready for writing. Within the school setting, proximal stability also may be improved through everyday routines, such as cleaning blackboards and table tops or pushing and moving classroom furniture or physical education equipment.

Alternative positions during writing activities can enhance proximal stability during writing. The prone position requires weight-bearing on the forearms for writing, which increases proximal joint stability and may enhance disassociation of the hand and digits from the forearm.

When preparing to write, some children may also benefit from developing more coordinated synergies of the intrinsic

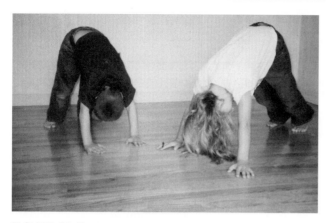

FIGURE 19-6 Two children participate in a yoga game to get ready for writing.

and extrinsic muscles of the hand to improve overall hand function. Typically, the hand needs to be stable and strong enough to provide support for fingers to manipulate tools. In-class hand-strengthening activities include carrying heavy cases with thick handles, practicing knot tying with thick rope, and participating in games with magnets.[8]

Prewriting, handwriting, and manipulative activities on vertical surfaces can assist children in developing more wrist extension stability to facilitate balanced use of the intrinsic musculature of the hand.[15] Activities requiring in-hand manipulation or the adjustment of an object after placement within the hand[39] may be appropriate for children with deficits in handwriting (see Chapter 10). *Translation*, moving the writing utensil from the palm to the fingers of the hand, *shifting* the shaft of the utensil within the hand for proper grasp, and *rotating* the pencil from the writing to the erasing position are all in-hand manipulation skills needed for writing tool management.

A study by Cornhill and Case-Smith of 48 first-graders demonstrated a moderate to high correlation between handwriting skills and in-hand manipulation, specifically translation and complex rotation.[29] Boehme suggested that vertical excursion of the writing line is produced by the flexion and extension movements of the digits, whereas horizontal excursion originates primarily from lateral wrist movements.[22] Hence, the balanced interaction of the intrinsic and extrinsic muscles of the hand appears to be key to the dynamic, efficient, and fluid movements required for handwriting.

Acquisitional

Handwriting may be viewed as a complex motor skill that "can be improved through practice, repetition, feedback, and reinforcement" (p. 70).[59] Graham and Miller recommended that handwriting instruction be (1) taught directly; (2) implemented in brief, daily lessons; (3) individualized to the child; (4) planned and changed based on evaluation and performance data; and (5) overlearned and used in a meaningful manner by the child.[49] When therapists and educators employ these conditions in a positive, interesting, and dynamic learning environment, children are more likely to become efficient, legible writers.[12,49,81] Therapeutic practice was more effective at improving handwriting performance than sensorimotor-based intervention.[32]

For occupational therapy practitioners, motor learning theories apply to handwriting instruction. Learning a new motor

skill has been described as progressing through three phases: cognitive, associative, and autonomous.[41] First, in the *cognitive phase,* the child is attempting to understand the demands of the handwriting task and develop a cognitive strategy for performing the necessary motor movements. Visual control of fine motor movements is thought to be important at this phase. A child learning handwriting in this phase may have developed strategies for writing some of the easier manuscript letters, such as *o, l,* or *t,* but may have more difficulty writing complicated letters, such as *b, q,* or *g.*

In the *associative phase,* the child has learned the fundamentals of performing handwriting and continues to adjust and refine the skill. Proprioceptive feedback becomes increasingly important during this phase, whereas reliance on visual cues declines. For example, in the associative phase a child may have mastered the formations of letters but is engaged in improving the handwriting product by learning to space words correctly, to write letters within guidelines, or to maintain consistent letter slant. Children continue to need practice, instructional guidance, and self-monitoring strategies of handwriting performance.

In the *autonomous phase,* the child can perform handwriting automatically with minimal conscious attention. Variability of performance is slight from day to day and the child is able to detect and adjust for any small errors that may occur.[96] Once the child has reached this level of handwriting, his or her attention can be expended on other higher-order elements of writing[44] or it can be saved to alleviate fatigue.[96]

Implications and strategies for handwriting instruction and remediation evolve from reviews of handwriting studies[17,49,88] as well as motor learning theory.[77] Many handwriting intervention programs are commercially available (see Appendix 19-C on the Evolve website for brief descriptions of and ordering information for these programs and a list of Internet resources). Each should contain a scope and sequence of letter and numeral formations along with successive instructional techniques. To date, no empirical evidence reveals one commercial handwriting program to be more effective than another.

The scope and sequence of the handwriting intervention program should focus on a structured progression of introducing and teaching letter and numeral forms. Frequently, letters with common formational features are introduced as a family, such as the lowercase letters *e, i, t,* and *l.* After the child has mastered these letters, she or he can use them immediately to write the words *eel, tile,* and *little.* Whether the chosen handwriting intervention method is a commercially available or a teacher- or therapist-prepared method, each child's program should be individualized to consist of the letters that he or she has not yet mastered. Thus, the focus of the child's program is to sequentially introduce new letters and use them with mastered letters, excluding letters the child is forming incorrectly or ones not known to the child, because this only reinforces unwelcome perceptual–motor patterns.[119] Combining newly acquired letters with already mastered letters allows the child to write in a meaningful context (i.e., the formation of words and sentences). This immediate reinforcement of writing words is more powerful and purposeful for the child than writing strings of letters repeatedly.

Instructional approaches of handwriting intervention programs vary but tend to comprise a combination of sequential

TABLE 19-7   Evidence on Modeling for Teaching Handwriting*

Author[†]	Methods	Treatment	Evidence
Hayes (1982)	45 kindergarten children and 45 third-grade students were observed	Effects of visual and/or verbal modeling in copying letter-like forms	Kindergarten students performed better with combined visual and verbal modeling. Third-grade students performed better with visual modeling only.
Kirk (1981)	54 kindergarten students were randomly assigned to four groups, each getting a different type of demonstration: visual only, verbal only, visual and verbal combined, or none	Effects on visual and/or verbal modeling, learning 12 uppercase and 12 lowercase letters	Combined demonstration has the best results. Any modeling is better than no demonstration at all.
Wright & Wright (1980)	120 first-grade students randomly assigned to two conditions	Flip books vs. static form as a letter model	No evident difference in handwriting performance.

*The evidence supports teacher modeling of letter formation prior to practice.
[†]Hayes, D. (1982). Handwriting practice: The effects of perceptual prompts. *Journal of Educational Research, 75,* 169–172; Kirk, U. (1981). The development and use of rules in the acquisition of perceptual motor skills. *Child Development, 52,* 299–305; Wright, C. D., & Wright, J. P. (1980). Handwriting: The effectiveness of copying from moving versus still models. *Journal of Educational Research, 74,* 95–98.

techniques including modeling (Table 19-7), tracing, stimulus fading, copying, composing, and self-monitoring.[6,17,81] When acquiring new letterforms, initially the child often needs many visual and auditory cues. However, the service provider fades the cues as soon as the child can successfully form the letter without them. Next, the child proceeds to copying letters and words from a model and then to writing letters and words from memory as they are dictated. Finally, the child advances to generating words and sentences for practice. In each phase, the child should be expected to assume responsibility for correcting his or her own work, also known as self-monitoring.[17] Older children can refer to a written checklist addressing spacing, size, alignment, letterforms, and slant during the self-assessment of their writing. However, younger children may need to verbally evaluate letter formation and overall appearance aloud to the service provider.

Acquiring handwriting skills and applying them in school means the educational team focuses not only on letter formation but also on the legibility and speed of the student's handwriting. In addition to correct letterforms, other components of legibility include spacing, size, slant, and alignment. Spacing between letters and words, text placement on lines, and sizing letters often need direct modeling and instruction.

An effective writing surface for assisting students with text placement and size is a color-coded, laminated sheet. When accompanied by verbal cues from the service provider, this sheet provides immediate visual cues to the child learning letterforms. Beneath the solid, red writing baseline, the color brown represents the "soil" or "ground"; the space above the solid baseline and dashed black middle guideline are green for the "grass"; and the space above the dashed guideline to the top solid writing line is blue for the "sky." For example, the letter *h* would start at the top of the sky, head downward, and end in the grass. This same pictorial scheme can be applied to lined paper for classroom assignments, allowing students strong cues for learning letter placement and size (Figure 19-7).[8] Various strategies for addressing handwriting problems related to legibility components, classroom writing assignments, and speed are listed in Table 19-8.

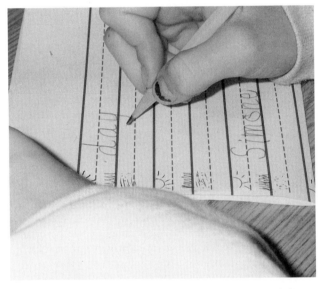

FIGURE 19-7   Lined paper with diagrams helps with letter size and the placement of text.

Sensorimotor

The parameters for this model of practice, when applied by the occupational therapist with children with handwriting problems, include providing multisensory input through selected activities to enhance the integration of sensory systems at the subcortical level.[99] When given various meaningful sensory opportunities at a level that permits assimilation, the child's nervous system can integrate information more efficiently to produce a satisfactory motor output (e.g., legible letters in a timely manner). All sensory systems, including the proprioceptive, tactile, visual, auditory, olfactory, and gustatory, can be tapped within a handwriting intervention program, which is thought to enhance learning. Incorporating a sensory integrative approach into handwriting intervention entails the use of a variety of sensory experiences, media, and instructional

TABLE 19-8 Strategies for Handwriting Problems

Handwriting Problems	Potential Solutions
Spacing between letters	Use finger spacing with index finger.
	Use fingerprint spacing by pressing on an inkpad before finger spacing.
	Teach the "no touching rule" of letters.
Spacing between words	Use adhesive strips (e.g., Post-it Notes) as spacers between words.
	Make spaces with a rubber stamp.
	Use a dot or a dash (Morse code) between words.
Spacing on paper	Use grid paper.
	Write on every other line of the paper.
	Draw colored lines to mark (e.g., green is left, red is right).
Placing text on lines	Use pictorial schemes on writing guidelines.
	Provide raised writing lines as tactile cues for letter placement.
	Remind students that unevenly placed letters are "popcorn letters."
Sizing letters and words	Use individualized boxes for each letter.
	Name letters with ascending stems, no stems, and descending stems—"birds," "skunks," and "snakes," respectively.
Near-point copying	Highlight the text on the worksheet to be copied.
	Teach the student to copy two or three letters at a time.
Far-point copying	Enlarge print for better viewing.
	Start with copying from nearby vertical models.
	Position the student to face the chalkboard.
Dictation	Attach an alphabet strip to a desktop for the student who cannot remember letterforms.
	Dictated spelling words can contain several but not all letters.
Composition	Be certain that students can form letters from memory.
	Provide magnetic words to write short poems or stories.
Speed	Allow students to begin projects early to finish with peers.
	Photocopy math problems from textbook to reduce copying.
	Preselect volume of work to be done that may be different from that of peers.

Modified from Amundson, S. J. (1998). *TRICS for written communication: Techniques for rebuilding and improving children's school skills.* Homer, AK: O.T. KIDS.

materials. In addition, providing novel and interesting materials for children to practice letterforms may keep students motivated, excited, and challenged, thereby enhancing student success and learning. Children with handwriting difficulties who have experienced frustration with commonly used paper-and-pencil drills may respond much more favorably to handwriting instruction using this unique multisensory format. A study by Woodward and Swinth indicated that 90% of school-based occupational therapists used this approach; altogether, 130 different multisensory modalities and activities were documented, with therapists using 5 or more activities per student.[117] Chalk and chalkboard were the most frequent format used, being selected by 87.3% of responding therapists.[32] A study of the effects of two interventions (sensorimotor and therapeutic practice) for children 6 to 11 years old with handwriting dysfunction found that children who received sensorimotor intervention improved in some sensorimotor components but also demonstrated a decline in handwriting performance.[117]

Writing tools, writing surfaces, and positions for writing are all integral parts of a sensorimotor approach. Examples of writing tools to be used are felt-tip pens (regular, overwriter, changeable-color), crayons (scented, glittered, glow-in-the-dark), paintbrushes, grease pencils or china markers, weighted pens, mechanical pencils, wooden dowels, vibratory pens, and chalk. Lamme and Ayris examined the effects of five different types of writing tools on handwriting legibility.[69] Results indicated that the type of writing tool did not influence legibility, but the educators involved in the study reported that

children's attitudes toward writing were more positive when children were able to use a felt-tip pen rather than a No. 2 pencil. This suggests that children's feelings about writing might improve when allowed to use a variety of writing tools. Writing with chalk, grease pencils, or a resistive tool also provides additional proprioceptive input to children, because more pressure for writing is required than with the traditional tools of paper and pencil. Unconventional writing tools can be easily incorporated into classroom assignments.

Writing surfaces may be in a vertical, horizontal, or vertically angled plane. Common vertical surfaces for writing include the chalkboard, painting easels, and poster board and laminated paper attached to the wall. These surfaces (e.g., desktop easels set at a slanted incline) facilitate a more mature grasp of the writing tool because a child's wrist extension may result in more arching of the hand and an open web space between the thumb and fingers.[16] Figure 19-8 shows a girl working on a homework assignment that is taped to a kitchen cupboard. An upright orientation may also decrease directional confusion of early writers when learning letter formations.[51] On the vertical plane, "up" means up and "down" means down, as opposed to working at a desktop where "up" means "away from the body" and "down" means "toward the body." Furthermore, standing in front of a chalkboard with the body in full extension and parallel to the writing surface may promote more internal stability of the trunk, increase neurologic arousal, and provide more proprioceptive input throughout the arm and shoulder and allow the hand to move independently or dissociate from the arm.[6]

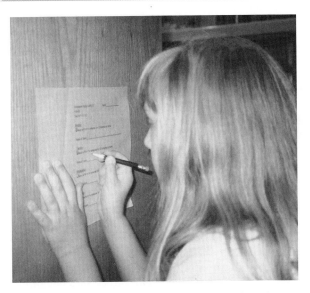

FIGURE 19-8 A girl works on a homework assignment that is taped to a vertical surface (i.e., kitchen cupboard).

Handwriting practice on a horizontal surface can be performed using a variety of materials that provide additional sensory input to the child's movement of the tool. Writing on plastic freezer bags partially filled with colored hair styling gel or trays filled with sand, dry pudding mix, clay, or a light coating of hand lotion provides unusual and reinforcing sensation. Writing on baking sheets or Styrofoam meat-packaging trays with isolated fingers or wooden dowels provides children additional tactile and proprioceptive input when forming letters, numbers, and words. Writing on textured wallpaper, nylon netting, finely meshed screen, or indoor–outdoor carpet squares also provides proprioceptive input.

Biomechanical

Ergonomic factors such as sitting posture, paper position, pencil grasp, writing instruments, and type of paper influence handwriting quality and speed. In this section, compensatory strategies—including adaptive devices, procedural adaptations, and environmental modifications to improve the interaction and fit between a child's capabilities and the demands of the handwriting task—are presented. This model emphasizes modifications to the student's context to improve handwriting and written production.

Sitting Posture

Although standing and lying prone may be encouraged as alternative writing positions, students continue to spend much of the school day seated at a desk. Therefore, the occupational therapist should immediately address the student's seated position in the classroom. While writing, the student should be seated with the feet planted firmly on the floor, providing support for weight shifting and postural adjustments.[16] The table surface should be 2 inches above the flexed elbows when the child is seated in the chair. In this position, the student can experience both symmetry and stability while performing written work. To facilitate appropriate seating for students, the occupational therapy practitioner may recommend adjusting heights of desks and chairs, providing footrests for children, adding seat cushions and inserts, or repositioning a child's desk to face the chalkboard in the classroom.

Paper Position

Paper should be slanted on the desktop so that it is parallel to the forearm of the writing hand when the child's forearms are resting on the desk with hands clasped.[72] This angle of the paper enables the student to see his or her written work and to avoid smearing his or her writing. Right-handed students may slant the top of their paper approximately 25° to 30° to the left with the paper just right of the body's midline. Conversely, a slant of 30° to 35° to the right and paper placement to the left of midline are needed for students using a left-handed tripod grasp.[4] For the student with a left-handed "hooked" pencil grasp lacking lateral wrist movements, slanting the paper to the left is appropriate.[16] The writing instrument should be held below the baseline, and the non-preferred hand should hold the writing paper.[4]

Pencil Grip

Benbow defined the ideal grasp as a dynamic tripod with an open web space.[14] With the web space open (forming a circle), the thumb and index and middle fingers make the longest flexion, extension, and rotary excursions with a pencil during handwriting.[16] Variations of grasps exist with some grips, making handwriting more difficult and less functional.[109] Educational team members may consider modifying a student's pencil grasp when the child (1) experiences muscular tension and fatigue, also known as writer's cramp; (2) demonstrates poor letter formation or writing speed; (3) demonstrates a tightly closed web space that limits controlled precision finger and thumb movements; or (4) holds the pencil with too much pressure or exerts too much pencil point pressure on the paper.[16]

In attempting to modify a grip pattern, characteristics of the child are an important consideration. The occupational therapy practitioner should encourage a mature grasp in young writers and recognize that modifying a grasp pattern may be more successful with younger children.[119] Once grip positions have been established, they are very difficult to change.[14] In fact, by the beginning of second grade, changing a child's grasp pattern may be stressful and not recommended.[16] Therefore, the educational team needs to carefully consider a child's age, cooperation, and motivation along with the child's acceptance of the new grip pattern or prosthetic device before attempting to reposition the child's fingers.

A variety of prosthetic devices and therapeutic strategies are available to assist the child in positioning the digits for better manipulation of the writing instrument.[8] The occupational therapist should be knowledgeable about hand functions to determine which adaptive devices and techniques are most appropriate for each individual child. Stetro grips, triangular pencils, moldable grips, and the Pencil Grip may facilitate tripod grasps. Writing muscle tension and fatigue may be reduced for some children by using a wider-barreled pencil. To gain more mobility of the radial digits, children may hold a small eraser against the palm with the ulnar digits, allowing for more dynamic movement of the pencil. Older children with hand hypotonicity may achieve a viable pencil grasp by holding the pencil shaft between the web space of the index and middle fingers with thumb opposition.[15] Other techniques to encourage the delicate stability–mobility balance of a functional pencil grasp include the use of external supports such as microfoam surgical tape, ring splints, and neoprene splints[14] and should be used with a working knowledge of hand anatomy and kinesiology. A rubber band sling that

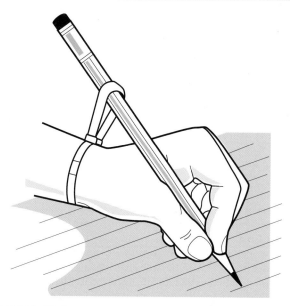

FIGURE 19-9 A rubber band sling allows for a slanted, relaxed pencil position.

encourages the student to use a slanted and relaxed pencil position for writing is shown in Figure 19-9.

Writing Tools

The type of writing instruments children use in the classroom also warrants consideration. In general, children should be allowed to choose among a variety of writing tools so parents and teachers may help the individual child determine which writing utensil is most efficient and comfortable. Traditionally, kindergarten and primary grade classroom teachers have promoted the use of a wide primary pencil for beginning writers. Carlson and Cunningham examined tool usage among preschool children performing drawing, tracing, and writing tasks.[23] They found that the readability of their written work was not enhanced by the use of a wider diameter pencil. This study suggests that the pervasive use of the primary pencil is probably not warranted for all kindergarten children because some children perform better with a No. 2 pencil, whereas others do well with a primary pencil. See Table 19-9 for evidence on writing instruments' effects on handwriting.

Paper

Various types of writing paper are available in the educational setting. Unlined paper and lined paper with a dashed middle guideline between the lower baseline and upper line are both commonly used in the early elementary grades. For the majority of children, most of the research confirms that lined paper improves the legibility of handwriting when compared with the use of unlined paper.[87] Children typically start out with wide-spaced (1-inch) guidelines. As handwriting proficiency improves, usually in grade 3 or 4, the child begins using paper with narrow-spaced (3/8-inch) lines.[12] The occupational therapist and educator can allow the student the opportunity to experiment with paper with different lines, sizes, and textures to determine which offers the child the best medium for handwriting. Several older studies examined the influence of the paper on handwriting outcomes. Lindsay and McLennan (1983) asked 6- to 9-year-olds to write an essay on lined and unlined paper to examine the effects of paper on legibility. The 6-year-olds had better legibility on unlined paper and the 9-year-olds had better legibility on lined paper. The 7- and 8-year-olds performed the same when writing on lined and unlined paper. Across all ages, the presence or absence of lines did not affect the quality or length of essays Other researchers examined the effects of wide lines on handwriting control in kindergarten through third graders in urban and suburban schools (Hill et al. 1982; Trap-Porter et al. 1983; Waggoner et al. 1981).[58,106,112] Wider lines facilitated production of manuscript for kindergarten through second-grade students and cursive production for second and third grade students. The wider lines also helped children in the suburban setting, but not those in urban school settings who had underdeveloped handwriting skills. The wide lines only helped third graders with cursive, not manuscript writing. These studies suggest that

TABLE 19-9 Evidence on Writing Instruments

Author	Method	Treatment	Evidence
Carlson & Cunningham (1990)	48 preschool children in the U.S. were observed	Use of the primary pencil vs. regular pencil	No statistical difference was found between the two in finger position, finger movement, or pencil control. Some children did better with the primary pencil, whereas others did better with a regular pencil.
Lamme & Ayris (1983)	35 first grade classrooms (n = 798) in the U.S. randomly assigned to use 1 or 5 implements in daily handwriting	Use of 5 types of instruments: primary pencil (with and without grip), regular pencil (with and without grip), and felt tip pen	No differences in legibility of a sentence copied emerged between groups. Children should be offered a variety of writing instruments to learn how to write.
Ziviani (1981 & 1983)	54 third graders in Australia were observed	Use of regular pencils and primary pencils with triangular grips	Primary pencils allow a more relaxed position of the forearm; however, students are more likely to "bow" their forefinger into an immature writing position.

Carlson, K., & Cunningham, J. (1990). Effect of pencil diameter on the graphomotor skill of preschoolers. *Early Childhood Research Quarterly, 5,* 279–293; Lamme, L. L., & Ayris, B. M. (1983). Is the handwriting of beginning writers influenced by writing tools? *Journal of Research and Development in Education, 17,* 33–38; Ziviani, J. (1981). Effects of pencil shape and size on motor accuracy and pencil posture of 8 year old children. ERIC Document Reproduction Service (ED 218 658); Ziviani, J. (1983). Qualitative changes in dynamic tripod grip between seven and 14 years of age. *Developmental Medicine and Child Neurology, 25,* 778–782.

requiring a student to use one type of paper or specific writing instrument may be unnecessarily restrictive.

Psychosocial

Psychosocial approaches used for children's handwriting intervention typically focus on improving the student's self-control, coping skills, and social behaviors. In the area of handwriting, this means that a child may produce neatly written text when addressing an envelope to his or her residence, knowing that the occupational therapist will later use the envelope to send the child a small "surprise." Receiving a surprise, such as a bookmark, from the therapist is socially reinforcing for the child. See Table 19-10 for evidence on positive behavioral techniques.

By sharing with children the importance of readable handwriting and the rationale for intervention, as well as providing positive, meaningful, everyday experiences using handwriting, behaviors by children that lead to more legible writing may increase. Simple games at school and home, such as tic-tac-toe, can be played using the newly acquired letterforms rather than the traditional X and O. When a child presents a neatly drawn and written (relative to the child's ability) Thanksgiving Day card at home, the parents can provide social reinforcement. In addition, teachers might reward the child with typically poor handwriting with a special certificate for improved handwriting on receipt of a readable spelling paper or written class assignment. By offering children choices, success, responsibility, and encouragement within the natural setting, therapists teach children to view handwriting as a functional and socially valid skill.

Using a psychosocial approach, the occupational therapy practitioner may also enhance children's social competence within the framework of a handwriting intervention group. Currently, the use of small groups as a service delivery model for school-based handwriting intervention is limited. Woodward and Swinth found that school-based occupational therapists used small groups for handwriting intervention infrequently (12.4%) when compared with other types of service provision in school-based settings.[117]

However, one successful group is a handwriting club of four to six students who work on improving handwriting, developing social skills, and monitoring their own work and behavior.[8] Poor social performance is common among children with learning disabilities. Behaviors that interfere with social relations include poor eye contact, physical intrusiveness, not greeting others, and unawareness of verbal and nonverbal social cues, to name a few.[116] The service provider may aptly provide group experiences and teach children needed social skills, such as complimenting others, self-regulating the tone and volume of the voice, accepting negative feedback, maintaining personal space, and giving and accepting apologies[116] while involved with the handwriting group.

In a handwriting club, for example, when children are lying in prone position and practicing letterforms on a chalk mat, each of them can decide the amount of personal space he needs to feel comfortable, as well as the amount of writing space required on the mat. In another example, a competitive game such as Kerplunk can be used as an in-hand manipulation preparatory activity. While the children remove plastic sticks supporting marbles from the game's cylinder, the occupational therapist reinforces the social skills of taking turns, self-regulating the behavioral state amid competition, and following the rules of a game.

Other strategies to enhance children's social performance within an intervention group may require a proactive role for the occupational therapist. Giving an overview of the intervention session at the beginning of the period and clearly delineating when activities are beginning and terminating can assist

TABLE 19-10 Evidence on Behavioral Techniques to Improve Handwriting

Author	Method	Treatment	Evidence
Hartley & Salzwedel (1980)	Case study: a 12-year-old boy with autism	Effects on behavioral techniques (e.g., fading, feedback, tracing) to improve handwriting	Only modest improvement.
Mabee (1988)	Multiple baseline across subjects design with three third-grade students	Effectiveness of "positive practice"	Small effect on students' performance.
McCoy & Leader (1980)	Case study: 5 visually impaired individuals	Cursive writing using physical, oral, and tracing cues	Successful.
McLaughlin et al. (1987)	Counterbalanced, multiple baseline design used with 36 junior high students receiving special services	Effect of positive practice and response cost	Number of errors decreased; however, number of legible words decreased as well. These techniques should be avoided because they cause an undesirable effect.
Sharpley, Irvine, & Hattie (1980)	56 fourth- and fifth-grade students in Australia	Effect of contingent rewards (praise and privilege) on handwriting performance	This method proved effective in improving performance. Performance declined if rewards were given unfairly among students.

Hartley, S., & Salzwedel, K. (1980). Behavioral writing for an autistic-like child. *Academic Therapy, 16,* 101–110; Mabee, W. S. (1988). The effects of academic positive practice on cursive letter writing. *Educ Treatment Children, 11,* 143–148; McCoy, K. M., & Leader, L. A. (1980). Teaching cursive signature to the blind: A task analytic approach. *Visual Impairment Blindness, 74,* 69–71; McLaughlin, T. F., Mabee, W. S., Byram, B. J., & Reiter, S. M. (1987). Effects of academic positive practice and response cost on writing legibility of behaviorally disordered and learning-disabled junior high school students. *Journal of Child Adolescent Psychology, 4,* 216–221; Sharpley, C. F., Irvine, J. W., & Hattie, J. A. (1980). Changes in performance of children's handwriting as a result of varying contingency conditions. *Alberta Journal of Educational Research, 26,* 183–193.

children who have difficulty with transitions between tasks and classes. Developing trust and a sense of cohesiveness among the children might be achieved by having the club or group members decide on a special name, logo, or handshake.[116] Finally, the interventionist should establish clear and reasonable rules and consequences, share them with the group members, and consistently and kindly manage the children's behavior. By placing the building of children's social skills within the framework of a handwriting intervention group, occupational therapy practitioners can help children become more socially competent with their peers and adults, as well as more efficient and fluent in their handwriting.

Evidence of Occupational Therapy Intervention on Handwriting

Some children are good candidates for improving their actual manuscript or cursive handwriting through remediation. However, other children are not. The occupational therapist and the child's clinical and educational teams need to consider compensatory strategies that allow the child with poor handwriting the greatest opportunity for functional written communication. Alternatives to handwriting include keyboarding and word prediction, adapting and reducing the amount of written assignments, dictating assignments, and having study buddies to assist with written expression. In school settings, the educational team must determine which type of written communication is or will be most functional for the child and develop a short-term plan (e.g., learning essential manuscript words) and a long-term plan (e.g., learning word processing).

Although occupational therapists assume that their interventions improve children's handwriting, there is a lack of controlled handwriting intervention studies in the professional literature. Two studies, however, indicated that occupational therapy intervention positively affected elementary students' handwriting.[24,89] Case-Smith investigated 29 children receiving occupational therapy services and 9 children who did not. Educational levels ranged from grades two through four.[24] Occupational therapy intervention with the children focused on visual–motor skill improvement and handwriting practice. The occupational therapists reportedly used eclectic theoretic approaches during intervention sessions. After 8.8 hours of direct occupational therapy, the intervention group made significant gains in handwriting legibility as measured by the Evaluation Tool of Children's Handwriting[7] when compared with the control group. Although handwriting speed was not significantly affected for the intervention group, the students, on average, increased from 32 to 37 letters per minute.

In the study by Peterson and Nelson, 59 first-grade students from families of low socioeconomic status participated.[89] Thirty children randomly assigned to an occupational therapy group received 10 hours of handwriting intervention. The control group (n = 29) received regular academic instruction for handwriting. The other children received handwriting intervention based on an integration of theoretic perspectives. Findings indicated that the children receiving handwriting intervention scored significantly higher on the Minnesota Handwriting Test[93] than did those in the control group.

Both handwriting intervention studies give evidence that occupational therapy interventions help to improve children's handwriting; however, both studies share limitations. One limitation is that the handwriting evaluators were not blind to the experimental conditions. Another limitation is that both of the handwriting instruments, the Evaluation Tool of Children's Handwriting[7] and the Minnesota Handwriting Test,[93] have only fair to good test reliability. Finally, the small sample sizes and specific geographic regions limit the generalizability of either study.

Service Delivery

According to the research, children with disabilities have less instructional time with literacy. The quantity and quality of literacy experiences are dramatically different from those of their peers.[83] Providing occupational therapy services to children with handwriting dysfunction should be based primarily on the needs of the individual child as determined by the educational or clinical team. Currently many educational teams use a continuum of service delivery that allows for more flexibility, fluidity, and responsiveness to an individual child's needs (see Chapter 24).

For example, at the beginning of second grade, Tara, a girl with a learning disability, is assessed by the occupational therapist for poor handling of classroom materials and tools (e.g., glue stick, scissors, computer mouse) and illegible handwriting. After a comprehensive occupational therapy evaluation, Tara's parents and the educational team decide to focus on assisting her to become a more proficient writer, with the occupational therapist and the regular education teacher spearheading the intervention program.

The therapist and the teacher met to develop classroom strategies to be implemented. These strategies included positioning Tara's desk directly in front of the chalkboard, reducing the length of her written assignments, and providing her with an alphabet strip attached to her desktop and placed at the recommended angle of her writing paper (Figure 19-10).

The educator also requested the help of the occupational therapist in implementing motivating exercises to prepare

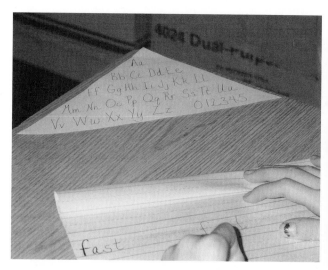

FIGURE 19-10 An angled strip is attached to a student's desktop.

("ready") the entire class for their daily creative writing period. The occupational therapist scheduled a time with the teacher and spent 10 to 15 minutes per week (for 4 weeks) teaching the entire class hand-dexterity games before a classroom writing activity. She also provided the teacher a written handout of games, so the teacher could ask questions and have a later reference.

Because of the extremely poor legibility of Tara's writing, the team chose to have her join an ongoing handwriting intervention group in the classroom. This group held 25-minute sessions twice a week for three consecutive weeks. During this direct service time, the occupational therapist further assessed individual children. She trained the teacher's assistant to coordinate the handwriting group and address some of the individual problems. The occupational therapist returned to the handwriting intervention session once every 2 weeks to supervise the service provider, monitor the children's progress, and modify the programs when needed. A regular consultation time was established with the educator to evaluate Tara's progress in class, strategize regarding new situations affecting her handwriting performance, and write a progress note to her parents.

In Tara's case, during the first 4 weeks after the initial team meeting, the occupational therapist implemented direct service, training of a teaching assistant, and consulting with the teacher. However, the provision of services was not locked into a set schedule (e.g., two 25-minute sessions per week of direct therapy). By using a continuum of service provision, the occupational therapist initially worked with the teacher, orchestrated an ongoing intervention program that another service provider could implement after training, and continued to make regular contact with Tara and the educational team members, including Tara's parents.

Consultation and training others to implement intervention strategies are often the most appropriate service delivery models to improve children's handwriting. Alternative service providers (e.g., educators, educational assistants, volunteers, high school students, and parents) are generally capable of and willing to implement techniques and programs if the occupational therapist assumes responsibility for organizing and monitoring the methods and programs used. To do this, the occupational therapist models the strategies for the services provider, clearly articulates the rationale for the methods and approaches used in the program, and designs a well-organized program that can be applied easily.

By supplying (1) specific written and oral directions of the program; (2) a container, such as a basket, full of materials for the handwriting intervention program (e.g., Thera-Band, in-hand manipulation games, sequenced writing lessons, clay trays, different writing tools); (3) data management sheets; and (4) a system to provide reinforcement and rewards, the program can be administered easily. A user-friendly program may increase the likelihood that the directions provided by the occupational therapist are followed. If the occupational therapist regularly observes sessions implemented by the service provider, discusses the rationale for using specific methods, and reviews the children's progress and the need for program changes, the training can be beneficial for the individual children receiving handwriting intervention. This training can also benefit other children in the classroom who may be struggling with handwriting.

SUMMARY

Handwriting is an important academic occupation for children. Children with mild neuromuscular impairments, learning disabilities, and developmental delays are often referred to occupational therapy for handwriting problems. The role of the occupational therapist includes evaluating the child's functional performance of prewriting and handwriting skills, along with the task demands and environmental features. The occupational therapist also assists the educational or clinical team in planning an integrated approach to promote a functional written communication means for the child.

Handwriting intervention programs should be comprehensive, incorporating activities and therapeutic techniques from the neurodevelopmental, acquisitional, sensorimotor, biomechanical, and psychosocial models of practice in the child's natural setting. Compensatory strategies may also be used to provide the child a successful and efficient means for functional written communication.

REFERENCES

1. Alston, J. (1983). A legibility index: Can handwriting be measured? *Educational Review, 35,* 237–242.
2. Alston, J. (1991). Handwriting in the new curriculum. *British Journal of Special Education, 18,* 13–15.
3. Alston, J. (1995). Assessing writing speeds and output: Some current norms and issues. *Handwriting Review,* 102–106.
4. Alston, J., & Taylor, J. (1987). *Handwriting: Theory, research and practice.* London: Croom Helm.
5. American Occupational Therapy Association. (2008). Occupational therapy practice framework: Domain and process second edition. *The American Journal of Occupational Therapy, 62,* 609–639.
6. Amundson, S. J. (1992). Handwriting: Evaluation and intervention in school settings. In J. Case-Smith & C. Pehoski (Eds.), *Development of hand skills in the child* (pp. 63–78). Rockville, MD: American Occupational Therapy Association.
7. Amundson, S. J. (1995). *Evaluation tool of children's handwriting.* Homer, AK: O.T. KIDS.
8. Amundson, S. J. (1998). *TRICS for written communication: Techniques for rebuilding and improving children's school skills.* Homer, AK: O.T. KIDS.
9. Anderson, P. L. (1983). *Denver handwriting analysis.* Novato, CA: Academic Therapy Publications.
10. Armitage, D., & Ratzlaff, H. (1985). The non-corrrelation of printing and writing skills. *Journal of Educational Research, 78,* 174–177.
11. Barbe, W. B., Milone, M. J., & Wasylyk, T. (1983). Manuscript is the write start. *Academic Therapy, 18,* 397–405.
12. Barchers, S. I. (1994). *Teaching language arts: An integrated approach.* Minneapolis, MN: West Publishing Company.
13. Beery, K. E. (1997). *The developmental test of visual-motor integration* (5th ed.). Austin, TX: Pro-Ed.
14. Benbow, M. (1995). Principles and practices of teaching handwriting. In A. Henderson & C. Pehoski (Eds.), *Hand function in the child: Foundations for remediation* (pp. 255–281). St. Louis: Mosby.
15. Benbow, M. (2006). Principles and practice of teaching handwriting. In A. Henderson & C. Pehoski (Eds.), *Hand function in the child: Foundations for remediation* (2nd ed.). St. Louis: Mosby.

16. Benbow, M., Hanft, B., & Marsh, D. (1992). Handwriting in the classroom: Improving written communication. In C. B. Royeen (Ed.), *AOTA self-study series: Classroom applications for school-based practice* (pp. 1–60). Rockville, MD: American Occupational Therapy Association.

17. Bergman, K. E., & McLaughlin, T. F. (1988). Remediating handwriting difficulties with learning disabled students: A review. *Journal of Special Education, 12,* 101–120.

18. Bergmann, K. P. (1990). Incidence of atypical pencil grasps among nondysfunctional adults. *American Journal of Occupational Therapy, 44,* 736–740.

19. Berninger, V., Mizokawa, D., & Bragg, R. (1991). Theory-based diagnosis and remediation of writing disabilities. *Journal of School Psychology, 29,* 57–97.

20. Berninger, V., Vaughan, K. B., Abbott, R. D., Abbott, S. P., Rogan, L. W., Brooks, A., et al. (1997). Treatment of handwriting problems in beginning writers: Transfer from handwriting to composition. *Journal of Education Psychology, 89,* 652–666.

21. Berninger, V., Yates, C., Cartwright, A., Rutberg, J., Remy, E., & Abbott, R. (1992). Lower-level developmental skills in beginning writing. *Reading and Writing: An Interdisciplinary Journal, 4,* 256–280.

22. Boehme, R. (1988). *Improving upper body control.* Tucson, AZ: Therapy Skill Builders.

23. Carlson, K., & Cunningham, J. (1990). Effect of pencil diameter on the graphomotor skill of preschoolers. *Early Childhood Research Quarterly, 5,* 279–293.

24. Case-Smith, J. (2002). Effectiveness of school-based occupational therapy intervention on handwriting. *American Journal of Occupational Therapy, 56,* 17–25.

25. Chandler, B. (1994). The power of information: School based practice survey results. *OT Week, 18,* 24.

26. Chase, C. (1986). Essay test scoring: Interaction of relevant variables. *Journal of Educational Measurement, 23,* 33–41.

27. Chu, S. (1997). Occupational therapy for children with handwriting difficulties: A framework for evaluation and treatment. *British Journal of Occupational Therapy, 60,* 514–520.

28. Connelly, V., Campbell, S., MacLean, M., & Barnes, J. (2006). Contribution of lower order skills to the written composition of college students with and without dyslexia. *Developmental Neuropsychology, 29,* 175–196.

29. Cornhill, H., & Case-Smith, J. (1996). Factors that relate to good and poor handwriting. *American Journal of Occupational Therapy, 50,* 732–739.

30. Daniels, L. E. (1988). The diagnosis and remediation of handwriting problems: An analysis. *Physical and Occupational Therapy in Pediatrics, 8,* 61–67.

31. Dennis, J. L., & Swinth, Y. (2001). Pencil grasp and children's handwriting legibility during different-length writing tasks. *American Journal of Occupational Therapy, 55,* 175–183.

32. Denton, P., Cope, S., & Moser, C. (2006). Effects of sensorimotor-based intervention versus therapeutic practice on improving handwriting performance in 6-to-11-year-old children. *American Journal of Occupational Therapy, 60,* 16–27.

33. Diekema, S. M., Deitz, J., & Amundson, S. J. (1998). Test-retest reliability of the evaluation of children's handwriting—manuscript. *American Journal of Occupational Therapy, 52,* 248–254.

34. Donoghue, M. (1975). *The child and the English language arts* (2nd ed.). Dubuque, IA: William C. Brown.

35. Deleted in proofs.

36. Duvall, B. (1985). *Evaluating the difficulty of cursive, manuscript, italic and D'Nealian handwriting* (No. CS 209 484). ERIC Document Reproduction Service No. ED 265 539.

37. Edwards, L. (2003). Writing instruction in kindergarten. *Journal of Learning Disabilities, 36,* 136–148.

38. Erhardt, R. P. (1982). *Developmental hand dysfunction: Theory, assessment, treatment.* Tucson, AZ: Therapy Skill Builders.

39. Exner, C. E. (1992). In-hand manipulation skills. In J. Case-Smith & C. Pehoski (Eds.), *Development of hand skills in the child* (pp. 35–45). Rockville, MD: American Occupational Therapy Association.

40. Feder, K., Majnemer, A., & Synnes, A. (2000). Handwriting: Current trends in occupational therapy practice. *Canadian Journal of Occupational Therapy, 67,* 197–204.

41. Fitts, P. M., & Posner, M. I. (1967). *Human performance.* Belmont, CA: Brooks/Cole.

42. Gardner, M. F. (1998). *Test of handwriting skills.* Hydesville, CA: Psychological and Educational Publications.

43. Graham, S. (1990). The role of production factors in learning disabled students' compositions. *Journal of Educational Psychology, 82,* 781–791.

44. Graham, S. (1992). Issues in handwriting instruction. *Focus on Exceptional Children, 25,* 1–14.

45. Graham, S., Berninger, V., Abbott, R., Abbott, S., & Whitaker, D. (1997). The role of mechanics in composing of elementary school students: A new methodological approach. *Journal of Educational Psychology, 89,* 170–182.

46. Graham, S., Berninger, V., Weintraub, N., & Shafer, W. (1998). The development of handwriting fluency and legibility in grades 1 through 9. *Journal of Educational Research, 92,* 42–52.

47. Graham, S., Boyer-Shick, K., & Tippets, E. (1989). The validity of the handwriting scale from the test of written language. *Journal of Educational Research, 82,* 166–171.

48. Graham, S., Harris, K. R., & Fink, B. (2000). Is handwriting causally related to learning to write? Treatment of handwriting problems in beginning writers. *Journal of Educational Psychology, 92,* 620–633.

49. Graham, S., & Miller, L. (1980). Handwriting research and practice: A unified approach. *Focus on Exceptional Children, 13,* 1–16.

50. Graham, S., & Weintraub, N. (1996). A review of handwriting research: Progress and prospects from 1980 to 1994. *Educational Psychology Review, 8,* 7–86.

51. Hagin, R. A. (1983). Write right or left: A practical approach to handwriting. *Journal of Learning Disabilities, 15,* 266–271.

52. Hammerschmidt, S. L., & Sudaswad, P. (2004). Teacher's survey on problems with handwriting: Referral, evaluation, and outcomes. *American Journal of Occupational Therapy, 58,* 185–191.

53. Hamstra-Bletz, L., & Blöte, A. (1990). Development of handwriting in primary school: A longitudinal study. *Perceptual and Motor Skills, 70,* 759–770.

54. Handley-More, D., Deitz, J., Billingsley, F. F., & Coggins, T. E. (2003). Facilitating written work using computer word processing and word prediction. *American Journal of Occupational Therapy, 57,* 139–151.

55. Hanft, B. E., & Place, P. A. (1996). *The consulting therapist: A guide for OTs and PTs in schools.* San Antonio, TX: The Psychological Corporation.

56. Hayes, J., & Flower, L. (1986). Writing research and the writer. *American Psychologist, 41,* 1106–1113.

57. Henry, D. (2005). Tools for tots: Sensory strategies for toddlers & preschoolers. Glendale, AZ: Henry OT Services.

58. Hill, D., Gladden, M., Porter, J., & Cooper, J. (1982). Variables affecting transitions from wide spaced to normal spaced paper for manuscript handwriting. *Journal of Educational Research, 76,* 50–53.

59. Holm, M. B. (2000). Our mandate for the new millennium: Evidence-based practice, 2000 Eleanor Clarke Slagle lecture. *American Journal of Occupational Therapy, 54,* 575–585.

60. Howle, J. M. (2002). *Neuro-developmental treatment approach: Theoretical foundations and principles of clinical practice.* Laguna Beach, CA: NDTA.

61. Jackson, A. D. (1971). A comparison of speed and legibility of manuscript and cursive handwriting of intermediate pupils.

Unpublished doctoral dissertation. *Dissertation Abstracts, 31,* 4383-A–4384-A.

62. Jarman, C. (1990). A national curriculum for handwriting? *British Journal of Special Education, 17,* 151–153.

63. Jenson, E. (1998). Teaching with the brain in mind. Alexandria, VA: Association for Supervision and Curriculum Development.

64. Karlsdottir, R., & Stefansson, T. (2002). Problems in developing functional handwriting. *Perceptual and Motor Skills, 94,* 623–662.

65. Kemmis, B., & Dunn, W. (1996). Collaborative consultation: The efficacy of remedial and compensatory interventions in school contexts. *American Journal of Occupational Therapy, 50,* 709–717.

66. Koziatek, S. M., & Powell, N. J. (2002). A validity study of the evaluation tool of children's handwriting—cursive. *American Journal of Occupational Therapy, 56,* 446–453.

67. Koziatek, S. M., & Powell, N. J. (2003). Pencil grips, legibility, and speed of fourth-graders' writing cursive. *American Journal of Occupational Therapy, 57,* 284–288.

68. Lamme, L. L. (1979). Handwriting in an early childhood curriculum. *Young Children, 35,* 20–27.

69. Lamme, L. L., & Ayris, B. M. (1983). Is the handwriting of beginning writers influenced by writing tools? *Journal of Research and Development in Education, 17,* 33–38.

70. Larsen, S. C., & Hammill, D. D. (1989). *Test of legible handwriting.* Austin, TX: Pro-Ed.

71. Laszlo, J. I., & Bairstow, P. J. (1984). Handwriting: Difficulties and possible solutions. *School Psychology International, 5,* 207–213.

72. Levine, K. J. (1991). *Fine motor dysfunction: Therapeutic strategies in the classroom.* Tucson, AZ: Therapy Skill Builders.

73. Levine, M. (1994). *Educational care: A system for understanding and helping children with learning problems at home and school.* Cambridge, MA: Educators Publishing Service.

74. Lewis, R. B., Graves, A. W., Ashton, T. M., & Kieley, C. L. (1998). Word processing tools for students with learning disabilities: A comparison of strategies to increase text entry speed. *Learning Disabilities Research and Practice, 13,* 95–108.

75. Lindsay, Ga. A., & McLennan, D. (1983). Lined paper: Its effects on the legibility and creativity of young children's writing. *British Journal of Educational Psychology, 53,* 364–368.

76. MacArthur, A., & Graham, S. (1987). Learning disabled students' composing under three methods of text production: Handwriting, word processing, and dictation. *Journal of Special Education, 21,* 22–42.

77. Magill, R. A. (1985). *Motor learning concepts and applications.* Dubuque, IA: William C. Brown.

78. McAvoy, C. (1996). Making writers. *Closing the Gap Newsletter, 15*(1), 9.

79. McGee, L. M., & Richgels, D. J. (2000). *Literacy's beginnings: Supporting young readers and writers* (3rd ed.). Boston: Allyn & Bacon.

80. McHale, K., & Cermak, S. (1992). Fine motor activities in elementary school: Preliminary findings and provisional implications for children with fine motor problems. *American Journal of Occupational Therapy, 46,* 898–903.

81. Milone, M. N., & Wasylyk, T. M. (1987). Handwriting in special education. *Teaching Exceptional Children, 14,* 58–61.

82. Mulligan, S. (2003). *Occupational therapy evaluation for children: A pocket guide.* Philadelphia: Lippincott Williams & Wilkins.

83. Musselwhite, C., & King-DeBaun, P. (1997). *Emergent literacy success: Merging technology and whole language for students with disabilities.* Park City, UT: Creative Communicating.

84. Myers, C. A. (1992). Therapeutic fine-motor activities for preschoolers. In J. Case-Smith & C. Pehoski (Eds.), *Development of hand skills in the child* (pp. 47–62). Rockville, MD: American Occupational Therapy Association.

85. Oliver, C. E. (1990). A sensorimotor program for improving writing readiness skills in elementary-age children. *American Journal of Occupational Therapy, 44,* 111–124.

86. Olsen, J., & Knapton. (2006). *The print tool evaluation and remediation package.* Cabin John, MD: Handwriting Without Tears.

87. Pasternicki, J. G. (1987). Paper for writing: Research and recommendations. In J. Alston & J. Taylor (Eds.), *Handwriting: Theory, research and practice* (pp. 68–80). London: Croom Helm.

88. Peck, M., Askov, E. N., & Fairchild, S. H. (1980). Another decade of research in handwriting: Progress and prose in the 1970s. *Journal of Educational Research, 73,* 283–298.

89. Peterson, C. Q., & Nelson, D. L. (2003). Effect of an occupational intervention on children with economic disadvantages. *American Journal of Occupational Therapy, 57,* 152–160.

90. Phelps, J., & Stempel, L. (1987). *The children's handwriting evaluation scale for manuscript writing.* Dallas, TX: Texas Scottish Rite Hospital for Crippled Children.

91. Phelps, J., Stempel, L., & Speck, G. (1984). *The children's handwriting evaluation scale: A new diagnostic tool.* Dallas, TX: Texas Scottish Rite Hospital for Crippled Children.

92. Reisman, J. (1991). Poor handwriting: Who is referred? *American Journal of Occupational Therapy, 45,* 849–852.

93. Reisman, J. (1999). *Minnesota handwriting test.* San Antonio, TX: Psychological Corporation.

94. Rosenbloom, L., & Horton, M. E. (1971). The maturation of fine prehension in young children. *Developmental Medicine and Child Neurology, 13,* 3–8.

95. Rubin, N., & Henderson, S. E. (1982). Two sides of the same coin: Variations in teaching methods and failure to learn to write. *Special Education: Forward Trends, 9,* 17–24.

96. Schmidt, R. A. (1982). *Motor control and learning.* Champaign, IL: Human Kinetic.

97. Schneck, C. M. (1991). Comparison of pencil-grip patterns in first graders with good and poor writing skills. *American Journal of Occupational Therapy, 45,* 701–706.

98. Schneck, C. M., & Henderson, A. (1990). Descriptive analysis of the developmental progression of grip position for pencil and crayon control in nondysfunctional children. *American Journal of Occupational Therapy, 44,* 893–900.

99. Simon, C. J. (1993). Sensory integration frame of reference. In H. L. Hopkins & H. D. Smith (Eds.), *Willard and Spackman's occupational therapy* (pp. 74–75). Philadelphia: J.B. Lippincott.

100. Sweedler-Brown, C. O. (1992). The effects of training on the appearance bias of holistic essay graders. *Journal of Research and Development in Education, 26,* 24–88.

101. Swinth, Y., & Anson, D. (1998). Alternatives to handwriting: Keyboarding and text-generation techniques for schools. In J. Case-Smith (Ed.), *AOTA self-study series: Making a difference in school system practice.* Bethesda, MD: American Occupational Therapy Association.

102. Talbert-Johnson, C., Salva, E., Sweeney, W. J., & Cooper, J. O. (1991). Cursive handwriting: Measurement of function rather than topography. *Journal of Educational Research, 85,* 117–124.

103. Tan-Lin, A. S. (1981). An investigation into the developmental course of preschool/kindergarten aged children's handwriting behavior. *Dissertation Abstracts International, 42,* 4287A.

104. Temple, C., Nathan, R., Temple, F., & Burris, N. A. (1993). *The beginnings of writing.* Boston: Allyn & Bacon.

105. Thurber, D. (1983). *D'Nealian manuscript—An aide to reading development* (Report No. CS 007 057). ERIC Document Reproduction Service No. ED 227 474.

106. Trap-Porter, J., Gladden, M., Hill, D., & Cooper, J. (1983). Space size and accuracy of second and third grade students' cursive handwriting. *Journal of Educational Research, 76,* 231–233.

107. Tseng, M. H. (1998). Development of pencil grip position in preschool children. *Occupational Therapy Journal of Research, 18,* 207–224.

108. Tseng, M. H., & Cermak, S. A. (1991). The evaluation of handwriting in children. *Sensory Integration Quarterly,* 1–6.

109. Tseng, M. H., & Cermak, S. A. (1993). The influence of ergonomic factors and perceptual-motor abilities on handwriting performance. *American Journal of Occupational Therapy, 47,* 919–926.

110. Tseng, M. H., & Chow, S. M. (2000). Perceptual-motor function of school age children with slow handwriting speed. *American Journal of Occupational Therapy, 54,* 83–88.

111. Volman, M. J. M., van Schendell, B. M., & Jongmans, M. J. (2006). Handwriting difficulties in primary school children: A search for underlying mechanisms. *American Journal of Occupational Therapy, 60,* 451–460.

112. Waggoner, J., LaNunziata, L., Hill, D., & Cooper, J. (1981). Space size accuracy of kindergarten and first grade students' manuscript handwriting. *Journal of Educational Research, 74,* 182–184.

113. Weil, M., & Amundson, S. J. (1994). Relationship between visual motor and handwriting skills of children in kindergarten. *American Journal of Occupational Therapy, 48,* 982–988.

114. Weintraub, N., & Graham, S. (1998). Writing legibly and quickly: A study of children's ability to adjust their handwriting to meet classroom demands. *Learning Disabilities Research and Practice, 13,* 146–152.

115. Weintraub, N., & Graham, S. (2000). The contribution of gender, orthographic, finger function, and visual-motor processes to the prediction of handwriting status. *Occupational Therapy Journal of Research, 20,* 121–140.

116. Williamson, G. G. (1993). Enhancing the social competence of children with learning disabilities. *American Occupational Therapy Association Sensory Integration Special Interest Section Newsletter, 16,* 1–2.

117. Woodward, S., & Swinth, Y. (2002). Multisensory approach to handwriting remediation: Perceptions of school-based occupational therapists. *American Journal of Occupational Therapy, 56,* 305–312.

118. Wright, J. P., & Allen, E. G. (1975). Ready to write! *Elementary School Journal, 75,* 430–435.

119. Ziviani, J. (1987). Pencil grasp and manipulation. In J. Alston & J. Taylor (Eds.), *Handwriting: Theory, research and practice* (pp. 24–39). London: Croom Helm.

120. Ziviani, J., & Elkins, J. (1984). An evaluation of handwriting performance. *Educational Review, 36,* 251–261.

121. Ziviani, J., & Watson-Will, A. (1998). Writing speed and legibility of 7- to 14-year-old school students using modern cursive script. *Australian Occupational Therapy Journal, 45,* 59–64.

Handwriting Assessments

CHILDREN'S HANDWRITING EVALUATION SCALE (CHES-C)

Description: Norm-referenced tool that assesses cursive writing of children in grades three through eight. Task consists of near-point copying of short paragraphs. Features similar to those of CHES-M.

Authors: Joanne Phelps, Lynn Stempel, and Gail Speck (1984)

Publication: CHES

Information: 6031 St. Andrews, Dallas, TX 75205

CHILDREN'S HANDWRITING EVALUATION SCALE FOR MANUSCRIPT WRITING (CHES-M)

Description: Norm-referenced test that examines rate and quality of children's handwriting for a near-point copying task. Children's handwriting in grades one and two is examined qualitatively by letterforms, spacing, rhythm, and general appearance.

Authors: Joanne Phelps and Lynn Stempel (1987)

Publication: CHES

Information: 6031 St. Andrews, Dallas, TX 75205

EVALUATION TOOL OF CHILDREN'S HANDWRITING (ETCH)

Description: Criterion-referenced test measuring a child's legibility and speed of children's handwriting in grades one through six. Domains (manuscript or cursive) include alphabet writing of lowercase and uppercase letters, numeral writing, near-point copying, far-point copying, manuscript-to-cursive transition, dictation, and sentence composition.

Author: Susan J. Amundson (1995)

Publication: O.T. KIDS, Inc.

Information: P.O. Box 1118, Homer, AK 99603

MINNESOTA HANDWRITING ASSESSMENT (MHA)

Description: Norm-referenced test that looks at quality and speed of manuscript handwriting for a near-point copying task. Models are in Zaner-Blöser or D'Nealian script for children in grades one and two.

Author: Judith Reisman (1999)

Publication: Therapy Skill Builders

Information: Psychological Corporation, 195000 Bulverde Road, San Antonio, TX 79259, (800) 872-1726

TEST OF HANDWRITING SKILLS

Description: Norm-referenced test that examines both manuscript and cursive handwriting through dictation, near-point copying, and alphabet writing from memory. Normative data are provided for children 5 through 11 years of age.

Author: Morrison F. Gardner (1998)

Publication: Psychological and Educational Publications, Inc.

Information: P.O. Box 520, Hydesville, CA 95547-0520

THE PRINT TOOL

Description: The Print Tool is a complete printing assessment for students age 6 and older. The Print Tool assesses capitals, numbers, and lowercase letter skills. The skills evaluated include memory, orientation, placement, size, start, sequence, control, and spacing.

Authors: Jan Z. Olsen and Emily F. Knapton (2006)

Publication: Handwriting Without Tears

Information: 8001 MacArthur Blvd, Cabin John, MD 20818, (301) 263-2700, Fax: (301) 263-2707, www.hwtears.com.

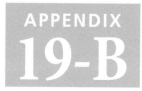

Handwriting Methods in Schools

D'NEALIAN HANDWRITING PROGRAM

Target: Manuscript, cursive
Author: Scott Foresman Co.
Vendor: Addison Wesley Longsman
Division of Scott Foresman Addison Wesley
1 Jacob Way
Reading, MA 01867
800-554-4411

ITALIC HANDWRITING SERIES

Target: Manuscript, connected script
Authors: B. Getty and I. Dubay
Vendor: Portland State University
Continuing Education Press
P.O. Box 1394
Portland, OR 97207-1394
800-547-8887, ext. 4891

PALMER METHOD OF HANDWRITING

Target: Manuscript, cursive
Author: McGraw-Hill
Vendor: McGraw-Hill
220 E. Danieldale Road
DeSoto, TX 75115
800-442-9685

ZANER-BLÖSER HANDWRITING

Target: Manuscript, cursive
Author: Zaner-Blöser
Vendor: Zaner-Blöser
P.O. Box 16764
Columbus, OH 43216-6764
800-421-3018

20

Influencing Participation Through Assistive Technology

Judith Schoonover • Rebecca E. Argabrite Grove • Yvonne Swinth

KEY TERMS

Assistive technology service
Universal design
Input
Output
Alternative and augmentative communication
Electronic aids for daily living
Learned helplessness
Self-determination
Electronic books

Computer-based communication system
Electronic communication aids
Non-electronic communication aids
Self-advocacy
Positioning and ergonomics
Digitized speech
Synthesized speech
Scanning methods

OBJECTIVES

1. Define and articulate the purposes of assistive devices and services and their relevance to the practice of occupational therapy.
2. Understand legal mandates regarding assistive technology service delivery.
3. Identify guiding frameworks/models that influence decisions about assistive technology.
4. Recognize and participate in a collaborative team approach for providing assistive technology services.
5. Describe application of assistive technology to enhance or improve childhood occupations across practice settings.
6. Apply a child and family-centered approach to evaluation, selection, and implementation of assistive technology.
7. Recognize cultural differences and their impact on acceptance of assistive technologies.
8. Recognize the continuum and interrelationship between no-tech and high-tech solutions.
9. Understand and apply evidence-based practices throughout the service delivery process.

"Not every child has an equal talent or an equal ability or equal motivation; but children have the equal right to develop their talent, their ability, and their motivation."

—*John F. Kennedy*

INTRODUCTION

Assistive technology (AT) has been an important tool since the origins of the occupational therapy profession, as well as throughout its history, to improve function and participation. Traditionally, therapists have used different types of adaptive equipment, such as reachers, buttonhooks, and pencil grips, to promote functional independence in their clients. However, within the past 10 to 15 years, with the rapid technological advances in society, specifically with the introduction of the microprocessor chip, occupational therapists have increasingly used a wide range of electronic devices, from simple switches to complex robotics, to support meaningful occupational engagement. Stoller described AT as "special devices or structural changes that promote a sense of self-competence, the further acquisition of developmental skills into occupational behaviors, and/or an improved balance of time spent between the occupational roles in an individual's life as determined by the individual's goals and interests and the external demands of the environment" (p. 6).[100]

"Occupational therapy practitioners' understanding of their clients' daily occupational needs, abilities, and contexts make them ideal collaborators in the design, development, and clinical application of new or customized technological devices" (p. 678).[3] Assistive technologies may unlock human potential and optimize human performance throughout the life span and across contexts, and allow individuals to assume or regain valued life roles. The selection of the "right tool for the job" bridges the gap between what people *want* to do and what they *can* do to participate in activities that are meaningful and life sustaining. Assistive technologies can serve a variety of needs and can be part of the educational and/or rehabilitative process depending on the environment in which services are provided. Congress has enacted a variety of legislation designed to support the procurement and use of AT for individuals with disabilities. This expansion in the use of AT opens new doors, creates opportunities, and enables individuals with disabilities to realize functional goals that were previously unattainable. Although the materials, structure, and form of devices used continue to change over time, the primary emphasis of AT across the life-span continues to be on functional outcomes for AT users above all other considerations.[28] With the influx of technology into the daily lives of all individuals comes the increased responsibility for occupational therapists to keep abreast of current trends so that the tools they recommend and implement can produce the best outcomes for the clients they serve.

Influencing Childrens' Growth and Development with Assistive Technology

Children have an "inborn drive to discover and learn" (p. 1)[19] that motivates them to understand the world around them, strive for independence, establish a sense of self, and connect socially with others. When a disabling condition is present, children may have difficulty with accessing play, learning, or self-care activities. Burkhart offered four "secrets" to support children's successful engagement: (1) create motivating activities, (2) develop opportunities for active participation, (3) present information and materials using multiple modalities, and (4) use authentic learning scenarios in natural contexts.[19] Research indicates that AT can be instrumental in helping young children with disabilities learn valuable life skills such as social skills, including sharing and taking turns, communication skills, attending, fine and gross motor skills, self-confidence, and independence.[7,54,76,105,107] As children grow, they may use technology to develop independence in many activities of daily living (ADLs) and instrumental activities of daily living (IADLs), complete school assignments, develop prevocational and vocational skills, increase opportunities for social participation, and play games or participate in leisure activities. The use of AT can create exciting opportunities for children to explore, interact, and function in their environments.

For children with disabilities, introducing the appropriate types of technology systems as early as possible may enable the child to participate in important learning situations that otherwise, because of his or her disabilities, may not be possible. For more than 20 years, researchers and clinicians have documented and discussed the unique opportunities that all types of AT offer for teaching and for advancing the life choices of children with disabilities.[9,10,33,43,54,61,85,101,105]

Because technology is constantly changing, this chapter presents problem-solving strategies, principles, and frameworks for decision making versus in-depth descriptions of specific devices or systems. The frameworks and guidelines for decision making that are presented should not be viewed as limiting strategies. Rather, they are meant to be a starting point. Each practitioner needs to adjust the concepts given the individual needs of the client and family, teaming issues, availability of resources, and many other factors unique to each situation.

Definition and Legal Aspects of Assistive Technology

AT comprises a broad range of devices, services, strategies, and practices used to address functional problems encountered by individuals who have disabilities.[28] *Assistive technology* is legally defined by Public Law (PL) 108-364 The Assistive Technology Act of 1998, as amended: "any item, piece of equipment or product system whether acquired commercially off the shelf, modified, or customized that is used to increase, maintain or improve functional capabilities of individuals with disabilities."

PL 108-364 further defines an AT service as any service that directly assists an individual with a disability in the selection, acquisition, or use of an AT device. The law includes several clarifications to enhance the definition of AT service: (1) evaluating needs and skills for AT; (2) acquiring assistive technologies; (3) selecting, designing, repairing, and fabricating AT; (4) coordinating services with other therapies; and (5) training both individuals with disabilities and those working with them to use the technologies effectively.

In a similar manner, the Individuals with Disabilities Education Improvement Act (IDEA) (PL 108-446) defines both AT devices and services as a means of providing a free and appropriate public education (FAPE). IDEA 2004 requires that individualized education program (IEP) and individualized family service plan (IFSP) teams consider a child's need for AT devices and services at least annually during the development of the IEP/IFSP. Additional information regarding other legislation related to AT can be found in Table 20-1.

In this chapter, *assistive technology* is used as a broad term that encompasses devices ranging from low technology to high technology. Low-tech devices (e.g., pencil-and-paper communication boards and built-up foam handles) are inexpensive, simple to make, and easy to obtain. High-tech devices (e.g., wheelchairs, augmentative communication devices, and computers) are generally expensive, more difficult to make, and more difficult to obtain. Mid-tech devices fall somewhere in between and may consist of hand-made or commercially available items.

This chapter discusses general information regarding the use of AT with children, followed by specific examples of application. Other chapters in this text specifically address the other areas of AT (see Chapters 16 and 21). Many of the principles and decision-making strategies discussed in this chapter can be generalized to all areas of AT.

Models for Assistive Technology Assessment and Decision Making

"When matching person and technology, you become an investigator, a detective. You find out what the different alternatives are within the constraints."
    —*From* Living in the State of Stuck: How Technology Impacts the Lives of People with Disabilities

The occupational therapy practitioner uses a variety of theories and practice models to guide the occupational therapy process (evaluation, intervention, and outcome monitoring). Practice models specifically related to AT help occupational therapists make decisions regarding its use and facilitate the integration of AT within the practice of occupational therapy.

Assessment tools and models to guide AT evaluation and service delivery have been developed by a number of professionals.[7,16,28,91,109,113] Each of these models provides a framework for evaluating needs, making decisions, and implementing intervention. Using a model for service delivery

TABLE 20-1   Other Legislation Related to Assistive Technology

Legislation	Application to AT
Rehabilitation Act of 1973 (Amended) http://www.hhs.gov/ocr/504.html	Section 504 requires federally funded activities and programs to offer reasonable accommodations to facilities and programs to ensure that people with disabilities have equal access and opportunity to derive benefits
Developmental Disabilities Assistance and Bill of Rights Act http://www.acf.hhs.gov/programs/ add/ddact/DDACT2.html	Provides grants to states for developmental disabilities councils, university-affiliated programs, and protection and advocacy activities for persons with developmental disabilities; provides training and technical assistance to improve access to AT services
Americans with Disabilities Act of 1990 http://www.usdoj.gov/crt/ada/cguide. htm#anchor62335 http://www.ada.gov	Prohibits discrimination on the basis of disability in employment, state and local government, public accommodations, commercial facilities, transportation, and telecommunications; Title II entities must communicate effectively with people who have hearing, vision, or speech disabilities; address telephone and television access for people with speech and hearing disabilities
Assistive Technology Act of 1990	First defined AT and established resource centers and information systems regarding obtaining and maintaining AT; some states supported training or establishment of central directories to facilitate access to AT; goals are to foster interagency cooperation, develop funding strategies, and promote access to AT throughout the life span
Assistive Technology Act of 1998 For a list of state projects funded under the Tech Act, visit: http://www.ataporg.org/ stateatprojects.asp	Title I state grant programs support public awareness, promote interagency coordination, provide technical assistance and training, and outreach support to statewide community-based organizations; Title II national activities provide increased coordination of federal efforts and authorize funding to support AT grants; Title III awards grants to states to help establish alternative funding
Medicaid http://www.cms.hhs.gov	Income-based program in which eligibility and services differ from state to state; federal government sets general program requirements and provides financial assistance to states by matching expenditures; largest funding source of AT benefits among all funding programs

From Cook, A., & Polgar, J. (2008). *Cook & Hussey's assistive technologies: principles and practice* (3rd ed.). St. Louis: Elsevier.

helps to ensure that the evaluation process is systematic and complete. Three models are highlighted in this chapter.

The Human Activity Assistive Technology (HAAT) model,[28] the Student Environment Task Tool (SETT) framework,[113] and the Matching Person and Technology (MPT) assessment process[90] follow the person-environment-occupation (PEO) model[65] and emphasize an occupation-based approach to AT practice. These models provide frameworks for decision making regarding the selection, implementation, and evaluation of AT.[28]

Human Activity Assistive Technology

The HAAT model (Figure 20-1) is a dynamic and interactive model in which three factors—the human, activity, and AT—form a collective whole that is then placed within the context of participation.[28] The human component includes physical, cognitive, and emotional elements. Activities are synonymous with occupations (e.g., self-care, productivity, leisure), and AT refers to a device and/or service. The context is strongly emphasized as a determining factor for outcomes.[28]

Student Environment Task Tool

A framework developed specifically for school settings is referred to as the SETT framework: student, environment, task, and tools. This framework is designed to support good decision making that promotes collaboration, communication, sharing of knowledge and perspectives, flexibility, and ongoing processes among educational team members.[113] It supports a student's participation in curricular and extracurricular

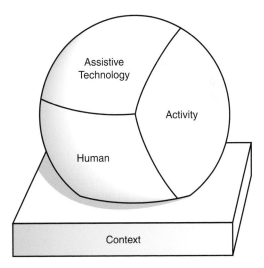

FIGURE 20-1   The Human Assistive Technology (HAAT) model.   (From Cook, A., & Polgar, J. [2008]. *Cook & Hussey's assistive technologies: Principles and practice* (3rd ed.). St. Louis: Elsevier.)

activities throughout the school day. SETT includes a series of questions that are designed to guide discussion, evaluation, and intervention. Teams may choose to use a few or all of the questions, depending on the needs of the student. Table 20-2 outlines the SETT questions. Many of these questions are consistent with the type of information that an occupational

TABLE 20-2 SETT Framework Questions

Context	Questions
Student	What does the student need to do?
	What are the student's special needs and current abilities?
Environments	What are the instructional and physical arrangements? Are there special concerns?
	What materials and equipment are currently available in the environments?
	What supports are available to the student and the people working with the student on a daily basis?
	How are the attitudes and expectations of the people in the environment likely to affect the student's performance?
Tasks	What activities occur in the student's natural environments that enable progress toward mastery of identified goals?
	What is everyone else doing?
	What are the critical elements of the activities?
	How might the activities be modified to accommodate the student's special needs?
Tools	What no-tech, low-tech, and high-tech options should be considered for inclusion in an AT system for a student with these needs and abilities doing these tasks in these environments?
	What strategies might be used to invite increased student performance?
	How might the student try out the proposed system of tools in the customary environments in which they will be used?

therapist gathers as part of the occupational profile and occupational performance analysis, and they appear applicable to a variety of settings.

Matching Person and Technology

The MPT model and assessment process are designed to help individualize the process of matching each person with the most appropriate AT. This model and process consider three factors: milieu (i.e., characteristics of the environment and psychosocial setting in which the person uses the technology), personality (i.e., personality, temperament, and preferences), and technology (i.e., functions and features).[90]

Child- and Family-Centered Approach

The social context of AT use can be considered the most influential and important, because it is often the social environment, including the attitude of others, that creates a disability more than the physical barriers in the environment.[28] Any person (e.g., parent, sibling, teacher) who interacts with an individual using AT, either directly or indirectly, is considered part of the social context. The simple presence of a disability can be socially stigmatizing, and the introduction of AT can add additional burden, particularly when individuals within the social environment do not support use of the technology. It is important to recognize key individuals

who provide assistance to the child using AT across environments (e.g., home, school, work), because technology use is facilitated when assistance is received from consistent individuals.

Each person's unique culture influences the manner in which he or she interacts with others and the importance of participation and engagement in various activities and life roles.[28] Some cultures do not value the independence that AT provides individuals with disabilities, or an AT device may be abandoned if it replaces an important life function of another family member. For example, the grandmother who views communicating for a child with cerebral palsy as one of her roles may resist the child's use of an augmentative communication system. Cultural factors must be considered in providing AT devices and services. Box 20-1 summarizes some sociocultural factors that the therapist may need to consider when evaluating, designing, and selecting AT systems for children.

Abandonment

> We are fascinated with technology. We expect it to make a difference in our lives, and particularly in education. We see its effects as beneficial. We look for it to change and improve what has come before. We await technological improvements in our lives, from better toaster ovens to improved, more efficient schools... (p. 3).[57]

Despite the many promises of technology, one third or more of individuals discontinue their use of their AT device.[90] Abandonment can mean the device is no longer needed, but more often it signifies a mismatch between the user and the device. When a device fails to live up to its promise of potential, freedom, and independence, disillusionment with the idea of AT may result. Failure to take into consideration the user's preferences, ideas and desires for an AT device is a primary reason for abandonment.[77,90] Users of AT, their families, and/or educational staff may have high expectations for an AT device and

BOX 20-1 Cultural Factors That Affect Assistive Technology Delivery

Use of time
Balance of work and play
Sense of personal space
Values regarding finance
Roles assumed in the family
Knowledge of disabilities and sources of information
Beliefs about causality
View of the inner workings of the body
Sources of social support
Acceptable amount of assistance from others
Degree of importance attributed to physical appearance
Degree of importance attributed to independence
Sense of control over things that happen
Typical or preferred coping strategies
Style of expressing emotions

From Cook, A., & Polgar, J. (2008). *Cook & Hussey's assistive technologies: principles and practice* (3rd ed.). St. Louis: Elsevier.

can be devastated when expectations are not fully met with far-reaching results.

Learned Helplessness and Self-Determination

Psychologist Norris Hansell theorized that there are seven essential and interrelated attachments necessary to create a sense of connectedness and quality of life.[49] These include having the supports necessary for existence (food, water, air, information); identity; connection with other persons; connection to groups; connection to a social role; money and purchasing power; and a system of meaning, each implying reciprocity with others. When this reciprocity is thrown off balance by internal or external circumstances, a sense of isolation, helplessness, and hopelessness can occur. "Human beings can be proactive and engaged, or, alternatively, passive and alienated, largely as a function of the social conditions in which they develop and function" (p. 68).[88] Ryan and Deci determined the needs for competence, relatedness, and autonomy as essential for social development and personal well-being.[88] AT can build bridges or create additional barriers between the user and the environment in which he or she wishes to participate.

Children with disabilities can become passive and unmotivated because of a lack of learning opportunities or a lack of independent control over their environment. This can result in decreased interest in or skills to interact with the environment.[35] When children perceive that they have little control over outcomes within their environments, the phenomenon of learned helplessness can result. Learned helplessness is a secondary disability and is the belief that one cannot exert personal control over outcomes experienced when interacting with the environment.[1,69] Children with learned helplessness exhibit low self-esteem, directly affecting how they interact and perform functional skills. They usually demonstrate a lack of initiation and an inability to cope with the events around them. In addition, when opportunities for integrating basic cognitive and perceptual skills are missed in early childhood, these children do not develop a foundation for learning higher-level concepts. Strategies and adaptations that allow these children the maximum amount of independence possible as early as possible decrease the chance for them to learn that they have no control over their environment.

The opposite of learned helplessness is self-determination. Self-determination is defined as "acting as the primary causal agent in one's life and making choices and decisions regarding one's quality of life free from undue external influence or interference" (p. 24).[110] Self-determination is an umbrella term that encompasses several common concepts used in describing children's personal, social, and skill development. These concepts include self-efficacy (outcome and efficacy expectations), self-esteem, and self-advocacy. Efficacy expectations are personal beliefs regarding one's capability to realize a desired behavior in a specific context (judgment of what one can do with the skills one has). Outcome expectations are personal beliefs about whether a particular behavior will lead to a particular consequence (being able to determine if one's goals are realistic). Self-esteem is the belief that one has in oneself, or self-respect. Self-advocacy refers to an individual's being able to speak for him or herself, make decisions for him or herself,

and know what his or her rights are, particularly when those rights have been violated or diminished. The individual is able to take ownership of his or her needs, rather than expecting someone else to take responsibility for them because he or she has a disability.[104,110] Appreciating and being able to function with a sense of interdependence are also crucial parts of self-determination.

Self-determination is a set of skills that can be taught and learned. Key characteristics and components include autonomy, self-awareness, choice making (i.e., often children with disabilities are not given the opportunities to make effective choices), decision making, problem solving, goal setting and attainment, internal locus of control, positive attributions of efficacy and outcome expectations, and self-knowledge.[110] With the increased emphasis on transition services and preparing children for life skills beyond school, occupational therapists should promote the development of self-determination for children of all ages. This includes ensuring that services develop skills of interdependence and independence, addressing the participation and productivity of children, recognizing that self-determination can mean different things to different people, and recognizing that self-determination is a quality-of-life issue that can be addressed across settings, environments, and opportunities. AT devices can help with the development, practice, and effective use of self-determining behaviors for children with disabilities.

SETTING THE STAGE FOR ASSISTIVE TECHNOLOGY SERVICE PROVISION

Practice Settings

"The institutional context refers to larger organizations within a society that are responsible for policies, decision-making processes, and procedures" (p. 43).[28] The International Classification of Function, Disability, and Health (ICF) categorizes economic, legal, and political components as services, systems, and policies. This institutional overlay has major implications for both the acquisition and use of AT, with regards to funding, legislation related to environmental and community access, as well as standards that govern product design, function, and safety standards.[28]

Differences in practice settings in which occupational therapy practitioners who use AT may be employed are outlined in Table 20-3. The role of the OT practitioner in each of these settings is governed by a combination of professional scope of practice, the expertise of other members of the team, and the agency or funding source.

Occupational Therapy Process and Assistive Technology in the Schools

According to the most recent statistics published by the U.S. Department of Education, Office of Special Education Programs, as required under the IDEA, an estimated 7.1 million children from birth to 21 years of age receive special education services.[108] Most children who need AT receive those services in school. AT devices and services are provided if necessary for a child to receive FAPE in the least restrictive environment (LRE). The need for AT must be considered, at least annually,

TABLE 20-3 Practice Settings In Which Assistive Technology (AT) Services Are Provided

Setting	Services Provided
Hospital or medical center	Primary role is evaluation that is typically provided on an outpatient basis for a series of assessments (1–2 visits); may require an inpatient stay of 2–3 weeks
	Referrals and recommendations made directly to agencies or third party payers
	Limited access to child for follow-up and training; limited opportunities to consult with parents and teachers
	May provide direct treatment, particularly for children under the age of 3 years or those who have an acquired disability (e.g., spinal cord injury)
Regional center	Developed in response to legislation, funded by the Department of Education or other agencies for individuals with disabilities
	Often have AT lending library for borrowing equipment on a short-term basis
	Team has broad-based experience with various diagnoses, resources for obtaining equipment, types of AT, and adapted methods of use
	Also involved in advocacy, consumer awareness, focus groups
	Limited follow-up care and minimal input into training the child, family, and educational team
Public school	Most children receive AT services at a school
	Daily problem solving related to AT use can occur and child receives support in the natural environment in which AT is to be used
	School-based team has easy access to child and understands educational curriculum but may lack expertise or experience with more complex AT systems
Home and community setting	May provide direct treatment, especially for children under the age of 3 years
	Direct training available to child and family
	Problem solving related to AT use can occur and child receives support in the natural environment in which AT is to be used
	Can provide carryover to other practice settings such as school or work
	May have limited opportunities to consult with others

Adapted from Beukelman, D.R., & Mirenda, P. (1992). *Augmentative and alternative communication: Management of severe communication disorders in children and adults.* Baltimore: Brookes.

for all children who receive services under IDEA. When AT is a necessary part of the student's program, then the school district is responsible to make sure that it is available to the child. It is not uncommon for the expertise of an occupational therapy practitioner to be requested when the team is considering AT for a student. Guides and models for considering AT for students in special education are available online (see Appendix 20-A on the Evolve website for Internet resources).

Baush, Ault, and Hasselbring indicated that appropriate AT devices and services can help a student improve, increase, or maintain performance to perform or develop functional skills (e.g., self-help, mobility, or communication), access curriculum (e.g., multimedia presentations or books on tape), become a more efficient learner (e.g., pencil grips and raised lined paper to improve writing legibility), or compensate for lack of skills (e.g., word prediction software to assist with spelling or reduce keystrokes).[8] The roles and responsibilities of IEP team members, including the occupational therapist, providing AT services within a school setting are listed in Box 20-2.

BOX 20-2 Roles and Responsibilities of School Assistive Technology (AT) Teams

1. Consider AT devices and services as an integral and necessary part of the IEP process as outlined by IDEA 2004.
2. Become familiar with different types of AT and a variety of tools that support student needs.
3. Assess each student's need for devices and services to support educational performance and access to curricular and extracurricular activities.
4. Seek additional resources and assistance from other educational professionals such as the members of an IEP.
5. Gather and analyze data about a student, his or her customary educational environments, goals, and tasks when considering AT needs. Student performance in core academic areas, social skills and behavior, communication, independent living, and organizational skills, along with demands of the task and environmental features, exist in a

dynamic relationship and may all be considered in combination during the AT assessment process.
6. Consider a range of AT options from no-tech to high-tech and use of existing resources, the procurement of new devices, or both.
7. Organize the physical space where AT is used, establish routines that support use of AT, and support consistent use of AT in all appropriate environments.
8. Communicate and document the AT process in the IEP, with rationale for the decisions made and scientific evidence to support devices and services. Supporting evidence may include AT assessments, device trials, student achievement with and without AT, student-based preferences, and teacher observations.

From Baush, Ault, & Hasselbring (2006). QIAT Consortium (2007). *Quality indicators for assistive technology services.* Retrieved August 2008 from *http://natri.uky.edu/assoc_projects/qiat/*.

The Transdisciplinary Team

The provision of AT services occurs across disciplines, and the training and experience of the service providers has not been widely studied[112] (Research Note 20-1) and the profession of "assistive technologist" does not exist.[95] Professionals specialize in AT on the basis of personal interest and self-study. Several universities offer certificate programs and advanced degrees in AT. In addition, the Rehabilitation Engineering and Technological Society of North America (RESNA) has established a mechanism for verifying a minimum level of competence for individuals serving as AT providers through an examination process that provides credentialing for persons working as assistive technology practitioners (ATPs). The ATP usually has a background in a rehabilitation discipline such as occupational therapy, physical therapy, speech-language pathology, or engineering.

As with many other specialty areas in pediatrics, the successful implementation of AT requires a cohesive and effective team that emphasizes shared vision and ownership. The team's input is critical to making decisions regarding AT because devices are used across the child's environments and address multiple performance goals that cross professional boundaries. Decisions that the transdisciplinary professional team and the family make together are most likely to meet the multifaceted needs of the child. The child and the family are considered members of the team in all forms of service delivery.

The specific members of the team may be different in various situations depending on the type of device being introduced to the child, the expertise of the individuals involved, and the specific setting. For example, in a clinical setting, the team may include the child and family, occupational therapist, physical therapist, speech-language pathologist, doctor, nurse, rehabilitation engineer, and social worker. In school-based practice, the team may include the child and family, occupational therapist, physical therapist, speech-language pathologist, educator, administrator, and psychologist.

In some settings, occupational therapy assistants and aides provide some of the AT services. Assistants are particularly helpful in training a child to use a system once the therapist has set up and established the program. Assistants and aides may also be involved in practicing use of the device with the child and helping others use the systems. Therapists working in AT service delivery must determine which activities are appropriate to delegate and which activities are specialized and require the training and skills of a therapist.

Assistive Technology Evaluation and Intervention: A Dynamic Process

The occupational therapist has a key role on the AT evaluation team. The unique perspective on occupation and engagement in meaningful activities that the occupational therapist offers the team is helpful in determining needs, problem-solving potential solutions, and evaluating outcomes. The assessment of client satisfaction has been one of the key factors in determining the effective implementation and usefulness of AT in the lives of individuals with disabilities.[30,31,90,92,104]

In addition to evaluation and intervention services, AT services may also include device procurement, training, skill acquisition, monitoring, and other services that support and enable the child's participation in home, school, and community activities. Because of the complexity of many AT systems, specifically those that are high-tech, the therapist needs a systematic procedure for follow-up and adjustments to help ensure the viability of the system over time. These steps of the process are dynamic rather than linear and sequential. For example, intervention may begin by addressing prerequisite skills for AT use before completing the AT evaluation and procuring a specific device. Once a system has been chosen and purchased, evaluation, monitoring, and decision-making processes continue throughout intervention.

Evaluation

When evaluating AT needs, the occupational therapist closely examines the child's abilities and difficulties, demands of the environment and task, and the child's goals. The first step of the evaluation is to identify key activities that the child or family needs or wants him or her to do. The Canadian Occupational Performance Measure is a useful tool to assist with the identification of client-centered goals and the importance of the goals.[64] The importance that an individual assigns to an activity helps predict whether he or she will accept technology that enables participation in that activity.[98]

A number of inventories, checklists, and processes have been developed to assist with evaluation.[95] When an evaluation

---

RESEARCH NOTE 20-1

Long, T. M., Woolverton, M., Perry, D. F., & Thomas, M. J. (2007). Training needs of pediatric occupational therapists in assistive technology. American Journal of Occupational Therapy, 61, 345–354.

ABSTRACT

The training of providers working with children who need AT devices or services has not kept pace with the variety and complexity of AT devices available. This article reports on a survey of pediatric occupational therapists who responded to questions about their training needs in the area of AT and delivering AT services. A large number of respondents reported less-than-adequate training in policies governing AT services and the organization and function of the service delivery system. Therapists reported a need and interest for accessible and affordable training in the areas of funding of technology and services; collaborating with families and other service providers; and accessing reliable, knowledgeable vendors.

IMPLICATIONS FOR PRACTICE
- Policy and practice context for providing AT services has become more complex, and practitioners are faced with, or unaware of, new and more sophisticated devices that might promote more opportunities for meaningful participation in their clients with disabilities.
- A majority of pediatric occupational therapists in this national sample rated their preparation in the area of AT as being less than adequate, and rated their confidence in terms of delivering AT and AT services as low.
- Training in identification of funding sources and use of high-tech devices is among the most pressing training needs.

is requested, observation should occur in the student's natural environment, which might include home, school (e.g., classroom, playground, lunchroom, bathroom, extracurricular areas), and community settings (e.g., work settings or other relevant locations). All the factors that are traditionally considered when conducting an occupational therapy evaluation, including frequency or duration needed to complete an activity, have a direct relationship to potential AT recommendations (Box 20-3). During the evaluation, it is important that any existing technology used by the child and its effectiveness in the customary environment be documented. A complete occupational therapy evaluation may or may not be a component of the AT process depending on the practice setting in which it occurs. Formal and informal assessments that may be used during the evaluation process are described in Table 20-4.

The AT evaluation may be completed by the team who will also provide the intervention (e.g., fitting and training of the device) or a team that has been formed specifically for the purpose of completing AT evaluations. Many hospitals, clinics, and some community agencies and schools have a designated AT team because of the complexity of many AT systems. The occupational therapist who does not work with AT on a regular basis may have difficulty maintaining expertise on all the systems and devices available because of the number of devices and the rapid development of new systems. When separate teams are responsible for evaluation and intervention, ideally these teams collaborate to make decisions and recommendations.

In addition to a comprehensive evaluation, a trial period with different types of AT is needed to achieve a good match between the AT device or system and the child and family. The trial period may be one of the most important aspects of the AT evaluation. These trials can help prevent the costly procurement of an incorrect device. The cost of AT includes not only the purchase of the device but also the ongoing expenses for maintenance, upgrades to the system, and repairs. Questions that the therapist should address throughout

assessment and intervention in relationship to cost include the following[105]:

- What financial resources are available to the family?
- When the AT device is in need of repair, does the family have access to services?
- Does the AT device significantly increase the child's level of independence and function?
- Can the AT device be adapted to enable higher levels of function as the child grows and matures?
- Can a less complex device meet the same needs just as well?

The team discusses these issues and others unique to each family in deciding whether the system is a reasonable and appropriate investment for the family that will result in increasing the child's functional independence. The team should present the child and family with objective and realistic information regarding investment in and use of AT.

Given a complete description of the options and alternatives, the family and the team make the final decision as to what AT is implemented and how it is incorporated into the child's program. Box 20-4 presents 11 criteria, developed by more than 700 AT consumers, that the team should use to evaluate different AT devices. In summary, AT evaluations should be conducted (1) as part of an ongoing process linked to educational and/or therapeutic planning, (2) by a team within the natural setting where the child needs to engage in his or her occupations, (3) with trials with potential AT devices, and (4) with meaningful follow-through involving all team members.[83]

Decision Making

Occupational therapy practitioners use problem-solving and clinical reasoning skills throughout the process of procurement, implementation, and follow-up with AT. Problem solving should involve defining the situation or problem, determining the short- and long-term goals, and brainstorming potential processes to reach the determined goals. The

---

BOX 20-3 Guiding Questions In Evaluating a Child for Assistive Technology

MOTOR
- What body parts are capable of reliable, accurate, and controlled movement?
- Can the child be positioned adequately in and maintain an upright sitting posture?
- Does the child have sufficient range of motion, finger dexterity, strength, and endurance?
- What is the child's overall endurance and strength?
- What is the child's level of independence in daily living skills?

SENSORY AND PERCEPTUAL
- Can the child attend to visual feedback on the monitor?
- Can the child respond to auditory feedback?
- What are the child's strengths and limitations in visual perception and visual motor skills?
- Is the child easily distracted by visual stimuli?

COGNITIVE AND COMMUNICATION
- What is the child's cognitive level?
- What is the child's attention span?
- What is/are the child's receptive and expressive language skills? potential?

- What are the child's face-to-face and written communication needs?
- Can the child sequence multiple-step directions?

PSYCHOSOCIAL
- Does the child seem motivated to use AT?
- What activities does the child enjoy?
- Does the child see AT use as meaningful and rewarding?
- Will the child and family tolerate the influence of this AT device?

CONTEXT
- Where will the child use the AT device?
- How can the AT device or interface be positioned for optimal use?
- Do classroom or home environments allow for safe and easy access to educational materials and use of the AT devices?
- Does the child have any previous experience with AT?
- Are the individuals who work with the child (family and professionals) willing to use AT?
- What are the short- and long-term goals with the AT device?

TABLE 20-4 Assistive Technology (AT) Assessments

Assessment Tool/System	Description
Wisconsin Assistive Technology Initiative (WATI) Assessment Package http://www.wati.org/Products/ products.html	Not designed as a test protocol but provides a process-based systematic approach to assessment. Package includes WATI Assessment forms including the Consideration Guide, Student Information Guide, Environmental Observation Guide, Decision Making Guide, AT Checklist, and Trial Use Guide.
Georgia Project for Assistive Technology (GPAT) http://www.gpat.org/default.htm	GPAT has developed evaluation tool kits. They contain a comprehensive list of types of tools that may be needed during an AT evaluation. It is not necessary to obtain all of the tools in the kit, and other tools may be equally appropriate.
MPT Assessment Instruments http://members.aol.com/IMPT97/ mptdesc.html	Each instrument is actually a pair of instruments—one designed for the provider of technologies (counselor, therapist, teacher, employer, trainer, etc.) and the other designed for the technology user. *Survey of Technology Use (SOTU)*—helps identify AT devices and systems an individual feels comfortable or successful using so new technology can be built around existing comfort or success *Assistive Technology Device Predisposition Assessment (ATD PA)*—helps people select AT *Educational Technology Predisposition Assessment (ET PA)*—helps students use AT to attain educational goals
Functional Evaluation for Assistive Technology (FEAT) http://www.nprinc.com/assist_tech/ feat.htm	Five scales are completed by various members of the AT team to allow for an ecologic assessment of needs: *Contextual Matching Inventory* (information about setting-specific demands) *Checklist of Strengths and Limitations* (used to gather data regarding person-specific characteristics) *Checklist of Technology Experiences* (additional information about the person-specific characteristics with regard to past/current use of technology) *Technology Characteristics Inventory* (examines device-specific characteristics such as dependability, product support) *Individual-Technology Evaluation Scale* (determines whether proposed AT offers legitimate potential for effectiveness)

BOX 20-4 Criteria for Evaluating Assistive Technology Devices

1. *Effectiveness.* How much the device improves the user's living situation and enhances functional capability and independence
2. *Affordability.* The extent to which a person can purchase, maintain, and repair a device without financial hardship
3. *Reliability.* The degree to which a device is dependable, consistent, and predictable in its performance and levels of accuracy for a reasonable amount of time
4. *Portability.* The influence of the device's size and weight on the user's ability to move, carry, relocate, and operate it in varied locations
5. *Durability.* The extent to which a device delivers continued operation for an extended period of time
6. *Securability.* How well a consumer believes that a device affords physical control and is secure from theft or vandalism
7. *Safety.* How well a device protects the user, care provider, or family member from potential harm, bodily injury, or infection
8. *Learnability.* The perspective of the device's ease of assembly, initial learning requirements, and time and effort to master use
9. *Comfort and acceptance.* The extent to which a user feels physically comfortable with the device and does not experience pain or discomfort with use; how aesthetically appealing the user finds the device and the user's psychologic comfort when using it in private or public
10. *Maintenance and repairability.* The degree to which the device is easy to maintain and repair (either by the consumer, a local repair shop, or a supplier)
11. *Operability.* The extent to which the device is easy to use, is adaptable and flexible, and affords easy access to controls and displays

From Scherer, M. J., & Lane, J. P. (1997). Assessing consumer profiles of "ideal" assistive technologies in ten categories: An integration of quantitative and qualitative methods. *Disability and Rehabilitation, 19,* 528-535.

therapist is often tempted to define the situation or problem and immediately jump to a possible technology for fixing the problem. However, if the therapist does not consider the short- and long-term goals before discussing potential solutions, the strategies implemented may not have a long-term benefit for the child. Many tools are available to support problem solving and decision making.

In addition to the assessment tools described in Table 20-4, The Council for Exceptional Children Technology and Media Division (TAM) website (http://www.tamcec.org/publications/index.htm) offers several tools, including an AT Consideration Wheel (Figure 20-2) that can help school teams consider a wide range of options, and a series of "fans" with user guides that feature technology devices on each blade, along with resources for locating the devices. Ablenet, a software company, has a CD-ROM available that provides information about low-tech devices and the use of simple communication aids for children with disabilities

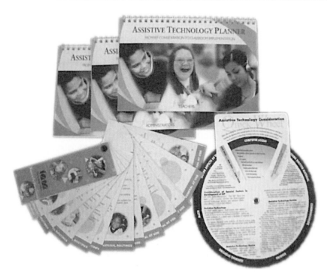

FIGURE 20-2   AT products available from the Technology and Media (TAM) Division of the Council for Exceptional Children, Reston, VA.   (Photo courtesy Judith Schoonover.)

(http://www.ablenet.com). Finally, new information that supports effective decision making for children with disabilities is continually being added to the National Center for Technology Innovation (NCTI) website (http://www.nationaltechcenter.org). Because of the rapid changes with technology in our society, practitioners working in this area of practice need to develop a strategy for keeping current with best practices related to effective decision making.

When working with children of any age, the team, including the occupational therapist, should consider short- and long-term goals in terms of what the child's needs are at present, 1 year later, 3 to 5 years later, and 7 to 10 years later. This can be difficult in working with young children, but the information can facilitate decision making, especially in addressing AT needs. In working with an adolescent, the focus becomes a successful transition plan, independence in the community, and participation in work roles. The procurement and use of the AT can be a critical part of a successful transition into future life roles for an adolescent.[18,63,99] The team should revisit and rewrite goals systematically as the child grows and matures, as contexts change, as child and family needs and desires change, and if the child's medical condition changes.

Lahm and Sizemore interviewed AT teams to identify factors that influenced decision making in selecting AT.[62] Important factors included client goals, environmental demands, family/client demands, and client diagnosis. Funding was considered but was lower in importance. Because an awareness of environmental demands was another important factor, evaluations should include strategies for gathering information about the environmental demands (e.g., phone interviews) to facilitate the best decision making.

Device Procurement

It can take up to several months to procure an AT device. When funding issues stall the process, members of the team may be involved in writing letters of justification to insurance companies and other third-party payers. Careful documentation

during the trial periods with different devices can help with this process. Documentation can include videos or pictures of the child using the system that demonstrates how the system helps improve his or her function.

Once the system has arrived, the team works to put the system together, test the system, and begin training. Some companies provide vendors that can help with the process, and others have videos that come with the system. However, it is not uncommon for a system to be delivered with minimal instructions. This can be daunting to the family if the system is delivered directly to the home and family members and other support providers are unsure how to use it. Comprehensive intervention and education are needed to help the child and family incorporate the device into their daily lives.

Funding

Occupational therapy practitioners working in the area of AT are often involved in helping procure the appropriate devices. In particular, they often provide the documentation used in applying for funding. Funding can come from various sources, including Medicaid, grants, private insurance, nonprofit agencies such as United Cerebral Palsy, private foundations, schools, and individual payment. In some states, funds are available through the Department of Developmental Disabilities, the Department of Health, or the Department of Social Services to help purchase AT devices. As students enter high school and begin the transition to work and career sites, the state's vocational rehabilitation agency may also assist with the funding of devices. In addition, there are some alternative sources of funding that the team may want to consider.[21] These include community service organizations, equipment loan programs, used and recycled equipment, and technical assistance projects. Often these alternative sources can take additional time and effort to research and contact. However, when a family or system has limited resources, pursuing creative funding options can result in the successful procurement of a device. When families cannot afford new devices or secure funding, they may explore AT reuse programs such as the *Pass It On Center* coordinated by the U.S. Department of Education's Office of Special Education and Rehabilitative Services (OSERS), because these programs often do not have eligibility requirements.[75] Occupational therapists should learn about the different funding options available within their state and region to contribute to the team's effort to obtain funding for AT devices.

Funding of AT in school districts often raises unique issues. The school district is the payer of last resort, but it is ultimately responsible for AT devices that the child needs to learn in the school environment.[21,106] Public or private insurance can be applied to obtain AT devices and services when they are determined to be medically necessary.[96] The use of these funds must be voluntary on the part of the parents and with their written consent. School districts can also work with community service organizations or associations (e.g., the Muscular Dystrophy Association) to purchase AT devices or pay for services. If the AT device is purchased with the parents' funds or insurance, then the device belongs to the child and the child's family. However, if the school district purchases the device, then the school district owns the device.[74,109]

Often the occupational therapist writes or assists with writing a letter of justification to support the funding of an

AT device. Strong supporting documentation that clearly demonstrates the necessity of the device to strengthen the child's engagement in occupation is an important part of the process. This documentation is based on the evaluation data gathered by the team and takes into consideration the language and priorities of the funding agency.[21] If the letter is written to a health insurance agency, then medical necessity must be emphasized; if it is directed to an education-related funding source, then it must address the child's ability to access and participate in educational programming. Requests to vocational agencies must address employment potential and skills.[21,93,109] Other key elements in the letter may include information about the child, the device, the evaluation procedures including results of any trials conducted, and the environment(s) in which it will be used; how the child will benefit from the device; alternative or potential outcomes of not being provided the device; supporting photos or measurements; and information about the cost of the device and other options considered.

Implementation of AT Services

An AT implementation plan should include: person(s) responsible, conditions of use, frequency of use, and duration of use. The team considers all of the tasks and contexts in which the AT will be used. Thus, for example, if a student requires a voice output communication system, it should be readily available at all times throughout his day (e.g., at lunch or recess to socialize, during instruction to ask or answer questions, during independent work to indicate needs and wants, and at home to interact with his/her family).

The introduction of an AT device, especially a complex device, can change the focus of a child's program. Time must be spent on training and practice within the child's natural environments (i.e., school, home) as the family and professionals make efforts to integrate use of the device into the child's everyday activities. Thus, the development of skills needed to use the device often becomes the focus of intervention. Involvement by every member of the team encourages skill generalization to various settings and situations of the child. When staff are encouraged to work as a team and time provided for them to communicate, the effectiveness of AT is likely to increase.[16] The AT devices should be readily accessible; if the device or strategy takes longer than 60 seconds to access and set up, it is less likely to be used. Examples of forms used to document an implementation plan (e.g., the *NATRI Assistive Technology Implementation Plan* and the *QIAT Plan for Evaluation of Effectiveness of AT Use*) can be accessed at the Evolve website.

Education Tech Points: A Framework for Assistive Technology Planning, as developed by Gayle Bowser and Penny Reed, identifies key points to assist educational teams in making decisions regarding the use of AT services and facilitates identifying resources that can be written into the child's IEP.[16] These points are beneficial for AT teams to consider regardless of the practice setting. Implementation and periodic review of the plan will help avoid the potential abandonment of recommended AT devices and services. Considerations related to AT implementation and day-to-day operations may include the following[16]:

- Who will ensure that the equipment is up and running?
- What will happen if the device needs repair?
- What will be provided in the interim if outside funding is sought to purchase a device?
- When and how much time will be provided for staff training and collaboration?

Measuring Progress and Outcomes

Not only does good AT decision making require an eye on the future, but evaluating the outcomes of AT takes a long-term commitment[32] to ensure that it continues to support the child's engagement and participation in purposeful activities. Often it is difficult to operationalize and define global outcomes specific to AT.[44] The goal of outcome measurement is to determine the efficacy and utility of AT devices and implications for abandonment. It is important that occupational therapists as members of AT teams select appropriate outcome measures to help determine whether devices and services have the intended effect.

Data collection is critical to evaluating AT's success. The team should be involved in a collaborative discussion regarding how data will be collected. Data collection should be simple and straightforward enough for all team members including family members to understand and complete with ease. Often, there are various ways to measure effectiveness or differing ideas on what the desired response or outcome of the child should be. For example, when designing a data sheet for switch use, one needs to consider which part of the body will be used to activate the switch, how much wait time will be allowed before a prompt is given, the type of prompt to be given (e.g., visual, verbal, hand-over-hand,), and how to define objectively what constitutes success for the given task (e.g., single switch activation, activation or deactivation of an electronic device, holding a switch for a specified amount of time). The occupational therapist can guide the team in a discussion of how to measure the child's performance.[95]

Data collected over time can support the continued use of AT devices already in place or justify the need for follow-up evaluation. Often data are collected on targeted goals and objectives and are dependent upon the service settings in which the device is used. Possible factors to measure include changes in the child's performance or level of function, change in level of participation, how often the device is used and under what circumstances, overall consumer satisfaction, goal achievement, quality of life, and cost analysis/savings. Table 20-5 outlines a number of assessments that may be used to evaluate outcome measures for AT.[5]

Often, once the child and family have a basic understanding of the AT system and begin to use it independently, the occupational therapist may discharge the child from direct services. However, discharge from a regular routine of intervention should include a follow-up plan. The therapist can perform follow-up in several ways, from a telephone call to an extended clinic visit or simple review and analysis of data collected. The type of follow-up and when it should occur depends on the complexity of the system and the skills of the child, family, and other professionals working with the child. A predetermined schedule for follow-up (e.g., at intervals of 6 months or less or sometimes 1 year or more) is a component of effective service delivery. Problems and delays in service can be prevented with planned periodic review.[16]

In addition to outcomes for individual users of AT, instruments are available to assist AT teams in conducting quality

TABLE 20-5 Assistive Technology (AT) Outcome Measures

AT-Specific Tools	General Tools
Efficiency of Assistive Technology and Services (EATS) Includes several assessments that target achievement of objectives (effectiveness) and individual perception of their value (utility) http://www.siva.it/research/eats/index.htm	Canadian Occupational Performance Measure (COPM) Client-centered measure used to detect self-perceived change in occupational performance over time Is completed by the caregiver for young child or child with limited ability to respond. http://www.caot.ca/copm/index.htm
Matching Person and Technology (MPT) Series of instruments that measure the fit between a person and technology http://members.aol.com/IMPT97/mptdesc.html	Occupational Self-Assessment (OSA) Self-rated measure of occupational performance and environmental adaptation Explores performance, habits, roles, volition, interests, and environment http://www.moho.uic.edu/assess/osa.html
Psychosocial Impact of Assistive Devices Scale (PIADS) Self-rating scale that measures the impact of rehabilitation products on quality of life in the areas of adaptability, competence, and self-esteem http://www.piads.ca	Occupational Therapy Functional Assessment Compilation Tool (OT FACT) Can compare and summarize longitudinal re-evaluation information following intervention Highlights skills and deficits, resulting disabilities and profiles of function in daily living, educational, vocational, and recreational activities http://www.r2d2.uwm.edu/otfact/
Quebec User Evaluation of Satisfaction with Assistive Technology (QUEST) Structured and standardized measure that allows one to rate degree of satisfaction with AT and importance ascribed to it http://members.aol.com/IMPT97/orderform.html#QUEST	School Function Assessment, AT Supplement (SFA-AT) Focus on how AT impacts a student's ability to complete functional tasks covered in the SFA http://www.r2d2.uwm.edu/atoms/idata/detail-idata.cfm?idata_id=43

From Argabrite Grove, R., Broeder, K., Gitlow, L., Goodrich, B., Levan, P., Moser, C., et al. (2007, April). *Assistive technology in the schools: From start to finish.* Pre-Conference Institute at AOTA's Annual Conference & Expo, St. Louis, MO.

assurance studies for the services that they provide. Quality Indicators for Assistive Technology (QIATs)[80] and the School Profile of Assistive Technology Services[81] are both used in school settings to support the development and delivery of AT services. Use of these indicators as guidelines can support outcomes for the child, the family, the classroom, and the system.

UNIVERSAL DESIGN AND ACCESS

Because it encompasses such a broad spectrum of services, the definition of AT is elusive. Perhaps because of this elusive nature, some therapists fail to recognize that the familiar tools in their "toolboxes" are really AT devices (Figure 20-3). Therapists working with children with special needs, their families, and educators often create, individualize, or adapt devices to enable independent participation for students with physical, communication, or developmental challenges to learning.[100]

Professionals and consumers have a common misconception that AT is complicated and expensive. Often, simple low-tech solutions are overlooked. Mistrett found that given a range of low- to high-tech solutions, families generally choose to use low-tech solutions more often, perhaps because their appearance is more like typically found toys and materials, and calls less attention to the disability.[72] Assistive technology can be viewed as a barrier rather than a bridge, or "just one

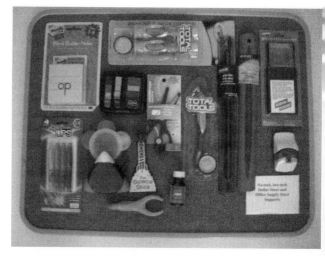

FIGURE 20-3 Examples of readily available, universally designed low-tech tools. (Photo courtesy Judith Schoonover.)

more thing to do," unless it is intuitive and its value is revealed in everyday successes. Special educator and AT consultant Judith Sweeney suggests that the best way to facilitate acceptance of AT is the EASY way: **E**conomy of cost and time; **A**dditional (or **A**dapted) use of familiar tools; tool selection based on **S**tandards that are already a part of what must be taught; and ownership, telling the student and teacher "the tool is **Y**ours."[103] Sweeney recognizes that it is imperative for the entire team to accept and promote use of the tools for students to be successful in their occupations.

AT can help to level the playing field for children with disabilities, enhancing physical, instructional, and social inclusion opportunities.

Access

Providing physical access to homes and schools may include both devices and services.[56] Modifications to buildings, rooms, and other facilities allow children with physical or sensory impairments to navigate both inside and outside of buildings using curb cuts, ramps, and door openers; labeling of key areas with pictures, text, and Braille; the provision of accommodations for individuals of varying sizes; or those who use wheelchairs to access restrooms, water fountains, pay phones, or elevators. Occupational therapy practitioners are trained to identify ways to improve performance and safety in the natural context to arrange resources, and to modify the environment to decrease or eliminate barriers.

Bus modifications for entry and exit and safe and appropriate seating can help with transportation to and from school and school-related activities including field trips, sports, and recreation. Within the building, doors, walkways, handles, light switches, and stairs can be modified to provide equal access to all students. Outside the building, seating and playground modifications can allow or enhance safe mobility and participation in recreational activities.[45]

Universal access has become an important concept that guides school and clinic purchase of new technology, particularly new computer systems. Most schools and clinics have established guidelines for ensuring universal access as they update and expand their computer systems. When all children, including those with disabilities, have equal access to technology, costly modifications for individuals can be avoided. Often the complexity of AT is not considered when general technology is purchased, so that computers do not support some of the software programs or adaptive peripherals needed by children with disabilities. A team of professionals, consumers, technology developers, and standards organizations must plan together to ensure that technology is accessible to all.

Universal Design

We must create spaces at all times that all can use, no matter their abilities, age or size.

—Ron Mace, Architect

Ronald Mace, founder and program director of The Center for Universal Design,[24] was an internationally known architect and visionary who used the term *universal design* to describe the concept of making all products and the built environment physically pleasing and usable to the greatest extent possible by everyone, regardless of their age, ability, or status in life. Mace used a wheelchair for mobility purposes, and his work relating to accessible design was instrumental in the passage of national legislation prohibiting discrimination against people with disabilities, the Fair Housing Amendments Act of 1988, and The Americans with Disabilities Act of 1990. The principles of universal design are outlined in Box 20-5.

According to The Center for Universal Design, "the intent of UD is to simplify life for everyone by making products, communications, and the built environment more usable by as many people as possible at little or no extra cost."[24] Universal design is a proactive approach that can eliminate many barriers, but does not replace the need for individualized AT. Although typical furnishings, toys, and instructional materials found in homes and classrooms may meet the needs of many, items that are "easier to handle, larger, less slippery, color

---

BOX 20-5 Principles of Universal Design

PRINCIPLE ONE:
Equitable Use
The design is useful and marketable to people with diverse abilities.

PRINCIPLE TWO:
Flexibility in Use
The design accommodates a wide range of individual preferences and abilities.

PRINCIPLE THREE:
Simple and Intuitive Use
Use of the design is easy to understand, regardless of the user's experience, knowledge, language skills, or current concentration level.

PRINCIPLE FOUR:
Perceptible Information
The design communicates necessary information effectively to the user, regardless of ambient conditions or the user's sensory abilities.

PRINCIPLE FIVE:
Tolerance for Error
The design minimizes hazards and the adverse consequences of accidental or unintended actions.

PRINCIPLE SIX:
Low Physical Effort
The design can be used efficiently and comfortably and with a minimum of fatigue.

PRINCIPLE SEVEN:
Size and Space for Approach and Use
Appropriate size and space are provided for approach, reach, manipulation, and use regardless of user's body size, posture, or mobility.

From North Carolina State University Center for Universal Design: *Principles of universal design*, Raleigh, NC, 2001, North Carolina State University Center for Universal Design. Complete guidelines can be found at http://www.design.ncsu.edu?cud/.

coded or in some ways more inviting and functional" (p. 5)[82] may be required for others.

Positioning and Ergonomics

Positioning and ergonomics conceptually include the physical positioning of the child for comfort, function, and work; location of the child within the environment; and location of supports in relationship to the child. A child's positioning should never be static in nature. Seating, positioning, and mobility devices are often the foundation for successful use of all other AT, and they may be used to improve body stability, provide proximal trunk and head support, allow for exploration of the environment, and reduce localized skin pressure.[78] The right seating and positioning equipment allow users to interact with their environment and perform tasks that are meaningful and life sustaining. "A task performance position is one that the person must be able to assume and maintain and in which the person can move" (p. 3).[55]

The environment cannot and should not come to the child; the child should be able to enter into and interact within the environment. One size does not fit all (Figure 20-4). With any population, there are variances in physical size and stature, and access methods can make it a challenge to provide adjustability to fit everyone comfortably. Computer use is rapidly becoming the rule (and the computer the tool of choice) rather than the exception in home, work, and school environments. Ergonomic working arrangements allow users to work in neutral, relaxed positions that consider energy conservation, which is important to maximize productivity for all users while protecting health and minimizing the risk of injury. Productivity is the result of a comfortable marriage of the user and the tool.

As technology becomes a more important part of children's lives at home and school, so does the need to pay attention to the health aspects of using computers. Proactive approaches to ergonomics programs should be embraced, particularly with regards to prolonged computer usage. American children typically spend between one and three hours a day at a computer, putting them at high risk for wrist, neck, and back problems.[29] If children, or those advocating on their behalf, learn at an early age how to adjust a workstation, they will make similar adjustments later in life. These habits and skills can be established as early as the preschool years. Many schools have chosen not to include ergonomics programs because of the costs often associated with implementation. Box 20-6 outlines some minor changes that have minimal or no costs associated with them.

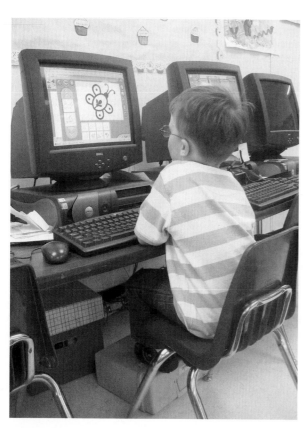

FIGURE 20-4 One size does not fit all. It is important to adjust learning environments to promote health and productivity. (Photo courtesy Judith Schoonover.)

BOX 20-6 ERGONOMICS: Budget-Minded Solutions/Tips for Home and School

Evaluate current equipment to determine whether it can be adjusted at all. If adjustable equipment is available, ensure that all users understand the need for it and how to adjust it. Educate and empower students to make their own workstation modifications by providing them with the tools and materials they require.

Recognize that lighting, glare, and proximity of computer monitor to the user can all have negative impact on vision. The computer monitor should be at or slightly below eye level and approximately 24 inches away. Provide document holders at eye level to minimize eyestrain when copying.

Good ergonomic habits are best learned when modeled.

One size does not fit all. Provide a number of seating options and footrests for the user to choose from.

Never use the "legs" that many keyboards have attached on the bottom surface of the keyboard because they place the keyboard at a positive slope (slant the keyboard towards the operator). This position forces the user to bend wrists to touch the keys rather than maintaining a neutral position. If a slanted plane is desirable for visibility purpose, place keyboard on binder so that user's wrists are supported.

Obtain or make footrests—investigate whether your school or a local high school can make footrests as part of their woodworking program.

Make adjustments to the equipment as needed—providing several heights of work surfaces or sizes of chairs may be warranted.

If a mouse tray is unavailable, make sure that the mouse is close to the side of the user's body. This is necessary to ensure that the upper arm can remain relaxed and posture can remain as neutral as possible. In some cases, a lap tray can be used.

Costs can be minimized by involving school maintenance staff, woodworking classes, parent organizations, or service clubs to make adjustments to equipment.

Stretching programs (i.e., to stretch neck, spine, shoulders) can be downloaded from many reputable websites at no charge. If no changes can be made to the workstation, ensure that all students are educated on taking appropriate breaks and are given stretches.

Modified from: Office ergonomics reminder sheet (2003). *Options Quarterly Online Newsletters.* Available at http://www.oiweb.com/pages/newsarchive03.html

PARTICIPATION: SUPPORTING LIFE SKILLS WITH ASSISTIVE TECHNOLOGY

Often, occupational therapy practitioners work with very young children or children with significant disabilities. Although prerequisite skills may be necessary for successful use of certain devices, many children use a range of AT to address life skills such as communication, mobility, self-help, play and leisure, and work.[114] For these children, low technology, such as the use of simple switches and cause and effect toys/appliances or software, may be the AT system of choice. Therapists may use these devices to help a child learn cause and effect or to build foundational skills for future AT systems. For some children with significant disabilities, simple devices that provide sensory input (e.g., fans, vibrators, music, lights) may be more motivating than some of the cause-effect toys or software (Figure 20-5). These devices can be hooked into an electronic aid to daily living (EADL) and then a switch can be used to turn them on and off. The EADL can run electronically operated toys or appliances and has functions that allow the child control of how the switch is used (e.g., a timer can be used so the child has to hit the switch every 30 seconds).

Often, low-tech solutions are controlled through a single switch. Typically, a touch switch that requires a press and release is used (Figure 20-6, *A*). However, for some children, this type of switch may not be motivating, or the student may not have the physical skills needed to access the switch. Figure 20-6, *B*, shows an example of a switch that helps a student learn cause-effect relationships. Some children may not have the physical skills to press or pull against resistance. These children may use a switch that is activated through a light touch (Figure 20-7, *A*). Switches can be mounted so that the position can be easily adjusted to improve access for a student

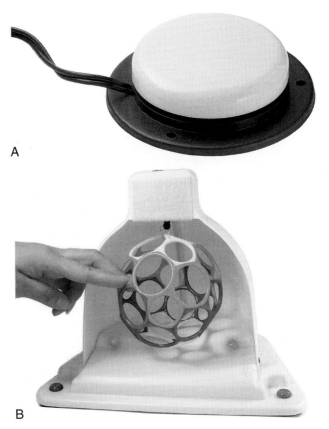

A

B

FIGURE 20-6   **A,** An example of a touch switch: the jelly bean switch. **B,** An example of a switch that is activated by pulling on the multicolored ball. (A, Photo courtesy Enabling Devices, B, Photo courtesy Ablenet; http://www.ablenetinc.com.)

(Figure 20-7, *B*). Although this switch requires minimal controlled movement, its cognitive demand is greater than that for the switches pictured. The touch-free switch may be too abstract for students with low cognitive skills.[26]

Through the use of low-tech tools, switches, and simple cause-effect activities, children with disabilities can participate in a variety of learning activities at home and in the classroom. Figure 20-8, *A*, shows an example of how a child with a disability can participate in a water play activity through a switch toy. Figure 20-8, *B*, shows how a child can participate in a gardening activity, and Figure 20-8, *C*, illustrates how a student with a disability can play a game with his peers. Switches may allow partial participation, in which the student uses a switch to complete one step of the task. For example in Figure 20-8, *B*, the student pressed the switch to turn on the Water-Pik; then another student used the Water-Pik to water the flowers.

Alternative and Augmentative Communication

If all my possessions were taken from me with one exception, I would choose to keep the power of communication, for by it I would soon regain all the rest.
—Daniel Webster, 1822

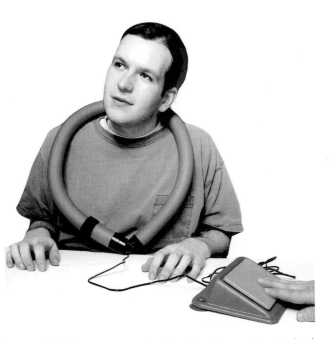

FIGURE 20-5   An example of a vibrating snake attached to a switch as a means to provide independent control of sensory input. (Photo courtesy Enabling Devices; http://enablingdevices.com.)

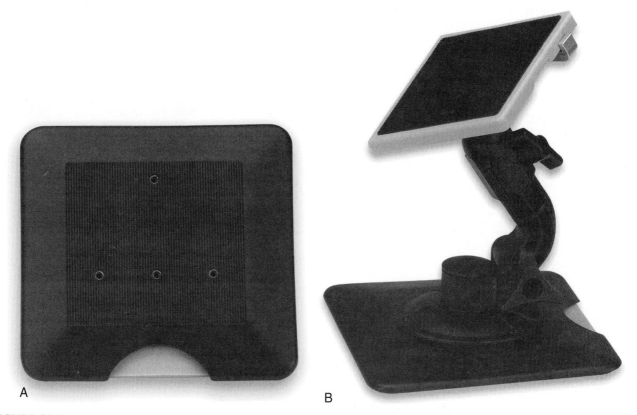

FIGURE 20-7   **A,** The Sensitrac flat pad switch. Switch is activated by a simple touch. **B,** The Sensitrac flat pad switch can be easily positioned for a child to access.   (Photos courtesy Ablenet.)

Verbal communication is an inherent function of human beings and lends quality and detail to our social interactions with one another. Communication is not designed to be a solitary activity, because the purpose of communication is to exchange and share information with another individual. Children with disabilities may present with a range of performance levels related to receptive and expressive language. It is important that we consider the continuum of AT options available to support communication at any level. As stated by the National Joint Committee for the Communications of Persons with Severe Disabilities, "all persons, regardless of the extent or severity of their disabilities, have a basic right to affect, through communication, the conditions of their own existence."[73] In addition to this basic right, the committee has outlined specific communication rights that should be ensured during all daily communication acts with persons with disabilities (Box 20-7).

Alternative and augmentative communication (AAC) is defined as communication that does not require speech and that can be individualized to the unique needs of the child. An AAC system uses a combination of all the methods of communication available to a child. This can include "any residual speech, vocalizations, gestures, and communicative behaviors in addition to specific communication strategies and communication aids" (p. 7).[34] The overall purpose of AAC is to enable the transmission of a message to another individual. According to Beukelman and Miranda, even students with severe disabilities can benefit from AAC use.[11] Research indicates that individuals with complex communication needs who do not gain successful access to AAC are at high risk for abuse, crime, unemployment, and limited social networks.[17,27]

AAC interventions, much like other AT tools, should be dynamic and include not only the individual child, but also his/her primary communication partners. Beyond the obvious function of self-expression, AAC can help to support the development of language, emerging literacy skills, enhance participation in educational settings, facilitate friendships, and support interactions with family members and people in the greater community.[28] When one family member relies on AAC, it always has an impact on the entire family unit.[47] For this reason, it is imperative to use a collaborative approach when evaluating and implementing AAC supports. Various members of the team will bring different levels of expertise to share: child and parents will have the best knowledge of daily communication needs and routines, teachers will have knowledge related to literacy and instruction, speech-language pathologists are experts in language development, and occupational and physical therapists provide services related to positioning, accessing, and physically using the AAC system.

Attitude and acceptance of AAC play a role in its impact on the quality and function of interactions. AAC systems must be designed with layout and components that match the desires, preferences, abilities, skills, and environmental contexts of the child. Many parents are fearful that AAC will interfere with speech development, when in fact it has been found to enhance it.[14] A family-centered approach should be used when

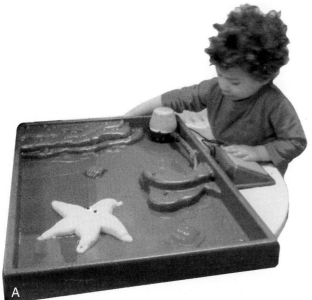

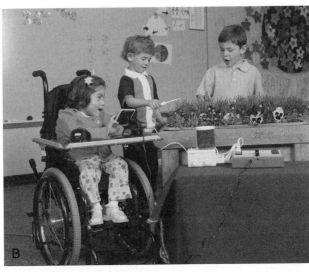

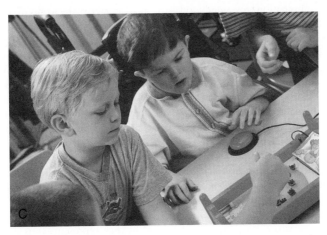

FIGURE 20-8   A, The child uses the switch to play with the water toy. **B,** The child uses the switches to participate in a gardening activity with her peers. **C,** The child uses the switch to turn on the Bed Bugs game.   (A and C, Photo courtesy Ablenet; B, Photo courtesy Enabling Devices.)

BOX 20-7   Basic Communication Rights

1. The right to request desired objects, actions, events, and persons and to express personal preferences or feelings
2. The right to be offered choices and alternatives
3. The right to reject or refuse undesired objects, events, or actions, including the right to decline or reject all proffered choices
4. The right to request and be given attention from and interaction with another person
5. The right to request feedback or information about a state, object, person, or event of restinte
6. The right to active treatment and intervention efforts to enable people with severe disabilities to communicate messages in whatever modes and as effectively and efficiently as their specific abilities will allow
7. The right to have communication acts acknowledged and responded to, even when the responder cannot fulfill the intent of these acts

8. The right to have access at all times to any needed augmentative and alternative communication devices and other assistive devices and to have those devices in good working order
9. The right to environmental contexts, interactions, and opportunities that expect and encourage persons with disabilities to participate as full communicative partners with other people, including peers
10. The right to be informed about the people, things, and events in one's immediate environment
11. The right to be communicated with in a manner that recognizes and acknowledges the inherent dignity of the person being addressed, including the right to be a part of communication exchanges about individuals that are conducted in his or her presence
12. The right to be communicated with in ways that are meaningful, understandable, and culturally and linguistically appropriate

From National Joint Committee for the Communication Needs of Persons with Severe Disabilities. (1992, March). Guidelines for meeting the communication needs of persons with severe disabilities. *ASHA, 34* (Suppl. 7), 1-8.

AAC is integrated into the child's daily experiences and inter- actions, to ensure caregiver support of its use.[68]

Communicative interaction has four purposes[67]: expression of wants and needs, information transfer, social closeness, and social etiquette. It is important for practitioners to also be aware of the three types of AAC communicators[36]: emergent communicators who have no reliable method of symbolic expression, context-dependent communicators who do have symbolic communication but are limited to specific contexts because they are only intelligible to familiar partners or may have insufficient vocabulary, and independent communicators who can communicate with anyone on any topic. Research indicates that children who use AAC are most frequently iden- tified as "responders," whereas typically developing peers con- sistently act as the "initiators" of communication.[25] These classifications can serve as a foundation for identifying and establishing an AAC system in conjunction with the use of strategies that facilitate communication (Box 20-8).

AAC devices can be viewed on at least two continua, including no-tech to high-tech systems and aided or unaided communication methods. Depending on their age, contexts, and skills, children may use a combination to aided and unaided communication and a combination of low- and high-tech devices. Unaided or body-based communication is no-tech and consists of vocalizations, gestures, facial expres- sions, sign language, pantomime, eye gaze, and/or pointing. All people use some combination of unaided communication. Children with disabilities often use gestures, facial expressions, and body language as allowed by their functional skills.

Aided communication systems are distinguished as either nonelectronic or electronic communication aids and require the child to be able to use a symbol system.[28] Nonelectronic aids are considered low-tech and include communication boards or books, picture-based systems, or paper and pencil. Picture-based systems are used increasingly with children in preschool, children with severe disabilities, and children with autism (Figure 20-9). Some children may find it easier to use visual-based systems of communication and to process content delivered using such sys- tems. Visual representation such as objects, photographs, realistic drawings, line drawings, and written words can be used to in- crease understanding, communication, and social connectedness,

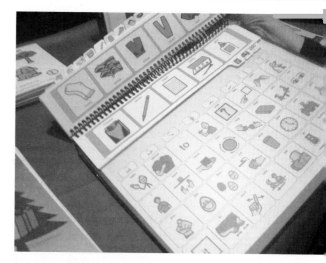

FIGURE 20-9 Example of a low-tech communication board. (Photo courtesy Judith Schoonover.)

and can take many forms depending on the environment and the circumstances under which they are used. Visual bridges[52] can be designed to assist students to communicate about themselves using a combination of written words, objects, photos, computer-gener- ated picture symbols, clip art, or other visual cues. Visual bridges can also be used during reading and writing activities. Emergent readers benefit from graphics paired with text to reinforce the meaning of print. Visual supports can be used during the develop- ment of schedules, augmentative communication systems, games, sequencing, and academics.

For individuals who have difficulty understanding two- dimensional visual representation systems such as photos, drawings, and graphics, Bloomfield suggests the use of True Object-Based Icons (TOBIs).[15] TOBIs are any drawing, pic- ture, or photo cut out in the actual shape or outline of the item they represent, thus providing visual information to the communicator (Figure 20-10). Tangible symbols are another

---

BOX 20-8 Strategies to Facilitate Communicative Interaction

1. Structure the environment to foster interaction.
2. Attend to the child. Solicit a shared focus.
3. Provide meaningful opportunities for communication.
4. Have realistic expectations for the child.
5. Provide appropriate language input.
6. Avoid yes/no questions and "test" questions.
7. Pace the interaction. Give the student time to communicate. WAIT.
8. Follow the child's lead. Respond to his or her attempts to communicate.
9. Provide models for the child's expressive modes of communication. Coach the child as needed.
10. Prompt if necessary. Remember to fade prompts to natural cues. Enjoy communication.

Adapted from Special Education Technology Center, Ellensburg, WA.

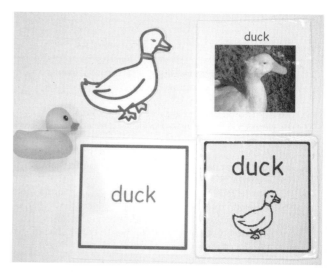

FIGURE 20-10 Multiple means of representation clock- wise from left: an object, a TOBI, a photo, a picture symbol, and a word. (Photo courtesy of Judith Schoonover.)

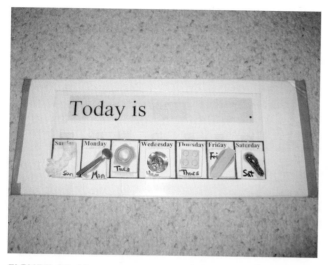

FIGURE 20-11 Example of a tactile symbol communication board. (Photo courtesy Judith Schoonover.)

example of providing symbolic representation of language, allowing communicators to relate to objects and experiences beyond their immediate context. Tangible symbols[87] are two- and three-dimensional manipulatives that can be objects, parts of an object, or an associated object that conveys meaningful information to the user or represents their communicative intent. For example, a small bit of chain might indicate time to swing, or a circle formed from a pipe cleaner may indicate "morning circle" (Figure 20-11).

Electronic communication aids or devices are generally considered more high-tech and may include speech generating devices, talking frames, cell phones, or computers. Speech-generating devices may produce digitized or synthesized speech output.[28] Digitized speech records a person's actual voice and allows flexibility in selecting a child, male, or female voice; however, it requires a

lot of memory for storage and is limited to only what is recorded and stored. Synthesized speech is generated electronically but has the advantage of text-to-speech capabilities. The intelligibility of synthesized speech can vary depending on the type of system.

For children with severe disabilities or young children, several different types of simple AAC devices can be used. One example can be seen in Figure 20-12, A. This device has a recorded message that is activated each time the user presses the switch (Figure 20-12, B). Another simple AAC device that is good for individuals who are ambulatory is shown in Figure 20-12, C; it is worn like a watch and can have several prerecorded messages. The messages are easy to change, and symbols can be used to help the user remember the messages (Figure 20-12, D). Devices like those in Figure 20-12, E, are good for children who may eventually use more high-tech AAC.

High-tech electronic communication aids generally are either computer-based systems or dedicated systems. Computer-based systems are often considered for children who are using or will be using some sort of computer-assistive technology in addition to a communication system. Computer-based systems are made up of computers that can perform as a communication system through the use of specialized software and other modifications, but can also carry out other functions such as environmental control. Ideally, computer-based systems should be able to be mounted on wheelchairs or easily portable in some other manner. Dedicated systems operate primarily as electronic communication aids (Figure 20-13) with hardware and software features specifically designed for communication purposes. These systems are available in various sizes and weights and provide auditory, visual, or printed output. All electronic communication devices are programmed with individualized overlays. The board's overlays can indicate as few as 2 and as many as 128 choices to the child.

A number of factors must be considered in designing a high-tech AAC system, the first of which is to assess the child's symbolic representation.[12] What type of symbol will the child be able

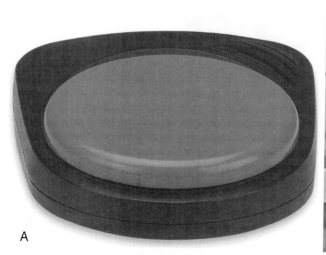

A

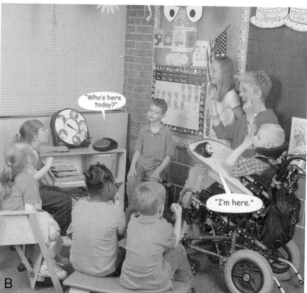

B

FIGURE 20-12 AAC devices. **A,** BigMac communication device. **B,** Using the BigMac to participate in circle time.

(Continued)

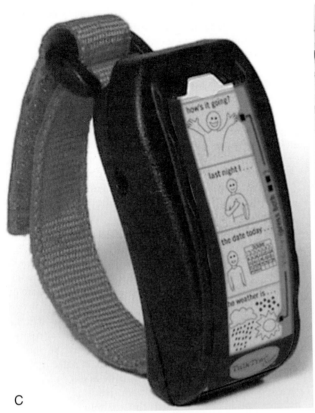

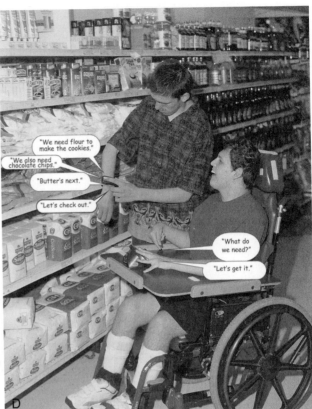

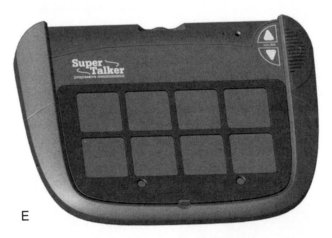

FIGURE 20-12, Cont'd **C,** Talk Trac communication device. **D,** Using the Talk Trac and Step-by-Step communication devices to go shopping. **E,** Supertalker. (Photos courtesy Ablenet.)

to use? Receptive understanding of functional objects, visual matching, and spelling and literacy skills related to word recognition are all cognitive skills that will help define the symbol system that is necessary. Examples of symbol systems include real objects, photographs, pictographs, Blissymbols (featuring grammar and syntax categorization by parts of language), and traditional orthography (use of letters and words). Examples of Blissymbols, Rebus, and PicSyms can be seen in Figure 20-14.

The control interface or manner in which a child interacts to provide input to the device may include use of a keyboard; single, dual, or multiple switch arrays; and joystick, mouse, or other alternative pointing devices.[28] A child may make selections either directly by pointing or touching, or he or she may use an indirect method such as auditory or visual scanning, directed scanning, or coded access. To allow a child to communicate faster than the rate of keying in text, encoding (or symbol) systems are used. This language uses sequenced multiple-meaning icons to retrieve words, phrases, or sentences. Like word prediction, many communication systems come with message prediction. Some of the more advanced systems can learn the communication "style" of the user and begin to predict with greater accuracy.

In addition to the input method, AAC devices use two visual display types (screens). A dynamic communication display offers

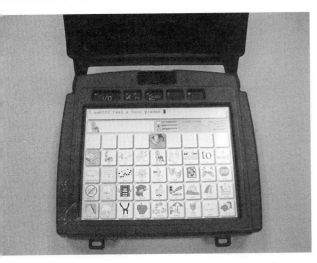

FIGURE 20-13   Example of a dedicated, dynamic display augmentative and alternative communication device.   (Photo courtesy of Judith Schoonover.)

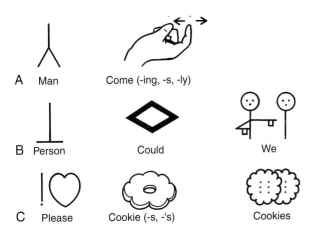

A   Man   Come (-ing, -s, -ly)

B   Person   Could   We

C   Please   Cookie (-s, -'s)   Cookies

FIGURE 20-14   Examples of symbol systems. **A,** Blissymbols. **B,** Rebus. **C,** Picsyms.

thousands of graphics (some that are electronically animated) and text options. The display changes (using the same message-formation process that produces natural speech) based on the choices of the user. They are often accessed via a touch screen; however, alternatives are available. Dynamic displays, such as the one in Figure 20-13, are helpful for children who may have difficulties with memory, but they do require a high level of visual attention, constant decision making, and the need for mastery of object permanence. Visual scene displays offer "hot spots" that are contextually embedded within graphics that provide more meaningful and individualized interactive displays (Figure 20-15). Drager[38] made a comparison of visual scene displays and more traditional grid layouts used by typically developing 2½-year-old children during communicative tasks during a birthday party. Findings indicated that performance was better using the visual scene display.

Once a device has been obtained, programming of the device and training of the child and all communication partners are essential for success. Collaborative efforts should be taken to identify vocabulary that includes conversational

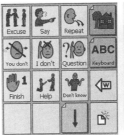
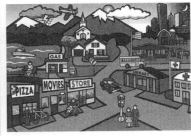

FIGURE 20-15   Visual scene display versus grid.   (From Blackstone, S. [2004]. Visual scene displays. *Augmentative Communications News, 16,* 1-5.)

messages (greetings, information sharing, and requests), core vocabulary (for literate or preliterate children to encourage language and cognitive development), and fringe vocabulary (unique to the individual child's activities, preferences, family, environments, favorite expressions, etc.).[28] Vocabulary needs will vary by context, communication mode, and individual characteristics.[13] Beukelman and Mirenda have developed core vocabulary and high-frequency word lists for a variety of settings and age groups, which can be found at http://aac.unl.edu/vbstudy. The child should be taught specific functions of communication such as requesting; rejecting/protesting; gaining attention; engaging in greetings, farewells, and other social niceties; commenting; achieving social closeness; asking for information; and confirming/denying.[37] Communication competence[67] should be the targeted outcome for any child using an AAC system (Box 20-9).

As with all other AT, communication systems are constantly being upgraded and changed. Continuing education courses and additional training can familiarize therapists with the terminology, communication strategies, and available hardware and software. AAC can help equalize opportunities for children to interact with peers, siblings and family members, and adults within relevant environments (e.g., school staff).

BOX 20-9   Communication Competence

Linguistic Competence: adequate mastery of the native language (i.e., vocabulary and grammar) plus mastery of the code (e.g., signs or symbols) required to operate the AAC system.

Operational Competence: mastery of technical skills required to operate the system, i.e., the motor and cognitive skills required to signal a message or to operate specific device features (e.g., pointing, signing, visual scanning, operating switches, controlling cursors, editing).

Social Competence: knowledge and skill in the social rules of communication, e.g., making appropriate eye contact, sharing the balance of talking and listening, and using communication for a range of different purposes (e.g., social chatting, requesting items, responding to others, contradicting people).

Strategic Competence: flexibility to adapt communicative style to suit the receiver (e.g., signing more slowly to strangers, turning up the volume on the communication aid).

From Light, J. (1989). Toward a definition of communicative competence for individuals using augmentative and alternative communication systems. *Augmentative and Alternative Communication, 5,* 137-144.

Computers

Use of personal computers by individuals of all ages is becoming more prevalent in school, home, and work settings. The computer is a flexible, motivating, and powerful instructional tool that can facilitate individualized teaching and learning. Computers with or without specialized software provide children with multiple means of communicating, playing, exploring, self-expression, interacting with the environment, learning cause and effect, and completing school and work-related tasks with greater degrees of independence. Most children with and without disabilities have had some exposure to a computer system by the time they enter school. At home, the computer might be used for recreation, entertainment, communication, work, and study. Social connections with others can be formed through e-mail, instant messaging, and social networking sites. For example, some adolescents with disabilities describe social networks and friendships that they have been able to develop using the computer, Internet access, and appropriate software programs.[104]

Swinth and colleagues found that children as young as 6 months of age could access a switch to play a simple cause-effect game on the computer.[106] A computer can motivate children to learn and develop a large repertoire of skills. It provides simulations of experiences that children with motor disabilities cannot otherwise experience. The computer is also infinitely patient with drill and practice and can provide the repetition needed for some children to learn. An almost endless variety of software programs, input devices, and output devices are available to customize computers to meet the individual needs of each child.[4] Young children can be introduced to a progression of systems that follows their developmental and functional needs. For a child who is born with a disability, success using simple systems precedes the use of more complex systems. Table 20-6 outlines benefits of computer use for children.

At school, children typically use word processing programs, the Internet, e-mail, and virtual classrooms in some aspect of their education. Software programs for children and adults cover most academic subjects as well as recreational and competitive activities. For example, math software and Internet sites include features such as virtual manipulatives or drills; creative writing software has recording features, sound, graphics, and animations; keyboarding software teaches typing as

TABLE 20-6 Benefits of Computers for Young Children

Benefit	Examples
Put child in control	Use child-directed software
	Allow child to move at his or her own pace
	Are accessible to children with limited motor control
	Use two-switch step scanning for simple cognitive interface
Engage the child cognitively	Use two-switch software whereby each switch has a distinct function
	Provide trial-and-error learning
	Provide logical consequences to the child's efforts
	Use of patterns and use of surprise
	Provide experiences with familiar objects and tasks
	Allow for active vs. passive learning
Provide opportunities for choice making	Sustain attention—increase opportunity for control and cognitive engagement
	Further expand awareness of consequences
	Provide error-free learning environment
Provide language immersion	Provide voice-output feedback describing child's actions
	Use simple but functional language
	Provide opportunities for sound play
	Offer predictable repeated lines with periodic surprise lines to go along with the action
	Relate three-dimensional experiences with objects and toys to two-dimensional screen
Provide opportunities for joint attention and shared interaction	Give opportunity for adult-child interaction
	Encourage pointing, showing, and shared enjoyment
	Provide opportunity for the child to take the lead and the adult to follow along and support
	Provide opportunities for child-child interaction
Facilitate communicative interaction	Allow the child to express ideas
	Provide voice-output and visual information that may be used to communicate to someone else
Provide multisensory feedback with consistency and repetition of language and cognitive concepts	Allow virtual manipulation of objects to develop cognitive skills
	Provide immediate feedback to child
	Allow child to control repetition as desired
	Reinforce emerging literacy skills
	Reinforce emerging mathematical skills or sequence, numbers and patterns within a play context—not adult directed
Ensure cognitive simplicity	Present concepts in small steps
	Help child maintain attention by providing immediate success
	Help child stay out of a random "guessing mode" or "trying to please mode," which could lead to inaccurate or confusing consequences

Burkhart, L. J. *Effective use of computers with young children.* Available at http://www.lburkhart.com/handcomp.html

software and website designers continue to add features that make their products and sites accessible to a growing range of people and abilities.

For all children, the judicious use of computers and software can help develop literacy or strengthen skills through the use of games, screen readers, and online books. "Virtual field trips" allow students to visit and explore environments that might otherwise be inaccessible, and computer simulations can provide preparation for social situations, academic tasks, prevocational training, and driver education. For children who are unable to recognize print in traditional formats, modifications to access the same text as that for their peers can decrease their dependence on the support of others in the environment to read or write for them. Often the computer is a magnet for children who have difficulty engaging in traditional classroom activities. When, as a result of motor, emotional, or attentional difficulties, children are challenged to produce art products or written work, the computer can assist in generating digital artwork or text that is neat and uniform in appearance. Producing more accurate, legible, or attractive work can increase self-esteem and self-expression and decrease frustration. The multimedia features of the computer can support learning rules, turn taking, and social skills.[94] As with any tool, the user must be aware of its features and trained in its applications and maintenance to receive full benefits. Competencies that school-based occupational therapists should possess include the ability to operate major computing systems used in public schools and troubleshoot system problems, establish networks using telecommunications systems, operate general application programs, apply teacher utility tools, and provide computer-based instruction.[48]

To successfully access a computer system, the user must be able to provide input into the system, receive output (or information) from the computer, and process that information to use it in a functional, meaningful manner. Various types of computers (e.g., Macintosh or personal computer [PC]) are available in the home, school, clinical, and work settings. Before recommending the purchase of software programs or adapted access devices, the memory and technology of the system must be evaluated to determine its compatibility with the program. Now, many software programs are both PC and Mac compatible. For example, alternative keyboards can be used on either machine without significant reconfiguration. However, because certain hardware and access devices remain specific to either the PC or the Mac, therapists should attend to these specifications.

Input

In considering different input systems, the "least change" principle should be applied. This means that a standard keyboard and standard workstation with some modifications are preferred over an expanded keyboard or other type of input device if the child can use them (Figure 20-16), exemplifying the concept of least restrictive environment (Table 20-7).

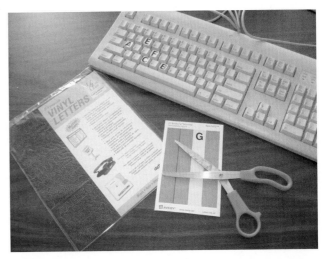

FIGURE 20-16 Example of low-tech keyboard modifications including color-coding and enlarging letters on keys. (Photo courtesy Judith Schoonover.)

TABLE 20-7 Problem Solving for Computer Access (Starting with a Standard Computer Workstation)

Problem	Potential Solutions
Difficulty pressing one or more keys	Change height of table or chair
	Change position of keyboard
	Change sensitivity of key or active delayed acceptance
	Use a keyguard
	Use an expanded keyboard with larger keys
	Use a stylus, mouthstick, or headstick
	Change size of letters on keyboard
Tendency to produce multiple characters rather than one	Change height of table or chair
	Change position of keyboard
	Change sensitivity of key or active delayed acceptance
	Deactivate auto-repeat
Difficulty holding down more than one key simultaneously	Use Sticky Keys feature or utility
	Use a mechanical key latch
Ability to use only one hand	Teach student to use one-handed typing techniques for standard keyboard
	Use a chord keyboard
	Reconfigure the keyboard to use one-handed pattern
	Use onscreen keyboard and mouse for typing

Continued

TABLE 20-7 Problem Solving for Computer Access (Starting with a Standard Computer Workstation)—Cont'd

Problem	Potential Solutions
Difficulty with the standard mouse	Use a trackball Use a trackpad Create a mouse track template Use MouseKeys feature of operating system
Slow or inefficient input	Increase keyboarding practice so that motor patterns are more automatic Set up templates for standard formats Use macros and abbreviation expansion for repeated words and phrases Use word prediction software programs
Drooling	Use a keyboard cover (Safe Skin) Use alternative keyboards that are not moisture sensitive
Difficulty seeing the screen or highlights	Ensure that the monitor is not facing a window or that the blinds are drawn Use an antiglare filter Reduce glare by turning down overhead lights Change size of font Change font (serif fonts are better for reading text; sans serif fonts are better for letter recognition) Change attributes of font (bold) Change color of background or text for greater contrast Set screen to monochrome Use a large screen or lower screen resolution Use a screen magnifier (hardware or software)
Difficulty reading text	Ensure that the monitor is not facing a window or that the blinds are drawn Use an antiglare filter Reduce glare by turning down overhead lights Change size of font Change font (serif fonts are better for reading text; sans serif fonts are better for letter recognition) Change attributes of font (bold) Change color of background or text for greater contrast Set screen to monochrome Use a large screen or lower screen resolution Use a screen magnifier (hardware or software) Use a voice output tool (screen reader)
Tendency to be distracted by sound	Turn off sound features of application Turn down volume from system control panel Use hearing protectors or noise-canceling ear protectors
Difficulty hearing feedback	Turn up volume (can use headphones) Use amplified speakers
Difficulty finding correct key on the keyboard	Use stickers or enlarged key letters to highlight correct keys Increase size or contrast of keyboard caps Use color coding for "landmark" keys Use Kids Keys Keyboard (for younger students) Mask non-applicable keys
Difficulty shifting between information on the screen, the keyboard, and the desktop	Use document clip to suspend printed page next to monitor Change position of keyboard Change position of monitor Use a touch screen and on-screen keyboard
Difficulty remembering keyboard functions	Develop a "cheat sheet" of keyboard shortcuts to keep close by Develop keyboard mnemonics to aid memory of keyboard functions
Decreased motivation	Recheck student goals to ensure student involvement in goal-making process Try a different software program to address goal Change the purpose for which the computer is being used Change the access method Decrease the amount of time on the computer Scale the activity to the student skills (up or down)

Swinth, Y. L., & Anson, D. (1998). Alternatives to handwriting: Keyboarding and text-generation techniques for schools. In J. Case-Smith (Ed.), *AOTA self-paced clinical course: Occupational therapy: Making a difference in school system practice*. Rockville, MD: AOTA.

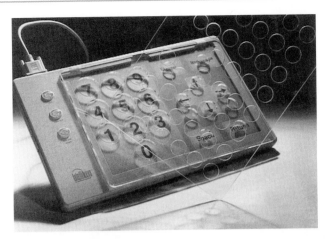

FIGURE 20-17 An example of a keyguard for an alternative keyboard. Keyguards also are available for standard keyboards. (Photo courtesy IntelliTools, Petaluma, CA.)

For some children, using an ergonomic keyboard rather than a standard keyboard will increase their proficiency on the computer. For a child with slight tremors, disabling the auto-repeat function, or using a keyguard (plastic covers for the keyboard with a single hole) may enable independent use of the standard system (Figure 20-17). Software programs are available to redefine the keyboard versus using the standard QWERTY keyboard that comes with most computers. One commonly used keyboard offers as one of its keyboard layouts a color-coded alphabetic layout for younger children or children with cognitive delays who cannot find letters using the QWERTY layout. Switches, adapted keyboards, and voice recognition systems offer alternative means for computer access to children with limited movement.

Alternate input systems come with their own software programs or a combination of unique hardware and software adaptations. Some alternate input systems allow for direct selection (the user selects letters, words, or phrases by touching or pointing to the desired key), and others allow indirect selection (an intermediate step is used when sending a command to the computer). Direct selection offers more choices to the child, requires less cognitive skill than indirect selection, and should be the first type of system considered. An example of direct selection is an expanded keyboard; indirect selection includes using letter scanning or Morse code and a switch. Various scanning methods are available including row-column scanning, step scanning, and automatic scanning. The method that the therapist chooses depends on the skills of the child using the system. In row-column scanning, the computer will scan down rows. Once the user selects the row in which the letter, number, or word resides, then the computer scans across the columns. In automatic scanning, the computer scans through all the choices at a predetermined rate.

Switches

Switches allow access to the computer with a single movement. Many of the switches that can be used to access low-tech solutions (see Figures 20-6 and 20-7) can also be used to access the computer. Many of the more complex switch systems use indirect selection. In considering a switch-driven system, consideration should be given to the motoric and cognitive requirements of the system.[26] For example, a child who is able to accurately and reliably hit a switch at 9 months of age does not have the cognitive skills to understand the concept of scanning. In addition, research suggests that the placement of the switch (e.g., a head switch versus a switch that is struck with the hand) may have a cognitive component that affects a child's accuracy.[46] A single (or dual) switch can be used to run systems such as Morse code and scanning. Morse code is faster than scanning, but requires the user to learn a new language.

Alternate Keyboards

Alternate keyboards include programmable membrane keyboards, miniature keyboards, chord keyboards, and onscreen keyboards. Each type of alternate keyboard varies in size, layout, and complexity. Membrane keyboards assist the child with decreased fine-motor control or cognitive delays to successfully make choices on the computer and allow for customization of overlays, and it provides voice output. Programmable keyboards (Figure 20-18) allow use of customized overlays and can be set up with "hotkeys" to allow the child to enter numbers, words, and phrases by hitting one key. Changing the overlay, software program, and customization setup is relatively simple, making it easy to create new activities that align with the classroom curriculum or the current interests of the child. Miniature keyboards are smaller than the standard keyboard. Miniature keyboards are typically lightweight and designed to be used by children with limited range of motion or poor endurance. Chord keyboards, like miniature keyboards, are designed to minimize finger travel. Use of these keyboards, similar to playing the piano, requires multiple simultaneous keystrokes to type letters and phrases. Onscreen keyboards (virtual keyboards) are software programs that provide the image of a standard or modified keyboard on the computer screen. The user can access these "keys" via different input systems such as a mouse, touch screen, trackball, joystick, or eye-gaze system.

Mouse Emulators

Mouse emulators are hardware or software systems with output that the computer reads like a standard mouse. Various devices are available that simulate mouse movement and/or clicking by using head and body movement to perform those operations. The continuum of mouse emulators included using the arrow keys on a standard keyboard, touch pads, trackballs, and head pointers. Interactive whiteboards and touch windows can also be considered mouse emulators. Using these systems, the child activates the computer by touching the interactive whiteboard, or the touch window that fits like a window over a computer monitor screen.

Voice Recognition

Voice (or speech) recognition systems, in which the computer recognizes and translates voice sounds into text or commands, can be an option for individuals with severe motoric limitations. The user must have fair-to-good articulation to successfully operate a voice recognition system, and typically understand basic editing and grammar commands. The child speaks into a microphone to enter text, control the mouse, and execute computer commands. Voice recognition systems generally are not used with children under 12 years of age because of the complexity of the system. These systems can be isolating to use as they often pick up ambient noise in the background and may require the user to work outside of the classroom.

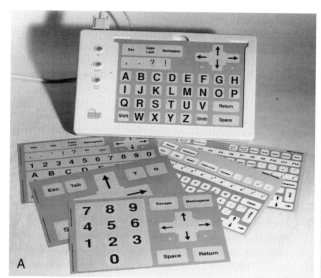

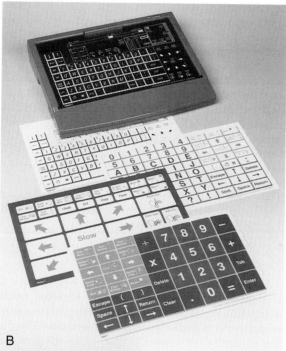

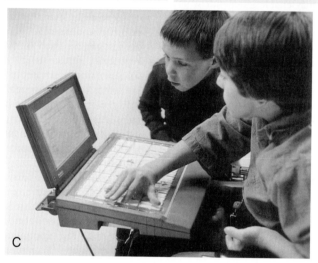

FIGURE 20-18 Examples of alternate keyboards. **A,** IntelliKeys with alphabet overlay. **B,** KeyLargo and overlay examples. **C,** KeyLargo used with a powerbook. (A, Photo courtesy Don Johnston, Inc., Wauconda, IL; B and C, Courtesy IntelliTools, Petaluma, CA. Note: KeyLargo is now available from Infogrip http://www.infogrip.com.)

Other Input Systems

Other types of input systems used with children include eye-gaze systems, Braille, TouchFree Switch, and a Tongue Touch Keypad. Eye-gaze systems require the child to visually focus on a desired position on the computer monitor. An optic light on the computer "reads" where the child gazes and makes the appropriate selection. To word process, eye-gaze systems use onscreen keyboards and other systems. Several programs allow a child who is blind or who has a significant visual impairment to input into the computer using Braille. The Touch Free Switch operates via a camera on top of the computer and is activated by a predetermined movement by the child. The Tongue Touch Keypad has nine tongue-activated keys that

the child activates. Once the user activates the keys, a signal is sent to an interface box connected to the computer.

Output Systems and Information Processing

Output is the product or outcome that is produced when using a computer. Just like input, computer output can also accommodate the needs of individuals with disabilities. Information (output) from the computer is displayed visually on the monitor or printed from the printer. For a child with a visual impairment, perceptual impairment, or cognitive impairment, adaptations to the monitor may need to be considered. Some printers provide Braille output, and several software programs provide voice output. Some of these programs read text, whereas others provide output regarding all the functions of the computer. Voice output systems can help support learning and computer use and exploration for students with learning disabilities, cognitive delays, autism, and visual impairments.

The computer's output and the child's successful processing of information are often closely related. If children with disabilities cannot successfully process and use the information received from the computer in a meaningful and functional manner, they will not use the system over time. With the increased screen resolution and the complexity of graphics now available in computers, some children with visual-perceptual difficulties find the visual information they receive distracting or overwhelming. For example, a child who has poor figure-ground skills may have difficulty with graphics that are cluttered and complex.

Software

Careful decisions must be made to find programs that match children's interests and skills. With the burgeoning number of software programs available, from simple to highly complex, many children with disabilities can use common software programs that are available to everyone. Often software programs require that the user make specific, discrete responses to visual, auditory, or tactile stimuli. The child must be able to attend briefly and have the interest and motivation to activate a toy or a computer purposefully. Computer activities and programs, including public domain software, can be used to teach basic skills, such as object permanence, sustained attention, and cause-effect relationships. Other computer programs teach skills in discrimination, matching, and directionality. The occupational therapist can determine whether and how the software customizes the video and audio display to meet students' individualized needs.

With all the different input and output methods and software programs available, computers offer many ways to help children develop functional independence in life roles. Children can have opportunities to use computers throughout their school years and into their work settings; they can also use computers as environmental control devices and for play and leisure exploration.

Electronic Aids for Daily Living

Originally, EADLs were known as environmental control units. These are systems that allow a child to control appliances in the environment. EADLs allow the child to interact with and manipulate one or more electronic appliances, such as a television, radio, CD player, lights, telephone, or fan. This can be accomplished using voice activation, switch access, a computer interface, or adaptations such as X-10 units (transmitters and receivers) that use a communications "language," allowing compatible products to interact with each other using the existing electrical wiring. The EADL should meet the child's primary needs, as well as any long-range goals. The system should also be fairly easy to assemble, learn to use, and maintain. As mentioned previously, EADLs can be integrated into a child's computer system. They also can be stand-alone systems. Some of these systems have discrete control interface (an electronic device is either turned on or off, such as lights, fans, or a television set), and others are capable of continuous control interface (devices that operate in successively greater or smaller degrees of control). Lowering and raising the volume on a television and dimming a light are examples of continuous control. A common EADL setup used with children is shown in Figure 20-19. Many EADL options are available for a variety of settings.

CHANGING THE LANDSCAPE IN EDUCATION: PLANNING FOR EVERY STUDENT IN THE 21st CENTURY

Universal Design for Learning

One aspect of universal access that is gaining increased attention in the schools is universal design for learning.[86] School administrators have placed increased emphasis on the development and implementation of a universally designed curriculum that allows all children equal opportunity to learn and demonstrate what they have learned. AT and accessible software are important elements of a universally designed curriculum.[51] Universal design for learning (UDL) involves developing and improving learning environments where all children are included. A UDL framework provides multiple means of (1) representation, to give learners various ways of acquiring information and knowledge; (2) expression, to provide learners alternatives for demonstrating what they know; and (3) engagement, to tap into learners' interests, offer appropriate challenges, and increase motivation.[53]

Instructional Technology

Sometimes students with disabilities *require* technology that is helpful or sometimes used by students without disabilities. For example, most classrooms have tools like calculators and word processors. Students with disabilities might *need* to use calculators or word processors, or use them with modifications to participate in math or writing activities. This *need* redefines common classroom tools as AT that may be a required service in the IEP; therefore, it is important to consider how important the tool is to the student's learning and participation.

Schools use many kinds of instructional technology, providing software in most academic areas and for students of all ages. Some examples include literacy software for children to develop letter-to-sound correspondence, math software for drill and practice of math facts, keyboarding software, and content-area software to reinforce concepts of science and social studies. Student assignments may include copying or producing written work using a word processor, research using the Internet, and email. A computer, computer-based device, or software program may be AT if it provides specific input or output that a user needs to access needed information. Features in software applications including adjustable user settings and alternate keyboard access can help reduce barriers and positively influence participation. Occupational therapy practitioners who are aware of the accessibility needs of their clients can advocate for the purchase of accessible instructional software. The National Center on Accessible Information Technology in Education promotes the use of electronic and information technology for individuals with disabilities in educational institutions at all academic levels, and features a searchable database of questions and answers regarding accessible educational and instructional technology on its website (http://www.washington.edu/accessit/). Features

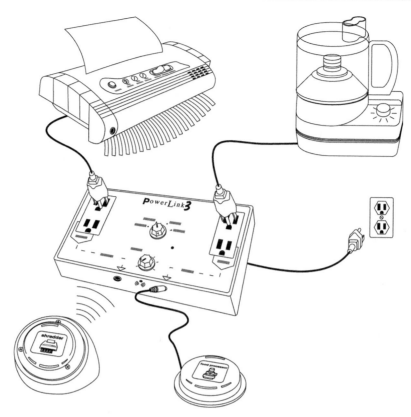

FIGURE 20-19   Schematic of an EADL setup with the Powerlink.   (Drawing courtesy Ablenet.)

to consider in evaluating accessibility of instructional software are outlined in Box 20-10.

Assistive Technology for Literacy Skills

The primary goals of IDEA 2004 and the No Child Left Behind Act (NCLB) of 2001 are improving student achievement and providing students with disabilities access to the general education curriculum; however, providing *access* does not guarantee increased participation, especially for children who have reading and writing difficulties.[23] Literacy skills include the complicated processes of reading, writing, and spelling as forms of communication; reading is the communication process of constructing meaning from written text, and writing is the communication process of composing meaningful text.

BOX 20-10   Key Features to Consider In Evaluating Accessibility of Instructional Software

- Does the documentation describe accessibility features such as keyboard access to functions and features, options to change display settings such as size and font, options to turn off animation or blinking, and information about how to turn on captioning for video content of the software program?
- Is documentation available in electronic text so that it can be converted easily to Braille or audio formats, and can be read easily by people who use a screen reader or screen magnification program?
- Are all commands and functions available from the keyboard? Keyboard commands or shortcuts provide a simplified method for navigating through menus and dialogues and making selections. These features are important for individuals who may not see the cursor on screen or who have difficulty with mouse control.
- If information is conveyed in color, is it also conveyed using text?

- Can users select features such as size, color, font, and contrast to aid those with visual or perceptual difficulties?
- If the software uses animation such as flashing or rotating or moving displays, is all information available when animation is turned off to support users who might become distracted or visually overwhelmed?
- Is information that is conveyed with sound such as music, narration, or tones also conveyed in another way?
- If a software program uses video to convey important information, is that information available in other formats such as a transcript or audio version? If the software program requires timed responses, can the response times be adjusted or disabled to meet user needs?
- Does the software program allow and support use of AT such as screen reading software, screen magnification software, voice recognition software, word prediction software, alternative keyboards or computer mice, and software that helps people who have difficulties reading and writing?

From National Center on Accessible Information Technology in Education. (2004). Accessible instructional software in education. *Accessible Information Technology Series #6.*

Literacy is more than learning to read, write and spell proficiently. It is learning to enjoy words and stories when someone else is reading to the child. It is learning to love books and all the worlds that can be opened by books. It is a way of achieving social closeness through sharing literacy experiences with friends or classmates. It is finding out about the way things are in places we have never visited or in places that have never existed. If we understand that literacy is all of these things and more we can also understand that everyone can achieve some degree of literacy if given opportunities and exposure (p. 3).[70]

Literacy begins with the recognition that words correspond to speech and that words are made up of sound. Repeated exposure to literacy experiences such as looking at books, exposure to signage, and writing demonstrates the importance of words. We live in a world that requires literacy. Traditional print such as books and newspapers, as well as information and communication technology including word processors, presentation software, the Internet, and e-mail, is used to relay information. In a text-based society, nonreaders are at risk for difficulties with managing information, and reduction in academic skill acquisition, societal integration, and quality of life. Limited literacy skills also affect the likelihood of successful competitive or supported employment.[60]

Children who struggle with learning to read and write need to be supported by individuals who can accurately assess their strengths and weaknesses, select, and apply AT tools and strategies effectively. AT can help children with disabilities in language acquisition. They can learn that words are something to pay attention to. They can learn about the world around them by simply listening to stories. Most important, they can increase their opportunities for social closeness. Koenig and Holbrook define functional literacy as "the application of literacy skills and the use of a variety of literacy tools to accomplish daily tasks in the home school, community, and work setting" (p. 265).[59] A multitude of software, word processors, text readers, and electronic books are available on the Internet to support children's literacy. An essential element related to the effectiveness of technology in supporting literacy is its interactive quality, which allows children to get involved with the content as they manipulate the media.[42] Literacy software programs interact with children, similar to a parent's reading to children and involving them in the book by turning the pages, looking at pictures, and asking questions. Technology allows children to control the process and "hook" their interest. Koenig reiterates the importance of starting early with children "regardless of the severity" of their disability.[58] All individuals can benefit from these experiences, although the benefits realized by each child will be different.

The National Center for Technology Innovation (NCTI) website (http://www.techmatrix.org/) serves as a database of published research and commercial products that are reviewed for universal design features that support student literacy. This site reviews products for features such as text-to-speech capabilities, in-line dictionary support, customizable views, and progress monitoring options, and allows the searcher to create a customized matrix by subject and/or type of learning support.

Reading Skills

Children most at risk for reading difficulties are those with less verbal skill, phonologic awareness, letter knowledge, and familiarity with the basic purposes of and mechanisms for reading.[20] Research on early reading development emphasizes the pairing of written words and sounds for helping children's decoding skills. For children with physical, visual, communication, or cognitive delays, traditional books may restrict their ability to interact with and access books. One of the methods that can be used to provide successful literacy experiences is through adapting books. Adapted books provide print access that follows the Universal Design for Learning (UDL) framework. Adaptations can include making books easier to use (turning pages or holding) and text easier to read (simplified, changed) and remember. The original story or subject is maintained, but may contain modified language, clear visual representations, and manageable page layouts to increase the potential for participation. Adapted books can be used by themselves, or with AT ranging from low-tech homemade devices to switches, voice output communication aides, Braille and large print materials, sign language, or adapted props.

Copyright laws allow the creation and use of books in an alternate format solely for the purpose of making the book accessible to persons with disabilities; however, it is important to review copyright laws and how they pertain to each situation in which an adapted book is being contemplated. A copy of the original book is required when using an adapted book. Books can be adapted to provide physical access to text by creating space between pages with page "fluffers" (foam, weather stripping, sponges, giant paper clips, clothespins), using book holders for stabilization (recipe book holders, card holders, acrylic display frames, easels), or by reproducing them so that they can be listened to or viewed with technology (Figure 20-20). Accommodations for print difficulties include change in font size and color, magnification, contrast, audio output, tactile display, icon-enhanced text, scaffolded information, and multimedia. Electronic books combine reading, writing, listening, and speaking and provide a multisensory approach with related pictures, sound, and video, and appeal to different learning styles. Through the appropriate provision and support, technology can allow children to control their own learning.

The ability to read is essential for many daily life activities and participation in varied environments at home, school,

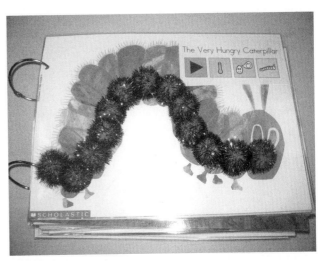

FIGURE 20-20 Example of an adapted book with tactile and rebus symbol support. (Photo courtesy Judith Schoonover.)

work, and in the community. Reading contributes to play and leisure, academics and world knowledge, communication and social awareness, following directions and schedules, shopping and meal preparation, and work-related tasks. When the ability to read print text is affected by visual, visual motor, visual processing, decoding, tracking, attentional, or cognitive difficulties, AT can provide alternatives to traditional print text. For example, Edyburn proposed a process of scaffolding digital text to meet the varied reading and cognitive needs of children by reducing the amount of text, as well as adding additional visual cues in the form of pictures or symbols. He used the term *cognitive rescaling* to describe "a process of altering the cognitive difficulty of information" (p. 10).[40] Other accommodations for print disabilities include the use of commercially available talking photo albums, specific reading software, e-text, audio recordings, screen readers, and multimedia.

Assistive Technology for Writing

The act of writing not only requires motor and sensory skills but also includes cognitive processes in the form of recognizable language and vocabulary, generation of ideas, organization of ideas, expression of ideas, and use of correct grammar, punctuation, and spelling. With handwriting as the most common reason for referrals to occupational therapy in school-based practice, practitioners are well aware that writing skills can be enhanced with no-tech or low-tech aids and devices. Simple adaptations, like smooth-writing pens that are comfortable to hold or adapted paper, can make the difference between needing physical assistance and working independently. Universally designed tools, such as a pen, become AT when needed to achieve targeted goals. Service delivery in the natural context, using tools that are intuitive, may mean borrowing or adapting tools that already exist in the classroom.

For individuals who may have motor difficulties that affect the ability to write for function, alternatives for written production should be explored such as the use of a keyboard and mouse (or alternative mouse) or a portable word processor or notebook computer. Beyond the physical components, writing can be conceptualized as a cognitive process that includes the following steps: prewriting/brainstorming ideas, drafting/composing and organizing initial ideas, editing, and, finally, publishing the final product.[28]

Standard word processing and multimedia software, often available in the classroom, features sizable and colored fonts, line spacing options, spell and grammar checking, opportunities for outlining and highlighting, use of tables to organize information, use of macros and abbreviation expansion, general accessibility features, and incorporation of multiple media to represent ideas. More specifically, concept-mapping software allows the user to conceptualize information graphically using a combination of pictures and/or text. It is helpful for planning, organizing, and drafting and frequently offers templates for getting started (Figure 20-21).

Other software products allow the child to complete a written assignment with visual and/or auditory feedback. Word prediction and word completion can reduce the number of keystrokes necessary and as a result may increase overall speed.[28] After a child types in the first few letters of a word, the program will attempt to predict whole words and presents a list of choices for the child to scan and select (Figure 20-22).

Many word prediction programs include customizable dictionaries that suggest alternative word selections, which can facilitate improvement in the quality of a child's written work. These features are beneficial to support spelling for children who have good word recognition skills. Spell-checking programs have proved to be helpful editing tools, specifically when integrated into a word processing program; however, grammar checkers have not.[66] Other options may include use of a traditional or electronic dictionary or thesaurus for children who have word retrieval deficits.

In combination with visual supports, some children benefit from the use of auditory feedback. Text-to-speech software converts printed digital text to synthetic speech. This feature is available in a number of software applications, free Internet downloads, and on recent versions of Windows and Macintosh operating systems. Synthesized text-to-speech screen readers support drafting and editing, which can help a child more readily detect errors because the text is read out loud. They also reduce the visual load for individuals with visual processing deficits, and are a valuable alternative for auditory learners. Users with print disabilities can also access contents of web pages, e-mail, e-books, or printed documents scanned with optical character recognition (OCR) software and converted to digital text. Pairing print with digital speech output is available in a number of applications. The age and gender of the "voice," reading rate, dynamic highlighting, and color of font and background can be manipulated to address the individual needs or preferences of the user.

Conversely, some children require speech-to-text (or voice recognition) options that allow them to dictate thoughts and commands to a program that produces written text for them. Speech input technology responds to the human voice by producing text or executing verbally dictated commands to navigate through computer applications.[28] Speech-to-text software was initially envisioned as a business tool, but has been found to be an effective strategy to support children's learning. Speech recognition presents words through speech, so to produce accurate dictation, the user must have appropriate oral mechanisms.[50] The process results in a multisensory written language experience. Voice quality, pitch, volume, and articulation have a direct impact on the quality of the product generated, as well as set-up and positioning of the user. In addition to specific dictation software products, recent versions of Windows and Macintosh operating systems include speech recognition features. A substantial training component is required to use this type of technology, and the environmental context in which it is used must be examined closely. Speech input can be accomplished by dictating to another individual or a tape recorder as a less costly alternative. This allows individuals with intelligible speech to express themselves, even when writing is problematic for attentional, motoric, or cognitive reasons.

Assistive Technology for Math

Mathematics is a part of typical school curriculum and is considered a functional life skill. Mathematical concepts include sorting, numbers, differences in attributes (color, shape, size), patterns, counting, sequence, graphing, and numeration. Ideally, a combination of individualized instructional strategies and numerous opportunities to use and manipulate concrete objects to count, sort, compare, and combine is used to

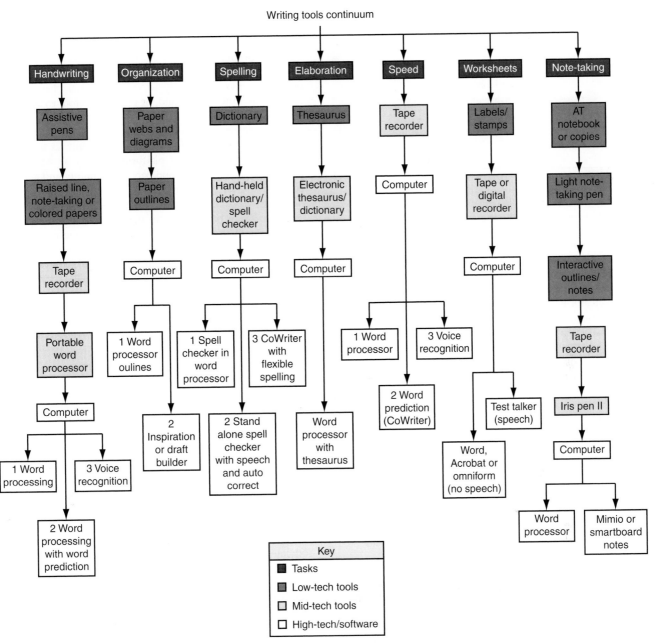

FIGURE 20-21 Writing tools continuum created with graphic organizer software by Judi Sweeney, Onion Mountain Technology (http://www.onionmountaintech.com). (Figure courtesy Judith Schoonover.)

reinforce concepts of same/different and greater than/less than/equal to. Children with sensory, cognitive, or physical disabilities may need additional support (e.g., grippers, non-skid materials) or alternatives to hands-on manipulation such as "virtual manipulation" (http://nlvm.usu.edu/en/NAV/vlibrary.html) to allow active participation in math exploration.[6]

Children with visual processing or visual motor deficits affecting their ability to see likenesses and differences in shape and form, difficulties with copying and writing, physical limitations, or cognitive challenges can benefit from a wide array of AT supports when instructional strategies, curriculum modifications, use of manipulatives, flashcards, and repetition are not enough. Math difficulties may affect future financial management skills, with resultant decrease in independence.

To determine whether a child needs AT in the area of mathematics, the IEP team should consider whether the child is able to effectively participate in math instruction and complete math requirements of the curriculum or work setting without the use of aids/devices. If not, then a determination must be made regarding which tools would most effectively reduce barriers to accessing the curriculum.

Common classroom math tools such as rulers, compasses, protractors, and calculators can be modified to make them easier to handle or keep in place. Low-tech math solutions may include use of a customized number line; TouchMath® (a multisensory teaching approach that links manipulation with memorization of math facts), enlarged or masked math worksheets; graph or grid paper for aligning problems;

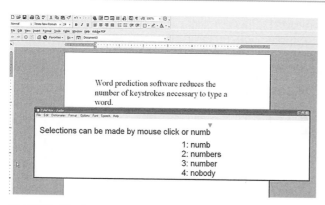

FIGURE 20-22 Example of word prediction software. (Image courtesy Judith Schoonover.)

alternatives for responding such as math stamps for drawing graphs, clocks, and number lines; and use of simple calculators (Figure 20-23). Providing alternative visual representation of math problems with graphics can increase the child's understanding.

A calculator is an electronic, mechanical, or onscreen device for the performance of mathematical computations. Calculators accept keypad input and display results on a readout screen, paper tape, or computer screen. Calculators speed up calculation time, provide feedback and an alternate way to "write" numbers, and may improve accuracy. Calculators come in many sizes with features such as big number buttons and large keypads, and range in operational capacity from simple to complex. Handheld calculators can help a learner who has problems writing numbers in the correct order; talking calculators vocalize data and resulting computations through speech synthesis; special-feature calculators allow the user to select options to speak and simultaneously display numbers, functions, entire equations, and results; onscreen computer calculator programs offer features such as speech synthesis, and some allow the user to adjust the display including size and color of the keys and numbers. Specialized calculators use realistic money bill and coin buttons

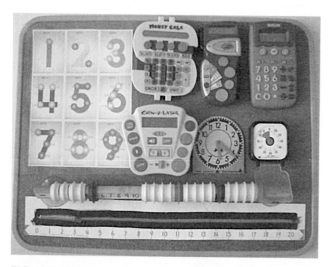

FIGURE 20-23 Examples of no-tech, low-tech math supports including TouchMath®, number lines and counters, coin calculators, a calculator with enlarged buttons, a Time Timer, and a standard Judy Clock math manipulative. (Photo courtesy Judith Schoonover.)

to count money or teach the value of different coins. Children can practice addition and subtraction with coin denominations. Individualizing the calculator for the user's unique needs may include providing tactile cues, enlarging or masking buttons, stabilizing or angling the calculator to improve access, using a colored filter over the display to change contrast between the numbers and the background, or providing a tool to access the buttons.

Access software or electronic math worksheets provide the opportunity to engage in the same curriculum as for typical peers by using a different platform to enter answers.[84] For example, instead of pencil and paper, a computer and a peripheral device such as a joystick, touch screen, interactive whiteboard, or alternate keyboard are used to record responses. These software programs help the user organize, align, and work through math problems using the computer. Numbers that appear onscreen can also be read aloud with a speech synthesizer. Microsoft Excel provides a computer equivalent to a paper ledger, with extensive graphing capabilities. Grids comprise columns and rows (intersections called *cells*). Each cell may contain labels, data, or formulas (mathematical equations that do all the work). Interactive math websites are available on the Internet. Textbook manufacturers may provide digital copies of textbooks on CD-ROM and most maintain websites with additional teaching resources and information.

Assistive Technology and Transition

Transition planning is essential to pave the way to successful change. Transitions are an inevitable part of life, yet the passages from preschool to elementary school, elementary school to high school, and high school into early adulthood can result in a loss of continuity. For an individual with disabilities, transitions can be especially challenging if the supports that provide access to participation are not available or prove unsuitable in the new environment. Critical information, as well as competencies, can be lost if positioning, teaching methodologies, and information regarding specialized technology are not passed along from one stage and setting to the next. IDEA mandates the provision of both AT services and transition services for students with disabilities. When a student with a disability requires AT to accomplish one or more functional skills, the use of that AT must be included in effective transition planning. Transition plans for AT users address the ways the student's use of devices and services are transferred from one setting to another. AT transition involves people from different classrooms, programs, buildings, or agencies working together to ensure continuity. Self-determination, advocacy, and implementation are critical issues for transition planning. Although the involvement of occupational therapy is important during the student's transition into adulthood, only 16% of all occupational therapists (compared with 29% who work in school settings) provide transition services for students ages 13 to 21.[2]

In addition to ensuring that AT devices and support services accompany students during transitions, service providers should assist clients and their families in becoming responsible users of AT. As Wehmeyer asserted, if students with disabilities are to actually achieve greater control over their lives, then it is important to provide (1) opportunities to exert control and make choices; (2) supports and accommodations needed; and

3) opportunities to learn new skills to increase participation.[111] The goal of self-management and independent use should begin the first time a child uses AT, steering him or her onto a path of optimal independence as an adult. Competencies should be developed in the area for which the AT device was chosen (e.g., communication, writing) as well as in how to use and care for the device, when to use it, and the social implications and responsibilities of using the device.[22] Development of self-determination skills to ensure that AT becomes an integrated part of typical routines will aid in successful transitions from home to school and from school to the community.[22]

For individuals beginning or ending their public school education, transition planning is included in legal mandates. Explicit documentation is needed during all transitions to ensure the individual transitioning has the support needed. Documentation can take the form of text, photos, and videos. For students who require AT devices or services to receive FAPE, transition plans should contain a statement of needed AT devices and services, and indicate agency responsibilities and linkages, if appropriate. The child should be allowed to take an AT device home or to other environments if it is necessary for FAPE. Various agencies may be involved, and the decision regarding who is responsible for providing the AT services needed for successful postgraduation activities should be determined in advance by the transition team.

Involvement of occupational therapy practitioners during the transition process assists the youth in the development of work, community, and independent living skills. Working as a member of the transition team, the occupational therapy practitioner may access and address student-related factors, including social, sensory, motor, and perceptual abilities; task-related factors, such as analysis of physical and perceptual requirements of the task; and environmental factors, such as analysis of noise level, clutter in the environment, and accessibility of work or living space. The QIAT Consortium has identified areas of best practice for AT transition[79] (Box 20-11), and although their guidelines focus mainly on the late high school transition to postsecondary and work placement, they serve as a reminder of the goals of the transition process and help identify key elements that need to be addressed in a transition plan.

BOX 20-11 **Components of Effective Transition Plans for Assistive Technology (AT) Users**

- Address the AT needs of the student, including roles and training needs of team members, subsequent steps in AT use, and follow-up after transition takes place.
- Empower the student using AT to participate in the transition planning at a level appropriate to age and ability.
- Recognize advocacy, as related to AT use, as critical to the plan's success.
- Identify the AT requirements in the receiving environment.
- Proceed according to an individualized timeline.
- Address specific equipment, training, and funding issues such as transfer or acquisition of AT, manuals, and support documents.

From QIAT Consortium (2007). *AT in transition.* Retrieved June 2, 2008, from http://natri.uky.edu/assoc_projects/qiat/documents/6%20QIAT%20QIs%20Transition.doc

---

Evidence-Based Practice and Assistive Technology

Although there is research available documenting the benefits and limitations of many AT devices,[39,41,89,102] AT outcome measurement and trials of AT services are limited. Because of the ever-changing nature of this field, the complexity of the devices, and the need for individualized decisions, it is difficult to build a large evidence base in this area of practice that is consistent with the available technology.[41] Some AT companies are adding research information regarding their products and AT outcomes to their websites. Whenever possible, AT research should guide and support decision making and provide further foundational knowledge about AT devices and services. When evidence is not available, occupational therapy practitioners working in this area must engage in data-based decision making with each client to document whether the use of the device results in increased participation across environments. Occupational therapists should be good consumers of AT research and should also measure and document AT outcomes as part of best practice services.

SUMMARY

Childhood is a time when children undergo continuous developmental changes and expand on skills that will eventually lead to functional abilities. Assistive technologies can diminish the impact of disabilities and allow children improved alternatives to participate.[72] Children who use AT at an early age have the advantage of developing with AT and using it to their benefit throughout their lives. Occupational therapy practitioners who work with children and youth should become familiar with the continuum of AT options (Table 20-8) and are ideally suited to evaluate and determine an appropriate match of AT tools to the child. The combination of occupational therapy and AT services together can promote success across all areas of occupation in which a child engages.[78]

To successfully blend the use of AT into occupational therapy practice, it is necessary to embrace a holistic approach of AT as both a device and a service. Considering the hopes and dreams of a child, his or her family, and the physical and social climate, occupational therapy practitioners can ensure that AT is matched appropriately to the child. Best-practice interventions should include AT and are dependent on the practitioner's ability to not only articulate what a child needs, but to also remain knowledgeable of current technologies, document the impact of interventions, collaborate with other team members, and influence decision making about participation across environmental contexts. The challenge is to increase collaborative practices, insist on opportunities for professional development, advocate for the provision of appropriate AT, and continue to define the role of occupational therapy in the provision of AT.

Various resources on the Internet can help occupational therapy practitioners stay current with all the changes in AT. Recent advances in AT allow many devices to grow and expand with the child during the developmental years and into adolescence and adulthood as they undergo transition into higher education and community work experiences. With the current pace of progress and research, future AT will offer greater ease of use, wider application, assistance in additional areas of function, and more availability as a result of lower costs (Case Study 20-1).

TABLE 20-8 Continuum of Assistive Technology Devices

Area of Need	No-Tech to Low-Tech	Mid-Tech	High-Tech
Learning	Schedules, checklists, color coding, highlighters, mnemonics	Tape recorders, graphic organization software	Simulation software
Math	Manipulatives, number lines, TouchMath	Coin-U-Lator, "talking calculator"	Personal digital assistants (PDAs)
Handwriting	Variety of writing tools, slant board, pencil grips	Portable word processor, tape recorder	Voice dictation software
Computer access	Adjustable-height table, letter stickers on keyboard	Macros, word prediction software, alternative keyboards	Voice recognition software, switch with scanning
Written composition	Word wall, editing checklists, picture dictionaries	Multimedia software, use of spell-checking and grammar-checking	Voice dictation software
Communication	"Wait time," picture schedules, eye gaze frame	Simple voice output device	Dynamic screen voice output device
Reading	Repetitive books, changing appearance of text	"Read back" feature of certain software programs	Electronic books
Hearing	Sign language, information in written form	Signaling devices	Personal amplification systems
Vision	Preferential seating, eyeglasses, modified materials	Word processing accessibility features, Braille materials	Screen reader, text reader, closed-circuit television
Recreation/leisure	Simple toy adaptations with Velcro, Universal cuff	Adapted sports equipment, computer games	Electronic aids to access computer, television, etc.
Mobility	Classes scheduled close together, walker	Manual wheelchair	Power wheelchair
Activities of daily living	Nonskid materials, built-up handles, organization	Adaptive devices for hygiene	Adaptive driving equipment
Environmental control	Light switch extension	Interface and switches for battery-operated toys	Environmental control units
Positioning	Blocks for feet, vestibular cushion	Alternative seating	Custom positioning inserts
Behavior support	Incentive chart, sensory breaks, Social Stories	Social skills videos	PDAs

From Schoonover, J., Levan, P., & Argabrite Grove, R. (2006). Occupational therapy and assistive technology in school-based practice: Supporting participation. *OT Practice, 11*(1), CE1-CE8.

CASE STUDY 20-1   AT Problem Solving

JEREMY

Jeremy is a 2-year-old with Down syndrome. His family wants to provide every opportunity for him to develop cognitive skills. They plan for him to attend regular education classrooms as he gets older. They were recently at a conference and heard about computers as tools for supporting learning and educational performance for some children with Down syndrome. They asked the early intervention team to recommend a computer system and software to use with Jeremy. What would you recommend?

LINNEA

Linnea is a third-grade student with spinal muscular atrophy. She is fully included in her neighborhood school with support from related services as needed. Recently, she has been complaining to her parents and therapists that her hand gets tired when writing and that her handwriting looks "sloppy." Her teacher also has noticed that she seems irritable and lacks concentration during class. Linnea, her family, and her therapists have discussed using computers for written communication in the past, but Linnea and her family have always been reluctant to explore this at length because she does not want to "look different." Linnea has had experience with computers since kindergarten. Her class goes to the computer lab three times a week, and she began learning basic keyboarding skills in second grade. Her classroom has two computers that students use for drill, practice, and special projects. How would you address Linnea's handwriting problems?

MARGY

Margy is 17 years old and has cognitive impairments and attention deficit–hyperactivity disorder (ADHD). During her last individualized transition plan (ITP), her family expressed the desire for Margy to get a job in the family carpet cleaning business. Margy enjoys greeting people, and others enjoy her bubbly and outgoing personality, so her dad and mom felt it would be good if she could work with the receptionist in the front office of their business. Her dad felt that she should have more responsibility than simply greeting customers. He said that Margy has always enjoyed working on the computer and recommended that she learn data entry on the computer to make productive use of her down time when she was not talking with a customer. The team agreed that this could be a reasonable expectation for Margy and worked to develop a plan to reach this goal. Describe a plan that evidences multidisciplinary input.

he responsibility of those who implement AT intervention is to rovide a health-promoting balance between occupational roles nd activities consistent with the individual's valued goals and nterests, as well as the demands of society.[100] The direct connec-ion between occupational therapy and AT allows us to unlock uman potential and optimize human performance through he promotion of participation in activities that are personally neaningful, relevant, and life sustaining.

REFERENCES

1. Abramson, L. Y., Seligman, M. E. P., & Teasdale, J. D. (1978). Learned helplessness in humans: Critique and reformation. *Journal of Abnormal Psychology, 87,* 49–74.

2. American Occupational Therapy Association. (2000). *AOTA 2000 member compensation survey.* Bethesda, MD: Author.

3. American Occupational Therapy Association. (2004). Assistive technology within occupational therapy practice. *American Journal of Occupational Therapy, 58,* 678–680.

4. Anson, D. K. (1997). *Alternative computer access: A guide to selection.* Philadelphia: F.A. Davis.

5. Argabrite Grove, R., Broeder, K., Gitlow, L., Goodrich, B., Levan, P., Moser, C., et al. (2007). *Assistive technology in the schools: From start to finish.* Pre-Conference Institute at AOTA's Annual Conference & Expo, St. Louis, MO.

6. Assistive Technology Training Online (ATTO) Project. Retrieved October 2006, from http://atto.buffalo.edu/registered/ATBasics/Curriculum/Math/printmodule.php.

7. Bain, B. K., & Leger, D. (1997). *Assistive technology: An interdisciplinary approach.* New York: Churchill Livingstone.

8. Baush, M. E., Ault, M. J., & Hasselbring, T. S. (2006). *Assistive technology planner: From IEP consideration to classroom implementation.* Lexington, KY: National Assistive Technology Research Institute.

9. Behrmann, M. M. (1984). A brighter future for early learning through high tech. *The Pointer, 28,* 23–26.

10. Behrmann, M. M., Jones, J. K., & Wilds, M. L. (1989). Technology intervention for very young children with disabilities. *Infants and Young Children, 1,* 66–77.

11. Beukelman, D. R., & Mirenda, P. (1992). *Augmentative and alternative communication: Management of severe communication disorders in children and adults.* Baltimore: Brookes.

12. Beukelman, D. R., & Mirenda, P. (2005). *Augmentative and alternative communication: Management of severe communication disorders in children and adults* (3rd ed.). Baltimore: Brookes.

13. Beukelman, D. R., McGinnis, J., & Morrow, D. (1991). Vocabulary selection in augmentative and alternative communication. *Augmentative and Alternative Communication, 7,* 171–185.

14. Blackstone, S. (2006). False beliefs, widely held. *Augmentative Communication News, 3,* 1–6.

15. Bloomfield, B. C. (2000). *Icon to, I Can: A visual bridge to independence.* TEACCH International Conference, Chapel Hill, NC, May 23–24.

16. Bowser, G., & Reed, P. (1998). *Education TECH points: A framework for assistive technology planning.* Winchester, OR: Coalition for Assistive Technology in Oregon.

17. Bryen, D. N., Cohen, K., & Carey, A. (2004). Augmentative communication employment training and supports: Some employment outcomes. *Journal of Rehabilitation, 70,* 10–18.

18. Burgstahler, S. (2003). The role of technology in preparing youth with disabilities for postsecondary education and employment. *Journal of Special Education Technology, 18,* 7–20.

19. Burkhart, L. (2002). *Getting past learned helplessness for children who face severe challenges: Four secrets for success.* Retrieved October 9, 2006, from http://www.lburkhart.com.

20. Burns, M. S., Griffin, P., & Snow, C. E. (Eds.). (1999). *Starting out right: A guide to promoting children's reading success.* Washington, DC: National Academy Press. Available online: http://www.nap.edu/html/sor/.

21. Carlson, S. J., Clarke, C. D., Harden, B., Karr, S., Rosenberg, G. G., Swinth, Y. L., et al. (2003). *Assistive technology and IDEA: Effective practices for related services personnel.* Rockville, MD: American Speech-Language-Hearing Association (ASHA).

22. Castellani, J., & Bowser, G. (2006). Transition planning: Assistive technology supports and services. *Technology in Action, 2.* Arlington, VA: Center for Technology in Education, Johns Hopkins University, and Technology and Media Division of the Council for Exceptional Children.

23. Castellani, J., & Jetts, T. (2005). Using technology to provide access to the general education curriculum-techniques to try. In C. Wilbarger (Ed.), *Technology and media for accessing the curriculum: Instructional support for students with disabilities.* Arlington, VA: Technology and Media Division (TAM) Council for Exceptional Children.

24. Center for Universal Design. (1997). *About universal design.* Retrieved August 30, 2008, from http://design.ncsu.edu/cud/about_ud/about_ud.htm.

25. Clarke, M., & Kirton, A. (2003). Patterns of interaction between children with physical disabilities using augmentative and alternative communication systems and their peers. *Child Language Teaching and Therapy, 19,* 135–151.

26. Cole, J., & Swinth, Y. L. (2004). Comparison of the touch-free switch to a physical switch, children's abilities and preferences: A pilot study. *Journal of Special Education Technology, 19*(2), 19–30.

27. Collier, B. (2005). When I grow up...Supporting youth who use augmentative communication for adulthood. In *Proceedings of the 2005 Alberta rehabilitation and assistive technology consortium conference.* Edmonton, Canada. Retrieved August 2008 from http://www.acrat.ca.

28. Cook, A., & Polgar, J. (2008). *Cook & Hussey's Assistive technologies: Principles and practice* (3rd ed.). St. Louis: Elsevier.

29. Cornell University. (1999). Computers in schools are putting elementary schoolchildren at risk for posture problems, says Cornell study. *Science Daily.* Retrieved August 2008 from http://www.sciencedaily.com/releases/1999/02/990202071806.htm.

30. Demers, L., Weiss-Lambrou, R., & Ska, B. (2002). The Quebec user evaluation of satisfaction with assistive technology (QUEST 2.0): An overview and recent progress. *Technology and Disability, 14,* 101–105.

31. Demers, L., Wessels, R. D., Weiss-Lambrou, R., Ska, B., & De Witte, L. P. (1999). An international content validation of the Quebec user evaluation of satisfaction with assistive technology (QUEST). *Occupational Therapy International, 6,* 159–175.

32. DeRuyter, F. (1995). Evaluating outcomes in assistive technology: Do we understand the commitment? *Assistive Technology, 7,* 3–16.

33. Dickey, R., & Shealey, S. H. (1987). Using technology to control the environment. *American Journal of Occupational Therapy, 41,* 717–721.

34. Doster, S., & Politano, P. (1996). Augmentative and alternative communication. In J. Hammel (Ed.), *AOTA self-paced clinical course: Technology and occupational therapy: A link to function.* Rockville, MD: AOTA.

35. Douglas, J., Reeson, B., & Ryan, M. (1988). Computer microtechnology for a severely disabled preschool child. *Child Care: Health and Development, 14,* 93–104.

36. Dowden, P., & Cook, A. M. (2002). Choosing effective selection techniques for beginning communicators. In J. Reichle, D. Beukelman, & J. Light (Eds.), *Exemplary practices for beginning communicators* (pp. 101–124). Baltimore: Brookes.

37. Downing, J. (2005). *Teaching communication skills to students with severe disabilities* (2nd ed.). Baltimore: Brookes.

38. Drager, K. (2003). Light technologies with different system layouts and language organizations. *Journal of Speech, Language, and Hearing Research, 46,* 289–312.

39. Edyburn, D. L. (2000). 1999 in review: A synthesis of the special education technology literature. *Journal of Special Education, 15,* 7–18.

40. Edyburn, D. L. (2002). Cognitive rescaling strategies. *Closing the Gap, 21,* 1–4.

41. Edyburn, D. L. (2003). Assistive technology and evidence-based practice. *ConnSENSE Bulletin.* Retrieved March 2008, from http://www.connsensebulletin.com.

42. Farmer, L. (1998). Turn on to reading through technology. *Library Talk,* (Sept./Oct.), 16–17.

43. Foulds, R. A. (1982). Applications of microcomputers in the education of the physically disabled child. *Exceptional Children, 49,* 143–162.

44. Gelderblom, G. J., & deWitte, L. P. (2002). The assessment of assistive technology outcomes, effects and costs. *Technology and Disability, 14,* 91–94.

45. George, C. L., Schaff, J. I., & Jeffs, T. L. (2005). Physical access in today's schools: Empowerment through assistive technology. In D. Edyburn, K. Higgins, & R. Boone (Eds.), *The handbook of special education technology.* Whitefish Bay, WI: Knowledge by Design.

46. Glickman, L., Deitz, J., Anson, D., & Stewart, K. (1996). Effect of switch control site on computer skills of infants and toddlers. *American Journal of Occupational Therapy, 50,* 545–553.

47. Goldbart, J., & Marshall, J. (2004). "Pushes and pulls" on the parents of children who use AAC. *Augmentative and Alternative Communication, 20,* 194–208.

48. Hammel, J., & Niehues, A. (1998). Integrating general and assistive technology into school-based practice: Process and information resources. In J. Case-Smith (Ed.), *Occupational therapy: Making a difference in school system practice.* Rockville, MD: AOTA.

49. Hansell, N. (1974). *The person-in-distress: On the biosocial mechanisms of adaptation.* New York: Behavioral Sciences Press.

50. Higgins, E. L., & Raskind, M. H. (2000). Speaking to read: the effects of continuous vs. discrete speech recognition systems on the reading and spelling of children with learning disabilities. *Journal of Special Education Technology, 15,* 19–30.

51. Hitchcock, C., & Stahl, S. (2003). Assistive technology, universal design, universal design for learning: improved learning opportunities. *Journal of Special Education Technology, 18,* 45–52. IDEA Practices. (2004). Retrieved August 2008 from http://www.ideapractices.org.

52. Hodgdon, L. A. (1995). *Visual strategies for improving communication, Volume I: Practical supports for school and home.* Troy, MI: QuirkRoberts Publishing.

53. Jackson, R. (2005). *Curriculum access for students with low-incidence disabilities: The promise of universal design for learning.* Wakefield, MA: National Center on Accessing the General Curriculum. Retrieved August 2008 from http://www.cast.org/publications/ncac/ncac_lowinc.html.

54. Judge, S. L. (2001). Computer applications in programs for young children with disabilities: Current status and future directions. *Journal of Special Education Technology, 16*(1), 29–40.

55. Kangas, K. M. (2000). The task performance position: providing seating for accurate access to assistive technology. *Physical Disabilities Special Interest Section Quarterly, 23*(September), 1–3.

56. Kelker, K., & Holt, R. (2000). *Family guide to assistive technology.* Cambridge, MA: Brookline Books.

57. Kerr, S. T. (1996). *Technology and the future of schooling: Ninety-fifth yearbook of the national society for the study of education, part II.* Chicago, IL: University of Chicago Press.

58. Koenig, A. J. (1992). A framework for understanding the literacy of individuals with visual impairments. *Journal of Visual Impairment and Blindness, 86,* 277–284.

59. Koenig, A. J., & Holbrook, M. C. (2000). Literacy skills. In A. J. Koenig & M. C. Holbrook (Eds.), *Foundations of education: Instructional strategies for teaching children and youth with visual impairments* (Vol. 2, pp. 265–329). New York: American Foundation for the Blind.

60. Koppenhaver, D. A., Evans, D., & Yoder, D. E. (1991). Childhood reading and writing experiences of literate adults with severe speech and motor impairments. *Augmentative and Alternative Communication, 7,* 20–33.

61. Lahm, E. A. (Ed.). (1989). *Technology with low incidence populations: Promoting access and learning.* Reston, VA: The Council for Exceptional Children.

62. Lahm, E. A., & Sizemore, L. (2002). Factors that influence assistive technology decision-making. *Journal of Special Education Technology, 17*(1), 15–26.

63. Lamb, P. (2003). The role of the vocational rehabilitation counselor in procuring technology to facilitate success in postsecondary education for youth with disabilities. *Journal of Special Education Technology, 18*(4), 53–63.

64. Law, M., Baptiste, S., Carswell, A., McColl, M. A., Polatajko, H., & Pollock, N. (2005). *Canadian Occupational Performance Measure* (4th ed.). Toronto, ON: Canadian Association of Occupational Therapy Inc.

65. Law, M., Cooper, B., Strong, S., Stewart, D., Rigby, P., & Letts, L. (1996). The person-environment-occupation model: A transactive approach to occupational performance. *Canadian Journal of Occupational Therapy, 63,* 9–23.

66. Lewis, R. (2005). Classroom technology for students with learning disabilities. In D. Edyburn, K. Higgins, & R. Boone (Eds.), *Handbook of special education technology research and practice.* Whitefish Bay, WI: Knowledge by Design.

67. Light, J. (1989). Toward a definition of communicative competence for individuals using augmentative and alternative communication systems. *Augmentative and Alternative Communication, 5,* 137–144.

68. Light, J. C., & Drager, K. (2002). Improving the design of augmentative and alternative technologies for young children. *Assistive Technology, 14,* 17–32.

69. Maier, S. F., & Seligman, M. E. (1976). Learned helplessness: Theory and evidence. *Journal of Experimental Psychology: General, 105,* 3–46.

70. Mirenda, P. (1993). Bonding the uncertain mosaic. *Augmentative and Alternative Communication, 9,* 3–9.

71. Deleted in proofs.

72. Mistrett, S. (2005). Assistive technology helps young children with disabilities participate in daily activities. In C. Wilbarger (Ed.), *Technology and media for accessing the curriculum: Instructional support for students with disabilities.* Arlington, VA: Technology and Media Division (TAM).

73. National Joint Committee for the Communication Needs of Persons with Severe Disabilities. (1992). Guidelines for meeting the communication needs of persons with severe disabilities. *ASHA, 34*(March), 1–8.

74. Neighborhood Legal Services, Inc. (2003). *Funding of assistive technology: The public school's special education system as a funding source: The cutting edge.* Retrieved October 10, 2008, from http://www.nls.org

75. Office of Special Education and Rehabilitative Services, U.S. Department of Education. *Reuse your assistive technology.* Retrieved July 2008 from http://www.ed.gov/print/programs/atsg/at-reuse.html.

76. Parette, H. P., & VanBiervliet, A. (1990). A prospective inquiry into technology needs and practices of school-aged children with disabilities. *Journal of Special Education Technology, 10,* 198–206.

77. Phillips, B., & Zhao, H. (1993). Predictors of assistive technology abandonment. *Assistive Technology, 5,* 36–45.

78. Post, K. M., Hartmann, K., Gitlow, L., & Rakoski, D. (2008). AOTA's Centennial Vision for the future: How can technology help? *Technology Special Interest Section Quarterly, 18*(March), 1–4.

79. QIAT Consortium. (2007). *AT in transition.* Retrieved June 2008 from http://natri.uky.edu/assoc_projects/qiat/documents/6%20QIAT%20QIs%20Transition.doc.

80. QIAT Consortium. (2007). *Quality indicators for assistive technology services.* Retrieved August 2008 from http://natri.uky.edu/assoc_projects/qiat/.

81. Reed, P. (2000). *School profile of assistive technology services.* Retrieved August 2008 from http://www.wati.org/AT_Services/schoolprofile.html.

82. Reed, P. (Ed.). (2003). *Designing environments for successful kids.* Oshkosh, WI: Wisconsin Assistive Technology Initiative.

83. Reed, P. (2004). *The WATI assessment package.* Retrieved October 2005 from http://www.wati.org/Materials/pdf/wati%20assessment.pdf.

84. Richardson, C. (2001). Technology supports for math. *T/TAC Linklines,* (November/December). Retrieved July 2009 from http://web.wm.edu/ttac/articles/assistivetech/mathsupports.html.

85. Robinson, L. M. (1986). Designing computer intervention for very young handicapped children. *Journal of the Division for Early Childhood, 103,* 209–213.

86. Rose, D. H., & Meyer, A. (2002). *Teaching every student in the digital age: Universal design for learning.* Alexandria, VA: Association for Supervision and Curriculum Development.

87. Rowland, C., & Schweigert, P. (2000). *Tangible symbol systems: Making the right to communicate a reality for individuals with sever disabilities* (2nd ed.). Portland, OR: OHSU Design to Learn Projects.

88. Ryan, R., & Deci, E. (2000). Self-determination theory and the facilitation of intrinsic motivation, social development, and well-being. *American Psychologist, 55,* 68–78.

89. Scherer, M. J. (1996). Outcomes of assistive technology use on quality of life. *Disability and Rehabilitation, 18,* 439–448.

90. Scherer, M. J. (2000). *Living in the state of stuck: How technology impacts the lives of people with disabilities.* Cambridge, MA: Brookline Books.

91. Scherer, M. J., & Craddock, G. (2002). Matching person & technology (MPT) assessment process. *Technology and Disability, 14,* 125–131.

92. Scherer, M. J., & Lane, J. P. (1997). Assessing consumer profiles of "ideal" assistive technologies in ten categories: An integration of quantitative and qualitative methods. *Disability and Rehabilitation, 19,* 528–535.

93. Schmeler, M. R. (1997). Strategies in documenting the need for assistive technology: An analysis of documentation procedures. In *AOTA Technology Special Interest Section Quarterly,* Vol. 7. Bethesda, MD: American Occupational Therapy Association.

94. Schoonover, J., & Feist, C. (2007). Using computers to design accessible learning environments. *AOTA. School System Special Interest Section Quarterly, 14*(March), 1–4.

95. Schoonover, J., Levan, P., & Argabrite Grove, R. (2006). Occupational therapy and assistive technology in school-based practice: supporting participation. *OT Practice, 11,* CE1–CE8.

96. Sibert, R. I. (1997). Financing assistive technology: An overview of public funding sources. *AOTA Technology Special Interest Section Newsletter, 7,* 1–4.

97. Deleted in proofs.

98. Spencer, J. (1998). Alternative meanings of assistive technology. In D. B. Gray, L. A. Quatrano, & M. L. Lieberman (Eds.), *Designing and using assistive technology: The human perspective.* Baltimore, MD: Brookes.

99. Stodden, R. A., Conway, M. A., & Chang, K. B. T. (2003). Findings from the study of transition, technology and postsecondary supports for youth with disabilities: Implications for secondary school educators. *Journal of Special Education Technology, 18* (4), 29–43.

100. Stoller, L. C. (1998). *Low-tech assistive devices: A handbook for the school setting.* Framingham, MA: Therapro, Inc.

101. Sullivan, M. W., & Lewis, M. (2000). Assistive technology for the very young: Creating responsive environments. *Infants and Young Children, 12*(4), 34–52.

102. Swanson, H. L. (1999). Instructional components that predict treatment outcomes for students with learning disabilities: Support for a combined strategy and direct instruction model. *Learning Disabilities Research and Practice, 14,* 129–140.

103. Sweeney, J. (2007). Getting assistive technology into the mainstream the EASY way. *Closing the Gap, 25,* 1–4.

104. Swinth, Y. L. (1997). *The meaning of assistive technology in the lives of high school students and their families.* Unpublished doctoral dissertation. Seattle, WA: University of Washington.

105. Swinth, Y. L. (1998). Assistive technology in early intervention: Theory and practice. In J. Case-Smith (Ed.), *Pediatric occupational therapy and early intervention* (2nd ed.). Woburn, MA: Butterworth-Heinemann.

106. Swinth, Y. L., & Anson, D. (1998). Alternatives to handwriting: Keyboarding and text-generation techniques for schools. In J. Case-Smith (Ed.), *AOTA self-paced clinical course: Occupational therapy: Making a difference in school system practice.* Rockville, MD: American Occupational Therapy Association.

107. Todis, M., & Walker, H. M. (1993). User perspectives on assistive technology in educational settings. *Focus on Exceptional Children, 46*(3), 1–16.

108. U.S. Department of Education, Office of Special Education Programs, Data Analysis System. (2006). *Children with disabilities receiving special education under Part B of the Individuals with Disabilities Education Act.* Retrieved July 2008 from https://www.ideadata.org/tables30th/ar_1-1.xls.

109. Washington Assistive Technology Alliance [WATA]. (1999). *Paying for the assistive technology you need: A consumer guide to funding sources in Washington State.* Retrieved November 2003 from http://uwctds.washington.edu/resources/legal/funding%20manual/index.htm.

110. Wehmeyer, M. L. (1996). Self-determination as an educational outcome: Why is it important to children, youth, and adults with disabilities? In D. J. Sands & M. L. Wehmeyer (Eds.), *Self-determination across the life span: Independence and choice for people with disabilities* (pp. 17–36). Baltimore: Brookes.

111. Wehmeyer, M. L. (2002). Promoting the self-determination of students with severe disabilities. *ERIC Digest.* Retrieved June 2008 from http://eric.ed.gov/ERICDocs/data/ericdocs2sql/content_storage_01/0000019b/80/29/d2/46.pdf.

112. Weintraub, H., Bacon, C., & Wilcox, M. (2004). AT and young children: Confidence, experience and education of early intervention providers. In *Research Brief,* Vol. 1. Tots n Tech Research Institute. Retrieved February 2008 from http://tnt.asu.edu.

113. Zabala, J. S. (2002). *2002 update of the SETT framework.* Retrieved September 2003 from (University of Kentucky) http://sweb.uky.edu/~jszabala/JoySETT.html.

114. Zabala, J. (2007). *10 Things everyone needs to know about assistive technology in schools in 2006.* Presented at the national conference of the Assistive Technology Industry Association (ATIA), Orlando, FL.

Christine Wright-Ott

KEY TERMS

Functional mobility
Community mobility
Developmental theory
 of mobility
Augmentative mobility
Manual wheelchairs

Power wheelchairs
Powered mobility
 evaluation
Seating
Positioning

OBJECTIVES

1. Understand the importance of mobility to child development.
2. Apply a mobility assessment model to children with different levels of motor function.
3. Identify alternative methods of mobility appropriate to meet the child's developmental and functional needs.
4. Describe wheelchair features and designs that meet the needs of children with various levels of motor control.
5. Identify power mobility devices currently available.
6. Describe power mobility assessment and intervention.
7. Describe new technology in assessing seating and positioning and new equipment available to children with unique seating and positioning needs.
8. Explain the biomechanical principles important to positioning and seating.

This chapter presents an overview of the importance of mobility for growth and development and the implications of impaired mobility. Responsibilities of the occupational therapist for evaluating and recommending appropriate mobility devices are emphasized. Guidelines and criteria for selecting mobility equipment are defined, and descriptions of mobility devices are provided. This chapter also describes the importance of positioning and other factors that influence successful use of assistive devices.

Mobility is fundamental to an individual's overall development and functioning in the occupations of self-care, work, and leisure and is essential to quality of life. The definition of *functional mobility* includes moving from one position or place to another (e.g., bed mobility, wheelchair mobility, and transfers [wheelchair, bed, car, tub or shower, toilet, or chair]), performing functional ambulation, and transporting objects. *Community mobility* is defined as moving oneself in the community and using public or private transportation (e.g., driving or accessing buses, taxicabs, or other public transportation systems). This chapter addresses primarily mobility as a means of locomotion, with an emphasis on evaluation and intervention principles.

DEVELOPMENTAL THEORY OF MOBILITY

The newborn has little independent control of any part of the body. Motor and sensory symmetry and midline orientation develop gradually, followed by controlled purposeful movements and the beginning of alternating coordinated movements. The first form of mobility that the infant experiences is rolling, first from side to supine, then prone to supine, and finally in either direction. The 6-month-old infant achieves mobility by pivoting in the prone position. The infant continually becomes more active against gravity (Figure 21-1). Most 8-month-old infants creep and move from sitting to quadruped positioning and back. By the ninth to tenth month, the infant has a strong desire to move upward. First infants pull to stand and cruise along furniture, such as a coffee table; then they hold onto someone or something as they take their first steps. The average age at independent walking is 11.2 months, and most children achieve independent upright ambulation between 9 and 15 months of age.[8,14]

With the developmental theory of mobility, developmental theorists accept that physical and psychologic developments are interrelated and that early experiences influence subsequent behavior. "Through their motor interactions infants and toddlers learn about things and people in their world and also discover they can cause things to happen" (p. 18).[12] During the first months of life, children seek physical control of their environment and continue to do so by building and enhancing their motor skills day by day.

During the first 4 years of life, the child gains independence through mastery of important life tasks such as locomotion, ability to manipulate, bowel and bladder control, language development, and social interactions. The most fundamental of these, with the widest influence in all spheres of development, are movement about the environment and use of language as a communicative and information processing system.

Children gain various learning experiences as they move about. Locomotion and other motor skills, which develop rapidly during the first 3 years of life, become the primary vehicles for learning and socialization and for the growth of a healthy

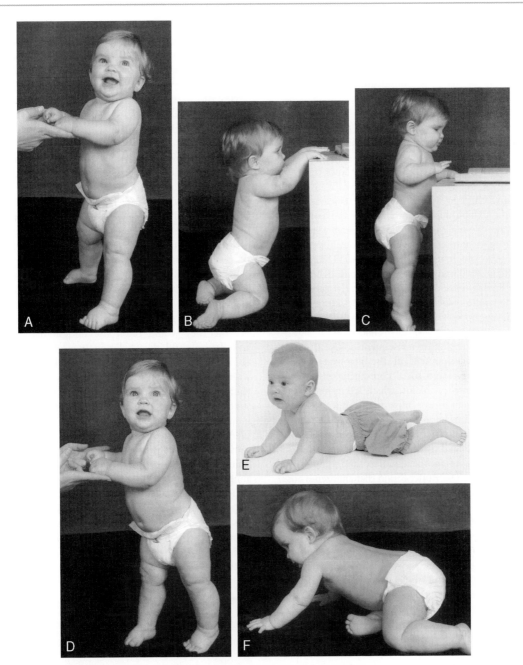

FIGURE 21-1 Development of locomotion. **A,** Infant bears full weight on feet by 7 months. **B,** Infant can maneuver from sitting to kneeling position. **C,** Infant can stand holding onto furniture at 9 months. **D,** While standing, infant takes deliberate step at 10 months. **E,** Infant crawls with abdomen on floor and pulls self forward, and then **(F)** creeps on hands and knees at 9 months. (From Hockenberry, M. J., Wilson, D., & Winkelstein, M. L. [2005]. *Wong's essentials of pediatric nursing* [7th ed]. St. Louis: Mosby; photos by Paul Vincent Kuntz, Texas Children's Hospital.)

sense of independence and competence. Piaget viewed self-produced movement as a crucial building block of knowledge. He theorized that the intercoordination of vision and audition with movements, including locomotion, laid the basis for the child's understanding of space, objects, causality, and self.[53] The ability of children to influence their environment and to affect or alter it through their own actions is intrinsically motivating. Early experiences are believed to foster curiosity, exploration, mastery, and persistence, and are therefore important for later intellectual functioning.

IMPAIRED MOBILITY

Children with physical disabilities who have difficulty achieving independent motor control are often deprived of opportunities for self-initiated or self-produced mobility. When these children do experience mobility, it is of a passive nature, as in being held or pushed in a stroller. Because they lack the necessary movements to explore and act on their environment, important learning opportunities are hindered. Mobility-impaired toddlers who cannot move across a room to reach out and touch an object or interact with a person are at a great disadvantage. They cannot experience the sensorimotor and developmental activities of their peers who have achieved upright mobility, such as pushing and pulling toys, opening and closing drawers, or moving around and under objects. Psychologists who have studied normal development have observed improvements in social-emotional, cognitive, perceptual, and motor functioning in infants when they first gain mobility.[71] Researchers who have studied the impact of early exploration on a child's development have also suggested that self-produced locomotion and active choice are important for the development of perception and cognition.[13,25,40,64] It appears that young children who actively seek to learn about their environment exhibit higher intelligence and cognitive ability at school age. Young children who at 3 years were high stimulation–seeking demonstrated increased cognitive, scholastic, and neuropsychologic test performance at 11 years.[55]

"When development along any line is restricted, delayed, or distorted, other lines of development are adversely affected as well" (p. 66).[11] Restricted experiences and mobility during early childhood can have a diffuse and lasting influence. Long-term physical restriction during infancy or early childhood can significantly alter and disrupt the entire subsequent course of emotional or psychologic development in the involved child.[36] Such deprivation of physical and social contingencies can lead to secondary developmental problems, which are motivational. Infants born with significant motor impairments quickly "begin to lose interest in a world which they do not expect to control" (p. 113).[9] This motivational effect is termed *learned helplessness,* a condition in which the child gives up trying to control his or her own world because of motor disability and diminished expectations of caregivers.[23,56] Butler found that children whose mobility is limited during early childhood develop a pattern of apathetic behavior—specifically, a lack of curiosity and initiative.[11] These character traits are believed to have a critical influence on intellectual performance and social interaction. The detrimental effects of limited early exploration were identified in a study comparing shortcut choices in a simulated maze of able-bodied teenagers with those of teenagers who had varying histories of mobility impairment. Despite equivalent levels of mobility, participants whose mobility was more limited early in development were poorer in the task than those whose mobility had deteriorated with age. The results suggest that early independent exploration is important in the development of spatial knowledge and that the detrimental effects of limited early exploratory experience may persist into the teenage years.[58]

In children with severe physical disabilities, newly gained independent mobility can have a positive effect on emotional, social, and intellectual states.[20,29] Paulsson and Christoffersen found that children with disabilities using mobility devices became less dependent on controlling their environment through verbal commands, more interested in all mobility skills, and more active in peer activities.[52] Butler found that children who had some means of ambulation could and would make choices, but those who did not ambulate were much less likely to exercise available options.[10] The lack of ambulation appeared to severely restrict the child's opportunities to practice decision making, thus giving him or her no reason to express an opinion or desire.

Intervention for young children with physical disabilities often includes the provision of adapted equipment: supported chairs, standers, bath seats, and adapted strollers. This equipment provides a means for properly and safely positioning a child, but does not provide a means for accessing the environment or experiencing the stages of development that occur with self-initiated mobility. Children who have a means for self-initiated mobility decide where, when, and how to move. It is the responsibility of the occupational and physical therapist to determine how young children with disabilities can access their environment, explore their surroundings, and experience developmentally appropriate activities. Mobility devices, which provide a physically disabled child with a means to access and explore the environment, not only provide a means for mobility but also facilitate psychosocial, language, and cognitive development. Such devices include prone scooters, handheld walkers, support walkers, manual and power wheelchairs, and alternative powered mobility devices. However, professionals lack agreement when and if mobility devices for very young children, particularly support walkers and powered mobility devices, are appropriate.

A support walker differs from a handheld walker in that it typically includes a seat with postural supports pelvis, trunk, and sometimes the head. In the past, therapists were reluctant to recommend support walkers for children with cerebral palsy because they would often use undesirable postures during ambulation,, and they believed it might increase the child's spasticity. However, many support walkers are now designed with features that complement the child's therapeutic goals (Figure 21-2).[49,51,76] In addition, several studies have demonstrated that resistive exercise does not increase spasticity in individuals with cerebral palsy.[7,21,26,44]

Although further study is needed, at least one study of persons with cerebral palsy concluded that a progressive strength-training program can improve muscle strength and walking ability without increasing spasticity.[2]

Professionals and third-party payers may resist providing a powered mobility device to a young child with physical disabilities, particularly before the age of 5 years. Indeed, most children born with congenital mobility impairments are not given their first wheelchair until the age of at least 3 years, and most of these do not receive a chair they can propel independently

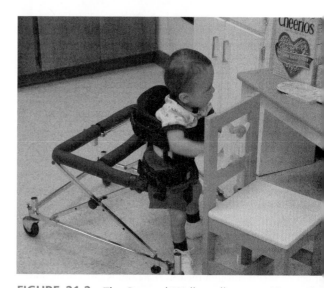

FIGURE 21-2 The Pommel Walker allows an 18-month-old child with a developmental delay to explore his environment. (Available from Freedom Concepts.)

until age 5.[27,29] Children with a physical disability under the age of 5 years are often denied the opportunity for using a powered mobility device because they are considered too young to have the cognitive skills to understand how to use it. However, "Clinical experience and research projects have established that powered mobility devices offer children at least as young as 17 months of age a safe and efficient method of independent locomotion" (p. 18).[12] Research continues to substantiate the fact that children as young as 18 months can achieve independent skills in powered mobility.[27,29]

Caregivers often believe that use of a power wheelchair will reduce the likelihood of their child's achieving independent mobility through ambulation. Research has not demonstrated that use of a powered mobility device prevents or delays the child's acquisition of motor skills. On the contrary, researchers have found positive changes in children's development after the introduction of a powered mobility device.[46,52,73] During mobility training, children with severe motor disabilities demonstrated improved head control and trunk stability, increased motivation, and greater self-confidence in movement.[10] Deitz, Swinth, and White concluded that for some young children with severe motor impairments and developmental delay, use of a powered mobility device may potentially increase self-initiated movement occurrences during free play.[19] Nilsson and Nyberg analyzed case studies of preschool children with profound cognitive disabilities participating in power wheelchair training experiences.[46] They concluded that the training experiences increased wakefulness and alertness, stimulated a limited use of arms and hands, and promoted the understanding of very simple cause-and-effect relationships.

In another study, children 15 months to 5 years of age with physical disabilities who participated in a 2-week mobility exploration day camp demonstrated a variety of positive behavioral changes.[73] The children experienced mobility by using the Mini-Bot, a standing powered mobility device, to explore the environment (Figure 21-3). They participated in daily 1½-hour sessions for 2 weeks. Behavioral changes that caregivers and occupational therapists observed in some children included increased eye contact, increased verbalization and communication, improved sleeping patterns, increased active arm use, and a more positive disposition.

The current trend is for mobility devices to be recommended at young ages, when typical children are first ambulating. Many professionals believe that if self-initiated mobility does not occur in the first year, the use of devices for mobility should be considered. Mobility appears to be a priority issue for children with disabilities and others in their environment. When researchers surveyed the occupational performance needs of school-age children with physical disabilities in the school system and community, most teachers, parents, and children identified mobility as their greatest area of concern.[54] However, it can be a challenging task for a therapist to suggest consideration of a mobility device, particularly a power wheelchair, to the family of a young mobility-impaired child. Many caregivers consider the suggestion as a symbol of giving up hope for independent ambulation. For this reason, use of a walker, support walker, or alternative powered mobility device may be more accepted by the families of very young children. The therapist must convey to the family the concept that all children need a means of mobility to access the environment for exploration to encourage development in the visual perceptual, language,

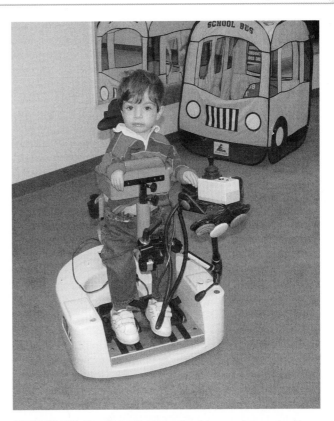

FIGURE 21-3 The Mini-Bot provides early, exploratory, self-initiated mobility experiences. A 2-year-old child with arthrogryposis stands and moves in the Mini-Bot using a joystick or switches. (Manufactured by Innovative Products, Inc.)

social, and cognitive domains. The mobility device is intended to assist the child in achieving independence in exploration until and if another method is acquired.

AUGMENTATIVE MOBILITY

Butler introduced the term *augmentative mobility* to describe all types of mobility that supplement or augment ambulation. "Given augmentative mobility, disabled children can experience more success in directly controlling their environment, thereby reducing or avoiding secondary social, emotional and intellectual handicaps" (p. 18).[12]

The concept of augmentative mobility for functional mobility can be expanded to include transitional mobility. Transitional mobility allows the child to use a mobility device to have self-initiated movement without the expectation that it must be functional. The child may not consistently move the mobility device in a desired direction but uses it as a means for exploring the effects of movement and learning how to move. The therapist can best provide transitional mobility by allowing the child to move the device in a large room with open space where the child is free to explore. These experiences can then help the child make the transition to a more functional level of purposeful mobility. Not all children are able to achieve functional mobility; in these instances, transitional mobility remains an important means for the child to explore the environment.

The team must consider several factors before selecting the type of mobility device that is appropriate for a child. These factors include the purpose or goals for using the device, environments for intended use, and the child's physical and psychosocial abilities and limitations. When selecting a mobility device, the team considers the advantages and disadvantages of the device, the modifications that may be needed for comfort and control, the congruence to intervention goals, and the cost-benefit ratio. Ideally, a mobility-impaired child should have more than one type of mobility device for use in indoor and outdoor environments. Any methods that are chosen for mobility require close cooperation among all professionals working with the child and family.

ASSESSMENT AND INTERVENTION

Classification of Mobility Skills

Children's mastery of functional mobility skills has been classified and categorized in several ways. Hays examined current existing diagnostic conditions of children without locomotion and divided them into four functional groups[34]:

1. *Children who will never ambulate.* This category includes children with cerebral palsy with severe involvement and spinal muscular atrophy types I and II. Generally, these children have no opportunity for independent mobility.

2. *Children with inefficient mobility who ambulate but are unable to do so at a reasonable rate of speed or with acceptable endurance.* This category includes children with cerebral palsy with less involvement and myelomeningocele with upper-extremity involvement. For these children, assisted mobility may provide an efficient means of mobility above that which they are capable of producing themselves. Warren uses the term *marginal ambulators* for this group.[70]

3. *Children who have lost their independent mobility.* This category includes victims of trauma and children with progressive neuromuscular disorders. The developmental implications may be less critical than in the first two groups, and the issue is acceptance of assisted mobility as an adaptation to the acquired disability.

4. *Children who temporarily require assisted mobility and often progress to independent mobility with age.* This category includes many children with osteogenesis imperfecta and arthrogryposis. Functional considerations in this group are both developmental and practical.

There are significant differences among these groups that may have implications for mobility and its integration into the child's overall concept of disability, as well as for evaluation and intervention. Group I children may achieve independent mobility through the use of a support walker and power wheelchair. Group II children may be able to independently propel a manual wheelchair, ambulate in a support walker indoors, and use a power wheelchair for community mobility. Children in groups III and IV will use a variety of mobility methods during the transition period.

Mobility Assessments

Evaluation of children has traditionally focused on the achievement of developmental milestones. Occupational therapists have discussed the limitation of such evaluations because underlying impairments (e.g., motor control deficits) cannot fully explain the extent and form of functional difficulties seen in children with disabilities.[17] Furthermore, the tasks that are most relevant for daily independence in mobility function have not been well defined in traditional developmental milestone tests. Using a top-down evaluation process, the therapist focuses on what the child needs or wants to do, the context in which he or she typically engages occupations, and the limitations that he or she may experience.[17,24] Therapists assess underlying performance abilities only to the extent that is needed to help clarify the possible sources of limitations in occupational performance. In mobility evaluation, occupational therapists focus on the child's overall pattern of locomotion and transfer skills in relation to a particular performance context.

Two instruments that evaluate children's functional abilities, including mobility, are the Pediatric Evaluation of Disabilities Inventory (PEDI)[32] and the Functional Independence Measure for Children (WeeFIM).[68] The PEDI rates two dimensions of performance: ability to perform functional skills and the level of caregiver assistance needed. The functional mobility subscale measures basic transfer skills (e.g., getting in and out of a car) and body transportation activities (e.g., walking up and down stairs). WeeFIM is based on the Functional Independence Measure (FIM) and is for children from 6 months to 7 years of age. This scale measures the child's independence in mobility: transfers, locomotion, and stairs and provides useful information for progress assessment, program planning, and communication with caregivers.

The Canadian Occupational Performance Measure (COPM)[42] is a semistructured interview that focuses on the identification of problems in self-care, productivity, and leisure. It provides a framework to help clients articulate the difficulties they are encountering in their daily lives and appears to be responsive to change after occupational therapy intervention.[42] In the case of mobility, the COPM can address the concerns of children and caregivers, help them identify what is important to them, and help them prioritize goals. The COPM also provides a baseline assessment for measuring outcomes on reassessment.

Tefft, Furumasu, and Guerette, at the Rehabilitation Engineering Research Center on Technology for Children with Orthopedic Disabilities at Rancho Los Amigos Medical Center, developed a cognitive assessment battery and a wheelchair mobility training and assessment program to help clinicians determine a young child's readiness to drive a power wheelchair.[61,62] The Pediatric Powered Wheelchair Screening Test (PPWST) and the Powered Mobility Program (PMP) were developed and validated for children ages 20 to 36 months with orthopedic disabilities who used a joystick to control the wheelchair.[30,31] Through this research, the cognitive domains of spatial relations and problem solving were found to be significant predictors of power wheelchair mobility performance.[63] The research team continues to study the validity of the assessment battery for children, with neurologic conditions such as cerebral palsy, who use a joystick or switches to drive power wheelchairs.

Occupational therapists evaluate several components of performance (e.g., motor, perceptual, and cognitive factors) that influence mobility. Human functions important to mobility include neuromotor status (vision, hearing, and seizure disorders), orthopedic conditions, and psychosocial variables.

therapists also consider both chronologic and developmental age and the child's environments. The therapist must make the mobility devices and positioning system available during the evaluation process so that the child and the caregivers have an opportunity to gain experience using potential mobility devices. These trials provide the caregivers and the child with information and experience that will assist them in becoming informed consumers and full participants in deciding which mobility device best meets their needs.

Mobility Evaluation Team Models

Selection of the most appropriate positioning and mobility device requires the skills of a therapy team working in close collaboration with the school team, prescribing physician, child, parent or caregiver, and assistive technology professional (ATP). The ATP is "a service provider who analyzes the needs of individuals with disabilities, assists in the selection of the appropriate equipment, and trains the consumer on how to properly use the specific equipment. This equipment may include manual and power wheelchairs, alternate computer access, augmentative and alternative communication devices, and other technology to improve the function and quality of life for an individual with a disability" (resna.org). The ATP is credentialed through the Rehabilitation Engineering and Assistive Technology Society of North America (RESNA). Occupational and physical therapists who make recommendations for assistive technology equipment often seek an ATP credential. This organization also provides certification for a Rehabilitation Engineering Technologist (RET) who designs, customizes, and modifies assistive technology (AT). The ATP is responsible for maintaining updated knowledge of available equipment and assisting in identifying choices of mobility devices according to the features that the child requires to use it optimally.

The physical or occupational therapist, together with the child and family, determines the needs of the child and establishes goals to identify the features and options in a mobility device or devices that will meet the desired outcomes and assist the family in setting appropriate functional goals and expectations for using the mobility device. The therapist is responsible for assisting the family in becoming informed consumers who can make decisions regarding a mobility device. Once the mobility device is selected and provided to the family, the therapist is responsible for periodically reevaluating the fit and function of the device to determine if it meets the stated goals and objectives.

Most funding agencies do not approve replacement of a mobility device, such as a wheelchair, within 3 to 5 years of the purchase date. If the equipment is not appropriate, the child and family may not have another option for several years. The limitations in reimbursement become critical when a misunderstanding during the evaluation or ordering process results in a device that does not meet the predetermined outcomes. It is imperative that the therapist, ATP, and family immediately decide how to best resolve these issues.

The occupational therapist selects among a variety of mobility evaluation models to evaluate a child for a mobility device. The most common is for the therapist to request a local supplier of durable medical equipment or ATP to bring the device under consideration to the therapy session. The ATP offers input about what features and options are available on the device and how to adjust it properly. The difficulty encountered with this model is that one supplier typically has a limited selection of devices available for demonstration, so only one device may be evaluated at each session. Therefore, the therapist does not have the opportunity to compare the child's performance in various types of mobility devices. Without direct comparison of the mobility devices, decisions about which devices are optimal for the child are difficult for the therapist to make. The decision is less risky when side-by-side comparisons of different devices are available during the evaluation. This method enables evaluation of performance with each mobility device under consistent child and environmental conditions.

Several AT centers and rehabilitation engineering centers throughout the country use a multidisciplinary team approach and side-by-side evaluation methods to assess seating and mobility needs, particularly with individuals who have severe disabilities. The teams consist of occupational therapists, physical therapists, rehabilitation engineers, speech pathologists, RETs, and ATPs working with the child's therapy team, school team, physician, and family. These centers offer the advantage of being able to consider all the needs of the child and offering a concentrated level of expertise.

MOBILITY DEVICES

Selection of a specific type of a mobility device depends on several factors. The therapy team must first decide on the purpose for using the mobility device or devices. Does the child need a means for exploring and accessing the environment (self-propelled manual, power wheelchair, or hands-free support walker) or do the caregivers need a convenient way to transport the child (stroller or manual wheelchair)? The next, most critical aspect of evaluating a mobility device is to consider the environments in which it is to be used by the child and caregivers. If the child's home has high pile carpet, propelling a manual wheelchair or using a walker with wheels smaller than 5 inches in diameter will be quite difficult. The force needed to move a wheelchair over various surfaces has been measured. Using concrete as the baseline, the increase in force needed to cross each surface is 3% for linoleum, 20% for low-pile carpet, and 62% for high-pile carpet.[1] The effort required by the individual to use the device will affect functional performance. If the mobility device is too complicated or the child must exert too much effort, it will not be used.

The occupational therapist must consider the features, adaptations, and hardware options needed for optimal use across all environments such as school, home, and community; the system must not reduce performance in functional activities such as eating, personal hygiene, transfers, and augmentative communication. Also important to consider are the needs and concerns of the caregivers and school personnel who will be transferring the child into and out of the device, transporting it, maintaining the equipment, and the costs versus benefits.

The occupational therapist must use the skills of an investigator during the mobility assessment process. Thoughtful planning and careful analysis of person-device-environment fit are necessary for the therapist to ensure that the child and

---

CASE STUDY 21-1 **Brian**

Brian is 5 years old and has severe spastic cerebral palsy. He is dependent on others for mobility in his manual wheelchair. He is fully included in a kindergarten classroom. His mother believes Brian will have more peer interaction if he can use a support walker in the classroom, which places him at his peer's height. She also believes he had better digestive function when he previously used a walker at a younger age. Brian was evaluated at his medical therapy session to determine what type of walker would provide him with mobility in the classroom. His parents expressed interest in a particular walker, and the therapist borrowed one from a medical equipment provider for Brian to use during the evaluation at the medical therapy unit. The family was excited when they observed Brian slowly propelling the walker forward. The therapist recommended the walker for purchase with custom modifications, which included a higher backrest, a headrest,

and a custom thigh-length seat to reduce adduction. The family ordered the walker and Brian began to use it in his classroom.

After 5 months of trying to use the support walker in the classroom, he could not take more than three steps in it. The therapist determined that he did not have the ability to maneuver the walker in the classroom because of a high degree of resistance from the carpeted surface. The therapist initially evaluated Brian in a room with linoleum, without consideration of the classroom environment. The therapist reevaluated Brian in another walker that had a large 20-inch wheel, which made it easier for him to maneuver over carpet. At this time, additional funding to purchase another walker is not available. He would have benefited from a side-by-side evaluation of several types of walkers with consideration of the characteristics of the environments in which he would use the walker.

---

family receive the optimal device. When a device is ordered without a comprehensive mobility evaluation, the child may end up with a wheelchair that will not fit into the family van with the user in it, tips over when the augmentative communication device is mounted on it, cannot be self-propelled outside because the family lives in a hilly area, or is too large to maneuver efficiently in the classroom environment. Case Study 21-1 provides an example of a child whose need for a mobility device—a support walker—was not evaluated properly.

Alternative Mobility Devices

Tricycles

Tricycles (Figure 21-4) are a means for mobility, although third-party funding is typically not available because tricycles are not considered a medical necessity. However, they can provide community mobility outdoors and on playgrounds. Many types of tricycles are available with adaptations, such as trunk supports, and hand-propelled models are available for children who do not have the ability to pedal with their legs (e.g., children with spina bifida). A unique and helpful feature for both the child and the care provider is a handle at the back of the Freedom Concepts tricycle, which enables the adult to steer the front wheel while the child pedals. This assists a child with limited upper extremity function who may not have the ability to hold onto the handle bars to steer the tricycle.

Prone Scooters

Prone scooters (Figure 21-5) require use of the arms and the ability to lift the head while moving. The advantages of using a prone scooter include access for participating in play activities on the floor, the ability to get on and off independently, and the ability to change direction more easily than with other types of manual mobility devices. Disadvantages include fatigue from maintaining neck and back extension, vulnerability of the head to hitting objects, the possibility of the hands getting caught in the casters or rubbed on rough surfaces, and difficulty viewing the environment above the ground level. Children with spina bifida may find the prone scooter functional

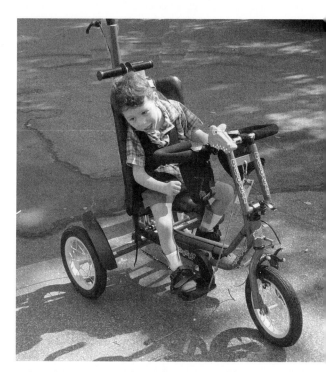

FIGURE 21-4 The Discovery Trike can fit a child as young as 12 months. An adult can assist the child by steering the front wheel with the push handle. (Available from Freedom Concepts.)

because they have the upper extremity function and strength to propel it and the scooter can support their legs.

Caster Carts

Caster carts offer another means of mobility to children with upper-extremity function (e.g., those with spina bifida) (Figure 21-6, *A*). Children can use caster carts indoors or on flat outdoor surfaces. Some children may be able to transfer on and off independently because of the close proximity to the floor. The device requires a considerable amount of energy

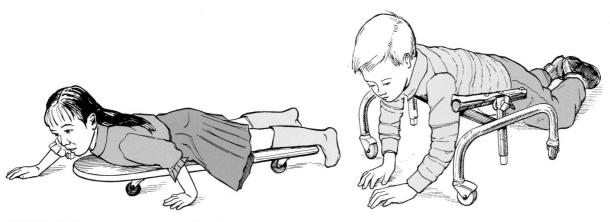

FIGURE 21-5 Prone scooter mobility devices.

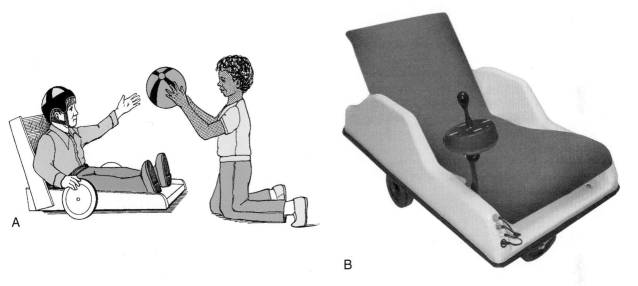

A

B

FIGURE 21-6 **A,** Caster cart mobility device. **B,** Joystick- or switch-controlled multi-directional scooter board. (Courtesy Enabling Devices, Hastings-on-Hudson, New York.)

expenditure for propelling long distances because of the small diameter of the wheels. Children with lower-extremity muscle contractures or tightness, such as in the hamstring muscles, may find it difficult to sit comfortably and securely because they are often unable to tolerate long-leg sitting. These children may feel more comfortable with a triangular-shaped wedge placed under the knees to support their legs in knee flexion. A battery-powered scooter from Enabling Devices allows a child to move either in a circular motion with one switch input or in all directions using several switches or a joystick (Figure 21-6, *B*).

Aeroplane Mobility Device

The *aeroplane mobility device* was designed by an occupational therapist for children with cerebral palsy who can move their legs but need support of the upper body (Figure 21-7). The device provides developmentally appropriate positioning, particularly for children with spasticity, because the child is positioned with hip abduction and extension with knee flexion, and the upper extremities are in a weight-bearing position. This position

often assists in reducing undesirable posturing in children who have spastic cerebral palsy, especially for children who exhibit extensor posturing in standing. Other advantages include ease in viewing the environment, the handmade nature of the device, and acceptance by parents, because it looks like a toy rather than an assistive device. The aeroplane mobility device is not available commercially but can be fabricated from wood. Disadvantages include lack of adjustability for growth, difficulty turning and moving backward, and heaviness.

Mobile Stander

If a child has upper extremity function to push and maneuver wheels, a *mobile stander* may provide another means for mobility. These devices allow the child to experience lower extremity weight bearing in a standing position. The child achieves mobility using large hand-held wheels for self-propulsion (Figure 21-8, *A*). If the child is unable to propel the wheels independently or functionally, but would like to achieve mobility in standing, a joystick-operated motorized stander such as the Standing Dani can provide mobility (Figure 21-8, *B*).

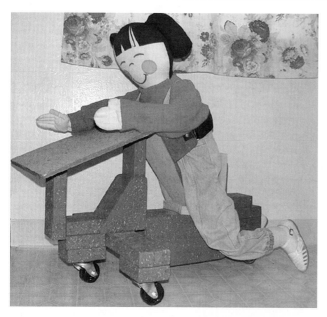

FIGURE 21-7 The aeroplane mobility device can be hand-made and is designed for children younger than 3 years of age.

Walkers

Children who have the ability to pull to a standing position maintain a grip on a handle, and steer with their arms may be able to use a *hand-held walker*. These walkers are designed for use either in front of *(anterior walker)* or behind *(posterior walker)* the child (Figure 21-9, *A*). Children with mild to moderate cerebral palsy or lower levels of spina bifida with leg bracing most commonly use hand-held walkers. Walkers can have three or four wheels and are available in various wheel sizes. The smaller the caster, the more difficult it is for use outdoors and over uneven surfaces. Posterior walkers are available with a feature in which the casters lock when the walker is pushed backward. This feature enables the child to stand and lean against the walker or the seat during rest periods. However, this feature makes maneuvering the walker more difficult because the child cannot move the walker in a reverse direction, which is needed when backing away and turning, without lifting it up to overcome the anti-rollback mechanism. Casters can be fixed rather than swiveled, which allows movement only in the forward direction so the user must lift the walker to turn it. Swivel casters allow the child to turn the walker without lifting it, but this feature requires more postural control from the child to direct the walker. The advantages of hand-held walkers are their low cost and convenient transportability.

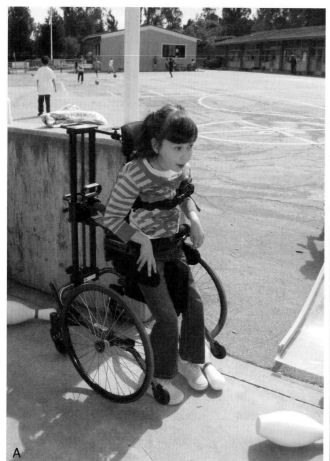

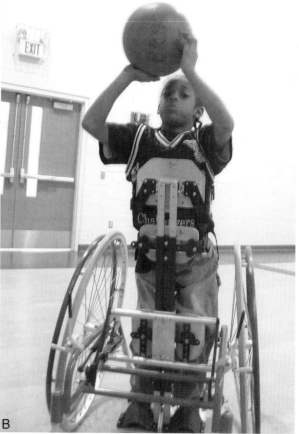

FIGURE 21-8 Mobile standers. **A,** The Dynamic Stander's large push wheels can be propelled by the child or easily removed to position the child close to a table or counter top. (Manufactured by Rifton.) **B,** The powered Standing Dani by Davis Made, a motorized standing device.

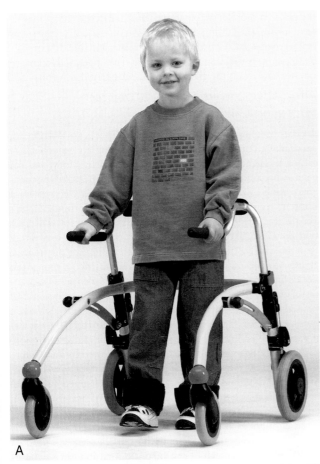

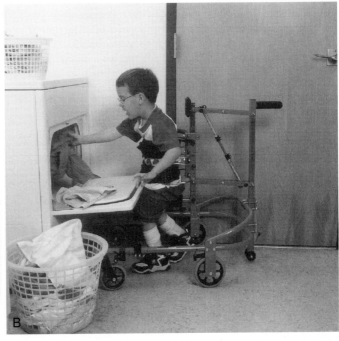

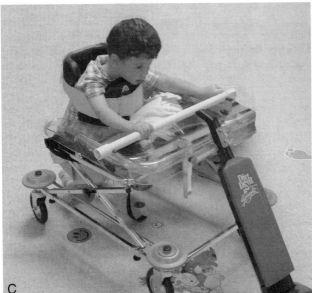

FIGURE 21-9 Walkers. **A,** The Crocodile posterior walker is designed for children from 2 to 14 years of age. (Manufactured by Snug Seat.) **B,** A young child helps with chores while using the Walkabout, a hands-free, weight-relieving walker. (Manufactured by Mulholland Positioning Systems, Inc.) **C,** A 2-year-old boy with spastic cerebral palsy uses the Pommel Walker in a forward pitch position, with a widely padded seat and a tray and hand grip to provide upper body support while pushing a toy vacuum. (Manufactured by Freedom Concepts.)

The disadvantages for some users include poor body alignment when pushing a walker and the fact that the hands are not free for performing tasks.

Support walkers are designed for children who have some ability to move their legs reciprocally but need support at the pelvis, chest, and possibly the upper extremities and head. It is critical to identify the purpose for using the support walker and in which environment it is to be used, to achieve maximum benefit for the child. If the purpose of the support walker is to provide self-initiated mobility for a child to access the indoor home environment, allowing the child to reach objects and people, then features should include wheels that are a minimum of 5 inches in diameter, which move more efficiently over carpets and thresholds than smaller wheels, and a design that does not include hardware, arm troughs, or a tray in front of the child, which would limit the ability to reach during exploratory activities (Figure 21-9, *B*). However, children with limited arm and hand function as a result of hypotonia or spasticity may require modifications to the support walker such as a tray, which limits getting close to objects and people, but encourages spatial awareness through movement (Figure 21-9, *C*).

Decisions regarding available options and features on a walker are made based on the child's physical function and the environment. Selection of appropriate features and adjustments that provide optimal positioning will increase functional use of these types of walkers. Children who adduct or scissor their legs as a result of spasticity may propel the walker more efficiently if a wider and longer padded seat is provided to reduce adduction and maintain leg alignment during ambulation. A young child with hypotonia or weakness may be more successful using a lightweight walker with all swivel casters over smooth flat surfaces such as linoleum (see Figure 21-2). Adjustable posterior tilt, a feature that positions the child slightly behind vertical, may also assist a weak child in maintaining an upright trunk and head position. Children with spastic cerebral palsy may need to be tilted in a slightly forward lean position, which along with a properly positioned pelvis (in neutral or anteriorly tilted position) assists in placing the feet behind the pelvis and trunk, thereby making it easier for the child to initiate movement in a forward direction. If the pelvis is not positioned optimally, the child's feet may move in front of the pelvis, allowing the child to only be able to push backwards.

Support walkers can provide children with the opportunity to explore their environment in an upright, hands-free position while providing capability for active range of motion. Therapists are being encouraged to promote more activity in children with cerebral palsy by using mobility-enhancing devices.[18] However, many support walkers have limitations in maneuverability, particularly indoors, because they require a large turning radius. The KidWalk is a new type of mobility system designed by an occupational therapist to promote use of the upper extremities during exploration.[51] It is designed with minimal hardware in front of the child so the child can use self-initiated mobility to be within arm's reach of people and objects to access and explore the environment and perform developmental activities such as pushing, pulling, opening and closing drawers, reaching, and carrying objects to achieve occupational therapy goals. The KidWalk allows a high degree of maneuverability, particularly over carpeted surfaces and thresholds, because of the placement of a large wheel located at the vector of the child's body, which also encourages rotation of the upper body over the pelvis, a more desirable movement. It incorporates a mechanism for weight shifting during ambulation and a dynamic swivel seat to encourage reciprocal leg movements and does not depend on upper body function to maneuver it. The upper body supports can be removed as the child develops balance and control.

Alternative Powered Mobility Devices for Young Children

A variety of alternative powered mobility devices are available for children who cannot achieve self-initiated mobility using reciprocal leg movements or by pushing large wheels. Motorized toy vehicles are available for children to provide early mobility experiences using a joystick; adapted models with special electronics for using up to four switches are also available. From the caregiver's perspective, the greatest advantage for use of these toy vehicles is that they look like a toy that any other child would use, rather than an assistive device. They are also an option for providing a child with the opportunity to learn how to drive a motorized device in preparation for using a power wheelchair. Disadvantages include difficulty using these vehicles indoors because of limited maneuverability; large size, which prevents the child from getting close to objects in the environment for reaching, exploring, and interacting with others; and sometimes noisy operation.

The MiniBot and the GoBot were developed by an occupational therapist (see Figure 21-3).[74,75] Each is a powered mobility device designed to enable physically challenged preschool children from 12 months to about 6 years of age to move in an upright position and explore the environment by getting close enough to objects and peers to reach and touch. It is intended for transitional mobility indoors or for use outdoors on flat surfaces. The child can be positioned in either a standing, semi-standing, or seated position. A joystick or multiple switches can be positioned at any location at which the child can reach the controls for driving the device. The MiniBot is not a power wheelchair; it is a therapeutic and educational tool intended to provide developmental opportunities equivalent to those experienced by able-bodied peers, such as pushing or pulling toys, kicking balls, moving quickly, moving slowly, and problem solving. The MiniBot is intended to increase the child's opportunities for hands-free exploration and provide new sensory experiences (particularly vestibular, visual motor, and spatial relations). The MiniBot is intended for children who would otherwise spend their early developmental years passively sitting in a stroller or manual wheelchair.

WHEELED MOBILITY SYSTEMS

Wheeled mobility systems include dependent mobility systems, independent manual mobility systems, and independent powered mobility systems. The first mobility system most children acquire is a stroller, which is considered to be a dependent mobility system because the user is depending on others for mobility. Parents often prefer the ease of use of a stroller and feel the appearance is more acceptable than that of a wheelchair when the child is very young.[15] A young child may be able to use a standard infant stroller, but if the seat does not provide supportive positioning, then a seating insert designed to provide support at the pelvis and trunk, such as the KidSert or Sit-to-Go, should be considered (Figure 21-10, *A*). Mobile positioning systems, which

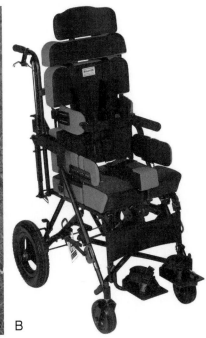

FIGURE 21-10   Strollers. **A,** The KidSert. **B,** The Mountee. (A and B, Manufactured by Convaid, Inc.)

provide more support than a stroller, while still being lightweight and easily foldable, are available through durable medical equipment providers. Some of these models, such as the Convaid Mountee, include bus or van anchors for transporting the child in a vehicle (Figure 21-10, *B*).

Other dependent seating and positioning systems offer an adjustable height chassis to position the child close to the floor or up to various table heights (Figure 21-11). The seating system is fully adjustable by the therapist to accommodate the needs of a variety of users so a custom seating system is not necessary. Dependent mobility systems can provide convenience for care providers and teachers, as well as optimal positioning for function. The seating system can also be removed on some models to transfer the seat to another type of base such as an outdoor base. The greatest disadvantage of a dependent mobility system is that the child must depend solely on others for mobility and has no means for self-initiated mobility and exploration. Dependent mobility systems that can be retrofitted into a larger wheel base should be considered if the team believes that the child will be able to self-propel within the next few years. Peers may also perceive an older child with a disability who uses a dependent mobility system such as a stroller, as being less able and less approachable than a child of similar age who sits in a wheelchair.

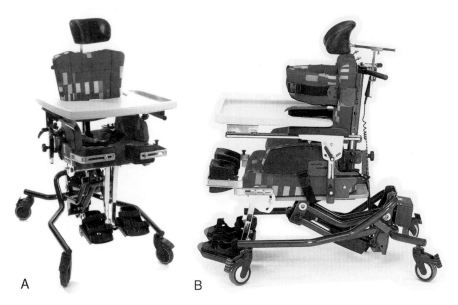

FIGURE 21-11   The Advance Contour Hi Low chair.

Manual Wheelchairs

Independent manual mobility systems include manual wheelchairs that allow the user to move independently by pushing two large wheels. A manual wheelchair is appropriate for a child who has the ability to functionally and efficiently propel it. It is also used as a means of transportation by caregivers or as a backup wheelchair when the child's power wheelchair is not working. Great strides in design and material selection have resulted in lighter frames than the standard 35-pound wheelchair (Figure 21-12, *A*). Weights can range as low as 14 pounds for lightweight, ultra-lightweight, and high-performance manual wheelchairs.[41] Manual wheelchairs for playing court sports such as tennis and basketball or racing are designed specifically for the sport.[16] These wheelchairs have a

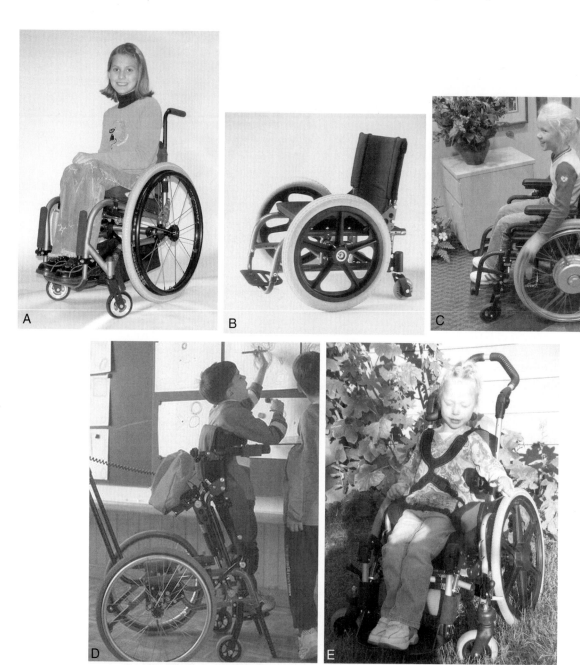

FIGURE 21-12   Manual wheelchairs. **A,** Chelsea, age 9 years with paraplegia at the L1 level, selects a TiLite TR for its features of lightweight, durability, and smooth ride. (Courtesy TiLite.) **B,** Quickie Kidz manual wheelchair features wider rear wheels for maximum pushing surface so that the chair can be propelled with either a push or pull motion. (Courtesy Sunrise Medical, Carlsbad, Calif.) **C,** Quickie Xtender provides power assist to a manual wheelchair by designing a motor unit into the hub of the quick release wheel. (Courtesy Sunrise Medical, Carlsbad, Calif.) **D,** The LEVO KID wheelchair provides a sit-to-stand feature in a manual wheelchair with the touch of a button. (Available through LEVO USA, Inc.) **E,** Kids ROCK wheelchair. (Manufactured by ART Group, a division of Sunrise Medical, Carlsbad, Calif.)

rigid frame and a high degree of camber in the rear wheels, and use small rollerblade-type casters in front.

Wheelchairs with large rear tires are most common, but models with large front tires and small back casters are available (Figure 21-12, *B*). Propelling a wheelchair with large front tires may be more efficient for the child because more surface area of the tire is exposed for gripping the wheel and pushing. However, the large front tires can limit access to the environment, such as when transferring and sitting at tables. The wheelchair with large front tires is also more difficult to push over curbs and uneven surfaces because of interference from the rear casters.

If the user has a single functional arm for wheelchair propulsion, such as a child with hemiplegia, an adapted manual wheelchair with a one-arm drive feature can provide independent mobility. The wheelchair is designed with two rims on the wheel the child uses to propel. One of the rims is connected through an axle to the other wheel. If either rim is pushed separately, it turns the wheelchair. If both rims are pushed simultaneously, the wheelchair moves forward or backwards. A manual wheelchair can also be propelled with the feet if the wheelchair has a low seat-to-floor height, known as *hemi-height*.

A power assist unit, designed into the hub of a special wheel attached to a manual wheelchair, provides the convenience of a manual wheelchair without the extra effort involved with propulsion (Figure 21-12, *C*). The LEVO Kid wheelchair includes a powered sit-to-stand feature, which can provide peer height interaction and the benefits of convenient standing throughout the day (Figure 21-12, *D*).

A new concept in mobility systems is the Kids ROCK active wheelchair, which provides dynamic seating for children with movement disorders such as children with cerebral palsy who posture into extension and find it difficult to be functional in a static seated position. The Kids ROCK active wheelchair allows the wheelchair seat to move when the child moves but maintains proper postural alignment and assists in reducing sacral sitting. When the child moves using hip and knee extension, the backrest reclines and the footrests move in an upward direction extending in a 35° range. When the child relaxes, the compressed springs move the backrest and footrests to the starting position (Figure 21-12, *E*).

Power Wheelchairs

Powered mobility wheelchairs have a motorized unit that the user operates by means of a joystick or alternative controls such as pneumatic sip-and-puff, ultrasonic head controls, proximity switches that operate by the user moving close to the switch but not touching it, or multiple push switches. If a child cannot propel a wheelchair long distances at the same speed and efficiency as demonstrated by the average person walking, then the therapist should consider recommending a power wheelchair to increase the child's independence and function. The advantages of a power wheelchair over a manual are increased speed capability, ease of maneuvering, and less energy expenditure required for moving, particularly for long distances. Some children who use a power wheelchair also have a manual wheelchair for use in environments that are not accessible to a power wheelchair or when the power wheelchair is being repaired.

Power wheelchairs are available in several styles with various options and are differentiated by the placement of the drive wheel, which may be mid-wheel (Figure 21-13, *A*), front-wheel (Figure 21-13, *B*), or rear-wheel drive (Figure 21-13, *C*). Attributes that are affected by the drive wheel position include maneuverability, stability, traction, and performance (speed, efficiency, obstacle climbing, and crossing a side slope). Maneuverability depends on the turning radius. Mid-wheel drive wheelchairs tend to have greater maneuverability because of the smaller turning radius.[37] Some mid-wheel power wheelchair manufacturers claim to have a 19-inch turning radius, versus a minimum 33-inch radius with a rear-wheel drive. However, mid-wheel drive wheelchairs require a third set of stabilizing caster wheels, which may extend up to 17 inches behind the user. This feature may make it difficult for users to turn around without catching the casters on objects, particularly if spatial awareness is not optimal.

Front-wheel drive works well over various types of terrain, uphill and downhill, because the power in front wheels pulls the user over obstacles. Children who have used a rear-wheel drive wheelchair may find maneuvering a front-wheel drive wheelchair more challenging because the back end of the wheelchair may fishtail at higher speeds. The recent trend in power wheelchair design is to provide a full suspension system in the front and rear casters or tires. This allows the user to move over a variety of terrains and drive up 3-inch curbs, even at slow speeds.

Standard rear-wheel drive wheelchairs are optimal for children who have limited vision and spatial awareness difficulty, because most of the wheelchair hardware is within their field of vision. Most wheelchair manufacturers provide a choice of several models that are intended for joystick operation and models that include sophisticated microcomputer electronics for alternative input methods for driving and for remotely operating environmental devices. Features of power wheelchair electronics can accommodate the needs of various users. Such features include adjustments for torque, tremor damping for children having difficulty directing the joystick, a short-throw joystick option for users with muscle weakness who do not have the strength to push the joystick to its end range, speed adjustments, and acceleration settings so that the wheelchair can be set to increase speed rapidly or gradually. Some manufacturers now offer electronics, such as the True Track Technology (Invacare Corp.), that enable the wheelchair to track straight on slopes and uneven surfaces. Speeds can be as high as 15 mph, but typically range from 3 to 10 mph. Distance traveled on one battery charge can be as far as 25 miles.

Several features can be made available on power wheelchairs to increase a child's function and level of independence. Technology-dependent children who require oxygen support can become mobile by using portable ventilator carts attached to the wheelchair.[5] Another useful feature for accessing the environment enables the child to independently move from a sitting to a standing position and drive around while standing (Figure 21-14, *A*). A powered elevating seat, which raises the child to various heights for greater accessibility in the environment, is also available (Figure 21-14, *B*). Additional features include power tilt-in-space, which tilts the seat backward to about 45° while maintaining the same seat-to-back angle (Figure 21-14, *C*), and power recline, which places the child in the supine position by reclining the back of the chair. These two features are useful for individuals who need frequent relief

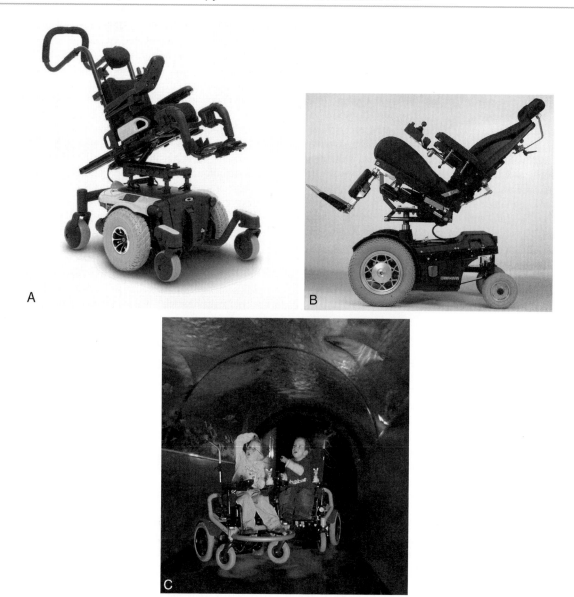

FIGURE 21-13 Power wheelchairs. **A,** Q610. **B,** Permobil 450. (Courtesy of Permobil, Lebanon, Tenn.) **C,** Skippi power wheelchair. (Manufactured by Otto Bock.)

of pressure under their buttocks, such as those with spinal cord injury and muscle weakness or for those with hip, back, and neck pain.

Power wheelchairs are typically controlled with a joystick. A proportional joystick allows the driver to increase acceleration and speed of the wheelchair in relation to the distance the joystick is moved. The farther the user pushes the proportional joystick, the more rapidly the wheelchair moves. A nonproportional joystick (digital or microswitch) does not affect the wheelchair's speed; any amount of force used to push the joystick results in the same speed. An attendant joystick is another option for a power wheelchair. It is typically a small joystick mounted to the back of the wheelchair and is accessed by the caregivers who need to drive the power wheelchair when accuracy is required, such as moving up a narrow ramp.

Power wheelchairs do not typically fold for transporting in a vehicle. Accessible vans that have been modified with a lift are required for transporting the user and power wheelchair in a vehicle. However, there is a pediatric power wheelchair, the Skippi from Otto Bock, that can be disassembled so that it can be transported in a vehicle without the need for a van (see Figure 21-13, *C*). If the child can be transferred to a car seat, a covered trailer can be hitched to the back of a vehicle for transporting a power wheelchair.

Three-wheeled scooters are another option for powered mobility. The individual who uses a scooter typically has good sitting balance, requires minimal positioning adaptation, and can understand and physically operate the tiller handle bar controls.

A manual wheelchair can be converted to a power wheelchair by purchasing an add-on unit that includes two motors that are placed on the tires to rotate them, batteries, an electronic control unit, and a joystick. The electronic controls for the add-on units are not as sophisticated or adjustable as those found on

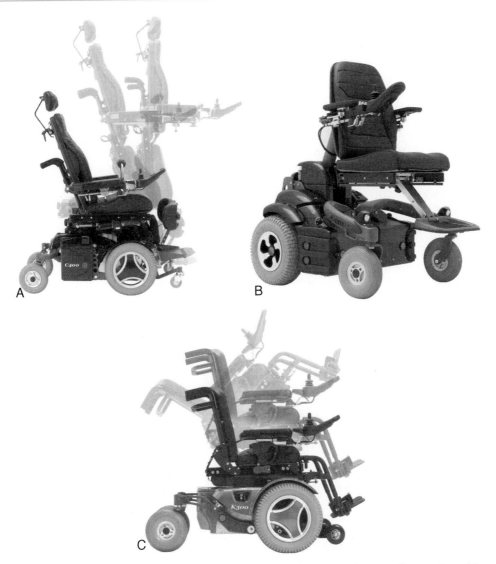

FIGURE 21-14 Useful features for a power wheelchair. **A,** The Chairman 2 K Stander. Standing can be achieved from a sitting position or gradually from supine. **B,** K450 from Permobil Playman Robo's seat will lower to the ground and elevate, covering a total of 25 inches height difference for vertical mobility. (Lebanon, Tenn.) **C,** Permobil K300 PS Jr. with tilt. Chairman 2 K front-wheel drive power wheelchair with the Corpus seating system and 45° of tilt in space. (A-C, Courtesy Permobil, Lebanon, Tenn.)

standard power wheelchairs. This makes it more difficult for some children with impaired motor responses to accurately operate the chair. Add-on units are also not highly recommended for individuals who use their wheelchairs outdoors and over rough terrain because they are not designed to withstand the forces that a power wheelchair must endure.

The power wheelchairs today offer sophisticated electronics that provide opportunities to integrate mobility with augmentative communication devices and electronic aids to daily living (EADLs) so the child can turn on lights, operate the television, and access a computer through the power wheelchair electronics.

Selection of Wheelchair Features

If a child will be independently propelling a manual wheelchair, it is critical that the wheelchair and seating be designed to allow use of proper biomechanics for efficient propulsion.

The therapist achieves this by selecting the proper size of wheelchair frame and an appropriate seating system. Most wheelchair manufacturers include wheelchair growth kits, which accommodate the need to widen or lengthen the frame without entirely replacing the wheelchair. The therapist must select a wheelchair that fits the child's present needs, rather than a wheelchair that is too large with the goal that the child will "grow into" it. A wheelchair that is too wide is more difficult for the child to propel. If the seat is too long, the child's pelvis cannot achieve a neutral position; it will be pulled into a posterior tilt, reducing upper extremity function and causing the child to sit on the sacrum with a rounded back, which contributes to the risk of sliding out of the seat.

The therapist simultaneously considers what type of seating or positioning system is needed and how it will interface with the mobility base for optimal function and performance. For example, in ordering a seat cushion, the child's functional mobility skills, the frame size of the manual wheelchair, and the desirable seat to floor height must be considered. If the cushion is placed on top of the wheelchair frame, the child may be positioned too far from the wheels for reaching and propelling them efficiently. To prevent this situation, the therapist will need to consider the height of the wheelchair seat when ordering the cushion; a workable alternative in this instance is a narrower cushion that can be recessed into the wheelchair frame.

Another common situation that reinforces the need to assess seating and wheelchair mobility simultaneously is recommending a backrest cushion for a child without considering the features of the wheelchair. The cushion may position the child too far forward of the axle's wheel. If the child's center of gravity is forward of the rear wheels instead of directly over the rear wheel axle, propulsion is more difficult and inefficient. Many wheelchairs have a standard axle plate where the hub of the wheel is mounted to the frame and the wheels cannot be relocated within the child's reach. However, if the therapist recommends an adjustable axle plate for the wheelchair in combination with the appropriate front caster size, the wheels can be relocated and mounted in the best location for the child to reach the wheels for propulsion.

Wheelchair features are recommended based on needs in the areas of mobility (being able to reach and propel the wheels of a manual wheelchair or reach the floor to propel with the feet), accessibility (moving through doorways, maneuvering in small spaces, and fitting under tables), transfer techniques (dependent or independent), seating and positioning, communication (which may include mounting a speech-generating device to the wheelchair), and transportation (if the child will be transported while sitting in the wheelchair; in a motor vehicle certain transportation options will need to be included on the wheelchair). The features available in a manual wheelchair that may affect the child's posture and function include the ability to mount an appropriate seating system and options such as tilt-in-space, recline, and capability for multiple axle positions for adjusting the wheel location.

Wheelchairs are available in standard or custom sizes as measured by the seat width and depth, height of the seat from the floor, and backrest height. The therapist must carefully consider features and options on wheelchairs and select the wheelchair to accommodate the child's growth and physical and functional needs as well as the needs of the caregivers. The therapist should begin selection of a wheelchair by evaluating and documenting the child's current physical and functional abilities, with consideration of physical changes that may occur and the positioning and mobility goals for the child. Wheelchair selection depends on the type of seating and positioning system the individual requires. For example, if a child needs to sit with a medial thigh pad or abductor to keep the knees apart, then a wider space between the leg rest hangers will be required. Wheelchairs are typically designed with equal clearance between the footrest hangers, but some models have a narrower, tapered footrest hanger. A tapered footrest hanger will not be appropriate for a child who needs to sit with an abducted leg position. The therapist must also consider the environments in which the child will use the wheelchair, what method the child will use for propelling the wheelchair, how the caregivers will transport it, and the sources of funding. The therapist is often responsible for providing a medical justification for the seating and mobility system.

Once the child's needs have been identified, the therapist matches them to the specific features available in a wheelchair. If a child cannot shift weight independently and is at risk for developing pressure-related problems, then a wheelchair with a pressure relief cushion and either a manual or powered tilt-in-space feature may be necessary to shift weight from under the buttocks to the back (see Figure 21-14, C). The manual tilt-in-space feature allows the caregiver to activate a lever that allows the frame of the wheelchair to be tilted backwards while the seating positioning system maintains the same seat-to-back angle. This differs from a reclining wheelchair, which opens the seat-to-back angle so that the person is lying supine with hip extension. Powered tilt-in-space is an option available on either manual or power wheelchairs so that the user has independent control of tilting the frame. The therapist must be aware of the impact that the tilt-in-space position may have on a child's field of vision. When tilted backwards, the child's visual field will be in an upward direction toward the ceiling. In this position the child will need to flex his or her head forward to view the surroundings. A tilted position may also stimulate the sleep mechanism rather than placing the child more upright in a "work-ready" position. A tilt-in-space feature can also provide a few degrees of anterior tilt to position the child slightly forward, which may encourage trunk and neck extension for a more work-ready position.

The therapist should consider the following wheelchair features:

- *Style of frame:* Folding manual wheelchair (has lots of flexibility; folds side to side or forward onto the seat); non-folding or rigid manual wheelchair (lightest weight, has "tightest" responsive ride, back folds down, and wheels are removable); modular folding (frames come apart, separating the seating system from the base, which folds for manual and power wheelchairs); modular non-folding (can be disassembled into several parts for manual and power wheelchairs).
- *Tilt-in-space:* Tilt adjusts the seat backward as an entire unit while maintaining the same seat-to-back angle. It can be manual or powered for independent operation by the user. Tilt ranges are 45° to 65°. Tilt can accommodate users with insufficient head and trunk control, individuals who require pressure relief under the pelvis, or those with back or hip pain. The greater the degree of tilt, the more weight is distributed from the pelvis to the back.
- *Recline:* Recline positions the user in a reclined position in which the seat-to-back angle opens from the seated angle to about 170°. It can be operated manually by a caregiver or operated with power by the user. Some children with gastrointestinal issues may need to recline after a meal. This feature may also assist the care provider by allowing a reclined position for diaper changes.
- *Footrest style:* Footrests support the user's feet and may act as a step for transfer in and out. Features include single plate or double plate, fixed, pull-up, swing-in or swing-out, and manual and powered elevating leg rests. The typical angle of footrests is 70° or 90° to accommodate fixed positions of the legs and feet. Many children sit more upright with 90° footrest hangers to accommodate tight hamstring muscles. If footplates are too far in front, placing a stretch on tight hamstrings, the pelvis will be pulled into a sacral sit position, thereby promoting a rounded trunk,

which will adversely affect the child's head position. Footrest hangers that are angled less than 90° make the length of the wheelchair frame longer, thereby decreasing maneuverability in tight places.

- *Armrest style:* Armrest styles can be full length, which makes it difficult to get close to a table or desk, or arm length, which incorporates a notched area in the frame of the armrest for getting under surfaces. Armrests can be height adjustable, fixed or removable, with pull-out or swing-away option. Some users may benefit from wider, contoured armrest pads for more arm support, particularly when using a joystick for driving a power wheelchair.
- *Backrest height:* A high backrest may be needed to support the seating and positioning needs of a client with a severe disability or for tilt and recline. A low backrest may be more functional for a client with good upper body function. A backrest that ends at the top of the shoulders is preferred so an adjustable height-contoured headrest can be positioned under the child's occiput.
- *Backrest adjustability:* An angle-adjustable back provides the ability to set the seat-to-back angle to accommodate the child's position. A child who extends or pushes backwards may benefit from a decreased back angle, whereas a child who is hypotonic and has difficulty maintaining a vertical head position may benefit from a greater than 90° seat-to-back angle.
- *Height and adjustability features* of push handles for the adult pushing the wheelchair.
- *Floor-to-seat height:* Seat height is important for transfers and getting under surfaces like tables. A lower seat height is typically preferred for younger children, particularly if a seating system will be integrated into the chair, which may raise the user higher.
- *Style and location of wheel locks or brakes.*
- *Type, size, and placement of wheels and casters* on a manual wheelchair for maximum efficiency during propulsion and to accommodate weight distribution: An adjustable axle plate can provide individualized wheel placement for the child to reach the tire. This may also assist children who are positioned forward of the push wheel because of a short seat depth, which places too much weight over the forward casters, thereby increasing resistance during propulsion. Tires can be pneumatic (air filled for a cushioned ride), semi-pneumatic (gel insert for flat-free maintenance), or solid (no maintenance but provides the stiffest ride and may add extra weight).
- *Additional features* include sit-to-stand in a manual wheelchair (see Figure 21-12, *D*) or a power wheelchair, whereby the child can move independently from a seated position to standing. The advantage of this feature is the ability to reach various heights, bear weight, and stretch throughout the day, and for some boys, the efficiency of standing without needing to transfer for toileting needs, as when using a urinal.

POWERED MOBILITY EVALUATION AND INTERVENTION

The therapist, teacher, child, and caregivers must first define the goals for using a powered mobility device. Are the goals to provide functional and independent home, school, and community mobility, or are the goals to provide transitional mobility experiences so that the child can have new opportunities to learn how to move, explore, and interact within the environment? Maneuverability features of the powered device are important in considering the various environments in which the device will be used (e.g., such as indoors in limited spaces such as a classroom or home, outdoors over rough terrain, or on a playground). What are the table heights the child's chair must fit under at school, the home, and community? If it is necessary for the child to reach various heights in the wheelchair, then a powered lift seat may be justified. Will the child need the ability to tilt in space or recline? How is the child transferred into and out of the wheelchair? How will the mobility device be transported? Will it need to be disassembled to fit inside the trunk of a vehicle? If the wheelchair is to be transported in a van, is head clearance sufficient for the child when entering the vehicle and can the wheelchair be secured to the van for transport? Will the environments need to be made accessible with ramps into doorways or powered lifts into vehicles?

The next consideration is to determine how the child will access or drive the power wheelchair, and which power wheelchairs provide the control interface methods that the child needs now and may need in the near future, if there is a change in motor performance. The therapist begins an evaluation of the child's ability to drive a power wheelchair by assessing the child's position to determine how to optimize motor function for efficient and accurate access of the controls. It may be necessary to use an evaluation seating system or interim modifications to the child's own seating system during the powered mobility evaluation. The child must feel secure, comfortable, and stable, particularly in the pelvis, trunk, and head, before attempting to operate a power wheelchair.

A joystick is the standard and often the preferred method for the individual who can maneuver it efficiently and accurately. The user can operate a joystick using a hand, foot, forearm, chin, head pointer, or even the back of the head, by using an adaptation that connects the joystick to a bracket that is attached to a moveable headrest. Some children may find it difficult to accurately use a joystick placed in its traditional location at the front end of the armrest. These children may have better motor control if the joystick is placed inside the armrest, in midline, or rotated several degrees toward the body (Case Study 21-2). A micro-joystick, or attendant joystick, which is smaller in size than a standard joystick, may be necessary for these types of situations and are available for most power wheelchairs. The small joystick is easier to position in midline or under the chin. Another feature that can assist in improving control or efficiency during joystick use is a support (such as a wide armrest or trough) under the elbow, forearm, or wrist. If the child has difficulty moving the joystick in the desired direction, the therapist can place a template with a cross shape cut out inside the control box to limit deviation of the joystick to the desired directions. The therapist can also position the joystick with proper hardware to another location, in which control be enhanced. During the evaluation for joystick operation, the therapist not only must evaluate the positioning needs of the child and placement of the joystick, but must consider the type of joystick, type of joystick knob, and desired location of the on-off switch for either independent access or may unintentional access by the user.

CASE STUDY 21-2   Trevor

Trevor, a 4-year-old child who is unable to communicate, was having difficulty driving the power wheelchair using a joystick placed at the end of his right armrest. The teacher questioned Trevor's ability to drive safely and accurately, believing that bumping into objects was purposeful. The occupational therapist observed Trevor's arm and hand movements and noted that he seemed to have difficulty pushing the joystick forward and to the right side. He tended to internally rotate his arm and pull it toward his body. The joystick was then mounted on an adjustable bracket that positioned it in midline, close to his chest. The midline position also enabled the joystick box to be rotated about 30° toward his body. After several more attempts at driving, Trevor's accuracy improved immediately. Once the most reliable placement was located, he became a functional driver.

Joystick knobs are available in various styles, shapes, and sizes to accommodate various hand and wrist positions. The most common shapes are round, T-shaped, and I-shaped. A child with weakness of the upper extremities may find it more efficient to use a U-shaped joystick so that the hand is supported in the palm and at the sides. Joysticks can be highly sensitive, such that they require only slight movement of one finger, which may be useful for a child with muscle disease. Selection of the most appropriate style of joystick and its placement directly affects the ability to accurately and efficiently drive a power wheelchair. Case Study 21-3 provides an example of a child whose position is evaluated for more accurate use of a powered mobility device.

Children with severe physical disabilities may be able to operate a power wheelchair but often are not given the opportunity because they are physically unable to operate a joystick. Alternative control interfaces or access methods are available for these individuals.

If a child does not have the physical ability to control a joystick with the hand, foot, or head, the therapist should consider alternative control interfaces or access methods such as switch operation, particularly for individuals with cerebral palsy. Switch access of a powered mobility device is typically achieved using three or four switches, one for each direction of movement. Various types of switches can be placed at the hand, head, elbows, or feet, where the child has the most reliable, accurate, and efficient movements. Before selecting the type of switch, the therapist should determine the movements that the child can use to access a switch. If the child can nod "yes" and "no," then he or she may have the ability to use switches around the back of the head.

The therapist may need to evaluate switch placement by allowing the child to first use switches to operate modified battery-operated toys.[72] The therapist first identifies the most reliable and efficient movements that the child can voluntarily use to access the switches. Switch placement should begin at the hands and proceed to the head, elbows, knees, feet, and any other location determined appropriate. An adjustable mounting bracket, such as that available through AbleNet Incorporated, is extremely helpful for positioning a switch in multiple locations.

Switches are either momentary or latched. Momentary switches require the user to maintain contact on the switch to activate it. The child needs to be able to maintain contact on the switch long enough to move the wheelchair in a desired direction. A latching mode allows the user to press the switch one time to activate it, rather than holding it in the "on" position. A second activation turns the switch "off." If the child needs to use switches to drive a power wheelchair, at least three switch sites are preferred: for driving forward and turning both directions. Reverse can be operated by a fourth switch or the adult. If the child can operate only one or two switches, the therapist may need to consider a scanning method; however, the scanning method requires a higher degree of cognitive function and concentration because of the complexity of the task.

An input method used frequently by individuals with spinal cord injuries is pneumatic sip-and-puff, which the user activates by gently inhaling or exhaling into a straw-like device held in the mouth. Another alternative method is the head-switch sensing array from Adapted Switch Labs, which consists of proximity switches embedded into a headrest that detect head movements for driving the wheelchair. These switches are operated not by making contact on the switch, but rather by getting close or proximal to the switch. The same switches can be embedded in a wheelchair lap tray so the child waves an arm above each switch to operate the wheelchair.

The Tongue Touch Keypad by New Abilities is a custom-made retainer in which small switches are embedded. The user activates each switch by touching it with the tongue. Multiple switch access is available in which push switches are placed around the body part that is able to reach the switches. The wheelchair is driven in one of four directions, depending on which switch is activated. It is even possible for the individual to drive a power wheelchair with one switch that operates a scanning light on a display. A recent development is the use of an interface tablet steering device to navigate a power wheelchair.[50]

Once the therapist has determined an accurate and reliable motor response, the child can assess the switch on a powered mobility device. However, the quality of motor control and accuracy is directly dependent on the child's body position and the extent to which the position influences stability, mobility, muscle tone, and energy expenditure. Therefore, an evaluation of power wheelchair mobility control must simultaneously include a seating evaluation to determine how the child's motor control is influenced by body position.

Several factors can interfere with a person's ability to drive a powered mobility device. If a child has difficulty, the occupational therapist should first consider if the wheelchair, electronics, and interface, such as switches, are working properly. The brakes must be released and the wheels must be engaged. If the child continues to have difficulty, the type and placement of the controls should be reevaluated. Simultaneously, the therapist evaluates the child's position to determine whether changes in the child's posture influence motor control. Other considerations include undetected visual and perceptual difficulties, impairment in hearing, processing and response time, seizures, motivation, and behavior. Children with visual impairment often find it difficult to drive a power wheelchair outdoors in bright sun, preferring to do so indoors in large areas such as a clinic or classroom.

Many children may not initially be successful using a power wheelchair because of the overwhelming amount and degree of sensory input that is required. Imagine being a child with

Amanda is a 9-year-old girl who has a diagnosis of cerebral palsy quadriplegia with athetosis (Figure 21-15). Her trunk stability is limited such that she cannot sit independently; she extends her hips and back, causing her to slide forward in her seat; she has minimal control of arm and hand movements but can voluntarily move her arms towards her side; she has fair to good head movements when her pelvis and trunk are stable. Efficient and reliable operation of a power wheelchair is not possible because the positioning seat belt slips, causing her to slide forward on the seat, adversely affecting motor control of her arms and head. She now sits in a custom seating system comprised of a contoured seat cushion, which is soft under the pelvis and moderately firm under her thighs to reduce extensor thrust posturing, a biangular back cushion with lateral hip and trunk pads, an occipital neck rest, and a sub-ASIS (defined below) padded bar.[43] The seat belt alone did not provide a stable pelvis that she needed to reduce extraneous body and head movements. The sub-ASIS bar is placed across the lap where the seat belt would be placed. It is hinged on one end of the seat cushion and connects to a bracket on the other end, which provides consistent but comfortable hip placement. It is positioned just below (sub) the anterior superior iliac spine (ASIS) of her pelvis, which provides a consistent pelvic position and, therefore, upper body position, rather than depending solely on a positioning belt, which loosens and allows her pelvis to slide forward on the seat, decreasing stability and increasing extraneous movements.

These seating components have increased her stability such that she can move her head accurately to activate three proximity switches from Adaptive Switch Labs (ASL) to drive a power wheelchair. She is able to independently access two switches placed on the side of her armrest to change modes of operation for speed and moving in reverse. A third switch placed on the right side of her armrest allows her to turn her wheelchair on and off independently. She accesses her augmentative communication device, a Vmax by DynaVox mounted to her power wheelchair, by using a head tracking–mouse emulation method that uses a camera to track her head movements. She wears a reflective dot on her forehead, which the camera tracks while she moves her head to position the cursor on the screen over a letter or symbol. Her communication device can also be programmed to work remotely with electronic devices around her house. She can use it as a universal remote for her television and DVD player and operate light switches in a room. She also has access to a telephone with an additional accessory on her Vmax.

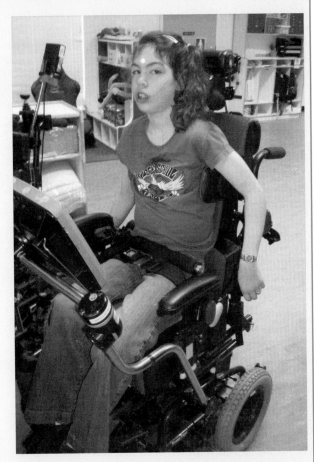

FIGURE 21-15   11-year-old girl in Power Tiger from ASL.

a severe disability who has difficulty with motor planning, coordination, visual perception, and communication, and is experiencing movement in a powered device for the first time. It would be overwhelming to experience the excitement and vestibular sensation of moving while trying to view the surroundings, which are quickly passing by, and simultaneously listen to an adult telling you how and where to move.

The therapist should assess a young child for powered mobility, whenever feasible, by providing a method that promotes exploration, problem solving, and self-learning for the child. Such a method requires an open space with activities and toys strategically placed around the room to facilitate experiences in movement and exploration.

The therapist should "limit physical and verbal commands as much as possible to avoid sensory overload on the part of the child" (p. 85).[60] If a child is trying to move toward an object, the therapist should state the desired outcome, such as "come closer," rather than specific commands, such as "push the joystick left" or "push the red switch and come over here." Feedback should also be positive, such as "you found the wall," rather than "oops, you crashed again."[73] If further assistance is needed to help the child understand the operation of the control, the therapist can facilitate the proper response by physically guiding the child's movements for the desired response. The therapist must understand that children respond to visual, auditory, and sensory demands at different rates. A child with spastic cerebral palsy or quadriplegia may require much longer to make a visual motor response than a child with athetoid cerebral palsy, a spinal cord injury or muscle disease.

The most common method for evaluating a person's ability to use a powered mobility device is to have the device available for trial use during the evaluation. A facility typically cannot afford to purchase power wheelchairs for evaluation purposes. Fortunately, ATPs often lend power wheelchairs to a clinical therapy unit for short-term evaluation purposes. The positioning and mobility equipment with the specific features that the child will need to operate the device should be available during the evaluation. Equipment used during an evaluation should be in optimal working condition. The therapist should begin the evaluation by test-driving the equipment to learn the forces and movements required to drive it, select the best speed for the client, and set any other adjustments, such as sensitivity of the controls.

It may also be beneficial to lend or rent a power wheelchair to children and their families for an extended evaluation. This allows more time for the child to learn how to use the controls and for the family to become familiar with the features of a power wheelchair to assist them in becoming more informed consumers. It also provides an opportunity for the family to experience the responsibilities of maintaining and transporting a power wheelchair.

Computer programs are also available for powered mobility assessment and training.[59] R. J. Cooper and Associates has developed a joystick and mouse training program and a wheelchair simulation program. The programs display a power wheelchair on the screen that the user must navigate through a maze or room. Hasdai, Jessel, and Weiss studied whether a driving simulator would help a child master skills that are comparable with those required to drive a power wheelchair.[33] Their results indicated benefits from using such a program to prepare children for powered mobility.

Researchers have explored the use of virtual reality for assessing and training powered mobility skills.[67] The user wears a helmet that has a screen display of a three-dimensional room through which the person must navigate by using a joystick. More research is needed to determine if virtual reality is an effective means for assessing and training powered mobility and to determine whether children will integrate the skills of wheelchair driving if they have not participated in the actual task.

SEATING AND POSITIONING

Positioning is critical to the successful use of any mobility device because posture and task performance are interrelated.[16] How an individual is positioned in a mobility device, whether it be standing or sitting, can have an effect on several physiologic factors, including visual and motor performance, postural control,[45] ranges of movement, muscle tone,[47] endurance, comfort, respiration, and digestion. These factors can affect functional performance activities such as hand function,[48] levels of independence in mobility, self-care, activities of daily living (ADLs) such as transfers, and social interaction with others.[35]

Understanding the Biomechanics of Seating

To identify the positioning needs of a child, the occupational therapist must first have a thorough understanding of the biomechanical forces and neurophysiologic factors that can influence posture and movement. Biomechanical considerations are critical to obtaining proper alignment of the pelvis, spine, and head when postures are flexible or when accommodating individuals who no longer have active or passive range of motion as a result of contractures. The position and stability of the pelvis provide a foundation for movements that occur above and below the pelvis. Box 21-1 presents exercises that stress the importance of good alignment in sitting. Neurophysiologic factors include the child's reaction to tactile input, body reactions to orientation in space, and movement.

Seating Guidelines

Optimal seating provides a stable place for the child's pelvis and spine, from which a range of controlled movements for achieving functional tasks can occur. Seating is not static. Rather, it is a series of active movements or postures an individual uses to accomplish a series of motor tasks, such as maintaining the pelvis, trunk, and head upright against gravity while using the movements of the eyes, arms, and hands to access the controls of a power wheelchair or push the wheels of a manual wheelchair. For this reason, a series of postures must be made available to the child, not by restraining the child with straps and harnesses, but rather by supporting and guiding the child's movements with an appropriate seating and mobility system. The occupational therapist needs to

---

BOX 21-1 Exercises to Understand the Biomechanics of Seating

SITTING IN POSTERIOR PELVIC TILT
While in a sitting position, place your hands on the anterior crest of your pelvis (the two hip bones). Bend forward by rounding your back. You will feel your pelvis rolling backward into a posteriorly tilted position. Hold your pelvis in this position and try to sit upright by extending your back. You may be able to move your head upright, but moving your trunk into a vertical position is dependent on placing your pelvis in a neutral or anteriorly tilted position. To view your environment with your pelvis in the posteriorly tilted position, you would need to either hyperextend your neck (an undesirable position) or slide your pelvis forward in the seat until your head achieves an upright position. Try maintaining a rounded or kyphotic back position and slide your pelvis forward in the seat. Feel the excessive pressure at the cervical and upper thoracic levels and the coccyx. Imagine being positioned like this for hours at a time and experiencing the discomfort, fatigue, and limited range of your upper extremities if you were in a wheelchair without a proper positioning system to improve or accommodate your posture.

PELVIC POSITION STABILITY
Place your buttocks at the edge of your seat, lean only onto one side of your pelvis, and lift your feet so they are unsupported. Hold your pencil at its top edge and try to write. It is difficult to perform accurate and efficient movements of your arm and hands because you do not have a stable base for the movements to occur. Imagine trying to accurately and safely operate the joystick of a power wheelchair in this position.

consider the biomechanical forces of an individual's movements to determine what may be contributing to undesirable postures and, therefore, limited function.

The goals of seating are to provide optimal alignment and stability to improve distal motor function while minimizing undesirable tone and reflexes that interfere with alignment and stability; distribute seated pressures to maintain skin integrity; improve physiologic function such as breathing, swallowing, and digestion; increase independence in ADLs, and provide comfort.

The key points in achieving functional seating are the position and stability of the pelvis. A pelvis in a slight anterior tilt or neutral position is preferred. The angle of hip flexion can also affect postural control in sitting. Children with extensor tone may have a reduction of muscle tone with less than 90° of hip flexion combined with hip abduction. Stability at the pelvis can be achieved through contact points around the pelvis. These include the surfaces under, at the sides, and on top of the pelvis. The therapist must determine how a child responds to various types of seat surfaces and contours under the pelvis such as a flat seat surface or a contoured seat (a seat cushion that provides a recessed pocket for the pelvis and blocks forward movement of the ischial tuberosities).

The three types of seating surfaces are planar, contoured, and custom molded. *Planar seating* consists of flat surfaces with no contours. This type of seating may be more appropriate for individuals with mildly affected development who require only minimal body contact with the support surfaces of the seat. *Contoured seating* systems allow the body to have more contact with the support surface because its shape conforms to the curves of the spine, buttocks, and thighs. A contoured seat can be fabricated by layering various densities of foam that respond to the shape and weight of the person, thereby contouring around the bony prominences and other body curves. The therapist can recommend a standard size contoured back and seat cushion that can be adjusted to fit individual needs (Figure 21-16, *A*). *Custom-molded seat cushions* are designed specifically for an individual by taking an impression of the body and making a mold, which is sent to the manufacturer for fabrication (Figure 21-16, *B*). Another method uses a computer-generated graphic picture taken from the impression, which is sent to the manufacturer, which then uses a computer-assisted milling machine to fabricate the cushions.

Cushions can also be custom molded using foam-in-bag technology, in which liquid foam is poured into an upholstered bag that is positioned around the person's body, providing a molded cushion that is then upholstered. This technique is more difficult to use because the individual's position must be held in place while the foam is being formed. If the child moves, the quality of the foam mold is negatively affected.

The therapist can also improve stability of the pelvis and trunk by ensuring that the femur is properly supported along its entire length, from the back of the pelvis to approximately 1 inch from the popliteal area under the knee. One exception is to use a much shorter seat depth for a client who can propel a wheelchair using the legs and feet. In this situation, a shorter seat with a slight anterior tilt would be preferred. Some individuals require support at the sides of the pelvis to maintain a symmetrical position and reduce pelvic shift to either side. Support at the sides of the pelvis can be contoured into the seat or added as lateral hip guides. Stability can be provided above the pelvis to reduce sliding in an upward and forward direction. The therapist typically accomplishes this by placing a positioning belt at a 45° angle to the seat or closer to the thighs. A new device for dynamically positioning the pelvis while allowing for functional pelvic movements is the Hip Grip Pelvic Stabilization Device from Body Point (Figure 21-17). Made of a contoured padded harness, the Hip-Grip attaches to the lower part of the wheelchair backrest and around the

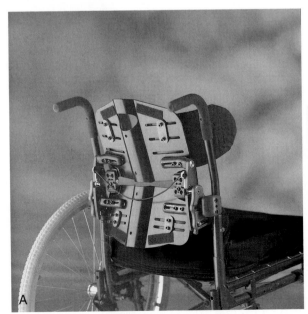
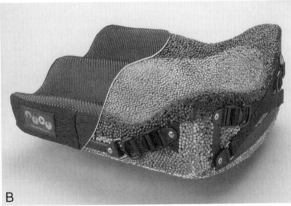

FIGURE 21-16   **A,** Infinity DualFlex 10 by Invacare. The Infinity DualFlex 10 is a modular seating system that accommodates a wide range of position needs. **B,** Ride designs cushion can be custom molded for an individual. (A, Courtesy Invacare, Elyria, Ohio.)

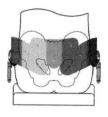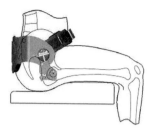

FIGURE 21-17 Hip Grip, a dynamic pelvic stabilization device. (Available through Bodypoint Inc.; http://www.body-point.com.)

sacral area of the pelvis. A positioning belt with sub-ASIS pads is secured in front of the pelvis. A rotational mechanism at the sides of the HipGrip maintains postural stability while allowing the user to move the pelvis in the anterior and posterior directions, as when reaching or propelling the wheelchair. Other components, such as footplates, lap trays, arm rests or arm troughs, a contoured backrest, and headrests, can provide additional support to the pelvis and trunk.

The use of orthotics, or devices for bracing the extremities or body, may also assist in achieving optimal positioning in the seated and standing positions. Ankle-foot orthoses are most commonly recommended to align the foot and ankle and assist in either reducing muscle tone or supporting a weak limb. A thoracic-lumbar-sacral orthosis (TLSO), or body jacket, may be another alternative for individuals with scoliosis to use for support in the seated position.

Young children who exhibit an increase in extensor movements and asymmetry when being evaluated for a seating system may benefit from using a "barrier" vest as proposed by Kangas.[39] The vest is made from Plastazote foam, which is not strong enough to totally support the child and does allow the child to have some movement. It is worn to decrease the child's sensitivity to individual points of contact from hands touching the body during handling or from pads on a seating system, which can set off the extensor body reaction. The child wears the vest for up to 6 months while developing greater postural stability.

Evaluation

The therapist should begin the initial assessment by observing the child using any existing seating and mobility systems to note posture, movements, comfort, satisfaction with the equipment, and other factors that may affect function. During the seating evaluation, the therapist will need to consider (1) the angle between the seat and the back surfaces, (2) the tilt of the system in space (orientation), and (3) the type of surface on which the child will be seated.[6]

The therapist should begin the evaluation by positioning the child on a low mat table so that he or she can complete a postural assessment to determine whether any limitations in ranges of movement exist that may interfere with the upright and seated positions. The therapist obtains further information by positioning the child in a sitting position while using the hands to support the child to identify key points of control and positions that provide a desirable

change in posture, muscle tone, and movements. These key points become the necessary components of the seating system. The positions, such as the angle of hip flexion and the orientation in space of the child, become the pitches and angles of the components necessary in the seating system and wheelchair hardware.[16]

Once the therapist gathers information from the postural assessment, other methods are also available that use evaluation equipment for assessment of the child's position to determine what components, angles, and sizes are needed in a seating system. Simulators are self-contained, adjustable fitting chairs that the therapist can adjust to fit a child or an adult, to determine what type of seating components and angles are appropriate.[65] The simulator allows the therapist to "evaluate the client in the system, alter angles of the seat to the back, try varying positions in space, and determine component sizes and accessories that are required before making recommendations for a particular system" (p. 73).[66]

The therapist and the ATP can use simulators to evaluate planar, contoured, and molded seating (Figure 21-18). The therapist first completes a postural evaluation of the individual to determine which seating components are necessary and then adjusts the simulator to the individual's size. The therapist selects angles, which include seat-to-back and tilt. Further adjustments can be made to determine how position influences movement and function. The advantages of using a seating simulator include (1) use as a single evaluation tool for various ages, sizes, and diagnoses; (2) source of information about the various types of seating systems, such as planar versus molded; and (3) options to motorize simulators to evaluate powered

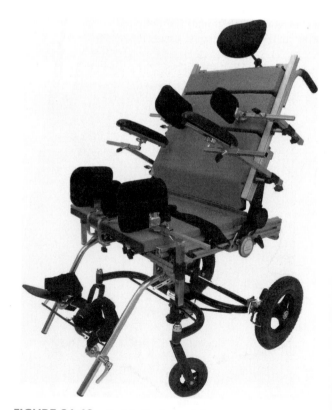

FIGURE 21-18 Prairie Seat simulator.

mobility access and the effect of positioning on motor control. The problem that the assessment team often encounters when using simulators is difficulty in transferring the information from the simulator into an actual seating system and knowing how that system will integrate into a mobility base. Children may also respond negatively to the simulator evaluation because its mechanical appearance and large size may intimidate them.

Another method for evaluating seating and positioning is use of a modular mockup or adjustable evaluation seat system that can be placed in a mobility base. These are typically available in planar or contoured seating devices rather than in custom-molded devices. The main advantage of using this method is that the child can use the actual mobility device while seated in the mockup seat. This is particularly important because positioning can influence body movements and therefore functional outcomes. The disadvantages are that more equipment must be available to fit a range of individuals, and pitches and angles cannot always be accurately assessed.

Children with hypotonia, such as those with muscle disease or cerebral palsy, have specific needs. A useful positioning system includes a biangular back design that supports the sacrum in a neutral position but angles the remaining backrest about 15° away from the back at the posterior superior iliac spine. This provides a resting position of the trunk behind the pelvis and accommodates the forces of gravity in the upright position (see Figure 21-16, B). Consideration of a tilt-in-space feature in the mobility base and an adjustable seat-to-back angle may also provide the hypotonic or weak child with greater tolerance for sitting upright.

Children with increased muscle tone and spasticity who adduct their legs and extend their hips and spine are often more difficult to position. The therapist must identify key points of control for positioning these children. For example, the therapist determines the desired degree of hip and knee flexion, hip abduction, and reduction of asymmetrical positioning that positively influences muscle tone and control of extremity movement. The critical factor for reducing the degree and frequency of extensor posturing is to determine what factors contribute to these undesirable movements. Kangas observed that certain children become more asymmetrical as hypertonus increases, and that this increase in muscle tone is stimulated when they feel pressure behind their head or neck from a headrest.[39] These children may also have better postural control in the upright position rather than reclined or tilted.[47] In other children who extend forcibly in combination with rotation of one side of the body forward, the resulting pelvic obliquity may place strain on the soft tissue when the child is positioned symmetrically with both legs forward. These children often prefer to have one leg abducted (almost off the seat cushion) and one leg forward. This often reduces the strength and frequency of hip extension and rotation of the upper body as the child extends.

The therapist must frequently reevaluate a child's position, particularly in a seated mobility device, to accommodate postural, developmental, and physiologic changes. Once a child receives a seating mobility system, the therapist should reevaluate its fit and function every 4 to 6 months. Positioning and mobility literature and support materials are available,[15,22,65,66] and more specific information and techniques on positioning are available through additional reading and workshops.

TRANSPORTATION OF MOBILITY SYSTEMS

Many manufacturers of wheelchair mobility systems do not recommend using them as a seat in a motor vehicle. However, most families do not recognize this warning and allow the child to travel while seated in the wheelchair in a motor vehicle or school bus. Manufacturers are now providing safer options for transporting a wheelchair with the child in it because of a voluntary ANSI/RESNA standard called WC-19, Wheelchairs Used as Seats in Motor Vehicles.[3] Wheelchairs are considered WC-19–compliant if they have four accessible and identifiable points to secure the chair to the vehicle, as well as seating, a frame, and other components designed to allow better fit of a lap and shoulder belt. The standard requires wheelchairs to be dynamically crash-tested at 30 miles per hour and 20g crash conditions, which are the standards used to test child safety seats.

It is important that occupational therapists recommend wheelchairs that are WC-19–compliant and educate clients and families on safe methods for transporting a wheelchair in a motor vehicle. Standards have also been developed to recognize the safety of a specialized seating system that may be used in another manufacturer's wheelchair bases. The ANSI/RESNA WC-20 standards are for seating devices for use in motor vehicles.[4] One standard requires that all students being transported in a wheelchair on a bus must face forward. Wheelchairs that are transported in a side-facing position are more likely to deform and collapse in a crash and the shoulder belt is ineffective.[57] School-based occupational therapists must work with transportation personnel to educate them on the importance of forward-facing positions for wheelchair riders, as well as the proper use of tie-downs. The lap belt must be snug and low on the pelvis and the shoulder belt positioned over the middle of the clavicle and across the sternum, where it connects to the pelvic belt over the hip. Any device such as an augmentative communication device or computer and lap tray must be removed and tied down separately.

FACTORS THAT INFLUENCE THE SUCCESSFUL USE OF MOBILITY DEVICES

Successful use of mobility devices depends on the fit of the child to the device, the features of the device, and the physical and social environments. Studies have shown a significant relationship between certain standardized tests of cognition and perception and use of powered mobility. Specific functional performance tasks correlate with the ability with use a power wheelchair. Preliminary findings indicate a relationship between specific cognitive scales and readiness for powered mobility, particularly in the areas of spatial relations and problem solving.[28,63,69]

Another factor that influences a child's ability to use a powered device is the ability of the professional or the caregiver to determine the most accurate and efficient means for the child to access the device. If a child is having significant difficulty in maneuvering a powered mobility device successfully, the therapist must first reevaluate the position of the child and the access method to determine whether it is the most effective means. The longer it takes a child to successfully demonstrate use of a control, the more likely it is that either the access method is inappropriate or the child's seating needs have not been met. Case Study 21-4 describes this type of situation.

The therapist must consider changes that the child will have in the future, both expected and unexpected, when recommending equipment. For example, the therapist must determine whether the system can be easily changed as the child gains new skills, grows, or changes physically. This is particularly important for the therapist to consider when ordering a power wheelchair. For example, a child with a progressive disability may be able to operate a joystick at the time the chair is ordered. However, electronic options need to be included, such as the ability to readily change the input method, if the child's functional status changes and use of a joystick is no longer feasible. It is more economical in most cases to initially order options on equipment rather than retrofit the equipment at a later date.

The therapist must also determine where and how augmentative communication equipment will be mounted to the child's wheelchair. Selection of the appropriate mounting bracket depends on the tube size of the wheelchair frame and locations on the wheelchair where it can be attached. A problem that therapists often encounter with manual wheelchairs is positioning the child or rear wheels too far forward of the center of gravity in the wheelchair, which often causes the wheelchair to tip forward when the communication device is mounted. The most frequent problem encountered with mounting augmentative communication devices on power wheelchairs is finding a place to mount the bracket on the frame and making certain it does not interfere with moving through doorways.

The therapy team and ATP have a responsibility to assist the family and child in becoming informed consumers by identifying seating and mobility issues and needs, then presenting several alternatives during the evaluation. The family should make the final decision on the specific type of mobility device after considering the options that the therapy team presents. The most important and significant contribution that the therapist can make is to evaluate access methods and help caregivers develop and implement strategies to meet identified goals. The therapist must reevaluate the outcome as the child progresses. This includes providing periodic evaluations of fit and function of the equipment.

SUMMARY

The literature indicates that independent mobility plays a facilitative role in cognitive, language, and social development.[38] Therefore, when mobility is severely delayed or restricted, emotional and psychosocial development are affected. Augmentative mobility devices can provide either functional or transitional mobility. These devices can provide children with physical disabilities greater opportunities to develop and become initiators and active participants in daily occupations and experiences. Occupational therapists emphasize methods of adapting the child's environments to maximize his or her functional mobility. The occupational therapist is responsible for ensuring that children with physical disabilities receive opportunities for mobility at the earliest age possible to promote participation and development more equal to their able-bodied peers.

Case Studies 21-5 and 21-6 include comprehensive information about the children's equipment and adapted environments. These descriptions demonstrate how mobility equipment is integrated with other AT and environmental adaptations to best meet the children's functional needs.

CASE STUDY 21-4   Stephanie

Stephanie was a 15-month-old girl with cerebral palsy who successfully used a switch-operated GoBot to maneuver and explore her surroundings. It took her about 5 hours to become proficient at using a set of four press switches with her hand and to understand the relationship to directionality. However, when she entered another therapy program, the therapist did not consider information on her ability to use switches for driving. Instead, the therapist placed her in a wheelchair training program using the only equipment available, a joystick-operated power wheelchair. After 6 months of training for 3 hours each week, Stephanie demonstrated no improvement in her ability to drive the power wheelchair. Upon reevaluation of her access method, the therapist provided her with four switches at her hand and evaluated a switch array behind her head. She was able to use both access methods but when questioned, preferred using switches behind her head. The head switch array provided her with immediate success in driving the power wheelchair. Had the therapist provided her with the appropriate control method (switch access instead of a joystick, which she could not operate because of her impaired motor function), she might have demonstrated the ability to use the power wheelchair in significantly less time.

CASE STUDY 21-5   David

David is an 11-year-old boy who was diagnosed with Duchenne's muscular dystrophy at 4 years of age. Shortly afterward, his little brother, Eric, was diagnosed with the same condition at 5 months of age. The two brothers and an older sister live with their parents in a small town.

Duchenne's muscular dystrophy is an inherited X-linked disease that affects the voluntary skeletal musculature, with progressive weakness and degeneration of the muscles that control movement. The muscle weakness begins in the proximal and axial musculature and slowly progresses distally. Frequently, children with Duchenne's muscular dystrophy require a wheelchair by 12 years of age. Breathing becomes affected during the later stages of the disease, leading to severe respiratory problems. Respiratory infections commonly cause death during the person's early twenties.

When receiving David's diagnosis, the family was introduced to a team of professionals who specialize in different aspects of musculoskeletal weaknesses. The family received support to help them deal with the initial shock and necessary information about the disease. Twice a year, the family continued to meet with the team for medical and orthopedic evaluations. Social and psychologic concerns were also addressed.

Last year, David had an Achilles tendon lengthening to release a tight heel cord. Today, he walks with a long-leg orthosis. It is important to lengthen the walking phase in boys with Duchenne's muscular dystrophy to delay hip and knee flexion deformities and equinovarus deformity of the foot and ankle. For 2 years, David used a standard lightweight manual wheelchair for traveling long distances or when he was fatigued. Currently, the therapy team and David's family are considering a power wheelchair for David, to allow him to conserve energy for social and educational activities. The team plans on spinal stabilization when David's scoliosis exceeds 25° and normal forced vital capacity (FVC) pulmonary function drops below 50%.

Eric is now 7 years of age. The progression of his disease is following the same course as David's, although somewhat slower. The early signs of Duchenne's muscular dystrophy are becoming prominent, such as the waddling gait, tendency to fall, and difficulty rising from a sitting or lying position.

At the time of Eric's diagnosis, the family lived in an apartment but soon decided to build a house. The occupational therapist provided recommendations for designing the house for wheelchair accessibility to maximize function and independence.

The family has been living in the house for 2 years, and they are pleased with the features that enable the boys to be independent. The outdoor surfaces (sidewalks and ramps) are firm, stable, and slip resistant. The floor plan is spacious, doorways are wide, and there are no thresholds. A few sliding doors have been installed to allow maximum door width and to eliminate floor swing space requirements. Controls, levers, and switches are placed low to be within reach from a wheelchair. The window's lower edge is only 20 inches above the floor for the same reason. The bathrooms are spacious, with both a bathtub and a shower. The boys love taking baths because they stay warmer and move more freely in the water. The sink is freestanding so the boys can get close to the sink. An automatic faucet has been installed, which turns on when the hands are placed under the faucet. A full-length mirror is on the wall.

The family continues to need a lot of support and assistance to adjust to new challenges. In addition to direct service to the family, the occupational therapist continues to work closely with the schools to ensure that accessibility is available.

CASE STUDY 21-6   Jason

Jason is a 7-year-old boy with cerebral palsy, which has affected his ability to speak, move his body with control, and eat. Although he demonstrates severe delays in his motor skills, he appears alert and attentive and understands what is said to him. From his early days, his family was motivated to ensure that Jason have a childhood as normal as possible. They were creative in designing simple devices and tools to accomplish these goals. His grandfather designed the first mobility device for him. It was a pushcart used to hold golf clubs, but he mounted a car seat to the frame and placed foam pieces in the seat to help align Jason's body and prevent him from leaning over. His mother would use it to push him around the neighborhood during her daily jogging routine. He also used a standard stroller but required a positioning system to assist him in sitting upright by providing support at the pelvis, trunk, and head. The first seating system was made of Tri-Wall, a three-layer-thick cardboard that can be used to fabricate temporary seat inserts for children. Another seat insert was fabricated from Tri-Wall and placed on a dining room chair so that he could eat at the family table instead of in a high chair.

By the time he was 12 months of age, Jason's family built him an aeroplane mobility device (see Figure 21-7) to use at home. When he outgrew this by 2 years of age, his therapist evaluated him for a support walker and found that he could effectively use the KidWalk by Prime Engineering (see Figure 21-9, D). He continued to use this device for indoor mobility and for playing in Little League for special needs children when he was 5 years of age. He and his teammates used an automatic device to hit the ball, and Jason ran around the field using his walker.

When Jason was 3 years old, his family decided that the walker alone did not adequately meet his community mobility needs. His therapist evaluated him for a power wheelchair, and he could operate the joystick once he was positioned with maximal support at his feet, pelvis, trunk, and head.

Continued

CASE STUDY 21-6   Jason—cont'd

His therapist and family determined the features he would need to operate a power wheelchair. He needed a molded seating system for support and alignment, and, to increase independence, the system needed to include the capability to elevate the seat from the floor to various heights. The therapist identified a power wheelchair with these features and recommended a custom-molded seating system.

The family made the home environment accessible to Jason in many ways. When he was 2 years of age, they decided that it was important for him to roll out of bed in the morning and try to roll on the floor. They placed a low-height mattress on the floor in the corner of his bedroom and made it his bed. They lined the sides of it with his stuffed toys to protect him from unintentionally hitting his arms against the walls. This arrangement allowed him to get out of bed on his own. They also extended the light switch in his room so that he could reach it from his walker or wheelchair.

Positioning in the bathtub when he was a toddler was a challenge, but his mother made a bath seat for him from a milk crate. She placed foam around the edges and the seat

for comfort. When he outgrew this, his family acquired a bath seat designed for children with disabilities. His occupational therapist recommended an adapted toilet seat with a high backrest. It provided Jason with the ability to begin toilet training at 2 years of age. His family also installed a flip-down bar in front of the toilet so Jason could stand at the toilet "like his dad."

During these early years, Jason's therapist introduced him to augmentative communication symbols and aids. By the time he was 12 months of age, he could point to symbols in his communication book using his fist and soon progressed to using an augmentative communication device with voice output by accessing it with a head tracking system on his head. The communication device was mounted on his power wheelchair. Today Jason is fully included in a second-grade class. He uses AT to do his schoolwork and has an attendant with him throughout the day. Both simple and sophisticated AT devices have enabled him to function within a regular education classroom and to participate in most of the activities of his peers.

REFERENCES

1. Americans with Disabilities Act & Accessible Information Technology Center. (2003). Bulletin #4. Retrieved July 2009 from http://www.adaproject.org
2. Andersson, C., Grooten, W., Hellsten, M., Kaping, K., & Mattsson, E. (2003). Adults with cerebral palsy: Walking ability after progressive strength training. *Developmental Medicine and Child Neurology, 45*, 220–228.
3. ANSI/RESNA Subcommittee on Wheelchairs and Transportation. (2000). *ANSI/RESNA WC, Vol.1/Sect. 19, Wheelchairs used as seats in motor vehicles.* Arlington, VA: RESNA.
4. ANSI/RESNA Subcommittee on Wheelchairs and Transportation. (2008). *ANSI/RESNA WC. Vol. 4/Sect. 20, Seating systems used in motor vehicles.* Arlington, VA: RESNA.
5. Backer, G., & Howell, B. (1997). Physical therapy goals and intervention for the ventilator-assisted child or adolescent. In L. Driver, V. Nelson, & S. Warschausky (Eds.), *The ventilator assisted child.* San Antonio, TX: Communication Skill Builders.
6. Bergen, A., Presperin, J., & Tallman, T. (1990). *Positioning for function: Wheelchairs and other assistive technologies.* New York: Valhalla Rehabilitation Publications.
7. Blundell, S., Shepherd, R., Dean, C., Adams, R., & Cahill, B. (2003). Functional strength training in cerebral palsy: A pilot study of a group circuit training class for children aged 4–8 years. *Clinical Rehabilitation, 17*, 48–57.
8. Bly, L. (1994). *Motor skills acquisition in the first year.* Tucson, AZ: Therapy Skill Builders.
9. Brinker, R. P., & Lewis, M. (1982). Making the world work with microcomputers: A learning prosthesis for handicapped infants. *Exceptional Children, 49*, 163–170.
10. Butler, C. (1986). Effects of powered mobility on self-initiated behaviors of very young children with locomotor disability. *Developmental Medicine and Child Neurology, 28*, 325–332.
11. Butler, C. (1988). High tech tots: Technology for mobility, manipulation, communication, and learning in early childhood. *Infants and Young Children, 2*, 66–73.

12. Butler, C. (1988). Powered tots: Augmentative mobility for locomotor disabled youngsters. *American Physical Therapy Association Pediatric Publication, 14*, 19.
13. Campos, J. J., & Bertenthal, B. I. (1987). Locomotion and psychological development in infancy. In K. M. Jaffe (Ed.), *Childhood powered mobility: Developmental, technical, and clinical perspectives. Proceedings of the RESNA First Northwest Regional Conference* (pp. 11–42). Washington, DC: RESNA Press.
14. Cech, D., & Martin, A. (1995). *Functional movement development across the life span.* Philadelphia: W.B. Saunders.
15. Cook, A., & Polgar, J. (2008). Technologies that enable mobility. In A. Cook & J. Polgar (Eds.), *Assistive technologies: Principles and practice* (3rd ed., pp. 408–442). St. Louis: Mosby.
16. Cooper, R. (1998). Biomechanics and ergonomics of wheelchairs. In R. Cooper (Ed.), *Wheelchair selection and configuration.* New York: Demos.
17. Coster, W. (1998). Occupation-centered assessment of children. *American Journal of Occupational Therapy, 52*, 337–344.
18. Damiano, D. L. (2006). Activity, activity, activity: Rethinking our physical therapy approach to cerebral palsy. *Physical Therapy, 86*, 1534–1540.
19. Deitz, J., Swinth, Y., & White, O. (2002). Powered mobility and preschoolers with complex developmental delays. *American Journal of Occupational Therapy, 56*, 86–96.
20. Douglas, J., & Ryan, M. (1987). A preschool severely disabled boy and his powered wheelchair: A case study. *Child Care, Health and Development, 13*, 303–309.
21. Eagleton, M., Iams, A., McDowell, J., Morrison, R., & Evans, C. L. (2004). The effects of strength training on gait in adolescents with cerebral palsy. *Pediatric Physical Therapy, 16*, 22–30.
22. Engstrom, B. (1993). *Ergonomics, wheelchairs and positioning.* Hasselby, Sweden: Posturalis Books.
23. Everand, L. (1997). Early mobility means easier integration. *Canadian Review of Sociology and Anthropology, 34*, 224–234.
24. Fisher, A. G. (1998). Uniting practice and theory in an occupational framework. *American Journal of Occupational Therapy, 52*, 509–519.

25. Foreman, N., Foreman, D., Cummings, A., & Owens, S. (1990). *Journal of General Psychology, 117,* 195–233.

26. Fowler, E. G., Ho, T. W., Nwigwe, A. I., & Dorey, F. J. (2001). The effect of quadriceps femoris muscle strengthening exercises on spasticity in children with cerebral palsy. *Physical Therapy, 81,* 1195–1223.

27. Furumasu, J., Guerrette, P., & Tefft, D. (1996). The development of a powered wheelchair mobility program for young children. *Technology and Disability, 5,* 41–48.

28. Furumasu, J., Guerette, P., & Tefft, D. (2004). Relevance of the Pediatric Powered Wheelchair Screening Test (PPWST) for children with cerebral palsy. *Developmental Medicine and Child Neurology, 46,* 468–474.

29. Furumasu, J., Tefft, D., & Guerette, P. (1996). Pediatric powered mobility: Readiness to learn. *Team Rehab,* 29–36.

30. Guerette, P., Tefft, D., & Furumasu, J. (2005). Pediatric powered mobility: Results of a national survey of providers. *Assistive Technology, 17,* 144–158.

31. Guerette, P., Tefft, D., Furumasu, J., & Moy, F. (1999). Development of a cognitive assessment battery for young children with physical impairments. *Infant-Toddler Intervention: The Transdisciplinary Journal, 9,* 169–181.

32. Haley, S. M., Coster, W. J., Ludlow, L. H., Haltiwanger, J., & Andrellos, P. (1992). *Pediatric Evaluation of Disability Inventory (PEDI).* San Antonio, TX: Psychological Corp.

33. Hasdai, A., Jessel, A. S., & Weiss, P. L. (1998). Use of computer simulator for training children with disabilities in the operation of a powered wheelchair. *American Journal of Occupational Therapy, 52,* 195–220.

34. Hays, R. (1987). Childhood motor impairments: Clinical overview and scope of the problem. In K. M. Jaffe (Ed.), *Childhood powered mobility: Developmental, technical, and clinical perspectives. Proceedings of the RESNA First Northwest Regional Conference.* Washington, DC: RESNA Press.

35. Hulme, J., Poor, R., Schulein, M., & Pezzino, J. (1983). Perceived behavioral changes observed with adaptive seating devices for multi-handicapped developmentally disabled individuals. *Physical Therapy, 62,* 204–208.

36. Hundert, J., & Hopkins, B. (1992). Training supervisors in a collaborative team approach to promote peer interactions of children with disabilities in integrated preschools. *Journal of Applied Behavior Analysis, 25,* 385–400.

37. Hune, K., Guarrera-Bowlby, P., Deutsch, J. (2007). The clinical decision-making process of prescribing power mobility for a child with cerebral palsy. *Pediatric Physical Therapy, 19,* 254–260.

38. Jones, M. A., McEwen, I. R., & Hansen, L. (2003). Use of power mobility for a young child with spinal muscular atrophy. *Physical Therapy, 83,* 253–262.

39. Kangas, K. (2001). Chest supports: Why they are not working. *Presented at the Seventeenth International Seating Symposium,* February 22–24, pp. 41–44.

40. Kermoian, R. (1997). Locomotion experience and psychological development in infancy. In J. Furumasu, *Pediatric powered mobility: Developmental perspectives, technical issues, clinical approaches* (pp. 7–22). Arlington, VA: RESNA Press.

41. Lange, M. (2008). Manual wheelchairs: Understanding these general categories can help therapists meet individual needs. *ADVANCE,* 31–33.

42. Law, M., Baptiste, S., Carswell, A., McColl, M. A., Polatajko, H., & Pollock, N. (2005). *The Canadian Occupational Performance Measure* (2nd ed.). Toronto, ON: CAOT Publications.

43. Margolis, S. A., et al. (1985). The Subasis Bar: An effective approach to pelvic stabilization in seated positioning. In *The Proceedings of the 8th Annual Conference on Rehabilitation Engineering,* pp. 45–47.

44. McBurney, H., Taylor, N. F., Dodd, K. J., & Graham, H. K. (2003). A qualitative analysis of the benefits of strength training for young people with cerebral palsy. *Developmental Medicine and Child Neurology, 45,* 658–663.

45. Myhr, U., & Wendt, L. (1991). Improvement of functional sitting position for children with cerebral palsy. *Developmental Medicine and Child Neurology, 33,* 246–256.

46. Nilsson, L., & Nyberg, P. (2003). Driving to learn: A new concept for training children with profound cognitive disabilities in a powered wheelchair. *American Journal of Occupational Therapy, 57,* 229–233.

47. Nwaobi, O. (1986). Effects of body orientation in space on tonic muscle activity of patients with cerebral palsy. *Developmental Medicine and Child Neurology, 28,* 41–44.

48. Nwaobi, O. (1987). Effect of unilateral arm restraint on upper extremity function in cerebral palsy. In *Proceedings of the Annual RESNA Conference* (pp. 311–313). Washington, DC: RESNA Press.

49. Paleg, G. (1997). Made for walking: A comparison of gait trainers. *Team Rehab Report,* 41–45.

50. Paleg, G. (2007). What's new in mobility accessories. *Rehab Management,* 24–27.

51. Paleg, G. (2008). Moving forward. *Rehab Management.* Retrieved July 2009 from http://www.rehabpub.com/issues/articles/2008-06_02.asp.

52. Paulsson, K., & Christoffersen, M. (1984). Psychological aspects of technical aids: How does independent mobility affect the psychological and intellectual development of children with physical disabilities? In *Proceedings of the Second Annual Conference on Rehabilitation Engineering* (pp. 282–286). Washington, DC: RESNA Press.

53. Piaget, J. (1954). *The construction of reality in the child.* New York: Basic Books.

54. Pollock, N., & Stewart, D. (1998). Occupational performance needs of school-aged children with physical disability in the community. *Physical and Occupational Therapy in Pediatrics, 18,* 55–68.

55. Raine, A., Reynolds, C., Venables, P. H., & Mednick, S. A. (2002). Stimulation seeking and intelligence: A retrospective longitudinal study. *Journal Personality and Social Psychology, 82,* 663–674.

56. Seligman, M. (1975). *Helplessness: On depression, development, and death.* San Francisco: W.H. Freeman.

57. Shutrump, S., Manary, M., Buning, M. (2008). Safe transportation for students who use wheelchairs on the school bus. *OT Practice,* 8–12.

58. Stanton, D., Wilson, P. N., & Foreman, N. (2002). Effects of early mobility on shortcut performance in a simulated maze. *Behavioral Brain Research, 136,* 61–66.

59. Taplin, C. S. (1989). Powered wheelchair control, assessment, and training. In *RESNA '89: Proceedings of the 12th annual conference* (pp. 45–46). Washington, DC: RESNA Press.

60. Taylor, S., & Monahan, L. (1989). Considerations in assessing for powered mobility. In C. Brubaker (Ed.), *Wheelchair IV: Report of a conference on the state of the art of powered wheelchair mobility, December 7–9, 1988.* Washington, DC: RESNA Press.

61. Tefft, D., Furumasu, J., & Guerette, P. (1993). Cognitive readiness for powered wheelchair mobility in the young child. In *Proceedings of the RESNA 1993 Annual Conference* (pp. 338–340). Washington, DC: RESNA Press.

62. Tefft, D., Furumasu, J., & Guerette, P. (1995). Development of a cognitive assessment battery for evaluating readiness for powered mobility. In *Proceedings of the RESNA 1995 Annual Conference* (pp. 320–322). Washington, DC: RESNA Press.

63. Tefft, D., Guerette, P., & Furumasu, J. (1999). Cognitive predictors of young children's readiness for powered mobility. *Developmental Medicine and Child Neurology, 41,* 665–670.

64. Telzrow, R., Campos, J., Shepherd, A., Bertenthal, B., & Atwater, S. (1987). Spatial understanding in infants with motor handicaps. In K. M. Jaffe (Ed.), *Childhood powered mobility: Developmental, technical and clinical perspectives.* In *Proceedings of the RESNA First Northwest Regional Conference* (pp. 62–69). Seattle, WA: RESNA Association for the Advancement of Rehabilitation Technology.

65. Trefler, E. (1999). Then and now: Saving time with simulators. *Team Rehab*, (February), 32–36.
66. Trefler, E., Hobson, D., Taylor, S., Monahan, L., & Shaw, C. (1993). *Seating and mobility.* Tucson, AZ: Therapy Skill Builders.
67. Trimble, J., Morris, T., & Crandall, R. (1992). Virtual reality: Designing accessible environments. *Team Rehab Report, 3,* 8–12.
68. Uniform Data System for Medical Rehabilitation. (1999). *Functional Independence Measure for Children (WeeFIM) (Outpatient version 5.0).* Buffalo, NY: State University of New York at Buffalo.
69. Verburg, G., Field, D., & Jarvis, S. (1987). Motor, perceptual, and cognitive factors that affect mobility control. In *Proceedings of the 10th Annual Conference on Rehabilitation Technology.* Washington, DC: RESNA Press.
70. Warren, C. G. (1990). Powered mobility and its implications. *Journal of Rehabilitation Research and Development. Clinical Supplement, 27,* 74–85.
71. Woods, H. (1998, Fall). Moving right along: Young disabled children can now experience the developmental benefits of moving and exploring on their own. *Stanford Medicine,* 15–19.
72. Wright, C., & Nomura, M. (1985). *From toys to computers, access for the physically disabled child.* San Jose, CA.
73. Wright-Ott, C. (1997). The transitional powered mobility aid: A new concept and tool for early mobility. In J. Furumasu (Ed.), *Pediatric powered mobility* (pp. 58–69). Washington, DC: RESNA Press.
74. Wright-Ott, C. (1998). Designing a transitional powered mobility aid for young children with physical disabilities. In D. Gray, L. Quatrano, & M. Lieverman (Eds.), *Designing and using assistive technology: The human perspective* (pp. 285–295). Baltimore: Brookes.
75. Wright-Ott, C. (1999). A transitional powered mobility aid for young children with physical disabilities. Presented at *ICORR 99 Sixth International Conference on Rehabilitation Robotics,* July 1999, Stanford, CA.
76. Wright-Ott, C., Escobar, R., & Leslie, S. Encouraging exploration. *Rehab Management.* Retrieved June 2002 from http://www.rehabpub.com/features/672002/3.asp.

SUGGESTED READING

Bertenthal, B. I., Campos, J. J., & Barrett, K. C. (1984). Self-produced locomotion: An organizer of emotional, cognitive, and social development in infancy. In R. N. Emde & R. J. Harmon (Eds.), *Continuities and discontinuities in development.* New York: Plenum Press.
Cook, A. & Polgar, J. (2008). *Assistive technologies: Principles and practice* (3rd ed.). St. Louis: Mosby.
Fuhrman, S., Buning, M., & Karg, P. (2008). Wheelchair transportation: Ensuring safe community mobility. *OT Practice,* (October), 10–13.
Tefft, D., Furumasu, J., Guerette, P. (1996). *Ready, set, go: Pediatric powered mobility with young children training video and manual.* Downey CA: LAREI.
Tefft, D., Furumasu, J., & Guerette, P. (1997). Pediatric powered mobility: Influential cognitive skills. In J. Furumasu (Ed.), *Pediatric powered mobility: Developmental perspectives, technical issues, clinical approaches* (pp. 70–91). Washington, DC: RESNA Press.
Werner, D. *Disabled village children: A guide for community health workers, rehabilitation workers and families.* Retrieved at http://disabledvillagechildren.projects.unamesa.org.

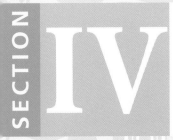
CHAPTER

22 Neonatal Intensive Care Unit

Jan G. Hunter

KEY TERMS

Preterm infants
Neonatal intensive care unit
Individualized developmentally supportive care
Preterm infant neurobehavioral organization
Synactive theory of development

Neonatal medical complications
Neuromotor and neurobehavioral development
Therapeutic positioning
Nutritive sucking
Nonnutritive sucking
Cue-based feeding

OBJECTIVES

1. Understand the scope of knowledge required for competent practice in the neonatal intensive care unit (NICU).
2. Compare the traditional occupational therapy approach of rehabilitation and developmental stimulation with current concepts of individualized developmentally supportive care in the NICU.
3. Define and compute postconceptional, chronologic, and corrected age.
4. Explain why preterm infants are so susceptible to heat loss and how heat loss can occur.
5. Define common medical conditions common to preterm and high-risk infants.
6. Identify potential negative effects of light, sound, and caregiving practices on infants in the NICU.

7. Describe protective interventions to reduce avoidable stimulation from excessive or inappropriate light, sound, and caregiving practices in the NICU.
8. Discuss factors that complicate parenting in the NICU.
9. Describe roles and potential interventions of the NICU therapist in providing family support through family-centered neonatal care.
10. Discuss factors that should be considered in evaluating an infant in the NICU, and identify published neonatal assessments.
11. Explain the synactive theory of development proposed by Heidi Als.
12. Describe neurobehavioral and neuromotor development in preterm infants.
13. Identify and describe the six neurobehavioral states.
14. Describe common positional deformities of preterm infants, and the potential influence of these iatrogenic deformities on future development.
15. Discuss the basic principles and techniques of developmentally supportive positioning in the NICU.
16. Explain the (limited) appropriate use for range of motion and splinting in the NICU.
17. Explain why nonnutritive sucking is beneficial to preterm infants.
18. Describe organized and disorganized nutritive sucking patterns observed during infant feeding.
19. Identify the differences between a traditional feeding approach and a cue-based feeding approach with NICU infants.
20. Summarize key factors that can facilitate successful breastfeeding in the NICU.

Kimberly underwent an emergency cesarean delivery at 26 weeks' gestation when intrauterine circulation problems developed between two of her three triplets. Savannah was born prematurely to a 15-year-old student who concealed her pregnancy from her parents. Tonya, with a history of three previous miscarriages, had a cerclage (a surgical procedure to keep the cervix closed during pregnancy), and was able to carry Darren until 32 weeks' gestation. Brittney was born at 28 weeks to a mother addicted to crack cocaine who received no prenatal care. Dylan, born at term to a febrile mother, became critically ill with pneumonia and developed respiratory failure during his first day of life. Myesha was delivered by an emergency cesarean section following a motor vehicle accident in which the placenta was partially torn from the uterine wall. Maria's prenatal ultrasound revealed an infant with multiple congenital anomalies.

These real-life examples represent the urgency and wide range of skilled medical care necessary to optimize both survival and functional outcome in preterm and high-risk infants. In all these cases, the infants were admitted to a neonatal intensive care unit (NICU) following delivery; all but one baby survived.

EVOLUTION OF NEONATAL INTENSIVE CARE

The NICU is a complex and highly specialized hospital unit designed to care for infants who are born prematurely or are critically ill (Figure 22-1). The first special care unit for preterm newborns, established by Dr. Pierre Budin in 1893, emphasized warmth, small feedings, and protection from infection. In the past 40 years, medical technology, knowledge, and interventions in the NICU have increased exponentially. An increased awareness of environmental and caregiving influences on the vulnerable newborn have enlarged the scope of NICU care to encompass developmental and family issues in addition to primary medical concerns.[40] This chapter discusses the knowledge and skills needed by the occupational therapist to work effectively and competently in high-tech neonatal care.

Nursery Classification and Regionalization of Care

The spiraling expense and complexity of medical care created a growing discrepancy between neonatal mortality rates at major medical centers and those at smaller hospitals. In the early 1970s, regionalization of perinatal care emerged to provide advanced levels of health care to any mother or infant within an identified perinatal region while avoiding unnecessary duplication of services. Patient care was generally provided at the nearest hospital, with transfer to a higher-level facility as needed for more complex problems. Area hospitals were designated as Level I, Level II, or Level III based on the comprehensiveness of available care; it has been recommended that numeric levels be replaced with more functional and descriptive designations of care level such as basic, specialty, and subspecialty.[6,86]

A Level I (basic) nursery (e.g., in a small community hospital) manages uncomplicated pregnancies with expected normal deliveries and well infants, although sufficient expertise and experience to stabilize ill newborns prior to transfer to a higher level facility is necessary. Level II (specialty) nurseries are designed to care for newborn infants who require some additional medical

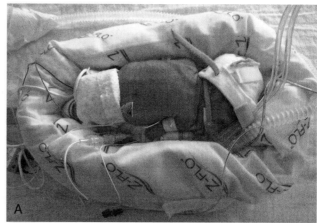

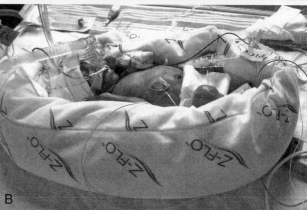

FIGURE 22-1 Newly born, extremely preterm twins in a NICU. These 24-weeks-gestation infants, in Z-Flo fluidized positioners and on radiant warmers, are receiving nasal continuous positive airway pressure (NCPAP), total parenteral nutrition (TPN), and phototherapy. (Courtesy Sundance Enterprises, Inc. White Plains, NY. http://www.sundancesolutions.com)

management, such as phototherapy for jaundice, intravenous antibiotics, or tube feedings. A neonatologist is usually on staff, but these units typically lack the equipment and additional expertise, such as a pediatric surgeon or cardiologist, to care for all medical emergencies and severe neonatal problems. Level III (subspecialty) nurseries have the necessary equipment and trained personnel in the NICU and other hospital departments to care for all potential neonatal conditions and emergencies. "Level IV" is an unofficial classification used to designate NICUs that offer current "rescue" technologies, although some interventions used initially for rescue (e.g. high-frequency ventilation [HFV] or inhaled nitric oxide [iNO]) have become a standard of care after continued proven success.

Since the 1980s, medical economics (NICUs are generally profitable), an increasingly competitive health care market, and the increased availability of neonatal technology and specialists have encouraged many community hospitals to expand their perinatal services, resulting in fragmentation of services with a wide disparity in level of care provided. With a focus on better outcomes, the current recommendation is that infants at less than 32 weeks' gestation or weighing less than 1500 grams be delivered at subspecialty perinatal centers able to provide necessary care to pregnant mothers and neonates of all risk categories.[4,6]

nclusion of Developmental Specialists n the NICU

nfant survival was the original indicator of NICU success. As he survival rate increased for younger, smaller, and sicker nfants, concerns emerged about the effects of the NICU envi-onment and about the long-term developmental outcome of NICU survivors. These concerns facilitated the entry of occu-ational therapists and other neonatal developmental specia-ists into the critical care arena of the NICU. There is, however, a wide discrepancy in specific roles, expectations, knowledge, and skills among neonatal therapists. Every experi-nced or aspiring NICU therapist must be committed to ontinuing education, mentoring, networking, and implemen-ation of evidence-based care practices to establish a more niform and credible standard of developmental care.

Practitioners and educators are interested in formalizing xpectations and competencies of NICU developmental care pecialists. The Advanced Competency in Developmental Care nitiative is a recognition program initiated in 2008 by the National Association of Neonatal Nurses (NANN; http:// www.nann.org). Experienced NICU practitioners in the United States or Canada of multiple disciplines are eligible to complete a comprehensive portfolio detailing their knowledge and exper-ise in neonatal developmental care; applicants whose portfolios re accepted must then pass a proctored online examination.

Sensory Deprivation versus Stimulation

Changing theories about sensory stimulation in the NICU have also promoted access for occupational therapists into the inten-sive care nursery. Understanding this evolution can help the new neonatal therapist utilize a state-of-the-art practice approach:

- *Minimal stimulation.* Special care nurseries in the 1940s and 1950s were strictly minimal stimulation units with low lights, quiet environments, and restricted access by families and even physicians.
- *Sensory deprivation theory.* The paucity of stimuli in these early nurseries precipitated a sensory deprivation theory in the 1960s and 1970s. Infants in the NICU were thought to be at increased developmental risk from deprivation of normal sensory stimulation that occurs naturally in the womb or at home after birth.
- *Sensory stimulation programs.* Sensory deficit proponents advocated compensation for perceived deprivation of beneficial sensory stimuli with selected regimens of patterned stimuli in a "one size fits all" approach. These supplemental stimulation programs utilized massage, stroking, passive range of motion, vestibular input, and/or auditory input. Concerns have been raised that extra stimulation may have benefited larger stable infants but possibly stressed more fragile babies; behavioral responses of individual infants were not reported in the studies of this era.
- *Sensory overload theory.* The sensory deficit model failed to recognize that the explosion of knowledge and technology in the 1960s and 1970s actually created an abundance of disorganized, noncontingent stimuli that was disturbing to infants in the NICU. Intensive care nurseries were large, brightly lit rooms filled with noisy monitors and equipment. Additional technology required increased staff, who engaged in more frequent handling of infants for

procedures and who greatly increased the general noise and activity level within the unit. The sensory overload theory began to emerge in the 1970s, and hypothesized that NICU infants were actually overwhelmed by a constant bombardment of inappropriate stimuli.

- *Environmental neonatology.* Increasing concerns about the significant quantity and variety of random stimuli prompted the rise in the 1980s and 1990s of "environmental neonatology," in which the short-term and long-term influence of animate and inanimate environmental factors on NICU infants is explored.
- *Individualized, relationship-based, family-centered developmental care.* Developmental care is a philosophy that recognizes that the interaction among the infant, family, and surrounding NICU environment is dynamic and ongoing. This approach strives to modify and structure the NICU environment and caregiving practices to support individualized needs of each infant and family, and to promote the involvement of family members as primary caregivers and integrated team members for support of their infant.

CHANGING FOCUS OF NEONATAL OCCUPATIONAL THERAPY

Traditional Occupational Therapy: Rehabilitation and Stimulation

Traditional neonatal occupational therapy in the 1980s (and still persisting in some NICUs) consisted solely of rehabilita-tion and developmental stimulation. Infants were identified as appropriate candidates for occupational therapy by specific risk factors (e.g., very low birth weight, prenatal drug expo-sure), diagnosis of pathology (e.g., congenital anomalies, severe asphyxia), or performance indicators (e.g., abnormal tone, poor feeding, chronic illness with developmental delay). Therapy targeted specific problems such as limited range of motion, high or low muscle tone, extreme irritability, poor feeding, or developmental delay (Figure 22-2, *A*).

Remediation and rehabilitation continue to be appropriate for NICU infants with pathology affecting development and function. Older chronically ill infants in the NICU may also need developmental therapy, although many of these infants are now transferred to step-down units or are discharged with home health services if they remain medically fragile and dependent on medical technology.

State-of-the-Art Occupational Therapy: Developmental Support

The unique knowledge and skills of neonatal occupational thera-pists support an expanded role beyond traditional rehabilitation to proficiency as developmental specialists. *Developmentally sup-portive care* begins at birth rather than once the baby is medically stable. This approach acknowledges that any infant young enough or sick enough to require intensive care has inherent developmen-tal risks and vulnerabilities, that parenting an infant in the NICU is stressful and difficult, and that both infant and family must receive individualized support throughout the NICU hospitaliza-tion for optimal outcome (Figure 22-2, *B*).[44,47]

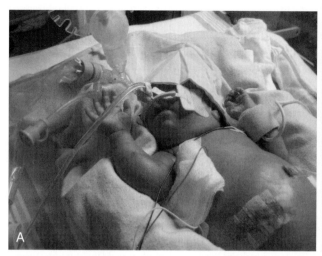
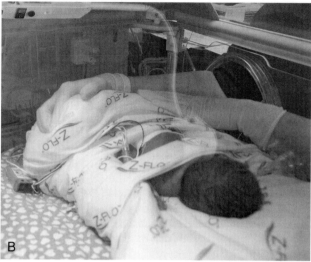

FIGURE 22-2 **A,** This infant has seizures, bowel pathology, and infections; "traditional" therapeutic positioning, pre-feeding oral stimulation and developmental therapy will be included as part of her OT treatment plan. (Courtesy of the Infant Special Care Unit, University of Texas Medical Branch, Galveston, TX. Photograph by Jan Hunter.) **B,** This infant was born at 22 weeks' gestation; multiple organ system vulnerabilities from extreme prematurity warrant protective developmental support from birth. (Courtesy Sundance Enterprises, Inc. White Plains, NY; http://www.sundancesolutions.com)

Developmental support includes a protective and preventive component of care that is not inherent in the traditional rehabilitation model. In contrast with the previous emphasis for direct "hands on" contact, protecting the fragile newborn from excessive or inappropriate sensory input is often a more urgent priority than direct interventions or interactions with the infant.[81] Trust, acceptance, and respect are gradually earned from protective NICU staff as each neonatal therapist consistently demonstrates competency in knowledge, skills, and interpersonal professional relationships.

The NICU is a specialized area of practice requiring advanced knowledge and skills.[81,82] Specialized knowledge requirements include familiarity with relevant neonatal medical conditions, procedures, and equipment; understanding the unique developmental abilities and vulnerabilities of term, preterm, and ill infants; familiarity with theories and clinical applications of neonatal behavioral organization, family systems, and NICU ecology; and appreciation of the manner in which these factors interact to influence infant and family behavior and development.

The remainder of this chapter is divided into four distinct but interrelated sections. The first section emphasizes development of a NICU medical foundation. The remaining three sections discuss the NICU environment, NICU family, and NICU infant; the infant is discussed last to symbolize the importance of a therapist's conscientious preparation before touching a NICU infant.

DEVELOPING A MEDICAL FOUNDATION

Abbreviations and Terminology

Learning the language of the NICU is essential for the neonatal occupational therapist. Documentation typically contains many abbreviations, as illustrated by the following medical summary:

Cody is a 39 wk pca wm born at 25 WBD, 24 WBE by SVD to a 19 y/o now G2P1Ab1, A+, VDRL– mom with h/o of IVDA, smoked 1 PPD, PIH, PTL, PPROM 72o PTD. Pt. had TCAN ×1 (reduced PTD), AGA at 545 gm, Apgars 11,35,610. Significant medical complications have included RDS, BPD, PIE, AOP, PDA (ligated), hyperbilirubinemia, anemia, MRSE and CONS sepsis, medical NEC, BIH, R gr. 3 and L gr. 4 IVH with frontal and temporal lobe PVL, ROP stage III OD (regressing) and stage III with plus disease OS (s/p laser OS). Pt. required HFOV with iNO, for 22 days, SIMV for 8 days, BiPAP for 14 days, NCPAP for 9 days, and remains on HFNC with FiO2 0.5 at .5L.

Understanding abbreviations and the terms they represent is a prerequisite to beginning a neonatal practice. Appendix 22-A at the end of the chapter lists some common NICU abbreviations.

Classifications for Age

Gestational age (GA) refers to the total number of weeks the infant was in utero before birth. Determination of gestational age may be based on dating the last menstrual period (LMP), by ultrasonography (USG), or by physical examination of the infant; it is generally considered accurate plus or minus 2 weeks. The range used for a full-term pregnancy is either 37 or 38 weeks to 42 weeks. Any infant born before 37 weeks is considered preterm; the infant born between 34 and 37 weeks is now called "late-preterm," with increasing recognition that such infants are still immature and vulnerable. An infant born after 42 weeks is post-term. Once the infant is born, the GA remains the same.

Postconceptional age (PCA) refers to the infant's age in relation to when conception occurred, and thus continually changes over time. PCA is obtained by adding the weeks since birth to the infant's gestational age. When the infant born at 27 weeks reaches his or her expected due date, the PCA is 40 weeks (27 weeks of gestation plus 13 weeks since birth).

PCA is commonly used until 40 to 44 weeks, equivalent to term or 1 month corrected age, respectively.

Chronologic age refers to the infant's actual age since birth. Chronologically, the infant born at 27 weeks' gestation is 3 months old on the expected due date and 12 months old on the first birthday. Chronologic age of preterm infants is usually "corrected for prematurity" to better correlate with developmental expectations and performance (e.g., the infant born at 27 weeks' gestation will not developmentally look the same at 3 months' chronologic age as the infant born at term).

Corrected age refers to how old the infant would be if born at term rather than prematurely. The number of weeks of prematurity is first determined (GA is subtracted from the term equivalent of 40 weeks) and then subtracted from the chronologic age. The infant born at 27 weeks' gestation was born 13 weeks prematurely (40 weeks − 27 weeks GA = 13 weeks early). The corrected age of this infant on the first birthday is 9 months because the actual birth was 3 months earlier than the expected due date. Corrected age is generally used until the first birthday in assessing developmental status.

Classifications by Birth Weight

Infants born above 2500 grams (5.5 pounds) are considered average in size. A birth weight of 1500 to 2500 grams is termed low birth weight (LBW). Very low birth weight (VLBW) is 1000 to 1500 grams, extremely low birth weight (ELBW) is less than 1000 grams, and ultra low birth weight (ULBW) is less than 750 grams.

Birth weight between the 10th and the 90th percentiles on a standardized growth chart is appropriate for gestational age (AGA). Birth weight below the 10th percentile is small for gestational age (SGA), and birth weight above the 90th percentile is large for gestational age (LGA). These categories apply equally to preterm, term, and postterm infants. Any infant growing normally in utero will be AGA. An infant of a mother with severe pregnancy-induced hypertension (PIH) who experienced intrauterine growth restriction (IUGR) may be born SGA, whereas the infant of a mother with diabetes is often LGA.

Thermoregulation

Preterm infants are predisposed to excessive heat loss and are vulnerable to cold stress from several causes. Extended postures, thin skin, and reduced insulating subcutaneous fat in very premature infants allow heat to transfer from the body to the air. A specialized brown fat used by newborns to metabolize heat is not produced until the last trimester of gestation. Pulmonary dysfunction, central nervous system (CNS) immaturity, and frequent caregiving interventions may also contribute to heat loss. The infant may lose heat by convection (heat loss to surrounding air), conduction (body contact with cooler solid surface), radiation (heat loss to cooler solid object not in direct contact with the infant, such as incubator walls), and evaporation (heat lost as liquid from the respiratory tract and permeable skin, which is converted into a vapor).[57,80]

Radiant warmers, incubators, initial use of humidity or emollients, prewarming of items that contact the baby (e.g. hands, stethoscopes, diaper wipes), positioning aids, clothes, and swaddling help conserve heat in NICU infants. Emerging technology shows promise for incorporating fabrics and products with phase-change molecules, which help maintain a desired temperature range through use of tiny in-woven capsules that respond to changes in heat or cooling. The neonatal therapist must diligently protect NICU infants from heat destabilization during all evaluations and interventions. Both cold stress and overheating can cause complications in NICU infants.

Medical Conditions and Equipment

Medical complications and technology both have profound effects on preterm and high-risk infants, with subsequent implications and precautions for neonatal therapists. Developing a basic medical foundation and learning NICU medical terminology is an ongoing process that progresses from a general familiarity with terms and definitions to gradually understanding the pathophysiology of diseases and the biomechanics of equipment. Table 22-1 lists common medical equipment in the NICU.

NICU ENVIRONMENT

"Mismatch" of Immature Infant in High-Tech Environment

Sensory components of the typical intrauterine and NICU extrauterine environments are significantly different (Table 22-2). Barring complications, the fetus develops in a warm, snug, dark environment in which basic needs are met and a normal sequence of development is supported. After birth, demands are suddenly made on the preterm newborn to breathe, regulate body temperature, move against the effects of gravity, adjust to bright light and unmuffled noise, cope with invasive or painful procedures, and endure frequent sleep disruption and deprivation.

The preterm infant's immature CNS is generally competent for protected intrauterine life but not sufficiently developed to adjust to and organize the overwhelming stimuli and demands of the NICU. This creates a "mismatch" of the neonate with the high-tech world now necessary for survival.

Continual overwhelming stimuli created by the NICU environment and caregiving practices may stress the highly sensitive preterm infant's already vulnerable and disorganized CNS. Excessive sensory stimulation can cause insults to the developing brain (e.g., from repeated hypoxic episodes related to stress) and create maladaptive behaviors that contribute to later poor developmental outcome.[33]

Because the sick preterm infant experiences significant stress (e.g., agitation, autonomic instability, excessive use of calories) when incoming stimuli exceed the ability of the immature CNS to respond and adapt, it becomes a priority to reduce avoidable stressors and help the infant remain calm and organized.[11,40] Developmental interventions that support neonatal physiologic stability and brain development include such practices as NICU light and sound modifications, therapeutic positioning, nurturing touch, non-nutritive sucking, alteration of caregiver timing and handling techniques, preservation of sleep, and increased family involvement.[44,47]

TABLE 22-1 Common Medical Equipment in the NICU

Equipment	Description	Purpose
THERMOREGULATION EQUIPMENT		
Radiant warmer	Open bed with overhead heat source	Typically used during medical workup of new admission or for critically ill infants requiring easy access for frequent or complicated medical care.
Incubator (Isolette)	Clear plastic heated box enclosing mattress and infant	Used to provide warmth (and sometimes humidity), allows calories to be used for growth and healing. Preferred location for attempting to reduce environmental stimuli, discourage unnecessary handling, and protect sleep. Infant may or may not be dressed and swaddled, depending on specific NICU protocol. Depending on design, access is through either portholes or a door on the front, or the entire top of the Isolette raises up.
Open crib	Bassinet-style bed; no external heat source provided; infant is dressed in clothes and swaddled in blankets	Used for larger and more stable infants; caregivers (including occupational therapist) must be careful to avoid cold stress during baths, assessments, and procedures.
OXYGEN THERAPY WITH ASSISTED VENTILATION		
Bag and mask ventilation	Bag attached to face mask is rhythmically squeezed to deliver positive pressure and oxygen	Used for resuscitation of an infant at delivery, during acute deterioration, or to increase oxygenation if necessary after an apneic spell.
CPAP	Steady stream of pressurized air given through an endotracheal tube, nasopharyngeal tube, nasal prongs, or small nasal mask; supplemental oxygen may or may not be used	Positive pressure is used to keep the alveoli and airways from collapsing (i.e., to keep them open) in an infant who is breathing spontaneously but has a disorder such as RDS, pulmonary edema, or apnea. CPAP is now commonly used from birth (when effective) to reduce potential problems from mechanical ventilation.
Mechanical ventilation (CMV, HFOV, HFJV)	Machine controls or assists breathing by mechanically inflating the lungs, increasing alveolar ventilation, and improving gas exchange. Conventional mechanical ventilation forces can contribute to lung damage; high frequency ventilation (oscillators and jets) use different mechanics to cause less barotrauma to the lungs	Used for infants with depressed respiratory drive, pulmonary disease with increased work of breathing and suboptimal oxygenation and ventilation (i.e., MAS, RDS), and frequent apnea despite CPAP; infant is usually orally or nasally intubated, but may have a tracheostomy if ventilator dependence will be prolonged.
ECMO	Sophisticated life-support system that uses a modified heart-lung bypass to provide nearly total lung rest and minimize barotrauma (lung damage that can occur with prolonged high ventilator settings)	Used as a "rescue" technology for qualifying infants in critical respiratory failure who are unresponsive to conventional medical management, or at times for preoperative support during cardiac surgery. Use of ECMO has decreased with advent of therapies such as high frequency ventilation and inhaled nitric oxide (pulmonary vasodilator drug).
OXYGEN THERAPY WITHOUT ASSISTED VENTILATION		
High-flow nasal cannula (HFNC)	Warmed and humidified oxygen or room air (21% oxygen) delivered at higher flow rates (> 1L/minute) by flexible NC with small prongs that fit into the nares; a HFNC can be set up from ventilators or many CPAP machines; Vapotherm is a separate respiratory therapy device attached to a nasal cannula that allows very high nasal flows of suspersaturated (saturated without condensation) air/oxygen blends	Used to improve gas exchange or reduce work of breathing. High flow rates may reduce the need for intubation and mechanical ventilation, or replace less well tolerated nasal CPAP. Very high humidity allows higher flow rates (compared with those possible with nasal cannula) without drying nasal mucosa.
Nasal cannula	Humidified oxygen delivered by flexible nasal cannula with small prongs that fit into the nares	Used for infants requiring supplemental oxygen without positive pressure support, generally for prolonged periods. Handling and portability are easier with a nasal cannula than with an oxyhood.
Oxygen hood (oxyhood)	Plastic hood with flow of warm humidified oxygen placed over infant's head and possibly upper trunk.	Used for infants who are breathing independently but need a higher concentration of oxygen than 21% room air; higher humidification allows oxygen delivery that is less drying to nasal mucosa than oxygen by a nasal cannula. Not as commonly used since HFNC's became available.

CPAP, continuous positive airway pressure; *ECMO,* extracorporeal membrane oxygenation; *HFJV,* high frequency jet ventilation; *HFNC,* high flow nasal cannula; *HFOV,* high-frequency oscillating ventilation; *NC,* nasal cannula; *MAS,* meconium aspiration syndrome; *RDS,* respiratory distress syndrome.

TABLE 22-2 Comparison of Intrauterine and Extrauterine Sensory Environments

System	Intrauterine	Extrauterine
Tactile	Constant proprioceptive input; smooth, wet, usually safe and comfortable; circumferential boundaries	Often painful and invasive; dry, cool air; predominance of medical touching with relative paucity of social touching
Vestibular	Maternal movements, diurnal cycles, amniotic fluid creates gently oscillating environment, flexed posture with boundaries to movements	Horizontal, flat postures; rapid position changes; influence of gravity, restraints, and equipment
Auditory	Maternal biologic sounds, muffled environmental sounds	Loud, noncontingent, mechanical, frequent (sometimes constant), harsh intermittent impulse noise
Visual	Dark; may occasionally have very dim red spectrum light	Bright lights, eyes unprotected Often no diurnal rhythm
Thermal	Constant warmth, consistent temperature	Environmental temperature variations, high risk of neonatal heat loss

Light in the NICU

Lighting Considerations for NICU Staff and Infants

Lighting requirements in the NICU are very different for NICU infants and their adult caregivers. NICU staff need variable light levels and sources for personal biorhythms (i.e., arousal and alertness, mood, temperature, hormone levels, sleep cycles) and for work-related tasks such as charting, infant assessments, and intricate procedures. Lighting needs generally increase with caregiver age.

Conversely, fragile immature infants generally need protection from NICU light sources. The visual system of the preterm infant is functionally and structurally incomplete before term birth, and requires dimness and sleep for continued optimal development.[30,61] The growth of the eye in utero is genetically coded and needs no light prior to 40 weeks; the infant's visual system continues to develop normally without external stimuli during the last trimester of gestation, with significant maturation and differentiation occurring in the retina and visual cortex.[30]

The eyelids remain fused until 24 to 26 weeks' gestation with little spontaneous eye opening until after 29 weeks, emphasizing that the eyes of the preterm infant are not yet ready to process visual input at this stage of development. Preterm infants are unable to protect themselves from room light because they are unable to close their eyelids tightly until after 30 weeks, their thin eyelids do not adequately filter light, and the iris does not significantly constrict until 30 to 34 weeks.[21]

Sensory interference can occur when one developing sensory system is stimulated out of turn or bombarded with inappropriate stimuli. For example, auditory system maturation typically occurs without strong competing sensory stimuli during the last trimester. Early birth with premature exposure to light may precipitate earlier visual system function, but preterm infants exposed to light in the NICU during the last trimester have an increased incidence of auditory processing dysfunction at school age. Premature stimulation of the visual system appears to compete and interfere with optimal development of the auditory sensory system during this critical period.[30] While early light exposure has not been shown to increase the incidence of retinopathy of prematurity,[68] ambient NICU illumination may be implicated in subtle visual pathway sequelae and visual processing problems that cannot be attributed to other major complications of preterm birth such as retinopathy of prematurity (ROP), strabismus, or myopia.[21,30,46]

Increased light intensity has been shown to increase heart rate and respiratory rate, and to decrease oxygen saturation for preterm infants in the NICU.[60] Light levels and abrupt fluctuations can disrupt sleep of the premature infant, an important consideration because much sensory system and early brain development only occurs during sleep in the last trimester.[31]

Circadian cycles are individual biorhythms over a period of approximately 24 hours. A third-trimester fetus has a functioning biologic clock (suprachiasmatic nuclei in the hypothalamus) capable of generating circadian rhythms in response to maternal day-night cues such as hormone secretion, activity patterns, and feeding cycles. These maternal circadian signals are disrupted when birth occurs prematurely.[47] Light impacts the infant's circadian system by a different neuronal pathway from that used for vision, and becomes important in regulating circadian biorhythms after preterm birth. It has been suggested the circadian system of a preterm infant is responsive to light very early (perhaps by 25 to 28 weeks' gestation), and that low-intensity light can entrain the developing circadian clock.[69,71]

Lighting Guidelines for the NICU

In contrast with the dark womb, many NICUs have chaotic and unpredictable lighting patterns. Neither continuous dim nor continuous bright light has been demonstrated to be optimal for the development of preterm babies, and often the youngest and sickest infants are exposed to the highest levels of light, such as during phototherapy or for medical procedures (Figure 22-3).[22] Guidelines for appropriate NICU lighting are available from regularly updated Recommended Standards for Newborn ICU Design.[88] Light intensity (illuminance) is measured with the metric unit lux (preferred term) or the English unit footcandle. One footcandle equals approximately 10 lux; more precisely, 1 footcandle equals 10.764 lux.

Flexibility in lighting options accommodates the variable needs of caregivers and of babies at differing stages of development and at various times throughout the day. Combinations of direct and indirect deflected lighting, adjustable ambient lighting at each bedside, no light source in an infant's direct line of sight, focused adjustable task lighting, and separate well-lit areas for tasks such as charting or medication preparation are beneficial.[88] At least one source of natural daylight visible from each patient care area provides psychological benefits to NICU families and staff, and assists with day-night cycled lighting.[3]

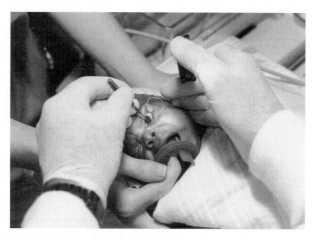

FIGURE 22-3 Neonatal intensive care unit infant is receiving eye examination by an ophthalmologist to check for development of retinopathy of prematurity. Swaddling and sucking on a pacifier dipped in 24% sucrose solution provide some relief for procedural discomfort. (Courtesy the Infant Special Care Unit, University of Texas Medical Branch, Galveston, TX. Photograph by John Glow.)

Because bright lights can disrupt sleep, current recommendations suggest a baseline (ambient) level for the patient care area of 10 to 20 lux.[88] This continuous dim lighting is probably best for infants younger than 28 weeks' gestation.[30] After 28 weeks gestation, there is some evidence that diurnally cycled lighting (dim lighting at night with daytime levels increased to 250-500 lux) has potential benefits for the infant (e.g., longer sleep, improved growth, more stable breathing, and decreased levels of stress hormones) and no evidence that cycled lighting in the NICU is harmful.[47,69]

The eyes of a preterm infant should always be protected from bright and direct light. The ability to visually attend emerges at 32 to 34 weeks' PCA and is enhanced in low ambient light.[47] Infants nearing term gestation and beyond need light and more complex visual stimulation for appropriate visual development and state regulation.

Sound in the NICU

Noise is undesirable sound.[5] The acoustic environment of the NICU is a function of both the building (e.g., ventilation systems and fire alarms), and of operations (e.g., activities of people, communication devices, medical equipment).[88] In a traditional NICU, environmental noise is constant throughout the day and night, is predominantly mechanical rather than social, and is noncontingent to individual infants. Sound inside the Isolette is characterized by continuous white noise and nonspeech sounds; harsh mechanical noises penetrate clearly and reverberate, whereas speech sounds are indistinct. NICU infants are exposed to vibration and noise during transport and when on high-frequency ventilation; noise and vibration combined may have a synergistic effect.[3]

Environmental noise can stress NICU infants with a resultant decrease in oxygenation and an increase in vasoconstriction, blood pressure, intracranial pressure, heart rate, and respiratory rate. High noise levels can contribute to apnea and bradycardia.[8] Noise disrupts sleep, which can impede an infant's growth, medical recovery, sensory system development, and early neural circuitry formation.[31,62]

An infant born prematurely is exposed to both low- and high-frequency sound without the protective noise attenuation of the mother's body. Hearing threshold of the infant has been reported as 40 decibels (dB) at 28 to 34 weeks' gestation, 30 dB at 35 to 38 weeks' gestation, and <20 dB at term; these thresholds are greatly exceeded in the NICU.[42] Loud or prolonged sounds may damage the delicate developing cochlea with resultant hearing loss, in the same frequency range as that of the damaging sound; preterm infants are at risk for hearing loss in both low-frequency (speech) and high-frequency ranges.

Critical human auditory system development occurs in the third trimester; sensory interference may occur when immature sensory systems are stimulated out of order or bombarded with inappropriate stimuli. Animal studies support a connection between atypical patterns of early sensory experience (i.e. chaotic environmental noise; excessive light exposure prior to term gestation when auditory system development should be occurring without competition) and disruption of early perceptual and behavioral development.[32,46]

Background noise in the NICU may interfere with the infant's ability to discriminate speech of parents and other caregivers.[13] Long-term difficulties in auditory processing can occur in the presence of normal intelligence and hearing sensitivity; behaviors associated with disturbed auditory processing have been noted in NICU graduates. Auditory processing problems may be manifested by poor listening skills ("huh?" "what?"), difficulty following multistep directions, poor discrimination of specific auditory signals amid other background or impulse noise, distractibility, short attention span, or poor reading and spelling skills.[39]

Environmental Modifications of Sound in the NICU

Guidelines for optimal sound levels in the NICU consider both intensity and duration of sound exposure, and are detailed in the current NICU Design Standards.[88] Structural modifications are the most effective method to minimize noise levels in the NICU, but caregiver modifications can help.[12] Staff members can move bed spaces of sensitive infants away from loud or high-traffic areas and hold conversations, including medical rounds, away from the bedside. Auditory alarms can be reduced in volume and silenced quickly to reduce infant exposure to piercing impulse noise; remote control devices to silence alarms, or visual alarms, are available. Respiratory tubing and water traps can be positioned to promote drainage; empty accumulated water frequently to prevent bubbling (60 to 70 dB). Isolette covers can significantly reduce the noise level within an incubator. Musical toys and tape recordings can reverberate inside the isolette; extreme caution and very low volume are recommended if these are used. Goals of a quieter NICU include prolonged periods of undisturbed sleep for the infant, providing an environment for discernment of an audible maternal voice at 31 to 32 weeks' gestation and beyond, and providing an improved and safer work environment for staff.[47]

Caregiving in the NICU

NICU caregiving patterns differ significantly from those in the fetal intrauterine environment and the normal home setting. The sense of touch is highly developed in utero, with gentle human touch normally providing consistent positive tactile input after term birth; touch in the NICU, however, is usually related to medical care rather than social nurturing.[51] NICU interventions are often intrusive or aversive, and are typically constant throughout a 24-hour span; observe the multiple procedures that are evident in the photographs of the NICU case study on the Evolve website.

Caregiving procedures may contribute to an infant's physiologic instability (e.g. increased heart rate, fluctuations in blood pressure, alterations in cerebral blood flow, and hypoxemia), motor stress, energy depletion, and agitation. Caregiving based primarily on external criteria, such as fixed schedules for vital signs and feeding, often ignores or delays the caregiver's response to the infant's cues that indicate that he or she needs care; caregiving thus becomes noncontingent to the infant's efforts to communicate.[24]

Preterm infants are extremely vulnerable to pain. Decreased ability to attenuate pain may allow even relatively benign procedures to be perceived as painful, especially if occurring just after handling or another painful experience.[66] Immediate consequences of severe or repetitive painful experiences in the NICU may include physiologic instability, medical complications, sleep disturbances, feeding problems, and poor self-regulation. Long-term changes of decreased pain thresholds and hypersensitivity to pain may also occur.[34,85] Repetitive or prolonged pain has been implicated in enhanced neuronal cell death in the immature brain, with concerns for future neurodevelopmental outcome.[10] Pharmacologic and non-pharmacologic management of pain is a top priority in NICU caregiving.[16,23]

Medical literature is unequivocal on the divergent effects of sleep deprivation and improved sleep on NICU infants.[31,44,47] A last-trimester fetus has undisturbed sleep in a protected environment; a NICU infant has frequent sleep disruptions in a stressful environment.

The brain of a 23-weeker is smooth with undeveloped synaptic connections, these connections will now be formed within the context of the NICU experience, rather than in an orderly sequential process in the womb. The primary ongoing event in brain and sensory system development during the last trimester is synaptogenesis, or the formation of billions of connections between neurons. Synaptogenesis at this stage is endogenous (occurs spontaneously within the brain in the absence of external stimulation), and forms the early brain architecture that is later refined by exogenous (external) stimuli. Endogenous synaptogenesis produces brain complexity and plasticity and occurs only during sleep, and only during REM sleep after 28 weeks' gestation.

Premies as children are known to have smaller brains than their term counterparts, plus increased risk for difficulties with learning, abstract thinking, behavior, coping, adaptability, and attention; brain "wiring" can be disturbed even in the absence of structural brain pathology. Undisturbed sleep is absolutely essential for normal development of the infant brain and sensory systems during the last trimester; interventions to protect and prolong sleep should be a top caregiving priority (Figure 22-4).

Modifications of Caregiving in the NICU

Developmentally supportive caregiving in the NICU strives to minimize avoidable stressors, facilitate infant medical and neurobehavioral stability, provide therapeutic positioning, facilitate and protect sleep, promote self-regulation, foster normal developmental sequences, and encourage family participation.[44,47] The individual infant's cues, sleep state, and ongoing medical

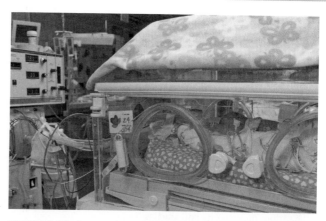

FIGURE 22-4 24-week-GA infant on high-frequency oscillating ventilation (HFOV). Efforts to protect sleep include placement of the infant in an incubator to decrease random handling and stimuli, clustered care, covering the Isolette to block overhead light (cover folded back for this picture), and supportive positioning in an individually contoured Z-Flo fluidized positioner. (Courtesy Sundance Enterprises, White Plains, NY; http://www sundancesolutions.com)

status should determine timing and sequencing of caregiving. Procedures and interventions for each infant should be based on necessity rather than nursery routines, avoiding unnecessary handling and movement. Caregivers prepare the baby for touch or movement by speaking softly and containing extremities during movement and lifting. Table 22-3 summarizes considerations for caregiving related to infant state of arousal.

Bath time is frequently stressful and exhausting to NICU infants. Bathing by immersion in warm water is usually more soothing than sponge bathing if the infant's body is well supported with extremities contained; "swaddled" bathing has proved successful even with irritable and disorganized infants. The swaddled infant is immersed to the shoulders in a tub of warm water, and the face is washed first with clean water. Next, one body section is unwrapped for bathing and rinsing, then rewrapped in the wet cloth before proceeding to washing another section of the body (i.e., right upper body, then left upper body, then legs and buttocks).[20] The warmth and proprioceptive weight of a wet blanket seem calming, and infants are usually quiet and alert throughout this bath, making swaddled bathing a successful and enjoyable caregiving experience for parents (Figure 22-5).

Even social touch and noninvasive caregiving procedures can disturb and stress vulnerable infants, requiring caregiver efforts at consoling and facilitating infant recovery. Examples of supportive measures are comfortable bedding, containment, parental skin-to-skin holding (kangaroo care), and reduction of environmental light and sound. Non-nutritive sucking is often successful for soothing and self-regulation; a pacifier dipped in a 24% sucrose solution can be used to help manage "minor" procedural pain.[25]

FAMILIES IN THE NICU

Families in Crisis

The admission of an infant to the NICU frequently puts that family in crisis, with an intense onslaught of confusing

TABLE 22-3 Newborn States and Considerations for Caregiving

Newborn State	Comments
SLEEP STATES	
Deep sleep (non-rapid eye movement [NREM])	Infant is very difficult if not impossible to arouse. Infant will not breastfeed or bottle-feed in this state, even after vigorous stimulation. Infant is unable to respond to environment; frustrating for caregivers.
Slow state changes	
Regular breathing	
Eyes closed; no eye movements	Term infants may exhibit a "slow" heart rate (80 to 90 beats per minute), which may trigger heart rate alarms and result in unnecessary stimulation by neonatal intensive care unit staff.
No spontaneous activity except startles and jerky movements	
Startles with some delay and suppresses rapidly	
Lowest oxygen consumption	At birth, preterm infants have altered states of consciousness: Early dominant states are light sleep, quiet, and active alert. "Protective apathy" enables the preterm infant to remain inactive, unresponsive, and in a sleep state to conserve energy, grow, and maintain physiologic homeostasis.
Light sleep (rapid eye movement [REM] sleep)	
Low activity level	
Random movements and startles	
Respirations irregular and abdominal	Full-term infants begin and end sleep in active sleep; preterm infants are more responsive (than term infants) to stimuli in active sleep.
Intermittent sucking movements	
Eyes closed; rapid eye movement	Infants may cry or fuss briefly in this state and be awakened to feed before they are truly awake and ready to eat.
Higher oxygen consumption	Lower and more variable oxygenation states.
AWAKE STATES	
Drowsy or semidozing	Infant may awaken further or return to sleep if left alone.
Eyelids fluttering	Quietly talking and looking at the infant, or offering a pacifier or an inanimate object to see and listen to may arouse the infant to the quiet alert state.
Eyes open or closed (dazed)	
Mild startles (intermittent)	
Delayed response to sensory stimuli	Less mature infants (30 weeks) demonstrate a drowsier than quiet alert state than older infants (36 weeks).
Smooth state change after stimulation	
Fussing may or may not be present	
Respirations—more rapid and shallow	
Quiet alert, with bright look	Immediately after birth, term newborns exhibit a period of quiet alertness, their first opportunity to "take in" their parents and the extrauterine environment.
Focuses attention on source of stimulation	
Impinging stimuli may break through; may have some delay in response	Dimmed lights, quiet talking, and stroking optimize this time for parents.
Minimal motor activity	Best state for learning to occur, because infant focuses all attention on visual, auditory, tactile, and sucking stimuli; best state for interaction with parents—baby is maximally able to attend and reciprocally respond to parents.
Active alert—eyes open	Infant has decreased threshold (increased sensitivity) to internal (hunger, fatigue) and external (wet, noise, handling) stimuli. Infant may quiet self, may escalate to crying, or with consolation by caretaker may become quiet, alert or go to sleep.
Considerable motor activity—thrusting movements of extremities; spontaneous startles	
Reacts to external stimuli with increase in movements and startles (discrete reactions difficult to differentiate because of general higher activity level)	Infant is unable to maximally attend to caretakers or environment because of increased motor activity and increased sensitivity to stimuli.
Respirations irregular	
May or may not be fussy	
Crying—intense and difficult to disrupt with external stimuli	Crying is infant's response to unpleasant internal and/or external stimulation—infant's tolerance limits have been reached (and exceeded). Infant may be able to quiet self with hand-to-mouth behaviors; talking may quiet a crying infant; holding, rocking, or putting infant upright on caretaker's shoulder may quiet infant.
Respirations rapid, shallow, and irregular	

From Gardner, S. L., & Goldson, E. (2006). The neonate and the environment: Impact on development. In G.B. Merenstein & S. L. Gardner (Eds.), *Handbook of neonatal intensive care*, (6th ed, pp. 279-280). St. Louis: Mosby.

emotions.[74] The delivery was often unexpected, and the family unit is now separated. The appearance of the infant can be frightening, and the NICU environment overwhelming. Unknown staff and unfamiliar terminology can hinder effective communication. Some mothers have continued physical complications or illness from the pregnancy or delivery. Financial considerations, transportation or travel issues, and conflicting needs of siblings can be worrisome. Parental shock, denial, and grief over loss of the ideal birth and perfect infant are compounded by concerns for the recovery of a critically ill infant; maternal depression increases stress and hinders coping.[76]

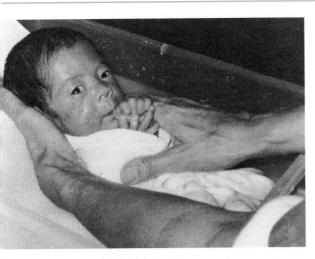

FIGURE 22-5   Swaddled bath. Swaddled preterm infant is immersed in a tub of warm water for a developmentally supportive bath.   (Courtesy the NICU, Medical Center of Plano, Plano, TX. Photograph by Dana Fern.)

The trend in NICUs is family-centered care.[56,88] Consistent implementation is a challenge that requires changing unit culture, including staff beliefs and practices. Unit-based developmental specialists can facilitate this change from traditional provider-centered, task-directed care to holistic individualized, relationship-based family-centered care.[9,44]

The many facets of understanding and working with families who have an ill or special needs child are discussed in depth in Chapter 5. Parental responsibilities have been described as providers, protectors, caregivers, educators, and facilitators of their child's development.[82] Many areas of normal parental control, however, are relinquished to medical staff members because the new mother and father are unprepared and uncertain how to parent an infant in the NICU. Policies in some units that prohibit access to the infant (e.g. restricted visiting hours; denial of entry during medical rounds or shift change) or that limit the presence of supportive family or friends can further limit and isolate parents. Conversely, family coping, satisfaction, confidence and competence can be facilitated through positive relationships with NICU staff who openly communicate and consistently include parents in decision making and caregiving throughout the infant's hospitalization.

Parents can be encouraged to ask questions about what they understand and want to know; staff responses need to be honest, consistent, and understandable. Parents are often frustrated when information appears contradictory; much of their anxiety stems from incomplete information or a perceived lack of truth. Printed resources can be available for parents in a waiting room, in a parents' library, or for individual checkout. Computers may be available with parent education and support resources, or with Internet access. Parent groups can also be helpful in providing information, comfort, and support; groups centered on activities such as scrapbooking seem to facilitate spontaneous sharing and support.

Family Inclusion in Developmental Support

Developmental support with NICU families is relationship-based. Nonjudgmental support adapted to parental coping mechanisms, learning styles, personalities, and cultural background is essential.

The former approach of "therapist as expert, child as client, parents as students" has evolved to family-centered mutual collaboration. Dialogue is reciprocal; the therapist talks with rather than to parents, and facilitates the family's active role with their infant and on the NICU team. Recognizing parental skills, celebrating successes, and facilitating parent's expertise are invaluable (see the NICU case study on the Evolve website).

Some family-friendly changes in NICU routines and practices automatically facilitate parenting. Twins with adjacent bedspaces (or co-bedded, with both twins in the same Isolette or crib) rather than in separate areas of the nursery helps create a family space. Staff efforts to make the infant as comfortable and as "normal" looking as possible (e.g., positional nesting, dressing in baby clothes, adding a hair bow, providing a cute name tag) help parents look beyond the diagnosis and technology. Diligence in using the infant's name and correct gender demonstrates to families that staff members acknowledge their baby as a real person, not just a sick premie. Caregiving can often be more flexible to accommodate parents' schedules. The inclusion of siblings, extended family members, and other support persons should be encouraged.

A behavioral and developmental assessment of an infant can be educational for the parents (Figure 22-6). The therapist can help parents gain competence and confidence in recognizing and responding to their infant's cues of stress or stability, providing therapeutic positioning and developmentally supportive handling (e.g., containing extremities in flexion, cupping infant's head and lower body in parent's palms in a "hand swaddle" or "facilitative tuck," letting the infant hold onto parent's finger), regulating sensory input to avoid overstimulation, facilitating functional oral feeding, and meeting the infant's long-term developmental needs.

If parents cannot come frequently to the NICU, a therapist can encourage phone calls, send pictures (printed or digital) or notes sharing significant events or behaviors, save photographs

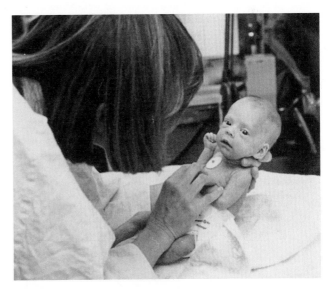

FIGURE 22-6   Assessment of this stable preterm infant includes evaluation of neuromotor and neurobehavioral functioning. The assessment can be a valuable teaching tool when performed jointly with the infant's parents.   (Courtesy of the Neonatal Intensive Care Unit, University of Connecticut Health Center's John N. Dempsey Hospital, Farmington, CT. Photograph by Gregory Kriss.)

for parent albums or scrapbooks, or keep a bedside journal in which staff members record observations or progress. A nontraditional work schedule that includes some evenings, weekends and holidays greatly increases the therapist's availability and benefit to families. Promoting parent-infant attachment, and helping the family know, love, and respond to their infant as a unique person, will yield greater benefits than any other intervention by the NICU therapist.

Skin-to-Skin Holding (Kangaroo Care)

Kangaroo care refers to the practice of parents holding their diaper-clad premature infant beneath their clothing, chest-to-chest and skin-to-skin (Figure 22-7). Kangaroo care originated in Bogota, Columbia, in response to overcrowded nurseries and insufficient medical equipment; but is now common throughout Western Europe and in the United States. Initiation, frequency, and duration of kangaroo care vary among individual NICUs according to age, weight, and acuity of the infant; skin-to-skin holding is more widely accepted for stable infants not on ventilators, but is also implemented with younger and sicker infants.[41,49]

Both infant and parents benefit from skin-to-skin holding.[15,19,48] Physiologic benefits to the infant from skin-to-skin holding include more stable heart and breathing rates, reduced apnea, stable body temperature, improved weight gain and growth, and decreased or less severe infections. Behavioral infant benefits include decreased agitation and less random motor activity, reduction in stress from environmental disturbances and medical interventions, improved state control with less crying and better self-regulation, and more mature sleep organization. Easier transition to breastfeeding, earlier hospital discharge, and a positive effect on neurodevelopmental outcome have also been noted.[48]

Skin-to-skin holding facilitates maternal milk production and longer duration of breastfeeding. Parents develop an increased awareness of their infant's cues of well-being or distress, and increased attachment and feelings of closeness to their infant. They demonstrate more positive touch of their infant, less focus on technical care, more confidence in their own caregiving ability, and decreased maternal stress.[15,19,48]

Discharge Planning

Discharge planning begins on the day of admission. Facilitating the infant's behavioral stability, sleep-wake cycle organization, and self-regulation capacities by consistent environmental modification and sensitive caregiving will ease the transition to home care for the infant and family. Including and supporting parents in active caregiving roles throughout hospitalization are essential.[18]

As the anticipated discharge date approaches, staff need to consistently model expectations for home caregiving, such as putting the infant on the back to sleep, removing positioning aids, and removing soft bedding and stuffed animals from the bed.[38,54] Protection of sleep and avoidance of overstimulation are also important at home. Following infant cues for feeding while ensuring adequate nutritional intake is a priority. Each NICU has specific transition to home guidelines that are worth the therapist's time to learn.

Many hospitals provide accommodations for parents to stay with their infant overnight in a NICU parent room before discharge. After downsizing closed some patient care areas, one innovative hospital allowed NICU parents to stay in unoccupied rooms and thus be readily available to help care for their infant breastfeeding during the night was common in their NICU.

Parents should be familiar with their infant's specific developmental strengths and needs. The therapist can provide information about community resources and parent support groups; an infant referral to a local early childhood intervention program should be completed when indicated, but is not routinely necessary for every NICU graduate. Arranging for parents to meet community resource personnel before hospital discharge and providing a follow-up telephone call from NICU staff after discharge can be helpful in reducing parental "separation anxiety" from the NICU.

It is extremely beneficial for neonatal therapists to actively participate in NICU follow-up clinics. Besides allowing reinforcement and continuation of developmental teaching, preventing some infants from "falling through the cracks," and continuing relationships with NICU families, the therapist gains valuable knowledge from countless opportunities to observe infant outcome from various diagnoses and clinical courses. Many infants do surprisingly well after prolonged NICU stays, while others develop unanticipated problems. Developmental sequelae seen in NICU graduates may stem from intrauterine problems (e.g., fetal infection or hypoxic events) that are often unknown until later developmental difficulties are observed. This information helps the therapist appreciate the unpredictable nature of NICU infant development and understand the variables that contribute to their developmental outcomes.

INFANTS IN THE NICU

Evaluation of the NICU Infant

The "Golden Rule" of occupational therapy evaluation and intervention with the NICU infant is "Above all, do no harm!" The following guidelines consider that goal.

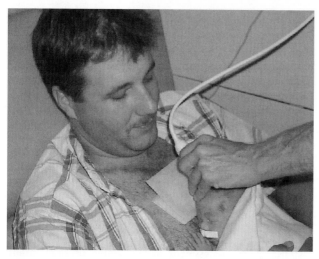

FIGURE 22-7 Father using skin-to-skin holding technique (kangaroo care) while preterm infant undergoes a head ultrasound to rule out intraventricular hemorrhage. (Courtesy the Infant Special Care Unit, University of Texas Medical Branch, Galveston, TX. Photograph by Jan Hunter.)

1. Safety for the infant takes priority over convenience for the therapist in all aspects of care. Review applicable medical conditions and equipment, be very aware of stress cues, and never perform an evaluation item simply to fill in a blank space on a form if the information obtained will not benefit the care plan for the baby.

2. Learn an evaluation tool thoroughly before touching an infant, and be constantly aware of changes in an infant's stress level. Many therapists use a structured assessment that is supplemented with data gathering and clinical observations. Administration of some structured neonatal assessments requires specialized training and/or certification to reliability (e.g., Neonatal Individualized Developmental Care and Assessment Program [NIDCAP]); others may be used after independent study of the manual and practice (e.g., Dubowitz Neonatal Neurological Exam).

3. Appreciate the nurse's role in protecting the infant, and use astute clinical observations of the infant and surrounding environment before any touching. Very fragile infants can be assessed entirely by skilled observations.

4. Weigh the value of any "hands-on" evaluation procedures against potential stressful effects on the infant. Co-assessments with other disciplines may reduce unnecessary duplication of items that require handling.

5. Time evaluation according to the infant's sleep cycle, feeding schedule, caregiving routine, and medical status. Respect the infant's signs of stress during handling; switch to an observational assessment if the infant does not readily return to a calm organized state even with caregiver assistance.

6. Performing an evaluation is easier than accurately analyzing the results; overinterpretation and mistaking immaturity for pathology are frequent errors of new neonatal therapists.

Preterm infants, especially those born at an extremely young GA, often differ in neuromotor and neurobehavioral progression from infants born at term. Routine ongoing reassessment in the NICU and in a follow-up clinic as infants mature and recover is essential for developing sound clinical judgment about the meaning of early clinical findings.

Neurobehavioral Organization of the Preterm Infant

Synactive Theory of Development

Preterm infants are continually affected by and responsive to environmental influences; Als has proposed a model for understanding these emerging capabilities of preterm infants to organize and control their behavior.[2] The synactive theory of development identifies five separate but interdependent subsystems (autonomic, motor, state, attention-interaction, and self-regulation) within the infant that are in constant interaction with one another and with the environment. Figure 22-8 illustrates the unfolding of these subsystems as the infant continues to mature before and after birth. Through recognizable approach and avoidance behaviors occurring in these subsystems, infants continually communicate their level of stress and stability in relation to what is happening to and around them (Table 22-4). Maturation and improved (or declining) health are reflected in sequential observation of subsystem development (Table 22-5).

Synactive theory forms the basis for individualized developmentally supportive and family-centered care. Caregivers are trained to be sensitive to each infant's fragility and stress behaviors, versus robustness and stability behaviors. The caregiver then uses these observations to modify the environment and caregiving practices to facilitate the infant's organization and

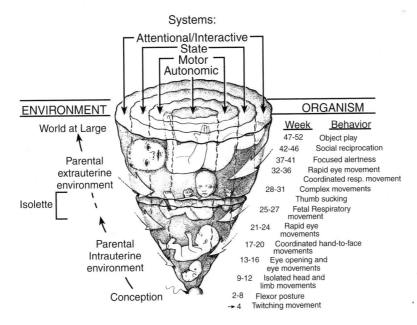

FIGURE 22-8   Beginning at conception, emerging and expanding capabilities of developing infant are illustrated in this model of synactive organization of behavioral development.   (From Als, H. [1982]. Toward a synactive theory of development: promise for the assessment and support of infant individuality. Infant Mental Health Journal, 3, 229-243.)

TABLE 22-4 Synactive Theory of Development: Neurobehavioral Subsystems, Signs of Stress and Stability*

Subsystem	Signs of Stress	Signs of Stability
AUTONOMIC	**Physiologic instability**	**Physiologic stability**
Respiratory	Pauses, tachypnea, gasping	Smooth, regular respiratory rate
Color	Changes to mottled, flushed, pale, dusky, cyanotic, gray or ashen	Pink, stable color
Visceral	Hiccups, gagging, spitting up, grunting, straining (as if producing bowel movement)	Stable viscera with no hiccups, gags, emesis, or grunting
Motor	Tremors, startles, twitches, coughs, sneezes, yawns, sighs, seizures	No sign of tremors, startles, twitches, coughs, sneezes, yawns, sighs, or seizures
MOTOR	**Fluctuating tone, uncontrolled activity**	**Consistent tone, controlled activity**
Flaccidity	Gape face, low tone in trunk, limp lower extremities and upper extremities	Muscle tone consistent in trunk and extremities and appropriate for postconceptional age
Hypertonicity	Leg extensions and sitting on air; upper-extremity salutes, finger splays, and fisting; trunk arching; tongue extensions	Smooth controlled posture Smooth movements of extremities and head
Hyperflexions	Trunk, lower and/or upper extremities Frantic, diffuse activity extremities	Motor control can be used for self-regulation (hand and foot clasp, leg and foot bracing, hand-to-mouth, grasping, tucking, sucking)
STATE	**Diffused or disorganized quality of states, including range and transition between states**	Clear states; good, calming, focused alertness
During sleep	Twitches, sounds, whimpers, jerky movements, irregular respiratory rate, fussy, grimaces	Clear, well-defined sleep states Smooth transition between states Good self-quieting and consolability
When awake	Abrupt state changes Eye floating, glassy eyed, staring, gaze aversion, worried or dull look, hyperalert panicked expression, weak cry, irritability	Focused clear alertness with animated expressions (e.g., frowning, cheek softening, "ooh" face, cooing, smiling) Robust crying
ATTENTION-INTERACTION	**Effort to attend and interact to specific stimulus elicits stress signals of other subsystems**	**Responsive to auditory, visual, and social stimuli is clear and prolonged**
Autonomic	Irregular respiratory rate, color changes, visceral responses, coughs, yawns, sneezes, sighs, straining tremors, twitches	Actively seeks out auditory stimulus; able to shift attention smoothly from one stimulus to another
Motor state	Fluctuating tone, frantic diffuse activity Eye floating, glassy eyed, staring, worried or dull look, hyperalert panicked expression, gaze aversion, weak cry, irritability Becomes stressed if more than one type of stimulus is given simultaneously Abrupt state changes	Face demonstrates bright-eyed purposeful interest varying between arousal and relaxation

SELF-REGULATION: Infant's efforts to achieve, maintain, or regain balance and self-organization in each subsystem as needed. Examples include motor strategies (e.g., foot clasp, leg and foot bracing, finger folding, hand clasping, hand to mouth, grasping, tucking, sucking, postural changes); state strategies (e.g., lowers state of arousal or releases energy with rhythmic, robust crying), and attention and orientation strategies such as visual locking. The success of various strategies may vary among infants.

*Modified from the multiple works of Heidi Als, PhD, on the synactive theory of development.

TABLE 22-5 Neurobehavioral Development of Preterm Infants by Gestational Age

Neurobehavioral System	Developmental Behaviors
INFANTS AT ≤30 WEEKS' GESTATION	
Autonomic	May exhibit periodic breathing, apnea, and bradycardia Color changes common with stimulation Eyelids are thin; infant has minimal ability to achieve or maintain protective tightening of eyelid against bright light Eyes flutter open, often with rapid uncoordinated eye movements or with diffuse unfocused gaze
Motor	Reflex smiling and startle response are present Muscle tone is low; limp extension of extremities and flat resting postures are predominant Uncontrolled spontaneous movements such as extremity twitches and tremors are common Active movements of extremities are jerky Infant is unable to coordinate sucking, swallowing, and breathing

Continued

TABLE 22-5   Neurobehavioral Development of Preterm Infants by Gestational Age—Cont'd

Neurobehavioral System	Developmental Behaviors
State	Light sleep states predominate, with rapid eye movements (REMs) and frequent tonguing/mouthing apparent
	States are not yet well defined; drowsy or awake "alert" periods are brief
	Visual acuity is poor, with little accommodation
	Apnea may result when visual stimuli are intense
Attention/interaction self-regulation	Hearing is well developed; preference for mother's voice is possible
	Usually easily stressed by environmental and caregiving stimuli
	Self-regulation efforts are immature and ineffective

INFANTS AT 30–33 WEEKS' GESTATION

Autonomic	May exhibit periodic breathing, apnea and bradycardia
	Reflexive ability to constrict iris emerges
	Able to keep eyelids shut, but eyelids still thin
Motor	Muscle tone improving and more flexion is apparent, motor tone better in lower extremities than in upper extremities
	Motor activity becoming smoother, but startles and tremors still common
	Improved head control is evident
State	Active sleep predominant, but quiet sleep increasing
	Increase in alert awake time
	States more distinct as sleep-wake organization emerges
	Arousal with feeding readiness cues may be observed
	Emerging coordination of sucking, swallowing, and breathing
Attention/interaction	Brightens to sound; preference for human voice
	May be able to briefly visually focus (with much effort) on specific stimulus
	Limited capacity for social contact
Self-regulation	Still often stressed by environmental and caregiving stimuli
	Self-regulation efforts (e.g., grasping, foot bracing, hand-to-mouth) increasing with variable effectiveness

INFANTS AT 34–36 WEEKS' GESTATION

Autonomic	Generally more stable heart rate, respiratory rate, and oxygen saturation
Motor	Muscle tone, activity level, and motor control continue to improve
	Able to right head forwards and backwards
	Decreased tremors
	Usually able to breast or bottle feed
State	Increase in quiet sleep with more regular respiration and decreased random activity
	Smoother transition between sleep and awake states
	Infant usually awakens to stimulation, although duration and quality of alertness may be variable
	Arousal and crying more frequent in response to discomfort, pain, or hunger
Attention/interaction	More consistent behavioral responsiveness to auditory stimuli
	Visual orientation (focus, brief tracking) present, but infant may become overstimulated or fatigued with the effort
Self-regulation	Increased capacity for social attentiveness and responsiveness
	May tolerate just one type of sensory or social stimulation at a time
	Improving efforts and success at self-consoling and self-regulation

INFANTS AT 37–40 WEEKS' GESTATION

Motor	Extremity flexor tone present; movements increasingly smooth and controlled
	Wide variety of movements are observed
	Takes feeds by breast or bottle
State	Well-defined range of states with smooth transitions
	Quiet sleep increases with equal periods of active sleep
	Sleep-wake cycles shorter with less mature sleep-wake organization than infant born at term
	Crying more closely approximates that of the term infant
Attention/interaction	Increasingly consistent behavioral responsiveness to auditory stimuli; prefers human voice
	Active "looking" behaviors increase during quiet alert periods
	Infant displays preferences for visual stimuli (usually human face) and tracks objects; best visual focus is at 8-10 inches
Self-regulation	More reciprocal social interaction
	Self-regulation efforts more organized and successful

Data from Hadley, M. A, West, D., Turner, A., & Santangelo, S. (1999). *Developmental and behavioral characteristics of preterm infants.* Petaluma, CA: NICU, Inc.; and Yecco, G. J. (1993). Neurobehavioral development and developmental support of premature infants. *Journal of Perinatal and Neonatal Nursing, 7,* 56-65.

well-being. Each infant's attempts to maintain or return to a calm, organized state are also noted and encouraged. The infant and family are seen as an integral unit, with parents supported in assuming an active role with their infant in the NICU.

Medical, developmental, and financial gains have been attributed to provision of developmentally supportive care.[64,87] Reported medical benefits include decreased severity of chronic lung disease, fewer days on assisted ventilation and supplemental oxygen, improved weight gain, reduced incidence of intraventricular hemorrhage (IVH), and reduced need for sedation. Earlier transition to oral feedings, improved cognitive and motor development as compared with control infants, and increased family involvement and confidence have been noted. Shorter hospital stays from these cumulative benefits can result in significant cost savings.

Preterm Neurobehavioral Organization: In-turning, Coming-out, and Reciprocity

Another description of preterm infant behavioral organization[28] facilitates "rule of thumb" guidelines for the occupational therapist seeking to determine appropriate interventions for specific infants. Infants in the "in-turning" stage are generally immature or critically ill; these infants need minimal handling with maximal environmental and caregiving protection. Infants in the "coming-out" stage remain fragile and vulnerable but have brief periods of availability to attend to their environment; graded unimodal stimulation may be appropriate in small doses based on observed infant tolerance. The more mature and stable infant in the "reciprocity" stage is able to attend and interact when in an appropriate quiet alert state, but the caregiver must still respect approach and avoidance signals. Advancing postconceptional age and medical status (acuity and chronicity) affect an individual infant's progression through these stages. Table 22-6

summarizes and compares the stages and characteristics of preterm behavioral organization of this theory and Als' synactive theory of development.

States of Arousal

State refers to the infant's degree of consciousness or arousal with quality and consistency of state control in preterm infants generally improving as age and maturation increase. State significantly affects other areas such as muscle tone, feeding performance, or reaction to stimuli.

State is most frequently classified into six categories: state 1 (deep sleep); state 2 (light sleep); state 3 (transitional state of dozing or drowsiness); state 4 (quiet and alert); state 5 (active alert); and state 6 (crying). The smoothness or abrupt fluctuation as the infant transitions between states, both spontaneously and during handling, provide information on neural organization and control.[11] The infant who cannot be aroused, who is excessively irritable, or who has wide swings between sleep and cry states with no interim alert periods may be demonstrating either immaturity or pathology. A gradual awakening with smooth transition from sleep to alertness and eventually back to sleep is one sign of maturation and neurologic integrity.

Smooth transition between states requires appropriate regulation and response to a variety of sensory input.[11] The ability to modulate state is affected by both intrinsic factors (pain, stress, immaturity, illness, intrauterine drug exposure) and extrinsic factors such as light, noise, and caregiving activities. Individual temperament may also be a variable in the infant's state of arousal; some infants are more active and demanding, whereas others are more relaxed.[24] Sleep is essential for body and brain growth and development; supporting and protecting undisturbed sleep should be a caregiving priority.[31]

TABLE 22-6 Stages and Characteristics of Behavioral Organization in Preterm Infant

Als	Gorski, Davidson, & Brazelton
Physiologic homeostasis—stabilizing and integrating temperature control, cardiorespiratory function, digestion, and elimination. Characteristics: becomes pale, dusky, cyanotic; heart and respiratory rates change—all symptoms of disorganization of autonomic nervous system.	"In turning"—physiologic stage of mere survival characterized by autonomic nervous system responses to stimuli (rapid color changes caused by swings in heart and respiratory rates); no or limited direct response; inability to arouse self spontaneously; jerky movements; asleep (and protecting the central nervous system from sensory overload) 97% of the time. Preterm infants (<32 weeks) are easily physiologically overwhelmed by stimuli.
Motor development may infringe on physiologic homeostasis, resulting in defensive strategies (vomiting, color change, apnea, and bradycardia). State development becomes less diffuse and encompasses full range: sleep, awake, crying. States and state changes may affect physiologic and motor stability.	"Coming out"—first active response to environment may be seen as early as 34 to 35 weeks (provided some physiologic stability has been achieved). Characteristics: remains pink with stimuli; has directed response for short periods; arouses spontaneously and maintains arousal after stimuli ceases; if interaction begins in alert state: maintains quiet alert for 5 to 10 minutes, tracks animate and inanimate stimuli; spends 10% to 15% of time in alert state with predictable interaction patterns.
Alert state is well differentiated from other states State changes may interfere with physiologic and motor stability.	"Reciprocity"—active interaction and reciprocity with environment from 36 to 40 weeks. Characteristics: directs response; arouses and consoles self; maintains alertness and interacts with both animate and inanimate objects; copes with external stress.

Modified from Als, H. (1986). A synactive model of neonatal behavior organization: Framework for the assessment of neurobehavioral development in the premature infant and for support of infants and parents in the neonatal intensive care environment. *Physical and Occupational Therapy in Pediatrics, 6,* 3-55; and Gorski, P. A., Davidson, M. F., & Brazelton, T. B. (1979). Stages of behavioral organization in the high-risk neonate: Theoretical clinical considerations. *Seminars in Perinatology, 3,* 61-72.

Sensory System Development and Sensory Stimulation

Sensory System Development

Development of fetal sensory systems occurs in a chronologic but overlapping order. The infant's sensory systems of touch, movement, taste, smell, and hearing are structurally complete but functionally immature at the age of viability. Box 22-1 summarizes highlights of fetal brain and sensory system development at advancing gestational ages, with corresponding implications for environmental and caregiving modifications.

Supplemental Sensory Stimulation

Much of the early research on supplemental stimulation with preterm infants was based on the sensory deprivation theory and the subsequent desire to provide additional stimuli. This research has been criticized because of the use of small samples, exclusive application to healthy preterm infants, wide age span of infants treated as a homogenous group, failure to take into account individual differences of infants, and methodologic discrepancies that preclude comparisons among studies.

When considering sensory stimulation in the NICU, protecting the fragile newborn from excessive or inappropriate sensory input is a more compelling priority than direct intervention or interaction with the infant. Stimulation is not therapeutic if it stresses the infant; an infant may respond to stimuli, but at a physiologic cost with no benefit. Therapists must continually modify sensory stimulation in the NICU according to each infant's postconceptional age, medical status, current state of readiness and responsiveness, and ongoing

---

BOX 22-1   Fetal Sensory System Development: Implications for Environmental and Caregiving Modifications

BASIC BRAIN DEVELOPMENT

First trimester: Formation of neural tube and prosencephalon. Disruption of normal development during this period can cause major malformations such as neural tube defects and agenesis of corpus callosum.

2-4 months' gestation: Proliferation of neuronal and glial cells, which are stored in the germinal matrix.

3-8 months' gestation: Migration of cells from germinal matrix to cerebral cortex.

5 months' gestation through childhood: Organization (alignment, orientation, layering) of cortical neurons; arborization (differentiation and branching of axons and dendrites to increase cell connection possibilities); increased complexity in brain surface convolutions (sulci) as different areas develop for specific functions.

8 months' gestation (peak time): Myelinization

MOST FETAL SENSORY SYSTEMS (TACTILE, VESTIBULAR, TASTE, SMELL) ARE FUNCTIONING AT THE AGE OF VIABILITY

Tactile: Even youngest NICU infant has sophisticated perioral sensation, and perceives pressure, pain, and temperature. Back and legs are very sensitive to touch, especially prior to 32 weeks when modulation improves.

Vestibular: System structurally complete but still functionally immature. Movement and position changes can be overstimulating and stressful.

Taste: Withdraws from bitter taste at 26-28 weeks. Calms to sweet taste at 35 weeks. Taste can be affected by sense of smell.

Smell: Responds to odors with approach or avoidance. Noxious odor can prompt physiologic instability and behavioral stress. Can recognize mother via smell.

NICU Implications

Coordinate care among disciplines to reduce handling, minimize sleep disturbances, accommodate feedings. Help support the infant during exams and procedures:

- Contain extremities (use hands, blanket, Snuggle-Up)
- Encourage sucking on pacifier or on own hand
- Brace feet against boundaries or palm of caregiver hand
- Have baby grasp tubing, strap, adult finger
- Shield infant's eyes from room or procedure light
- Observe for signs of overstimulation; can you pause and help infant reorganize before proceeding

- Contain infant's extremities flexed against his/her body during smooth, slow position changes.
- Use soft, fluid boundaries; amount of support needed will vary, but is greater for younger, sicker infants.
- Firm, steady touch (i.e. containment) is better tolerated than light, moving touch (stroking).
- Young infants may tolerate holding better skin-to-skin (vs. swaddled), and without vestibular stimulation (rocking).
- Protective gloves may have unpleasant taste; wash and rinse first if inserting finger into infant's mouth.
- Oral medication—consider gavage, mixing with feeds.
- Protect infant from noxious smells (i.e. disinfectant).
- Mother's breast pad, or Snoedle, near infant may be calming and facilitate feeding.

AUDITORY/VISUAL SENSORY SYSTEM FETAL DEVELOPMENT (AT AGE OF VIABILITY) WITH NICU IMPLICATIONS

Auditory System

24 weeks: Ear (outer, middle, inner) and cortical auditory center essentially formed and functional.

26 weeks: Can elicit brainstem evoked potentials.

Note: Preterm infants have increased incidence of sensorineural hearing loss. Auditory processing problems also occur; some animal studies implicate "sensory interference" (inappropriate timing and intensity of exposure to sensory stimuli related to critical periods of development).

NICU Implications

Preterm infants are sensitive to NICU noise. Auditory overstimulation can cause physiologic stress.

"People" noise is the hardest to reduce and control.

Isolettes can be protective (note: mechanical noises penetrate incubators better than the speech sounds).

Efforts to reduce noise can occur at many levels:

- Environmental modifications (sound-absorbing ceiling tiles, carpet, padding bottoms/lids of trash cans, padded Isolette covers, no radios, etc.)
- Activity relocation (clerk, main phone, medical rounds, all moved away from bedside areas)
- Caregiving practices (silence alarms quickly, speak softly, close Isolette doors quietly)
- Technology (visual alarms, vibrating beepers).

Neonates demonstrate preference for mother's voice. Relaxing music may be effective with older infants.

Continued

BOX 22-1 Fetal Sensory System Development: Implications for Environmental and Caregiving Modifications—Cont'd

Visual System

WEEKS	DEVELOPMENT
22	All retinal layers are present
25	Can distinguish rods and cones
	Light elicits blink reflex
25–26	All neurons of visual cortex are present
26–28	Eyelids open (no longer fused)
27	May have brief spontaneous wakefulness
	Unable to visually focus
28–30	Eyes may remain open occasionally
	Eye movements typically rapid and jerky
30–32	Closes eyes to bright light
	Brief quiet alert state
	Visual attention still often stressful
	Vision is monocular
32–35	Demonstrates visual preference
	Visually tracks horizontally past midline
	Efforts at visual attention may fatigue infant
36–40	Retinal vascularization and optic nerve development are complete
	Visually tracks in horizontal, vertical, and circular directions
	Head and eye movements not well coordinated
	Preference for curved lines and shapes (vs. angular, straight); can see colors

NICU Implications

Visual system is the least mature of all sensory systems at preterm birth; must consistently protect infant while visual maturation continues.

- Eyelids are thin and do not block out all room light. Decrease NICU room light, cover bedspace, and/or shield eyes of individual infants from direct or bright lighting (including during procedures).
- Avoid abrupt increases in lighting levels.
- Lower light helps reduce staff noise, activity, stress.
- Studies suggest benefits in altering NICU light levels to provide day-night cycles.
- Supplemental visual stimulation does not seem to accelerate visual system maturation, can fatigue young premies, and can create significant neurobehavioral stress, including apnea and bradycardia.
- Allow infant to indicate readiness for visual stimulation (in quiet alert state, already attending to environment).
- Lower light levels facilitate eye opening for attention.
- Black-and-white designs are overstimulating for immature infants; the human face is the best model for visual stimulation when baby is mature and stable.
- Black-and-white may be therapeutic for infants with significant visual impairments.
- Brainstem visual evoked potentials in preterm infants are difficult to interpret because of visual system immaturity

cues of stress or stability. In other words, the therapist provides graded sensory input when the infant is ready and seeking, not because it is "time for OT." Early stimulation for these younger preterm infants may be safest if it replicates normal parenting activities such as being held, listening to the caregiver's soft voice, or looking at the caregiver's face. Young infants tolerate stimulation best if it is unimodal (one sensory input at a time). Ideally, family members provide this contact (Figure 22-9).

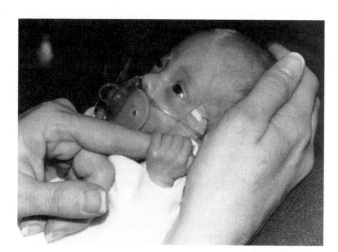

FIGURE 22-9 The support provided by containment, sucking, and grasping helps this preterm infant establish eye contact with her mother for a time of quality interaction. (Courtesy the NICU, Medical Center of Plano, Plano, TX. Photograph by Vicky Leland.)

Auditory Stimulation

Recommended guidelines for auditory stimulation in the NICU can be summarized as follows[24,29]:

- Although the evidence that supports the use of recorded music or speech in the NICU is minimal, ample opportunities should be provided for the infant to hear live and interactive parent voices at the bedside.
- Earphones and other devices attached to the infant's ears for sound transmission should never be used.
- Any auditory stimuli should be played only for brief periods, be less than 55 dB, and at a reasonable distance from the infant's ear. Audio recordings should not be used routinely or left unattended in the environment of the high-risk infant.
- Supplemental auditory stimulation can be used if the older infant remains soothed and stable with adequate protected sleep, but should be discontinued if the infant becomes distressed (stressed, restless, agitated).

Visual Stimulation

Current guidelines for visual development include the following[26,30]:

- Cluster care to provide extended periods of very low light and REM sleep for normal visual system formation.
- Protect eyes from direct light exposure and avoid abrupt light fluctuations.
- Adequate oxygen saturation levels are necessary to allow retinal dark currents that form early neural pathways.
- Reduce or avoid strong competing sensory stimuli.
- Help minimize suppression of retinal currents from sedative and analgesic drugs by using non-pharmacologic methods when possible to reduce stress and control pain.

- For infants at or past term age equivalency, provide both light and visual stimuli to continue optimal visual development.

Traditional Developmental Stimulation

Traditional developmental stimulation is generally not appropriate until the infant is both nearing (or past) term equivalency and sufficiently medically stable to be seeking attention and interaction. Infants vary significantly; the therapist needs to be sensitive to each infant's cues.

Stable infants approaching or exceeding term postconceptional age may demand more attention with varying success; it is worrisome if prolonged crying is ignored. The occupational therapist may provide mobiles, mirrors, or toys for visual stimulation, and musical toys or tape recorders with lullabies or audiotapes of family members singing or reading stories. Baby swings or vibrating bouncy infant seats can provide gentle vestibular input and a different view of the world. Even the variety of being placed in a standard infant seat may calm some infants. Portable infant carriers may be options for stable infants who can be temporarily separated from (or have portable) medical equipment. Supporting families to be available, involved, and knowledgeable is the best way for the therapist to meet the infant's developmental and emotional needs, both in the NICU and after discharge.

Infant Massage

Massage is an art and a science, best performed by a caregiver specifically trained in infant massage techniques, precautions, and warning signs. Massage is an active engagement between the infant and the caregiver; it is done "with" (rather than "to") the baby. As with any type of stimulation, the therapist should closely monitor the infant's physiologic and neurobehavioral responses, with handling modified accordingly.

Traditional infant massage can be physiologically stressful and behaviorally disorganizing to preterm infants younger than about 32 weeks postconception, or those who are not yet medically stable. These younger or medically fragile infants may benefit more from the gentle human touch of a static "hand swaddle" (facilitative tuck). Preterm infants with the prerequisite degree of medical stability for more traditional infant massage are often approaching hospital discharge; therapists can teach parents infant massage techniques for home use.

Massage has increasingly been recommended as an intervention to promote growth and development of preterm and low-birth weight infants in the NICU. While authors of a Cochrane Review (published by a non-profit organization that explores the evidence for and against the effectiveness and appropriateness of treatments) concluded that evidence of developmental benefits from massage for preterm infants is weak and does not currently warrant wider use of preterm infant massage,[83] an increasing number of NICU nurses and therapists show interest in and cautious use of limited infant massage.

Evidence-Based Potentially Better Practices (PBPs) to Support Neurodevelopment in the NICU

Developmentally supportive care is a philosophy and approach to caregiving intended to improve neurodevelopmental outcome in preterm and sick infants who lack the maturity, health, or competence necessary to easily cope with life in the NICU. Incorporating rapidly growing scientific knowledge from multiple disciplines, *developmental care* is an inclusive term applied to environmental modifications, changes in caregiving practices, and efforts to increase family involvement.

A collaborative hospital project within the Vermont Oxford Network "bundled" general recommendations for environment-related care practices that potentially support neurodevelopment, with an emphasis on "potential" and not "definitive" benefit (Table 22-7).[44,47] Caregiving interventions were bundled because they are all necessary and more effective as a group than if implemented separately, and omission of any one of these practices may lessen the ultimate benefit. The extensive literature review, application to sensory systems, evidence-based conclusions, and implementation strategies make these two articles valuable developmentally supportive care resources for the NICU therapist or caregiver.

It is revealing that 9 of 11 potentially better practices in Cluster I (see Table 22-7), and 11 of the total 16 potentially better practices (PBPs) (when Clusters I and II are combined) protect and promote infant sleep. Sleep is absolutely critical to early brain and sensory system development,[31] but is not easily accomplished.[44] Facilitating infant sleep in the NICU should be a priority for all caregivers, including therapists (Figure 22-10).

Neuromotor Development and Interventions

Reflex Development

Neonatal reflex development is well documented in medical and therapy literature. Although some therapists include reflex testing in their standard NICU assessment, complete reflex testing is extremely stressful for young or acutely ill NICU infants and is unnecessary as an early routine evaluation. Self-regulatory reflexes such as suck and grasp can indicate primitive reflex integrity in young or ill infants. Selective reflex testing may be appropriate with older stable infants prior to discharge,[7] or if the infant has known or suspected neuromuscular pathology (e.g., spina bifida, congenital neuropathy). Many reflexes (e.g., grasping, sucking, head righting) can be observed within the context of normal handling, which provides functional information with less stress than generalized "formal" reflex testing.

Muscle Tone

Hypotonia is normal for extremely preterm infants. Muscle tone gradually increases with age, and in caudocephalic (feet-to-head) and distal-proximal (extremities-to-trunk) directions. Active muscle tone, observed during spontaneous movement or elicited by righting reactions when the infant is handled, develops before passive flexor tone is seen at rest.[11] An extremely preterm infant at term equivalency will typically demonstrate greater extension and less physiologic flexion than a newborn full-term infant. Twitches, tremors and startles are common in preterm infants,[34] but movements typically become smoother and tremors less prevalent as term equivalency nears.

In addition to PCA, state of arousal and medical status are significant variables in assessing muscle tone. A preterm infant may be active and feisty when awake, but hypotonic if assessed while drowsy or asleep. Muscle tone in an acutely ill infant cannot be accurately evaluated; the underlying muscle tone usually changes as the infant recovers. Many medications have

TABLE 22-7   Potentially Better Practices to Support Neurodevelopment in the NICU

System	Potentially Better Practice	Benefits
Cluster I: Full implementation recommended for all NICU admissions beginning at 23 weeks' gestation		
T-1	Containment and body flexion	T, S
T-2	Positive oral stimulation; non-nutritive suck	T
T-3a	Gentle touch, hand grasping/facial stimulation	T
T-4	Decrease painful/negative stimulation	T, S
C-1	Exposure to mother's scent	C, S
C-2	Minimize exposure to noxious odors	C, S
A-1	Noise abatement	A, S
V-1	Minimize ambient light exposure	V, S
V-2	Avoid direct light exposure	V, S
S-1	Develop strategies that preserve normal infant sleep cycles	S
	Support family involvement in care practices that promote sleep	
	Non-emergent care provided at appropriate times to minimize the disruption of sleep (with diurnal implementation, as possible, after 30 weeks gestation)	
S-2	Minimize exposure to narcotics and other medications that may disrupt or disturb sleep cycles	S
Cluster II: Full implementation recommended for all NICU admissions beginning at 31–32 weeks		
T-3b	Infant massage/diurnal implementation	T
T-3c	Skin-to-skin care	T, C, S
A-2	Exposure to audible maternal voice/diurnal implementation	A
V-3	Cycled lighting: minimum of 1-2 hours	A, V, S
V-4	Provide more complex visual stimulation: after 37 weeks (term gestation)	V

A, auditory development; *C*, chemosensory development; *S*, preservation of sleep; *T*, somatesthetic/kinesthetic/proprioceptive development; *V*, visual development. Note: A potentially better practice may impact multiple developing sensory systems (T/C/A/V/S).
Data from Laudert, S., Liu, W. F., Blackington, S., Perkins, B., Martin, S., MacMillan-York, E., Graven, S., & Handyside, J. (on behalf of the NIC/Q 2005 Physical Environment Exploratory Group). (2007). Implementing potentially better practices to support the neurodevelopment of infants in the NICU. *Journal of Perinatology, 27*, S75-S93; and Liu, W. F., Laudert, S., Perkins, B., MacMillan-York, E., Martin, S., & Graven, S. (for the NIC/Q 2005 Physical Environment Exploratory Group). (2007). The development of potentially better practices to support the neurodevelopment of infants in the NICU. *Journal of Perinatology, 27*, S48-S74.

neuromotor side effects. For example, phenobarbital for seizures may initially make the infant lethargic, theophylline or caffeine for apnea may make the infant jittery, and midazolam for sedation may cause tremors.

The influence of evolving muscle tone on resting posture and quantity or quality of movement has implications for positioning and caregiving needs. The therapist should monitor atypical findings or asymmetrical responses; unusual movement patterns often resolve with maturation and physical recovery.

Posture and Movement Patterns

A fetus in the womb is typically flexed and contained with midline orientation of the head and extremities. Healthy term newborns maintain this general posture as a result of (1) physiologic flexion (i.e., posture is biased toward flexion with temporary "contractures" of the knees/hips/elbows due to limited intrauterine space), and (2) important neural connections that are being formed and reinforced during the last trimester of pregnancy emphasize flexion and midline as the "normal" baseline resting posture.[36]

The womb allows a much more controlled and predictable progression of this neuronal development than does the NICU. Flexion and symmetry are reinforced in developing neuronal pathways in utero; active fetal extension is always followed by a return to flexion because of flexible uterine constraints. Due to the effects of gravity, prematurity, illness, weakness, low tone, primitive reflexes, and immature neuromotor control,[76] the resting posture of a NICU infant without therapeutic positioning will be flat, extended, asymmetrical with the head to one side,

and with the extremities abducted and externally rotated (Figure 22-11). Active extension of the trunk and extremities still occurs, but without boundaries, the infant does not spontaneously return to a flexed midline posture. Over time, these are the postures and movement patterns that become reinforced in developing neuronal connections—a flat, externally rotated and asymmetrical resting posture becomes the "baseline" for that infant; active extension and arching become unopposed dominant motor patterns. It is well documented that lack of appropriate NICU positioning can create short-term and long-term functional problems for NICU infants, even in the absence of overt brain pathology (Figure 22-12).

Therapeutic Positioning

Positioning in the NICU tends to simulate the flexed/contained/midline posture of the infant in utero; external supports provide a temporary substitute for the immature infant's diminished internal motor control. Traditionally, NICU positioning has been a neuromotor developmental intervention to minimize positional deformities and to improve muscle tone, postural alignment, movement patterns, and ultimately developmental milestones.

Therapeutic positioning is an excellent example of how evolving knowledge and advances in technology drive changes in developmental clinical practice. In the 1970s, few or no attempts were made to provide boundaries or positional support for infants in the NICU. In the 1980s, increased awareness of infant developmental vulnerability and environmental stressors resulted in the use of blanket rolls for boundaries, with

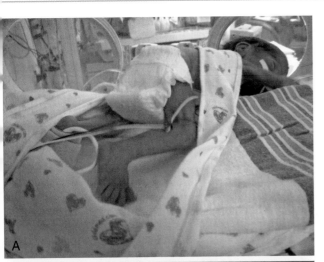

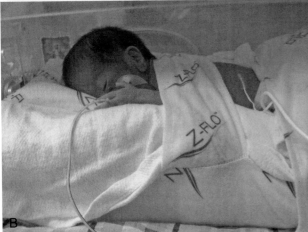

FIGURE 22-10 Continuously restless infant (1000 grams, small for gestational age) unable to settle in cloth bunting. She relaxed and fell asleep in minutes after being positioned on a Z-Flo full-body positioner with a smaller Z-Flo pad used as a prone roll. (Courtesy Sundance Enterprises, Inc., White Plains, NY; http://www.sundancesolutions.com)

variable effectiveness (Figure 22-13, *A*). Commercial positioning devices became widely available in the 1990s (Figure 22-13, *B*), promoted in part by the presence of NICU therapists who understood the importance of facilitating normal posture, tone, and movement patterns while minimizing hospital-acquired positional deformities. The goal was to improve the infant's emerging neuromotor control and long-term developmental outcome. These commercial NICU positioners were made of various combinations of cloth, foam, water-based gel, beanbags, and bendable rods. NICU infant positioning improved, but some problems persisted (e.g., some infant still "frogged" within positioner, continued lateral head flattening).

Z-Flo fluidized neonatal positioners (Sundance Enterprises, Inc., http://www.sundancesolutions.com) were introduced for NICU use in 2007 (Figure 22-14). Made of microscopic lubricated microspheres (encapsulated air bubbles) encased in polyurethane, Z-Flo positioners[55]:
- Allow individually contoured support for each infant regardless of size, deformity and medical conditions
- Adapt to and accommodate NICU medical equipment

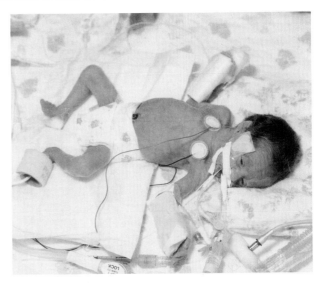

FIGURE 22-11 Hypotonic posture of premature infant. Without therapeutic positioning, "W" configuration of arms, "frogged" posture of legs, and asymmetrical head position may lead to positional deformities. (Courtesy the Infant Special Care Unit, University of Texas Medical Branch, Galveston, TX. Photograph by John Glow.)

- Facilitate skin integrity by reducing body pressure points, friction, and shear
- Respond three-dimensionally to infant movement, while tether straps maintain the integrity of the positioning unit.

This allows the positioners to provide both positional support and the opportunity for spontaneous movement of the infant within flexible boundaries. Active infant movement is potentially important for normal muscle tension on bone and necessary for mineralization and bone density.

Aside from effectiveness of developmental positioning, NICU clinical observations suggest Z-Flo use may also provide physiologic benefits of energy conservation (e.g. reduced agitation/restlessness, weaning supplemental oxygen concentration, better weight gain), calmer behaviors, reduced need for pain medication, and improved sleep. Parents appreciate the perceived increased comfort of their infant on Z-Flo neonatal positioners.

Range of Motion

Passive range of motion (PROM) may be appropriate for infants who demonstrate structural or neuromuscular limitation of movement and would tolerate a rehabilitation approach. PROM incorporated into therapeutic handling is preferable to conventional ranging techniques for most infants. Hypertonicity may relax more with sustained stretch and therapeutic positioning than with repetitive PROM. Infants usually do not need PROM after treatment for osteomyelitis because they begin to move the affected extremity spontaneously once the pain and swelling have subsided. PROM occasionally may be appropriate for an infant who is sedated or chemically paralyzed for prolonged periods. However, experience suggests that prevention of positional deformities with therapeutic positioning may be sufficient intervention for infants whose movement is temporarily restricted. Therapists should never consider PROM to be a routine NICU intervention, because it is unnecessary and often stressful to the general preterm population.

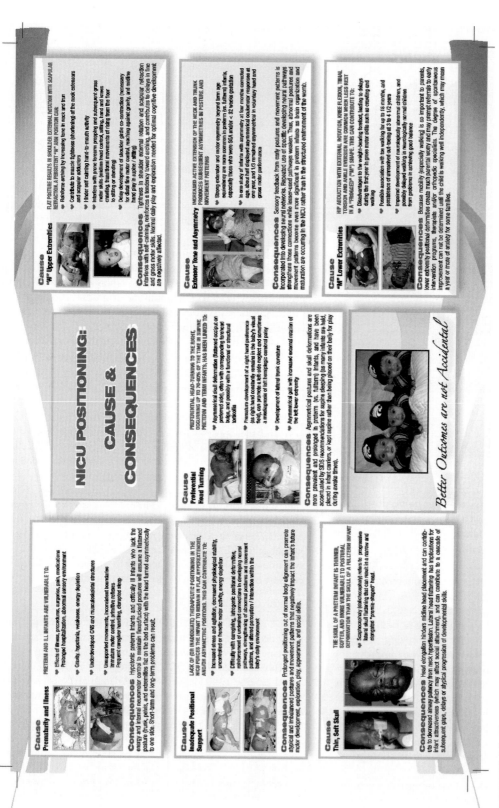

FIGURES 22-12 Illustrated developmental cause and consequences lack of therapeutic positioning and subsequent positional deformities in the NICU population. Hospital-acquired positional deformities are largely avoidable with good positioning. References can be found on the Sundance Solutions website listed in the credit. (Reprinted with permission of Sundance Enterprises, Inc., White Plains, NY.; http://www.sundancesolutions.com; a PDF of this poster can be found at http://sundancesolutions.com/literature/sundanceCandC.pdf)

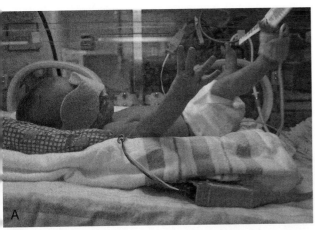

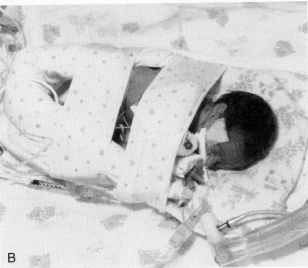

FIGURE 22-13 **A,** Blanket rolls are often too shallow and too wide to provide secure boundaries and postural support. (Courtesy of the Infant Special Care Unit, University of Texas Medical Branch, Galveston, TX. Photograph by Jan Hunter). **B,** Commercial positioning devices such as the Snuggle-Up. (Children's Medical Ventures) made positioning easier; this small preterm infant is supported in sidelying position with midline orientation and flexion of extremities. (A and B, Courtesy of the Infant Special Care Unit, University of Texas Medical Branch, Galveston, TX. Photograph by John Glow.)

Splinting

Splinting also is rarely needed with NICU infants. Although occurring with specific diagnoses, rigid contractures are actually uncommon, and infants are notably pliable over time. Therapists usually achieve significant rapid improvement with gentle stretch, therapeutic positioning, the effects of gravity, and spontaneous movement of the infant. Conversely, spontaneous movement is inhibited while the infant is wearing a rigid splint.

Protecting skin integrity and encouraging active movement are priorities in designing a neonatal splint. Thermoplastic material may create pressure points; adding sufficient padding may alter fit. It can also be difficult to maintain correct joint alignment on a rigid splint when extremity movement of ¼ inch can significantly change hand placement.

Less is better, and creative combinations of foams are often sufficient. Figure 22-15 illustrates bilateral hand splints made from foam pencil grips, foam straps, and a little Velcro. Alignment is corrected by tension on either strap, spontaneous movement is facilitated rather than repressed, risk for pressure is minimal, and both splints fit either hand—eliminating the potential right hand–left hand misapplication. The serial photographs were posted at bedside and given to the Spanish-speaking parents for follow-up with the local early childhood intervention program. When appropriate, splints like these rarely cause problems; the therapist, however, is always responsible for monitoring, adaptation, and education.

Feeding

A Word about Breastfeeding

Although this section focuses on bottle feeding, breast milk is the optimal nutrition for NICU infants. Any breast milk the infant receives is valuable. Mothers of preterm or ill infants who are educated about the benefits of breast milk often choose to pump milk for their infants; many are unable to maintain sufficient lactation for successful or exclusive breastfeeding at discharge. Early initiation of frequent breast pumping with a hospital-grade double electric breast pump, skin-to-skin holding as soon and as often as possible, non-nutritive sucking at breast (breast pumped first, although the breast is never truly empty and milk may "let down"), and establishing the basics of breastfeeding before offering a bottle are all useful in maintaining a milk supply. Late preterm infants (34 to 36 weeks' and 6 days' gestation) are especially vulnerable to being discharged before breastfeeding is established, with increased risk of significant medical complications. Breastfeeding educator (breastfeeding specialist) courses are widely available for nurses and therapists, often through government programs such as state health departments or women-infant-children (WIC) clinics. These courses are highly recommended to build knowledge, confidence, and competence. Websites such as that of The Academy of Breastfeeding (http://www.bfmed.org) can also provide useful information. Some therapists may eventually choose to continue breastfeeding specialization by pursuing credentials to become an International Board Certified Lactation Consultant (IBCLC) (http://www.ilca.org).

Bottle Feeding

Parents often ask when their baby can go home. For most NICU babies, the last obstacle to hospital discharge is accomplishing oral feeding. Historically, sufficient time was allowed for the preterm infant to gain endurance and for suck-swallow-breathe coordination to mature. Currently, oral feedings are often initiated at earlier ages or pushed more aggressively.[75] Late preterm infants (35 to 37 weeks' gestation) are expected to orally feed as competently as term infants, but may struggle because the CNS is underdeveloped. Physiological and neuromotor immaturity, lack of endurance, poor state regulation, and medical complications can interfere with oral feeding.[1,50] Infants with anomalies or persistent illness who are unable to achieve oral feeding within a "reasonable" time may be sent home with feeding gastrostomies. Oral feeding is complex, with an increased risk of silent aspiration in the NICU population; each infant's feeding readiness and safety should guide caregiver efforts.[70,79]

Non-nutritive Sucking

Non-nutritive sucking (NNS) or "dry" sucking, such as on a fist or pacifier, is present but disorganized in infants younger

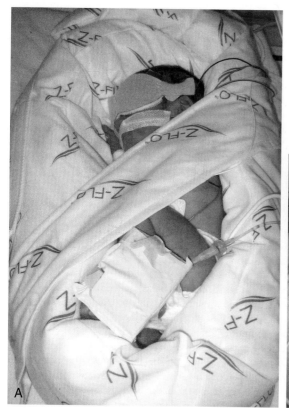
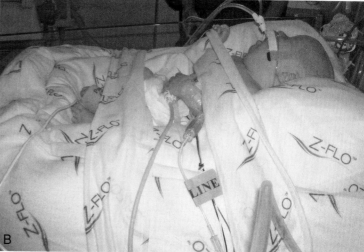

FIGURE 22-14 **A,** NICU infant in drug withdrawal needing firm circumferential boundaries. The Z-Flo tube's elasticized Velcro closure and the adjustable cross strap maintain the integrity of the positioner, while Z-Flo's fluidized properties allow the infant to move within the boundaries. His peripheral intravenous line and feeding tube are easily accommodated. **B,** Complex positioning on Z-Flo for a critically ill infant with a genetic syndrome including a short proximal esophageal atresia and a hypoplastic diaphragm. He has a gastrostomy tube; the large oral tube is hooked to wall suction for drainage of secretions, with variable effectiveness. The infant required frequent deep manual suctioning and was often extremely agitated with significant oxygen desaturations. Positioning increased calming and sleep, facilitated correct placement of the oral tube with more effective suctioning and less aversive vagal response from the infant, reduced the need for manual suctioning, and delayed intubation. An esophagostomy (spit fistula) was surgically placed the next week.   (A and B, Courtesy Sundance Enterprises, Inc., White Plains, NY; http://www.sundancesolutions.com)

than 30 weeks; sucking rhythm generally improves by 30 to 32 weeks' postconception. Because non-nutritive sucking does not interrupt breathing, it is usually (but not always) established before an infant has the neurologic maturation to coordinate sucking with swallows and breathing. Clinically, the presence of a rhythmic non-nutritive suck does not guarantee that an infant will orally feed well, and some infants with a poor non-nutritive suck may actually feed without difficulty.

NNS has been described as a self soothing activity. Benefits of NNS have been summarized as increased oxygenation, faster transition to nipple feeding, and better bottle-feeding performance. Infants who engage in NNS experience less time in fussy and awake states, quicker settling after feedings, less defensive behaviors during tube feeding, and a significantly decreased hospital stay. No short-term negative effects were identified.[65] NNS on a pacifier dipped in a 24% sucrose solution is advocated for the relief of procedural pain.[77]

Nutritive Sucking Patterns

Nutritive sucking is stimulated by the presence of fluid that must be swallowed; suck and swallow must be coordinated with breathing. Infants with organized sucking patterns (mature or immature) who can coordinate sucks and swallows with breathing are generally safe feeders when behavioral cues are respected. Transitional or disorganized feeding patterns are common in preterm or ill NICU infants learning to orally feeding; these infants have difficulty coordinating sucks and swallows with breathing, and benefit from caregiver interventions such as slow-flow nipples and pacing to force breaks for breathing. Dysfunctional feeders demonstrate abnormal movements of the jaw and tongue; oral feeding is often possible but with atypical oral mechanics.[58] Identification of the infant's sucking pattern will guide the therapist's expectations and interventions.

Mature sucking is an organized feeding pattern typical of healthy term infants. Sucking bursts are initially continuous for 10 to 30 sucks, with a smooth 1:1:1 suck-swallow-breathe rhythm in which respiration appears continuous and uninterrupted. Brief respiratory pauses between sucking bursts may be noted. Sucking bursts are usually longest at the beginning of a feeding (continuous sucking), followed by intermittent sucking with more opportunities for breathing as the feeding continues. Aside from normal infant feeding techniques (e.g. adequate postural support, calm environment, burping), no

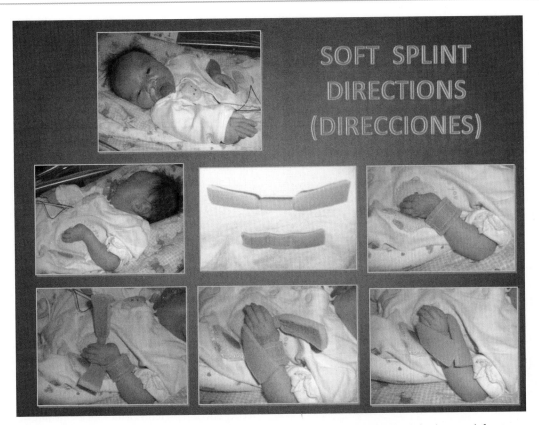

FIGURE 22-15 Newborn infant with congenital muscular dystrophy, a right humeral fracture, and obvious hand deformities. Bilateral soft splints (fabricated from foam pencil grips, small Velfoam straps, and Velcro) had no pressure points. Movement was not restricted; corrected alignment actually increased the infant's active movement. (Courtesy the Infant Special Care Unit, University of Texas Medical Branch, Galveston, TX. Photographs and slide by Jan Hunter.)

therapeutic interventions are necessary. Some term newborns eat well from the start; others seem to need a few days to recover from birth, gain endurance, and develop hunger.

Instead of having the 1:1:1 suck-swallow-breathe coordination seen in term babies, infants with an immature sucking pattern cluster three to five sucks together while holding their breath, swallow the accumulated bolus, then cluster several rapid recovery breaths. Observed in healthy preterm infants as young as 32 ½ weeks, this pattern is slower and not as efficient as mature sucking, but is organized as sucks and swallows alternate with breathing in a coordinated manner. Breath-holding during sucking is believed to be related to the infant's instinct to protect the airway from penetration by the liquid bolus. Therapists and nurses should allow these infants to set their own pace, and avoid stimulating sucking while they are in the breathing pause of the cycle. If the rest pause becomes prolonged, a slight gentle outward tug on the nipple may encourage the infant to re-latch and continue sucking; conversely, twirling the nipple in the infant's mouth can make the nipple difficult to grasp. Forced oral feeding (caregiver is "working" harder than the baby, or passively milking formula into the mouth of a non-participatory infant) increases the risk of disorganization and aspiration. Endurance may be limited, with the remainder of a feed given by gavage tube if the infant becomes fatigued.

A transitional (disorganized) pattern, observed in some preterm infants and older medically fragile infants (up to 45 weeks' PCA), is characterized by difficulty coordinating suck and swallow with breathing. An infant tries to use the continuous sucking burst of a mature pattern, but does not yet have a smooth rhythm of suck-swallow with breathing. Sucking bursts are generally 6 to 10 sucks, but frequent and significant variation in the length of sucking bursts may occur during the same feeding. Intermittent or increasing disorganization, air hunger with apnea after longer sucking bursts, and insufficient endurance to complete the feed are common. Disorganized transitional sucking is a frequently observed feeding pattern in NICU infants. Suck-swallow-breathe coordination can be facilitated by providing secure postural support, reducing stimuli, using a slow-flow nipple, and pacing to allow breathing pauses (Figure 22-16).[45] An infant with chronic lung disease may benefit from temporarily increased supplemental oxygen during feeding. A cue-based feeding approach, discussed further on, allows an infant to drive the frequency and duration of oral feedings without being force-fed.

Dysfunctional sucking is a disorganized feeding pattern of variable efficiency characterized by abnormal movements of the tongue and jaw and has been linked to future speech and language delays.[59] Oral motor interventions will vary with each infant, but may include such options as pre-feeding oral

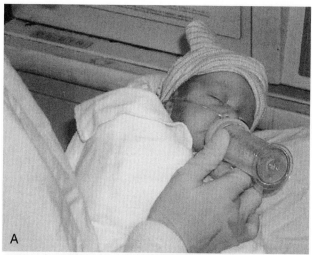

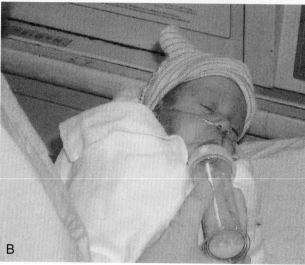

FIGURE 22-16 *A,* Preterm infant with transitional sucking pattern is fed in modified side-lying (breast-feeding) position. *B,* Infant's feeding is externally paced as the caregiver tips the bottle to force a breathing break. (Courtesy the Infant Special Care Unit, University of Texas Medical Branch, Galveston, TX. Photographs by Jan Hunter.)

stimulation for a "warm-up," use of different nipples, jaw support, inward and downward pressure on the tongue to inhibit excessive protrusion, and thickened formula for easier oral bolus control.

Stripping from the Nipple in Nutritive Sucking

Liquid is removed (stripped) from the nipple by a combination of suction (negative pressure) and compression (positive pressure).[27,89] Suction refers to negative intraoral pressure generated as the infant (1) enlarges the oral cavity by lowering the jaw and (2) prevents air entry by sealing the lips around the nipple and elevating the soft palate to close off the nasopharynx. Compression occurs when the nipple is squeezed against the premaxilla (gums) and palate by the tongue and lower jaw and is exerted by repetitive peristaltic motions of the tongue that strip fluid from the nipple. Compromise of either of these sucking pressure components, as in a very hypotonic infant or one with a cleft lip and palate, will impact stripping. An infant may demonstrate

rhythmic sucking, with relatively little milk removed from the bottle. Special nipples and bottles may be useful.

Nutritive Sucking and Respiration

Oral feeding compromises oxygenation and ventilation during nutritive sucking because the airway briefly closes during every reflexive swallow.[35] This compromise is more significant during continuous sucking than during intermittent sucking, and worse with an indwelling nasogastric tube than without the tube.[73]

Preterm and ill infants frequently demonstrate physiologic and neurologic immaturity, respiratory compromise, disorganized sucking, and inadequate endurance.[17,43] This disorganization often persists in the infant with chronic lung disease because the need to breathe supersedes the infant's efforts to suck.[67]

Improvement in feeding-induced apnea, often associated with multiple swallows without breathing, appears to correlate more with advancing age (maturation) than with practice.[35] Traditionally this has been interpreted to mean that additional time to mature is more beneficial than more frequent opportunities to "practice" oral feeding for younger preterm infants.

Nutritive Sucking and Aspiration

In addition to the suck-swallow reflex, a term neonate has anatomic and physiologic "safety features" that offer some natural protection against aspiration. These include proportionately large soft tissue structures (i.e., tongue, epiglottis, and vocal folds), relatively small openings, shorter passageways of smaller diameter, and a higher resting position of the larynx under the base of the tongue, providing an "umbrella" or "watershed" protective effect. A preterm infant with less mature development and function of these structures may not have the same degree of protection from aspiration during feeding; trace aspiration may occur frequently in NICU infants, and frank aspiration often is silent (i.e., no clinical signs of choke, cough, color change) in this population.[14] Initiation of bottle feeding at 30 to 33 weeks' PCA has been suggested,[63,75] but the possibility of silent aspiration during bottle feeding at 30 to 32 weeks' PCA has not been studied with definitive modified barium swallow studies and therefore the ultimate safety of these early feedings is not known.

Feeding Readiness and Cue-Based Infant-Driven Feeding

Historically, traditional NICU criteria for starting oral feedings require the relatively stable preterm infant to reach a certain age or weight. Feedings are based on a set number of calories and fluid volume per kilogram of body weight, and are given on a set schedule around the clock. But infants mature at different rates, and developing biorhythms may not coincide with the NICU clock. Too often, the result has been feedings that were "forced," with the caregiver using multiple manipulations to empty the bottle within 22 to 25 minutes. If the infant is not actively participating in the feed, however, the risk of aspiration increases.

In contrast, more NICUs are currently implementing a cue-based or infant-driven approach to oral feeding.[50,52] This individualized approach to feeding readiness considers such factors as the infant's medical status, neurobehavioral organization (i.e., vigor, sleep-wake cycle, ability to achieve some stable alert periods, autonomic/motor/state stability), and feeding readiness cues (e.g., awakening or fussing prior to feedings, spontaneous rooting and sucking behaviors, gagging with gavage tube insertion).[37,53] Descriptive scales can be included on nursing flow sheets to more consistently and objectively document both feeding readiness and performance at each feeding.[84]

Because cue-based feedings depend on active infant participation rather than caregiver manipulations, the risk of aspiration is decreased. This approach allows opportunities for the infant to feed orally without pressure or compromised nutrition; the frequency, duration, and volume of feedings will vary according to the infant's tolerance. For example, an infant who does not arouse with caregiving or initiate sucking on the nipple will receive a supplemental feeding by nasogastric tube; an infant who does well initially before becoming disorganized and tachypneic may feed orally for a few minutes, with the remaining volume given by nasogastric tube. Staff members can offer oral feedings more often but avoid prolonged sessions of trying to force-feed preset volumes. Ideally, cumulative exhaustion is avoided, with improved weight gain and smoother transition to oral feeds.

Because the infant participates during cue-based feedings, parents often experience greater success feeding their baby. Teaching parents how to reduce extraneous external stimuli, read and respect their infant's individual cues, provide secure postural support, and facilitate rest pauses or breathing breaks as needed (external pacing) will boost their confidence and help oral feeding be successful after discharge.

SUMMARY

The NICU is a complex hospital unit in which specialized care is provided to infants who are born prematurely or born with significant medical problems. Occupational therapists who work in the NICU must be armed with specialized knowledge about neonatal medical conditions, intensive care equipment, necessary precautions related to handling the neonates, preterm infant development, and interventions that promote behavioral organization and interaction. This chapter described the NICU environment and emphasized how certain lighting and sound conditions affect preterm neonate neurobehavioral systems. Occupational therapy services emphasize the developmental supportive care, developmentally appropriate interactions, and interventions that facilitate the neonate's neurobehavioral organization. Occupational therapists are sensitive to the family's response to preterm birth, and they coach parents in how to care for the neonate and help to prepare the family for the neonate's discharge from the NICU. Best practice services emphasize preventive interventions and protect the infant from unnecessary stress. Services are also directed to the parents as primary caregivers to promote their skills in handling and interacting with an infant who may be vulnerable and medically fragile when discharged from the NICU. Occupational therapists interested in working in a NICU are encouraged to obtain advanced training on preterm development, neonatal neurobehavioral systems, developmentally supportive interventions, and protective measures important to this vulnerable population.

REFERENCES

1. Adamkin, D. H. (2006). Feeding problems in the late preterm infant. *Clinics in Perinatology, 33*, 831–837.
2. Als, H. (1986). A synactive model of neonatal behavior organization: Framework for the assessment of neurobehavioral development in the premature infant and for support of infants and parents in the neonatal intensive care environment. *Physical and Occupational Therapy in Pediatrics, 6*, 3–55.
3. Altimier, L. (2007). The neonatal intensive care unit environment. In L. Altimier (Ed.), *Mosby's neonatal nursing online course manual*. St. Louis: Elsevier.
4. Altimier, L., Brown, B., & Tedeschi, L. (2006). *NANN guidelines for neonatal nursing policies, procedures, competencies, and clinical pathways*. Retrieved August 2009 from http://www.NANN.org/publications
5. American Academy of Pediatrics, Committee on Environmental Health. (1997). Policy statement: Noise, a hazard for the fetus and newborn (RE9728). *Pediatrics, 100*, 724–727.
6. American Academy of Pediatrics and the American College of Obstetrics and Gynecology. (2002). *Guidelines for perinatal care* (5th ed.). Washington DC: AAPACOG.
7. Amiel-Tison, C. (2002). Update of the Amiel-Tison neurologic assessment for the term neonate or at 40 weeks corrected age. *Pediatric Neurology, 27*, 196–212.
8. Bachman, T. E. (2006). Noise in the NICU: Still asking questions. *Neonatal Intensive Care, 19*(1), 21–23.
9. Ballweg, D. D. (2001). Implementing developmentally supportive family-centered care in the newborn intensive care unit as a quality improvement initiative. *Journal of Perinatal and Neonatal Nursing, 15*, 58–73.
10. Bhutta, A. T., & Anand, K. J. (2002). Vulnerability of the developing brain: Neuronal mechanisms. *Clinics in Perinatology, 29*, 357–372.
11. Blackburn, S. T. (2003). Neuromuscular and sensory systems. In *Maternal, Fetal, and Neonatal Physiology: A Clinical Perspective* (2nd ed, pp. 546–598). St. Louis: Saunders.
12. Byers, J. F., Waugh, W. R., & Lowman, L. B. (2006). Sound level exposure of high-risk infants in different environmental conditions. *Neonatal Network, 25*(1), 25–32.
13. Chang, E. F., & Merzenich, M. M. (2003). Environmental noise retards auditory cortical development. *Science, 300*, 498–502.
14. Comrie, J. D., & Helm, J. M. (1997). Common feeding problems in the intensive care nursery: Maturation, organization, evaluation and management strategies. *Seminars in Speech and Language, 18*, 239–261.
15. Conde-Agudelo, A., Diaz-Rossello, J. L., & Belizan, J. M. (2003). Kangaroo mother care to reduce morbidity and mortality in low birthweight infants. *Cochrane Database of Systematic Reviews*, (2), CD002771.
16. Conkright, L., Lamping, M., & Altimier, L. (2007). Neonatal Pain Management. In L. Altimier (Ed.), *Mosby's neonatal nursing online course manual*. St. Louis: Elsevier.
17. Craig, C. M., Lee, D. N., Freer, Y. N., & Laing, I. A. (1999). Modulations in breathing patterns during intermittent feeding in term infants and preterm infants with bronchopulmonary dysplasia. *Developmental Medicine and Child Neurology, 41*, 616–624.
18. Ellison, G., Bowers, B., & Kenner, C. (2007). Transition to home. In L. Altimier (Ed.), *Mosby's neonatal nursing online course manual*. St. Louis: Elsevier.
19. Feldman, R., & Eidelman, A. I. (2003). Skin-to-skin contact (Kangaroo Care) accelerates autonomic and neurobehavioural maturation in preterm infants. *Developmental Medicine and Child Neurology, 45*, 274–281.
20. Fern, D., Graves, C., & L'Huillier, M. (2002). Swaddled bathing in the newborn intensive care unit. *Newborn and Infant Nursing Reviews, 2*, 3–4.
21. Fielder, A. R., & Moseley, M. J. (2000). Environmental light and the preterm infant. *Seminars in Perinatology, 24*, 291–298.
22. Figueiro, M. G., Appleman, K., Bullough, J. D., & Rea, M. S. (2006). A discussion of recommended standards for lighting in the newborn intensive care unit. In R. White & G. I. Martin (Eds.), *New standards for newborn intensive care unit (NICU) design*. Journal of Perinatology, 26, S5–S26.

23. Gardner, S. L., Enzman-Hagedorn, M. I., & Dickey, L. A. (2006). Pain and pain relief. In S. L. Merenstein & G. B. Gardner (Eds.), *Handbook of neonatal intensive care* (6th ed., pp. 223–272). St. Louis: Mosby.

24. Gardner, S. L., & Goldson, E. (2006). The neonate and the environment: Impact on development. In S. L. Merenstein & G. B. Gardner (Eds.), *Handbook of neonatal intensive care* (6th ed., pp. 273–349). St. Louis: Mosby.

25. Gibbins, S., Stevens, B., Hodnett, E., Pinelli, J., Ohlsson, A., & Darlington, G. (2002). Efficacy and safety of sucrose for procedural pain relief in preterm and term neonates. *Nursing Research, 51*, 375–382.

26. Glass, P. (2002). Development of the visual system and implications for early intervention. *Infants & Young Children, 15*, 1–10.

27. Glass, R. P., & Wolf, L. S. (1998). Feeding and oral-motor skills. In J. Case-Smith (Ed.), *Pediatric occupational therapy and early intervention* (2nd Ed. pp. 127–166). Boston: Butterworth Heinemann.

28. Gorski, P. A., Davidson, M. F., & Brazelton, T. B. (1979). Stages of behavioral organization in the high-risk neonate: Theoretical clinical considerations. *Seminars in Perinatology, 3*, 61–72.

29. Graven, S. N. (2000). Sound and the developing infant in the NICU: Conclusions and recommendations for care. *Journal of Perinatology, 20*, S88–S93.

30. Graven, S. N. (2004). Early neurosensory visual development of the fetus and newborn. *Clinics in Perinatology, 31*, 199–216.

31. Graven, S. (2006). Sleep and brain development. *Clinics in Perinatology, 33*, 693–706.

32. Gray, L., & Philbin, M. K. (2004). Effects of the neonatal intensive care unit on auditory attention and distraction. *Clinics in Perinatology, 31*, 243–260.

33. Gressens, P., Rogido, M., Paindaveine, B., & Sola, A. (2002). The impact of neonatal intensive care practices on the developing brain. *Journal of Pediatrics, 14*, 646–653.

34. Grunau, R. (2002). Early pain in preterm infants: A model of long-term effects. *Clinics in Perinatology, 29*, 373–394.

35. Hanlon, M. B., Tripp, J. H., Ellis, R. E., Flack, F. C., Selley, W. G., & Shoesmith, H. J. (1997). Deglutition apnea as indicator of maturation of suckle feeding in bottle-fed infants. *Developmental Medicine and Child Neurology, 39*, 534–542.

36. Heijst, J. J. V., Touwen, B. C. L., & Vos, J. E. (1999). Implications of a neural network model of sensori-motor development for the field of developmental neurology. *Early Human Development, 55*, 77–95.

37. Hunter, J., & L'Huillier, M. (2007). Bottle feeding in the NICU. In L. Altimier (Ed.), *Mosby's neonatal nursing online course manual*. St. Louis: Elsevier.

38. Hunter, J. G., & Malloy, M. H. (2002). Effect of sleep and play positions on infant development: reconciling developmental concerns with SIDS prevention. *Newborn and Infant Nursing Review, 2*, 9–16.

39. Jerger, J., & Musiek, F. (2000). Report of the consensus conference on the diagnosis of auditory processing disorders in school-aged children. *Journal of the American Academy of Audiology, 11*, 467–474.

40. Kenner, C., & McGrath, J. M. (Eds.). (2004). *Developmental care of newborns & infants: A guide for healthcare professionals*. St. Louis: Mosby.

41. Kledzik, T. (2005). Holding the very low birth weight infant: Skin-to-skin techniques. *Neonatal Network, 24*, 7–14.

42. Krueger, C., Wall, S., Parker, L., & Nealis, R. (2005). Elevated sound levels within a busy NICU. *Neonatal Network, 24*(6), 33–37.

43. Lau, C., Smith, E. O., & Schanler, R. J. (2003). Coordination of suck-swallow and swallow respiration in preterm infants. *Acta Paediatrica, 92*, 721–727.

44. Laudert, S., Liu, W. F., Blackington, S., Perkins, B., Martin, S., MacMillan-York, E., et al. (on behalf of the NIC/Q 2005 Physical Environment Exploratory Group). (2007). Implementing potentially better practices to support the neurodevelopment of infants in the NICU. *Journal of Perinatology, 27*, S75–S93.

45. Law-Morstatt, L., Judd, D. M., Snyder, P., et al. (2003). Pacing as a treatment technique for transitional sucking patterns. *Journal of Perinatology, 23*, 483–488.

46. Lickliter, R. (2000). The role of sensory stimulation in perinatal development: Insights from comparative research for care of the high-risk infant. *Journal of Developmental and Behavioral Pediatrics, 21*, 437–447.

47. Liu, W. F., Laudert, S., Perkins, B., MacMillan-York, E., Martin, S., & Graven, S. (for the NIC/Q 2005 Physical Environment Exploratory Group). (2007). The development of potentially better practices to support the neurodevelopment of infants in the NICU. *Journal of Perinatology, 27*, S48–S74.

48. Ludington-Hoe, S. M., Johnson, M. W., Morgan, K., Lewis, T., Gutman, J., Wilson, P. D., et al. (2006). Neurophysiologic assessment of neonatal sleep organization: Preliminary results of a randomized, controlled trial of skin contact with preterm infants. *Pediatrics, 117*, e909–e923.

49. Ludington-Hoe, S. M., Morgan, K., & Abouelfettoh, A. (2008). A clinical guideline for implementation of kangaroo care with premature infants of 30 or more weeks postmenstrual age. *Advances in Neonatal Care, 8*, S3–S23.

50. Ludwig, S. (2007). Oral feeding and the late preterm infant. *Newborn & Infant Nursing Reviews, 7*(2), 72–75.

51. Lynam, L. (2003). The impact of the microenvironment on newborn care: A facility report: Christiana Care Health System. *Neonatal Intensive Care, 16*, 13–20.

52. McCain, G. C. (2003). An evidence-based guideline for introducing oral feeding to healthy preterm infants. *Neonatal Network, 22*, 45–50.

53. McGrath, J. M., & Braescu, A. V. (2004). Feeding readiness in the preterm infant. *Journal of Perinatal and Neonatal Nursing, 18*, 353–368.

54. McMullen, S. L., Lipke, B., & LeMura, C. (2009). Sudden infant death syndrome prevention—a model for NICUs. *Neonatal Network, 28*(1), 7–12.

55. Miller, M. E. (2003). The bone disease of preterm birth: A biomechanical perspective. *Pediatric Research, 53*(1), 10–15.

56. Moore, K. A., Coker, K., DuBuisson, A. B., Swett, B., & Edwards, W. H. (2003). Implementing potentially better practices for improving family-centered care in neonatal intensive care units: Successes and challenges. *Pediatrics, 112*, e450–60.

57. Noerr, B. (2004). Thermoregulation. In M. T. Verklan, & M. Walden (Eds.), *Core curriculum for neonatal intensive care nursing*. St. Louis: Elsevier.

58. Palmer, M. M. (1993). Identification and management of the transitional suck pattern in premature infants. *Journal of Perinatal and Neonatal Nursing, 7*, 66–75.

59. Palmer, M. M., Crawley, K., & Blanco, I. A. (1993). Neonatal oral-motor assessment scale: A reliability study. *Journal of Perinatology, 13*, 28–35.

60. Peng, N., Mao, H., Chen, Y., & Chang, Y. (2001). Effects of light intensity on the physiological parameters of the premature infant. *Journal of Nursing Research, 9*, 333–343.

61. Penn, A. A., & Schatz, C. J. (1999). Brain waves and brain wiring: The role of endogenous and sensory-driven neural activity in development. *Pediatric Research, 45*, 447–458.

62. Philbin, M. K. (2000). The influence of auditory experience on the behavior of preterm newborns. *Journal of Perinatology, 20*, S77–S87.

63. Pickler, R. H., & Reyna, B. A. (2003). A descriptive study of bottle-feeding opportunities in preterm infants. *Advances in Neonatal Care, 3*, 139–146.

64. Pickler, R. H., Reyna, B. A., & McGrath, J. M. (2004). NICU and beyond benefits: Benchmarking with measurable outcomes. In C. Kenner & J. M. McGrath (Eds.), *Developmental care of newborns & infants: a guide for health professionals* (pp. 411–421). St. Louis: Mosby.

65. Pinelli, J., & Symington, A. (2005). Non-nutritive sucking for promoting physiologic stability and nutrition in preterm infants. *Cochrane Database of Systematic Reviews*, (4).

66. Porter, F. L., Wolf, C. M., & Miller, J. P. (1998). The effect of handling and immobilization on the response to acute pain in newborn infants. *Pediatrics, 102*, 1383–1389.

67. Pridham, K., Brown, R., Sondel, S., Green, C., Wedel, N. Y., & Lai, H. C. (1998). Transition time to full nipple feeding for premature infants with a history of lung disease. *Journal of Obstetric, Gynecologic, and Neonatal Nursing, 27*, 533–545.

68. Reynolds, J. D., Hardy, R. J., Kennedy, K. A., Spencer, R., van Heuven, W. A. J., & Fielder, A. R., (for the LIGHT - ROP Cooperative Group). (1998). Lack of efficacy of light preventing retinopathy of prematurity. *New England Journal of Medicine, 338*, 1572–1576.

69. Rivkees, S. A., Mayes, L., Jacobs, H., & Gross, I. (2004). Rest-activity patterns of premature infants are regulated by cycled lighting. *Pediatrics, 113*, 833–839.

70. Ross, E. S., & Browne, J. V. (2002). Developmental progression of feeding skills: An approach to supporting feeding in preterm infants. *Seminars in Neonatology, 7*, 469–475.

71. Scher, M., Johnson, M., & Holditch-Davis, D. (2005). Cyclicity of neonatal sleep behaviors at 25 to 30 weeks' postconceptual age. *Pediatric Research, 57*, 879–882.

72. Deleted in proofs.

73. Shiao, S. Y. P. K., Brooker, J., & DiFiore, T. (1996). Desaturation events during oral feedings with and without a nasogastric tube in very low birth weight infants. *Heart and Lung, 25*, 236–245.

74. Siegel, R., Gardner, S. L., & Merenstein, G. B. (2002). Families in crisis: theoretical and practical considerations. In S. L. Merenstein & G. B. Gardner (Eds.), *Handbook of neonatal intensive care* (6th ed., pp. 863–913). St. Louis: Mosby.

75. Simpson, C., Schanler, R. J., & Lau, C. (2002). Early introduction of oral feeding in preterm infants. *Pediatrics, 110*, 517–522.

76. Spear, M. L., Leef, K., Epps, S., & Locke, R. (2002). Family reactions during infants' hospitalization in the neonatal intensive care unit. *American Journal of Perinatology, 19*, 205–213.

77. Stevens, B., Yamada, J., & Ohlsson, A. (2004). Sucrose for analgesia in newborn infants undergoing painful procedures. *Cochrane Database of Systematic Reviews*, (3).

78. Deleted in proofs.

79. Thoyre, S. M., Shaker, C. S., & Pridham, K. F. (2005). The early feeding skills assessment for preterm infants. *Neonatal Network, 24*, 7–16.

80. Uebel, P. (2007). Neonatal thermoregulation. In L. Altimier (Ed.), *Mosby's neonatal nursing online course manual*. St. Louis: Elsevier.

81. Vergara, E., Anzalone, M., Bigsby, R., Gorga, D., Holloway, E., Hunter, J., et al., 2005 Neonatal Intensive Care Unit Task Force. (2006). Specialized knowledge and skills for occupational therapy practice in the neonatal intensive care unit. *American Journal of Occupational Therapy, 60*, 659–668.

82. Vergara, E. R., & Bigsby, R. (2003). *Developmental and therapeutic interventions in the NICU*. Baltimore: Brookes.

83. Vickers, A., Ohlsson, A., Lacy, J. B., & Horsley, A. (2004). Massage for promoting growth and development of preterm and/or low birth-weight infants. *The Cochrane Library*, (2).

84. Waitzman, K. A., & Ludwig, S. M. (2007). Changing feeding documentation to reflect infant-driven feeding practice. *Newborn & Infant Nursing Reviews, 7*(3), 155–160.

85. Walden, M., & Franck, L. S. (2003). Identification, management, and prevention of newborn/infant pain. In C. Kenner & J. Lott (Eds.), *Comprehensive neonatal nursing: Physiologic perspective* (pp. 844–856). Philadelphia: Saunders.

86. Warner, B. (2007). Regionalization. In L. Altimier (Ed.), *Mosby's neonatal nursing online course manual*. St. Louis: Elsevier.

87. Westrup, B., Kleberg, A., von Eichwald, K., Stjernqvist, K., & Lagercrantz, H. A. (2000). A randomized, controlled trial to evaluate the effects of the newborn individualized developmental care and assessment program in a Swedish setting. *Pediatrics, 105*(1 Pt 1), 66–72.

88. White, R. D. (2007). Recommended standards for newborn ICU design. Report of the Seventh Consensus Conference on Newborn ICU Design. *Journal of Perinatology, 27*, S4–S19. Available at: http://www.nd.edu/~nicudes/index.html

89. Wolf, L. S., & Glass, R. P. (1992). *Feeding and swallowing disorders in infancy: Assessment and management*. Tucson, AZ: Therapy Skill Builders.

Medical Abbreviations Commonly Used in the Neonatal Intensive Care Unit

A

A: apnea
Ab: abortions (includes spontaneous)
ABG: arterial blood gas
ABR: auditory brain stem response
AD: right ear
AEP: auditory evoked potential
AGA: appropriate for gestational age
A-line: arterial line
AOP: apnea of prematurity
APIP: Assessment of Preterm Infant Behavior (Als)
AROM: assisted rupture of membranes
AS: left ear
As & Bs: apnea and bradycardia
ASD: atrial septal defect
AU: both ears

B

B: bilateral, or bradycardia
BAEP: brain stem auditory evoked potential
BAER: brain stem auditory evoked response
BIH: bilateral inguinal hernia
BPD: bronchopulmonary dysplasia
BPM: beats per minute (pulse)
BSER: brain stem evoked response (same as ABR, AEP, BAER, or BAEP)
BW: birth weight

C

CAN: cord around neck (nuchal cord)
CBC: complete blood count
CDH: congenitally dislocated hip
CHD: congenital heart disease
CHF: congestive heart failure
CLD: chronic lung disease
CMV: cytomegalovirus
CNGF: continuous nasogastric feeding
CNS: central nervous system
COGF: continuous orogastric feeding
CPAP: continuous positive airway pressure
CPT: chest physical therapy
C/S: cesarean section
CSF: cerebrospinal fluid
CTF: continuous tube feeding
CXR: chest x-ray

D

D_5W: 5% glucose solution
$D_{10}W$: 10% glucose solution
DIC: disseminated intravascular coagulation
DTGV: transposition of the great vessels

E

ECMO: extracorporeal membrane oxygenation
ELBW: extremely low birth weight (<1000 g)

F

FEN: fluids, electrolytes, nutrition
FHR: fetal heart rate
FiO_2: fraction of inspired oxygen (percentage of oxygen concentration)
FT: full term

G

G: gravida (pregnancies)
GA: gestational age
GBS: group B streptococcus
GER: gastroesophageal reflux
GERD: gastroesophageal reflux disease

H

HAL: hyperalimentation (same as TPN)
HC: head circumference
HFV: high-frequency ventilation
HFJV: high-frequency jet ventilation
HFOV: high-frequency oscillating ventilation
HIE: hypoxic-ischemic encephalopathy
HMD: hyaline membrane disease
HR: heart rate
HSV: herpes simplex virus
HTN: hypertension
HUS: head ultrasound

I

ICH: intracranial hemorrhage
ICN: intensive care nursery
IDM (or IODM): infant of a diabetic mother

IDV: intermittent demand ventilation
IH: inguinal hernia
IMV: intermittent mandatory ventilation
I/O: intake/output
IPPB: intermittent positive pressure breathing
IRV: inspiratory reserve volume
IUGR: intrauterine growth retardation
IV: intravenous
IVDA: intravenous drug abuse
IVF: in vitro fertilization; intravenous feeding
IVH: intraventricular hemorrhage

K

Kcal: kilocalories

L

L (or LC): living children
LA: left atrium
LBW: low birth weight (<2500 g)
LGA: large for gestational age
LMP: last menstrual period
L/S ratio: lecithin/sphingomyelin ratio
LTGV: physiologically corrected transposition of the great vessels
LV: left ventricle

M

MAP: mean airway pressure
MAS: meconium aspiration syndrome
MCA: multiple congenital anomalies
MDU: maternal drug use
MRSA: methicillin-resistant *Staphylococcus aureus*
MRSE: methicillin-resistant *Staphylococcus epidermidis*

N

NB: newborn
NBAS: Newborn Behavioral Assessment Scale (Brazelton)
NC: nasal cannula
NCPAP: nasal continuous positive airway pressure
ND: nasoduodenal
NEC: necrotizing enterocolitis
NG: nasogastric
NGT: nasogastric tube
NICU: neonatal intensive care unit
NIDCAP: Neonatal Individualized Developmental Care and Assessment Program (Als)
NNNS: Neonatal Network Neurobehavioral Scale
NNS: non-nutritive sucking
NO: nitric oxide
NP: nasopharyngeal
NPCPAP: nasopharyngeal continuous positive airway pressure
NPO: nothing by mouth
NS: nutritive sucking
NTE: neutral thermal environment

O

O_2 sats: oxygen saturation
OD: oral-duodenal; right eye
OG: oral gastric
OGT: oral gastric tube
OS: left eye
OU: both eyes

P

P: pulse; para (births)
P_1: primipara (first birth)
$PaCO_2$: arterial partial pressure of CO_2 (concentration of CO_2 in peripheral arteries)
PaO_2: arterial partial pressure of O_2 (concentration of O_2 in peripheral arteries)
PCA: postconceptional age
PDA: patent ductus arteriosus
PEEP: positive end-expiratory pressure
PFC: persistent fetal circulation (more correctly called *persistent pulmonary hypertension of the newborn [PPHN]*)
PICC: percutaneously inserted central catheter
PIE: pulmonary interstitial emphysema
PIH: pregnancy-induced hypertension (preeclampsia, eclampsia)
PIP: pulmonary insufficiency of the preterm; peak inspiratory pressure
PO: by mouth
PPD: packs per day (refers to smoking)
PPHN: persistent pulmonary hypertension of the newborn (previously called *persistent fetal circulation [PFC]*)
PROM: premature rupture of membranes
PPROM: prolonged premature rupture of membranes
PS: pulmonic stenosis
PPS: peripheral pulmonic stenosis
PT: preterm
PTL: preterm labor
PVL: periventricular leukomalacia

Q

q: every
qh: every hour
qid: 4 times a day

R

RA: right atrium
RBC: red blood cell
RDS: respiratory distress syndrome
ROM: rupture of membranes
ROP: retinopathy of prematurity (formerly called *retrolental fibroplasia [RLF]*)
RPR: rapid plasma reagin (can be used to test for syphilis)
RRR: rate, rhythm, respiration
RV: right ventricle

S

SA: substance abuse
sats: oxygen saturation levels
SCN: special care nursery
SGA: small for gestational age
SIMV: synchronized intermittent mandatory ventilation
s/p: status post
SROM: spontaneous rupture of membranes
SVD: spontaneous vaginal delivery

T

TA: truncus arteriosus
TAPVR: total anomalous pulmonary venous return
TCAN: tight cord around neck
TCM: transcutaneous monitor
$TcPO_2$: transcutaneous oxygen pressure
TLC: total lung capacity
TOF: tetralogy of Fallot
TORCH: congenital viral infections (toxoplasmosis, rubella, cytomegalovirus, and herpes)
TPF: toxoplasmosis fetalis
TPN: total parenteral nutrition
TPR: temperature, pulse, respiration
TRDN: transient respiratory distress of the newborn
TTN: transient tachypnea of the newborn

U

UAC: umbilical artery catheter
UAL: umbilical artery line
ULBW: ultra low birth weight (<750 g)
URI: upper respiratory infection
USG: ultrasound
UTI: urinary tract infection
UVC: umbilical venous catheter

V

VDRL: Venereal Disease Research Laboratory
VEP (VER): vision evoked potential (response)
VLBW: very low birth weight (<1500 g)
VSD: ventricular septal defect

W

WBC: white blood cell
WBD: weeks by dates (for gestational age)
WBE: weeks by examination (for gestational age)

Early Intervention

Christine Teeters Myers　•　Linda Stephens　•　Susan Tauber

OBJECTIVES

1. Explain family-centered early intervention philosophy and principles.
2. Define the components of an individualized family service plan (IFSP).
3. Explain models of evaluation, and describe specific assessments.
4. Describe developmentally appropriate and family-centered intervention approaches.
5. Define areas of emphasis in occupational therapy.
6. Explain strategies and activities used by occupational therapists in working with infants and children.
7. Describe the early intervention legislation and program regulations.

WHAT IS EARLY INTERVENTION?

The term *early intervention* connotes different meanings to different professionals. In this chapter, *early* refers to the critical period of a child's development between birth and 3 years of age. *Intervention* refers to program implementation designed to maintain or enhance the child's development in natural environments and as a member of a family. *Early intervention* describes services for children from birth to 3 years of age who have an established risk, have a developmental delay, or are considered to be environmentally or biologically at risk. The goal of early intervention is "to prevent or minimize the physical, cognitive, emotional, and resource limitations of young children disadvantaged by biologic or environmental risk factors" (p. 11).[2]

Legislation Related to Early Intervention

The 1980s brought widespread acceptance and support for family-centered care for children with special needs.[62] Family-centered care is based on the principle that an infant is dependent on his or her parents and other family members for daily care and meeting his or her physical and emotional needs. At the same time, the birth of an infant with special health care needs affects the entire family emotionally, socially, and economically. In 1986, amendments to the Education of the Handicapped Act (EHA) established incentives for states to develop systems of coordinated family-centered care for infants with disabilities. These incentives were strengthened in 1990, when the EHA was further amended and retitled the Individuals with Disabilities Education Act (IDEA).[36] Through Part C of IDEA, all children from birth through 2 years of age who have developmental delays are entitled to services. Revisions to IDEA were made again in 1997 and 2004; the newest version is P.L. 108-446, or the Individuals with Disabilities Education Improvement Act of 2004.

Part C of IDEA delineates the policies and regulations that participating states must follow in establishing early intervention services and systems. Table 23-1 summarizes the differences between Part C, which defines early intervention services for children between birth and 3 years of age, and Part B, which defines school programs for eligible students between 3 and 21 years of age (see Chapter 24). Part C is an entitlement program, and Part B defines mandated services. An entitlement simply acknowledges one's rights to something; a mandate establishes programs and services that are obligatory by law.

The purpose of Part C of IDEA is to give each state support in maintaining and implementing comprehensive, coordinated, multidisciplinary, interagency systems of early intervention services for infants and toddlers with disabilities and their families. A description of Part C regulations can be found at the U.S. Department of Education website (http://idea.ed.gov/).

Occupational Therapy Services in Early Intervention Systems

Part C of IDEA considers occupational therapy to be a "primary service" for eligible infants and toddlers from birth through 2 years of age who qualify for early intervention services. As a primary service, occupational therapy can be provided as the only service a child receives or in addition to other early intervention services. By its legal definition,

TABLE 23-1 Comparison of Educational Programs by Age Group

	0–2 Yr	3–5 Yr	6–21 Yr
Legislation	IDEA, Part C	IDEA, Part B	IDEA, Part B
Program	Early intervention	Special education	Special education
Type	Entitlement	Mandate	Mandate
Eligibility	Noncategorical	Categorical	Categorical
Services provided	16 primary services, including occupational therapy, physical therapy, speech language pathology, and special instruction	Related services only as support to special education	Related services only as support to special education
	Interdisciplinary and transdisciplinary assessment	Interdisciplinary and discipline-specific assessment	Discipline-specific assessment as related to education
	Individualized Family Service Plan	Individualized education program	Individualized education program
	Family-centered	Family-focused in theory, child-focused in practice	Child-focused with emphasis on curricular standards
	Service coordination	Service coordination recommended but not mandated	Service coordination recommended but not mandated
Location	Natural settings	Home, center, or school-based	School-based

IDEA, Individuals with Disabilities Education Act.

occupational therapy includes services to address the functional needs of the child related to adaptive development; adaptive behavior and play; and sensory, motor, and postural development. It includes adaptation of the environment and selection, design, and fabrication of assistive and orthotic devices to facilitate development and promote the acquisition of functional skills. The therapist designs these services to prevent or minimize the influence of initial or future impairment, delay in development, or loss of functional ability.

As described in the following sections, occupational therapists provide early intervention services as part of a team, coach team members and families to support occupational therapy interventions, use a family-centered approach that respects cultural differences, consult with families and children, and provide services in natural environments.

CURRENT PRACTICE IN EARLY INTERVENTION

Partnering with Families

The early intervention system recognizes that families can be and often are knowledgeable consumers and effective change agents for the child. It also acknowledges that families have specific needs related to a child with disabilities and that families may be the recipients of services.[45,67] The early intervention team includes not only the family but also professionals who help each family identify its unique resources, priorities, and concerns. The team then identifies outcomes and goals that enable the family to function more effectively and help the child as a member of the family unit.[41]

The term *family-centered* encompasses several aspects: Importance is placed on family strengths, not deficits; families deserve to have control and make choices regarding the care their child receives; and families and providers work together to ensure provision of optimal early intervention services.[16] Within a family-centered model, occupational therapists

develop goals collaboratively with parents or primary caregivers. Using a family systems perspective, the therapist recognizes the influence and interrelationships of the family within various systems, such as extended family, neighborhood, and early intervention programs. By thinking broadly about families and their subsystems, the therapist can help parents communicate their concerns and identify their priorities for the child.

Families are both participants in and consumers of early intervention services. Traditionally, occupational therapists provided early intervention services with a medical orientation. That is, occupational therapy was provided in a clinic or center, and sessions usually were conducted one-on-one with the therapist and child or in a small group with peers who were also receiving early intervention services. With the changes to IDEA 1997, which required services to be provided in the natural environment, occupational therapists had to expand their thinking about early intervention. Service provision now occurs primarily in the home or other community-based settings and families have a greater role in carrying out therapeutic activities. The nature and extent of family involvement may vary and will depend on family needs, values, lifestyles, and variables within the structure of the early intervention program itself. The degree of family involvement may fluctuate and change in response to external or internal factors that affect family functioning and coping. Some examples are degree of acceptance of the child's disability, job status of one or both parents, a new infant in the family, and changes in the family's support networks, such as grandparents, friends, or church groups.

To provide appropriate intervention within the family-centered model, the occupational therapist must be aware of and respect differences in beliefs and values based on culture. "Perhaps no set of programs or services interacts with cultural views and values more than early intervention because of the focus on the very young child with a disability and the family" (p. 116).[29] The therapist who provides intervention in the home has an intimate view of such things as customs, eating habits, and child-rearing practices that may vary among cultures. The family's beliefs and views of disability and its cause,

heir view of the health care system, and their sources of medical information affect their attitude toward early interven-
ion.[70] Based on individual cultural backgrounds, the family
may view the therapist as either a helper or one who interferes.
Research suggests that early intervention providers may not
develop individualized family service plan (IFSP) goals that
consider cultural diversity (e.g., family income, location of res-
dence).[56] Given the importance of the IFSP in directing program implementation, this finding indicates that early
ntervention service providers need to make certain they
nclude all family-identified priorities, not just those that relate
to child development (see Box 23-1).

Many of the areas in which occupational therapists provide
ntervention and suggestions involve caregiving and are closely
tied to values and beliefs about parenting and cultural views of
children. Practices regarding feeding, toileting, and bathing
may vary among cultures. The therapist is urged to evaluate
various health beliefs to determine whether the effects are beneficial, harmless, harmful, or uncertain before making recommendations for change.[30]

Occupational therapists must be sensitive to the multiple
factors that affect family involvement. It may be tempting to
label a family as "difficult" or "noncompliant"; however,
families of children with disabilities may be under a great deal
of stress and may be doing their best at any particular time.[33]
For example, a parent who is homeless or jobless may not be

concerned about occupational therapy for the child. Another
parent may believe that certain skills or goals are more important than those identified by the occupational therapist. Family
priorities need to be respected.

Building an ongoing relationship with families will enhance
the early intervention process. Effective listening and interviewing skills are essential, as is the ability to communicate with sensitivity the therapist's own concerns about the child's occupations.
Families who have children with special needs highly value services in which professionals provide clear, understandable, complete information; demonstrate respect for the child and family;
provide emotional support; and provide expert, skillful intervention.[57] Box 23-2 lists principles of family-centered intervention.

Partnering with Professionals

The success of an early intervention program depends largely
on the integration of the child's individual program components into a comprehensive system by a cooperative team of

---

BOX 23-1   Questions to Foster Cultural Competence

1. *What do I know about the family's culture and beliefs about health?* This represents the basic knowledge of cultural health practices and beliefs. Conclusions or judgments should not be formed about why these practices are present.

2. *Does the family agree with these beliefs?* Although a client may affiliate with a specific cultural group, the OT must investigate whether the cultural beliefs of health and the client's beliefs of health are similar.

3. *How will these beliefs influence the intervention and outcomes of services provided?* The OT must acknowledge and respond to the influences of cultural beliefs and practices within the intervention plan. To design a plan that conflicts with cultural beliefs would not only be counterproductive to client-centered services but would be disrespectful of the family's belief system. If a family, in deference to the authority of the OT, follows an intervention that conflicts with cultural practices, the family may risk receiving support and affiliation with their cultural group.

4. *How can the intervention plan support culturally endorsed occupations, roles, and responsibilities to promote the family's engagement in occupation?* The OT must consider the important occupations from a cultural perspective. Evening meals may include specific behaviors that possess strong cultural symbols for one family but another family may view an evening meal as merely taking in food with no prescribed rituals.

Modified from Schultz-Krohn, W., & Pendleton, H. M. (2006). Application of the occupational therapy framework to physical dysfunction. In W. Schultz-Krohn & H. M. Pendleton (Eds.), *Pedretti's occupational therapy: Practice skills for physical dysfunction.* St. Louis: Mosby.

BOX 23-2   Principles of Family-Centered Intervention

The following principles have been generally accepted in the implementation of family-centered care:

1. Infants and children are uniquely dependent on their families for their survival and nurturance. This dependence necessitates a family-centered approach to early intervention.

2. Programs should define family in a way that reflects the diversity of family patterns and structures.

3. Each family has its own structure, roles, values, beliefs, and coping styles. Respect for and acceptance of this diversity constitute a cornerstone of family-centered early intervention.

4. Early intervention systems and strategies must honor the racial, ethnic, cultural, and socioeconomic diversity of families.

5. Respect for family autonomy, independence, and decision making means that families must be able to choose the level and nature of early intervention involvement in their lives.

6. Family and professional collaboration and partnerships are the keys to family-centered early intervention and to successful implementation of the IFSP process.

7. An enabling approach to working with families requires that professionals reexamine their traditional roles and practices and develop new practices when necessary (practices that promote mutual respect and partnerships).

8. Early intervention services should be flexible, accessible, and responsive to family-identified needs.

9. Professionals should provide early intervention services according to the normalization principle (i.e., families should have access to services provided in as normal a fashion and environment as possible and that promote the integration of the child and family within the community).

10. No one agency or discipline can meet the diverse and complex needs of infants and children with special needs and their families. Therefore a team approach to planning and implementing the IFSP is necessary.

From McGonigal, M. J., & Garland, C. W. (1988). The individualized family service plan and the early intervention team: Team and family issues and recommended practices. *Infants & Young Children, 1,* 10-21.

professionals. Teamwork is critical because of the interrelated nature of the problems of the developing child and the need for skills and resources from many professionals to meet the needs of the child and family. Occupational therapists working with infants and toddlers are early interventionists who have both specialized knowledge of childhood occupations and generalized knowledge regarding young children with special needs. The emphasis of intervention should be the child within the family unit, rather than the child alone, and intervention should be carried out through collaboration among all professionals involved.

The occupational therapist may participate in various service delivery models. Direct, individual, child-centered services often are not the most appropriate in early intervention, and many programs provide services using a consultative model instead.[49] Role release represents a common practice in early intervention using consultation. In role release, one professional, sometimes called the primary service provider, may be trained to take over functions that traditionally have been performed by another professional (Figure 23-1).[5,48,55] Optimally, role release should be practiced as part of a transdisciplinary team model, where frequent collaboration among team members is supported.[46] By ensuring regular face-to-face meetings, team members may build relationships characterized by mutual trust and respect, thus decreasing potential feelings of ownership over particular therapeutic approaches. Limited contact among team members may result in difficulties in implementing role release and ultimately inadequate services for children and families. Coaching, a practice used in both direct and consultative early intervention, has the potential to support role release and is discussed later in the chapter.

Opportunities for participating in collaborative activities and teaming may be challenging, depending on the type of early intervention program. Greater possibilities existed for informal teaming when therapists provided intervention in centers versus the current practice in most states of providing intervention individually in homes and other community settings. In a study by Campbell and Halbert, early intervention service providers identified the need to improve communication and collaboration.[7] Suggestions included a once-a-month meeting for team members to exchange information, a communication book available for all team members, and cotreatments with providers from different disciplines.

Provision of Early Intervention Services

Assessment and Intervention Planning

Teti and Gibbs traced the interest in infancy and infant assessment back to the 1800s and the Child Study Movement and the efforts of Stanley Hall, founder of the normative study of child development.[65] Normative study of development is the basis for norm-referenced assessment, which assesses a particular behavior or attribute of children of a particular age group, establishing a mean age at development and an accompanying developmental curve against which other children can be evaluated.

An assumption of the developmental theory is that there is continuity of function from the infancy stages of sensorimotor development through the early childhood stages of verbalization and representational play. However, environmental and physiologic factors influence the continuity of development. The knowledge that environmental factors influence the infant's development, and the belief that neurodevelopment in the infant is plastic and malleable, support the concept of early intervention.[63,65]

The developmental approach to infant assessment involves a multidimensional, holistic method in which individual developmental domains are assessed and their influence on behavior as a whole is considered. For example, infants with motor impairments are restricted in their ability to explore their environment, a critical component of sensorimotor development, which in turn can affect other developmental areas of cognition, language, and socialization.

The functional approach, which is analogous to an occupational approach, focuses on the child's performance as it interacts with environmental activities, contexts, and conditions. To implement a functional approach, the therapist gathers information about the types of activities in which the child is to participate, methods of the child's participation, and expected goals for each activity. Using this information, the therapist analyzes competencies and barriers to the child's independent participation in relevant activities.

The functional approach relies on an ecologic framework that emphasizes skills and behaviors. This contrasts with the developmental approach, which documents the child's skills by developmental domain (e.g., motor or cognitive). The functional approach documents the child's behaviors by referencing skill clusters that describe occupations (e.g., feeding or playing).

Early intervention evaluation consists of a series of steps and is an ongoing, collaborative process of collecting, analyzing, and gathering information about the infant and the family to identify specific needs and develop goals in the IFSP.[47] The evaluation, combined with a treatment program and ongoing reassessment, is a problem-solving process that continues throughout the period during which the infant or toddler is eligible for Part C services. Therapists can use developmental evaluations for screening, diagnosing or evaluating, and program planning. These processes are described in Chapters 7 and 8.

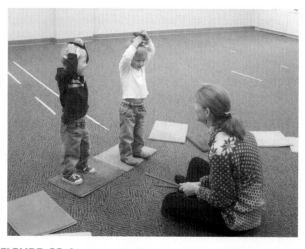

FIGURE 23-1 A music therapist helps children enhance their body awareness, a goal that is a primary responsibility of the occupational therapist.

Evaluation and Planning

The process of evaluation is the gathering and interpreting of information on the child's health status and medical background, current developmental levels of functioning, and family resources to maximize the child's development. Two major goals in the evaluation of infants and toddlers are (1) determination of eligibility for early intervention programs and (2) development of outcomes and goals to guide the early intervention program. The second goal is addressed in the planning aspect of early intervention services, as discussed further on.

Eligibility Determination

Infants and toddlers who have established risk because of their diagnosis are automatically eligible for Part C services. This category includes diagnoses associated with developmental delay, such as cerebral palsy, Down syndrome, or spina bifida. Infants and toddlers without a specific diagnosis who are suspected of having developmental delay are entitled to an evaluation, which must be timely and comprehensive and must include input by a multidisciplinary team. The occupational therapist may be a member of the evaluation team. The team should be responsive to the family's needs and desires when determining the time and location of the evaluation and which individuals should be present. The family's involvement is central to the evaluation process, and a complete evaluation involves observation of interaction between the caregiver and the child. Information caregivers share about the child influences how assessments are implemented and results are interpreted. The focus of the evaluation should be on the process itself (i.e., engaging the child and eliciting representative performance). In addition to test scores, the evaluation should result in a list of strengths and weaknesses.[49]

The developmental areas that the team evaluates to determine eligibility are cognition, communication, motor, social-emotional, and adaptive. Play is another area of importance for the team to assess but is not part of most assessment instruments. However, play assessments demonstrate how well the child integrates separate skill areas and how he or she playfully interacts with social and physical environments. Therapists may use informal assessment through observing the child playing with caregivers, siblings, or peers. The Transdisciplinary Play-Based Assessment, Second Edition (TPBA-2) is an example of a commonly used play assessment that incorporates the early intervention team, rather than just one provider.[43]

Used frequently by early intervention teams, criterion-referenced assessments, including curriculum-based assessments, provide information about a child's ability to perform a certain set of skills within a particular age range. Criterion-referenced tests are favored over norm-referenced tests, which compare a child's abilities with those of their same-age peers, because children receiving early intervention services often have invalid scores because of a lack of flexibility in administering standardized protocols. The Hawaii Early Learning Profile (HELP); the Assessment, Evaluation and Programming System for Infants and Children, Second Edition (AEPS); and the Carolina Curriculum for Infants and Toddlers with Special Needs, Third Edition are well-used developmental curriculum-based assessments.[3,38,54] Other recently developed scales are listed in Appendix 7-A.

Standardized assessments should never be the sole source for determining eligibility for early intervention services.[1]

Furthermore, few reliable, comprehensive standardized assessments are available for children between birth and 2 years of age. A standardized test provides merely a sampling of a child's abilities and behaviors observed at a particular time and situation, from a particular perspective, and with a particular instrument.[26] Assessment results that do not reflect the child's typical functioning or behavioral characteristics are neither meaningful nor accurate. Therefore, professional judgment is a critical element of assessment. The test instruments chosen and the use of professional judgment may vary from state to state and may be specified by policies of the state lead agency.

Miller made the following recommendations for evaluation of infants and young children[50]:

- The therapist should base the assessment on an integrated developmental model. Parents and professionals must observe the child's range of functions in different contexts to identify how the child can best be helped, rather than just coming up with a test score.
- Assessment involves multiple sources and multiple components of information. Parents and professionals contribute to forming the total picture of the child.
- An understanding of typical child development is essential to the interpretation of developmental differences among infants and young children.
- The assessment should emphasize the child's functional capacities, such as attending, engaging, reciprocating, interacting intentionally, organizing patterns of behavior, understanding his or her environment symbolically, and having problem-solving abilities.[25]
- The assessment process should identify the child's current abilities, strengths, and areas of need to attain desired developmental outcomes (Figure 23-2).
- The therapist should not challenge young children during the assessment by separating them from their parents or caregivers. The parents' presence supports the child and begins the parent-professional collaborative process.
- An unfamiliar examiner should not assess young children. The therapist should give the child a "warm-up" period. Assessment by a stranger when the parent is restricted to

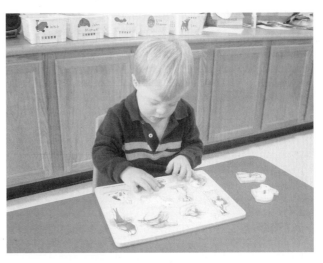

FIGURE 23-2 The therapist can assess perceptual motor skills through observation of puzzle completion.

the role of a passive observer represents an additional challenge.

- Assessments that are limited to easily measurable areas, such as certain motor or cognitive skills, should not be considered complete.
- The therapist should not consider formal or standardized tests the determining factor in the assessment of the infant or young child. Most formal tests were developed and standardized on typically developing children and not on those with special needs. Furthermore, many young children have difficulty attending to or complying with the basic expectations of formal tests. Formal test procedures are not the best context in which to observe functional capacities of young children. Assessments that are intended for intervention planning should use structured tests only as part of an integrated approach (Figure 23-3).

Once the team has defined a child's eligibility for early intervention services, further assessment is important for the therapist and family to determine what intervention strategies and services are of greatest value to the child and family. At this point, evaluation becomes a comprehensive decision-making process to identify social-emotional, cognitive, motor, and communication problems; develop goals; and define an early intervention program plan.

Development of the IFSP

The IFSP is a map of the family's services and informs anyone who will be working with the child and family which services will be provided, where they will be provided, and who will provide them. IDEA specifies that services must be provided in the infant's natural settings. Development of the IFSP follows completion of the initial evaluation and assessment. The IFSP defines the environments in which the child is to be served and provides a statement of justification if services are not provided in natural environments. Occupational therapy intervention, as with other early intervention services, is based on identified concerns and expected outcomes in the IFSP. It is a process in which professionals and families share information to assist the family in making decisions about the types

of services they believe will benefit them and the child. The IFSP also specifies who the provider will be; the location of the services; the frequency, intensity, and duration of services; and the funding sources. Box 23-3 lists the required components as they are stated in IDEA. The development of the IFSP occurs during a meeting facilitated by the service coordinator and attended by the family and at least one member of the evaluation team. The service coordinator's role is to assist the family in accessing information and resources and coordinate implementation of the IFSP. Other service providers or anyone else the family would like to invite may also be in attendance. IFSP forms vary from state to state and among early intervention programs. Despite the differences in forms, each must include specific information as denoted by IDEA. The IFSP is a dynamic plan. To ensure that it meets the changing needs of the child and family, it is reviewed every 6 months or more often if deemed necessary. The family meets with other team members at least once a year. During this meeting, outcomes are examined and families may opt to make changes, including in the type of services the child receives.

Writing Goals and Objectives

The occupational therapist on the early intervention team focuses on outcomes from a family-centered perspective and identifies the child's occupational performance as it relates to

---

BOX 23-3   Required Components of the Individualized Family Service Plan

The IFSP shall be in writing and shall contain the following (IDEA, sec. 636):

1. A statement of the infant's or child's present level of motor, cognitive, communication, social-emotional, and adaptive development, based on objective criteria
2. A statement of the family's resources, priorities, and concerns related to enhancing the development of the infant or child
3. A statement of the major outcomes expected to be achieved for the infant or child and the family, and the criteria, procedures, and timelines used to determine the degree to which progress toward achieving the outcomes is being made and whether modifications or revisions of the outcomes or service are necessary
4. A statement of specific early intervention services necessary to meet the unique needs of the infant or child and the family, including the frequency, intensity, and method of delivering services
5. A statement of the natural environments in which early intervention services shall appropriately be provided, including a justification of the extent, if any, to which the services will not be provided in a natural environment
6. The projected dates for initiation of service and the anticipated duration of the services
7. The identification of the service coordinator from the profession most immediately relevant to the infant's or family's needs who will be responsible for the implementation of the plan and coordination with other agencies and persons
8. The steps to be taken to support the transition of the child with a disability to preschool or other appropriate services

---

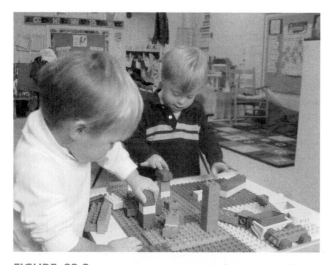

FIGURE 23-3   Important assessment data are gathered through structured observations of the child's play in his or her everyday environment.

From Campbell, S. K., Vander Linden, D. W., & Palisano, R. J. (2006). *Physical therapy for children*. St. Louis: Saunders.

BOX 23-4 Questions to Discuss with Families When Establishing Activities for Services in Natural Environments

- What activities made up your week days and weekends?
- What activities are going well and not going well?
- What activities would you like support for?
- What activities does the child prefer to participate in?
- What activities provide natural learning opportunities?
- What activities provide opportunities for child initiation?
- What activities provide opportunities for peer interaction?
- Are there new activities that you would like to try?

daily family routines. Box 23-4 lists questions to discuss with families. An outcome is a statement of changes desired by the family that can focus on any area of the child's development or family life as it relates to the child.[42] It reflects family priorities, hopes, and concerns in a broad statement that the whole team addresses. Before an outcome is developed, the early intervention team should collect information about the natural environments in which families and children spend their time, such as different areas of the home or the community (e.g., childcare center, playground, library). The team should also assist the family in identifying the activities that they typically do or would like to do in those environments, such as a family who eats breakfast at the kitchen table and would like the child to participate in eating as a morning routine.[48,58] Early intervention providers may then provide strategies for caregivers to use to support child or family participation in an identified activity.

Once routines, activities, and suggested strategies have been identified, outcome statements may be written (see Figure 23-6). Because occupational therapists focus on child and family function and context, outcomes reflect performance areas and contexts rather than performance components.[11] For example, it is not appropriate to write an outcome to "improve pincer grasp," but instead to link a fine motor problem to daily function of both the child and the family unit. Examples of outcomes are "to feed himself finger food" and "to play with toys." Often, outcome statements for children in early intervention are concerned with social participation. This includes those behaviors and skills needed to "fit in" and have been defined as "active engagement in typical activities available to and/or expected of peers in the same context" (p. 338).[12] Typical outcome statements might be "to go to the grocery store with her parent" or "to play with other children." Other outcome statements are parent focused and may include learning strategies to support the child or validation and understanding of the role of a parent of a child with special needs.

After an outcome is developed, the next step is to describe what is happening now and what will happen when the outcome is achieved. Strategies are listed to address the outcome with people and resources that are needed. All relevant team members should be included. For example, if the outcome is "to feed himself finger food at a family meal," the current problems might be "unable to hold food in hand and bring

to mouth, cannot sit at a table, cries during meals unless parent is feeding him." The team will recognize progress when the child can sit at the table independently and pick up and eat small pieces of food. To achieve this outcome, a number of strategies are proposed. The strategies are usually addressed according to the practice areas of specific disciplines. For instance, the physical therapist addresses stability for sitting (Figure 23-4) and the speech language pathologist provides strategies for communication, whereas the occupational therapist addresses sensory issues and hand use (Figure 23-5).

Outcomes focused on participation in community activities may be particularly meaningful for families and young children.[8] Involvement in activities that occur in a setting outside the home, such as a local restaurant, church, or library, may be a caregiver's main concern. Strategies could include adaptations to the environment or activity to support involvement and interventions to support development. An example of a worksheet that may be used to help families and other team members determine how to incorporate ideas and strategies into routines in community settings is provided (Table 23-2).

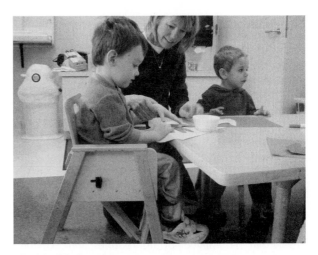

FIGURE 23-4 Adapted seating promotes good postural alignment for fine-motor play at a table.

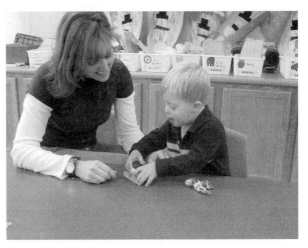

FIGURE 23-5 The occupational therapist and child use an activity to enhance fine-motor skills.

Planning for Interventions within Naturally Occurring Family Routines and Activities
(Adapted by WPDP for the Wisconsin Birth to 3 Program from FACETS materials, Lindeman & Woods)

Outcome: Katy will use playground equipment, play in the sandbox, and explore the outdoors.

Why is this important? We like to take our kids to the park and want both of our daughters to enjoy this activity. We want Katy to have things she can do with her sister, on her own and with other kids whether she is at the neighborhood park, in out backyard, or in some other outdoor location on family visits.

How will you know you have met your outcome? Katy will have 3 things she likes to and can do at the park with her sister, and one thing she likes to do and will do by herself at home and in the park.

Routine: Playing outside at the park or family backyard

Skills, Supports, and Adaptations Needed to Work on This Outcome

What's already working?
- Katy loves to be outside and is motivated to play
- Family is very supportive
- Park is within walking distance

What skills does Katy need to work on this outcome?
- Walk on rough surfaces
- Climb stairs
- Hold on to a swing rope
- A willingness to explore a variety of textures with her hands
- Focus attention
- Take turns, follow directions
- Use signs or words to indicate needs and respond to questions

What environmental supports/adaptations would enhance this outcome?
- Encourage the use of a walking stick, as needed, on rough surfaces
- Use sandbox toys with varied textures, sounds, and colors
- Encourage Katy's sister to plan and lead games/activities at the park
- Use an adapted child swing

What skills/support does the family need to work on this outcome?
- Suggested activities
- Reassurance of safety

Possible Learning Opportunities/Activities:
What possible opportunities exist within the routine or environment for meeting this outcome?
- Walking over the wood chips around the playground equipment
- Climbing up the ladder and going down the slide
- Playing games in the sandbox
- Swinging
- Playing a direction following game
- Walking around the pond to look for frogs or fish
- Going on a treasure hunt
- Crossing a bridge
- Searching in the grass for clovers

Who Can Help? *(Brainstorm a list of possibilities.)*
Who are the family members, professionals/providers, and others who can help child/family achieve this outcome?

Mother, Father, Sister	Educator
Other children at the park	SLP
PT	Family friends

Possible Locations:
Where could child/family work on this outcome?
- Neighborhood park
- Family's backyard
- Other outdoor locations visited by the family

FIGURE 23-6   Sample Outcomes Sheet from an IFSP. (From Wisconsin Birth to 3 Information. [n.d.] *Planning for Interventions within naturally occurring routines and activities.* Retrieved September 2008 from http://www.waisman.wisc.edu/birthto3/KATY_ROUTINES.pdf).

Transition Planning

Another aspect of planning is working with the early intervention team on the child's transition from early intervention to preschool (Part C to Part B services). The transition process for young children with disabilities and their families is often characterized by stress because of the many factors involved, such as a change of environment (i.e., receiving early intervention services at home and then moving to a preschool classroom), a change of providers (i.e., the child and family may have a close relationship with early intervention providers, but will receive services from school personnel after the transition), and a difference in philosophy between early intervention programs and schools (i.e., family-centered in early intervention versus child-centered in schools).[59] Stress may be decreased when transitions are well-planned and support to families and children is provided throughout the process.[29]

Occupational therapists have an important role in transition planning because their background in understanding how different contexts may influence occupational performance is a distinctive part of occupational therapy intervention.[51] Outcomes and strategies written on the IFSP may be used as guides for addressing the needs of the child and family during the transition process, such as having a child participate in a small play group (Case Study 23-1) to help them adjust to the social expectations of preschool. Potential ways in which occupational therapists may support families and children during transition include: preparing caregivers for changes in roles and routines that will occur after the move to preschool, teaching caregivers how to work with their children to develop specific skills needed in preschool, and visiting the preschool classroom before the transition to assess needs for environmental adaptation or modification. The therapist might also support a smooth transition by making sure the child's adaptive equipment is sent to the new setting and providing team members in the new setting a videotape of the child and caregivers doing self-care routines.[69]

TABLE 23-2   Plan of Strategies Worksheet

Plan of Strategies to Promote Tunisha's Participation in Library Story Hour

Ways to Position Tunisha

When the other children . . .	Tunisha can . . .
Sit on the floor	Sit in her floor sitter chair
	Sit with you, between your legs
	Be propped up in a bean bag chair
	Lie on her stomach
Sit at a table	Sit in a chair pushed up to the table and with a strap at her hips
	Sit in her stroller pushed up to the table
Stand	Sit in her stroller
	Stand in front of you, with you holding her at her hips (takes two hands)
	Stand in front of a table with you behind her so that your leg is between her legs (to keep them apart)

Helping Tunisha Manipulate Objects or Materials

When the activity requires objects . . .	Tunisha can . . .
Storybook stick props; rhythm band instruments; other objects	Hold objects that are large when placed in her hand (e.g., instead of using a stick on the storybook props, staple Tunisha's prop to a paper towel cardboard tube)
	Hold objects that can be placed on her hand or arm so that she doesn't have to grasp (e.g., bells fastened to her wrist, puppets)
	Hold objects using her Velcro glove
Markers, crayons, paint brushes	Hold the object with her Velcro glove
	Use fat crayons (the ones with the knobs at the top)
	Finger paint instead
	Draw with an adult or another child helping her hold the object and move her arms

Adapted from Campbell, P. (2004). Participation-based services: Promoting children's participation in natural settings. *Young Exceptional Children, 8*(1), 20-29.

CASE STUDY 23-1   Jeremy

BACKGROUND

Jeremy's pediatric neurologist referred him for a transdisciplinary assessment at 18 months of age because of motor delays caused by his mitochondrial encephalopathy. An early intervention team, which consisted of an occupational therapist, a physical therapist, a speech-language pathologist, and an early childhood intervention specialist, assessed him in an arena assessment. Both parents participated in the assessment. Although Jeremy had received occupational therapy and physical therapy since he was 6 months old, his parents thought he would benefit from inclusion in a small group of children with special needs and children who were typically developing in which he could receive his therapies and special instruction in an integrated manner.

ASSESSMENT

The team chose to administer the Battelle Developmental Inventory, Second Edition (BDI-2), and the HELP.[53] The latter was administered through observation, direct administration of test items, and interview with the parents. The team modified portions to accommodate for Jeremy's physical limitations. Most important, the therapists engaged him in play activities and used their interpretation of his interactions and movements to estimate his functional abilities.

Overall, Jeremy had very low muscle tone and poor physical endurance. He needed support for sitting and could bear only some of his weight when supported in standing. He was unable to roll or crawl. Head control was poor, with head stacking in a supported sitting position and lack of head righting in the prone position. He used his left hand very well to play with toys when he was positioned appropriately but did not use his right hand and protested when the therapist attempted to evaluate passive range of motion. Jeremy was alert and interested but was reluctant to leave his mother's lap. Communication skills and cognition appeared to be on age level, whereas social skills seemed immature.

INTERVENTION

Jeremy started in an inclusive playgroup two mornings a week. He received occupational therapy, physical therapy,

Continued

CASE STUDY 23-1 **Jeremy—cont'd**

and speech language pathology on a consultative basis, with direct special instruction while in the play group. The team members took care to close coordination and carryover of all skills. All services and special instruction were aimed at helping Jeremy improve social interaction with peers, improve self-help skills, and develop physical abilities to the greatest extent possible. The team obtained adapted seating and eating utensils for him and modified group activities to enable him to participate actively and as independently as possible.

INDIVIDUAL FAMILY SERVICE PLAN REVIEW

After 6 months, the service coordinator, intervention team, and family members met to review the goals on Jeremy's IFSP and to update and modify it as needed. The family and the team were pleased with Jeremy's progress and thought that he was benefiting from his intervention program. Jeremy was gaining confidence in a small group, developing good social and communication skills, and no longer tiring as easily. Jeremy's service coordinator arranged for him to participate in a special grant program at a local child care center. He was enrolled in a class for 2-year-old children that met a few hours a week and had the support of an assistant who had been trained to facilitate the inclusion of children with special needs in the typical childcare setting. Although this facilitator had several other children to work with and was not in Jeremy's class all the time, she was available at any time that he needed help or that the teacher had a question or concern. After a few months, Jeremy started attending this program two times a week; meanwhile, he continued to receive therapy services on a consultative basis at home and at the center.

ANNUAL REASSESSMENT

One year after entrance into the early intervention program, the intervention team reassessed Jeremy in preparation for the development of a new IFSP. They did not perform this assessment in a formal testing session but over a period of weeks as

Jeremy participated in various activities with the group. In addition to the BDI-2, Jeremy's team also updated the HELP.

Results of the reassessment indicated a bright, happy, verbal 2-year-old child. Although he had gained in physical abilities, Jeremy needed a stroller-type wheelchair with special inserts for appropriate seating. The removable seat also acted as a floor sitter so that Jeremy could be close to the same level as his peers when they played on the floor. The teacher observed that Jeremy had shown considerable improvement in his play skills and that they were definitely more appropriate when he was positioned upright rather than lying on the floor. He demonstrated spontaneous interactions with his peers, took turns with little prompting, and began to share toys.

Jeremy continued to participate in the class at the childcare center and no longer had the facilitator's support. The occupational therapist and the physical therapist continued to provide on-site consultation. Through a problem-solving approach with close cooperation among the family, childcare personnel, and therapists, Jeremy thrived in the class. Strategies that supported his participation included providing wheelchair access to the playground (they had been carrying him), teaching principles of lifting and carrying, and making the stroller available to transport him from room to room so that the teacher had her hands free to keep up with other active 2-year-old children.

SUMMARY

Jeremy is an example of a child who was able to benefit from a combination of programming that included an inclusive playgroup and a typical childcare setting. His program required close cooperation among the family, early intervention personnel, and community resources. His parents look forward to his graduation to the class for 3-year-old children and increasing his typical class time to 3 days a week. They have already visited the neighborhood school and plan for him to attend a regular kindergarten class when he is 5 years of age where he will be supported by therapies at school. Jeremy is bright, and with the right kind of support and technology, he can fully participate in school and in the community.

Payment for Occupational Therapy Services

States determine how therapists are paid for their services. In some states, therapists are employed by the state agency that oversees the early intervention program, whereas in others the therapist is self-employed or employed through a private agency. In a typical scenario, the therapist bills for the time spent in direct, face-to-face contact with the child, family, or other caregiver. Billing for time spent in team meetings, on the phone with team members or family, and other indirect activities may or may not be reimbursed. Because state funding for early intervention programs is subject to annual budget shortfalls and at continuous risk for being cut, therapists are typically reimbursed through federal programs (i.e., Medicaid) or private insurance first with families paying part of the cost of early intervention services.[24] Often the payment amount is determined on a sliding scale based on a family's income.

Although therapists working in early intervention must travel throughout the community to provide services in natural environments, travel is rarely reimbursed.

Working in Natural Environments

Settings

Part C of IDEA specifies that early intervention services are provided in the child's natural environment. *Natural environments* are defined as settings that are natural or normal for children without disabilities and include the home and community settings. To enable the child to remain an integral part of the family and for the family to be integral parts of the neighborhood and community, services should be community based and in locations convenient to the family.[18,37,66] Ideally, the therapist should offer the family a range of options so they

an choose those that best fit their priorities, lifestyle, and
values. These options should include those that provide the
least restrictive settings in situations that would be natural
environments for a typically developing child of the same
age. Some examples are a playgroup, mother's morning out
program, childcare center, playgrounds, grocery stores, or
fast-food restaurants (Figure 23-7). In addition, the outcomes
on the IFSP should support the provision of services in the natural
environment, with outcomes linked directly to family routines and
contexts (Figure 23-8).[39,40]

The key to successful intervention is collaboration between
therapists and caregivers within the home or childcare setting.
Intervention in natural environments includes using toys and
materials that can be found in the natural environment and will
remain available to the family or other caregivers on a consistent
basis. Therapists who rely on clinical equipment, whether they
bring it to home visits or use it in their centers, may be trying
to influence the child's performance by using toys and equipment most comfortable for the therapist.[28] Specialized equipment, such as suspended swings, therapy balls, or a child-sized
table and chair (Figure 23-9), may be optimal for a clinic-based
program for addressing sensory or motor deficits, but may not
be available to families at home, caregivers at a child care facility,
or another environment in the absence of the therapist. If early
intervention is provided in a clinical setting, it is equally important for the therapist to offer opportunities for the family and
other caregivers to learn and practice the interactions and principles to promote generalization in the natural environment.
Best practice in occupational therapy infers expanding direct

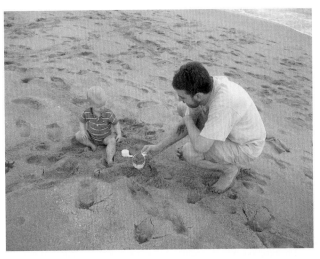

FIGURE 23-8 Family involvement supports the child in the natural environment.

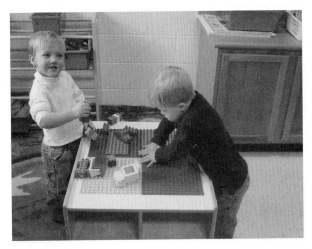

FIGURE 23-9 The occupational therapist uses preschool materials to achieve the child's fine-motor goals.

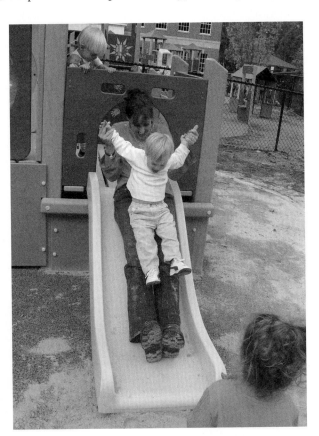

FIGURE 23-7 The therapist encourages a child to participate in sensory motor activities on the playground.

treatment to include primary caregivers (parents, grandparents,
childcare providers). This involves learning to accept and respect
differences in philosophies, priorities, and practices.[27]

The Division of Early Childhood of the Council for Exceptional Children supports the philosophy of inclusion in natural
environments with the following statement: "Inclusion, as a
value, supports the right of all children, regardless of their
diverse abilities, to participate actively in natural settings within
their communities. A natural setting is one in which the child
would spend time if he or she had not had a disability" (p. 4).[15]

The philosophy of inclusion extends beyond physical inclusion to mean social and emotional inclusion of the child and
family.[10,67] The implications for occupational therapists are
that they provide opportunities for expanded and enriched
natural learning with typically developing peers. Self-contained
or segregated settings are more restrictive and do not prepare
children for participating or being a part of their natural and
spontaneous environment.[61]

Occupational Therapy in Natural Environments

By providing early intervention services in natural environments, occupational therapists may take advantage of the actual contexts in which the occupations and co-occupations of children and families occur. Natural learning environments are those in which planned and unplanned, structured and unstructured, and intentional and incidental learning experiences occur.[20] Mothers' Morning Out and mother-infant playgroups exemplify such planned activity. Petting a puppy in the park is an unplanned activity. Hippotherapy and doing puzzles are structured activities, whereas playing on the playground is an unstructured one. Putting on one's clothes is an intentional task; falling into a pile of autumn leaves is an incidental learning experience. Learning opportunities are composed of a variety of life experiences that make activity setting an appropriate description for natural learning environments.[20]

Literature on early intervention supports service delivery in natural environments and includes studies on natural intervention strategies, generalization of skills, inclusion, home-based services, and consultation with service providers.[61] Research suggests that opportunities for learning in natural environments were most effective for addressing the developmental needs of young children when the opportunities were "interesting and engaging and . . . provided children contexts for exploring, practicing, and perfecting competence" (p. 90).[21]

Natural intervention strategies are those that use incidental learning opportunities that occur throughout the child's typical activities and interactions with peers and adults (Figure 23-10), follow the child's lead, and use natural consequences. Intervention strategies that occur in real-life settings over those that take place in more contrived clinic-based settings are more effective in promoting the child's acquisition of functional motor, social, and communication skills (Figure 23-11).[5,32,49] At one time, segregated settings such as special preschools and pediatric therapy clinics were seen as the only or preferred setting for children with disabilities to receive therapy services because inclusive opportunities were limited or did not exist. A resulting advantage of providing occupational therapy in natural environments is that children tend to be more comfortable in familiar settings such as their

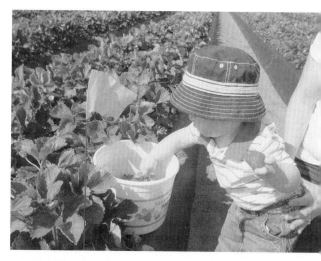

FIGURE 23-11   Participation in community-based family activities promotes developmental skills.

home and are more apt to be responsive and interactive with the therapist.

Generalization of skills is the ability to respond appropriately under spontaneous and natural conditions such as responses to people, environments, objects, and stimuli. Generalization of skills and behaviors occurs more readily when the intervention setting is the same as the child's natural environment(s) (Figure 23-12).[35] This requires the therapist's ingenuity to develop strategies that will be acceptable and supported by the caregiver(s).[8,28] Recognizing and accepting the family's uniqueness in cultural and child-rearing practices, occupational therapists are able to facilitate the child's ability to generalize new skills to a variety of settings (Figure 23-13).

Inclusive early childhood programs provide opportunities for therapists to collaborate with primary caregivers including parents, grandparents, and childcare providers. Including siblings in therapy sessions can reinforce meaningful relationships between siblings who often feel left out during the care for their brother or sister with special needs. Inclusive settings

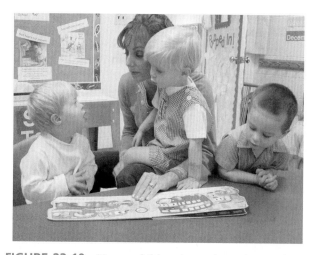

FIGURE 23-10   Young children learn through peer interaction and peer imitation.

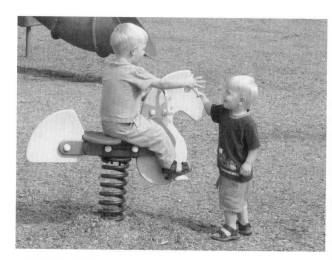

FIGURE 23-12   Play with peers in natural environments helps the child generalize newly learned skills.

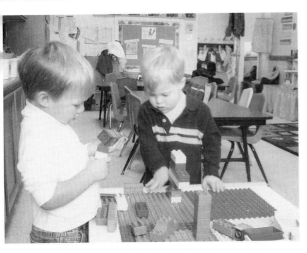

FIGURE 23-13 Peer play helps the child generalize newly learned skills.

provide a variety of enriching learning opportunities. Early childhood programs, for example, enhance opportunities for play and interactions with typically developing peers in real-life situations in the classroom. Therapists can benefit from collaborating with childcare providers through opportunities for peer role modeling and teaching (Figure 23-14). Participation in community programs gives the family common experiences for relating to friends and neighbors and helps them view their child as one with differing abilities rather than one with disabilities. To be successful, the inclusion program should ensure that (1) the child's individual needs are met with appropriate aids and support services, (2) the child with special needs benefits from the typical program, and (3) the needs of the typical children are not compromised.

Home-based services are another example of services in the natural environment. Therapists have the benefit of seeing the child with special needs within the context of the family and in

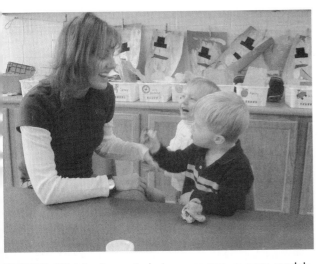

FIGURE 23-14 In an inclusive program, a peer models, encourages, and supports the child with developmental delays.

activities of daily living and a multitude of interrelated roles.[28,61] Therapists are trained to be good observers, a skill that is a distinct advantage in natural environments. Home therapy programs designed during home-based visits tend to be more successful because therapists are more realistic in suggesting goals that are based on the resources available, can problem-solve issues unique to the home environment, and can better individualize the program to meet the family's interests and needs.

Challenges to Implementing Therapy in Natural Environments

Providing therapy in natural environments presents several challenges from the perspective of therapy providers, families, and governing bodies (particularly state and local agencies). Therapists may engage in role release through coaching and provide support to caregivers within the child's natural environments. A transdisciplinary model requires developing effective communication skills to make available the same repertoire of intervention strategies among providers and to support the family's integration of the strategies into their daily routine.[23,61]

Occupational therapists must be able to work within multiple environments creatively and flexibly and take advantage of teachable moments. For example, the occupational therapist may have plans to use the playground for sensory integration strategies and the classroom in the childcare center for addressing fine motor skills, only to find it is a rainy day and the children cannot go outdoors. When she arrives at the classroom, the occupational therapist sees that the children are engaged in a rainy day activity of playing dress-up, which she immediately uses as the context for her intervention. Being able to revise treatment requires quick thinking and creativity.

Providing services within natural environments requires therapists to travel. Travel time between cases can be lengthy because of traffic in urban settings and distances in rural settings, resulting in increased mileage costs and lower caseloads.

Third-party payers (insurance companies, Medicaid, managed care organizations) may consider therapy in community settings as an indirect service, which is not reimbursable.[27] Early intervention payers often reimburse only for direct or hands-on time with the child and generally will not reimburse for parent sessions, team meetings, or training of essential staff.[28]

Therapists must be familiar with state legislation related to early intervention and become advocates for their families. An early intervention therapist may assume the role of political activist as legislation may be amended. Interpretations of the laws often differ from region to region, which can affect service delivery.

Occupational therapy services are provided in various settings that represent a continuum from the most restrictive (e.g., hospital settings) to the least restrictive (e.g., community settings). The setting should reflect family preferences and should be consistent with the needs of the child and the goals identified on the IFSP. For example, a child with significant and acute medical problems may be best served in the hospital-based program, whereas another with similar problems may be best served in the home. A child with autism may function best in a preschool program with typically developing peers. Occupational therapy in this natural environment would focus on functional behaviors and skills such as facilitating

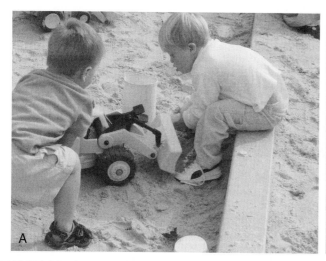

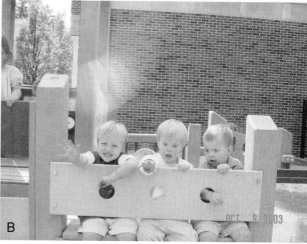

FIGURE 23-15 **A,** Sensory motor play in the sandbox. **B,** Children learn many skills through imitation of their peers.

transitions from one activity to another, engaging with and responding to peers and teachers, practicing activities of daily living, or participating in sensory or tactile activities (Figure 23-15, *A*). The occupational therapist can include the typical peers as role models and as partners in play (Figure 23-15, *B*). Another child with the same diagnosis, however, may not be ready for a group environment and would be best seen in one-on-one therapy in an environment with fewer distractions, such as in a home. Early intervention legislation requires interagency cooperation; thus, families can choose the most appropriate settings and services from either private or public providers.

OCCUPATIONAL THERAPY INTERVENTION

Occupational therapists promote a child's independence, mastery, and sense of self-worth and self-confidence in their physical, emotional, and psychosocial development. These services are designed to help families and other caregivers improve children's functioning within their environments. Intervention characterized by engagement in meaningful occupations of the child and family in the natural environment is used to expand the child's functional abilities.

Addressing Family and Child Needs in Natural Environments

Family-Centered Intervention

In family-centered intervention, the occupational therapist addresses the needs of the entire family, rather than concentrating only on specific deficits in the child. The therapist should be guided by family concerns and the amount of involvement that various family members choose to have in the child's intervention program. One important way for the therapist to increase the effect of their services is to make the program relevant to the family's lifestyle and time

commitments. Activities should be those that target behaviors and skills that the child can generalize to his or her daily routines at home, school, and community. Parents vary in their ability to implement structured therapy activities with their children. Family demands and support networks are always considerations in discussing home programs with parents. One mother stated the following: "There are times when even an acceptable amount of therapy becomes too much—when your child needs time just to be a child, or when you need time to be with the rest of the family. It is okay to say 'no' at those times, for a while. Your instinct will tell you when" (p. 51).[64]

Sometimes it is more important to support the role of parent than to assume that the parent can take on the role of the therapist. Daily routines in a family with a child who has a disability can take an excessive amount of time and energy, which does not allow for carrying out a therapy home program. Suggestions that the family can incorporate into the daily routine are the most successful. For example, the caregiver can provide tactile stimulation and range of motion at bath time; an older sibling can encourage the infant to reach for toys while their mother cooks dinner.

Occupational therapists can provide support for families by listening to them, giving positive feedback regarding parenting skills, encouraging recreational activities for the family, and helping them access community resources.[22] Often the therapist can help the family by providing intervention to make daily routines go more smoothly. Examples are suggestions for positioning and handling to make feeding more efficient and for adapting a bath seat to make bathing less taxing. Research on supporting caregiver-child relationships is summarized in a table on the Evolve website.

An understanding of and respect for the individual differences between families are important because recent research suggests that there is great variation among families receiving early intervention services (Research Note 23-1). DeGrace reminds occupational therapists that customs and beliefs of families serve as the basis for daily routines and that therapists should "be aware of their biases, and sensitive to the ethnic

RESEARCH NOTE 23-1

Hebbeler, K., Spiker, D., Bailey, D., Scarborough, A., Mallik, S., Simeonsson, R., et al. (2007). Early intervention for infants and toddlers with disabilities and their families: Participants, services, and outcomes. *Final Report of the National Early Intervention Longitudinal Study (NEILS). Menlo Park, CA: SRI International.*

ABSTRACT

Beginning in 1996, the Office of Special Education Programs of the U.S. Department of Education sponsored research regarding early intervention (Part C). This longitudinal, descriptive study was based on an ecologic model in which young children receiving early intervention services (EI) are considered to be influenced by a variety of factors such as environment, genetics, and cultural attitudes. In particular, there was a special consideration of the interactions between child and family. Questions that guided the study were focused on determining characteristics of children and families who received services, the types of services received, the costs of services, the outcomes experienced by children and families, and the relationship among outcomes, services, and child-family characteristics. A nationally representative sample of 3338 children was included in the study, which drew data from a variety of sources over time: family interviews (telephone and mail), service records (i.e., IFSP), service provider surveys, and kindergarten teacher surveys.

IMPLICATIONS FOR PRACTICE

- There was great variation in the types of children and families that received EI services, yet over half of families were coping with multiple risk factors beyond disability or developmental delay in their children, including poverty, low level of maternal education, a single-parent household, and having another child with special needs. The authors of NEILS point out that this diversity supports the requirement for individualized services in EI, which take into account how to best support families and are flexible to the needs of families and children at different points in time.
- Many of the children who received EI did not receive special education services in preschool or kindergarten, suggesting that for some children, disability and delay identified before 36 months may be transitory in nature. Occupational therapists need to be aware that many young children with mild impairments may need services for only a short time. In this case EI can be considered a prevention program addressing specific developmental challenges in infancy and toddlerhood and preventing or reducing the need for additional services in the future.
- Areas of concern identified by parents and kindergarten teachers of children formerly in EI included communication problems and social-emotional problems. Occupational therapists would benefit from training to address simple communication and behavioral issues within the context of different service delivery models, and an understanding of when these issues need to be addressed by a professional with specialized knowledge.

- At the time of data collection (late 1990s), families were receiving typically two to four different services with a median of 1.5 hours of scheduled service time per week. This limited amount of service time spread among several professionals supports the need for occupational therapists to incorporate families into intervention by addressing how intervention strategies will fit into family routines and daily activities within the natural environment.
- A majority of the families who participated in EI identified positive outcomes associated with the program such as knowing how to care for their child, helping their child learn and develop, knowing how to work well with professionals and how to obtain help and support from relatives and friends. However, ratings from low-income and minority families were lower in these areas, suggesting that EI providers, including occupational therapists, should be thoughtful of the specific needs of diverse families.

and cultural ways of living of those we serve" (p. 348).[14] She encourages therapists to think beyond routines and consider family rituals, multifaceted experiences that support the building of family relationships and occupations (e.g., saying goodnight, buying new school shoes) as key elements in family-centered intervention. In this way, occupational therapy goals then center on meaningful aspects of family life, such as celebrations, family traditions, and daily rituals.

Intervention Approaches

Several authors have described family-centered approaches for providing inclusive early intervention services within the natural environment.[10] One approach that takes advantage of adult learning styles is coaching. Natural environments offer opportunities for therapists to coach caregivers to gain self-confidence and assume responsibility in their child's daily care, and coaching other service providers to carry out occupational therapy interventions. As described by Rush, Shelden, and Hanft, the process of coaching is characterized by the coach (the early interventionist), who "has specialized knowledge and skills to share about growth and development, specific intervention strategies, and enhancing the performance of young children with disabilities," and the learner (the caregiver), who "has intimate knowledge of a child's abilities, challenges, and typical performance in a given situation . . . daily routines and settings, lifestyle, family culture . . . desirable goals for [the learner] and the child" (p. 38).[60] The coach supports the learner and the child to achieve outcomes through a process described by Rush et al. (Figure 23-16)[60]:

- *Initiation*: The coach or the learner identifies a need, and a joint plan is developed that includes the purpose of the coaching and specific learner outcomes.
- *Observation*: The coach may use four possible types of observation: (1) the learner demonstrates an existing challenge or practices a new skill while the coach observes; (2) the coach models a technique, strategy, or skill while the learner observes; (3) the learner consciously thinks about how to support the child's learning while performing the

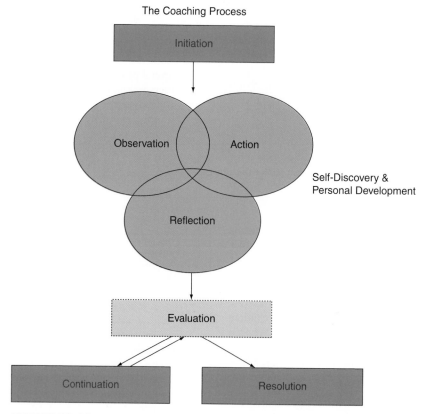

The Coaching Process

FIGURE 23-16 The Coaching Process. (Modified from Rush, D. D., Shelden, M. L., & Hanft, B. E. [2003]. Coaching families and colleagues: A process for collaboration in natural settings. *Infants & Young Children 16*[1], 33-47.)

activity; and (4) the coach and the learner observe aspects of the environment to determine how they may influence the situation.

- *Action*: This includes activities that take place at times other than when the coach and the learner are in contact, such as the learner's practicing the new skill or strategy or engaging in a situation that may be discussed with the coach.
- *Reflection*: The coach uses questioning and reflective listening, and provides reflective feedback and joint problem solving to help the learner understand how to analyze practices and behaviors. The coach then reviews the discussion or observes the learner to assess the learner's understanding. The learner's strengths, competence, and mastery are acknowledged.
- *Evaluation*: The coach evaluates the effectiveness of the coaching process with both the learner and also himself or herself. Evaluation with the learner may not take place every time the coach and the learner have discussions; however, the coach should self-evaluate to determine if changes need to be made, if the coach is assisting the learner to achieve identified outcomes, or if the coaching needs to continue.
- *Continuation*: The results of the coaching session are summarized and a plan is developed for what should occur before and during the following session.
- *Resolution*: Both the coach and the learner agree that identified outcomes have been achieved. The learner

has increased competence and confidence to support the child's learning opportunities in the natural environment.

Coaching may be especially helpful in a service delivery model, where one early intervention team member is the primary provider for the child and family (Case Study 23-2). In this model, the other team members provide coaching on a consultative basis for the family, and they also provide coaching to the primary service provider. As in any team process, coaching requires that team members use good communication skills, and trust and respect one another. Opportunities for communication and collaboration are crucial to the success of coaching, thus necessitating support from early intervention programs and agencies for additional meeting time and covisits. It is important for team members to understand that coaching is not a linear process, but rather a process in which feedback is used to refine solutions as needed (Box 23-5).

The occupational therapist may work with caregivers to plan and carry out therapeutic interventions for the infant and child by integrating developmentally appropriate activities into daily routines and activity settings identified by the family, rather than focusing on the acquisition of isolated skills. For example, it would be inappropriate for the occupational therapist to concentrate on coaching caregivers on how to develop precise fingertip prehension without consideration of how this skill contributes to the overall function of the child in the environment or how it fits into

CASE STUDY 23-2 Alana

BACKGROUND

Alana is a 2-year, 3-month-old child who was diagnosed with developmental delay. She has recently begun receiving early intervention services because of delays in motor, self-care/adaptive, and social-emotional domains. Findings from her initial assessment suggested that Alana's delays may be related to problems with sensory processing. Specifically, Alana demonstrates sensory-seeking behaviors. Karen, the occupational therapist, is Alana's primary service provider because of expertise in addressing sensory processing challenges. Alana's mother, Carmen, has requested that services be provided in the family's home at this time, so Karen has been making home visits once weekly. During the IFSP, the family identified that Alana has difficulty falling asleep. They would like the early intervention team to address this issue.

INTERVENTION

At the first home visit, Carmen mentioned that Alana had been difficult to get to bed at night. Karen hypothesized that Alana's struggle to calm down in the evening and fall asleep was most likely because of her sensory processing difficulties. Karen initiated a coaching relationship with Carmen by asking her if she would like to work together to explore ways to help Alana sleep better. Carmen enthusiastically agreed.

Karen asked Carmen to explain what she and her husband, Ramon, had already tried with Alana during bedtime. Carmen explained that they typically gave Alana a bath, let her watch a video, and then moved into her room for some quiet time before going to bed. However, Alana, who recently switched from a crib to a toddler bed, refused to stay in bed. Instead she would pull her toys out, jump on her mattress, and run around her room, becoming increasingly active as the night wore on. Eventually, several hours later, Alana would crash on her bed and fall asleep. Carmen felt that the sleep problems were causing tension between her and Ramon since they were getting less sleep and became easily frustrated with each other.

Karen told Carmen about her suspicion that there was a relationship between Alana's sensory processing and her difficulty falling asleep. She provided Carmen with two suggestions of strategies that incorporated increased sensory input to put into action before the next visit: (1) give Alana more opportunities for play that incorporated movement, such as climbing and crawling, before initiating the bedtime routine, and (2) use a textured bath mitt or loofah during the bath. Karen decided that it would be beneficial to observe Alana's bedtime routine, so she scheduled her next visit in the evening. When she arrived, she asked Carmen what happened when the sensory-based suggestions were implemented. Carmen reflected on the last several days and replied that it was difficult to give Alana more play time because of the late hour that the family arrived home after picking her up from daycare. Carmen did feel that the loofah was calming to Alana in the bath, but Alana was still taking a long time to settle down for bed.

During her observation of the bedtime routine, Karen noted aspects of the routine that could be strengthened to support Alana's sensory needs, and behaviors that were not necessarily sensory based, but more likely a result of typical development in the toddler stage, such as Alana's refusal to go to bed. She observed that Alana enjoyed her bath and sought out sensory experiences like splashing and rubbing soap on her arms and legs. Karen watched how Carmen gave the loofah to Alana to use rather than Carmen using it. Karen modeled to Carmen how to use the loofah to provide deep pressure to Alana's arms, legs, and back while in the tub and how to use the towel to do the same while drying off. After the bath Karen followed Carmen and Alana into the bedroom and Carmen turned on the video. Alana was running around the room in circles while the video, a cartoon with very little action, played. Karen asked Carmen if she had a video with characters that danced and sang. Carmen changed the video and soon Alana was dancing along with the characters. Karen explained that the dancing provided both movement and muscle work, which is what Alana was seeking.

After 15 minutes Carmen turned off the video and they went to Alana's room. Carmen shut the blinds and pulled the dark shades so that the room was dimly lit. Although Alana was calm when entering her room, she became increasingly active as the room got darker and the house grew quieter. Karen asked Carmen if she had an extra nightlight and Carmen placed one in the corner of Alana's room. Karen turned on Alana's small radio to the classical station at a soft volume. Karen explained that Alana may need extra visual and auditory input to help stay calm. After looking at books in bed, Carmen told Alana it was time to go to sleep. Alana began to protest, but Karen quickly suggested that they play the "Cloud Game" before going to sleep. She took Alana's pillow and placed it on Alana's back with Alana lying on her stomach. Karen pressed the pillow down firmly and told Alana "the clouds are carrying you off to sleep." Karen traded places with Carmen and encouraged Carmen to continue providing the deep pressure to Alana until Alana indicated she was ready to go to sleep.

After they left the room, Carmen called Ramon into the kitchen so that they could speak with Karen. They were both excited that Alana was asleep and how much easier it had been when using the strategies Karen suggested. Carmen and Ramon planned to try the techniques until the next visit when they would evaluate how the bedtime routine was working.

FOLLOW-UP

Karen arrived at Alana's home the next week and was greeted by Ramon. He told Karen that Alana continued to show improvement in going to sleep and was even asking to go into her bed so she could play the "Cloud Game." Karen, Carmen, and Ramon decided that further intervention regarding Alana's sleep was not needed and ended the coaching relationship for that particular need.

BOX 23-5 Example of How Coaching Is Not a Linear Process

Initiation: You are going to serve as the primary coach for a family. You discuss any barriers to the coaching process and ground rules. Based on the individualized family service plan, the family identified some ways you could support them in promoting their child's development.

Reflection: The family tells you how they would like for their child to sit in the cart at the department store so that they can do their shopping and so that he can see what's going on around him. You ask what they've been doing and how well it's worked. You and the family brainstorm some ideas to try.

Action: You go with the father and child to the department store. The father practices putting the child in the seat of the cart and strapping him in as the two of you had discussed.

Observation: You observe how the father positions the child and notice that the child's bottom is not scooted all the way to the back of the seat.

Reflection: You ask the father how the child's position matches what the two of you had discussed. He shares his thoughts. You provide feedback on the position and suggest that he scoot the child's bottom to the back of the seat.

Observation: You observe how well the child sits in the seat and his ability to be actively engaged with his father and participate in the shopping trip.

Reflection: You ask the father how well he thought the shopping trip went and what caused him to think that. You ask him what, if anything, he might do differently next time. You ask the father how the cart seats at the grocery store are different and what he might need to do differently to position the child in the cart.

Evaluation (Continuation-Plan): You and the father develop a plan that includes actions and practice that will occur during shopping trips until your next coaching conversation.

From Hanft, B.E., Rush, D.D., & Shelden, M.L. (2004). *Coaching families and colleagues in early childhood.* Baltimore: Brookes.

---

the developmental needs of the child. Developmentally based curricula such as the HELP, AEPS, or Transdisciplinary Play-Based Intervention, Second Edition provide activities matched to the developmental sequences within each domain.[44] However, the therapist should guard against using a "cookbook" approach in intervention for specific developmental deficits.

After identifying a need in a specific domain, such as fine motor skills, the therapist can work with caregivers to identify learning opportunities in the natural environment that require a child to use those skills. To promote generalization of the fine motor skills, the therapist and caregivers should use play activities that involve the "just right" challenge to the child across domains (i.e., activities that include skill building in the cognitive and social domains). For example, playing with puzzles is a motor task that also involves cognitive skills such as concept of size, shape, and dimension, and visual perceptual skills such as visual closure. Most developmental skills and play occupations are learned in the context of social interaction, including give and take with another child or adult, eye contact, praise, and delight at successful attempts. A team whose members have overlapping functions can effectively address developmental needs (Figure 23-17).

Working with Medically Fragile Children

Young children who have special health care needs make up approximately 11.2% of the age group birth through 5 years.[34] Children who are medically fragile represent a subset of these and often require the use of specialized medical equipment (e.g., ventilator, gastrostomy tube) and receive services from two or more medical specialists (e.g., neurologist, developmental pediatrician).[52] They and their families may have additional challenges when receiving health care services, including early intervention. For instance, families of these children in the birth through 5 age group reported that their health care providers did not listen carefully or spend enough time with them at visits, and had significantly more hospitalizations, doctor visits, and nonphysician visits (e.g., occupational therapy)

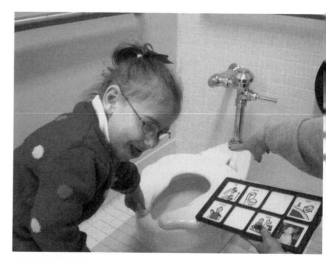

FIGURE 23-17 The occupational therapist integrates speech goals into toilet training.

than families who did not have children with complex health care needs.[34] More time is spent coordinating the care of young children with complex health care needs than that of other children in early intervention.[52] A recent study found that 87% of families of young medically fragile children (birth through 5) identified that they usually or always felt like a partner in their child's care; however, the percentage decreased as the poverty level increased and as the child's functional abilities decreased.[13]

Occupational therapists working with medically fragile children in early intervention should be prepared to address family needs related to daily routines, such as helping families determine optimal positioning during catheterization or timing attempts at oral feeding in a child with a gastrostomy tube. Occupational therapists should identify that the child's primary caregivers know the child best, thus respecting family opinions regarding the child's care. In addition, occupational therapists need to be flexible with family schedules, given the frequency with which a young child with complex health care needs may require hospitalizations or doctor visits. Occupational therapists should work closely with the team to determine the optimal approach for involving families, particularly those who live in poverty or represent diverse cultures. A thoughtful, family-centered approach that takes into account specific, individualized needs of the child and family is necessary.

Areas of Intervention

Play

One of the most important areas of a child's development is involvement in the occupation of play. Play is open-ended, self-initiated, self-directed, and unlimited in its variety. Play can be exploratory, symbolic, creative, or competitive in nature (see Chapter 18). Skills that will be the foundation for engagement in other occupations, such as the ability to manipulate objects, problem-solve, and attend to tasks, may be developed and practiced during play. Research on play with young children is summarized in Table 23-3.

Learning how to play may also be a goal of intervention, particularly for children with significant disabilities. Children with special needs may not develop play skills because of long hospitalizations or medical treatments, or because of the limitations imposed by a physical impairment. Other children may experience deficits in play because of cognitive limitations or difficulties in social interactions.

Because play is usually embedded in the daily routine of young children, therapists should coach caregivers on how to use different toys or play activities to support the child's learning of new skills. The occupational therapist should work with families to determine the natural environments where play takes place or where caregivers or children want play to occur, such as in the backyard, the child's bedroom, or a community playground. Childcare providers may also receive support to learn strategies and approaches that will enhance play. The therapist may suggest ways in which the provider can encourage age-appropriate play with peers, and play with toys and other materials (e.g., sand and water table) at the childcare facility.

Objects and materials typically found in the natural environment should be the focus of play, rather than items brought into the home by the therapist (e.g., therapy ball). Therapists can show caregivers how to create games and toys out of everyday objects, such as plastic containers and wooden spoons. Because play is intrinsically motivating for young children, therapists and caregivers should seek natural learning opportunities within play activities that the child enjoys. For example, a toddler with hemiplegic cerebral palsy is observed playing with stuffed animals and using her affected arm to stabilize her trunk when reaching into a bin to take them out. This activity supports a motor-based occupational therapy goal for the child to incorporate her affected arm in play and may be repeated for practice with gradual adaptation (e.g., the toddler gives her animals a bear hug before putting them back in the bin). This is a learning opportunity that uses play as initiated by the child with her own toys.

Sometimes therapists are so intent on remediating certain deficits that they ignore the importance of play. A toy becomes only a motivator, or a diversion, so that a specific skill or component of that skill can be mastered.[6] Although this may sometimes be necessary, the therapist must also teach caregivers to facilitate play skills in the child and use play as a way of enhancing development. To use play as an intervention strategy for caregivers, the occupational therapist must model playfulness in interactions with the child. Whether it is a game of peek-a-boo or knocking down a pretend wall and falling into the foam blocks, the activity should elicit a sense of enjoyment and fun (Figure 23-18).

Motor Performance

The occupational therapist is often concerned with delayed function or atypical function in the motor domain, particularly fine motor skills including grasp and release of objects, bilateral manipulation, and in-hand manipulation; hesitancy to touch and explore with the hands; and lack of hand-to-mouth pattern and other skills. Some relevant research for occupational therapists on motor skills and young children is presented in Table 23-4. Intervention begins with analyzing the quality of movement and determining underlying factors, such as tactile discrimination and kinesthetic awareness.

To analyze motor performance, the therapist observes how functional a child is in a particular skill, such as stacking blocks. Although this is not an essential functional skill, it is a play activity that assists in development of sufficient hand skill for manipulating, placing, and releasing objects. These skills enable the child to use tools with control and with the arms unsupported. When this type of skill appears delayed or deficient, the therapist analyzes which underlying components are interfering with performance (Figure 23-19). For example, the therapist notes the influence of muscle tone and proximal stability when the child attempts stacking 1-inch cubes. The therapist must then determine the following:

- Does muscle tone increase?
- Are spasticity, tremor, or associated movements (mirroring) present?
- Does total body tone change with effort?
- Can the child stack the cubes while sitting unsupported on the floor?
- Does the child slump or demonstrate lack of postural stability?
- Can the child easily disassociate the movement of the arm from the body?
- Is the child's hand-eye coordination delayed?
- Does inattention or a lack of understanding interfere with performing the task?
- Does the child have difficulty with the motor planning needed for precise release of one block on top of another?
- Does tactile hypersensitivity cause the child to be reluctant to handle the block or result in flinging or throwing any object held in the hand?

The best indication of the child's fine motor abilities may be through observation of spontaneous activity. For instance, a child with autistic spectrum disorder or another disorder that interferes with the child's ability to interact with others may be unable to imitate or follow directions for a task. Therefore inability to stack blocks may reflect not a deficit in fine motor ability but rather inexperience or disinterest in the activity. Motivation must always be taken into account in analyzing a child's ability to perform an activity. In addition to observing

TABLE 23-3 Relevant Research on Play Skills and Young Children

Authors, Date	Research Design	Research Questions or Hypothesis	Sample (number and description)	Measures/Data Collection	Intervention	Findings
Saunders, Sayer, & Goodale (1999)	Correlational	1. There is a positive correlation between playfulness and coping skills 2. Age or gender will affect children's playfulness and coping ability	n = 19 Age range 36 to 63 mo from Head Start and preschool programs	The Test of Playfulness (Version 2.0), The Coping Inventory	n/a	Moderately strong and significant correlation between playfulness and coping. Coping and playfulness ratings on the basis of age and gender were not significant.
Okimoto, Bundy, & Hanzlik (2000)	Nonrandomized study using 2 matched groups	1. Young children with typical development will score significantly higher on the ToP than young children with cerebral palsy (CP) and developmental delays (DD) before intervention 2. The ToP scores of young children with CP and DD whose mothers are given information on improving their communication patterns will increase significantly more than those of young children with CP and DD who received direct NDT 3. Young children with CP and DD whose mothers are given information on improving their communication patterns will score significantly higher on the ToP at posttest than before the intervention	n = 19 Two matched groups of 19 Caucasian mother-infant pairs (one group with CP and DD and one group without) The mother-infant pairs were randomly assigned either to a group in which the mothers received intervention to improve mother-child interactions (n = 10) or a group in which the children received NDT while their mothers assisted (n = 6).	The Test of Playfulness, (Version 3.0)	One-hour intervention to improve mother-child interactions	The mean scores of the children who were typically developing were significantly higher on the ToP than the mean scores of those with CP and DD. There was no significant difference between the mean gain score of the children whose mothers received the intervention and that of the children who received NDT. There was a significant difference in pretest and posttest ToP scores for the intervention group.

Citation	Design	Purpose/Research Questions	Sample	Data Collection/Measures		Results
Pierce (2000)	Grounded theory	To describe the work done by mothers as they manage the spaces and objects of the home to support the development of infants and toddlers at play	n = 18 (typically developing infants and their mothers)	Data were collected monthly in the home, beginning at age 1 mo and continuing through 18 mo. Data included written observation records, maternal interviews, and videotapes of the infants at play.	n/a	The results describe the everyday tasks of mothers of infants and toddlers, such as selecting toys and household objects for play, positioning infants for play, maintaining and making play objects available, furnishing the home with childcare equipment, controlling infant access to home spaces, and monitoring for safety.
Tanta, Deitz, White, & Billingsley (2005)	Single-subject, alternating-treatments design	1. What is the difference in the amount of initiation of and interaction exhibited by preschool-aged children with play delays when interacting with peers with higher developmental play skills as compared to when interacting with peers with lower developmental play skills?	n = 15: 5 participants and 10 peer playmates (ages ranged from 3 yr, 8 mo to 6 yr, 3 mo)	Preschool Play Scale	For 5 or 6 days (depending on the participant), there was one 11-min session of free play with a peer whose play skill level was higher than the participant's or with a peer whose play skill level was lower than the participant's.	For preschoolers with developmental play skill delays, play with familiar peers who had higher-level skills generally resulted in higher levels of both initiation and response.
Daunhauer, Bolton, & Cermak (2005)	Descriptive and cross-sectional	1. What are the time-use patterns of young children who are institutionalized in an Eastern European orphanage? 2. How do the time-use patterns of children who are institutionalized compare with those of children the same age attending child care in the United States?	n = 32 (age range from 8 to 36 mo; 16 in Romanian orphanage, 16 in full-time child care in the United States)	Rating form developed for the study	n/a	The Romanian institutionalized group spent more time alone and the U.S. child care group spent more time with a caregiver. The Romanian group most frequently engaged in passive leisure activities such as lying down or sitting, whereas the U.S. childcare group spent the least amount of time performing passive leisure activities. The Romanian group spent less time in adult-led activities than the U.S. childcare group.

Continued

TABLE 23-3 Relevant Research on Play Skills and Young Children—Cont'd

Authors, Date	Research Design	Research Questions or Hypothesis	Sample (number and description)	Measures/Data Collection	Intervention	Findings
Daunhauer, Coster, Tickle-Degnen, & Cermak (2007)	Repeated measures and correlational	1. Will institutionalized children demonstrate more developmentally competent play when interacting with a caregiver than when playing alone? 2. What are the qualities of interactions between the caregivers and institutionalized children associated with the children's most developmentally competent level of play?	n = 26 (age range from 10 to 38 mo residing in a Romanian orphanage) 11 caregivers (1 man, 10 women) were videotaped during interactive play sessions with a child (ages ranged from 25 to 46 [M = 33.00])	Caregiver–Child Interaction Rating Scale (CIRS)	Two 6-min independent play sessions: one with the exploratory toys and one with the symbolic toys, followed by an additional 6-min interactive session with a known caregiver who was instructed to play with the child as he/she normally would.	The children demonstrated significantly more competent play when interacting with a caregiver than when playing independently. Structured, directive, and encouraging qualities of caregivers were positively associated with successful child engagement.

Summary and Practice Applications:

In the series of studies presented above, the role of caregivers and others for supporting children's play activities in the infant through preschool years is described. The studies by Okimoto et al. (2000) and Daunhauer et al. (2007) specifically point to the importance of caregivers in helping young children with disabilities or at-risk for developmental delays to develop play occupations. Tanta et al. (2005) suggest that similar-age peers may also have the potential to support play skill development in at-risk populations although more research is needed. In sum, the research findings on play in young children indicate that many factors relate to engagement of play, particularly for young children with developmental delays.

Occupational therapists working in early intervention should involve caregivers in play-based interventions and routines.

Special attention should be given to the type of interactions caregivers have with their children during play and modeling or coaching strategies may be used by occupational therapists to assist caregivers in developing strong play interaction skills.

Play in the natural environment should incorporate typically developing peers when possible, such as a community playground.

Data from Saunders, I., Sayer, M., & Goodale, A. (1999). The relationship between playfulness and coping in preschool children: A pilot study. *American Journal of Occupational Therapy, 53,* 221–226; Okimoto, A. M., Bundy, A., & Hanzik, J. (2000). Playfulness in children with and without disability: Measurement and intervention. *American Journal of Occupational Therapy, 54,* 73–82; Pierce, D. (2000). Maternal management of the home as a developmental play space for infants and toddlers. *American Journal of Occupational Therapy, 54,* 290–299; Tanta, K. J., Deitz, J.C., White, O., & Billingsley, F. (2005). The effects of peer play level on initiations and responses of preschool children with delayed lay skills. *American Journal of Occupational Therapy, 59,* 437–445; Daunhauer, L. A., Bolton, A., & Cermak, S. A. (2005). Time-use patterns of young children institutionalized in Eastern Europe. *Occupational Therapy Journal of Research: Occupation, Participation, and Health, 25,* 33–40; Daunhauer, L. A., Coster, W. J., Tickle-Degnen, L., & Cermak, S. A. (2007). Effects of caregiver–child interactions on play occupations among young children institutionalized in Eastern Europe. *American Journal of Occupational Therapy, 61,* 429–440.

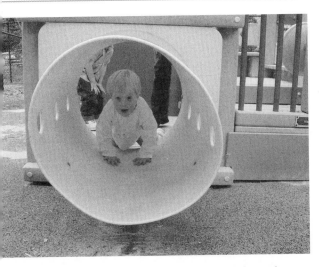

FIGURE 23-18   Exploratory, sensory motor play enhances development of body scheme, coordination, and a range of motor skills.

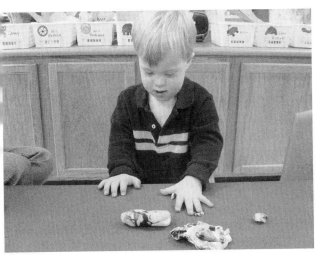

FIGURE 23-19   Observation of play with age-appropriate materials is used to assess fine motor skills.

spontaneous activity, the occupational therapist could ask caregivers to suggest motor-based activities that are meaningful to the child and then gradually modify them to increase the challenge. Through careful observation, the occupational therapist can establish what underlying factors may be interfering with the development of motor skills.

Once the analysis is complete, the occupational therapist works with caregivers to determine how various age-appropriate toys, games, sensorimotor experiences, and other strategies may be incorporated into the child's daily routine to remediate motor skill deficits. For instance, a family who enjoys hiking may encourage their toddler to pick up fallen leaves on the trail and put them in a small bag, an activity that encourages refined grasp and release skills. A provider in an infant's childcare room may take extra time to play with the infant using colorful rattles to encourage activation of the arm for reaching.

Because engaging in motor activities may be especially challenging for young children with special needs, it

behooves the occupational therapist to be creative when designing intervention strategies with caregivers. New motor skills are learned through practice.[9] The more a child enjoys the motor activity, the more likely he or she will perform it repeatedly. Also, an intervention strategy that fits easily into a caregiver's routine is more likely to be repeated. In this way, practice becomes incorporated into the everyday life of the child and family.

Sensory Processing

Infants and toddlers who have difficulty processing sensory information lack the ability to cope with environmental demands or to achieve internal control. As infants, they may be irritable, cry frequently, be difficult to comfort, or have difficulty with changes in routine. Alternately, they may sleep extensively with little awake time, seem oblivious to noises that others attend to, or have delays in motor development. As these infants move into toddlerhood, their deficits in sensory processing may continue and influence their engagement in everyday occupations such as dressing, grooming, and eating meals. Occupational therapists have an important role in addressing sensory processing challenges in young children (see Chapter 11).

Dunn described four main types of sensory processing difficulties in young children[17]:

- *Low registration*: These children notice less in their environment. Although they appear more easygoing than other children, they may have behaviors that interfere with their learning such as not responding to their name when called and having a more difficult time completing tasks.
- *Sensation seeking*: These children need a greater amount of sensory input than others and will seek out intense sensory experiences. They may have difficulty completing tasks because they become easily distracted by sensory experiences and may find ways to give themselves sensory input, such as through frequent movement or humming.
- *Sensation avoiding*: These children tend to notice things in the environment more than others, becoming easily overwhelmed by sensory input. They are often alone, isolating themselves from others and preferring to be in quiet places.
- *Sensory sensitivity*: These children detect sensation more than others, tending to become distracted and often upset by sensory events that are not easily noticed by others.

The occupational therapist recognizes that sensory processing difficulties have a pervasive influence on the child's development. There are two main ways in which the occupational therapist may intervene. First, the therapist may use appropriate tactile, vestibular, and proprioceptive input that elicits organized behavior and adaptive responses on the part of the child. For example, it was determined that a 1-year-old child displayed tactile sensitivity. He refused to hold toys, refused to bear weight on his arms, was irritable when held, pulled away from touch, and avoided exploring his environment. The occupational therapist worked with the caregivers to plan intervention that included proprioceptive and tactile input and midline play with textured toys. She and the child's mother reviewed the daily routine and determined that additional tactile stimulation be provided at bath time with water play, foamy soap, and terrycloth rubs. Soon the child was clapping

TABLE 23-4 Examples of Research on Motor Skills and Young Children

Authors, Date	Research Design	Research Questions or Hypothesis	Sample (number and description)	Measures/ Data Collection	Intervention	Findings
Dankert, Davies, & Gavin (2003)	Quasi-experimental, two-factor mixed design	1. Do preschool children with developmental delays demonstrate significant improvements on the Development Test of Visual-Motor Integration (VMI) following occupational therapy for 1 school year when compared with their performance on the VMI before therapy? 2. Will preschool children with developmental delays exhibit a rate of gain consistent with typical peers following occupational therapy for 1 school year?	$n = 12$ (G1: treatment group; preschool children with developmental delay; 8 males; $M = 53.34$ mo) $n = 16$ (G2: treatment group; preschool children with no developmental delays; 5 males; $M = 52.63$ mo) $n = 15$ (G3: control group; preschool children with no developmental delays; 8 males; $M = 53.40$ mo)	VMI and the two supplemental Visual Perception and Motor Coordination tests	Children in G1 received direct occupational therapy consisting of at least one 30-minute individual session per week. Children in G1 and G2 received one 30-minute group session per week. Individual therapy sessions for children in G1 addressed all areas of need as defined on their IEPs except for visual motor skills. Group therapy addressed visual motor skills and included: (a) fine motor activities, (b) gross motor activities, and (c) visual motor and visual perception activities.	Preschoolers with developmental delays (G1) demonstrated significant improvement in VMI Scores and the Visual Perception test scores, but not on the Motor Coordination test. On the Motor Coordination test, children without disabilities demonstrated statistically significant larger gains than those exhibited by the children with developmental delays. Significant differences between G1 and G3 remained on all three measures after therapy.
Dreiling & Bundy (2003)	Between-group design	This study compared outcomes for students with motor delays who were served through either direct-indirect intervention or consultation with parents and preschool staff.	$n = 11$ (students in the consultation group 7 males, 4 females; $M = 4.5$ yr) $n = 9$ (students in the direct-indirect intervention group; 5 males, 4 females; $M = 4.7$)	Goal Attainment Scaling	Consultation services included spending 1 full day a week for 40 weeks observing the students during various activities; consulting with the staff regarding therapeutic strategies; meeting with the full preschool team for 1 half-day twice a month; meeting with parents on an as-needed basis for consultation. Direct-indirect intervention included providing direct services for 1½ hours during a full week every 3 weeks for 40 weeks; instructing the team in how to implement the intervention in the occupational therapist's absence; and participating in a half-day planning session weekly with the team.	Both models of intervention were found to help students meet their goals at the rate expected. Students in the consultation group met or exceeded expectations on 56% of goals, whereas students in the direct-indirect intervention group met or exceeded expectations on 50% of goals. There was no difference between the outcomes for students receiving intervention in the consultative model and those receiving direct intervention.

| Marr, Cermak, Cohn, & Henderson (2003) | Descriptive | What are the types of fine motor activities and what is the time spent in those activities in Head Start and kindergarten classrooms? | n = 10 (Head Start classrooms) n = 10 (kindergarten classrooms) | Activities of two children per classroom (identified by the teacher) were recorded for 1 entire school day. | n/a | The children in Head Start classrooms spent a higher percentage of the day in fine motor, nonacademic activities, whereas the children in kindergarten spent more equal amounts of time in fine motor, nonacademic, and academic activities. The children in Head Start spent more time engaged in self-care, equal time in manipulative activities, and less time in pencil and paper activities when compared with children in kindergarten. |

Summary and practice Applications:
The research studies on development of motor skills provides preliminary support for the use of different service delivery models such as consultation through home programs and in preschools (Dankert, et al., 2003; Dreiling & Bundy, 2003).

Although several studies above suggest that consultation may be an effective approach for preschool-age children, more research is needed to determine if children in early intervention programs benefit more from this approach than individual therapy. Future research on the use of transdisciplinary models and parent support activities, such as coaching, would greatly enhance occupational therapy's involvement in early intervention.

Data from Dankert, H. L., Davies, P. L., & Gavin, W.J. (2003). Occupational therapy effects on visual-motor skills in preschool children. *American Journal of Occupational Therapy, 57,* 542–549; Dreiling, D., S., & Bundy, A. C. (2003). A comparison of consultative model and direct-indirect intervention with preschoolers. *American Journal of Occupational Therapy, 57,* 566–569; Marr, D., Cermak, S., Cohn, E. S., & Henderson, A. (2003). Fine motor activities in Head Start and kindergarten classrooms. *American Journal of Occupational Therapy, 57,* 550–557.

his hands spontaneously—a skill he had not attempted before and a nice adaptive response (Case Study 23-3).

A second approach to addressing sensory processing difficulties has been described by Dunn.[17] In this approach, occupational therapists focus on context, including both the physical context and the social context (e.g., relationship between child and caregivers), making modifications and adaptations to natural environments when needed. Because sensory experiences are rooted in the daily routines of children, occupational therapists need to work with caregivers to determine when the child demonstrates difficulties. The therapist may then provide strategies for modification or adaptation of the routine to support the child's engagement. Generally, children who have low registration and those who are sensation seeking will benefit from intense sensory experiences integrated into the daily routine, whereas children who are sensation avoiding need less sensory input throughout the day, and children with sensory sensitivity will benefit from structured patterns of sensory experiences incorporated into daily routines. Specialized assessment tools, such as The Infant/Toddler Sensory Profile, may be used to help determine intervention needs.[16]

Dunn provides the example of Millie, a 30-month-old toddler who is sensory avoiding.[17] After hearing concerns from her parents, the therapist visits Millie at a daycare center to observe her play behaviors and notices that Millie has difficulty playing in groups. It appears that Millie becomes overwhelmed during open playtime and tends to watch the other children instead of engaging in play. To support Millie at daycare, the therapist, parents, and daycare providers discuss potential strategies and decide to provide her with a separate yet visually accessible play space, enabling her to participate in play and limiting the sensory input.

Infants and toddlers with sensory processing difficulties can be challenging for caregivers, particularly infants and toddlers who fall into the sensory sensitivity category because their behavior may be unpredictable. The caregiver-child relationship with an infant who has behaviors such as crying when

---

CASE STUDY 23-3   Alex

BACKGROUND

Alex's pediatrician referred him to occupational therapy at 11 months of age because of suspected sensory processing problems. He had a diagnosis of developmental delay and had been receiving physical therapy because of gross motor delays. Alex cried often in a distressful manner. Problem areas for Alex, as reported by his mother, included uncooperative behaviors, rages or temper tantrums, whining and fussing, feeding problems, fearfulness, poor balance, and a dislike for being on his tummy. Although he sat independently at 6 months of age, he did not reach for and grasp an object until 8 months of age. He rolled from back to stomach at 9 months of age, and he was not yet crawling at 11 months.

ASSESSMENT

Alex was a pleasant infant who preferred not to be touched or held. He interacted with the examiner with caution after a brief period of ignoring her. His mother remained in the room and participated in the assessment. The examiner obtained a sensorimotor history by interview with Alex's mother. His mother had noticed that he had difficulty with being touched and pulled away when touched. Sometimes he stiffened and arched his back when held. Alex's mother reported that he was irritable when held and resisted having his hair or face washed. Alex seemed oversensitive to noises and was bothered by such things as a vacuum cleaner and hair dryer. Although his aversion to sound had improved, he remained apprehensive of toys with noises. Alex seemed to be fearful in situations with auditory and visual stimulation, such as a shopping mall. Alex enjoyed swinging and other movement stimuli.

When handled, Alex exhibited a mildly defensive reaction to touch. He became disorganized when removing a mitt from his foot and became upset when a piece of tape was placed on the back of his hand. He seemed unable to plan the movements needed to remove the mitt or tape. Although he seemed to be visually oriented, visual tracking was delayed and inconsistent. Alex enjoyed the vestibular input as he was held and moved up and down or in circular motions. He also enjoyed upside-down positions. His mother completed the Infant/Toddler Sensory Profile, and Alex's sensory responses placed him in the sensory sensitivity category.[16]

The examiner observed that Alex avoided and resisted changing his body position (e.g., going from sitting to quadruped) and resisted the proprioceptive input of weight bearing on his upper extremities. Extensor muscle tone was increased with lower-extremity weight bearing, so much so that it was difficult to flex his hips passively for sitting. Alex went into plantar flexion and lower-extremity extension when this parent bounced him on his bare feet.

At a chronologic age of 11 months, Alex received a scaled score of 7 (8 to 12 is the normal range) on the fine motor subtest of the Peabody Developmental Motor Scales. He used his right hand more efficiently than his left but was able to bring his hands to midline to bang cubes. However, he resisted clapping his hands. Alex removed pegs from a pegboard and briefly manipulated a piece of paper. He was able to transfer a cube from his left hand to his right when the cube was placed in his left hand. Alex had difficulty removing rings from a stand. He also displayed difficulty in deliberately releasing cubes to give to the examiner or to put them in a cup.

SUMMARY AND INTERPRETATION

Alex was a delightful infant who experienced significant difficulties in receiving and modulating sensory information. This was evident particularly in his irritability and intolerance to touch and auditory stimulation. Inadequate adaptive motor function seemed to be related to his hypersensitivity. Alex's tactile sensitivity probably contributed to his fine motor delays. Given his hypersensitivity to touch, it is understandable that he was limited in his abilities to explore and manipulate objects, especially those that were new to him and in an unfamiliar environment.

CASE STUDY 23-3   Alex—cont'd

INTERVENTION

The team recommended weekly occupational therapy for Alex, which became part of his IFSP. The occupational therapist provided services in his child center once a week and at home once a month. The therapist used a sensory integrative approach with developmentally appropriate play, with emphasis on increased functional hand use. The play activities incorporated vestibular, proprioceptive, and tactile input (as tolerated). Intervention included working with Alex's parents and child care providers to incorporate sensory strategies into the daily routine such as frequent brushing of the extremities and the back with a towel or lotion followed by deep proprioceptive input, play with textured toys, activities that encouraged the use of both hands at the midline, and activities that encouraged the bearing of weight on his upper extremities (e.g., climbing over pillows). The therapist provided his mother with reading material and a videotape to help her learn about sensory integration and understand how sensory processing affects behavior.

Alex responded well to the intervention approach and began to show indications of more efficient sensory processing and the ability to modulate sensory input. Within a few weeks, Alex began to mold to his mother when she held him and was less irritable and more relaxed in situations with auditory stimulation. After 3 months of therapy, Alex's mother reported increased cuddling and noticeable improvement in eating. He attempted a greater variety of foods and few aversions, feeding time was shorter, and it was no longer necessary to use the television as a diversion to get him to eat. Alex began to interact more with his siblings and explore his environment. Best of all, he no longer had temper tantrums when his mother left the room. His childcare provider reported that Alex tolerated the prone position and weight bearing on his hands; he had recently begun to crawl. Play skills and hand use also appeared to increase.

---

picked up or cuddled, sleeping only for short periods, feeding poorly, and smiling infrequently may be characterized by weak caregiver attachment because they can interfere with the bonding process.[68] Occupational therapists should work closely with caregivers to address not only changes in the daily routine to support the young child, but also to investigate ways to support the caregiver-child relationship, such as modeling for caregivers how to engage their infant in simple play activities without providing extra sensory stimulation.

Self-Care/Adaptive

Occupational therapists have longstanding experience in the area of activities of daily living (ADLs), also referred to as self-care or adaptive skills. In children, the focus is on participation in eating and feeding, dressing, toileting, and sleeping. Physical difficulties may interfere with the ability to perform self-care skills, such as bringing the hand to the mouth during feeding and cooperating in dressing by extending an arm or a leg. Psychosocial behaviors that influence the acquisition of self-care skills are temperament, self-regulation, caregiver-child interaction, motivation, and adaptability. Sensory processing problems may cause aversive behaviors, such as the child with tactile hypersensitivity who gags on some foods or refuses to wear certain articles of clothing. The evaluation of self-care skills should occur in the natural environment in which the skills occur, such as the child's home, daycare center, or preschool (Figure 23-20). Information on interventions for improving self-care skills and feeding may be found in Chapters 15 and 16, respectively.

Adapted Equipment and Positioning

The occupational therapist in early intervention can make an important contribution to the overall functioning of children through the recommendation and provision of appropriate adapted equipment (see Chapters 16 and 21) (Figure 23-21). A floor sitter may enable the child with cerebral palsy to play on the floor near his or her typically developing peers. An adapted insert for a chair may make it possible for a child to begin to use the hands for an art project or to self-feed. As the neurologically involved child approaches preschool age and is not yet ambulating, the parents may have to face the prospect of obtaining a wheelchair. The occupational therapist can assist in recommending appropriate equipment and in being sensitive to the effect that envisioning their child in a wheelchair may have on the family. The child with a neurologic impairment who can stay in an infant stroller or a highchair does not appear as different as the 3-year-old child who must have a wheelchair and special equipment.

SUMMARY

Occupational therapists use holistic approaches with children and their families that emphasize functional, developmentally appropriate approaches. By recognizing that children are part of a family system, the therapist designs programs that fit into the family's daily routine; consider sensory, motor (gross and fine), social, and cognitive aspects of performance; and emphasize play as the child's primary occupation.

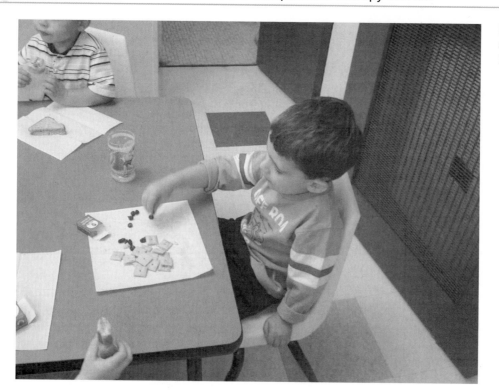

FIGURE 23-20 The therapist assesses feeding skills during the lunchtime routine in preschool.

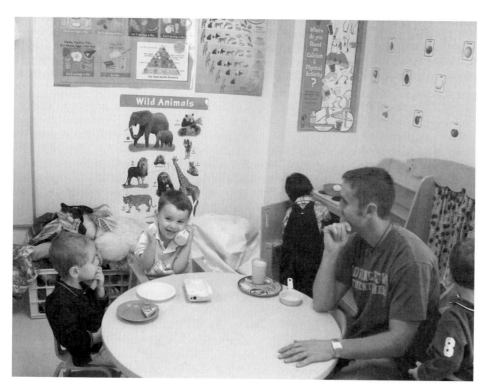

FIGURE 23-21 Adapted seating enables a child with postural instability to play with a peer at the table.

REFERENCES

1. Andersson, L. L. (2004). Appropriate and inappropriate interpretation and use of test scores in early intervention. *Journal of Early Intervention, 27*(1), 55–68.

2. Blackman, J. A. (2002). Early intervention: A global perspective. *Infants & Young Children, 15*(2), 11–19.

3. Bricker. (2002). *Assessment, evaluation, and programming system (AEPS) for infants and children* (2nd ed.). Baltimore: Brookes.

4. Bruder, M. B. (1993). The provision of early intervention and early childhood special education within community early childhood programs: Characteristics of effective service delivery. *Topics in Early Childhood Special Education, 13*, 19–37.

5. Bruder, M. B., & Bologna, T. (1993). Collaboration and service coordination for effective early intervention. In W. Brown, S. K. Thurman, & I. F. Pearl (Eds.), *Family centered early intervention with infants and toddlers: Innovative cross-disciplinary approaches* (pp. 103–127). Baltimore: Brookes.

6. Burke, J. (1998). Play: The life role of the infant and young child. In J. Case-Smith (Ed.), *Pediatric occupational therapy and early intervention* (2nd ed., pp. 189–206). Boston: Butterworth-Heinemann.

7. Campbell, P., & Halbert, J. (2002). Between research and practice: Provider perspectives on early intervention. *Topics in Early Childhood Special Education, 22*, 213–226.

8. Campbell, P. (2004). Participation-based services: Promoting children's participation in natural settings. *Young Exceptional Children, 8*(1), 20–29.

9. Cech, D. J., & Martin, S. (2002). Motor learning and motor control. In D. J. Cech & S. Martin (Eds.), *Functional movement development across the lifespan* (2nd ed., pp. 86–117). Philadelphia: W.B. Saunders.

10. Chai, A. Y., Zhang, C., & Bisberg, M. (2006). Rethinking natural environment practice: Implications from examining various implications and approaches. *Early Childhood Education Journal, 34*, 203–208.

11. Cohn, E. S., & Cermak, S. A. (1998). Including the family perspective in sensory integration outcomes research. *American Journal of Occupational Therapy, 52*, 540–546.

12. Coster, W. (1998). Occupation-centered assessment of children. *American Journal of Occupational Therapy, 52*, 337–344.

13. Denboba, D., McPherson, M. G., Kenney, M. K., Strickland, B., & Newacheck, P. W. (2006). Achieving family and provider partnerships for children with special health care needs. *Pediatrics, 118*, 1607–1615.

14. DeGrace, B. W. (2003). Occupation-based and family-centered care: A challenge for current practice. *American Journal of Occupational Therapy, 57*, 347–350.

15. Division of Early Childhood. (1993). DEC position statement on inclusion. *DEC Communicator, 19*, 4.

16. Dunn, W. (2002). *The Infant-Toddler Sensory Profile.* San Antonio, TX: Psychological Corp.

17. Dunn, W. (2007). Supporting children to participate successfully in everyday life by using sensory processing knowledge. *Infants & Young Children, 20*, 84–101.

18. Dunst, C. J. (1991). Implementation of the individualized family service plan. In M. J. McGonigel, R. Kaufmann, & B. Johnson (Eds.), *Guidelines and recommended practices for the individualized family service plan* (2nd ed., pp. 67–78). Bethesda, MD: Association for the Care of Children's Health.

19. Dunst, C. J. (2002). Family-centered practices: Birth through high school. *Journal of Special Education, 36*(3), 139–147.

20. Dunst, C. J., Trivette, C. M., Humphries, T., Raab, M., & Roper, N. (2001). Contrasting approaches to natural learning environment interventions. *Infants & Young Children, 14*(2), 48–63.

21. Dunst, C. J., Bruder, M. B., Trivette, C. M., Hamby, D., Raab, M., & Mclean, M. (2001). Characteristics and consequences of everyday natural learning opportunities. *Topics in Early Childhood Special Education, 21*, 68–92.

22. Edwards, M. A., Millard, P., Praskac, L. A., & Wisniewski, P. A. (2003). Occupational therapy and early intervention: A family-centered approach. *Occupational Therapy International, 10*, 239–252.

23. Effgen, S. K., & Chiarello, L. A. (2000). Physical therapist education for service in early intervention. *Infants & Young Children, 1*, 63–76.

24. Grant, R. (2005). State strategies to contain costs in the early intervention program: Policy and evidence. *Topics in Early Childhood Special Education, 25*(4), 243–250.

25. Greenspan, S. I. (1992). *Infancy and early childhood.* Madison, CT: International Universities Press.

26. Greenspan, S. I., & Meisels, S. (1994). Toward a new vision for the developmental assessment of infants and young children. *Zero to Three, 14*(6), 2–41.

27. Hanft, B. E., & Anzalone, M. (2001). Issues in professional development: Preparing and supporting occupational therapists in early childhood. *Infants & Young Children, 13*(4), 67–78.

28. Hanft, B. E., & Pilkington, K. O. (2000). Therapy in natural environments: The means or end goal for early intervention? *Infants & Young Children, 12*(4), 1–13.

29. Hanson, M. J. (1990). Honoring the cultural diversity of families when gathering data. *Topics in Early Childhood Special Education, 10*, 112–131.

30. Hanson, M. J. (1998). Ethnic, cultural, and language diversity in intervention settings. In E. Lynch & M. Hanson (Eds.), *Developing cross-cultural competence* (2nd ed., pp. 3–22). Baltimore: Brookes.

31. Hanson, M. J., Beckman, P. J., Horn, E., Marquart, J., Sandall, S. R., Greig, D., et al. (2000). Entering preschool: Family and professional experiences in this transition process. *Journal of Early Intervention, 23*, 279–293.

32. Harris, S. R. (1997). The effectiveness of early intervention for children with cerebral palsy and related motor disabilities. In M. J. Guralnick (Ed.), *The effectiveness of early intervention* (pp. 327–347). Baltimore: Paul H. Brookes.

33. Hastings, R. P. (2002). Parental stress and behavior problems of children with developmental disability. *Journal of Intellectual and Developmental Disability, 27*(3), 149–160.

34. Houtrow, A. J., Kim, S. E., & Newacheck, P. W. (2008). Health care utilization, access, and expenditures for infants and children with special health care needs. *Infants & Young Children, 21*, 149–159.

35. Humphry, R. (2002). Young children's occupations: Explicating the dynamics of developmental processes. *American Journal of Occupational Therapy, 56*, 171–179.

36. *Individuals With Disabilities Education Act of 1990 Amendments* (P.L. 102–119), 20 U.S.C. et seq., 1400–1485.

37. IDEA. (2004). *Individuals With Disabilities Education Improvement Act of 2004* (P.L. 108–446), 120 U.S.C. § 1400 et. seq. Sec. 632(4) (G),(H).

38. Johnson-Martin, N. M., Attermeier, S. M., & Hacker, B. J. (2004). *The Carolina curriculum for young children with special needs* (3rd ed.). Baltimore: Brookes.

39. Jung, L. A. (2007). Writing individualized family service plan strategies that fit into the ROUTINE. *Young Exceptional Children, 10*(3), 2–9.

40. Jung, L. A., & Grisham-Brown, J. (2006). Moving from assessment information to IFSP's: Guidelines for a family-centered process. *Young Exceptional Children, 9*(2), 2–11.

41. Kaiser, A. P., & Hancock, T. B. (2003). Teaching parents new skills to support their young children's development. *Infants & Young Children, 16,* 9–21.

42. Kramer, S., McGonigel, M., & Kaufman, R. (1991). Developing the IFSP: Outcomes, strategies, activities, and services. In M. McGonigel, R. Kaufmann, & B. Johnson (Eds.), *Guidelines and recommended practices for the individualized family service plan* (2nd ed.). Bethesda, MD: Association for the Care of Children's Health.

43. Linder, T. W. (2008a). *Transdisciplinary play-based assessment: A functional approach to working with young children* (2nd ed.). Baltimore: Brookes.

44. Linder, T. W. (2008b). *Transdisciplinary play-based intervention: Guidelines for developing a meaningful curriculum for young children* (2nd ed.). Baltimore: Brookes.

45. Mahoney, G., & Filer, J. (1996). How responsive is early intervention to the priorities and needs of families? *Topics in Early Childhood Special Education, 16*(4), 437–457.

46. McCormick, L. (2006a). Professional and family partnerships. In M. J. Noonan & L. McCormick (Eds.), *Young children with disabilities in natural environments* (pp. 27–45). Baltimore: Brookes.

47. McCormick, L. (2006b). Assessment and planning: The IFSP and the IEP. In M. J. Noonan & L. McCormick (Eds.), *Young children with disabilities in natural environments* (pp. 47–75). Baltimore: Brookes.

48. McGonigel, M. J., & Garland, C. W. (1988). The individualized family service plan and the early intervention team: Team and family issues and recommended practices. *Infants & Young Children, 1,* 10–21.

49. McWilliam, R. A. (1996). How to provide integrated therapy. In R. A. McWilliam (Ed.), *Rethinking pull-out services in early intervention* (pp. 49–69). Baltimore: Brookes.

50. Miller, L. J. (1994). Journey to a desirable future: A value-based model of infant and toddler assessment. *Zero to Three, 14*(6), 23–26.

51. Myers, C. T. (2006). Exploring occupational therapy and transitions for young children with special needs. *Physical and Occupational Therapy in Pediatrics, 26*(3), 73–88.

52. Nolan, K. W., Young, E. C., Hebert, E. B., & Wilding, G. (2005). Service coordination for children with complex health care needs in an early intervention program. *Infants & Young Children, 18,* 161–170.

53. Newborg, J. (2005). *Battelle developmental inventory* (2nd ed.). Chicago: Riverside.

54. Parks, S. (2006). *Inside HELP: Administration manual.* Palo Alto, CA: VORT.

55. Pilkington, K. O., & Malinowski, M. (2002). The natural environment II: Uncovering deeper responsibilities within relationship-based services. *Infants & Young Children, 15*(2), 78–84.

56. Ridgely, R., & Hallam, R. (2006). Examining the IFSP's of rural, low-income families: Are they reflective of family concerns? *Journal of Research in Childhood Education, 21,* 149–162.

57. Rosenbaum, P., King, S., Law, M., King, G., & Evans, J. (1998). Family-centered service: A conceptual framework and research review. *Physical & Occupational Therapy in Pediatrics, 18,* 1–20.

58. Rosenkoetter, S. E., & Squires, S. (2000). Writing outcomes that make a difference for children and families. *Young Exceptional Children, 4,* 2–8.

59. Rous, B., Hallam, R., Harbin, G., McCormick, K., & Jung, L. A. (2007). The transition process for young children with disabilities: A conceptual framework. *Infants & Young Children, 20,* 135–148.

60. Rush, D. D., Shelden, M. L., & Hanft, B. E. (2003). Coaching families and colleagues: A process for collaboration in natural settings. *Infants & Young Children, 16,* 33–47.

61. Shelden, M. L., & Rush, D. D. (2001). The ten myths about providing early intervention services in natural environments. *Infants & Young Children, 14*(1), 1–13.

62. Shonkoff, J. P., & Meisels, S. J. (1990). Early childhood intervention: The evolution of a concept. In S. J. Meisels & J. P. Shonkoff (Eds.), *Handbook of early childhood intervention* (pp. 3–31). Cambridge, MA: Cambridge University Press.

63. Shonkoff, J. P., & Philips, D. A. (Eds.). (2000). *From neurons to neighborhoods: the science of early childhood development.* Washington, DC: National Academy Press.

64. Simons, R. (1985). *After the tears.* New York: Harcourt Brace Jovanovich.

65. Teti, T. M., & Gibbs, E. D. (1990). Infant assessment: Historical antecedents and contemporary issues. In E. D. Gibbs & D. M. Teti (Eds.), *Interdisciplinary assessment of infants* (pp. 3–10). Baltimore: Brookes.

66. Turnbull, A. P., Turbiville, V., & Turnbull, H. R. (2000). Evolution of family-professional partnerships: Collective empowerment as the model for the early twenty-first century. In J. P. Shonkoff & S. J. Meisels (Eds.), *Handbook of early childhood intervention* (2nd ed., pp. 630–650). Cambridge, MA: Cambridge University Press.

67. Turnbull, A. P., Turnbull, H. R., & Blue-Banning, M. (1994). Enhancing inclusion of infants and toddlers with disabilities and their families: A theoretical and programmatic analysis. *Infants & Young Children, 7*(2), 1–14.

68. Weatherston, D. J., Ribaudo, J., & Glovak, S. (2002). Becoming whole: Combining infant mental health and occupational therapy on behalf of a toddler with sensory integration difficulties and his family. *Infants & Young Children, 15*(1), 19–28.

69. Wisconsin Birth to Three Training and Technical Assistance. (n.d.). *Fundamentals of service coordination for the Wisconsin birth to three program.* Retrieved September 16, 2008, from http://www.waisman.wisc.edu/birthto3/KATY_ROUTINES.pdf

69. Wooster, D. A. (2001). Early intervention programs. In M. Scaffa (Ed.), *Occupational therapy in community-based practice settings* (pp. 271–290). Philadelphia: F.A. Davis.

70. Zhang, C., & Bennett, T. (2003). Facilitating the meaningful participation of culturally and linguistically diverse families in the IFSP and IEP process. *Focus on Autism and Other Developmental Disabilities, 18*(1), 51–59.

SUGGESTED READINGS

Buysse, V., & Aytch, L. (Eds.) (2007). *Early school success; Equity and access for diverse learners* (executive summary from the FirstSchool Diversity Symposium. Chapel Hill: University of North Carolina, FPG Child Development Institute. Retrieved from http://www.fpg.unc.edu/~firstschool/assets/FirstSchool_Symposium_ExecutiveSummary_2007.pdf.

Cook, R. E., & Sparks, S. N. (2008). *The art and practice of home visiting: Early intervention for children with special needs and their families*. Baltimore: Brookes.

Hanft, B., & Shepherd, J. (2008). *Collaborating for student success: A guide for school-based occupational therapy*. Bethesda, MD: AOTA Press.

Jackson, L. L. (Eds.) (2007). *Occupational therapy services for children and youth under IDEA* (3rd ed.) Bethesda, MD: AOTA Press.

Klein, M. D., Cook, R. E., & Richardson-Gibbs, A. M. (2001). *Strategies for including children with special needs in early childhood settings*. Albany: Delmar Cengage Learning.

Kuhaneck, H. M., Spitzer, S. L., & Miller, E. (2010). *Activity analysis, creativity, and playfulness in pediatric occupational therapy: Making play just right*. Sudbury, MA: Jones and Bartlett.

Lynch, E., & Hanson, M. (1998). *Developing cross-cultural competence* (2nd ed). Baltimore: Brookes.

Marr, D., & Nackley, V. (2007). *Sensory* stories. Framingham, MA: Therapro.

Parham, L. D. & Fazio, L. (2008). *Play in occupational therapy for children* (2nd ed.). St. Louis: Mosby.

Shonkoff, J. P., Meisels, S. J., & Zigler, E. F. (2000). *Handbook of early childhood intervention* (2nd ed.). Cambridge: Cambridge University Press.

Williams, M. S., & Shellenberger, S. (1996). *How does your engine run? A leader's guide to the Alert Program for Self-Regulation*. Albuquerque, NM: TherapyWorks.

24 School-Based Occupational Therapy

Susan Bazyk • Jane Case-Smith

The task of a sound education, Plato argued twenty-five centuries ago, is to teach young people to find pleasure in the right things. If children enjoyed math, they would learn math. If they enjoyed helping friends, they would grow into helpful adults. If they enjoyed Shakespeare, they would not be content watching television programs. If they enjoyed life, they would take greater pains to protect it (p. 39).[21]

Education systems around the world have the responsibility of preparing children for adulthood and, as such, most professionals agree that schools must provide the intellectual and practical tools needed for successful participation in classrooms, families, future workplaces, and communities.[27] Occupational therapy practitioners help people of all ages engage in and enjoy meaningful and purposeful life activities—in schools, this means helping children participate in the academic, social, extracurricular, independent living, and vocational activities needed for student success and transition.[2,79] Given occupational therapy's focus on a broad range of occupational performance areas (education, social participation, play, leisure, work, activities of daily living), it is not surprising that occupational therapists enjoy a long tradition of providing services in schools and early intervention settings, making these the primary work environments for occupational therapists.[45]

Practice in schools is influenced by an educational versus medical model requiring a set of knowledge and skills unique to both occupational therapy and school settings. School-based therapists must combine a sound understanding of occupational therapy's domain of practice with a current understanding of the school context, which is guided by federal laws and regulations. In a recent U.S. survey, school-based occupational therapists identified the greatest need for knowledge and skills in the areas of federal/state regulations, role of occupational therapy, evaluation and intervention approaches, writing individualized education program (IEP) goals, collaboration, and evaluation for assistive technology.[10] This chapter provides information to prepare occupational therapists for school-based practice.

SPECIAL AND GENERAL EDUCATION LEGISLATION

Federal policy, which is shaped by trends in health and education practice, directly influences services for children. Although occupational therapy's early work with children occurred primarily in medical rather than educational settings, a rapid shift to practicing in schools took place with the enactment of the Education of All Handicapped Act (EHA) of 1975 (P.L. 94-142). At the time this law was enacted, more than 1 million children with disabilities were excluded from the public school system, and for those who did receive education, more than half did not receive appropriate services. This legislation, now known as the Individuals with Disabilities Education Act (IDEA 2004) (i.e., P.L. 108-446), requires that states provide free appropriate education (FAPE) in the least restrictive environment (LRE) for students with disabilities attending public schools. Further, the law stipulates that individually designed special education and *related services* must be provided to students 3 to 21 years of age, if the student needs such services to benefit from her or his education (§300.17). As a related service provider, occupational therapy is defined in the law and accompanying federal regulations as "such developmental, corrective, and other supportive services as are required to assist a child with a disability to benefit from special education, and includes... occupational therapy" (IDEA 2004, Final Regulations, §300.34, 2006). IDEA increased the demand for occupational therapy practitioners employed in schools exponentially because of the legal mandate to provide services should a child require occupational therapy to benefit from special education.

Once legislation such as IDEA becomes law, the agency responsible for the program (e.g., U.S. Department of Education) develops regulations to guide implementation at the national, state, and local levels. In addition, federal laws are reauthorized routinely to allow for review and revisions based on the needs of children and their families. For example, IDEA is reauthorized every 5 to 7 years. Although keeping up with evolving policies can be an overwhelming task, it is critical for occupational therapy practitioners working in educational settings to maintain an understanding of current policies to provide appropriate services and take advantage of new opportunities for practice.[45,60] Figure 24-1 depicts a timeline of important legislation, policy changes, and practice developments influencing school practice. This section provides a brief overview of key legislation influencing occupational therapy practice in schools. This is followed by a more detailed discussion of the evolution of IDEA and No Child Left Behind (NCLB) and the major shifts in occupational therapy practice that have resulted.

Individuals with Disabilities Education Act (IDEA)

Most children with disabilities receiving occupational therapy in schools obtain services under IDEA, with a smaller number served under Section 504 of the Rehabilitation Act of 1973. IDEA establishes educational programs that ensure two significant rights for children with disabilities—FAPE in the LRE.[63] Four additional principles guiding the education of children with disabilities were adopted with the original law in 1975 and have remained unchanged, but with subsequent amendments (Box 24-1).

Each of these concepts has significant implications for the public education system, children with disabilities and their families, and occupational therapists. A "free appropriate public education" refers to special education and related services

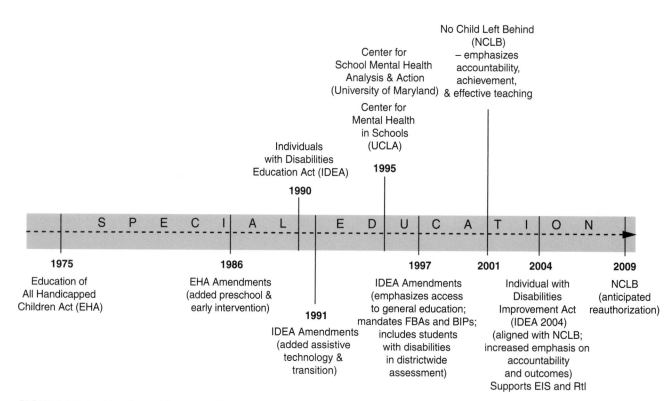

FIGURE 24-1 Timeline of important legislation and developments influencing occupational therapy's role in schools.

BOX 24-1   Principles of the Individuals with Disabilities Education Act (formerly EHA [P.L. 94-142])

1. *Free Appropriate Public Education* (FAPE). Every eligible child is entitled to an appropriate education that is free to families (supported by public funds).
2. *Least Restrictive Environment (LRE).* Children with disabilities are most appropriately educated with their nondisabled peers. Special classes, separate schooling, or other removal of children with disabilities from the regular educational environment is to occur only when the nature or severity of the disability of a child is such that education in regular classes with the use of supplementary aids and services cannot be achieved satisfactorily [§612 (a)(5)(A)].
3. *Appropriate Evaluation.* All children with disabilities must be appropriately assessed for purposes of eligibility determination, educational programming, and individual performance monitoring.
4. *Individualized Education Program.* A document that includes an annual plan is developed, written, and (as appropriate) revised for each child with disabilities.
5. *Parent and Student Participation in Decision Making.* Parents and families must have meaningful opportunities to participate in the education of their children at school and at home.
6. *Procedural Safeguards.* Safeguards are in place to ensure that the rights of children with disabilities and their parents are protected, and that students with disabilities and their parents are provided with the information they need to make decisions. In addition, procedures and mechanisms must be in place to resolve disagreements between parents and school officials.

---

that (1) meet the standards of the state education agency (SEA); (2) are provided at public expense; (3) are under public supervision and direction; (4) include an appropriate education at preschool, elementary, and secondary levels; and (5) are provided in accordance with an individualized education program (IEP). "Free" means at no cost to parents, but of course does not preclude the incidental fees that are normally charged to students without disabilities. The word "appropriate" is more difficult to define because it does not necessarily refer to a grade level or the chronologic age of a child. The IEP, as the centerpiece of IDEA, is used by parents to ensure the development of an "appropriate" special education program to meet their child's unique needs. This program is based on results of a comprehensive, multidisciplinary assessment. As part of the educational team, occupational therapists have essential roles in these processes.

Least Restrictive Environment

IDEA mandates that students with disabilities be offered special education and related services in the LRE. This means that children with disabilities are educated with children who are not disabled, to the maximum extent appropriate (§300.114). Whatever the disability, the first student placement that should be considered according to IDEA is the general education classroom, with appropriate aids and supports.[42] This policy is clearly stated in IDEA; the "removal of children with disabilities occurs only when the nature or severity of the disability of a child is such that education in regular classes with the use of supplementary aids and services cannot be achieved satisfactorily" (32 C.F.R., §612[5][A]). The overriding rule is that placement decisions must be determined on an individual basis, based on the child's unique needs and IEP.

The amount of support provided to students integrated in general education varies from a full-time aide to periodic, consultative services by an occupational therapist or special educator. When a child cannot be educated in the regular classroom, an alternative placement is considered. Accordingly, schools are required by law to ensure that a continuum of alternative placements is available to meet the needs of children

with disabilities. This continuum includes a range of alternative placements such as instruction in regular classes, special classes, special schools, home instruction, and instruction in hospitals and institutions. Most children with disabilities spend at least a portion of their day in general education classrooms.

Evolution of IDEA

Although the original goal of FAPE in the LRE for children with disabilities has not changed, each reauthorization of IDEA has prompted reflection and a reevaluation of educational services, which, in turn, has brought about important shifts in the delivery of special education and related services.

In 1986, amendments allowed states to provide preschool and early intervention services for children with disabilities from birth to age 5. To reflect current language, the law's name was changed to the Individuals with Disabilities Education Act in 1990. This amendment authorized additional services (i.e., assistive technology services and devices and transition planning). The reauthorization in 1997 was significant in placing greater emphasis on delivering related services to children with disabilities within the context of the student's general education curriculum.[59,65] As a result, there has been a gradual shift in service delivery from traditional "pull-out" approaches to the integration of occupational therapy services into the student's classroom and other relevant school environments (e.g., lunchroom, playground, restroom).[78] This shift has required occupational therapists to become knowledgeable about the curriculum adopted in specific classrooms and within their school district so that they can better specify how a student's disability affects functioning within the educational environment and develop relevant intervention strategies. The IDEA Amendments of 1997 also focused on student outcomes by requiring students with disabilities to be included in state and districtwide assessments.

IDEA was most recently reauthorized in 2004 as the Individuals with Disabilities Education Improvement Act. The primary goals of IDEA 2004 are to increase the focus of education on results; prevent problems through early intervening; and improve students' academic achievement, functional outcomes, and postsecondary success.[45] By focusing on accountability and improving educational outcomes, Congress intentionally aligned IDEA 2004 with the No Child Left Behind Act (NCLB) of 2002. The long-term goal of special education and related services according to IDEA is to prepare students with disabilities for further education, employment, and independent living.

Section 504 of the Rehabilitation Act and the Americans with Disabilities Act

Section 504 of the Rehabilitation Act of 1973 and Title II of the Americans with Disabilities Act of 1990 (ADA) complement IDEA to ensure nondiscrimination against children with disabilities in public schools.[87] Section 504 requires schools receiving federal funds to provide qualified students with disabilities access to public education. The ADA ensures that the educational program is accessible to individuals with disabilities and may include providing specific accommodations. The definition of "disability" under Section 504 and ADA includes any student with "a physical or mental impairment that substantially limits one or more major life activities, who has record of such an impairment, or is regarded as having such an impairment" (34 C.F.R. 104.3(j)(2)(i)). Some examples of impairments that may substantially limit major life activities are mental illness, specific learning disabilities, arthritis, cancer, diabetes, and hearing impairment. Major life activities include caring for oneself, education and learning, performing manual tasks, seeing, hearing, speaking, working, walking, and breathing. Because this definition is broader than IDEA's definition of disability, students who are not IDEA-eligible may be 504-eligible for accommodations to access to the learning environment. "Under Section 504, occupational therapy can be provided alone or in combination with other educations services and may be provided directly to students or as program supports to teachers working with the student" (p. 1).[3] Student eligibility for Section 504 services are documented in guidelines developed by each state and local school agency.

Sometimes students with diagnoses such as attention deficit–hyperactivity disorder (ADHD), for example, are not eligible for special education programs. However, these students may struggle to fully participate in classroom activities and often benefit from occupational therapy services. Occupational therapy in the schools can be provided to these students under Section 504. Because the definition of disability is broader in this civil rights act, a child may be eligible for occupational therapy, even when he or she is not eligible for special education services. Although school personnel are not required to develop IEPs for students served under the Rehabilitation Act, a team should develop a written plan that states goals, services, and accommodations needed to meet those goals.[45]

Although additional federal and state funds are not provided for these laws, school districts that do not provide accommodations to students who are eligible through Section 504 and ADA can lose federal funding. Occupational therapy practitioners may assist the school team in determining the most effective and efficient solutions for meeting students' needs under Section 504 and the ADA.

No Child Left Behind

NCLB, signed into law in 2002 (Public Law 107-110), made major changes to the Elementary and Secondary Education Act of 1965. The original intent of this law was to ensure that all children have an equal opportunity to participate in and receive a good education in school.[66] This law, which is considered a key component in the education reform movement, covers all public schools in all states.

NCLB is mainly understood to be a *general education law* emphasizing increased accountability for results. Under this law, states are working to close the achievement gap by establishing high achievement standards for all students, especially those who are disadvantaged because of poverty or disability.[81] Based on yearly testing, annual state and district report cards indicate whether the state, district, and schools are making adequate yearly progress (AYP) toward proficiency (i.e., achieving grade level). Parents whose children are attending Title I (low-income) schools that do not make AYP for several years are given the option to transfer their child to a better performing school or obtain free tutoring.[82] In addition to proficiency testing, NCLB raised the requirements for public school teachers in all states to meet the standards of "highly qualified"—holding at least a bachelor's degree and having passed a state test of subject knowledge.

This synthesis of legislation provides the foundation for understanding the evolving role of occupational therapy practitioners working in schools. In the following sections, occupational therapy's traditional role serving children with disabilities is presented, followed by a discussion of emerging roles in general education and school mental health based on current legislation. For example, changes brought about by the reauthorization of IDEA and the enactment of NCLB have been instrumental in providing opportunities for expanding occupational therapy's role to serving *all* children attending school.[45]

OCCUPATIONAL THERAPY SERVICES FOR CHILDREN WITH DISABILITIES

Occupational Therapy Domain in School-Based Practice

Education is identified as one of the key performance areas in the Occupational Therapy Practice Framework: Domain and Process, 2nd edition (Framework-II) (2008) and refers to the "activities needed for being a student and participating in the learning environment" (p. 620).[1] The occupation of education includes academic (math, reading, writing), nonacademic (recess, lunch, self-help skills), extracurricular (sports, band, cheerleading, clubs), and prevocational and vocational activities.[49] Consequently, in addressing a student's education, attention to a broad range of occupational performance areas is often required to help children succeed in their student role including play, leisure, social participation, activities of daily living, and work.

Occupational therapists working in schools must skillfully combine their professional knowledge and skills with the definition of occupational therapy in federal and state education legislation. School districts are mandated to provide *related services*, including occupational therapy, when a student who receives special education requires such services to benefit from special education. "Related services" means "transportation, and such developmental, corrective, and other supportive services including speech-language pathology and audiology services, interpreting services, psychological services, physical and occupational therapy, recreation, including therapeutic recreation, social work services, school nurse services... counseling services, including rehabilitation counseling, orientation and mobility services, and medical services, except that such medical services shall be for diagnostic and evaluation purposes only as may be required to assist a child with a disability to benefit from special education, and includes the early identification and assessment of disabling conditions in children" (§300.320(a)(4)). Special education and related services may be provided in a number of settings including schools, homes, hospitals, juvenile justice centers, and alternative education settings.[2]

Occupational therapy services must be *educationally relevant*, by contributing to the development, or improvement, of the child's academic and functional school performance. The regulations of IDEA define occupational therapy broadly as "(A) improving, developing or restoring functions impaired or lost through illness, injury or deprivation, (B) improving ability to perform tasks for independent functioning when functions are impaired or lost, and (C) preventing, through early intervention, initial or further impairment or loss of function" [§300.34(c)(6)]. Occupational therapy services can promote self-help skills (e.g., eating, dressing); positioning (e.g., sitting appropriately in class); sensory-motor processing; fine motor performance; psychosocial function; and life skills training.[64] Services must be provided by a qualified occupational therapist or service provider under the direction or supervision of a qualified occupational therapist. Although regulations focus on what constitutes "highly qualified" teachers, requirements beyond adhering to state licensure laws have not been created for occupational therapy.[44]

Occupational Therapy Process in School-Based Practice

The reauthorization of IDEA (2004) increased the focus of special education and related services on results—including academic achievement, functional outcomes, and postsecondary success. Expected outcomes for students with disabilities leaving high school include higher education, employment, and independent living (§602(d)). In collaboration with other members of the education team, occupational therapists contribute to the referral, evaluation, intervention, and outcome processes. With these important outcomes in mind, a key question guiding the special education process should be: "What does the child need or want to do to be successful as a student now and to prepare for future roles?"[79] The special education process is depicted in Figure 24-2. This section describes the occupational therapy processes of referral, evaluation, and intervention.

Referral

Each local education agency (LEA) has a "Child Find" system that locates, identifies, and evaluates all children who have disabilities and need special education.[69] A referral of a child suspected as having a disability may be made by any source, including parents, teachers, or other individuals. An occupational therapist evaluation may be requested at the time of initial referral *if* the team perceives that information provided by an occupational therapist will contribute to the evaluation process. This suggests how critical it is for school administrators and other team members to have an accurate understanding of the domain and scope of occupational therapy practice—that occupational therapists address the education, activities of daily living, play, leisure, work, and social participation areas of function related to the student's academic and nonacademic expectations. If team members have a narrow understanding of the scope of occupational therapy practice (e.g., occupational therapists address handwriting issues), then it is likely that the role of occupational therapy in that setting will be narrow as well.[48] Effort spent in informing principals, teachers, school psychologists, and other personnel about the role of occupational therapy in regular and general education ensures that students who may benefit from occupational therapy services are identified.

Evaluation

"Evaluation means procedures used in accordance with §§300.304–300.311 to determine whether a child has a disability and the nature and extent of the special education and related services that the child needs" (§300.15).

After obtaining parental consent, a full and individual evaluation is completed by a multidisciplinary team to determine whether the child is eligible for special education and, if so, it identifies educational and related service needs (§300.301). This multidisciplinary evaluation is needed even when the child has an obvious disability (e.g., cerebral palsy, Down syndrome) and has received therapeutic services in the past (e.g., in an early intervention program). In addition, this team determines the nature and scope of the full and individual evaluations for each child and decides if related services evaluations, including occupational therapy, are needed. The role of the occupational therapist in the evaluation process depends on how well he or she has explained the role and the team's understanding of the domain and scope of occupational therapy.

IDEA and the OTPF define evaluation and assessment consistently.[1] *Evaluation* refers to the process of gathering and interpreting information about the student's strengths and educational needs. *Assessments* refer to the tests or measures used to obtain data about specific areas of function. IDEA specifies that school personnel evaluate referred or eligible students in all areas of suspected disability. Furthermore, a variety of assessment tools or evaluation strategies must be used to obtain relevant academic, functional, and developmental information about the student (§300.304(b)(1)). The evaluation must be completed within 60 days of initial parent consent, unless the state specifies otherwise.

Top-down or occupation-based approach. Although one of the main purposes of evaluation according to IDEA is to determine eligibility, which is based on qualifying as a child with a disability, the law has placed greater emphasis on assessing the child's participation needs in relevant school contexts. This thinking is in agreement with current social

Early Intervening Services for Students Pre K through Grade 12
Screening or Child Find efforts identify students who may require interventions and supports within general education. Progress monitoring determines whether adequate progress is made or whether a referral for an evaluation to determine the need for special education is necessary.

Referral
"Child Find" activities are conducted in order for the state to identify, locate, and evaluate all children who may need special education and related services. A referral may be made by any source including parents, school staff, or other individuals. Findings of early intervening services are reviewed as a part of the referral process.

Evaluation
The child is evaluated in all areas related to the suspected disability. Results will be used to determine the child's eligibility for special education and related services.

Eligibility
Based on evaluation results, a group of qualified professionals and the parents decide if the child is a 'child with a disability' according to IDEA and eligible for special education and related services.

IEP
Within 30 days after a child is determined eligible for special education and related services, an IEP team (including the parents and students when appropriate) must develop an IEP. The child receives services as soon as possible following parental consent of the IEP.

Services
The school ensures that the child's IEP is being implemented as written. Teachers and service providers are responsible for carrying out her or his specific responsibilities as outlined on the IEP including accommodations, modifications, and supports.

Annual Review/Re-Evaluation
The IEP is reviewed by the IEP team at least once a year, or more often if the parents or school requests a review. At least every three years the child must be reevaluated to determine if the child continues to be a "child with a disability" as defined by IDEA and what the child's educational needs are.

FIGURE 24-2 Special Education Process. (Adapted from Office of Special Education and Rehabilitative Services U.S. Department of Education. [2000, July]. *A Guide to the Individualized Education Program*, 5–7.)

views regarding the evaluation of children and those adopted within the profession of occupational therapy. A top-down approach to evaluation is believed to more accurately reflect the true nature of occupational therapy and has been referred to as *occupation-based evaluation*.[69] A *top-down approach* to evaluation begins with gathering information about what the person needs and wants to do across a variety of occupational performance areas and settings (Figure 24-3).[18,30] Box 24-2 provides a description of the School Function Assessment[19] representing a top-down strategy used to initiate the evaluation process. Performance component function is assessed to the extent that it is thought to limit participation in occupation. An occupational therapist's ability to implement this approach is dependent on using appropriate evaluation strategies and assessment tools, developing the knowledge and skills needed to implement these strategies, and then actually using them in practice.

International social views of children's health also focus on participation in context. The World Health Organization (WHO), for example, recently published the *International Classification of Functioning, Disability and Health for Children and Youth (ICF-CY)*, in 2007.[86] This document emphasizes that the health of children is dependent upon their participation in context—both within their stage of development and in relevant environments. Similar to IDEA and OTPF, this model focuses on how multiple factors (i.e., individual abilities, activity, and context) influence the child's function.[69]

Evaluation Strategies

"Occupation-based evaluation approaches help the IEP team make decisions about the student's ability to participate and perform in the school setting and identify the ways that the disability affects the student's participation in school activities

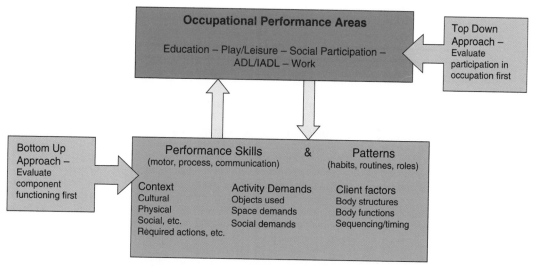

FIGURE 24-3   Top-down versus bottom-up approaches to evaluation and intervention.

BOX 24-2   The School Function Assessment: A Top-Down Measure of Student Participation

SCHOOL FUNCTION ASSESSMENT (SFA)

What? The SFA is a comprehensive assessment of function and participation for students in K to grade 6.

Purpose:

1. To measure the student's performance in functional tasks that support participation in academic and social aspects of elementary school (focuses primarily on nonacademic tasks).

2. Facilitate collaborative programming during IEP development and provide a means of documenting progress. Its three sections provide scales for identifying a child's level of participation, assessing the need for task support, and evaluating performance in school activities. In addition to academic outcomes, students must demonstrate socially appropriate behaviors and functional performance that enables them to participate in nonacademic school activities (e.g., eating lunch, playing with peers on the playground). Occupational therapists often focus on functional performance in nonacademic areas in addition to providing support for academic performance.

This *criterion-referenced* tool assesses the school functions that are primary domains of concern for occupational therapists, physical therapists, and teachers. The *physical subscales* identified in the SFA are travel, maintaining and changing positions, recreational movement, using materials, set-up and cleanup, eating and drinking, hygiene, clothing management, written work, movement up and/or downstairs, and computer and equipment use. The *cognitive and or behavioral subscales* identified in the SFA are functional communication, memory and understanding, following social conventions, task behavior and completion, compliance with adult directives and school rules, positive interaction, behavior regulation, personal care awareness, and safety.

To rate the SFA, the child is judged in relationship to the performance of the other students in his or her grade level or classroom. A child's participation is understood through observation of how peers perform and function relative to the curriculum and environment and what level of participation the teacher expects. The SFA is designed so that multiple team members (parents, teachers, and therapists) knowledgeable about the student's performance can contribute to the data-gathering process, yielding a more comprehensive understanding of the child. Through her everyday observations of the student, the team identifies the activities in which the student struggles or fails. Based on the team's observation, the child and the context become well understood, often leading to an interpretation of the problem that sheds new light on the child's behaviors.

---

and routines" (p. 35).[69] The occupational therapy evaluation focuses on areas of strength and weakness in educationally relevant occupational performance areas (education, social participation, activities of daily living, play, leisure, and work) related to the student's suspected disability (Table 24-1). Obtaining an *occupational profile* initiates the evaluation process by exploring the student's educational history, interests, values, and needs. The student may be interviewed using questions such as the following:

- What kinds of things are going well for you?
- What are some of your challenges?
- What would you like to see changed?

The therapist can also interview the teacher about his or her classroom expectations for the student. The parents are asked to identify their priorities for the child. Information obtained from the occupational profile assists the therapist in developing initial impressions about the student's difficulties, which may be useful in directing the rest of the evaluation process.

In addition to interviews, other useful evaluation strategies include document or chart review to obtain background information and observations of the student in a variety of school contexts (e.g., classroom, cafeteria, playground, locker room). The evaluation process involves an examination of the dynamic relationship among the student's *participation and*

TABLE 24-1 School-Related Occupational Performance Addressed During Evaluation and Intervention

Occupational Area	Examples of Participation in School-Related Occupational Performance	Examples of OT Intervention	School-Related Outcomes
Education	Access to and participation in classroom curriculum Organizational skills Attending to instruction Fine motor skills and hand function Written communication/handwriting	Assist with adapting assignments with high or low technology; adapt child's positioning so child can perform handwriting as effectively as possible Management of books and notebooks, desk, homework assignments, and backpack Enable child to use self-regulatory activities to foster attending; provide strategies to enhance work completion Provide classroom materials and activities to promote fine motor skills development and in-hand manipulation skills Consult with curriculum committee in the selection of a handwriting curriculum; direct services in groups or individually to assist students in letter formation; provide modifications to complete written communication, including use of technology	Achieves in the learning environment including academic (e.g., reading, math), nonacademic (e.g., recess, lunch, relationships with peers), prevocational and vocational activities (e.g., professional and technical education).
Social participation	Successful interaction with teachers, other school personnel, and peers Ability to adapt to environmental demands	Foster appropriate interaction with peers during group interventions; attend to social interaction during lunch and recess and foster the development of friendships Provide strategies for coping with test anxiety; adapt procedures to reduce stressful school expectation	Develops appropriate social relationships at school with peers, teachers. and other school personnel within classroom, extracurricular activities, and preparation for work.
Play/leisure	Plays with peers during recess Participates successfully in class games Develops structured leisure interests for out-of-school time (e.g., sports, art, dance)	Assist in making play environments (e.g., playground) accessible; consult with school administration to ensure recess is play-based; assist students in exploring leisure interests; consult with parents to promote structured leisure participation during after-school time.	Identifies and engages in age-appropriate toys, games, and play activities; participates in meaningful selection of art, music, sports, and after-school activities.
Work	Prevocational	Advocate for embedding productive occupations into the school day (e.g., putting supplies away; cleaning work spaces); involve students with disabilities in work activities within the school environment (wiping down lunch tables); develop group programs to foster work skills	Develops interests, habits, and work skills needed to work or volunteer in the community after graduation from school.
Activities of daily living (basic and instrumental)	Dressing (putting on and taking off coat; dressing for gym) Eating lunch and/or snack Toileting (bowel and bladder management) Basic hygiene and grooming Using communication devices Meal preparation in class Using computers Shopping Doing laundry	Provide direct intervention using a chaining approach to teach dressing or self-feeding Teach appropriate transferring strategies for wheelchair to toilet Provide group activities to promote participation in independent living skills such as shopping, cooking, and cleanup	Attends to basic self-care needs in school (e.g., eating, toileting, managing shoes and coats); uses public transportation to travel in the community; develops health management routines; develops home management routines to the maximum extent possible (e.g., cleaning, shopping, meal preparation, safety and emergency responses, and budgeting)

Adapted from Kentucky Department of Education. (2006). *Resource manual for educationally related occupational therapy and physical therapy in Kentucky public schools*; and Swinth, Y. (2007). Evaluating evidence to support practice. In L. L. Jackson (Ed.), *Occupational therapy services for children and youth under IDEA* (3rd ed.) Bethesda, MD: American Occupational Therapy Association; and Swinth, Y., Chandler, B., Hanft, B., Jackson, L., & Shepherd, J. (2003). *Personnel issues in school-based occupational therapy: Supply and demand, preparation, certification and licensure.* (COPSSE Document No. IB-1). Gainesville, FL: University of Florida, Center on Personnel Studies in Special Education.

performance skills, educational context, and *specific educational/activity demands* that may be contributing to the problems.[79] For example, to fully understand a student's difficulty with written communication during test-taking, the therapist may want to observe the student while taking a test, compare work with that of peers in the same environment, and explore curricular demands with the teacher.

Evaluation of *school environment* includes the classrooms, cafeteria, playgrounds, gymnasium, and other spaces (Figure 24-4). For children using wheelchairs or walkers, the focus of this part of the assessment may be accessibility. For children with sensory processing problems, the focus may be the degree and types of sensory stimulation in the environment. Classrooms tend to be highly visually stimulating environments, and they can be disorganizing and overwhelming to students with sensory processing problems (Figure 24-5).

To analyze *educational and/or activity demands,* the expected performance (as defined by the teacher and curriculum) must be understood fully. When teachers expect neat, precisely aligned, and well-formed handwriting, a student with poor handwriting will have a significant problem in meeting that teacher's standard. As another example, some teachers show high tolerance for disruptive behavior and allow students to move freely about the room. A student with a high activity level and sensory-seeking behaviors would have greater success in a classroom where movement was allowed, rather than one in which students were expected to remain in their seats. Often a student's goals and services are based more on the discrepancy between the student's performance and classroom-teacher expectations than on performance delays as determined by norms that reference the student's age. In addition, occupational

therapists need to become familiar with their states' learning and achievement standards—accessible from the state's department of education website.

Assessment Measures

The occupational therapist may also decide to administer informal or formal assessment measures to obtain a full evaluation of the child's occupational performance related to curricular and extracurricular needs. However, according to IDEA, the use of assessment tools is not required if observations and interviews have provided the needed information for decision making. Because the number of standardized pediatric assessments available today has grown significantly over the past 2 decades, it is important for occupational therapists practicing in schools to make informed decisions when selecting assessments.

Three basic constructs of pediatric assessments have been identified—developmental, functional, and health-related quality of life (HRQL).[38] These are described in Table 24-2. Although developmental assessments may be particularly helpful when working with infants and preschoolers to identify developmental delays, these are less useful with the school-aged population, where the emphasis shifts to functional performance and participation in context. Developmental assessments measure a child's behavior and skills rather than the ability to function as a student.[80] With a developmental approach, intervention emphasizes normalizing the underlying processes to achieve greater function.[17] Current intervention approaches, however, suggest that in addition to addressing characteristics of the person, physical and social aspects of the environment, and features of the activity, influence function and need to be addressed.[18]

In contrast to developmental assessments, functional assessments measure abilities and limitations in performance of necessary daily activities.[22] The School Function Assessment (SFA)[19] and a growing number of functional, top-down assessments are now available. Although a number of occupation-based assessments have been published in the past decade, one survey found that school-based occupational therapy practitioners primarily used developmental assessments of gross and fine motor skills (e.g., Bruininks-Oseretsky Test of Motor Proficiency, Peabody Developmental Motor Scales, Beery Test of Visual Motor Integration).[12] When the findings of this survey were compared with previous research, similar trends in the use of motor and visual perception tests were found.

One of the major obstacles to using functional assessments is the dominance of the developmental model.[18] Functional assessments have only been available during the past 10 years, and time is needed for therapists to become educated and skilled in using them. Most functional assessments (e.g., the SFA) are often designed so that multiple team members (parents, teachers, and therapists) knowledgeable about the student's performance can contribute to the data-gathering process, yielding a comprehensive understanding of the child. In a study of the validity and reliability of the SFA, findings suggest that occupational therapists and teachers view students' functioning similarly.[22]

Recent evidence has indicated that in addition to using adult informants, children can also participate more actively in the evaluation process and goal setting if the procedures used are developmentally appropriate.[57] The Perceived

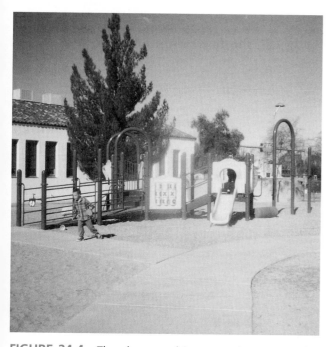

FIGURE 24-4 The playground is one environment to be evaluated, emphasizing accessibility and safety. Although schools are constructing playgrounds with wheelchair accessibility, many remain only partially accessible. Playgrounds should include equipment that requires a range of skills and a range of sensory input.

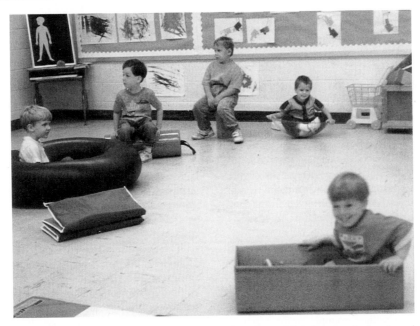

FIGURE 24-5   Preschool classrooms tend to have high levels of visual and auditory stimuli.

TABLE 24-2   Types of Assessment Tools

Type	Description of Purpose and Implications	Assessments
Developmental	Assess underlying performance areas to determine the: Presence of a developmental delay Presumed cause of the functional limitations Areas assessed: gross motor, fine motor, sensory, self-care, social, visual perceptual, communication, adaptive/cognitive Setting: secluded testing room Problem is perceived to be within the child Assessments tend to be norm-referenced, comparing the child's performance with that of a normative sample Intervention focuses on development of isolated skills	Peabody Developmental Motor Scales, 2nd Edition (PDMS-2) Bruininks-Oseretsky Test of Motor Proficiency (BOT-2) Beery-Buktenica Developmental Test of Visual-Motor Integration, 5th Edition (VMI)
Functional	Assess function in context; focus is on personal capacities, not failure of organ function Areas assessed: hygiene, handwriting, play, social participation, material management Setting: natural environment; parent or teacher may provide the data Assessments tend to be criterion-referenced, determining how a child performs in relation to a set of standards Intervention focuses on successful participation in all school activities and settings	WeeFIM System (Functional Independence Measure for Children) School Function Assessment (SFA) Children's Assessment of Participation and Enjoyment (CAPE) and Preferences for Activities of Children (PAC)–CAPE/PAC Miller FUNction and Participation Scales (FUN Scale) Social Skills Rating System (SSRS) OT Pal–Occupational Therapy Psychosocial Assessment of Learning School Version of the Assessment of Motor and Process Skills (School AMPS) Sensory Processing Measure (SPM)
Child-reported health-related quality of life (HRQL)	Assess how the child feels about her/his life, abilities, and overall sense of well-being Aim is to complement functional assessments by providing a more complete picture of the person Areas assessed: person's feelings about participating in childhood roles and overall sense of well-being	The Perceived Efficacy and Goal Setting System (PEGS) The School Setting Interview (SSI) Child Health Questionnaire (CHQ) Youth Quality of Life Instrument (YQOL)

Data from Coster, W., Deeney, T., Haltiwanger, J., & Haley, S. (1998). *School function assessment.* San Antonio: Psychological Corporation; Davies, P. L., Soon, P. L., Young, M., & Clausen-Yamaki, A. (2004). Validity and reliability of the school function assessment in elementary school students with disabilities. *Physical & Occupational Therapy in Pediatrics, 24,* 23-43; Haley, S. M. (1994). Our measures reflect our practices and beliefs: A perspective on clinical measurement in pediatric physical therapy. *Pediatric Physical Therapy, 6,* 142-3; and Schneider, J. W., Gurucharri, L. M., Gutierrez, A. L., & Gaebler-Spira, D. J. (2000) Health-related quality of life and functional outcome measures for children with cerebral palsy. *Developmental Medicine & Child Neurology, 43,* 601-608.

Efficacy and Goal Setting System (PEGS)[58] is one example of such a measure. The PEGS was designed to help children with disabilities reflect on their ability to perform everyday activities and identify goals for occupational therapy intervention. Another assessment tool developed to gather information directly from the child is the School Setting Interview (SSI).[43] The information gathered from these measures on children's thoughts and feelings about their ability to fulfill childhood roles can complement results obtained from functional assessments by providing a more complete picture of the person.[72] In addition, occupational therapists may consider using some type of HRQL measures to obtain a clear sense of the child's life satisfaction.

Documentation

The final step in the evaluation process involves effectively communicating the findings and recommendations in a written report. Occupational therapy documentation should reflect a top-down presentation of the student's strengths and limitations regarding participation in academic and nonacademic activities across all student environments. Performance component issues (e.g., body structure and function) that affect participation should be reported using language understandable to all team members, including parents.

Eligibility

After the evaluation process, the team reviews all of the data to determine eligibility for special education and related services. A student is eligible for special education under IDEA if she or he meets two criteria: (1) is a child with a disability under one of the disability categories or under the developmental delay category; and (2) needs special education services. The *disability categories* include: mental retardation, a hearing impairment (including deafness), a speech or language impairment, a visual impairment (including blindness), a serious emotional disturbance, an orthopedic impairment, autism, traumatic brain injury, another health impairment, a specific learning disability, deaf-blindness, or multiple disabilities (34 C.F.R. §300.8). The phrase *child with a disability* for children aged 3 through 9 years may, at the discretion of the SEA and LEA and in accordance with §300.111(b), include a child who demonstrates developmental delays, as defined by the state and as measured by appropriate diagnostic instruments and procedures, in one or more of the following areas: physical development, cognitive development, communication development, social or emotional development, or adaptive development; and who, by reason thereof, needs special education and related services.

If the team determines that a child is eligible for special education, the IEP process begins—the IEP team meets to develop a special education plan and determine if related services are necessary. Occupational therapy evaluation data provides the IEP team with "information related to enabling the child to be involved in and progress in the general education curriculum, or for preschool children, to participate in appropriate activities" (§614(b)(2)(A)(ii)). The determination of need for occupational therapy services should not be based on evaluation alone but should be driven by the student's educational program and annual goals.

A child with a disability who is *not* eligible for special education under IDEA may be eligible for services under Section 504 of the Rehabilitation Act of 1973. Using information from multiple sources, a multidisciplinary team determines if the child has a disability (as defined in Section 504) that substantially limits a major life activity.

Individualized Education Program

The IEP represents both the formal planning *process* and the resulting *legal document* that establishes the services and programs that will enable the student to participate in school activities and receive an "appropriate education." According to IDEA (34 C.F.R. §§300.320–300.324), the IEP is a written statement for each child with a disability that outlines the student's educational and functional needs and the supports and services required to meet those needs. It is developed, reviewed, and revised in a meeting in accordance with the guidelines of the IDEA.

The *IEP team* is made up at minimum of the child's parents; one regular education teacher of the child; one special education teacher of the child; one special education provider, when appropriate; a representative of the public agency who had knowledge and qualifications; an individual who can interpret the instructional implications of the evaluation results (may be one of the other members); other individuals who have knowledge or special expertise regarding the child (e.g., related services personnel) as appropriate, and the child with a disability when appropriate (34 C.F.R. §300.321(a) and (b)(1)). Although related services personnel are generally considered "discretionary" team members (§300.321(a)(6)), if an occupational therapist formally identified as a member of a particular IEP team or if occupational therapy is being discussed at the meeting, it is fitting and desirable that the therapist attend the meeting.[45]

The collaborative planning procedure that guides the process of developing an IEP involves many components. The school-based occupational therapist contributes to many of those components when participating as a member of a student's IEP team. Although the exact components may vary from state to state, depending on the special education policies and procedures adopted by the state, the following items represent at least the minimum for all states because they are mandated as general requirements by IDEA (34 C.F.R. §300.320(a))(Table 24-3).

The *first steps* involve interpretation of the most recent evaluation of the child, consideration of the child's performance on any general state or districtwide assessment programs, and identification of the student's strengths and needs. It also involves discussion with the parents, educational team, and sometimes the student regarding priorities and goals. During this initial phase, it is important to "create a team 'vision' about who the student is and what a student needs to succeed in school" (p. 1).[49] This information is documented on the IEP as the present levels of academic achievement and functional performance and the description of how the student's disability affects participation in general education. For a preschool student, consideration is given to whether the disability affects participation in any activity appropriate for a preschooler. Typically, all team members participate in developing this statement, which includes a summary of all evaluation results, thus giving a total picture of the student's academic and functional performance. Occupational therapists should

TABLE 24-3 Process Depicting the Development of the Individualized Education Program (IEP)

Step	Description
VISION OF CHILD'S NEEDS	
1. Determine present levels of academic achievement and functional performance	Interpretation of the full and individual evaluation (FIE)
2. Describe how the student's disability affects participation in general education	Consider how disability influences access and participation in academic and functional activities
	Identification of the student's strengths and needs
	Discuss parent, student, and team member priorities for the child
MEASURABLE GOALS	
Develop measurable and attainable annual goals (both academic and functional)	One-year goals
	All team members contribute to goal development
	Goals may be linked to state curriculum content standards
	Plan for measuring progress toward annual goals
	Related services goals must be "educationally relevant"
	For children with disabilities who take alternate assessments aligned to alternate achievement standards, a description of benchmarks or short-term objectives
SPECIAL EDUCATION AND RELATED SERVICES	
Determine the special education, related services, supplemental aids and services, modifications, and supports	Represents services student needs to accomplish IEP goals
	Team determines all needed services
	Services meet academic, functional, and extracurricular needs
	Services based on peer-reviewed research to the extent practicable
	Projected date for initiating services, anticipated frequency, location, and duration of the services
STATEMENT OF ACCOMMODATIONS	
Needed to measure academic achievement and functional performance on state and districtwide assessments	Statement of why the child cannot participate in the regular assessment and why the particular alternate assessment selected is appropriate for the child
PLACEMENT IN LEAST RESTRICTIVE ENVIRONMENT	
	Educate students with disabilities with their nondisabled peers to the maximum extent appropriate
	Consider general education environment first
	Placement determined annually
	Must offer a range of service delivery options
TRANSITION PLAN	
Beginning at 16 yr	Based on age-appropriate transition assessments related to training, education, employment, and independent living skills
	Identifies transition services needed to assist the child in reaching goals that may include vocational training, supported employment, independent living, work experience, community participation, or planning appropriate high school classes in preparation for college

be ready to share evaluation results, which are included in the student's present levels of performance. Therapists should specify how the student's performance influences participation in the general education curriculum, including functional activities. For example, sharing the student's time delay before initiating work, percentage of time engaged in off-task behavior, or how writing speed relates to educationally relevant performance in written expression. In the case of a preschool student, the therapist should document whether the performance results suggest problems that will affect the student's access to typical preschool activities. Table 24-4 provides examples of educationally relevant present levels of performance and statements of need.

The next step involves the development of *measurable annual goals* (both academic and functional) designed to enable the student to have access to and make progress in the general education curriculum and meet the child's other educational needs that result from the child's disability (34 C.F.R. §300.320(a)(2)(i)(B)). The goals are statements of measurable and attainable behaviors a student is expected to demonstrate within 1 year. Many states are linking goals to their state curriculum content standards.[44] This ensures that the goals are related directly to the learning objectives mandated by the SEA for all students. IDEA 2004 eliminated the requirement of writing short-term objectives (benchmarks) in the IEP except for children with disabilities who take alternate assessments

TABLE 24-4   Educationally Relevant Levels of Performance and Educational Need

Present Performance Level	Educational Need
Forms all letters correctly in isolation	Increase speed and spacing so written words and sentences are legible
Highly sensitive to unexpected touch; will push other children when in line or moving through the hallways	Strategies and supports to tolerate being close to peers; accommodations to leave class early to avoid crowded hallways
Eyes remain fixed when reading	Accommodations and instruction to read text without skipping or rereading words
Desk and workspace cluttered; unable to locate assignments and homework	Learn to use an organizational system
Enjoys recess but tires after 5 minutes on the playground	Frequent rest breaks and strategies to understand and communicate fatigue to teaching staff
Has adequate skills for hands-on prevocational work experiences; personal hygiene not sufficient for work settings	Awareness and training for increased independence and carryover in self-care areas

Data from Knippenberg, C., & Hanft, B. (2004). The key to educational relevance: Occupation throughout the school day. *School System Special Interest Section Quarterly, 11*(4), 1-4.

aligned to alternate achievement standards (§300.320(a)(2)(ii). Congress opted to eliminate short-term objectives as a way to reduce paperwork and also because parents are informed of short-term progress through the use of quarterly and other periodic reports. Although short-term objectives are not required for all students receiving special education, a *plan for measuring progress* must be documented, specifying how the child is meeting IEP goals and when periodic progress reports will be provided (such as through the use of quarterly reports concurrent with the issuance of report cards) (34 C.F.R. §300.320(a)(2)). It should be noted that the frequency of reporting progress must be at least as often as the progress reports received by the parents of nondisabled students. The actual progress attained toward the goals must be included. Occupational therapists are responsible for measuring progress toward annual goals and objectives when they are one of the services listed to support that student's goal. Often, several members of the IEP team share data keeping for a student's progress toward general education goals.

Goal writing is a collaborative process and is completed at the IEP meeting with the input of *all* team members including the parents, and in some cases the student. Goal writing in most districts is facilitated by an online process that enables the IEP to be developed on a shared website. Student needs are prioritized and academic and functional goals are selected based on identifying skills that are needed to progress in the general educational environment. Team members, including occupational therapists, must relate their activities and recommendations to the general education curriculum and extracurricular activities. Therefore, all team members must be knowledgeable about the classroom curriculum and behavioral expectations and the state educational standards. Target behaviors are those actions and skills that students typically do or need to develop, such as participating in physical education, writing an essay, eating lunch independently, playing with friends during recess, and participating in after-school clubs.[49] Although occupational therapists may identify limitations in discrete performance skills that negatively impact school participation, such separate clinical goals should not be suggested to the IEP team. Goals need to address academic achievement and functional performance. Furthermore, the occupational therapist may feel that a particular skill is a priority for a child. However, when viewing the whole child, the team may not concur. If this is the case, some negotiation among IEP team members may be needed to select the priorities for the child so that appropriate goals and objectives can be developed for the student. A description of how to develop goals is provided in Box 24-3.

Once the IEP goals have been developed, the team determines the special education, related services, supplemental aids and services, modifications, and supports to be provided by the school. These pertain to the student's advancement toward the annual goals and access to the general education curriculum, and participation in nonacademic and extracurricular activities. The IEP team determines if related services are "required to assist a child with a disability to benefit from special education" (34 C.F.R. §300.34(a)). "One of the most important clarifications that teams should understand is that students with disabilities do not attend school to receive related services; they receive services so they can attend and participate in school" (p. 6).[34] Therefore, the role of the school-based occupational therapist is not to provide a full rehabilitation program but to support the child's efforts within the academic environment and only if necessary.[32] In general, occupational therapy services under IDEA are not provided when a student has a temporary impairment (e.g., a fractured bone) or when an impairment does not interfere with the student's performance in school. For example, a bright first grader had mild left hemiparesis cerebral palsy. This student participated in all aspects of the educational program, including physical education, with few adaptations. The disability did not interfere with the student's educational program. Therefore, she was not eligible for occupational therapy in school, despite the fact that she did not have the full use of her left hand (Figure 24-6).

It is important, however, for the occupational therapist to effectively communicate the domain and scope of occupational therapy services to the entire IEP team so that an informed decision will be made regarding service provision. On the basis of evaluation findings, the occupational therapist articulates to the IEP team recommendations regarding the need for occupational therapy services to enable the child to benefit from his or her education. The IEP team makes the decision based on the student's educational program and unique needs. "Occupational therapy services are appropriate when the unique skills and expertise of the occupational therapist are needed to support the priorities identified by the team" (p. 78).[40]

If the occupational therapist is to provide services to the student, it must be noted specifically in this section of the IEP along with the projected date for initiating services and anticipated frequency, location, and duration of the services.

BOX 24-3   Evaluation of Performance As It Relates to Participation in School

Following a top-down approach to evaluation, specific evaluation of performance components is assessed to the extent that it is thought to limit participation in school function. At this stage, the goal is to identify reasons for the student's difficulties. Standardized tools and structured observation are used. Typical areas of assessment—*(1) motor performance, (2) sensory processing, (3) perceptual processing, (4) cognitive abilities,* and *(5) social-emotional abilities*—are described below.

Motor Performance. Children in school are expected to travel independently within the school and move safely within the classroom, playground, and hallways. They must manipulate their schoolbooks, writing and cutting tools, paper, and materials; use tools such as scissors; produce legible handwriting; eat and drink independently; and use a computer. Related to their self-maintenance, they must use the toilet, wash their hands, put on and take off their jackets, and demonstrate other hygiene skills. Standardized tests to measure motor performance include the Peabody Developmental Motor Scales (2nd ed.) (PDMS)[31] and the Bruininks-Oseretsky Test of Motor Proficiency (2nd ed.) (BOTMP).[11] Although both of these developmental assessments offer a method for evaluating a child's motor performance, the items do not necessarily relate to school function and, therefore, a cautious interpretation of the scores is needed. Visual-motor tests (e.g., Developmental Test of Visual-Motor Integration[8]) that require paper and/or pencil skills relate to school functions, such as handwriting and tool use. These tests measure the child's skills in tracing and copying designs. As a functional assessment, the School Function Assessment (SFA) has sections that measure physical performance, using a comprehensive representation of the movements and manipulation skills required to function at school.

Sensory Processing. A child's sensory processing can be assessed using standardized interviews, inventories, or observational tests. Inventories such as the Sensory Profile[25] rate sensory processing in natural situations. The Sensory Profile School Companion[26] assesses the student's response to sensory experiences that reflect participation in the classroom. The Sensory Processing Measure[35] assesses sensory processing in six environments outside of the classroom. Observational assessments of children's sensory processing are used to supplement the parents' or teachers' reports on the child's response to sensory input (e.g., Sensory

Integration Inventory—Revised, for Individuals with Developmental Disabilities[75]).

Perceptual Processing. Assessment of a child's visual perceptual processing is particularly important to his or her school function. Standardized instruments to measure visual perception include the Developmental Test of Visual Perception (2nd ed.) (DTVP-II)[39] and the Motor-Free Visual Perception Test-3.[15] Aspects of visual perception that relate to school function (e.g., reading, handwriting) include spatial relations, figure-ground perception, and form constancy. Other perceptual skills important to understanding performance in school activities include body scheme and body awareness, orientation to time and place, and spatial awareness (see Chapter 12).

Cognitive Abilities. Problem solving, organizational skills, and attention are essential performance areas of school function. The SFA Activity Scales rate behavior and cognition using 10 scales. Each has high relevance to a child's success in the school environment. Another assessment of cognitive ability is the DOTCA-Ch (Dynamic Occupational Therapy Cognitive Assessment for Children)[47] developed to assess the cognitive areas of orientation, spatial perception, praxis, visuomotor construction, and thinking operations of 6- to 12-year-old children.

Social Interaction and Behavior. Behaviors are often the focus of the IEP because they determine the child's ability to function in a structured environment (e.g., classroom), to attend, demonstrate responsibility, positively interact with others, cope with new situations, and fit into the social norms of the classroom. Socially appropriate behavior is highly related to the student's academic achievement and his or her ability to succeed in environments outside school (e.g., community, work). Important elements of behavior that are often the focus of occupational therapy are attention and persistence, task completion, compliance, self-esteem and self-image, peer and adult interaction, problem solving, and safety. Students frequently have difficulty transitioning from one activity to another and adapting to new situations. Adaptive behaviors are analyzed to determine the antecedents to aggressive or disruptive behaviors, or to withdrawal behaviors. As in every other performance area, standardized tools are available. Examples are the Behavior Evaluation Scale-2[58] and the Social Skills Rating System (SSRS).

Documentation of the type of occupational therapy service delivery should ensure that a *range of service* approaches be available to the student—both *direct* (to the child) and *indirect* (on behalf of the child) services. Based on the individualized needs of the student, direct intervention may be necessary during one week, whereas indirect consultation provided to the teacher on the student's behalf may be useful during the next week. In addition, flexibility in documenting time and frequency is also recommended (i.e., 2 hours per month or 1 hour per grading period), rather than specifying set weekly visits. "For example, a high school student may need 3 hours the first month to set up a prevocational program and to train the instructional team. Much smaller periods of time, such as 1 hour per month, may be needed when the OT returns in subsequent weeks to evaluate the effectiveness of the program and revise as needed" (p. 3).[68] Recommendations for duration of services, generally written as beginning and ending dates, and location of services (e.g., cafeteria, classroom, playground, hallways) must also be specified.

The occupational therapist may also participate in suggesting appropriate modifications and support based on the assessment results. As an example, the occupational therapist may suggest limiting the amount of information on the student's worksheets because of a student's poor visual figure-ground processing. If the team were to agree to the recommendation, it would be documented on the IEP. Similarly, a statement of any individual appropriate *accommodations* that are necessary to measure the academic achievement and functional performance of the child on state and districtwide assessments consistent with §612(a)(16) of the IDEA, must also be determined by the IEP team.[63] In addition, if the IEP team determines that the child must take an alternate assessment instead of the regular state or districtwide assessment of student achievement, a statement of why the child cannot participate in the regular assessment and why the alternate assessment is appropriate for the child must be documented. The occupational therapist may contribute in the team discussion about appropriate testing modification.

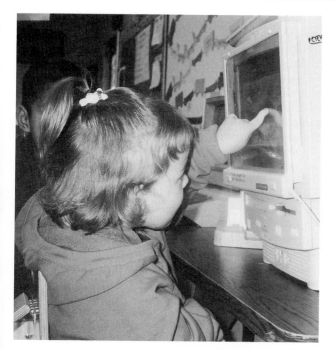

FIGURE 24-6 A child with left hemiparesis uses a touch window on the classroom computer. Despite her left-side motor impairments, she did not qualify for related services under IDEA because she was fully functional and met all standards for kindergarten performance.

For example, the occupational therapist may suggest testing a student with sensory sensitivities in a separate room. For a student with motor limitations and difficulty with handwriting, the occupational therapist may suggest using an electronic text format of the test that would allow the student to use a keyboard. Each state determines the allowable modifications.

Once the IEP team has determined *what* the child needs in terms of special education services, the team can determine *where* the services should be provided. *Placement decisions* are made annually based on where the IEP team has determined that the student's IEP goals can be met.[88] In accordance with LRE as defined in the IDEA, children with disabilities are required to be educated with their nondisabled peers to the maximum extent appropriate (34 C.F.R. §300.114(A)(2)(i)). This means instruction must be available in a continuum of placement options ranging from regular education classrooms to specialized classrooms, residential facilities, and home-based programs. Removal to separate classes is permissible only "if the nature or severity of the disability is such that education in regular classes with the use of supplementary aids and services cannot be achieved satisfactorily" (34 C.F.R. §300.114(A(2)(ii)). On the basis of student's IEP goals, the team should consider whether supplementary aids and services provided within a general education classroom would allow the student to receive an appropriate education or whether such a placement would impede her or his learning and/or the learning of other students. If a child will not be participating fully with children without disabilities in a regular classroom, in nonacademic and extracurricular activities, there must be an explanation on the IEP as to the extent the child will not be participating.

Finally, once the child turns 16, or before that if determined appropriate by the IEP team, the IEP must include a written *transition plan*. Transition is the process of beginning to plan for the student's completion of education and post-graduation life. This plan is based on age-appropriate transition assessments related to training, education, employment, and, when appropriate, independent living skills. The transition plan should include a statement of the services needed and should clearly connect the student's goals for after-school life and a planned course of studies in high school. The transition services (including courses of study) needed to assist the child in reaching those goals may include vocational training, supported employment, independent living, work experience, community participation, or planning appropriate high school classes in preparation for college. When the student reaches age 16, a statement of interagency responsibility is also included in the IEP. Occupational therapists may be involved in this process by providing input on the student's functional capabilities related to vocational planning and community living.

The development of IEPs can be a daunting task because of the changing legal requirements with each reauthorization of IDEA and the changing face of each IEP team. Occupational therapists need to develop the skills to work effectively with a multitude of parents and professionals. Although IEP teams have characteristics that make them like other types of working teams, there are also unique characteristics to IEP teams that need to be considered by the various members. It has been suggested that IEP teams differ from other teams in the following ways[20]:

1. There is a legal framework of required relationships among partners. Federal, state, and local laws and policies spell out in some detail who must participate and what they must do. This is especially true for the school district, which has many legal responsibilities regarding the education of students with disabilities.

2. The team members share both responsibility and accountability for the success of the student in meeting his or her goals.

3. The process is "results-oriented," meaning that what matters is not how happy everyone is with the process, but the success of the student's educational program.

As a result of these differences, development of the IEP involves high levels of collaboration and, at times, negotiation among and consensus building by all team members. The written IEP document is developed in a formal meeting, so the contents reflect the consensus of the team. Parents and other team members, including occupational therapists, contribute equally to the process. The team members discuss the student's strengths and needs and then develop goals, outcome statements, and plans through a collaborative process. By developing the student's IEP using a team process that includes the family, the team assures the family that the IEP belongs to the student and is unique to that student's educational needs.

Occupational Therapy Services

Once the IEP team agrees that occupational therapy services are necessary to support the student's goal achievement, the occupational therapist can propose how to provide services. IDEA 2004 recognizes that services and supports need to be delivered in different ways for children with disabilities to benefit from education. The nature of occupational therapy practice in schools is complex because of the considerable variability in service provision including the target of services (*who*), types of services and how these are delivered (*what and how*), scheduling of services (*when*), and place of delivery (*where*).

Although the primary "client" is the child, intervention may also target general and special education teachers, other related service providers (e.g., music therapists), administrators (e.g., principals), and paraprofessionals involved in supporting the child's IEP.[14,41] Intervention with a variety of "clients" occurs as a direct result of employing a *range of service delivery* options. Traditionally, services in schools were provided directly to the child in an isolated therapy setting similar to clinical practice. This type of service delivery involves primarily one "client" —the child. However, IDEA does not mandate any one service model and allows for a range of services including those provided *directly* to the child (direct), *on behalf of the child* (indirect), and as *program supports* or modifications for teachers and other staff working with the child (indirect) (§614(d)(IV)). Services provided on behalf of the child or to

provide program supports, require the therapist to work directly with a range of other "clients" including regular and special educators, parents, or paraprofessionals. For instance, a therapist may consult with the classroom teacher to help modify instructional materials and methods for a student with physical or organizational needs requiring close interaction with the teacher. Decisions about how occupational therapy services are made based on the child's needs, the educational program, and expected outcomes.[14,67] Examples of the range of services provided by an occupational therapy practitioner are working individually with children, consulting with the teacher about a student, co-leading a small group in the classroom, providing an in-service training program for educational personnel, and/or working on a curriculum or other school-level committee.[77] For example, an occupational therapist may co-lead groups with a special education teacher as discussed in Box 24-4 (Figure 24-7).

In addition to determining the most effective range of services for a child, therapists are also encouraged to *provide services in a flexible manner* depending on the student's stage in

---

BOX 24-4   "Brownie Busters": An Occupation-Based Work Group for Children with Multiple Disabilities

PROGRAM DEVELOPMENT

The purpose of the "Brownie Busters" program is to (1) provide a community-based functional curriculum for students with multiple disabilities attending elementary school, (2) provide tasks that are meaningful to elementary school students while teaching them skills needed for future employment and independence in their homes and neighborhood community, and (3) encourage collaboration among school team members, including the teacher, teacher's assistant, occupational therapist, and parents.

The foundation for the development of the 6-week Brownie Busters work group was based on literature regarding the development of work skills in children with multiple disabilities, indicating that (1) preparation for employment needs to begin at an early age,[46] (2) participation in meaningful activities within an educational or work context reinforces interest,[6,53] and (3) programs for students with moderate intellectual disabilities should emphasize skills that are both functional and longitudinally relevant.[58] An occupational therapist working in a large Midwestern municipal school district developed and facilitated the 1½-hour weekly groups over a period of 6 weeks. The classroom teacher, the teacher's assistant, and the parent volunteer served as helpers during the groups.

The overall purpose of the Brownie Busters work group was to have the students make and sell brownie-making kits to teachers, students, and staff at their school. The groups were designed to promote the development of several independent living and work skills including planning a work task; functional reading (reading labels and recipes); safety issues related to walking in the community; grocery shopping; simple cooking (learning about ingredients, measuring ingredients, pouring ingredients, mixing ingredients); using an oven; sanitary food handling; and selling a product.

PARTICIPANTS

The work group consisted of eight elementary students ages 9 to 12 with multiple disabilities including mild to moderate intellectual impairment and language delays. The diagnoses of the students included with cerebral palsy, Down syndrome, and autism.

GROUP SESSIONS

The group sessions involved weekly discussions of basic work skills, a trip to the grocery store, and making the brownie mixes, putting them in jars, decorating the jars, and selling them. Each session also involved clean-up.

QUALITATIVE RESEARCH FINDINGS

Qualitative research methods were used to explore the meaning of group participation from the children's perspective. Each of the eight group members were interviewed during weeks 2 and 6 of the program by the occupational therapist, to explore the personal meaning ascribed to the group experience. Participant observations served as the second form of data and consisted of weekly observations of the group. Based on a qualitative analysis of the interviews and participant observations, three essential themes unfolded—*shopping*, *special ingredients*, and *doing everything*. When asked what comes to mind or what they liked the most when they think of the occupational therapy groups, all of the participants talked about walking to and shopping at the neighborhood grocery store, about ingredients needed for the project, and about doing the tasks necessary for making the brownie jars. By being actively involved in the shopping process, students learned firsthand about how to locate the baking ingredients needed for the brownies. The students began to take on the role of "shopper" by looking for items needed for baking and using a shopping list. Students also learned about each "special ingredient's" unique properties by handling, measuring, and tasting them. Finally, students expressed joy in "doing everything" and began to function like workers— doing the task, sharing, demonstrating care with the ingredients, using sanitary strategies for handling of food, and preparing the jars to sell. Findings support the importance of occupation-based practice in fostering the link between doing and becoming.

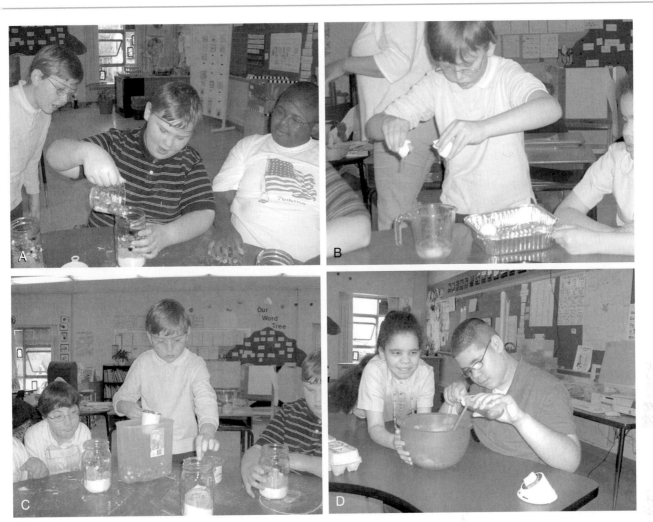

FIGURE 24-7   Brownie Buster group pictures.

the therapy process and particular needs. For example, the occupational therapist may choose to work directly with a student for several weeks to teach the student how to implement the *ALERT Program of Self-Regulation*,[85] followed by consultation with the teacher or paraprofessional to ensure generalization of the strategies in the classroom.

Another factor influencing occupational therapy service provision is a consideration of the different *approaches to intervention*—to promote health, prevent disability, restore function, adapt/modify task, or maintain function. Traditionally, occupational therapy's role in the schools has focused on restoring function and adapting the task or environment to promote participation for children with disabilities. However, the reauthorization of IDEA and NCLB has created new opportunities for occupational therapy to contribute to health promotion and prevention in *all* children. The shift to preventive models of service delivery will likely broaden the definition of "client" for occupational therapists to include all children in general education.

Given the variability, provision based on the unique needs of each child given the who, what, when, where, and why determining needed services, occupational therapists must enter school practice aware of this complexity and the personal and interpersonal skills required to succeed in such an environment. For example, therapists need good organization and time management to develop and maintain their work schedules given the variability of school settings and types of service needs of their particular caseload. Therapists must be as effective and efficient as possible in meeting the complex demands of their job. Providing group interventions to children with and without disabilities, for example, offers an opportunity to serve several children at once and allows the therapist to assess and promote social participation among the group members at the same time.

In addition to the required documentation for the IEP and follow-up progress reports, routine documentation of service provision is not mandated by IDEA. The occupational therapist should develop a method of documentation of services to record the student's progress toward goals, response to interventions, other changes in performance, and strategies that were promising or ineffective.[14]

Scientifically Based Instructional Practices

School-based occupational therapists apply a wide array of intervention methodologies based on a variety of theoretical frames of reference (e.g., sensory integration, motor learning, behavioral, biomechanical). According to IDEA 2004, and consistent with NCLB, schools are required to use "qualified personnel" and "ensure that such personnel have the skills and knowledge necessary to improve the academic achievement and functional performance of children with disabilities, including the use of scientifically based instructional practices, to the maximum extent possible" (§601(c)(5)(E)). *Scientifically based practices* refer to those that have a strong research base, indicating that the interventions will most likely produce the targeted outcomes for students with disabilities. In a recent evidence-based review of occupational therapy school-based practice, Swinth et al. reviewed a number of one group cohort and single-subject design studies; however, a limited number of reports of controlled trials were found.[79]

Integrated Service Delivery

Although IDEA does not specify service delivery types, it does indicate that all related services be *provided in the least restrictive environment* to foster participation in the general education curriculum. Because occupational therapy services support both academic goals (e.g., handwriting and literacy) and functional goals (e.g., organizing materials, self-feeding during lunch), the service context can include a wide range of natural settings including classroom, playground, cafeteria, restroom, and hallways. In addition to promoting the integration of students with disabilities with their nondisabled peers, interventions provided in natural settings during daily routines are more likely to be applied consistently.[2] Because therapists must work closely with teachers to identify intervention opportunities that have the greatest contextual application and generalizability, consultation should be a part of each therapy visit. "Although therapists may pull students out of the classroom for brief periods to explore strategies or to introduce a new skill, time away from instruction is minimized" (p. 3).[68]

Full inclusion refers to a child's access to and participation in all activities of the school setting. Supports and adaptations are provided as needed to enable the child with disabilities to participate in activities with his or her peers. These services are typically provided in the child's neighborhood school. For example, Josh, a child with spina bifida and mild learning disabilities, attends his local, home elementary school in a rural community. Josh is in the regular classroom for the entire day, with a classroom aide assisting him with self-care tasks as needed. The school's special education teacher helps the classroom teacher in adapting Josh's assignments when needed.

Inclusion can consist of a variety of learning options. A student may spend a portion of the day in a resource room and a portion in regular education classes. For instance, Brian, who is in the sixth grade, participates in the regular-education classroom for all of his classes except math and reading. For these subjects, he receives instruction from the resource room teacher because his performance in these classes is significantly lower than that of his peers, and he requires a special curriculum to progress in these areas.

Modifications and accommodations are made to support Brian's learning needs so that he can participate in learning activities. Often, the regular classroom teacher groups students for science and social studies projects so that each of the students is given a task that he or she can manage. Because Brian has difficulty with manipulation, the teacher gives manipulation tasks to the other students in the group and often selects Brian

to search the Internet or oversee final-project assembly. Tests are read to Brian, and he is allowed to dictate his answers. Greg attends full-day, inclusive kindergarten with occupational therapy, physical therapy, and special education supporting his participation in the regular education curriculum (Figure 24-11).

Of note, effectively integrating therapy into the general or special education classroom using both direct and indirect services requires an important set of knowledge and skills. Integrated therapy models imply high levels of collaboration, therapy sessions embedded within the classroom, and working directly with the teacher (e.g., co-teaching). When providing indirect services, occupational therapists use consultation and training of others to implement intervention strategies.

In an integrated therapy model, the practitioner provides intervention in the child's natural environment (e.g., within the classroom, on the playground, in the cafeteria, on and off the school bus) emphasizing nonintrusive methods. The therapist's presence in the classroom benefits the instructional staff members, who observe the occupational therapy intervention. Working within the classroom benefits the therapist in gaining a thorough understanding of the classroom environment and the behavioral and achievement expectations of its students. This integrated model of therapy also allows the student to participate in the classroom activities, with therapy support. Integrated therapy ensures that the therapist's focus has high relevance to the performance expected within the student's classroom. It also promotes the likelihood that adaptations and therapeutic techniques will be carried over into classroom activities.[89] Giangreco described an integrated therapy model as one in which teams that include related services (1) establish a shared set of goals and objectives based on family priorities and participation in the general curriculum; (2) support the teachers' goals; and (3) provide a just-right level of related service support with guidance from the team.[33] Occupational therapists are responsible for ensuring that their services are integral to the education program.[70]

Educational proponents of inclusion who support integrated models of therapy suggest that pull-out services are appropriate only when students need to work on a skill that is far below the tasks presented to other students in the classroom or when the intervention activities cannot appropriately occur in a typical classroom (e.g., therapeutic use of equipment such as a swing). When intervention activities create a distraction that prevents other students from learning or the teacher from teaching, they should be performed outside the classroom.[29] McWilliam cautions that pull-out therapy is less effective than integrated services.[56]

One method to promote integrated services is *block scheduling,* in which therapy sessions are scheduled in longer blocks of time than usual, so that the therapist has time to work within the classroom setting during the times when meaningful activities occur.[71] The overall total therapy time in a given month may remain the same, but the students are seen every other week rather than weekly. If several students are seen in the same classroom, the therapist may continue weekly services for each by combining the students' time. The therapist remains in the classroom for the entire morning or afternoon and moves between students during each of the activities presented. Block scheduling gives the therapist opportunities for *co-teaching* or *team teaching.* In this method, a therapist and a classroom teacher jointly design and implement learning experiences within the classroom setting. The therapist's time is scheduled for the co-planned activities, rather than for individual sessions.

Not only do the targeted students benefit from the interventions, but the other students in the class also benefit from the multidisciplinary input. For example, the classroom teacher and occupational therapist may co-plan a handwriting session. The session may include both the third-grade curriculum and practice of the mechanics of handwriting. Other examples of activities to promote fine motor skills related to school functions are listed in Table 24-5. Activities to improve handwriting skills are listed in Table 24-6.

In integrated services, the occupational therapist may plan a program that involves specific activities for a student, to be carried out with the help of other personnel (e.g., teaching assistant, aide). To enable the person who is chosen to implement the program, the therapist uses modeling and coaching as the child attempts the activities in his or her natural routine. The therapist may give the teacher materials helpful for implementing the intervention (e.g., tongs to practice dynamic grasp, sensory bag, tweezers, clothespins) or help to adapt the environment so that the child can participate (e.g., establish a sensory corner, set up a tent, obtain bean bag chairs, therapy balls, prone standers). Regular contact is necessary to update programs and supervise the manner in which the activities are

TABLE 24-5 Recommended Fine Motor Activities to Improve School Functions

Goal	Activities
Strengthening	PlayDoh, Silly Putty, clay
	Hide and then find tiny pegs, beads, marbles in Silly Putty or PlayDoh
	Crumple paper or tissue paper to fill a bag
	Nuts and bolts
	Roll and pull taffy
	Build with magnets
	Use clothespins on rope
Visual-motor/eye-hand coordination	Cut shapes
	Lite Brite
	Make a necklace
	String macaroni
	Play Jenga
	Use a toy hammer and nails
	Draw with templates
	Use tweezers to pick up small objects
	Lacing projects
Manipulation skills	Place stickers on paper
	Use eye dropper to squirt colored water on paper; place dried peas in a small container with tweezers
	Use a small musical keyboard
	Hold coins and place one at a time into slot
	Use turkey baster to blow ping-pong balls
	Use chopsticks to pick up marshmallows

Adapted from Fine/Visual Motor Activities and Developed by School Therapists, compiled by Deanna Iris Sava, 2004. Retrieved on April 28, 2004, at http://www.otexchange.org. Fine Motor List.

TABLE 24-6 Activities to Prepare Children for Writing

Goal	Strategies/Activities
Improve posture	Adjust the seat and table height
	Recommend standing during writing work
	Use of a therapy ball with a stand
	Use of a "sit n'move" cushion
Improve hand dominance and grasping patterns	Practice cutting
	Use a nuts and bolts game
	Use a toy hammer and nails
	Lacing
	Stringing beads
	Drawing with templates and stencils
Improve use of appropriate force	Using clothespins
	Hiding small objects in PlayDoh
	Practice writing on NCR paper
	Practice writing on sandpaper
	Practice using a mechanical pencil without breaking the tip
Improve tripod grasp	Tweezer games
	Clothespin games
	Manipulation of nuts and bolts
	Twisting on/off lids
	Using small crayons or small chalk
	Lacing
	Using a pencil grip
Improve letter forms	Use color codes to identify top and bottom of each line
	Have the student fill in missing parts of letters
	Practice dot-to-dot pictures and letters
	Draw letter in sand or sugar
	Print over tactile surfaces such as sandpaper
Improve spacing and alignment	Use graph paper and ask the student to leave one box open as a space between words
	Use a popsicle stick between words
	Have student review his or her work and self-correct
	Use paper with raised lines
	Use paper with different colors for each line (e.g., earth paper)
	Have child draw letters in small boxes

From Amundson, S. (1999). *Tricks for written communication.* Homer, Alaska: OTKids, Inc; and Ginsberg-Brown, C., & Schotzer, T. (2004). *Pre-referral form: Intervention strategies.* Retrieved on April 28, 2004, from http://www.otexchange.org.

implemented. Examples of activities that the occupational therapist may initiate and then help staff to implement are positioning a student for written activities and implementation of assistive technology (e.g., adapted keyboard).

When working with students in a classroom, the therapist needs to have a clear understanding of the classroom expectations. This includes knowledge of classroom rules, routines, and dynamics, and knowledge of the general education curriculum and special education adaptations. Each classroom teacher has unique teaching and classroom management styles. Intervention techniques conducted in the classroom that may be acceptable to one teacher may not be acceptable to another teacher; they may even be considered intrusive.

Griswold recommended that therapists offer interventions that fit the existing classroom structure and culture.[37] For example, a teacher who values child-directed learning and hands-on learning centers may respond well to a therapist's suggestions for activities to be included in the learning centers (Figures 24-8 and 24-9). Another teacher who uses a strong teacher-directed classroom may prefer to engage in team-teaching activities with the therapist.

Therapists also need to be sensitive to the regular education schedule and not disrupt the child's and the classroom schedule, if possible. Teachers may prefer to have the therapist in the classroom at certain times or on certain days. These preferences

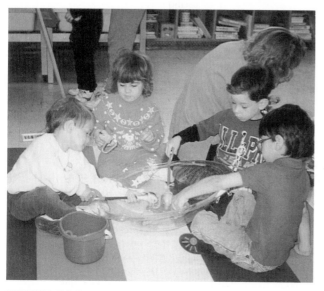

FIGURE 24-8 The occupational therapist may help the teacher establish learning centers for sensory exploration.

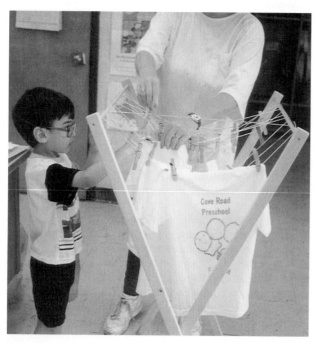

FIGURE 24-9 A fine-motor learning center may include hanging up T-shirts and pictures using clothespins.

should be negotiated with the teacher before intervention, and attempts should be made to schedule times for providing services to the child that coincide with targeted goal areas. For example, handwriting interventions can be integrated into the student's language arts time and keyboarding skills can be addressed during the student's computer or language arts class.

The support that an occupational therapist provides within the school should make both the child and the teacher's jobs easier, without placing unreasonable burdens on either the student or the teacher. Although the teacher's and the therapist's jobs are to support the child's role as a student, at times there is a mismatch between what teachers (and parents) want and what occupational therapists want. Conflicts in point of view can be minimized or avoided if consistent communication is maintained between teachers and support personnel. The responsibility for maintaining open pathways of communication rests equally on all members of the team.

Consultation

"The key to effective collaboration in educational settings is learning to use one's professional knowledge and interpersonal skills to blend hands-on services for students with team and system supports for families, educators, and the school system at large."[41] School-based collaboration involves an interactive team process among students, families, teachers, and related service providers to enhance the academic achievement and functional performance of all students.[41] Occupational therapists are challenged to skillfully blend their role in providing direct hands-on services for students with team and system supports. In consultation, the therapist and the teacher (or other professional) form a cooperative partnership and engage in a reciprocal problem-solving process. One of the goals of consultation is to enhance the skills of the consultee and to improve the targeted performance area of the student. At times, the focus of consultation is on implementation of a specific program for the student. At other times, the focus is more directly on enhancing the teacher's knowledge and skills. Although occupational therapists practicing in schools must learn how to function within an educational model, it is also important to acknowledge therapists' medical background and knowledge base. The occupational therapist's translation of medical information can be used by the multidisciplinary team to make meaningful decisions and provide appropriate services.[14]

To provide effective consultation, the occupational therapist needs (1) in-depth knowledge and understanding of the problem, (2) knowledge of appropriate interventions, and (3) effective communication and interaction skills. The occupational therapist also must thoroughly understand the educational system so that the intervention strategies that he or she recommends are feasible within the system. Understanding the educational system also helps the therapist to ensure that appropriate classroom and student supports are identified. An understanding of the system and school policies is particularly important when the therapist identifies curricular or environmental modifications that would benefit the student's educational program.

Collaborative consultation emphasizes that the consultant and the consultee have equally important roles. The parties agree on and work toward common goals to make decisions. Although the consultant and the consultee work jointly on an equal basis, they have different roles.[90] The consultant structures and guides the overall process, whereas the consultee rovides information about the problem and the expectations. The consultee generally (1) retains responsibility for the student, (2) judges treatment acceptability, and (3) implements the intervention. Because the consultee implements the intervention, it is important that he or she can accurately apply it, recognize the expected or desired response, and judge when modifications to the strategy are needed. It is the responsibility of the consultant to ensure that the consultee is well informed and sensitive to the issues. Therefore, the consultant's responsibilities include (1) presenting a new or more in-depth understanding of the student's problem, (2) identifying and presenting interventions for possible implementation, (3) assisting in selecting the most appropriate and realistic solutions, and (4) developing an evaluation plan. These differing responsibilities suggest that a complementary, interdependent working relationship is needed.[90]

Hanft and Place described types of decision making required in the consultation role.[41] The most appropriate intervention strategies are selected first. These decisions are based on (1) the student's and teacher's goals, (2) the student's problems, (3) the consultee's skills and interaction style, and (4) the flexibility and constraints of the environment. Examples of typical strategies recommended by occupational therapists are listed in Table 24-7.

With appropriate intervention strategies in mind, the occupational therapist selects a method for implementing the strategies. Methods range from very directive (e.g., modeling, teaching) to indirect strategies, where the therapist primarily offers encouragement and support. The occupational therapist also provides specific information to help the teacher in problem solving. The method selected is based on the teacher's knowledge about and experience with children with disabilities and also learning style. One teacher may be quite experienced in working with children with physical disabilities and need little support; another teacher may have minimal experience in working with students with physical disabilities and need more support. An example of occupational therapy services focusing on consultation is described in a Case Study 24-1.

In each model, clarity, specificity, and accuracy of the information are important. In general, a combination of methods works best. For example, the therapist can model joint compression and hand massage before writing activities or one-handed techniques in dressing. Providing written handouts and verbal cues is also helpful in guiding the teacher's facilitation of student's performance. The therapist can ask the teacher to try an intervention, to give the therapist feedback on its success, so that adjustments can be made or the strategies refined. Feedback is important to the success of the interventions over time; the student and the environment continually evolve. The third decision that the therapist must make is selection of interaction style. The occupational therapist selects an interaction style likely to be most effective with the consultee. Interaction styles are defined using different parameters. Examples of interaction styles are achiever, analyst, supporter, and persuader.[24]

These four styles reflect that individuals vary along a continuum of high to low people orientation and of high to low risk-taking. Table 24-8 describes each style and the implication for consulting with an individual with each style.

As Hanft and Place have suggested,[41] the consultant's style varies from being very directive to being primarily supportive, based on the consultee's needs and style. Also, the degree of

TABLE 24-7	Intervention Strategies When Consulting
Intervention Strategies	**Examples**
Reframe the teacher's perspective	Explain the functional consequences of the perceptual problems observed in children with spina bifida.
	Identify that a child with autism is hypersensitive to tactile and auditory stimuli.
	Suggest that a child's difficulty in sitting quietly is related to his or her low arousal level and need for sensory input.
Improve the student's skills	Recommend that a student use carbon paper to monitor the amount of force applied with the pencil.
	Recommend that a student practice letter formation, using wide-lined paper and beginning at the top of the letter.
	Recommend that a teacher provide standby assistance when the child practices carrying a lunch tray in the cafeteria.
Adapt the task	Recommend that a student begin to use a computer keyboard.
	Introduce compensatory methods for putting on a jacket.
	Teach one-handed techniques during toilet training.
	Recommend that a student use earphones with music during written tests.
Adapt the environment	Establish a quiet area with a tent in which students can hide and remove themselves from the stimulating environment.
	Suggest that excess visual stimulation be removed from the wall in front of a student.
Adapt the routine	Recommend that a student have opportunities for exercise three times each day.
	Recommend that a student be given extra time to complete certain written assignments.
	Suggest that the student receive speech therapy after occupational therapy so that he or she can be focused and attentive during the session.

specificity and detail depend on the consultee's preference and ability to generalize concepts and principles. It is important that occupational therapists identify their own style, so that they can recognize when styles may conflict and when changes in the predominant approach are needed.

Annual Review and Reevaluation

The student's IEP must be reviewed by the IEP team at least once a year, or more often if the parents or school requests a review. Outcomes are measured by student achievement of the IEP goals, including participation on state and districtwide assessments.[2] At the time of review, it is important to keep in mind one of the primary goals of IDEA 2004—to improve student academic achievement and functional outcomes in

CASE STUDY 24-1 William

This case study emphasizes teamwork and consultation with a student preparing to enter high school. William was 13 years old and in middle school. He was the oldest of three children and loved nothing more than being with his younger brother and sister. At age 2, William had suffered a severe traumatic brain injury when he was in a car accident. He emerged from a 3-week coma with no movement on his right side and no speech. Although he regained some function in his right arm and leg, his movement remained quite impaired. William demonstrated partial range in his right shoulder and elbow but was unable to move his wrist and fingers. He used a one-hand drive wheelchair for mobility and could stand with assistance and take several steps. However, independent ambulation was not a goal.

William was essentially nonverbal in preschool. However, by age 13 he used two- and four-word phrases appropriately. He impulsively responded to every query by saying "no" when he generally meant "yes," and he required a long time to think of words. The words he could produce were quite simple, his cognitive limitations were severe, and learning required many repetitions. William's primary asset was his social nature. He was friendly and cheerful; he offered everyone a smile. He tried new activities, even when they caused him discomfort. Staff in the school and his peers reported that they enjoyed being around William.

PARTICIPATION IN THE SCHOOL ENVIRONMENT

Information about William's level of participation at school was gathered from his mother and his teacher. His mother reported that he was easy-going and happy. At times he demonstrated some frustration, because he had become more aware that he was different from other children. His mother's greatest concerns related to his judgment. He did not seem to understand when he was in danger and when he could hurt someone else. His mother reported that he had begun to develop some peer relations. In the past, he would spend time at school by himself. However, in middle school he had established some friendships and spent more time interacting with his peers.

William's teacher reported that he was a "doll, as sweet as he could be." His academic work was at a low level, and he required extra time to complete all work. However, he had made steady, slow progress in his reading and writing.

His teacher was concerned with his safety. She worried about his judgment, particularly outside the classroom. Currently his reading program emphasized safety words and concepts.

William had great difficulty in handling his school materials. He printed with cueing. However, his letters were poorly formed. He used a keyboard, also with verbal prompts. He independently turned on the computer and operated preschool-age storybook programs. Most of his work required assistance to keep him focused and to read difficult words. Both handwriting and keyboarding required great amounts of time and effort.

PERFORMANCE IN SCHOOL ACTIVITIES

Self-Maintenance. William ate independently in the cafeteria after his cartons were opened and his food was cut up. Eating was a favorite activity. He required minimal assistance to put on his jacket because he continued to neglect his right arm and only dressed his left side. William required assistance during two-handed activities and needed minimal assistance in transferring from his wheelchair to the toilet.

Manipulation of Materials and Writing. William required intermittent assistance to manage his school materials. He tended to neglect materials on his right side, and activities needed to be placed on his left side. He was unable to use scissors or other tools that required two hands. To help him write, William's paper was stabilized on his desk with a clipboard and Dycem. In writing, his letters were large and poorly formed. He copied letters but did not compose.

Posture and Mobility. William's posture had deteriorated in the previous year; he leaned to the right with a rounded trunk. Poor posture had begun to interfere with eye-hand coordination and his ability to move his left arm. In addition, the occupational therapist was concerned about the potential for development of scoliosis.

Behaviors. William was cooperative and pleasant. He followed instructions, although at times he did not attend well to classroom instructions. In addition, William continued to need one-on-one supervision for many activities, primarily because of his low cognitive level and his difficulty in problem solving the steps of a task. However, he initiated social interaction and consistently responded to others. He was motivated to try new activities and demonstrated persistence, particularly in one-on-one situations. Judgment remained a problem and seemed to relate to his impulsiveness and deficits in problem solving.

OCCUPATIONAL THERAPY SERVICES

The occupational therapist contributed to all of these performance issues. She worked with William in a small group of his peers, generally on computing skills and functional mobility within the school environment. She used several typing programs that could be graded easily for beginners. William's favorite was "Slam Dunk" because he was an avid basketball fan. His family also purchased this program for practice at home.

The occupational therapist adapted William's wheelchair to improve his posture by moving his tray to a higher position and recommending a new strapping system that included a chest strap. A lateral pad on the right was tried, but it was not effective when he slumped forward in trunk flexion.

Once a month, William's therapy group planned and completed a community outing. A variety of field trips were planned, including a trip to a restaurant, a movie, a shopping trip, and a visit to a nearby factory and the post office. The purpose of these field trips was to increase William's ability to function in the community. Safety concepts were practiced and reinforced, including crossing the street, mobility around stairs and escalators, and care of his right arm. Appropriate social interactions with strangers and service persons were practiced. Basic concepts regarding handling money, ordering food and service, and requesting assistance were also emphasized.

These community outings were extremely helpful in identifying issues that would need to be addressed in the coming years, when William's ability to function in the community would become an important goal. Transition into community living and vocation can be addressed at age 14, and these experiences helped the team establish realistic goals for the next year's IEP.

Courtesy Janet Rogers.

TABLE 24-8   Consultation by Interaction Style

Style	Primary Characteristics of Consultee	Implications for the Consultant
Achiever	Consultee is directive, likes to make decisions, is a risk taker, likes to be in charge, needs an end goal, and may not be sensitive to personal issues in desire to accomplish a goal.	Consultant needs to be directive and assertive; should keep recommendations short, make measurable, achievable recommendations; allow the achiever to feel in charge; should be incisive.
Analyst	Consultee is precise, detail oriented, low in people orientation, and therefore satisfied to work on own; needs lots of data to act, and needs to know that solutions are correct. Consultee implements recommendations with high precision; not a risk taker.	Consultant needs to give detailed, precise directives, and have patience with the analyst's need for information. Consultant should not push this person into decisions and should respect the person's analytical ability. Include data collection in the plan. Consultant should encourage decision making in a timely way. The consultant should minimize risks.
Persuader	Consultee is enthusiastic, good at influencing others, relates well to almost everyone. Consultee is highly people oriented and is a high-risk taker; will sell solutions to the consultant. Consultee does not need details—likes to take action.	This consultee is fun to consult with, but follow-up is necessary. Often this person will try whatever is readily available in the environment. Consultant needs to be aware that the consultee is easily influenced and may jump tracks midstream. Consultant should market ideas with enthusiasm and optimism.
Supporter	Consultee is encouraging and supportive of everyone, has high people orientation skills, and prefers that people get along rather than achieve specific goals. Consultee is good at holding together a team; may not be efficient in implementing recommendations because this person easily becomes overcommitted.	Consultant's job is easy because this person is agreeable and flexible. Consultant should listen attentively and make clear recommendations that include a rationale. It is important to be positive because this consultee is often sensitive. Follow-up is needed because often the supporter has taken on too much. Consultee may be slow to respond to recommendations because of other commitments.

Adapted from DeBoer, A. (1991). *The art of consulting.* Chicago: Arcturus.

addition to postsecondary success. The long-term goal is for students with disabilities to leave high school prepared to work, attend higher education, and live independently.

Termination of related services may be decided at any annual review if the team determines that the related service is not necessary for the student to benefit from her or his IEP. The occupational therapist may recommend termination when the student has acquired the needed skills and uses them during school, when needed adaptations and supports are in place, or when services have failed to produce the desired outcomes despite numerous approaches and lengthy attempts.[68] At least every 3 years, the child must be reevaluated to determine if he or she continues to be a "child with a disability" as defined by IDEA and then to redefine the child's educational needs.

NEW DIRECTIONS IN SCHOOL-BASED PRACTICE: PREVENTION-BASED MULTITIERED SERVICES AND SCHOOL MENTAL HEALTH

Prevention-Based Multitiered Services

The reauthorization of IDEA in 1997 ended a long period during which special education and general education were viewed as separate programs serving separate populations.[75] IDEA 1997 placed greater emphasis on the inclusion of students with disabilities in general education by embedding special education and related services in the classroom and extracurricular activities when possible. General and special education practices have further aligned as a result of IDEA 2004 and NCLB, providing school personnel including occupational therapists with increasing opportunities to expand their role in schools, particularly in the area of prevention.[13]

These shifting roles can be visualized as a movement from a two-tiered to multitiered model of service delivery (Figure 24-10). The traditional two-tiered system represents students falling into one of two categories—children with disabilities who meet eligibility criteria as outlined in IDEA or Section 504 and receive services *or* students in general education who do not receive services. A concern with this system is that some children in general education with learning or behavioral difficulties do *not* qualify for services under IDEA. In such instances, children may experience frustration and failure before becoming eligible for special education and related services.[13] In contrast, a multitiered model of supports and services commits to the success of *all* students by providing early identification and intervening services.

To address increasing concerns among parents, teachers, and policymakers that some students have not received needed help in a timely manner, two provisions in IDEA 2004 enable schools to help students struggling with learning or behavior before they are referred to special education.[63] These are *early intervening services* (EIS) and *response to intervention* (RtI).

Comprehensive EIS are designed to help students in general education who are *not* eligible for special education but who need additional academic and behavioral supports to succeed in school (34 CFR §300.226). Schools are allowed to spend up to 15% of special education funds for EIS, including professional development for teachers and other staff and to fund direct services, such as small group instruction, behavioral evaluations and supports, or information on the use of adaptive and instructional software. *Related services* are specifically included in IDEA 2004 (§300.208) as possible EIS. In addition, under NCLB, occupational therapists may function as *pupil services personnel* (professionals who provide services to students) in providing EIS.

The second provision in IDEA 2004 developed to prevent school failure is the response-to-intervention (RtI) process.

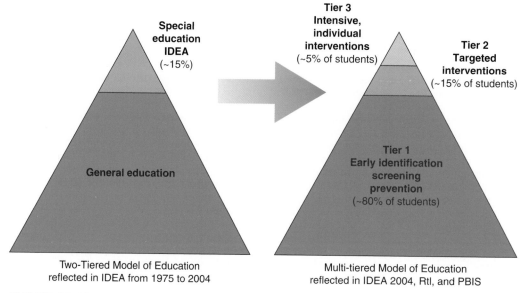

FIGURE 24-10　Tiered model of education.

Federal regulations (34 C.F.R. §§300.307–309) require that states adopt criteria for determining that a child has a specific learning disability.[83] RtI is a research-based model of school-wide support services that focuses on providing high-quality instruction and intervention matched to student needs followed by systematically looking at their response to education/intervention.[61,73] Although originally explored as an approach assisting students with specific learning disabilities, evidence has supported its effectiveness for any student with academic or behavioral problems.[5,52]

The overall purpose of RtI is one of prevention and early intervention—to identify and address student problems early to reduce the need for more intensive services later. Typical practices underpinning an RtI model include (1) high-quality general education instruction based on scientific evidence, (2) continuous progress monitoring of student performance, (3) universal screening of academics and behavior, and (4) the use of multiple tiers of instruction that are progressively more intense based on the student's response to intervention.[83] Most states and local districts use a multitiered model of interventions and supports made up of three levels—*Tier 1* (universal or core instruction); *Tier 2* (targeted intervention); and *Tier 3* (intensive intervention). In a three-tiered model, the first tier provides school- or classroom-wide interventions made up of high quality instructional, behavioral, and social supports for *all* students.[73] Whole-class screening is used to assess whether academic and behavioral performance is appropriate for the student's age and grade. For the group of struggling students, Tier 2–targeted interventions may be developed by student support teams (SSTs) to address specific needs. Interventions and supports at this level may include small group interventions or more intensive instruction such as tutoring. At this level, interventions reflect more intensive 1:1 services and supports provided within general education or special education.

With the growing movement to a three-tiered system of service provision, it is important for occupational therapists to envision, articulate, and advocate for their role within each of the tiers. For example, occupational therapists should educate student-support teams on how their services can meet the academic and behavioral needs of students in general education.[45] At Tier 1 (schoolwide services), occupational therapists can assist the general education team in helping students access and participate in the curriculum by paying careful attention to areas of function within our scope of practice—education, social participation, play/leisure, activities of daily living, and work. For instance, the occupational therapist may participate in universal screening of handwriting to identify students who are struggling (depending on whether the state allows screening).[3] This might be followed by providing a teacher in-service training presentation on multisensory strategies for teaching handwriting and joining a curriculum committee to assist in identifying an appropriate handwriting curriculum. To help foster student attendance and positive behavior, the occupational therapist might assist educators in implementing the *ALERT Program* in their classroom.[85] In addition, the occupational therapist might join a school team working on a student conduct and behavior management program to become aware of issues in this area and offer strategies from an occupational therapy perspective.

At Tier 2 (targeted interventions for those at risk), the occupational therapist might develop a social skills group for students struggling with behavior management and social interaction with peers. Tier 3 interventions call for more individualized interventions for those not responding to Tier 2 interventions. At this level, students may receive such services as a part of RtI or may be referred for special education.

With opportunities to expand occupational therapy's role in general education, therapists might be questioning how they can create time to provide prevention and early intervening services. Traditionally, an occupational therapist's job expectations have been based on a *caseload* model of counting the number of children receiving direct intervention as a part of their IEP.[4] This model often neglects to account for essential indirect services including collaborative consultation, team meetings, and in-service trainings.[76] In contrast, the concept of *workload* encompasses all of the direct and indirect services performed to benefit students making a workload approach helpful for conceptualizing work patterns that optimize effectiveness and impact.[4] Occupational therapists must have the flexibility of organizing their work patterns to serve students in their LRE, collaborate with teachers and other school personnel, attend meetings, supervise and train occupational therapy assistants, plan interventions, and collect data. Careful documentation of workload using a time study may help state regulatory boards become knowledgeable about the range of occupational therapy services and encourage them to adopt a workload versus caseload system of documenting service provision. Kentucky, for example, has adopted a workload model, defining workload as "the amount of minutes per day, week, or month a therapist needs to work to adequately perform his/her duties" (p. 43).[75]

OCCUPATIONAL THERAPY'S ROLE IN SCHOOL MENTAL HEALTH

The School Mental Health Movement

Although mental health services for children have historically been provided in hospitals and community mental health centers, the EHA of 1975 was the first federal initiative that required schools to meet the mental health needs of students with emotional disturbance, playing a key role in blurring the lines of responsibility for where such services should be provided.[7,53] Because IDEA focuses solely on students with identifiable disabilities that interfere with educational achievement, only a small percentage of children needing mental health services actually receive such care in school. Nonetheless, most children receiving mental health services obtain care in schools, making schools the "de facto mental health system for children in this country" (p. 62) (see Figure 24-1).[53]

A national movement to develop and expand school mental health (SMH) services has grown during the past 2 decades as a result of the high prevalence of mental health conditions among youth and the awareness that more youth can be reached in schools.[54,84] Approximately one in five children ages 9 to 17 have a diagnosable emotional or behavioral disorder, with the most common being anxiety, depression, conduct disorders, and attention-deficit/hyperactive disorder (ADHD) (see Chapter 13).[51] Prominent federal initiatives (Surgeon General's Report on Children's Mental Health, 1999, and President's New Freedom Commission on Mental Health, 2003) have identified fragmented services and gaps in care, forcing federal, state, and local child-serving agencies to address the mental health needs of children attending school.[84] As a result of federal support, two national technical assistance centers were developed in 1995 to promote mental health in schools—the Center for Mental Health in Schools at the University of California at Los Angeles (UCLA) and the Center for School Mental Health Analysis and Action (CSMA) at the University of Maryland. Despite the recent emphasis on SMH, the field can be viewed as underdeveloped and emerging—far too many children continue to be underidentified and underserved in schools.[51] Schools must be active partners in the mental health of children because it is currently accepted that a major barrier to learning is immature or limited social-emotional skills and not necessarily cognitive impairment.[50]

Multitiered Public Health Model of School Mental Health

Although the mental health field has traditionally been viewed as the domain of mental health specialists, it is now acknowledged that addressing mental health issues is far too complex to relegate to a few professionals. Experts are calling for a paradigm shift to better prepare *all* school personnel (teachers, administrators, psychologists, social workers, and related service providers) to proactively address the mental health needs of *all* students.[50] Teachers and other front line personnel, including occupational therapists, play a crucial role in the development of children from both an academic and personal, social, and emotional perspectives.

The failure to adequately provide mental health services for children has been viewed as a major public health concern, causing leaders in the field to propose a *public health model* of service delivery to address the needs of all children.[23,50] A public health model supports a systemwide shift from an individual, deficit-driven model of intervention to a schoolwide strength-based model focusing on prevention, early intervention, and integration of services for all children. Similar to RtI, three major tiers of service are promoted—*universal or schoolwide intervention, selective/targeted interventions,* and *intensive individualized interventions* (Figure 24-11).

The Role of Occupational Therapy

With occupational therapy's rich history of addressing mental health in all areas of practice, along with the call for all school personnel to proactively address children's mental health,[7] the role of occupational therapy in SMH seems clear.[7] Occupational therapy practitioners have specialized knowledge and skills in addressing psychosocial and mental health needs of individuals and thus are well positioned to contribute to all three levels of prevention and intervention. A continuum of occupational therapy early intervening services (EIS) aimed at social emotional and mental health promotion, prevention of problem behaviors, early detection through screening, and intensive intervention is recommended. Depending on state guidelines, these services could involve occupational therapy practitioners working directly with students, providing professional development for school personnel, or working collaboratively with teachers and parents.

Occupational therapists can use a number of traditional approaches to guide service provision within a public health model including meaningful occupations and sensory strategies. The findings of a recent evidence-based literature review, for example, indicate that activity-based interventions help improve children's peer interactions, task-focused behaviors, and conformity to social norms.[46] An example of an activity-based approach to foster successful completion is analyzing and modifying homework requirements for a child experiencing anxiety. Other traditional occupational therapy approaches used to evaluate and address the psychosocial needs of children include sensory-based interventions and social learning theory.

In addition to traditional occupational therapy intervention approaches, other approaches developed in the fields of psychology and education are often used by occupational therapists—social-emotional learning (SEL) and positive behavior supports (PBSs).

Social-Emotional Learning

In 1994, *social and emotional learning* was developed as a conceptual framework to focus on the emotional needs of children and address the fragmented programs meant to address those needs.[36] SEL is defined as "the process of acquiring the skills to recognize and manage emotions, develop caring and concern for others, make responsible decisions, establish positive relationships, and handle challenging situations effectively."[16] Programs developed to enhance SEL help children recognize their emotions, think about their feelings and how one should act, and regulate their behavior based on thoughtful decision making.[28] As a national leader in the field, the Collaborative for Academic, Social, and Emotional Learning (CASEL) focuses on the development of high-quality, evidence-based SEL programs, promoting these as a necessary part of preschool through high school education. Under the leadership of CASEL, the state of Illinois, by developing social and emotional learning standards for schools, has become an example for the nation.

Positive Behavior Support

PBS interventions and supports are designed to prevent problem behaviors by proactively altering a situation before problems escalate, and by concurrently teaching appropriate alternatives. This approach recognizes that a number of relevant factors can influence a student's behavior, including those existing within the child, and those reflected in the interaction between the child and the environment.[74] Schoolwide PBS systems support *all* students along a continuum of need based on the three-tiered prevention model depicted in Figure 24-11. For students receiving services under IDEA, PBS is mandated for those whose behavior impedes the child's learning or that of others (§614(d)(3)(B)(i)).

Within a three-tiered public health model, occupational therapy practitioners can provide a continuum of services geared toward mental health promotion, prevention, early identification, and intervention. Intervention strategies should be integrated into the student's classroom schedule, school routines, and curriculum. An example of an interdisciplinary social skills group for young students involving an occupational therapist, speech language pathologist, and special educator is presented in Box 24-5. In addition, sample occupational therapy activities for each tier of the public health model of SMH are depicted in Table 24-9. These activities should be designed in accordance with scientifically based evidence to the extent possible.

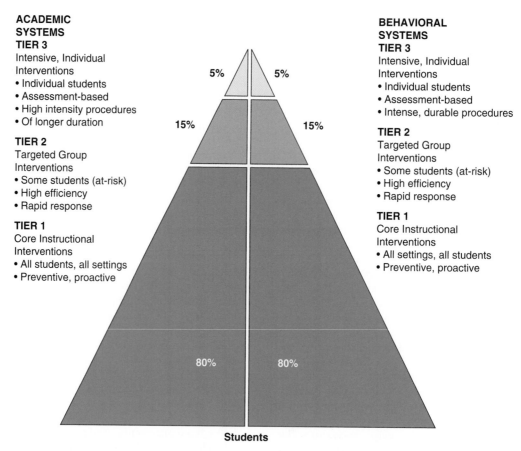

FIGURE 24-11 Academic and behavioral tiered levels of intervention. (Data from National Association of State Directors of Special Education & Council of Administrators of Special Education [CASE]. [2006]. Retrieved from http://www.nasdse.org/Portals/0/Documents/Download%20Publications/RtlAnAdministrators Perspective1-06.pdf.)

BOX 24-5 Occupational Therapy Services Focusing on Social-Emotional Learning: Teaching Social Skills

The children enter the room one by one or in pairs, locate the clothespin with their name printed on it, and clamp it to the "Engine Chart." This program is based on the concepts from *How Does Your Engine Run?* (Williams & Shellenberger, 1996), a guide developed to help children monitor their internal signals that indicate readiness to work, play, listen, attend, and participate in the activities of life. The 11 kindergartners, first graders, and second graders greet each other and wait for this social skills group to start. Three special education teachers, a speech-language pathologist, and an occupational therapist run the program.

Michelle has to be coaxed from behind the door, and Randy is having a bad day, so he is spoken to quietly by a teacher. After the students have "signed in," I step to the front of the room and hold up a strip of paper with the sentence "My engine is in _____ because _____." Annie starts. "My engine is in high today because my mother is taking me for ice cream after school. I am really excited," she beams. Each student takes a turn describing his or her engine speed and the emotions behind that speed. Today, most of them have engines running "just right." Two children are happy, one is calm, one is tired, several have to be cued by their teachers or peers, and one (Randy) is "really mad" at having to "do work." Most have accurately identified how they at least appear to others. Next we sing the "Engine Song," complete with actions, and review the "High Five Listening Song" (two songs I developed for groups like this).

Michelle is one of several group members with autism. She used to play in isolation and entertain herself with "video talk." Randy has a physical disability and uses a wheelchair. When he joined the group, he tended to expect others to anticipate his needs and talked more to adults than to his classmates. Annie takes medication to help her pay attention. She has had trouble with peer relationships and tried to enforce all school rules in an aggressive manner. Before joining the group, Jeff had no peer relationships, bossed his classmates around, demanded attention, and lacked awareness of many social rules, such as sharing a toy or wiping his mouth after eating.

The group was formed when the special education team met in the fall to discuss the best ways to meet the social and learning needs of their students. Children chosen for the social skills group were all included with typical peers for at least part of the school day but demonstrated significant problems with social awareness, peer relationships, self-regulatory behaviors, and language expression, which interfered with their childhood occupations of student and friend. Every child in the group received speech and language services, and all but one received special education support. Seven children received occupational therapy.

Part of my contribution as an occupational therapist was to help the team develop a uniform terminology for the students and adults to describe their behavior to others. We used the Alert Program described in *How Does Your Engine Run?* as a foundation. By tying emotions and arousal level to three speeds—high, low, and just right—we helped the children relabel some of the behaviors they thought of as "bad." When the group formed, we sent a letter home so that the parents could use the same terms. Because team members delivered additional services to the children in their classrooms using "push-in" rather than "pull-out" models, general education teachers also became familiar with our program's terms and goals.

Much of the fall was spent with the students manufacturing engine speed cards and sensory tools to assist with self-regulation. They documented their sessions using a fill-in-the-blank format to inform their parents of the group activities. Occasionally a parent would drop in to observe or assist with the group. When the team members felt satisfied that the children were ready to use the terms and strategies to work on social skills development, the children were divided into three groups, each led by an adult. A teacher and I were "floaters" to help with visuals, sensory supports, or discipline.

Pertinent IEP objectives were printed on recording sheets so that each group leader could refer to them. After I directed a 15-minute sensory-based opening, each group leader was responsible for leading a 20- to 25-minute activity based on a monthly theme, such as asking a friend to play, sportsmanship, anger management, or self-control. Each week the children went to a different group leader, and on the fourth week of each month, I took the entire group for some form of sensory activity or to develop a group social story to review taught skills or to preview the next month's theme.

Because of the children's differences in communication skills, cognition, and attention levels, we chose themes based on the character education concepts used schoolwide and on real-life problems the children displayed in their day-to-day interactions with peers. Each group facilitator used a variety of methods and media to illustrate the theme. The speech-language pathologist used role-playing in her planned groups and developed a board game based on "wh" questions to teach conversational skills. The teachers chose books, videos, and games to teach sportsmanship, turn taking, and anger management. Software programs, such as Boardmaker and PixWriter, were used to create visuals and social stories that were integrated into the children's mainstream classrooms. Lesson plans developed during the team planning sessions were circulated so that the floating teacher or I could fill in when a group member was absent. All lesson plans, documentation, stories, and ideas were placed in a notebook so that our work could be duplicated the following year. During whole-group handwriting lessons that I directed in two of the mainstream classes, the special education teacher and I incorporated themes and behavioral expectations into the warm-up and writing activities, modeling for students the importance of using their "engine" strategies in all settings.

As the year drew to a close, the group leaders evaluated the effectiveness of the group and agreed that all the children had displayed documented improvements. Michelle's "video talk" had reduced in frequency with the "high five" signal, and she pouted less when corrected. Annie still played primarily by herself, but she was not as bossy. Randy relied less on adults, had better social relationships with his peers, and probably no longer needed the group. Other group members appeared more thoughtful, conscientious, or aware of the impact of their behavior on others. At a recent IEP meeting, the parent of a child who is prone to unexpected outbursts said that for the first time her daughter could verbalize how she was feeling and why. In addition, two of the mainstream classroom teachers used the same strategies and terminology in their classrooms, with positive results for the entire class.

From Schoonover, J. (2002). Excerpt from Swinth, Y., & Hanft, B. (2002). School-based practice: Moving beyond 1:1 service delivery. *OT Practice, 7*(16), 12–14, 16–20.

TABLE 24-9 Sample Activities Provided by Occupational Therapy Under a Public Health Model of School Mental Health

Tier	Activities
TIER 3 Intensive interventions for high-risk students	Analyze the student's unique sensory needs and develop intervention strategies to promote sensory processing and successful function in multiple school contexts (e.g., classroom, cafeteria) Identify ways to modify or enhance school routines to reduce stress and the likelihood of behavioral outbursts Provide individual or group intervention to students with serious emotional disturbance (SED), through either special education or Section 504 to enhance participation in education, social participation, play/leisure, and activities of daily living Assist teachers in modifying classroom expectations based on the student's specific behavioral or mental health needs Collaborate with the school-based mental health providers to ensure a coordinated system of care for students needing intensive interventions Assist in the implementation of the Functional Behavior Assessment (FBA) and development and implementation of the Behavioral Intervention Plan (BIP)
TIER 2 Selective or targeted intervention; at-risk students	Assist in early identification of mental health problems by providing formal and/or informal screenings of psychosocial function to at-risk students (e.g., Social Skills Rating Scale) Recognize symptoms of illness at their onset and create intervention or modifications to prevent acute illness from occurring Evaluate social participation with peers during all school activities including recess and lunch Analyze the sensory, social, and cognitive demands of school tasks and recommend adaptations to support a student's participation Provide early intervening services or Section 504 accommodations for students demonstrating behavioral or learning difficulties due to mild mental health disorders or psychosocial issues Consult with teachers to modify learning demands and academic routines to support a student's development of specific social-emotional skills Provide parent education on how to adapt family routines or activities to support children's mental health, especially with high-risk children Develop and run group programs to foster social participation for students struggling with peer interaction Provide psychoeducation in-services training programs to educate teachers about the early signs of mental illness and appropriate accommodations Provide an in-service to school personnel, including the mental health providers, about occupational therapy's unique role in the promotion of mental health and intervention for mental health dysfunction
TIER 1 Schoolwide, universal	Evaluate lunch and recess environments for factors that may impede social participation for any student Assist teachers and other school personnel in developing and implementing schoolwide PBS for various contexts—classroom, hallways, lunchroom, playground, and restrooms (e.g., establish clear rules, foster a positive classroom environment) Informally observe *all* children for behaviors that might suggest mental health concerns or limitations in social-emotional development; bring concerns to the educational team. Provide in-service training to teachers and staff on the following topics: Sensory processing—How to adapt classroom practices based on students' varying sensory needs to enhance attending and behavior regulation (e.g., The Alert Program) Social emotional learning (SEL)—how to embed SEL activities within classroom routines and activities (e.g., identifying feelings, thinking about how feelings influence behavior, perspective taking) Psychoeducation—Educate teachers about the early signs of mental illness and proactive strength-based prevention strategies Tips for promoting successful functioning throughout the school day, including transitioning to classes, organizing work spaces such as desk and locker, handling stress, and developing strategies for time management Consult with teachers to help them recognize the student's most effective learning styles; ensure that students are able to meet classroom demands and create modifications if needed Clearly articulate the scope of occupational therapy practice as including social participation, social-emotional function, and mental health (all tiers)

SUMMARY

Occupational therapists must skillfully combine a sound understanding of occupational therapy's role with children with a current understanding of the evolving school context. Over the past 10 years, special and general education services have gradually aligned as a result of IDEA 2004 and NCLB, providing occupational therapists with opportunities to expand their role, particularly in the direction of prevention and early intervention. Providing services in natural contexts, collaborating effectively with school personnel and parents, shifting from caseload to workload models, developing prevention strategies, and advocating for a role in general education are among the important roles of occupational therapists. By embracing these changes and developing the knowledge and skills to work in new ways, occupational therapists can help all children participate successfully in and enjoy school.

REFERENCES

1. American Occupational Therapy Association. (2008). Occupational therapy practice framework: Domain and process (2nd ed.). *American Journal of Occupational Therapy, 62,* 625–683.
2. American Occupational Therapy Association. (2004). Occupational therapy services in early intervention and school-based programs. *American Journal of Occupational Therapy, 59,* 681–685.
3. American Occupational Therapy Association. (2006). *FAQ on response to intervention for school-based occupational therapists and occupational therapy assistants.* Bethesda, MD: American Occupational Therapy Association.
4. American Occupational Therapy Association. (2006). *Transforming caseload to workload in school-based early intervention occupational therapy services.* Bethesda, MD: American Occupational Therapy Association.
5. Ardoin, S. P., Witt, J. C., Connell, J. E., & Koenig, J. L. (2005). Application of a three-tiered response to intervention model for instructional planning, decision making, and the identification of children needing services. *Journal of Psychoeducational Assessment, 23,* 362–380.
6. Bazyk, S. (2005). Exploring the development of meaningful work for children and youth in Western contexts. *WORK: A Journal of Prevention, Assessment, & Rehabilitation, 24,* 11–20.
7. Bazyk, S. (2007). Addressing the mental health needs of children in schools. In L. Jackson (Ed.), *Occupational therapy services for children and youth under IDEA* (3rd ed.). Bethesda, MD: American Occupational Therapy Association.
8. Bazyk, S., Schefkind, S., Brandenburger Shasby, S., Olson, L., Richman, J., & Gross, M. (2008). *FAQ on School Mental Health for school-based occupational therapy practitioners.* American Occupational Therapy Association.
9. Beery, K. E., Buktenica, N. A., & Beery, N. A. (2004). *Beery-Buktenica Developmental Test of Visual-Motor Integration* (5th ed.). San Antonio, TX: Psych Corp.
10. Brandenburger-Shasby, S. (2005). School-based practice: Acquiring the knowledge and skills. *American Journal of Occupational Therapy, 59,* 88–96.
11. Bruininks, B. D., & Bruininks, R. H. (2005). *BOT-2: Bruininks-Oseretsky Test of Motor Proficiency* (2nd ed.). San Antonio, TX: Psych Corp.
12. Burtner, P., McMain, M. P., & Crowe, T. K. (2002). Survey of occupational therapy practitioners in southwestern schools: Assessments used and preparation of students for school-based practice. *Physical and Occupational Therapy in Pediatrics, 22*(1), 25–39.
13. Cahill, S. M. (2007). A perspective on response to intervention. *Special Interest Section Quarterly: School System, 14*(3), 1–4.
14. Carrasco, R. C., Skees-Hermes, S., Frolek-Clark, G., Polichino, J. E., & Ralabate, P., et al. (2007). Occupational therapy service delivery to support child and family participation in context. In L. L. Jackson (Ed.), *Occupational therapy services for children and youth under IDEA* (3rd ed.). Bethesda, MD: American Occupational Therapy Association.
15. Colarusso & Hammill. (2002). *Motor-free Visual Perception Test* (3rd ed.). Austin, TX: Pro-Ed.
16. Collaborative for Academic, Social, and Emotional Learning (CASEL). (2006). Retrieved April 15, 2008 from http://www.casel.org
17. Coster, W. J. (1995). Development. In C. A. Trombly (Ed.), *Occupational therapy for physical dysfunction* (4th ed., pp. 255–264). Baltimore: Williams & Wilkins.
18. Coster, W. J. (1998). Occupation-centered assessment of children. *American Journal of Occupational Therapy, 52,* 337–344.
19. Coster, W., Deeney, T., Haltiwanger, J., & Haley, S. (1998). *School Function Assessment.* San Antonio, TX: Psychological Corp.
20. Council for Exceptional Children. (1999). *IEP team guide.* Arlington, VA: Council for Exceptional Children.
21. Csikszentmihalyi, M. (1993). Activity and happiness: Towards a science of occupation. *Occupational Science: Australia, 1,* 38–42.
22. Davies, P. L., Soon, P. L., Young, M., & Clausen-Yamaki, A. (2004). Validity and reliability of the School Function Assessment in elementary school students with disabilities. *Physical & Occupational Therapy in Pediatrics, 24,* 23–43.
23. Davis, N. J. (2002). The promotion of mental health and the prevention of mental and behavioral disorders: Surely the time is right. *International Journal of Emergency Mental Health, 4,* 3–29.
24. DeBoer, A. L. (1991). *The art of consulting.* Chicago: Arcturus Books.
25. Dunn, W. W. (1999). *Sensory Profile.* San Antonio, TX: Psychological Corp.
26. Dunn, W. W. (2006). *Sensory Profile School Companion.* San Antonio. TX: Pearson.
27. Elias, M. J. (2003). *Academic and social-emotional learning: Educational practices series-11.* Geneva: International Academy of Education.
28. Elias, M. J., Zins, J. D., Weissberg, R. P., Frey, K. S., Greenberg, M. T., & Haynes, N. M., et al. (1997). *Promoting social and emotional learning: Guidelines for educators.* Alexandria, VA: Association for Supervision and Curriculum.
29. Elliot, D., & McKenny, M. (1998). Four inclusion models that work. *Teaching Exceptional Students, 30*(4), 54–58.
30. Fisher, A. G., & Short-DeGraff, M. (1993). Nationally speaking—Improving functional assessment in occupational therapy: Recommendations and philosophy for change. *American Journal of Occupational Therapy, 47,* 199–200.
31. Folio, M. R., & Fewell, R. R. (2000). *Peabody Developmental Motor Scales (PDMS-2).* Austin, TX: Pro-Ed.
32. Giangreco, M. F. (1995). Related services decision-making: A foundational component of effective education for students with disabilities. *Physical and Occupational Therapy in Pediatrics, 15*(2), 47–67.
33. Giangreco, M. F. (1996). *Vermont interdependent services team approach: A guide to coordinating education support services.* Baltimore: Brookes.
34. Giangreco, M. F. (2001). *Guidelines for making decisions about IEP services.* Montpelier, VT: Vermont Department of Education.
35. Glennon, T. J., Miller Kuhaneck, H., Parham, D., Henry, D. A., & Ecker, C. (2007). *Sensory Processing Measure (SPM).* Los Angeles: Western Psychological Services.
36. Greenberg, M. T., Weissberg, R. P., O'Brian, M., Zins, J. E., Fredericks, L., & Resnik, H., et al. (2003). Enhancing school-based prevention and youth development through coordinated social, emotional, and academic learning. *American Psychologist, 58,* 466–474.

37. Griswold, L. (1993). Ethnographic analysis: A study of classroom environments. *American Journal of Occupational Therapy, 48,* 397–402.

38. Haley, S. M. (1994). Our measures reflect our practices and beliefs: A perspective on clinical measurement in pediatric physical therapy. *Pediatric Physical Therapy, 6,* 142–143.

39. Hammill, D. D., Pearson, N. A., & Voress, J. K. (1993). *Developmental Test of Visual Perception* (2nd ed.). Austin, TX: Pro-Ed.

40. Handley-More, D., & Chandler, B. E. (2007). Occupational therapy decision-making process. In L. L. Jackson (Ed.), *Occupational therapy services for children and youth under IDEA* (3rd ed.). Bethesda, MD: American Occupational Therapy Association.

41. Hanft, B. E., & Place, P. A. (1996). *The consulting therapist: A guide for OTs and PTs in Schools.* San Antonio, TX: Therapy Skill Builders.

42. Hanft, B. E., & Shepherd, J. (2008). *Collaborating for student success: A guide for school-based occupational therapy.* Bethesda, MD: American Occupational Therapy Association Press.

43. Hoffman, O. R., Hemmingsson, H., & Kielhofner, G. (2000). *The school setting interview: A user's manual.* Chicago: University of Illinois, Department of Occupational Therapy.

44. Holbrook, M. D. (2007). *A seven-step process to creating standards-based IEPs. Project forum at NASDSE.* Retrieved June 29, 2008 from http://www.projectforum.org/docs/SevenStepProcessto CreatingStandards-basedIEPs.pdf

45. Jackson, L. L. (Ed.). (2007). *Occupational therapy services for children and youth under IDEA* (3rd ed.). Bethesda, MD: American Occupational Therapy Association.

46. Jackson, L. L., & Arbesman, M. (Eds.). (2005). *Occupational therapy practice guidelines for children with behavioral and psychosocial needs.* Bethesda, MD: American Occupational Therapy Association Press.

47. Katz, N., Parush, S., & Traub Bar-Ilan, R. (2005). *DOTCA-Ch: Dynamic Occupational Therapy Cognitive Assessment for Children.* Pequannock NJ: Maddak.

48. Kentucky Department of Education. (2006). *Resource manual for educationally related occupational therapy and physical therapy in Kentucky public schools.* Frankfort, KY: Kentucky Department of Education.

49. Knippenberg, C., & Hanft, B. (2004). The key to educational relevance: Occupation throughout the school day. *School System Special Interest Section Quarterly, 11*(4), 1–4.

50. Koller, J. R., & Bertel, J. M. (2006). Responding to today's mental health needs of children, families and schools: Revisiting the preservice training and preparation of school-based personnel. *Education and Treatment of Children, 29,* 197–217.

51. Koppelman, J. (2004). *Children with mental disorders: Making sense of their needs and systems that help them (NHPF Issue Brief, No. 799).* Washington, DC: National Health Policy Forum, The George Washington University.

52. Kovaleski, J. F., Tucker, J. A., & Stevens, L. J. (1996). Bridging special and regular education: The Pennsylvania initiative. *Educational Leadership, 53,* 44–47.

53. Kutash, K., Duchnowski, A. J., & Lynn, N. (2006). *School-based mental health: An empirical guide for decision-makers.* Tampa, FL: University of South Florida, The Louis de la Parte Florida Mental Health Institute, Department of Child & Family Studies, Research and Training Center for Children's Mental Health.

54. Masia-Warner, C., Nangle, D. W., & Hansen, D. J. (2006). Bringing evidence-based child mental health services to the schools: General issues and specific populations. *Education and Treatment of Children, 29,* 165–172.

55. McCarney, S. B., & Leigh, J. E. (1990). *Behavior Evaluation Scale-2.* Columbia, MO: Hawthorne Educational Services, Inc.

56. McWilliam, R. A. (1995). Integration of therapy and consultative special education: A continuum in early intervention. *Infants & Young Children, 7*(4), 29–38.

57. Missiauna, C., & Pollock, N. (2000). Perceived efficacy and goal setting in young children. *Canadian Journal of Occupational Therapy, 67,* 101–109.

58. Missiauna, C., Pollock, N., & Law, M. (2004). *Perceived efficacy and goal setting system (PEGS).* San Antonio, TX: Psychological Corp.

59. Muhlenhaupt, M., Miller, H., Sanders, J., & Swinth, Y. (1998). Implications of the 1997 reauthorization of IDEA for school-based occupational therapy. *School System Special Interest Section Quarterly, 5*(3), 1–4.

60. Nanof, T. (2007). Education policy, practice, and the importance of OT in determining our role in education and early intervention. *School System Special Interest Section Quarterly, 14*(2), 1–4.

61. National Association of State Directors of Special Education (NASDSE). (2006a). *Response to intervention: Policy considerations and implementation.* Alexandria, VA: Author.

62. National Council on Disability. (2000). *Back to school on civil rights.* Retrieved June 8, 2008 from http://www.ncd.gov/news room/publications/2000/pdf/backtoschool.pdf.

63. National Dissemination Center for Children with Disabilities (NICHCY). (2007). *Building a legacy: A training curriculum on IDEA 2004.* Retrieved June 12, 2008 from http://www.nichcy.org/training/contents.asp#description.

64. NICHCY. (2008). *Related services.* Retrieved August 25, 2008 from http://www.nichcy.org/EducateChildren/IEP/Pages/RelatedServices.aspx.

65. Nolan, K., Mannato, L., & Wilding, G. (2004). Integrated models of pediatric physical and occupational therapy: Regional practice and related outcomes. *Pediatric Physical Therapy, 16,* 121–128.

66. Opp, A. (2007). Reauthorizing no child left behind: Opportunities for OTs. *OT Practice, 12,* 9–13.

67. Pape, L., & Ryba, K. (2004). *Practical considerations for school-based occupational therapists.* Bethesda, MD: American Occupational Therapy Association.

68. Polichino, J. E. (2001). An education-based reasoning model to support best practices for school-based OT under IDEA 97. *School System Special Interest Section Quarterly, 8*(2), 1–4.

69. Polichino, J. E., Frolek Clark, G., Swinth, Y., & Muhlenhaupt, M. (2007). Evaluating occupational performance in schools and early childhood settings. In L. L. Jackson (Ed.), *Occupational therapy services for children and youth under IDEA* (3rd ed.). Bethesda, MD: American Occupational Therapy Association.

70. Rainforth, B. (2002). The primary therapist model: Addressing challenges to practice in special education. *Physical and Occupational Therapy in Pediatrics, 22*(2), 29–51.

71. Rainforth, B., & York-Barr, J. (1997). *Collaborative teams for students with severe disabilities: Integrating therapy and educational services* (2nd ed.). Baltimore: Brookes.

72. Rosenbaum, P. L., & Saigal, S. (1996). Measuring health-related quality of life in pediatric populations: Conceptual issues. In B. Spilker (Ed.), *Quality of life and pharmacoeconomics in clinical trials* (2nd ed.). Philadelphia: Lippincott-Raven.

73. RTI Action Network. (n.d.). *What is RTI?* Retrieved July 2009 from http://www.rtinetwork.org/Learn/What

74. Safran, S. P., & Oswald, K. (2003). Positive behavior supports: Can schools reshape disciplinary practices? *Exceptional Children, 69,* 361–373.

75. Spencer, K. C., Turkett, A., Vaughan, R., & Koenig, S. (2006). School-based practice patterns: A survey of occupational therapists in Colorado. *American Journal of Occupational Therapy, 60,* 81–90.

76. Swinth, Y. (2007). Evaluating evidence to support practice. In L. L. Jackson (Ed.), *Occupational therapy services for children and youth under IDEA* (3rd ed.). Bethesda, MD: American Occupational Therapy Association.

77. Swinth, Y., Chandler, B., Hanft, B., Jackson, L., & Shepherd, J. (2003). *Personnel issues in school-based occupational therapy: Supply and demand, preparation, certification and licensure (COPSSE*

Document No. IB-1). Gainesville, FL: University of Florida, Center on Personnel Studies in Special Education.

78. Swinth, Y., & Hanft, B. (2002). School-based practice: Moving beyond 1:1 service delivery. *OT Practice, 7*(16), 12–20.

79. Swinth, Y., Spencer, K. C., & Jackson, L. L. (2007). *Occupational therapy: Effective school-based practices within a policy context (COPSSE Document No. OP-3)*. Gainesville, FL: University of Florida, Center on Personnel Studies in Special Education. Retrieved May 16, 2008 from http://www.coe.ufl.edu/copsse/docs/OT_CP_081307/1/OT_CP_081307.pdf.

80. Trombly, C. (1993). The issue is – Anticipating the future: Assessment of occupational function. *American Journal of Occupational Therapy, 47,* 253–257.

81. U.S. Department of Education. (2008). *U.S. Secretary of Education Margaret Spellings announces proposed regulations to strengthen No Child Left Behind*. Retrieved June 14, 2008 from http://www.ed.gov/news/pressreleases/2008/04/04222008.html.

82. U.S. Department of Education. (2008). *No Child Left Behind—2008: Summary of proposed regulations for Title I*. Retrieved June 19, 2008 from http://www.ed.gov/policy/elsec/reg/proposal/summary.pdf.

83. U.S. Office of Special Education Programs. (2007). *Presentation: Response to intervention and early intervening programs*. Retrieved August 24, 2008 from http://idea.ed.gov/explore/view/p/%2Croot%2Cdynamic%2CPresentation%2C28%2C.

84. Weist, M. D., & Paternite, C. E. (2006). Building an interconnected policy-training-practice-research agenda to advance school mental health. *Education and Treatment of Children, 29,* 173–196.

85. Williams, M. S., & Shellenberger, S. (1996). *"How does your engine run?": A leader's guide to the Alert Program for self-regulation*. Albuquerque: TherapyWorks.

86. World Health Organization. (2007). *ICF-CY: International classification of functioning, disability and health - children and youth version*. Geneva: WHO Press.

87. Wright, P. W., & Wright, P. D. (2008). *Key differences between Section 504, the ADA and the IDEA*. Retrieved August 27, 2008 from http://www.wrightslaw.com/info/sec504.summ.rights.htm

88. Yell, M., & Katsiyannis, A. (2004). Placing students with disabilities in inclusive settings: Legal guidelines and preferred practices. *Preventing School Failure, 49*(1), 28–35.

89. York, J., Giangreco, M. F., Vandercook, T., & McDonald, C. (1992). Integrating support personnel in the inclusive classroom. In S. Stainback & W. Stainback (Eds.), *Curriculum considerations in inclusive classrooms: Facilitating learning for all students* (pp. 101–116). Baltimore: Brookes.

90. Zins, J. E., & Erchul, W. P. (1995). Best practice in school consultation. In A. Thomas, & J. Grimes (Eds.), *Best practices in school psychology—III* (pp. 651–660). Washington, DC: The National Association of School Psychologists.

Service for Children with Visual or Hearing Impairments

Elizabeth Russel • Patricia S. Nagaishi

Conductive hearing loss
Sensorineural hearing loss
Hearing impairment
Manual communication (sign language)
Total communication
American Sign Language
Listening and spoken language
Auditory-verbal (therapy)
Cochlear implants

Visual acuity
Visual impairment
Functional vision
Cortical visual impairment
Legal blindness
Low vision
Echolocation
Braille
Vision therapy
Orientation and mobility training
Low vision training
Deaf-blind

1. Define terms related to visual and hearing impairment.
2. Discuss the possible effects of visual and hearing impairments on a child's development.
3. Explain the impact of hearing impairment and visual impairment on engagement in occupations, including activities of daily living, education/learning, play, social participation, instrumental activities of daily living, and preparation for work.
4. Discuss the evaluation of a child with hearing and visual impairment, and assessments that are helpful in the development of intervention plans.
5. Describe intervention strategies for children with hearing and visual impairments that promote their participation in occupations.
6. Describe special techniques and strategies that can be used with children with hearing and visual impairments.
7. Illustrate principles of evaluation and intervention within case studies.

Hearing and vision enable us to understand what is happening in the world around us. Persons with normal sensory function cannot truly understand the experience of being hearing or vision-impaired. However, participating in sensory awareness activities can increase understanding of the difficulties associated with hearing or vision loss. Such sensory awareness activities may include eating a meal blindfolded and listening to recordings that simulate what songs sound like to an individual with a certain type of hearing loss.

However, sensory awareness activities do not give the total picture of what it is like to have a hearing- or vision-related disability because individuals with normally functioning senses have a vast wealth of visual and auditory memories to call upon that are not available to children with hearing or visual impairments, most of whom have congenital conditions. As with other aspects of development, the development of hearing and vision (i.e., making sense of the sounds and sights around us) is experience-dependent.

The sense organs (i.e., eyes, ears, skin, nose, tongue) are all extensions of the brain. The brain's primary function is to receive information, or sensory stimuli, from the world for processing and coding. This information is integrated and associated with past experiences. Because the nature and intensity of stimulation to the sense organs vary greatly, one experience may take precedence over others. If a particular sense organ is not working properly, the others do not totally compensate for the loss. However, one sensory system may take precedence over another weak or damaged system; for example, vision may take precedence in the child with a hearing impairment.

Vision is the sense we use for understanding the relationships between people and objects. It puts the environment in perspective and is an efficient integrator of multisensory information that contributes to the development of perceptual abilities and concept formation. Vision, then, involves the body and all of the other senses, and integrates and makes use of all sensory information.[26] We use vision to scan the environment (e.g., obtain information about distance, movement, spatial relations) and to discriminate features of objects and symbols (e.g., size, shape, color, orientation of letters). Children with visual impairment often have delayed language because it is difficult for them to grasp relationships and associations between people and objects. In a discussion of vision, it is important to differentiate between *sight*—the ability to discriminate small objects—which is measured as visual acuity (or the resolving power of the eye to see small detail at a specified distance [i.e., 20/20 acuity is considered normal]), and *vision*—the process of taking in, processing, and integrating visual and other sensory information to form a perception.[99]

Scheiman describes an optometric model of vision comprising three interrelated components.[99] The first component consists of acuity, refraction, and eye health; the second component includes visual efficiency skills; and the third component involves visual information processing. Scheiman contends that occupational therapists must understand the complexity and importance of vision because of the significant impact visual impairment has on occupational engagement and participation in the lives of the individuals they see in all areas of practice.

Titcomb and Okoye discuss *vision* as a dynamic, complex system of visual skills, neural processing and integration, cortical interpretation, and adaptive visual-motor function.[113] Visual skills are dynamic and develop with the central nervous system as a result of interactions with the world. Visual skills include *fixation, tracking/pursuits, saccade, accommodation, convergence,* and *binocular vision*. In addition, *stereopsis* (binocular depth perception), form perception, and field of vision, depend on the coordination of accommodation and convergence.[113] Visual and sensorimotor integration involves integration of visual skills with the other sensory systems (e.g., vestibular, proprioception, auditory, tactile), which enables the child to develop functional skills (e.g., orienting responses, protective reactions, spatiotemporal orientation, eye-hand and eye-foot coordination, perceptual skills, and academic skills). At the same time, sensorimotor functions support the development of visual skills. Impairment can occur in any or all components in varying degrees of severity.

In addition to its function as the foundation for speech and spoken language, *audition* is the sense that conveys sound. Sound gives information on distance and direction or localization. For example, we can hear a dog bark and, without seeing the dog, judge where and how far away it is. *Auditory perception* is the attachment of meaning to sound patterns. Sound has qualities of *duration, intensity, frequency, loudness,* and *pitch* that make up auditory acuity.

As with vision, impairment can occur at the level of acuity, processing, integration, awareness, and/or perception. Although oral language development is an obvious difficulty for a child with a hearing loss, other complex challenges arise because language is critical to socialization and to development of the child's inner logic. The capacity for language is innate, but it requires environmental stimulation to trigger its development.[17,66,83] As the child learns language, he or she can exert greater control over the environment.

Children with visual or hearing impairment can experience substantial difficulties that affect their development and learning. Although these children face many shared difficulties, the differences are striking. For this reason, this chapter deals separately with children with hearing impairment, visual impairment, and multisensory impairment. Occupational therapy services for children with visual or hearing impairment focus on activities of daily living (ADLs) (e.g., feeding, dressing, toileting), education/learning, play, social participation, instrumental activities of daily living (IADLs) (e.g., community mobility, shopping, meal preparation), and preparation for work. In addition, occupational therapists help children achieve performance skills, including sensory processing and perceptual skills, gross motor skills and postural control, and fine motor coordination and dexterity. The goal of occupational therapy is to help the child and family engage in typical occupations. These services need to have meaning and purpose to the child and his or her family and they need to occur in the natural contexts the child and family experience. Occupational therapists also provide consultation to parents, teachers, and caregivers as part of the child's overall developmental and educational plan, and in conjunction with the professionals primarily involved with the child's.

In the provision of occupational therapy for children with sensory loss, the importance of play cannot be overemphasized. Play is the means by which the child develops skills, learns how to solve problems, to cope with the environmental demands, to face the unknown, and to adapt by changing their behaviors according to situation demands.[38,70,79] Play is also a "vehicle of meaning" for children who engage in it for its own sake, which promotes health.[79] For children whose distance senses and perceptions of the environment are limited, the development of play skills, particularly active play involving use of the vestibular and proprioceptive systems, and the promotion of playfulness, should be the highest priority (see Chapter 18 for a full discussion of play).

VISUAL IMPAIRMENT

For the purposes of this chapter, *visual impairment* is defined as the loss of or deficits in visual function (i.e., vision, visual perception, interpretation of visual input) due to pathology or processing problems in one or more components of the visual system (e.g., structures of the eye, visual pathways, and the brain) that limits the individual's ability to engage in and participate in daily occupations. The leading causes of visual impairment in young children are cortical visual impairment (CVI), retinopathy of prematurity (ROP), and optic nerve hypoplasia.[26,32,71] Other common causes include microphthalmia, anophthalmia, childhood glaucoma, retinoblastoma, and congenital cataracts, whereas less common causes include severe myopia, albinism, and nystagmus.[26] Diagnostic information, identification of children with visual impairment, common pediatric eye disorders, and a list of other specialists who may be involved in working with children with visual impairments are presented in Appendix 25-A on the Evolve website.

Because the effects of visual impairment are evident in the acquisition of early milestones for mobility and manipulation, children with visual impairments are often referred for developmental evaluation and intervention by pediatricians. However, children with developmental disabilities (e.g., cerebral palsy, Down syndrome) are among the most likely to receive services from occupational therapists, and 50% to 66% of children with developmental disabilities also have a significant ocular disorder or visual impairment.[71,84] Thus the primary referral concerns may focus on developmental areas (e.g., fine motor skills, locomotion, self-care) and may not necessarily specifically identify vision-related issues, even though the visual impairment is among the contributing factors affecting the child's development. Therefore it is important for occupational therapy practitioners to recognize, understand, and address how the child's visual functioning influences occupational functioning.

Whatever the impetus for referral, children with visual impairment are often identified in the first year of life and begin to receive services from local early intervention programs. Services may be provided in a variety of settings and program models, including home-based, or center-based, public or private, combination home- and center-based, generic special education, or disability-specific programs.[21,84] Locations may include the home, daycare center, preschool/school, residential facility, or hospital.

Just as do children with other disabilities or impairments, children with visual impairment demonstrate a wide range of abilities and functional outcomes. The picture becomes more complex when the developing child with visual impairment has other associated problems or is multi-impaired. Therefore it is important that the etiology, age at onset, degree of visual impairment, and the presence of co-existing conditions be taken into consideration when occupational therapy evaluation and intervention services are provided.

In a national collaborative study that examined the developmental trajectories of a group of 186 children with visual impairment, Hatton, Bailey, Burchinal, and Ferrell found that children with visual impairment and co-occurring disabilities (e.g., intellectual disability [ID] or developmental delay [DD]) had lower developmental age scores as measured by the Battelle Developmental Inventory (BDI), and showed a slower rate of development when compared with children with visual impairment who did not have ID, regardless of the levels of visual functioning demonstrated by the children (Research Note 25-1).[44] However, the level of visual function was highly correlated with the presence of ID in that more than half of the children with severe vision loss also had ID, whereas children with mild to moderate vision loss did not. The authors considered that these findings suggest that a more severe underlying central nervous system disorder is responsible both for the visual impairment and for ID in these children.

Among the children with no ID, those with the least vision had significantly lower BDI scores across all domains and slower rates of motor and personal-social development when compared with those with the most vision. The degree of visual impairment, therefore, is a factor in the development of these children, and those with better vision are more likely to have favorable developmental outcomes.[44]

The degree of visual impairment, however, is only one variable that must be considered in the individual child's developmental trajectory. On the basis of the variability in functional performance of children with visual impairment, Warren argued that an individual differences approach is more meaningful for studying visual impairment in young children than is a comparative approach that relies on knowledge of chronologic age norms for sighted children.[117,118] Some children with visual impairments function at least within the average range or even at the high end of developmental age norms for sighted children. Therefore the evaluation of development in relation to the demands (i.e., expectations and challenges) of the environment in which the child with visual impairment functions and how these interactions change over time is presented as a more useful framework.[118] This perspective is consistent with the transactional model of early intervention[95] and with the person-environment-occupation (PEO) framework of occupational therapy discussed in Chapter 2. Whether the child with a visual impairment is singly impaired or multi-impaired, occupational therapists view the child and family in relation to their ability to participate and engage in

RESEARCH NOTE 25-1

Hatton, D. D., Bailey, D. B., Burchinal, M. R
Ferrell, K. A. (1997). Developmental growth c
of preschool children with vision impairments. C
Development, 68, 788-806.

ABSTRACT

This study described the development of 186 children (12-73 months) with vision impairments who were asse using the Battelle Developmental Inventory (BDI). Gro curve analysis was used to describe developmental patt over time and the extent to which their development va as a function of etiology, visual function, and co-occur disabilities based on the results from 566 BDI assessmc Children with co-occurring disabilities (intellectual disab [ID]) had lower developmental age scores and slower of growth. Children with minimal visual function (20/ or worse) had significantly lower developmental ages ad time in all domains measured by the BDI—personal-so adaptive, motor, cognition, and communication—and slc rates of growth in the personal-social and motor doma Amount of functional vision and ID did not interact, w suggested that these factors had additive, rather than m plicative, effects on development in early childhood.

IMPLICATIONS FOR PRACTICE

- The presence of co-occurring disabilities, ID, in chilc with visual impairment had a significant impact on th development, and these children also tended to have more severe visual impairment, suggesting an additive effect of the visual impairment on development.
- In addition, among those without ID, the developm of children with minimal visual function (20/800 or worse) was significantly different, particularly in the personal-social and motor domains, from that of chilc whose visual function was 20/500 or better, whose developmental trajectory may be similar to that of typ sighted children.
- A comprehensive developmental assessment is useful identifying a profile of strengths and needs across all domains because there is variability in the developmen children with visual impairment alone, and with child with visual impairment and co-occurring disabilities.
- Occupational therapists must take into consideration amount of visual function and the presence of co-occurring disabilities when planning and implementin intervention and working with these children and the families.

occupations and activities that are meaningful to their every lives. To illustrate these points, three case vignettes are p sented in Case Study 25-1 to highlight the heterogeneity s within the population of children who are visually impai and are referred to throughout this section.

As can be seen in the first of these vignettes, Natalia high risk factors and very little vision, and one might b expected poor visual and developmental outcomes, but was functioning at age-appropriate levels in all areas and co participate fully in a general education environment. In

CASE STUDY 25-1   Natalia, Nicholas, and Hannah

The following vignettes are composites from actual cases and illustrate the wide range of visual and occupational functioning that can be seen in children with visual impairment or blindness.

NATALIA

Natalia lived with her parents and younger brother in a small upstairs apartment. She had a history of extreme prematurity (24 weeks' gestation, birth weight 1 pound, 10 ounces) and received NICU care for several neonatal conditions, including stage 3 retinopathy of prematurity. She underwent several eye procedures for retinal detachment. Her visual status at the time of referral was minimal light perception in the right eye and no vision in the left eye. At the time of her referral to the preschool assessment team, she had received Part C early intervention services that included occupational therapy, physical therapy, vision services, and a center-based early intervention program.

At age 3 years, Natalia was demonstrating age-appropriate skills in all areas, and her gross motor and fine motor skills were progressing as expected for children with visual impairment. She could navigate the home environment independently and the classroom environment with auditory and tactile cues, and was learning cane skills. She demonstrated good tactile discrimination abilities and appropriate grasp patterns to explore and manipulate objects, and she used auditory cues to locate or search for toys. She placed small items into openings, nested or stacked cups, activated cause-effect toys, and placed forms into a formboard. By the first grade, she was in a general education class with specialized vision services, orientation and mobility training, and adapted physical education as related services. She was doing well in learning Braille reading and writing skills, performing at grade level in all academic areas, acquiring high-level cane skills, and engaging in age-appropriate social interactions and communication with peers.

NICHOLAS

Nicholas was diagnosed with Leber's congenital amaurosis at 3 months of age. His birth history was unremarkable. He presented with light perception in both eyes. He lived with his mother, and he was cared for by his grandmother while his mother worked. He began receiving early intervention services soon after the diagnosis, starting with a home-based early intervention program with an early childhood special education teacher, and consultation provided by a teacher of students with visual impairment, occupational therapist, and speech-language pathologist. He transitioned to a center-based early intervention program at about 22 months of age.

At the time of his assessment, at age 39 months, Nicholas exhibited significantly delay in all areas of development. He displayed negative reactions to auditory and tactile experiences at a much greater frequency and intensity than expected for most children with blindness, so he had a severely constricted range of manipulative and play skills. He typically engaged in repetitive actions with favored objects, and did not explore or cast aside most other objects or toys that were introduced. He did not display problem-solving skills, point to body parts, use language to interact socially, or respond to questions or requests, and was dependent in his self-care. He was easily disoriented when walking through space and lost his balance when walking even when holding onto an adult's hand. He could sing favorite songs from circle time and he could spell words that he had learned from memory. He preferred to be alone and would turn away or protest if another child approached him. These observations and findings were atypical for the developmental trajectory of most children with visual impairments, and the nature of the behaviors displayed suggested the presence of an autistic spectrum disorder. Further evaluation by a psychologist with expertise in assessing young children with vision impairment and developmental disabilities was recommended.

After this evaluation was completed, Nicholas was diagnosed with autism. He attended a self-contained special education preschool class and received occupational therapy, educational vision services (provided by the teacher for students with visual impairment and orientation and mobility specialist), and speech-language therapy as related services. By the time he reached second grade, Nicholas was attending an inclusion class. He demonstrated strengths in his ability to memorize information, orientation and mobility skills to negotiate the school campus, and in reading and spelling; he was working on fine motor skills needed for self-care and classroom activities; and experienced the greatest challenges in communication and social interactions with peers.

HANNAH

Hannah was 4 years, 3 months old when she was first referred for evaluation to determine eligibility for special education. She had arrived in the United States from a European country with her family about 4 months before being seen. Hannah was born at term and had early difficulties with sucking for feeding and remained in the hospital for about 3 weeks. Her parents became concerned about Hannah's vision when she was 5 months old, and she was evaluated by a pediatric neurologist and an ophthalmologist.

She was noted to have some cranial abnormalities and optic atrophy. Vision in the right eye was hyperopic, while vision in the left eye was myopic with very poor vision associated with the optic atrophy. Results of the visual evoked potential (VEP) test indicated cortical visual impairment. Hannah also had a history of infantile seizures for which she was placed on medication for several months. Since discontinuation of the medication, she remained seizure free.

Up until the referral, Hannah had not received any early intervention services or attended a preschool. Assessment findings indicated that Hannah had significant delays in all areas of development, with relative strengths using her available vision (together with auditory, vestibular, and proprioceptive cues) to track moving objects of interest, accurately reach for a desired object, negotiate the environment, and perform tasks such as manipulating cause-effect toys,

Continued

engaging in reciprocal ball play, and using a spoon to feed herself. Her use of tactile exploration and manipulation of a variety of objects was limited and she was beginning to say single words. Hannah attended a private preschool for children with blindness and visual impairments, and significant progress in her learning, language and communication, manipulative, and self-care skills was seen, although her overall functioning was still below age expectations. She received vision, orientation and mobility, occupational therapy, and speech language pathology services at the school. She transitioned to an inclusion kindergarten classroom at a public school and continued to receive vision and orientation and mobility services, and pre-Braille instruction, speech therapy, and occupational therapy. She was engaging in play and interactions with peers; increasing her knowledge of color, number, and letter concepts; taking care of her toileting needs; and participating in art and manipulative activities with some adaptations and modifications in tools and materials.

---

second vignette, by contrast, Nicholas, who also had very little vision, exhibited atypical and delayed development (both with respect to same-age children who are visually impaired and those who are sighted) and was found to have autism. Hannah had significant delays in all areas of development and had not received any intervention until after 4 years of age, but she had functional vision (i.e., a degree of usable vision that is available for learning and daily activities) that she was able to use quite well together with other sensory input that contributed to her positive response to intervention and substantial progress in a short period of time that enabled her to transition to an inclusion kindergarten class.

Developmental Considerations and the Impact of Visual Impairment

It is important that the occupational therapist understand the development of the visual system, and the development of visual functioning, to evaluate the ability of children to engage in age-appropriate occupations and to design appropriate interventions. Vision is a quick, efficient integrating sense that allows immediate feedback and appreciation of both near and distant information about the environment in multiple locations.[53,112] At 25 to 24 weeks' gestation, the major structures of the eye and the visual pathway to the level of the visual cortex are in place, but the eyelids are fused and the visual system remains immature.[39,40] Therefore infants born extremely premature are at high risk for retinopathy of prematurity (ROP) because the retina and visual cortex undergo further maturation during the last trimester of pregnancy.[39] However, improvements in neonatal and ophthalmic care may result in improved visual outcomes for children with ROP,[102] although extremely low birth-weight children may be at higher risk for visual acuity problems.[107] By 24 to 28 weeks, the eyelids are no longer fused and an immature visual response emerges, but the awake and sleep states are not well differentiated. By 30 to 34 weeks, sleep and awake states become differentiated, the eyes may open, and brief visual fixation may occur. By 36 weeks, the visual evoked response is similar to that of a full-term infant, and the awake state can be sustained for longer periods.[40]

At birth, the infant's visual acuity is approximately 20/200 (i.e., the infant can see at 20 feet what an adult with normal vision can see at 200 feet): at 1 year, it is about 20/50, and by 2 years normal 20/20 acuity is present.[26] The maturation of the visual system in typical infants continues after birth and is a function of the transactions that occur between the infant and the environment and concurrent changes in the synaptic density of the visual cortex and other parts of the brain.[40] Vision enables an infant to explore the environment and negotiate space, to learn about the properties of objects, to interact and communicate with caregivers, and to develop the visual-perceptual skills needed for more complex activities such as reading and writing, and for play and self-care occupations. In addition, vision is major contributor to praxis, which allows an individual to organize ideas and actions and to anticipate, monitor, and adapt to the demands of the environment.[97,106] Because many of the conditions that affect vision are congenital or have a prenatal etiology, a major system for processing and interpreting information is compromised at birth, with substantial impact on the child's subsequent development in all areas. The following discussion focuses on areas relevant to occupational therapy, except for visual perception, which is discussed in Chapter 12.

Participation in Co-occupations of Caregiving

Through engagement in the daily caregiving activities and routines of feeding, bathing, sleep, and playful interactions, the infant and the caregiver co-regulate their signals and responses, and each actively participates in these interactions. Also, through these interactions the infant and the caregiver develop their relationship, and infant behaviors such as eye gaze and visual regard of faces, and the mother's interpretations of these behaviors, are seen as important to this process. However, according to Warren, the basic infant behaviors that elicit caregiver responses, such as smiling and vocalizing, do not depend on vision, and vision is not required for infants to perceive the caregiver's responsive behaviors, such as vocalizing, cuddling, or feeding.[118] In their study of mothers' interpretations of their infants' behaviors, Baird, Mayfield, and Baker found that both sighted infants and their sample of infants with visual impairments engaged in similar proportions of facial expressions that were considered meaningful by their mothers, and smiling was the predominant facial expression interpreted.[6]

Indeed, positive and strong attachment relationships can occur in infants with visual impairment.[117] A caregiver who is coping with learning that the infant has a visual impairment may have difficulty responding to the infant's cues, but at the same time, the infant may display fewer behaviors that elicit positive responses from the caregiver, setting up a cycle of interactions that are out of sync or not mutually and emotionally satisfying. Furthermore, an infant who is visually impaired may be securely attached to a primary caregiver, but have attachment behaviors that are different from those seen and expected in sighted children.[28] Vision loss itself is not necessarily a causal factor, but it may create a condition of risk for early social-emotional development and attachment.[118]

On the other hand, young children with visual impairment may experience sleep disorders that could impact the bedtime and sleep-wake routines in the household, and their behavior and performance.[28] One study examined the sleep patterns of two groups of toddlers with visual impairment ranging in age from 10 months to 39 months: one group without associated disabilities, and one group with associated disabilities.[31] The investigators found that when compared with the control group of typical sighted peers, the children with visual impairment had more difficulty falling asleep (i.e., longer time) and sleeping through the night (i.e., longer time spent awake, and greater number of nocturnal awakenings), and the sleep behaviors were not related to the presence of associated disabilities. Thus it is important that occupational therapists take into consideration the daily routines of the child and family, including sleep-wake cycles as part of the evaluation and intervention processes.

Exploration and Play

Children with visual impairment, particularly those who have significantly decreased visual functioning, have a qualitatively different experience with, and level of access to, objects and people in their environment.[111] Vision provides children access and motivation to explore and seek out interactions with the physical and social worlds that not only contribute to the acquisition of motor skills, but also promotes development in all areas.

As discussed previously in the study by Hatton and colleagues, many children with visual impairment demonstrated delayed achievement of certain milestones, such as crawling and walking.[44] In a survey of 200 families with children with visual impairment, Celeste found that the total sample demonstrated delayed gross motor development for nearly every milestone, but the greatest delays occurred for milestones related to locomotion, such as cruising around furniture, walking independently, and negotiating stairs.[13] Among the subgroups in the sample, children with the least vision (i.e., light perception only or no light perception) had the poorest motor outcomes, followed by children with visual impairments who were born prematurely. Other studies have shown differences among children with visual impairment in their motor function that varied with etiology, severity of visual impairment, and presence and extent of additional disabilities. A summary of selected studies comparing motor function (and visual motor function, which is discussed in the next section), degree of visual impairment, and severity of co-occurring conditions is presented in Table 25-1.

Warren suggested that lack of vision may have an indirect rather than a direct effect on locomotion, because studies have shown significant variance among infants with visual impairment, with some achieving milestones for crawling and walking well within the normal range.[118] Specifically, vision may serve as a motivator for infants to explore interesting sights out of reach, and perhaps more important, according to Warren, is the extent to which infants are provided with opportunities and encouragement to explore. A study that examined physical activity in children with visual impairments from a family perspective found that younger children in the sample were more active than older children, and the levels of physical activity differed among parents and siblings when the children with visual impairments were active (up to 21% for parents, and 11% to 53% for siblings). Even though parents indicated that their involvement was important for participation of their children in physical activity, their actual level of involvement was low.[5] Factors such as transportation to physical activity settings, busy family schedules, peer involvement, and safety concerns were cited as facilitators or barriers to the children's participation in physical activity.

Learning, Education, and Academic Performance

Children with visual impairment learn in a range of educational environments, from general education settings to residential facilities. According to the 27th Individuals with Disabilities Education Act Annual Report to Congress,[114] data for 2003 indicated that most preschoolers with visual impairment were served in early childhood special education settings (28%) and early childhood settings (26%), whereas school-age children with visual impairments were served in the regular classroom (55% spent up to 21% of the day outside the regular class). The development of cognition, concept development, and language in young children needs to be viewed both from a developmental perspective and in terms of the unique needs of the child with visual impairment. Knowledge of typical developmental processes is critical not only for comparison with sighted children, but to provide a context for clinical decision making to determine developmentally appropriate evaluation and intervention.[29] For example, children develop an understanding of the properties of the world and how things relate and work, develop logical thought and learn to problem-solve, and also learn to regulate and organize executive functions such as memory, attention, and information processing. They learn by exploring and engaging in sensorimotor actions with objects, developing associations among objects, experiencing the relationship between self and others and objects in space, establishing perception and mental representations, solving complex problems, and ultimately using symbolic representation and manipulation for abstract thinking.

As stated earlier, developmental patterns in children with visual impairment may vary in terms of rate and sequence of acquisition in that they may achieve some developmental milestones within the same typical range as for sighted children, or acquire other skills earlier, and show later acquisition for still other milestones.[32] This is true for the development of cognition and communication, and depends on factors such as age at onset, degree of visual functioning, presence of other disabilities, and the nature of the child's experiences in different contexts. For example, Hatton et al. found that communication scores were significantly higher than those for other domain scores.[44] Children with the least visual function tended to score proportionately higher on this domain, whereas those with other developmental disabilities showed smaller gains over time for both the cognitive and communication domains. Other studies have shown no significant differences in the cognitive/learning and communication development or school performance of children with

TABLE 25-1 Comparison of Motor Functioning, Degree of Visual Impairment, and Severity of Co-occurring Disabilities

Authors, Date	Research Design	Research Questions or Hypotheses	Sample	Dependent Variable Measures	Findings and Limitations
Hatton, Bailey, Burchinal, & Ferrell, 1997[44]	Longitudinal, repeated measures, descriptive study	To what extent do etiology, visual function, and co-occurring disabilities affect the developmental trajectories of young children with visual impairments?	• 186 children (106 boys, 80 girls), 12 to 73 months of age, with visual acuities of 20/70 or worse in the best eye; 29% had light perception at best • 60% white, 25% African-American, 11% Latino, 4% other • 40% had additional disabilities • Sample was drawn from a state agency serving children with visual impairment in a southern state, and a prospective national study of children with visual impairments in eight states	Developmental status—Battelle Development Inventory (BDI)	• Mean scores in the motor domain were significantly lower than the mean scores in the adaptive, communication, personal-social domains • Children with higher visual function had higher estimated means at 30 months on the motor scale and showed significantly more gain over time than children with the least vision • Children with co-occurring intellectual disability (ID) had lower developmental levels and developed at a slower rate for the overall BDI score and in all developmental domains when compared with children with visual impairment without co-occurring disabilities Limitations of the study: • Data obtained from two sources, with different evaluators; • Children from the prospective study were younger than children from the state agency, with no extensive overlap of data for participants by age • Interrelatedness of eye condition, visual function, and presence of ID make it difficult to sort out the unique contributions of each variable
Ghasia, Brunstrom, Gordon, & Tyschsen (2008)*	Observational, cross-sectional design	• To determine whether children at different levels of Gross Motor Function Classification System (GMFCS) have different levels of or types of visual disability • To analyze findings relative to anatomic and physiologic descriptors (e.g., type of CP, spasticity)	• Patients referred to the Cerebral Palsy Center, St Louis Children's Hospital at Washington University Medical Center from 2000 to 2006 • 50 children and adolescents with CP (mean age 5.9 years, range 2-19.5 years); 33 boys and 17 girls; mean	• Gross Motor Function Classification System (GMFCS) used to grade patients along a 5-unit ordinal scale ranging from level 1 (mild) to level 5 (most severe) • Ophthalmic examination and classification: multiple ophthalmic and orthoptic measures	• Children with more severe CP (i.e., level 5 GMFCS) were at greater risk for high myopia, absence of any fusion, dyskinetic strabismus, more severe gaze dysfunction, and optic neuropathy or cortical visual impairment (CVI) relative to children with mild CP (i.e., level 1 GMFCS), in whom such deficits were rare or absent

Freeman, Salt, Prusa, Malm, Ferret, Buffolano, et al. (2005)[35]	Prospective comparison study	Are 3-year-old children with congenital toxoplasmosis (CT) more at risk for adverse developmental or behavioral outcomes than uninfected children?	• 178 parents of children infected with CT and 527 parents of uninfected children from 9 centers in Europe
			• Included all children identified by prenatal or neonatal screening at 3 years of age
			• Prenatal history, pediatric exams at 6 and 12 months, ophthalmoscopy before 4 and at 12 months, cranial ultrasound neonatal screening at 3 years of age
				• Questionnaire including separate assessment tools for behavior, speech and language, cognition, and motor skills that had been validated with standardized clinician assessments; included child-completed fine motor tasks to draw a line, circle, and cross, and to draw a man	• Based on parent responses, 24/178 (13.5%) of children infected with CT had adverse motor outcomes compared with 58/525 (11%) of children not infected with CT
					• There were no significant associations between children's infection status and motor development (nor any of the other developmental areas)
					• Limitations:
					  ○ Response rate was lower for uninfected children than infected children
					  ○ Use of parts of the standardized assessment tool, or a modified version, for all outcomes except behavior (to enhance response with a reasonable length and completion time)

(from previous entry, continued)

gestational age of 31 weeks (range 24-40 weeks)
• Neurologic examination and classification by attending neurologist and pediatric nurse practitioners; Committee for the Definition of Cerebral Palsy criteria used for motor function assessment and assignment to physiologic and anatomic subtypes

including acuity (best corrected), papillary examination, sensorimotor examination, automated retinoscopy

• Children with milder or less severe CP resemble the 1%-4% of typical children in the general population who have infantile or refractive strabismus, while children with severe CP have vision deficits that are either uncommon or never seen in neurologically normal children
• Limitations of the study:
  ○ Possible sampling bias: Children with CP referred for evaluation may be more severely impaired than those who were not referred
  ○ Difficulty conducting repeated measures to catalog and describe accurately the spectrum of visual deficits in this group; limited, nonstandardized ophthalmic CP nomenclature

Continued

TABLE 25-1 Comparison of Motor Functioning, Degree of Visual Impairment, and Severity of Co-occurring Disabilities—Cont'd

Authors, Date	Research Design	Research Questions or Hypotheses	Sample	Dependent Variable Measures	Findings and Limitations
Kutzbach, Summers, Holleschau, & McDonald (2008)[60]	Observational cohort series	To determine the effect of visual impairment on the development, behavior, and education of children with albinism	• 78 children with albinism, 42 boys, 36 girls, ages 4-18 years (mean age = 9.14 years) recruited at the 11th annual meeting of the National Organization of Albinism and Hypopigmentation in Minneapolis in July 2006 and from the University of Minnesota International Albinism Center • 46 (59%) with oculocutaneous albinism type 1 (OCA1); 8 (10.2%) with OCA 2; 1 (1.3%) with ocular albinism type 1; 1 (1.3%) with Hermansky-Pudlak syndrome; and 22 (28.2%) with unknown type • Binocular best-corrected visual acuity (BCVA) measured by a certified orthoptist using the letter visual	• Parent questionnaire for birth, development, and school performance; delay in gross motor development determined by parent report of participant not walking before 16 months of age • Standardized testing administered to 44 children: Woodcock-Johnson III for those 6 years of age and the Young Children's Achievement Test for children 4-6 years • Physician evaluation for attention deficit–hyperactivity disorder (ADHD), using DSM IV and parent Connors Rating Scale • Pediatric neurologist or pediatrician evaluation of balance and fine and gross motor skills (e.g., timed and nontimed tests: stands on one	• Walking was delayed in 12 (15%) of the children in the sample (2 of the 12 had pervasive developmental disorder, 2 others were born prematurely) • Of the 78 children attending school, 26% received either occupational therapy or physical therapy services • Half of the children receiving occupational and/or physical therapy services also had ADHD • Balance and fine motor and gross motor skills were generally normal • Subtle signs of balance and/or motor difficulties were noted in 12% to 25% of the children, depending upon the test • There was no significant relationship between any of the neurodevelopmental variables and visual acuity; children had visual deficits without clinically significant problems with motor coordination, balance, and ambulation • Authors suggested that there is adequate central nervous system compensation for decreased visual acuity in developing children with albinism

Author	Study description	Sample	Methods/Measures	Findings/Limitations
			acuity test appropriate for age of the child	foot; hops on one foot, four-foot tandem gait; throws ball overhand; finger sequencing, finger repetition, hand mirror movements Limitations: • Sample may not be representative of the population of individuals with albinism due to recruitment bias • Inability to detect a relationship between BCVA and neurodevelopmental parameters may have been due to factors such as early intervention and related services received under IEPs, reliability of parental report
Ross, Lipper, Abramson, & Presier (2001)[91]	Descriptive study based on medical record review and pediatric, psychological, and visual evaluations	To assess the mental and motor development of young children with retinoblastoma (RB) to determine whether they are at greater risk of developmental delays than the normal population and whether medical characteristics were related to developmental outcome	• 54 children between 6 and 40 months of age with RB who attended the Ophthalmology Oncology Center at New York Presbyterian Hospital • 23 (43%) boys, 31 (57%) girls; 21 (39%) white; 17 (31%) African-American; 13 (24%) Hispanic; 3 (5%) Asian • 21 with unilateral RB, 33 with bilateral RB • Pediatric examination, a test of visual acuity	• Psychological evaluation including the Bayley Scales of Infant Development II	• Most of the children with RB had normal motor (and mental) development • 21 of 26 children were referred for intervention services to address visuomotor skills, and were more likely to fail Bayley test items requiring eye-hand coordination • Children with bilateral RB performed significantly less well on motor ability than children with unilateral RB, and were more likely to be referred for visuomotor therapy; they were also more likely to have received multiple treatments for their disease Limitations: None discussed by the investigators but • Relatively small sample and those referred to the center may not represent the full range of outcomes • Wide age range, one-time evaluation

Freeman, K., Salt, A., Prusa, A., Malm, G., Ferret, N., & Buffolano, W., et al. (2005). Association between congenital toxoplasmosis and parent – reported developmental outcomes, concerns, and impairment in 3 year old children. *BMC Pediatrics, 5,* 25. Retrieved from http://www.biomedcentral.com/1471-2431/5/25; Ghasia, F., Brunstrom, J., Gordon, M., & Tychsen, L. (2008). Frequency and severity of visual sensory and motor deficits in children with cerebral palsy: Gross motor function classification scale. *Investigative Ophthalmology & Visual Science, 49*(2), 572-580; Hatton, D. D., Bailey, D. G., Burchinal, M. R., & Ferrell, K. A. (1997). Developmental growth curves of preschool children with vision impairments. *Child Development, 58,* 788-806; Kutzbach, B. R., Summers, C. G., Holleschau, A. M., & MacDonald, J. T. (2008). Neurodevelopment in children with albinism. *Opthalmology. 115,* 1805-1808; Roman-Lantzy, C. (2007). *Cortical visual impairment. An approach to Assessment and intervention.* New York: AFB Press.

visual impairment secondary to different etiologies (e.g., congenital toxoplasmosis, albinism, retinoblastoma) when compared with normative samples or of typical peers.[35,60,90,92]

This does not mean, however, that children with visual impairment who perform within the typical range based on standardized test scores do not have qualitative differences or needs that may affect occupational performance and require intervention. For example, several studies have reported cognitive functioning in the normal range among children with visual impairment, but some children displayed a pattern of differences in visual motor performance (refer to Table 25-1). In one study, although the mean scores for mental and motor development as measured using the Bayley Scales of Infant Development II fell within the average range for a group of 54 young children with retinoblastoma (RB), visual motor performance differed relative to extent of RB (unilateral or bilateral).[92] The children with bilateral RB had significantly lower mean scores for motor development (although still within the average range), and they were more likely to be referred for intervention to address visuomotor difficulties than the children with unilateral RB.

Another study examined the cognitive function in children with visual impairment caused by congenital toxoplasmosis[90] and compared intelligence quotient (IQ) scores (using the WPPSI-R) between two groups—one group of 48 children with normal visual acuity in the best eye, and a second group of 16 children with impaired vision (<20/40) in their best eye. Mean verbal, performance, and full scale intelligence quotient (IQ) scores were in the normal range for group 1; and for group 2, mean verbal IQ was in the normal range whereas performance and full scale IQ scores were in the borderline range (77.8 and 81.2, respectively). However, scores for group 2 were lowest for object assembly (puzzles), geometric design, mazes, and picture completion (i.e., tasks that require visual discrimination of fine lines and eye-hand coordination [except for picture completion]). Thus when gathering information from other disciplines (e.g., review of evaluation reports from psychologists, and speech and language pathologists), an occupational therapist should be familiar with the measures used and consider not only global scores, but also the pattern of specific results related to relevant subtest scores and the nature of the tasks involved in his or her own evaluation of the child's occupational performance.

Potential unidentified visual deficits among older children who display academic problems also need to be considered. Goldstand, Koslowe, and Parush found that among a sample of 71 seventh graders (mean age of 12.7 years; 46 proficient readers, 25 nonproficient readers) in middle school in Jerusalem, over half the group failed the Modified Clinical Technique (MCT) optometric vision screening measure for Total Vision and Visual Efficiency, and a little over a third failed the category of Visual Health.[41] Those who passed the MCT screening had significantly better mean academic scores, and significantly better performance on a visual information processing measure (the MVPT) compared with children who failed the MCT, but no difference in performance on the VMI was found. Nonproficient readers had significantly poorer visual efficiency skills when compared with proficient readers, but no differences were found for visual information-processing scores and VMI scores between the two groups.

These findings suggest that visual deficits may be common among school-age children, and that many of these children

are in school with uncorrected visual problems. These children were not receiving any supports or accommodations, nor were they receiving remedial intervention or related services (e.g. occupational therapy, speech-language pathology, physical therapy), suggesting relatively mild learning problems. However, screening for and recognizing visual problems among children who are struggling in school can be an important role for the occupational therapist, who can make a referral to a vision care specialist for comprehensive evaluation and diagnosis. Once a child with visual problems is identified, the occupational therapist can develop appropriate compensatory and instructional strategies, accommodations, and other supports to help the child access the curriculum and improve academic performance.

Use of Information from Other Sensory Systems

It is a common assumption that children with visual impairment are able to compensate for the loss of vision through increased use or heightened performance of the remaining senses. What is important to remember, however, is that the child who is visually impaired (i.e., from birth or early infancy) is in the *process* of building experiences that affect the developing brain and therefore must learn differently than do typical children. However, infants and young children with visual impairment do make sensory associations to form perceptions through their experiences, and if the remaining sensory systems are working well and the infant is otherwise healthy, the capacity to become competent and independent can be realized.[106] Furthermore, the research suggests that visual impairment does not have a negative impact on early development of tactile and auditory perception in that infants with visual impairment demonstrate basic discrimination abilities similar to those of sighted infants.[118] As Glass noted, infants with visual impairment may have a heightened behavioral response to auditory stimuli.[40] In addition, normal newborns respond more or less to sound of a given intensity, depending on the intensity of the corresponding light level (visual input).

Although infants with visual impairment are able to discriminate and thus respond accordingly to caregivers' voices or touch, their ability to connect auditory input to signify external objects in a specific location and to use this information to reach for objects appears to take longer to develop.[118] It is not a simple matter for an infant to know that a sound goes with an object that would be desirable to play with and that it can easily be located. Ross and Tobin posited that an infant may expend energy trying to interpret sounds at the expense of exploratory motor behavior.[94]

The development of fine motor skills depends on visual monitoring, and loss or distortion of visual input makes it more difficult for children to acquire these skills, although information from the tactile system can offer some compensatory strategies.[106] Children with visual impairment can manipulate objects to detect their form and shape, and therefore their concepts of objects are developed using haptic perception. In addition, their ability to coordinate reaching with sound depends on precise tactile system perception used for exploration and concept development[63] and the use of audition to locate an object in space. Although object concept behaviors in children with visual impairment are similar to hose in sighted infants through the first year and a half, performance on tasks that involve complex spatial displacements that cannot easily be tracked by audition or touch is more difficult; therefore, spatial understanding may be more of a problem than object conceptualization for children with visual impairment.[118]

The use of remaining sensory systems does not substitute for the efficiency of the visual system in integrating the child's experiences, and therefore the child with a visual impairment takes longer to develop his or her conceptual understanding of the world.[29,87] Learning is much more efficient for sighted children, who have the benefit of seeing the whole first and then can discover the different parts. As Fazzi and Klein explain, children with visual impairment must learn about things in parts based on different, discrete sensory inputs without seeing what the whole looks like first.[29] In their example, a child with a visual impairment may experience something with a furry body, a wet nose and tongue, a moving tail, loud barking, and must then integrate these pieces of sensory information to form the complete concept of "dog." Without adequate opportunities to experience all parts, the child's "picture" of the whole may be incomplete or inaccurate.

Although the child with visual impairment may gain specific information about an object's unique properties, the remaining senses do not necessarily provide him or her with sufficient information about the contexts in which the object exists.[106] For example, a child may learn about the cup he uses for drinking but may not come to understand for years that his plastic tumbler, his father's coffee mug, and the crystal wine glass used for special occasions are all variations of a class of objects used for drinking, especially if he has not had direct tactile experience with these items. If a child has limited experiences and does not have systematic introduction to objects in context, he or she will have a narrow range of schemes to work with, and these available schemes may not be fully validated by others.[87]

The importance of opportunities for multiple and varied experiences with explicit and targeted teaching is illustrated in the case vignettes in Case Study 25-1. Natalia, who had little or no vision, was provided with multiple opportunities for exploration by her family during everyday activities and she also received early intervention services, which promoted her ability to acquire concepts and language with little difficulty. Hannah, on the other hand, had some functional vision, but did not receive any intervention until she was a preschooler and required more intensive supports in a special day class. As she transitioned into an inclusion kindergarten class she was increasing her knowledge of letter, number, and shape concepts and participating in manipulative activities with adaptations and modifications, and thus her development in this area was occurring at a slower rate. Nicholas (who had only light perception) exhibited limited exploration of objects because he was hypersensitive and had a narrow range of preferences.

Sensory Modulation

Children with visual impairment and blindness often demonstrate stereotypical or repetitive behaviors, such as hand flapping, eye poking, or self-rocking. However, occupational therapists need to be mindful that these behaviors are also seen in children with other conditions, such as autistic spectrum disorder, severe or profound intellectual disabilities, and other developmental disabilities. Therefore the presence of these behaviors (with the exception of eye poking) may not be due to blindness per se but rather to the underlying cause of the blindness, particularly in children with multiple disabilities. These stereotypic behaviors have been hypothesized to be sensory-seeking activities that may compensate for the vision loss, but another explanation may be that the behaviors emerge as a result of the severely limited repertoires of movement and behavior available to children with visual impairment.[106] Among the children presented in the case vignettes, Nicholas displayed eye-pressing behaviors that was attributed to his visual impairment, but he also displayed repetitive behaviors including side-to-side rocking while standing (which may or may not have been due to the visual impairment) and repetitive actions with favored objects, whereas Natalia and Hannah did not display such behaviors.

Some children with visual impairment also present with behaviors that suggest tactile defensiveness, postural instability, or gravitational insecurity. That is, a child may withdraw his or her hand from an object or art media, may object to being touched, may be fearful of moving through space, or may be afraid to get on playground equipment such as swings or the jungle gym. The intensity of the child's responses in these situations varies as does the degree to which the responses interfere with the child's ability to engage in everyday occupations. Children with visual impairment who present with these behaviors may have restricted interactions with the environment and fewer typical motor and manipulative experiences that allow them to develop the postural control, gross and fine motor skills, and praxis at similar levels of competence and quality as those of typical sighted children.

It therefore becomes important for the occupational therapist to evaluate the child's behaviors carefully. For example, a child who may appear to demonstrate tactile hypersensitivity may not truly have a sensory modulation disorder or generalized hypersensitivities, but rather may need additional cues and strategies for managing new tactile experiences. The child may tolerate other tactile experiences, such as being held or wearing clothing made of different fabrics, and once the child becomes familiar with the object or material, the "defensive" reactions no longer occur. This scenario is different from that in which a child consistently demonstrates tactile hypersensitivity even to familiar tactile experiences or exhibits strong reactions to tactile stimuli beyond what could be attributed to caution or hesitance. For example, in the case vignettes, both Natalia and Hannah did not display overresponsiveness to tactile sensations (although Hannah's repertoire was narrower than Natalia's). Each reached for toys using auditory and tactile cues or available vision and auditory cues and both generally adapted quickly to new or unfamiliar experiences. Nicholas was extremely overreactive to touch (and other sensory input) and appeared to have sensory modulation difficulties.

Children with visual impairment whose motor experiences are limited may be fearful about moving through open space (e.g., crawling across the room, walking across the playground), moving on equipment such as tricycles or swings, or climbing on play structures or going down a slide. Children with visual impairment often display characteristic postural and movement patterns (Box 25-1) that may give the

---

BOX 25-1 Postural and Motor Characteristics Seen in Children with Visual Impairment.

Children with visual impairment may display the following:
- Overall low muscle and postural tone, including instability in shoulder girdle and hips
- Head tilted to one side (visual or auditory accommodation)
- Head forward, or hyperextended, resting on neck
- Head movements (e.g., swaying)
- Maintains wide base of support when standing or when walking
- Tendency to move in straight planes (e.g., decreased trunk rotation)
- High guard posture when walking

Data from Strickling, C. A. (1998). *Impact of vision loss on motor development. Information for occupational and physical therapists working with students with visual impairments.* Austin, TX: Texas School for the Blind and Visually Impaired; and Strickling, C. A., & Pogrund, R. L. (2002). Motor focus. Promoting movement experiences and motor development. In R. L. Pogrund, & D. L. Fazzi (Eds.), *Early focus: Working with young children who are blind or visually impaired and their families* (2nd ed., pp. 287-325). New York: AFB Press.

---

appearance of or contribute to movement challenges, depending upon the demonstrated level of functioning. In addition, caregivers (e.g., parents, daycare staff, teachers) who are concerned about safety may become overprotective and prevent or restrict children with visual impairment from engaging in movement and exploratory activities and experiencing the bumps and bruises that go with them, thus transmitting their fear to the child.

All three children in the case vignettes displayed some of these characteristic posture and movement patterns in various degrees. However, Natalia was very confident in her movements to negotiate familiar environments and had frequent opportunities to negotiate stairs and changes in surfaces indoors and outdoors, so that she could function independently in and around her home. Hannah also was able to do well in familiar environments, but often maintained a high guard posture with her arms, moved cautiously, and relied on adult supports including verbal cues to help guide her. Nicholas, on the other hand, was fearful of movement even in familiar environments, and often preferred to stay in one place, seated on the floor. When attempting to move in open space, such as when getting from one part of the classroom to another, he maintained a wide base of support, took small steps and became disoriented unless an adult was there to provide physical assistance (holding one hand). For a child such as Nicholas, caregivers should provide safe, graded movement experiences in a variety of contexts to build his confidence and expand his repertoire of play, mobility, and self-care skills and social participation.

Each of these children had varying ability to use their functional vision and sensory input to support exploration of the environment and movement through space. Without vision, the child must use vestibular, proprioceptive, and auditory information to orient to gravity, move through space, and maintain postural alignment.[106,110] To integrate these sensory systems, the child must have opportunities to actively engage in and experience movement in a variety of situations.

Activities of Daily Living and Instrumental Activities of Daily Living

Children with visual impairment may also have difficulty performing ADLs, such as dressing and self-feeding. The impact of visual impairment on the development of locomotion, gross and fine motor skills, and praxis for play may also affect the child's ability to stand and lift the leg to put on a pair of pants, or to direct the spoon to the plate to scoop up food, or to get into and out of the bathtub. In addition, if tactile hypersensitivity is present, the child's ability to engage in dressing, grooming, and toileting activities may be limited, or if oral hypersensitivity is present, the progression to more textured foods and eating a variety of foods may be problematic. These reactions can disrupt a daily caregiving routine for both the child and the caregivers, as well as interface with interactions with others and limit participation in learning activities at school. Negative associations with these activities can have long-lasting effects on the child's relationships with others and on occupational performance.

As children grow older and move into adolescence, participation in instrumental activities of daily living (IADLs) such as meal preparation, care of pets, use of communication devices including Braille writers, also needs to be considered. Preparation for and promotion of the development of skills needed for these more complex activities occurs through the developmental process in early childhood, but also need to be targeted specifically so that appropriate strategies and supports can be incorporated.

Social Participation and Communication

Patterns of interaction for young children with visual impairment and their caregivers differ from those of sighted children, although much of preverbal and nonverbal communication continues to occur in the absence of full functional vision.[118] Again, it is the nature of the experiences that appears to be the key factor in the development of children with visual impairment.

The quality of social participation is influenced not only by the visual impairment but also the degree to which the child has acquired specific social skills. One study examined the quality of social participation in different contexts (i.e., one-to-one, small group, and large group), for 64 children (4 to 18 years, mean age = 11.9 years) with visual impairment based on teacher ratings using an observational checklist assessing several components of social skills.[11] The investigators found that visual impairment was a significant predictor for the quality of one-to-one interactions along with verbal skills, body language, and recognition and expression of emotions, whereas intellectual disability and visual impairment were significant predictors for large group interactions with verbal skills, body language, play skills, and cooperation skills as important factors. As with small group interactions, intellectual disability was a significant predictor of social participation, with 59% of the variance explained by verbal skills and play skills. Thus while vision impairment may be a significant contributor to the quality of social interaction experienced by children, the acquisition of specific social skills may be even more important.

Young children with visual impairment may experience difficulty initiating and sustaining play and social interactions with peers. Without visual information to size up the context of the interaction and to pick up cues to respond to or imitate actions, the child with visual impairment may not have strategies to support the fluid give and take of a play scenario or social interaction.[28] The child may need explicit facilitation using physical, tactile, and verbal cues to keep up with changes that are often unpredictable, such as when play partners move to a different part of the playground, or switch from sand play to ball play. In addition, the child with visual impairment may need to rely on tactile and auditory means for social referencing, and typical peers may need help to understand that the child's physical contact or listening is not meant to be intrusive or nonresponsive.

As children grow older, the complexity of interactions increases, and the contextual aspects of language and communication become important. Vision plays a significant role in the interpretation of facial expressions and body language and in the imitation and sustaining of the give and take of these interactions. According to Smith Roley and Schneck, making eye contact, imitating facial gestures, shifting gaze, and perceiving the contextual features of visual images are often not part of the repertoire or experience of children who have vision loss at an early age.[106] The English language has many visual references that describe images, and Western culture expects individuals with visual impairment to communicate using the language of those who have sight.

Children with congenital visual impairment cannot "see" many features or qualities of objects using the other sensory channels such as a "red" button or "green" grass, nor can they see "a beautiful sunset" or "that one over there." Consequently, they can only try to imagine what it means when such descriptors or phrases are used.[106] In addition, children with visual impairment may not demonstrate the animation and nuances of facial expression because they have not experienced seeing and imitating these expressions. Because they need to concentrate on what is being said when there is competing activity and noise in the surroundings, they may be perceived as not paying attention to the speaker or as being bored or unfriendly.

These misperceptions may negatively affect the self-concept and perceived competence among children with visual impairment. Shapiro, Moffet, Lieberman, and Drummer examined the self-perceptions of 43 children and youths (27 boys with a mean age of 12.37 years, and 16 girls with a mean age 14.0 years) with visual impairment who attended a 1-week summer sports camp.[104] Based on participant responses for items in three dimensions in the Self-Perception Profile for Children (8-14 years) or the Self-Perception Profile for Adolescents (15-21 years), the investigators found that mean scores for physical appearance were rated highest, followed by social acceptance, and then athletic competence for both precamp and postcamp measures. The investigators suggest that the children and youths took pride in their appearance, but may not have felt they had adequate skills to participate in the sports available at the camp. The higher scores for social acceptance relative to athletic competence suggested that the campers believed they had acquired the social skills necessary for interactions in social contexts, but not necessarily for participation in group physical activities.

As can be seen, then, not only do difficulties such as delayed motor skills or limited range of manipulative interactions and play with objects affect the ability of children with visual impairment to engage in play activities with peers or to participate in social activities (e.g., eating lunch with friends, or participating in team or group sports), but the degree to which social skills are effective in different social contexts may also vary. These motor and social skills difficulties can affect the child's ability to develop friendships or to fit in with the social demands and expectations of his or her peer group, and thus impact one's perceived social competence. Beginning early in the child's life, it is important to provide a range of opportunities in a variety of contexts with targeted strategies to support social development.

Occupational Therapy Evaluation

In many respects evaluation of the occupational performance of children with visual impairment encompasses the same components as in evaluation of children with other disabilities. Participation in play, self-care, school occupations, and preparation for work are areas of focus for evaluation depending on the age and needs of the child. Evaluation of the performance skills (e.g., motor, process, and communication/interaction skills) that support or limit the child's ability to engage in specific activities in these areas, and the activity demands, client factors, and contexts in which the child performs these activities, is also part of a comprehensive assessment. For example, a toddler with a visual impairment who has difficulty playing with toys may need evaluation of fine motor skills, tactile and proprioceptive processing, and postural control in sitting, with observations conducted in the home and in daycare or early intervention settings.

Standardized assessment tools for evaluating overall development in major domains (e.g., the Bayley Scales of Infant and Toddler Development, 3rd edition [Bayley III],[9] or the Peabody Developmental Motor Scales, 2nd edition [PDMS-2][34]) should be used with caution because these measures were not standardized on children with visual impairment and the administration procedures do not include adaptations for this group. Therefore comparison of performance to that of sighted peers and use of the standard scores based on the normative sample are usually not appropriate. A few tools, such as the Battelle Developmental Inventory, 2nd edition (BDI-2),[77] are both standardized and criterion-referenced and include administration instructions for children with motor or sensory impairments.

Criterion-referenced measures such as the Hawaii Early Learning Profile (HELP) for infants and toddlers[80] and preschoolers,[116] or play-based assessment tools such as the Transdisciplinary Play-Based Assessment, 2nd edition (TPBA-2),[65] may be more useful because they yield a profile of individual strengths and limitations or concerns that can be used to formulate an intervention plan. In addition, tools such as the Oregon Project Skills Inventory, 5th edition,[3] take into consideration what is known about the unique developmental trajectories of certain skills (e.g., walking independently, reaching to sound) in children with visual impairment. Other assessment tools specifically designed for children with visual impairment or that evaluate visual skills are described in Appendix 25-A on the Evolve website.

Skilled observation and parent or caregiver questionnaires can be useful for gathering information about the child's temperament, self-regulation capacities, sensory processing and sensory modulation behaviors, and interaction with caregivers. In addition, interviews with the parents, teachers, or other caregivers can provide information about daily routines, contexts, and expectations and resources available to support the family's and the child's participation in activities. As children get older, in addition to the areas and skills discussed previously, the focus of evaluation for the occupational therapist may involve collaboration with the special education or regular education teacher, and education vision specialists (e.g., teacher for students with visual impairment, or orientation and mobility specialist), and vision care specialists (e.g., developmental optometrist) to assess barriers in school and play settings and determine the need for adaptations for performing classroom activities or organization of desk space or the use of assistive technology.[57,85,86] For adolescents, the occupational therapist, in collaboration with teachers, vision specialists, and the family, may evaluate the individual's ability to travel in the school, community, or work setting, in addition to leisure interests and activities and levels of school functioning. Evaluation of age-appropriate ADL and IADL performance in different settings may also be included.

An assessment tool that specifically addresses the impact of visual impairment on quality of life for students with low vision has been developed and may be of interest to occupational therapists.[19] This questionnaire was based on the Impact of Vision Impairment Profile developed for adults,[61,62,119] and consists of five domains: school/specialist instruction, social interaction, community, family, and vision impairment/peer interaction. The questionnaire is helpful in identifying needs and planning intervention and its items emphasize participation in routine school and daily activities relative to social interaction, academic success, orientation and mobility skills, community acceptance, and other social opportunities.

In some instances a child who has developmental delays or difficulties may be referred for occupational therapy but has not yet been diagnosed with a visual impairment. If a child shows signs or symptoms of a vision problem (Table 25-2) and a visual impairment is suspected, the occupational therapist can assist in the diagnostic process through screening or evaluation of oculomotor skills (e.g., visual tracking, fixation, shifting gaze), focusing skills (e.g., shift from near to far), and eye teaming or binocularity (e.g., strabismus). The occupational therapist may also measure the child's visual perceptual skills (e.g., visual discrimination, visual spatial relations) and visual motor integration. Some developmental measures (e.g., Bayley III, HELP) include items that require visual attention, visual tracking, visual memory, and other vision-related areas. Specific visual perception and visual motor tests are also available (see Chapter 12).

Occupational Therapy Intervention

The overall outcome of occupational therapy intervention for children with visual impairment is to support participation in the contexts in which they function on a daily basis. For a 6-month-old premature infant with retinopathy of prematurity, for example, the occupational therapist may focus on establishing oral motor skills for feeding and self-soothing

TABLE 25-2 Signs and Symptoms of Visual Problems*

Category	Signs and Symptoms
Physical	Eyes shake or randomly wander
	Eyes are not able to follow moving object, face of parent
	Pupils of the eyes are excessively large or small
	Pupils of the eyes are not black; a cloudy film appears to be present
	Eyes are not in alignment (e.g., they are crossed or turn outward)
	Blurred vision or double vision
	Sensitivity to light
Behavioral	Needs to move closer to objects of interest; sits excessively close to the television
	Squinting, eyestrain, frequently rubs eyes
	Covers or closes one eye when looking at detail
	Excessive head movement
	Complains of discomfort or headaches when reading or doing close work
	Turns or tilts head when looking at detail
	Responds significantly better to objects on one side of the body than on the other
	Avoidance of or becomes tired after close work
	Poor attention span
	Complains of moving print
Performance	Appears clumsy, or frequently bumps into objects when walking and running
	Cannot find necessary items for activities
	Difficulty learning left and right
	Has trouble learning the alphabet, recognizing words, learning basic math concepts of size, magnitude, position
	Difficulty with reading—reads slowly, skips lines, trouble with navigating page
	Difficulty with drawing, copying, writing—alignment, accuracy, reversals, organization on page, etc.
	Difficulty copying from board
	Has trouble keeping up with assignments
Social	Lack of interest in the environment
	Anxiety, social isolation
	Decreased self-confidence

*If a child shows any of the listed signs or symptoms, a referral to an eye care specialist is indicated.

Data from Takeshita, B. (n.d.). *Developing your child's vision.* Los Angeles: Center for the Partially Sighted; Scheiman, M. (2002). Optometric model of vision, parts one, two and three. In *Understanding and managing vision deficits: A guide for occupational therapists* (2nd ed., pp. 17-84). Thorofare, NJ: Slack; and Goldstand, S., Koslowe, K. D., & Parush, S. (2005). Vision, visual-information processing, and academic performance among seventh-grade school children: A more significant relationship than we thought? *American Journal of Occupational Therapy, 59,* 377-389.

strategies for calming; other recommendations may include positioning strategies for feeding and caregiver-infant interactions and selecting toys that enhance the use of available vision, along with auditory and tactile channels. For a 10-year-old boy who has cerebral palsy with spastic hemiparesis and legal blindness (i.e., best corrected visual acuity of 20/200 or worse, or a visual field of 20 degrees or less in the better eye[122]), the school-based occupational therapist may focus on maintaining self-care skills; establishing organizational skills for using desk space and completing assignments; devising strategies that support the use of low vision aids; and promoting social participation in games with peers with modifications and adaptations.

Occupational therapy models of practice that are particularly useful for evaluation and intervention with children who have visual impairments include sensory integration, motor acquisition and motor learning, visual information processing/visual perception, and person-environment-occupation (PEO) frameworks. Neurodevelopmental and biomechanical models of practice may also be useful, particularly for children with multiple disabilities. All types of occupational therapy interventions—therapeutic use of self; therapeutic use of occupations and activities; consultation; and education—may be incorporated in different combinations and at different points during intervention in a dynamic process that changes based on the needs of the child and family; the progress and response to interventions; and the demands of the contexts involved.

The occupational therapist may be the primary interventionist for children who have visual impairments with other conditions; however, if the visual impairment is the primary or sole condition, it is more likely that an educational vision specialist (i.e., teacher of students with visual impairment; orientation and mobility specialist) is the primary interventionist, and the occupational therapist may provide consultation as needed. Generally the occupational therapist is a member of a team of professionals (e.g., general education teacher and/or special education teacher, educational vision specialist, speech language pathologist, vision care specialist) who, along with the family, collaborate to identify the child's and family's needs and develop an intervention program to address those needs with one or more individuals providing services.

The occupational therapist and the occupational therapy assistant often provide services to achieve the following goals:

- *Develop self-care skills.* The occupational therapist may consult with and educate those who work with the child with visual impairment to identify skill levels and explain problems affecting the child's development of self-care skills. The occupational therapist may specifically address underlying foundations and specific skills needed to perform self-care tasks, and also work collaboratively with the family and the team to incorporate behavioral or learning strategies; suggest adaptations or modifications to the environment; recommend seating or other equipment; and incorporate strategies that support independence (e.g., placing a tactile cue in specific areas of clothing to distinguish front from back or to identify color; using a divided plate or the clock orientation to serve food items).

- *Enhance sensory processing, sensory modulation, and sensory integration.* Developmentally age-appropriate activities and materials that provide tactile, auditory, proprioceptive, and vestibular input can benefit the child with visual impairment and enhance or promote development of body concept, postural control, and tactile discrimination for recognizing and manipulating objects; self-regulation; spatial relation perceptions; and grasp, release, bilateral hand use, and praxis. Suspended equipment, scooterboards, tilt boards, obstacle courses, and other movement or balance equipment are useful, but it is also important to provide interventions using playground equipment (e.g., slides,

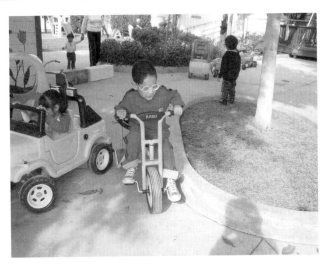

FIGURE 25-1   Child with low vision tracking around a curb on a playground tricycle.   (Courtesy Jill Brody, OTR/L, Blind Children's Center, Los Angeles.)

jungle gyms, tricycles, swings) in the natural settings in which the child functions on a regular basis (Figure 25-1). In addition to a traditional sensory integration approach, some programs specifically incorporate the visual and/or auditory system as part of intervention. For example, an occupational therapy program that was designed to fully address oculomotor control and visual processing within a sensory integration approach—the Vestibular-Oculomotor "Astronaut Training" Protocol—focuses on vestibular, proprioceptive, and oculomotor aspects of sensory processing and postural adaptation in time and space[52] and may be appropriate for some children. It is important, however, that safety be maintained in the use of equipment and that, as appropriate, the child be allowed to control the movement and amount of input within his or her range of adaptive responses. (Additional discussion of intervention strategies using a sensory integrative approach with children with visual impairments can be found in Smith Roley & Schneck[106] and Schaaf and Smith Roley[97]).

The child with visual impairment does not see the approach of people and objects and may therefore exhibit hypersensitivity to touch. In many instances children who have some or variable vision may have more difficulty with this than children with total blindness because children with some functional vision or low vision (i.e., best corrected visual acuity of 20/70 in the better eye[36,122]) receive unpredictable visual input from light patterns and movements. For children with total blindness, the visual input is essentially consistent. Firm touch generally is better than light touch, which can be interpreted as painful or aversive. The child with visual impairment often is more comfortable and less defensive when a verbal cue accompanies or precedes the tactile cue. Strategies to help children modulate their reactions to tactile input include activities that encourage the child to explore and play with various materials using graded textures (e.g., sand, dried lentils, beans, and rice); activities that include vibration or proprioceptive input; and incorporation of a sensory diet at home and in the classroom.

Support of the child's sensory modulation may be needed before an activity that the child finds aversive, such as art time, sand play, or eating. The child with hypersensitivity may benefit from recommendations for clothing, sleepwear, and linens. Also, if oral sensory defensiveness is a factor, strategies such as introduction of graded food and liquid textures and tactile/proprioceptive activities involving the mouth (e.g., using straws with thickened liquids; blowing activities with bubbles or whistles) can be implemented. During these activities, it is important for the child with visual impairment to experience contingent responses to his or her behaviors, taking into consideration individual needs and preferences, rather than being a passive recipient of adult actions (noncontingent experiences).[16] For example, a child should not experience tactile stimulation in isolation (e.g., rubbing of different textured cloths on the arms); rather, the tactile experiences should be provided in the context of real life activities (e.g., using a nubby towel to dry oneself after a bath) so that the child associates tactile experiences with actions and events.

- *Enhance postural control and movement in space.* Providing a variety of movement experiences throughout the daily routines early in life is important. Caregivers can be encouraged to use different carrying positions or carriers while engaging in everyday activities so that infants experience movement (and vestibular and proprioceptive input) under secure conditions. Instead of passive positioning in prone, in which motivation to lift the head is minimal, when visual impairment is significant, caregivers can be encouraged to engage in games that include tilting the child toward and away from them while talking to and having fun with the child, or positioning toys of interest in front of or to either side of the child and encouraging the child to reach for them.[86,111] The occupational therapist and the orientation and mobility specialist can work closely to facilitate and establish the child's ability to move through space through the use of push toys, riding toys, and moving over surfaces of different heights, density or firmness, and textures (Figure 25-2). Occupational therapists may also

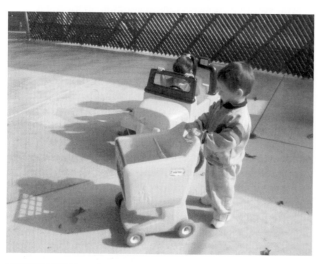

FIGURE 25-2 Child with severe visual impairment using a push toy as a mobility aid. (Courtesy Jill Brody, OTR/L, Blind Children's Center, Los Angeles.)

use neurodevelopmental facilitation techniques to help the child use trunk rotation instead of moving in straight planes, develop balance and righting reactions on unstable equipment, and improve transitional movements. In addition, motor learning principles may be applied to provide children with opportunities to practice a variety of movement strategies during different play activities with feedback on their performance and results of their actions.

- *Develop body awareness and spatial orientation.* Many of the aforementioned activities can also help the child develop body awareness and directionality. Obstacle courses can teach the child spatial concepts such as left-right, up-down, over-under, in-out, beside, around, and behind. It is important to describe the movement or direction the child experiences to help him or her establish the association that will give meaning to the spatial concepts. Body awareness and spatial awareness are critical components that contribute to the child's development of mobility and language.[96,97,106,111]

- *Develop tactile-proprioceptive perceptual abilities.* The child with visual impairment needs to maximize tactile discrimination abilities to learn about the features and properties of objects; to adjust grasp according to the size, shape, and weight of an object; and to grade the amount of pressure, force, or speed needed to manipulate toys or to use tools. Tactile discrimination is also important for learning to read Braille. Finger painting, finding and identifying objects hidden in sand or beans or other media, and experiencing gradations of textures among everyday objects and materials, clothing, and surfaces are examples of activities that can increase tactile awareness and discrimination. In addition, manipulating objects, to operating or using toys functionally (e.g., pushing button on a toy phone, playing with shape sorter toys with auditory feedback), helps children develop functional skills using tactile-proprioceptive and auditory information.

  Children also need opportunities to explore and feel real-life objects to build multisensory associations and perceptions that ultimately will become integrated and provide foundations for progression to more abstract representations (e.g., a real orange that is round, cold, fragrant, has an outside texture that can be peeled, can be separated into segments, tasted; a plastic orange and orange wedges used in kitchen and food play; a flat orange-shaped puzzle piece that fits into a puzzle board; a raised outline of an orange on paper for coloring). These experiences can help a child with visual impairment establish a mental image of the label "orange" and the color "orange" that is unique to each child based on characteristics that are meaningful to him or her.

- *Improve manipulation and fine motor skills.* At first the world has to come to the child with visual impairment. A variety of toys and objects should be maintained within reach (e.g., tied to the crib, on the high chair or tabletop, on the floor). In addition, activities should be incorporated that promote upper extremity weight bearing and exploration of toys to promote development of the arches of the hand, which are often not as well developed in children with visual impairment.[110,111] By assessing the sensory features of the toys or objects, the occupational therapist can select objects and media appropriate for the child's ability to process the information and for his or her skill level. For example, objects may vary in texture, or in texture and sound, or may have multisensory features (e.g., sound, texture, flashing lights) and media that are typically available in school settings (e.g., sand, paint, glue, PlayDoh) should also be incorporated. Providing opportunities for the child with visual impairment to practice in-hand manipulation with activities that involve rotation and translation of small objects can improve the dynamic use of tools. Some of the activities described previously (e.g., that address sensory integration and hypersensitivity) can also be used for sensory preparation of the hands before manipulation of objects.

- *Maximize use of functional vision.* The occupational therapist should always facilitate the child's use of whatever vision is available to him or her during intervention and everyday activities. The more a child uses visual pathways, the better vision develops.[7] Visual awareness and discrimination activities, such as color or shape recognition and matching, are important for children with functional vision. Activities such as use of a flashlight in a darkened room for tracking games or localizing targets may also improve visual skills. The occupational therapist can also promote the child's use of low vision aids recommended by the vision care specialist such as large print books or magnifiers and any other assistive technology that may be appropriate (e.g., closed-circuit Television [CCTV], computers with special software).

All these goals require the occupational therapist to educate and consult with family members, who should be encouraged to provide the child with visual impairment many opportunities for engagement in activities as they would a child without disability. Verbal and physical interaction should also be encouraged because the child may not always demonstrate behaviors that elicit interaction. Occupational therapists may consult with parents on ways to create a safe environment in which the child can play independently and make recommendations for adapting the environment to optimize independent functioning of the child. The family should also be informed about the importance of early intervention and their options for services.

Additional team goals to which the occupational therapist contributes include the following:

- *Encourage socially acceptable behaviors.* Children with visual impairment are at a disadvantage in social situations, particularly at school, where typical children are active and often participate in a variety of physical games. It is difficult for children with visual impairment to signal their interest in playing with peers, and reliance on others to help them with these interactions limits their ability to experience social competence.[28,53] It is important to provide the child with real-life activities, with specific instruction in symbolic play, perhaps with one other child at first and introducing other children as the child gains skills. Role playing, turn taking, and use of facial expressions with high affect and animation are strategies that can be used to facilitate social interactions. The child with visual impairment may need verbal or tactile cues to face people when speaking, to smile, and to maintain an upright posture with the head in midline. He or she must also learn to determine how others are reacting based on voices rather than gestures, facial expressions, or body language.

- *Encourage language and concept development.* The child with visual impairment must consciously be taught to develop cognitive schemes that the sighted child picks up in a relatively casual manner. This is done with verbalization and the use of the child's intact sensory systems, as described in other sections of this chapter. Those things that cannot be touched or heard (e.g., clouds) need to be described and explained. To reiterate, it is also beneficial to provide real-life, hands-on, multisensory experiences in a variety of meaningful contexts to help children with visual impairment establish the foundations for understanding concrete, functional, and abstract concepts.[29]

- *Strengthen cognitive skills, such as object permanence, cause and effect, object recognition, and ability to match and sort.* A variety of toys are available to help infants and toddlers and preschoolers develop these skills. Capitalizing on toys that are of high interest and motivating can be incorporated to build intentionality, effective search strategies, and means-end understanding within everyday routines.[29] In addition, shape sorters, formboards and simple puzzles, or blocks that provide auditory feedback (e.g., music, animal sounds) when inserted into appropriate openings or when connected are useful, but it is also important to help children with visual impairment to develop strategies such as using one hand to locate the opening tactually and placing the shape with the other hand. For older children, these goals can be accomplished through games (e.g., to promote memory, classification, sorting) using different media and many simple craft activities. The unique abilities and limitations of the child must be considered in addressing academic goals.

- *Maximize auditory perceptual abilities.* The child with visual impairment must learn to identify sounds and their meanings and react to them appropriately. Sounds come from several basic sources: toys, speech, and the environment. Active, rather than passive, listening should be emphasized. Helpful activities include locating a variety of sounds in the environment, identifying sounds, and following directions from persons and recordings. In addition, the child with visual impairment must also use hearing as the primary distance sense and source for spatial information that guides his or her movement in the environment.[4] Helping children with visual impairment to use one or two sound references in their environments (e.g., the clock ticking on the wall; a bell attached to the classroom door) will be useful to enable them to know automatically where they are and where they want or need to go in a given space. Incorporate mobile objects that have sound (e.g., balls with bells inside; toy cars that make sounds) and encourage children to discover interesting sounds and vary the volume. It is just as important for children with visual impairment to register soft sounds and to filter out irrelevant auditory information, so use of toys and activities should involve grading the intensity of sensory input accordingly to avoid overwhelming or distracting the child.

Also important for the child with visual impairment is the development of echolocation skills. *Echolocation* is the ability to hear and interpret sound waves, which is important for orientation and travel in the environment.[4] By using clear sound signals (e.g., a clap, tongue clicking, tapping, or a hand-held clicker) the child uses echoes produced to determine the location of objects and important features (e.g., size, general shape, density) and to detect buildings, play structures, doorways, stairs, and potential obstacles (e.g., poles, trees). Echolocation serves as a means to extend the reach of the cane to gather information at much greater distances. Some children with visual impairment develop echolocation skills on their own without any instruction, whereas other children will need targeted intervention. The occupational therapist can collaborate with the orientation and mobility specialist to support recommended strategies that promote the development of echolocation skills.

Issues in Critical Thinking and Decision Making

Some key considerations for working with children with visual impairment influence the process occupational therapists engage in to think critically, interpret data, and make decisions regarding how to approach evaluation and intervention to address the unique, yet diverse profile of abilities and needs presented by this population.

Having information regarding the nature of the child's visual impairment, additional or co-existing conditions, and the degree of functional vision available provides a starting point at the time of referral or soon thereafter for anticipating possible areas of concern and what assessment tools and methods may be appropriate. For example, given Natalia's history of extreme prematurity and retinopathy of prematurity and her limited visual function, the occupational therapist's knowledge of possible developmental consequences as a result of prematurity and those associated with visual impairment may lead the therapist to anticipate neuromotor difficulties and delayed acquisition of skills. Conducting a team assessment at Natalia's home was invaluable in providing an opportunity to see her in a natural setting, as it became evident that she was demonstrating age-appropriate functioning. In addition to play-based and criterion-referenced measures, administration of items from a standardized test (even though standard scores could not be used) was possible with relatively few adaptations (e.g., tapping a cube to introduce block items, providing tactile cues to locate materials, allowing time to touch items), which provided an indication of how well she incorporated strategies that enabled her to perform adult-presented activities with materials that were not necessarily the same as those she interacted with at home. Her performance in many ways was similar to that of typical, sighted children, it was also apparent that early intervention services could provide rich opportunities to promote development. Use of the Oregon Project Skills Inventory provided additional information to confirm that she demonstrated skills that were at age expected levels for children with visual impairment and that she had visual and compensatory skills that would serve her well for orientation and mobility, cane use, and Braille. The occupational therapist's findings, together with those of the other team members, led to the determination that occupational therapy was no longer indicated (as had been provided through the early intervention program) and that services provided by the orientation and mobility specialist and the teacher for students with visual impairment were the most appropriate to support access to her educational program.

Because of Nicholas' Leber's congenital amaurosis (LCA and his visual function—light perception in only both eyes—and delayed development, the occupational therapist decided that standardized testing was not appropriate. A team assessment was conducted, and it was evident from observations of his performance and behavior that Nicholas had behaviors that could not be attributed to the visual impairment alone. The parent interview and skilled observations, therefore, were particularly informative to the team. The occupational therapist conducted separate observations at the center-based early intervention program and in the home to interpret how Nicholas performed and behaved in different contexts. The team's observations led to the possibility that autism may be a co-existing condition, notably because Nicholas' use of language was a rote skill (even though it was initially perceived by some as advanced) versus a means to socially interact with others that was atypical for children with visual impairment He also displayed atypical imitation and play skills. It was important, then, to determine to what extent skills and behaviors were typical, expected for a child with visual impairment, or characteristic of autism (refer to Table 25-3 for a comparison of behaviors).

A review of some relevant studies is provided here to highlight the complexity that may be involved in this process. For example, studies that have examined the presence of autism in children with visual impairment because of different causes have shown inconsistent findings. One study found that five preschool boys with LCA met the criteria for autism with a distinct profile and higher scores on measures such as the Childhood Autism Rating Scale (CARS) when compared with a group of five boys with visual impairment from other causes.[88] In contrast, another study with a larger sample of 24 children with LCA (13 boys, 11 girls; 2 to 11 years of age) found that only 4 of the children displayed autism of a mild/moderate degree based on scores on the modified CARS (excluding visual responsiveness items).[30] Given that very few children in their sample had delays in their social and emotional responsiveness or in their social relationships, the investigators suggested that some of the behaviors that may be rated as autistic-like were likely the result of the impact of severe visual deficits on their early interactions and that the risk for such behaviors could be minimized with intervention. In another study, Goodman and Ashby found that some children with delayed visual maturation (DVM) who displayed autistic-type behaviors showed improvement in language, play, social interest, and social competence that appeared to be associated with their increased visual function (i.e., their visual unresponsiveness resolved, as is expected in children with DVM).[42] Other studies suggest that children with visual impairment who also have autism were more likely to have an underlying neurologic impairment.[25,74] In addition, the visual impairment was more severe in those students with autism than among the students with visual impairment only.

Because Nicholas had significant difficulties with sensory modulation, the occupational therapists used a sensory integration approach. Clinic-based services facilitated his ability to manage activities on dynamic equipment and to negotiate surfaces of different heights (i.e., relative to hyperresponsivity to gravity and to tactile sensations, and postural instability). Therapy activities also promoted praxis, and his manipulative skills in play and functional activities. The school-based

TABLE 25-3   Comparison of Characteristic Behaviors in Children with Visual Impairment and Autism to Typically Developing Children and Children with Visual Impairment

	Typical	Visually Impaired or Blind	Visually Impaired or Blind and Autistic Disorder
Communication	Uses jargon, follows simple commands Vocabulary increases as expected for age Uses language for social interactions Initiates, sustains back-and-forth communication	Speech may be echolalic, duration is short May display delayed language if experiences are limited, but is not distorted Enjoys give and take of communication	Uses words without attaching meaning to them Echolalia may be difficult to alter or diminish, or may lead to verbal perseveration with idiosyncratic meanings Difficulty initiating and maintaining back-and-forth interactions with others
Social interactions	Takes turns with adult during vocal play, other play actions Imitates, engages in pretend play with elaborated schemas Enjoys and initiates play with others Engages in cooperative play	Engages in social give and take, seeks to share information with others May display delayed imitation and pretend play, but can be taught Needs feedback to understand social situations, cues	Limited response, orientation to sound Limited social interest Repetitive play actions, may not use toys in their intended ways Prefers to play alone, limited social curiosity Anxious or uncomfortable in social situations
Repetitive, stereotypical behaviors	Shows typical development of reaching, manipulation of objects, sensorimotor play actions Repetitive actions reflect developmentally appropriate interest in practice, mastery Expands, creates scenarios in play	May show stereotypical behaviors (i.e., in novel or unfamiliar situations, but amenable to redirection and engagement in meaningful activities and can learn to control behaviors when older)	Repetitive play actions, restricted repertoire that is not elaborated May perseverate on a particular feature of an object or play action May display rigidity in routines, difficulty with transitions, can be difficult to redirect

Adapted from Gense, M. H., & Gense, D. J. (2005). *Autism spectrum disorders and visual impairment. Meeting students' learning needs.* New York: AFB Press.

occupational therapist recommended a sensory diet to support his participation in learning and play activities, strategies to expand his interactions with peers, and activities to promote fine motor and self-care skills (in the home and community as well). Collaboration with other related service providers, including the orientation and mobility specialist, the teacher for students with visual impairment, the special education teacher, the behavior specialist, the speech-language pathologist, and the parents and grandparents, was also critical to move him forward as his readiness and ability to cope with increased demands improved and his repertoire of skills expanded.

Hannah was older at the time of referral and had no early intervention services. She had refractive errors (hyperopia in the right eye, myopia in the left eye), and optic atrophy and cortical visual impairment (CVI). She also had a history of seizures. Thus neurologic involvement was evident and the impact of CVI on development needed to be considered. That is, occupational therapists (and other team members) need to be aware of and understand characteristic behaviors that are typically seen in children with CVI, who have different visual behaviors from those seen in children with other types of visual impairment.[8,91] These include delayed response (visual latency) in looking at objects and the need for movement (either the object or the viewer) to elicit sustained visual attention. Therefore they display difficulty assimilating visual novelty and visual complexity

(e.g., bringing an object close to their eyes as a strategy to block out irrelevant background stimuli), nonpurposeful gaze; absence of visually directed reach; and inconsistency in what they see and how visual input is interpreted.[8,26,91] This knowledge and use of skilled observation of visual behavior are extremely important to evaluate and interpret observations and findings, and to determine appropriate interventions.

Team assessment with Hannah included play-based observations, criterion-referenced measures, and classroom observations at the private preschool. (Functional vision assessment by a teacher for students with visual impairment had been conducted with all three children.) Hannah was observed to use available vision to reach for objects with reasonable accuracy, engage in reciprocal ball play, use her body adequately to negotiate the environment, and use a spoon to feed herself. However, her repertoire and level of play skills, limited communication, and limited problem-solving skills indicated overall delayed development when considering her chronologic age and her visual impairment. Her family had limited resources since emigrating to the United States, but they negotiated with the various agencies and the school district to obtain services. The classroom observations showed that she had responded quickly to the intervention services and preschool program. Occupational therapy focused on increasing her use of tactual exploration of objects, and increasing her repertoire of manipulative and play skills. She responded better when she was in control of the tactile input she received, and because she enjoyed vestibular activities, swinging was incorporated to increase her arousal level and enhance her motivation to try games with different objects. Collaboration with the teacher for students with visual impairment, the speech-language pathologist, and her parents occurred to promote concept development, receptive and expressive language skills, and social participation. Her cognitive abilities and overall developmental level, and the length of time before intervention was initiated were considered in determining appropriate accommodations.

As can be seen from these case vignettes, team assessment and collaboration were significant components of the service models implemented with these children. Team models vary in different settings, and whether the occupational therapist is part of a team or not, communication with other service providers involved with the child with visual impairment and his or her family is extremely important. Consistent and open communication is necessary to avoid duplication of services, share knowledge and expertise toward common goals, be aware of any contraindications, and to plan and provide individualized programs to meet the unique needs of the child.[21,55]

Occupational therapy practitioners vary in the degree of awareness and knowledge of the impact visual impairment may have on a child's functioning, and thus it becomes critical that the occupational therapist obtains information from those with expertise, and informs the other providers about the occupational therapist's role and contribution to the child's program. Although implementing a team evaluation process is highly valuable, it is not always possible or practical. Nevertheless, an occupational therapist who conducts an evaluation can review and incorporate information from evaluation reports from others working with the child (e.g., psychologist, vision care specialist, teacher for students with visual impairment) into his or her analysis and interpretation of findings. This enables the occupational therapist to obtain a comprehensive profile of the child's abilities and needs in different contexts, particularly if the occupational therapist is not able to conduct a home visit or classroom observation.

Special Techniques and Strategies

Children with severe visual impairments may rely on Braille materials and talking books (e.g., those that can be listened to using devices such as compact discs [CDs] and MP3 players) for their education. Braille is a system of six raised dots arranged in a cell to represent the letters of the alphabet, numbers, and words. It is produced on a special slate with a stylus or on a machine called a braillewriter. The system was developed by a young, blind French student, Louis Braille, in 1824, and was found to be more efficient than attempting to read the raised Roman alphabet. The complete Braille code consists of letters of the alphabet and contractions and words in short form.[57] Advances in technology now make it possible to use computer software and devices that incorporate Braille and/or audio formats. These devices can increase the amount and quality of written output, and provide opportunities for interactive learning.

Optometrists provide vision therapy using various low vision aids, occlusion (patching), specific exercises, and other activities.[14,100] Vision therapy (also known as orthoptics, vision training, visual training, eye training) involves an organized therapeutic regimen that includes functional activities used to treat conditions that interfere with visual function.[100] The purpose of vision therapy is to provide activities and devices to increase visual efficiency and visual information processing skills. Occupational therapists often team with optometrists to reinforce these goals.

Various types of lenses are available for individuals with visual impairment, from the relatively common ones used to correct refractive errors to telescopic lenses (for viewing distant objects) and microscopic lenses (for viewing near objects) that are used as low vision aids for certain types of vision problems. Hand-held magnifiersinclude those that have the lens in sturdy housing (i.e., stand magnifiers) that are placed directly onto the reading material, and those that can be worn around the neck. Electronic magnification systems include CCTV systems, hand-held cameras that interface with a display monitor, head-mounted systems with a camera and display unit in front of each eye, small electronic systems that combine a camera and display for portable use, and miniature LCD magnifiers.[33]

Some occupational therapists are involved with low vision training (or vision therapy) to teach the child with visual impairment to use his or her available vision[8,100] in collaboration with a low vision specialist (i.e., optometrist). This may involve specific activities recommended by the low vision specialist that address problems with accommodation, vergence, visual fixation and focusing, oculomotor skills or other vision-related problems, many of which can be incorporated into the play-based or therapeutic activities that the occupational therapist already implements. In addition, a variety of adaptations and accommodations can be incorporated, including adjusting the intensity, position, and type of light (illumination) in the environment; minimizing glare; enhancing or maximizing contracts between objects and background or surfaces; adjusting size of objects or print; spacing and positioning of objects; color selection; and the amount of time to complete tasks.[26]

Orientation and mobility training or instruction teaches basic skills and techniques for travel in the environment such as trailing, human (sighted) guide technique, and protective techniques.[4] In the *human guide technique*, the child who is blind takes the guide's arm and walks a half step behind and to the side of the guide to follow the guide's movements. For young children, an adapted grasp may be used, such as holding the guide's wrist (and progressing to the guide's elbow as they get older), or the child may hold the guide's index finger. This is preferred over the adult's holding the child's hand and pulling or leading the child. The human guide technique is safe and efficient and enables the child to interpret the guide's body movement (i.e., on uneven surfaces) and changes in direction.[4] Specific verbal and tactual cues are incorporated to negotiate stairs, narrow passages, or if the child with visual impairment needs to change sides.

Trailing is a technique whereby the child with visual impairment holds his or her arm at a 45-degree angle in front and to the side of the body to follow a surface (e.g., wall) with the hand. Trailing serves several functions, including protection during movement, a method for gathering information and locating landmarks and destinations, and for alignment.[4] The use of trailing can be enhanced when taught together with using a cane.

Protective techniques can be taught to toddlers and preschoolers (depending upon motor development, physical coordination, and attention span) and involve upper body and lower body techniques in which the arm is flexed with forearm held across the body with palm facing out at about shoulder height or at an angle in front of the face, or extended downward and diagonally across the body at the hip with palm facing the body, respectively. Another protection technique, which can be used in bending down to retrieve a dropped object, is to extend the arm palm out in front of the head. The child with visual impairment can search for a lost object by touching the ground to establish a beginning point and then searching in an ever-widening concentric circle pattern. A technique for exploring a room involves searching the parameters of the room first, then mentally dividing it into grids to be searched methodically. This method can be used to introduce the child with vision impairment to a new classroom or new home setup. The use of landmarks and cues (e.g., the grass at the edge of the sidewalk) is beneficial for independent movement in the environment. These techniques help to protect against obstacles during movement, although the degree of protection is limited if it is the only technique used, and if used frequently the child may become fatigued.[4] As with trailing, these techniques are more beneficial if used in conjunction with the long cane.

The orientation and mobility specialist is typically the one who teaches human guide, trailing, and protection techniques. However, occupational therapists, as well as caregivers and others who work with children with visual impairment, should learn the basic techniques to reinforce appropriate use and to support the child's interaction with the environment. *Cane technique* is a specialized procedure that requires training from a professional, but occupational therapists can promote skills and prepare young children with visual impairment for using a mobility device, particularly when co-existing conditions also affect mobility. The occupational therapist can recommend activities and provide intervention to improve balance, coordination, postural control, praxis, and prehension. The occupational therapist (and physical therapist) can also provide input and education regarding the advantages and disadvantages of the use of commercially available infant walkers or other apparatus (e.g., infant swings, jumpers) based on the postural, motor, and sensory processing of the child. Mobile toys, such as shopping carts, push toys with long handles, ride-on toys, or large balls, can be incorporated to provide movement experiences and serve as an early navigation tool as long as they are used with safety, function, and social acceptability in mind.[4]

The orientation and mobility specialist performs evaluations to determine a child's readiness for use of a cane. Various types of mobility devices are available, including long canes (e.g., with dual handles, or dual grips); and polyvinyl chloride devices (e.g., with curved tips, rollers, or wheels). Specialists disagree regarding the introduction of cane use with preschoolers, arguing for and against early use; however, a child with visual impairment who is determined to be ready and is motivated to learn to use a cane (such as Natalia was) will likely benefit from early introduction to its use and move toward independent mobility.

Preparation for Adulthood

The adolescent with visual impairment may face significant challenges in selecting an appropriate occupation,[63] although with current technology, many more opportunities are available than in the past.[96] Although individuals with visual impairment as a group may experience unemployment or underemployment, an appropriate match between the personality and talent areas of the adolescent and the occupational choice can lead to a successful and enduring career. Lack of exposure to vocational options is a problem that the occupational therapist can address through community orientation and various activities that provide the individual with a variety of prevocational experiences.

Certain mannerisms and behaviors often interfere with optimal social interaction in the work environment. Behaviors that the occupational therapist and all professionals involved with the adolescent with visual impairment should work to modify include the following:

- Standing in the personal space of others
- Rocking the body
- Blinking, rubbing, or rolling the eyes
- Stamping or shuffling the feet
- Lack of eye contact with the person who is speaking

Ideally, these behaviors are addressed earlier in the adolescent's life, but may need reinforcement of or changes to age-appropriate strategies.

IADLs, such as cooking, cleaning, and recreation, become increasingly important as the child with visual impairment reaches adolescence. The American Foundation for the Blind (http://www.afb.org) provides a comprehensive list of aids and appliances that can help the adolescent with visual impairment engage in such activities.[1] These may include a sugar meter that dispenses half a teaspoon of sugar at a time; an elbow-length oven mitt that protects against accidental burns; kits for marking canned goods; and self-threading needles. Recreational and leisure activities such as games with Braille cards, or low vision cards, or board games (e.g., Scrabble, Monopoly) with Braille markings are available. Because many adults with severe visual impairment lead sedentary lives, it is important to instill the benefits of physical activity early in children's lives to promote healthy habits and routines. Organizations such as the United States Association for Blind Athletes (USABA) (http://www.usaba.org), Special Olympics (http://www.specialolympics.org), and community recreation programs offer sports and other physical activities in which children and youth with visual impairment can participate, train, and compete.

HEARING IMPAIRMENT

The occupational therapist encounters children with hearing impairment in neonatal intensive care units or in hospitals, clinics, early intervention programs, and community and school settings. Prematurity increases the risk of hearing impairment,[45] and often infants leave the neonatal unit with a suspected hearing loss (see Chapter 22). Universal newborn hearing screening (NBHS) programs are now operative in all states in wellborn nurseries and neonatal intensive care units.[50] Statewide statistics on universal newborn hearing screening are available at http://www.infanthearing.org. This NBHS program is having wide-ranging effects on early detection and intervention.

Although universal newborn hearing screening is resulting in significantly earlier detection and treatment of hearing losses in children, early intervention systems and personnel continue to have concerns about correct identification of children with hearing losses. Not the least of these problems is the lack of follow-up for many of the infants who fail the initial screen. Almost half of infants who do not pass the initial screen either do not have a follow-up assessment to determine if hearing loss exists or fail to obtain the needed intervention services.[50] Also current screening technologies fail to identify some hearing losses, especially those with milder or isolated frequency losses and those losses acquired later in life. For this reason, the Joint Commission on Infant Hearing (JCIH) recommendations include guidelines for surveillance and screening in the medical home. The 2007 JCIH report detailed a listing of 11 risk indicators associated with permanent congenital, delayed-onset, or progressive hearing loss in children (Box 25-2). Occupational therapists need to be familiar with these risk factors and to be always vigilant for any signs of hearing loss no matter how mild, because any loss represents information that the child does not have available for processing and adapting to the environment and performing to maximal capacity.

A recent national study of parents revealed that a large number of children with hearing loss do not get the help they need, and that parents and professionals do not recognize the hearing loss or underestimate the impact of mild or unilateral hearing losses.[56] Many parents do not bring an infant back for a detailed hearing evaluation after they fail the initial hearing screening, mistakenly thinking that the child is hearing well. Also, many parents are told the child does not need treatment because the loss is mild or in only in one ear. These children may be at risk for multiple difficulties with school skills, social skills, and speech and language development. Occupational therapists providing services to children within early intervention or school settings should always be aware that there might be a mild or unilateral hearing loss that could be contributing to the difficulties the child is experiencing. Counseling the parents about the impact that even mild losses can have on children and referral for appropriate testing and treatment are indicated.

With the emphasis on least restrictive environments and natural environments, and the advances in technology, including technologies used in newborn hearing screening, digital hearing aids, bone-anchored implants, and cochlear implants, the percentage of children with hearing impairment who learn spoken language and are totally integrated into regular education classrooms has markedly increased, whereas the percentage attending residential schools has decreased dramatically.[45,73,78] An annual survey of youth with hearing impairments is performed each year by Gallaudet University and is available online at http://www.gri/gallaudet.edu.[37] The 2006-2007 data indicate that 26% of children with hearing impairments are attending special or center schools, with 42.4% attending regular school settings with hearing students, 20.4% attending self-contained classrooms on regular education campuses, and 12.1% receiving resource room assistance. The percentage of children receiving the various educational support services is now also being tracked by the Gallaudet survey. In the 2006-2007 survey, 9.7% received occupational or physical therapy as instructional support services.

The occupational therapist has a strategic role in supporting students' activities of daily living, education/learning, play, social participation, and preparation for work. The increase in early intervention programs and earlier identification of hearing impairment allow for more therapist involvement in intervention for young children with hearing impairments. Just as do children with visual impairment, the child with hearing impairment demonstrates a wide range of abilities and functional outcomes. It is important that factors such as age at onset, degree and type of loss, presence of coexisting conditions, and quality of parent support and educational program be taken into consideration when occupational therapy assessment and intervention services are provided.

Developmental Considerations and the Impact of Hearing Impairment

To occupational therapists, the most important characteristic of the child with hearing impairment is the delay of early language development and the difficulty this causes in all other

---

BOX 25-2 Risk Indicators Associated with Permanent Congenital, Delayed-Onset, or Progressive Hearing Loss in Childhood

- Caregiver concern regarding hearing, speech, language, or developmental delay
- Family history of permanent childhood hearing loss
- Neonatal intensive care of >5 days, or any of the following regardless of length of stay: ECMO, assisted ventilation, exposure to ototoxic medications (gentamicin and tobramycin) or loop diuretics (furosemide/Lasix), and hyperbilirubinemia requiring exchange transfusion
- In utero infections, such as CMV infection, herpes, rubella, syphilis, and toxoplasmosis
- Craniofacial anomalies, including those involving the pinna ear canal, ear tags, ear pits, and temporal bone anomalies
- Physical findings, such as white forelock, associated with a syndrome known to include sensorineural or permanent conductive loss
- Syndromes associated with hearing loss or late-onset hearing loss, such as neurofibromatosis, osteopetrosis, and Usher syndrome; other frequently identified syndromes include Waardenburg, Alport, Pendred, and Jervell and Lange-Nielson
- Neurodegenerative disorders such as Hunter syndrome, or sensory motor neuropathies, such as Friedreich ataxia and Charcot-Marie-Tooth syndrome
- Culture-positive postnatal infections associated with sensorineural hearing loss, including confirmed bacterial and viral (especially herpesviruses and varicella virus) meningitis
- Head trauma, especially basal skull/temporal bone fracture requiring hospitalization
- Chemotherapy

CMV, cytomegalovirus; *ECMO,* extracorporeal membrane oxygenation.
From Joint Committee on Infant Hearing. (2007). *Year 2007 position statement: Principles and guidelines for early hearing detection and intervention.* Available from http://www.asha.org/policy.

areas of development.[66,67,69,73,78,98] What at first appears to be a fairly simple problem becomes complicated when considered in light of the importance language plays in our society. The inability of the child to be understood by others and to express himself or herself to others significantly limits social participation.

Researchers have demonstrated that delaying intervention until 3 or 4 years of age lessens the child's potential since this is the formative period of language development.[66,68,78,81] Most research indicates that the first 18 months of life are the most critical for the development of language.[20] Hearing loss decreases stimulation of neural connections and results in subsequent loss of available auditory synapses used to develop auditory perception and spoken language skills in young children. Physiologic measurements of the infant's critical synapses have found that "mapping" of auditory input is complete by the end of the first year.[59] Sharma measured central auditory pathways and demonstrated that these pathways are normalized following early cochlear implantation, before 3.5 years.[105] If the child is denied cortical stimulation by organic means (because of impaired auditory stimuli), he or she may need to conceptualize by other means (e.g., visual, experiential, tactile). Unfortunately, despite the emphasis on early identification, the diagnosis of hearing impairment and the subsequent beginning of intervention are often delayed.[56] Newborn hearing screening programs across the nation are addressing this issue with the hope that this will lead to earlier diagnosis and intervention.

More children are now receiving cochlear implants. The 2006-2007 Gallaudet survey reports that 12.6% of children with hearing impairment now have cochlear implants, an increase from 9.4% in the 2002-2003 survey.[37] The numbers of children receiving cochlear implants is expected to rise dramatically over the next few years, with increasing awareness of this technology and increased funding by public and private insurance programs.

Cochlear implantation not only positively affects development of language but is also linked to improvements in nonverbal skill development. Yucel and Dermin examined visual attention skills in children receiving cochlear implants and found that hearing impaired children had fewer correct responses than normal hearing peers.[123] Age of the cochlear implantation (under age 4 vs. over age 4) made a significant difference in visual attention skills; children who received implants over 4 years of age were more careless and impulsive in their attention to visual tasks.

Babbling is an early indicator of language development. Babbling is vocal play that involves use of the vocal cords and muscles of the mouth, tongue, and larynx; all children do this and the early vocalizations of infants sound alike regardless of parental language. Children who are able to hear, receive the stimulus of hearing themselves, and their parents' vocalized responses. In contrast, children with hearing impairment get insufficient feedback, and babbling does not progress to language development. The infant with deafness generally babbles normally until approximately 5 months of age.[109] However, after 5 months, the typically developing infant develops a growing repertoire of sounds, whereas the child with hearing impairment demonstrates language delay.

Language assists in environmental manipulation and gives the child labels for objects and concepts. Language allows children to share their thoughts and ideas with others. Children with hearing impairment can have difficulty learning abstract concepts and multiple meanings of words. Language also plays a critical role in socialization and in adult-child and child-child interactions.[23,64] Age-appropriate social skills, such as turn taking and the ability to control impulsivity, can be adversely affected by a lack of language skills.

The co-occupations of caregiving between mother and child also can be affected. For example, the typically developing infant smiles and quiets to the sounds of his mother, whereas the infant with a hearing impairment does not respond to his mother's soft voice.[67] Parental communication is limited because the child needs to be close to and visually focused on the mother to hear her. Strong and positive attachments can occur, but the mother may have to learn adaptive techniques to gain the child's attention. As with the visually impaired child, the infant and/or mother may display fewer behaviors that elicit positive responses, setting up a cycle that can lead to interactions that are out of sync and not emotionally satisfying.

Researchers have found differences in mother-child interactions when both mother and child have hearing impairments and when a hearing mother has a hearing-impaired child.[23,68,69] Ease of communication was significantly different in these two groups. When both mother and child had hearing impairments, signing was a natural method of communication, done in a rich and fluent manner. In contrast, hearing mothers of children with hearing impairments often struggled, not only with adjusting to the knowledge that the child had a disability but also with learning an entirely new language. More than 90% of children with hearing impairments have hearing parents.[64] The mismatch in communication strategies in these dyads becomes a pivotal issue in the mother-child relationship. Mohay discussed strategies that parents with hearing impairments use to communicate with their children with hearing impairments and suggested that strategies such as using touch to gain the child's attention and interrupting the child's line of gaze with movements of the body or hands can be taught to hearing parents to facilitate communication.[72] When the child receives appropriately-fitted auditory devices early on, parents can learn how to engage their child through natural auditory means (providing an auditory stimulus before visually gaining the child's attention to look for it), thus establishing the auditory link to later learning of spoken language.

Social participation and communication are also affected by the fact that hearing impairment causes the loss of knowledge associated with the "incidental" reception of sound. Aside from direct communication with others, a great deal of social and environmental information is gained from background sound. This incidental or background sound prompts a person to look in a certain direction or at a specific person or object. Thus hearing loss affects the child's ability to use vision despite the need to compensate for the loss of hearing with the use of vision.

Visual attention is especially needed when there is direct communication between the child and another person using signing, speech reading, and/or cued speech (i.e., a system of hand signs and positions designed to help speech readers distinguish between sounds that look alike on the lips).[66] Regardless of what method is chosen for communication, visual attention must be closely focused on the individual communicating with the child. This need to focus on the person communicating with the child eliminates the ability to use vision to monitor other individuals and aspects of the physical environment. Also, the individual wishing to communicate must first obtain the child's visual attention to be successful.

Of particular interest to occupational therapy practitioners are recent findings that in comparison with children with normal hearing, children with deafness demonstrated significant delay in sensorimotor integration, balance, and the ability to carry out complex motor sequences.[103] See Research Note 25-2 for further details of this study.

RESEARCH NOTE 25-2

Schlumberger, E., Narbona, J., & Manrique, M. (2004). Non-verbal development of children with deafness with and without cochlear implants. Developmental Medicine and Child Neurology, 46, 599-606.

ABSTRACT

This study explored the effect of hearing in the development of sensorimotor integration and nonverbal skills. The study examined 54 children with severe to profound bilateral hearing loss compared with 40 children with normal hearing. The children with hearing loss were further separated based on whether they had received cochlear implants or not. Group A consisted of children with hearing impairments who had not received implants, whereas group B was composed of a matched sample of hearing impaired children who had received cochlear implants. Group C were children with no hearing loss. Children with known neurologic or learning disabilities were excluded from the study. All children received a battery of nonverbal neuropsychological tests and a balance assessment. To identify maturational changes over time, all groups were analyzed by two groupings—under 7 years of age and 7 years and above.

Age at walking for the total group with hearing loss was 14 months compared with 11.8 for the hearing group. Balance was better for the hearing group than for the total group with hearing loss although there was no significant difference between the hearing group and the implanted segment of the group with hearing loss. Repetitive alternating and sequential movements showed increased velocity with increasing age in all three groups. On the whole children with normal hearing were faster than children with hearing loss; Group C scored significantly higher than group A in most of the measures. Motor test variables were divided into two factors—simple movement and complex movement. Simple movements were those that could be done easily after a few repetitions; complex movements were those that were more difficult to learn and required more muscle groups. For children over 7, there was a significant difference in complex movements between children with normal hearing and both groups of children with hearing impairment.

General conclusions were that hearing does affect development of motor control, spatial integration, and attention. This effect is not overwhelming but accounts for subtle differences between children with hearing impairments and children with normal hearing. In addition there is evidence that early cochlear implantation has a positive effect on nonverbal development.

IMPLICATIONS FOR PRACTICE

- Occupational therapists are in a unique position to evaluate and treat sensorimotor and sensory integration problems in children with hearing losses.
- Even subtle motor issues can intensify dysfunction for a child with hearing impairment. Although the most obvious difficulties seen in children with hearing impairment involve language and social development, nonverbal aspects of development need to be evaluated by occupational therapists and addressed in treatment plans to optimize function.
- It is important to consider including adaptations and compensatory techniques for problems such as lack of balance or difficulties with attention

Occupational Therapy Evaluation

As with the child with visual impairment, occupational therapy evaluation of the child with hearing impairment involves examination of occupational performance to determine what supports or limits the child's ability to participate in home, community, and school settings. Activity demands, client factors, and contexts in which the child performs occupations are also part of a comprehensive evaluation. For example, a child with a hearing impairment who has difficulty playing with toys may need evaluation of the toys available in the environment and the performance skills needed to use them. The evaluation may also include process skills related to using toys appropriately and asking for help.

Given that children are frequently diagnosed with hearing impairment at a later age and the difficulty differentiating hearing loss (especially at lower levels of loss) from other behavioral and cognitive impairments, occupational therapists may discover a mild problem that was previously undiagnosed. For example, when a pediatrician recommends evaluation of a child who is showing problems with attention deficit, distractibility, delayed language, or behavioral issues, the occupational therapist may identify that a hearing loss contributes to these problems. Some children with auditory impairments also show signs of autism spectrum disorder. A thorough evaluation of behavior is needed to determine whether delayed speech (e.g., communicating to meet basic needs but not for social interaction) is due to a hearing impairment or an additional disability (such as autism spectrum disorder).[121]

Although each child's language development is unique, certain findings indicate the possibility of hearing loss and suggest referral to appropriate professionals (Box 25-3). Decreased socialization and interaction may be subtle indicators of hearing loss.[54]

In most cases parents are the keenest observers of their child. Therefore, special attention should be given to a child whose parent reports that he or she does not awaken to loud noises, respond when called, or attend to noisy toys, or turns up the sound on a television or computer. In addition, therapists should follow up when a parent reports that the child gestures to communicate wants to the exclusion of words. Occupational therapists may recommend testing or referral to hearing specialists when parents complain that their child is distractible, inattentive to commands, and doesn't respond to verbal direction or responds inappropriately to verbal stimuli.

BOX 25-3 Findings That Indicate the Possibility of Hearing Loss

Possible hearing impairment must be considered in the following instances:

- A newborn does not awaken to sounds as expected.
- A newborn does not exhibit a startle (*Moro*) reflex in response to sharp clap 3 to 6 feet away.
- A 3-month-old infant has not developed auditory orienting responses, as indicated by not becoming alert to noises made by certain toys.
- An 8- to 12-month-old child does not turn to a whispered voice.
- An 8- to 12-month-old child does not turn to sounds, such as a rattle, 3 feet to the rear.
- A 1-year-old child does not understand a variety of words, such as "bye-bye" and "doggie."
- A 2-year-old child is not using words.
- A 2-year-old child is unable to identify an object with a verbal cue alone, such as "Show me the ball."
- A 3-year-old child has largely unintelligible speech.
- A 3-year-old child omits final consonants.
- A 3-year-old child does not use two- and three-word sentences.
- A 3-year-old child mainly uses vowel sounds.
- A child of any age speaks in a voice that is too loud, too soft, of poor quality, or of a quality that does not fit his or her age and gender.
- A child always sounds as if he or she has a cold.

Referral to a hearing specialist is also appropriate when a child with a history of recurrent ear infections or upper respiratory infections presents with a possible conductive hearing loss.

With some modifications in instructional methods, developmental screenings and assessments of fine motor, gross motor, visual motor, sensory integration, and self-care skills can be administered to children with hearing impairments. Program or facility-wide screening efforts with assessments such as the Developmental Activities Screening Inventory (DASI-II) or the Denver Developmental Screening Test (DDST-II) may be used to indicate if children with auditory impairments have developmental issues concomitant with the identified hearing loss. Sensory, psychosocial, and behavioral concerns can be screened with instruments such as the Temperament and Atypical Behavior Scale (TABS), the Checklist for Autism in Toddlers (CHAT), or the Infant/Toddler Sensory Profile. Addressing any associated delays or concerns can increase the effectiveness of the early intervention and/or school program for the child with auditory impairment.

The therapist also can use norm-referenced and criterion-referenced developmental assessment instruments (e.g., the Battelle Developmental Inventory [BDI], the Bayley Scales of Infant and Toddler Development, 3rd edition [BSID-III], the Developmental Assessment of Young Children [DAYC]) as part of a comprehensive evaluation of the child with hearing impairment. However, the language areas of these tests must be modified, and standard scores should not be used. If reported, scores must acknowledge any modifications made to the test. The therapist notes if the child is using a hearing aid, cochlear implant, speech reading, cued speech, or sign language. Test results should include if the child uses sign language and how the therapist testing the child communicates. In some instances, a registered interpreter is required to test a client with hearing impairment accurately.

A functional developmental assessment, such as the Transdisciplinary Play-Based Assessment, 2nd edition (TPBA-2), is helpful in determining the child's strengths and limitations[65] and avoids problems with test validity. The TPBA can be useful with the child with hearing impairment because the assessment is administered in a natural setting. When using this assessment the play facilitator should be skilled in the communication system used by the child. This allows other team members who are not skilled in the child's communication system to observe the assessment and obtain the information they need through the facilitator. Another advantage of TPBA is that the assessment team may view a video recording of the session to identify emerging signs, cues, and beginning language and/or communication attempts that may be too subtle to be noted initially.

Vestibular dysfunction needs to be assessed in all children with hearing impairments either formally or informally. As many as 70% of children with congenital hearing loss have some degree of vestibular impairment.[3] Children whose loss is caused by meningitis almost always have vestibular impairment. Vestibular impairment is often expressed as lack of coordination, difficulty with visual development, low muscle tone, or delayed reflex maturation. Recognition of the difficulty can assist greatly in intervention planning for children with hearing impairment.

Skilled observation and parent and caregiver questionnaires can be useful for gathering information about the child's temperament, self-regulation capacities, sensory processing, and sensory modulation behaviors, and caregiver-child interactions. Interviews with parents, teachers, and other caregivers provide information about daily routines, contexts, expectations, and resources available to support the child's participation in activities. As the child gets older, the focus of the evaluation may be participation in school and education/learning. Written instructions should be used only if the child has the appropriate level of written comprehension. The language demands of any written test must be considered when interpreting the results. Therapists should also note the method of communication used (i.e., oral, sign, cues, and/or pantomime). In adolescents, the occupational therapist, in collaboration with the educator and vocational counselor, may evaluate the individual's driving performance, communication skills with others who have no knowledge of signing or cueing, work skills, and on the job behaviors.

Diagnostic information and a description of specialized tests and interventions for children with hearing impairment can be found in Appendix 25-B on the Evolve website.

Occupational Therapy Intervention

The overall targeted outcome of occupational therapy intervention for children with hearing impairment is participation in their everyday contexts. Approaches include establishing skills and abilities; maintaining performance capabilities; using compensatory strategies, adaptations, or modifications; and preventing barriers to occupational performance. For example, with a 16-year-old with severe hearing loss and mild intellectual disability, the occupational therapist may address communication and interaction skills, such as using appropriate gestures to gain attention and adaptations for obtaining needed information. For a 9-month-old who is rejecting the placement of hearing aids, the early intervention occupational therapist may focus on sensory processing and modulation skills and use various desensitization techniques. With an 8-year-old with profound hearing loss who shows difficulty with fine motor coordination, the school occupational therapist may address motor performance skills and also process skills (e.g., attention to task and temporal organization) to improve the child's signing abilities. For the 4-year-old with cochlear implants receiving auditory training, the school occupational therapist may address delays in nonverbal skills while at the same time reinforcing age-appropriate language skills such as vocabulary development and interaction with hearing peers (Case Study 25-2).

Occupational therapy models of practice that are particularly useful in the evaluation and intervention process with children who are hearing impaired are sensory integration, visual information processing/visual perception, person-environment-occupation, cognitive, and psychosocial (coping and social skills development) frameworks.

The occupational therapist's goals must be well coordinated with the goals of those involved with the child, including the parent, early infant specialist, special educator, speech language pathologist, and audiologist. Generally, the occupational therapist is not the primary participant in intervention for the child with hearing impairment; therefore, the intervention goals for the child with hearing impairment are embedded in the team's goals for the child. As with any other child, the occupational therapist incorporates use of self and selects activities to encourage participation in occupations meaningful to the child and family. However, with the child with hearing impairment,

---

CASE STUDY 25-2 | Tori

Tori is a 4-year-old girl who developed a hearing loss at 2 years of age after having bacterial meningitis (streptococcal pneumonia). At that time she was hospitalized for 2 weeks. Her mother's pregnancy and delivery, and Tori's early development, were described as normal. Tori has no other disabilities. She lives with a single mother and a 6-year-old sibling in an apartment in an urban environment.

Initial testing indicated a moderate-to-severe flat sensorineural loss bilaterally. Tori first received hearing aids at 2 years, 9 months, but they were not programmed appropriately, so she heard minimal sound or speech. She had recurring middle ear problems, including negative pressure, increased fluid, and ear wax buildup. Preschool testing indicated a more profound hearing loss, with better hearing thresholds in the left ear. She currently shows a severe-profound sensorineural loss and wears appropriately fitted bilateral behind-the-ear aids during all waking hours. She is awaiting insurance approval for a cochlear implant. She also uses an FM system in the classroom 4 days a week. She currently attends a preschool program specifically for hearing impaired children with an auditory-verbal focus. The classroom includes typical children.

Her mother and staff members at the preschool describe Tori as a pleasant, somewhat reserved child who is distractible and has a short attention span. She is secure in her attachment to her mother, who reports no behavioral issues except in the area of feeding/eating.

The following observations and findings were obtained through a team (including occupational therapy, physical therapy, speech therapy, educator, nurse, and psychologist) evaluation using the Transdisciplinary Play-Based Assessment-2 (TPBA-2)[66]; the Leiter International Performance Scale[90]; and observations of Tori in the home, classroom, and play area.

Tori demonstrated a full repertoire of age-appropriate motor skills. She walked, ran, and climbed well. She engaged in rapid running and jumping inside and outside, apparently attempting to integrate stimuli. She preferred

W-sitting with frequent postural changes and frequently engaged in head shaking (possibly a form of sensory self-stimulation).

Tori exhibited a definite right preference and used a neat pincer grasp and age-appropriate pencil grasp. She sorted objects by color and shape. She enjoyed puzzles, drawing, and art activities. Her attention to task was limited and she was easily distracted by visual and physical stimuli.

Tori understood multistep directions. She used gesturing, some signing, and physical prompting for expression but was resistant to initiate conversation with verbal speech. She responded using single words and struggled with questioning techniques and conversational turn taking. With a peer or in a small group she was unable to verbally express herself adequately to become part of the dyad or small group, not waiting her turn to answer or ask a question.

Tori undressed herself with minimal assistance, removed her own shoes, and attempted to put on her shoes. She inserted her hearing aids and turned them on with minimal assistance. She was independent in toileting. She fed herself with fork and spoon but preferred to be fed by her mother.

Tori demonstrated difficulty chewing hard foods and bi-textured foods, gagging and spitting out pieces. She was a very slow eater, frequently needing cues to continue, and did not want to try new foods. Her diet was limited to soft foods and she mostly ate carbohydrates. She demonstrated low oral motor tone with open mouth posture, decreased tone in the upper lip and cheeks, low tone in the jaw affecting chewing skills, and oral hypersensitivity to touch. She had low chewing endurance.

Tori adjusted to new situations with relative ease and often sought out attention from other children. She engaged in interactive and pretend play and showed definite play preferences.

She struggled with integrating intense stimuli, occasionally exhibiting aggressive behavior towards peers or throwing herself on the ground. These behaviors were seen most often when fatigued.

---

*Special thanks to Beth Jacobs, MA, OTR/L for her contributions to this case study.

the type of communication system chosen by the parents and educators may affect the focus and nature of the type of activities selected to facilitate this participation. Because of the frequent delay in diagnosis until the age of 18 to 30 months,[58] all intervention, including occupational therapy initially may need to focus on developing and/or improving performance skills that are lagging as a result of auditory language deprivation.

Examples of typical occupational therapy objectives include the following:

- *Enhance sensory processing, sensory modulation, and sensory integration.* The child with hearing impairment must learn to use all available sensory input to the fullest. Problems in sensory processing, sensory modulation, behavior modulation, levels of alertness, regulation, tactile sensitivity, and sensory integration can greatly interfere with function. The therapist can enhance kinesthetic, tactile, and visual processing through multisensory activities. Sensory integrative techniques are useful for developing the kinesthetic system (Figure 25-3). The tactile and proprioceptive systems are important in the use of sign language. Tactile activities, such as having the child locate objects hidden in sand or identify objects behind a shield, are among many that can be used. Tracking exercises, perceptual-motor activities, and many games and crafts can enhance the visual system.

- *Maximize use of vestibular function.* Vestibular activities such as therapy ball, trampoline, and balance beam activities can be helpful in strengthening the available vestibular function. Activities that increase proprioceptive, tactile, muscle strength, or motor planning skills can be used to strengthen skills or develop appropriate compensation techniques to overcome any loss of vestibular function.

- *Maximize use of residual hearing.* The child with hearing impairment is denied normal cortical stimulation by auditory channels and needs to learn to maximize the auditory stimulation available, and to increase auditory awareness, processing, and perception skills. Auditory games and auditory input accompanying other activities (especially active rather than passive activities) can facilitate maximum use of available auditory abilities. Auditory activities, such as hiding a toy somewhere in an obstacle course and asking the child locate the toy through audition while the toy emits an auditory stimulus can enhance the child's auditory awareness.

- *Encourage age-appropriate self-care skills.* Often the occupational therapist acts as a consultant, recommending strategies for improving the child's self-care independence. Of special importance for the child with hearing impairment is inserting and removing, caring for, and maintaining the hearing aid and/or the external components of the cochlear implant. Adapted techniques or assistive devices may be needed. At times self-care skills involve concepts that require concrete cues the child must learn. For example, the idea of left shoe and right shoe can be shown visually with color coding.

- *Enhance fine motor coordination skills.* The movements of the hands of a fluent signer require opposition, finger and thumb flexion and extension, and finger and thumb abduction and adduction. These movements are performed by isolated digits and in total patterns, but they are all done in rapid succession and with remarkable coordination (Figure 25-4). The hand's coordination seems to be related

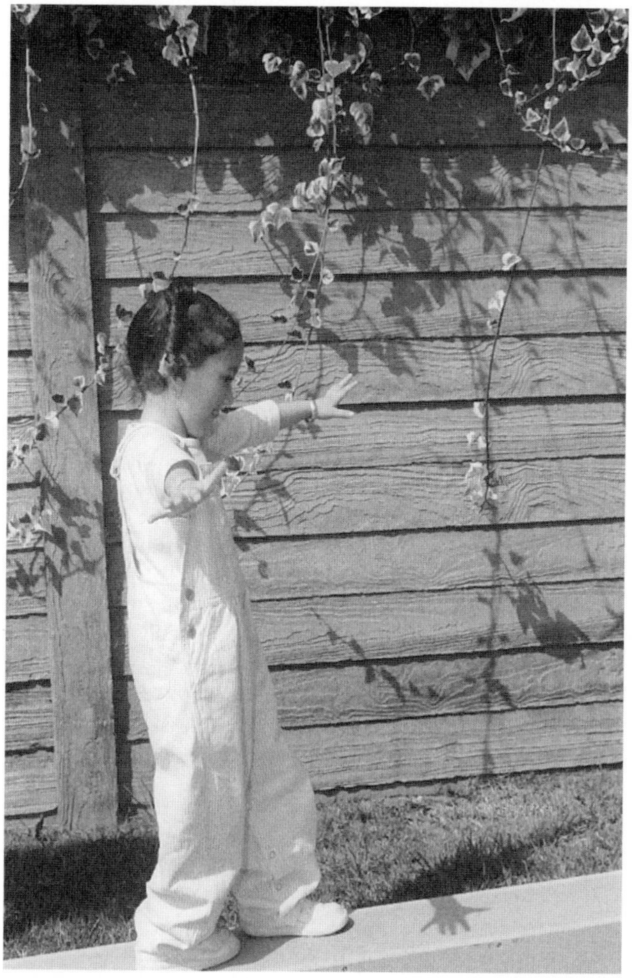

FIGURE 25-3 Child with behind-the-ear hearing aids working on balance and equilibrium skills. (Courtesy Beth Jacobs, OTR/L, John Tracy Clinic, Los Angeles.)

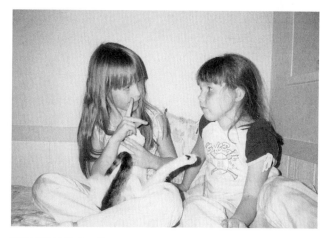

FIGURE 25-4 Sisters communicating using sign language, discussing playing with their pet cat—a favorite shared occupation.

to its sensory abilities, particularly tactile discrimination. This skill does not always come naturally to a child with hearing loss and therefore has to be learned. Occupational therapy's emphasis on hand skills can do much for the child with hearing loss, particularly for children who have an identified delay in fine motor skills.

- *Maximize oral-motor coordination.* The fine motor skills necessary for eating (e.g., jaw control, tongue lateralization, and lip closure) are similar to those needed for speech (Figure 25-5). The hearing-impaired child may have decreased oral-motor sensory abilities, coordination, strength, and endurance. The occupational therapist, in conjunction with the educator and the speech-language pathologist, can use various oral-motor games and activities to facilitate the development of oral-motor skills, and oral language.

- *Maximize visual processing, integration, and perception.* A child with hearing loss may rely on the visual system to some degree to perceive communication. Children with no usable hearing must rely totally on vision for perception of sign language and finger spelling. Children using auditory methods of communication may rely primarily on audition to learn spoken language, or may rely on vision for speech reading and/or cued speech. It is important that visual or auditory scanning and visual or auditory figure-*ground perception be well developed. The child must learn t*o attend simultaneously to multiple sources of visual and/or auditory input (see Chapter 12 for discussion of visual perception).

- *Encourage socialization and peer interaction.* This part of occupational therapy intervention cannot be done in

isolation and is of utmost importance to the child with hearing impairment. Involving the child in group activities with his or her peers encourages socialization. A child with a hearing impairment may not be aware of or may not process all the nuances of spoken language. Hearing impairment is not a visible disability. Others may mistakenly perceive a child with hearing impairment as being rude if he or she does not answer questions or respond to social overtures, when in fact the child has simply not received the correct stimuli. Therefore development of the child's ability to adapt to the environment and understand social interaction and communication should also be stressed.

Special Techniques and Strategies

The therapist who works with a child with a hearing impairment becomes intimately involved with the special techniques and/or equipment used with that child (e.g., sign language, cued speech, speech reading, auditory techniques, hearing aids and cochlear implants). In the field of hearing loss, controversy revolves around the two predominant views of communication and education: spoken language and signed language. Education in spoken language involves the use of advanced auditory technologies (e.g., digital hearing aids, cochlear implants, and FM systems), and strategies to develop spoken language (which usually includes emphasizing auditory learning activities, and may include speech reading, cued speech, and auditory-verbal training).[15,48,81] Education in signed language usually involves strategies to develop signed language, which may include American Sign Language (ASL), or a variety of manually coded language systems (e.g., Signing Exact English [SEE]). Education programs may also use forms of manually coded languages in conjunction with spoken language, speech reading, and auditory training (total communication). The bilingual-bicultural approach advocates using ASL until it is well established and then introducing English later, as a second language.[45]

Proponents of spoken language maintain that if a child is taught to sign, he or she may never learn to use oral language successfully as the primary mode of communication. Proponents of sign language and total communication argue that signing encourages communication and language development and that the child with hearing impairment needs sign for early concept development.[73]

The decision on what techniques and equipment will be used with a child is the prerogative of the child's family and is part of the team negotiations through the individualized family service plan (IFSP) or individualized education program (IEP). It is important that the occupational therapist realize and understand the theory behind the decision and also know how best to facilitate the use of the techniques or equipment chosen. The communication system used to teach children with hearing impairment is tracked by the Gallaudet survey and indicates trends over time. The 2006-2007 data indicates the following: speech only, 51.6% (increase from 1994 when 43%); sign with speech, 35.5% (decrease from 1994 when 54%); and sign only 11.2% (increase from 1994 when 3%).[37]

At first glance, teaching the child *speech reading* would seem to be a good choice. However, many of the sounds made in English look alike. For example, *p*, *m*, and *b* are all made with the same lip movement (i.e., lips together). Another

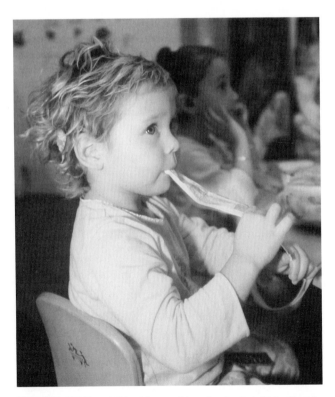

FIGURE 25-5   Child with a cochlear implant participating in an oral motor group to facilitate oral language skills.   (Courtesy Beth Jacobs, OTR/L, John Tracy Clinic, Los Angeles.)

example of look-alike movements would be *f* and *v*, which both are formed with the teeth to the lower lip. Cued speech addresses the need to differentiate between these letters that look alike in lip movement.

With the advent of more effective technology to assist hearing (e.g., digital hearing aids, cochlear implants), programs are using more auditory training techniques (i.e., emphasizing teaching the child to hear). One such program is auditory-verbal training.[27] In this program the child is cued to focus on what he or she is hearing with the therapist/parent using a hand cue of briefly covering the mouth when they start to speak. This therapy program emphasizes children receiving cochlear implants or hearing aids as soon as possible followed by intensive individual therapy to facilitate hearing speech during the critical language years before the auditory pathways deteriorate. These programs, however, entail the child having some level of hearing and special training and commitment for the therapist and family.

Another option is sign language, which is not easily understood and involves many different methods. For example, in the United States, finger spelling, or *dactylology,* is done with one hand, and each configuration represents a letter in the English alphabet. Finger spelling is used by itself or in conjunction with other forms of sign language. Although it is not too difficult for the hearing person to learn to finger spell, when receiving, or listening, the tendency is to see the individual letters and not the words. With finger spelling, it is important that the hand be close enough to the face so that the person with hearing impairment can see both the lip movements and the finger spelling at the same time. For fluency and readability, the hand must be held in a comfortable position, not stiffly.

Sign language can be divided into two categories: ASL and manually coded languages, which include systems such as SEE and other related systems.[10,43,49,81,120] ASL is a language in itself and is not directly translatable to English. ASL has many abbreviations and phrases contained in a single sign, and its own syntax, which is different from that of the structure of English.[108] ASL is the native language of the American Deaf Culture.[98,115] See Research Note 25-3 for a discussion of deaf culture and difficulties in participation in community life.[75] There is no written language associated with ASL. However, SEE does conform to the structure and form of the English language as it was created to facilitate reading and writing skills in children with hearing impairments.

Using sign and speech together may seem appealing but has proved to be difficult, with research indicating that it is not easy to combine speech and sign at the same time. The sign, the speech, and/or the language will suffer because each system is produced at a different rate.[10] If professionals have a difficult time with sign language, then parents have an even tougher task ahead of them, particularly if they are attempting to learn ASL, a language that is not based on English syntax at all. Parents and therapists who are novices at sign languages often resort to using single signs with the child, rather than being able to provide the child with a grammatically correct sentence, as would a native user of sign language.

If signing is used, it is important that the therapist become as fluent as possible in the particular system used by the child. Many occupational therapists learn only the simplest and most frequently used words and phrases. However, the more the

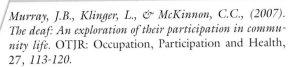

RESEARCH NOTE 25-3

Murray, J.B., Klinger, L., & McKinnon, C.C., (2007). The deaf: An exploration of their participation in community life. OTJR: Occupation, Participation and Health, 27, 113-120.

ABSTRACT

The purpose of this qualitative study was to explore the perceptions of seven individuals who defined themselves as culturally deaf regarding their participation in both hearing and deaf communities. Semistructured interviews using American Sign Language (ASL) interpreters were completed and data analyzed to ascertain whether developing themes fit the Person-Environment-Occupation Model. Difficulty with communication was cited as the major barrier to community participation within both the deaf and the hearing communities. This barrier to communication led to disadvantages in educational, social/interaction, and work/employment areas. Competitive employment was limited thus restricting financial resources, with limited social interaction resulting in fewer social resources. The Person-Environment-Occupation Model proved to be a helpful model for conceptualizing results of this study.

IMPLICATIONS FOR PRACTICE
- Occupational therapists have to be cognizant of the difference between constructions of deafness as a disability versus a linguistic minority.
- Therapists need to develop an understanding of the deaf community and the impact of the use of ASL as a primary means of communication
- Goals for hearing-impaired children who will be using ASL as a primary language are to facilitate social and educational interaction of the children they treat within both the hearing and the deaf community; therapeutic interventions necessitate inclusion of adaptive techniques to lessen the impact of the disadvantages in education, social, and work situations.
- Occupational therapists can facilitate advocacy by their clients and families to eliminate barriers to communication.

therapist knows of the child's sign system, the more effective the communication/interaction will be and consequently the more effective the intervention. Many good texts are available on the different types of signing. However, it is best to attend a class or practice with a friend who knows signing because it often is difficult to interpret the configuration and movement patterns of the hands correctly.

The occupational therapist is sometimes involved with the child during the initial stages of learning sign. In this case, it is best to select the first signs to be taught from those that represent familiar objects, real life situations, and familiar actions. The adult should begin with what is available to the child (e.g., things to feel, handle, or do) and provide parents with a likes-dislikes checklist to determine what is appropriate for the individual child. Often a food item is used first because of its value as a reward. The adult should work at the eye level of the child,

BOX 25-4 Suggestions for Communicating with Hearing-Impaired Children

- Face the child squarely at eye level.
- Check to make sure the auditory equipment is working properly.
- Position yourself so that the child can easily see your face and hands at the same time.
- Make sure you have the child's attention.
- Avoid backlighting. If the child has to look into the light, he or she may be unable to see your lips.
- Use a normal tone of voice. Do not exaggerate mouth movements, because this may confuse the speech reader.
- Speak in natural but clear speech, no more than 3 feet from the child's microphone.
- If the child signs, speak the word and give the sign at the same time, rather than consecutively.
- Use appropriate pauses between words, especially when finger spelling is used.
- Sit close to the child rather than across the room.
- Keep instruction simple and to the point.
- Be consistent, especially with a young child.

obtain eye contact, make the sign preferably within a grammatically correct sentence, if possible, and then physically manipulate the child's hands through the sign. Some basic suggestions for the use of total communication are listed in Box 25-4. These suggestions are also useful in any interaction with a hearing-impaired child since they facilitate engaging the child's attention, whether that attention will be used for visual or auditory input.

An occupational therapy perspective, in addition to the education perspective, can add to the process of learning sign language. Occupational therapy's emphasis on occupation can assist the team by ensuring that the child and family are taught signs that label the activities that have particular meaning and purpose to them (i.e., their occupations). An occupational therapy profile can be used to gain an understanding of the child's and family's occupational experiences, patterns of daily living, interests, values, and needs and may add to the team's knowledge of the child and family and the language that is uniquely important to them.

If spoken language is the communication system of choice, the occupational therapist will need to seek training in and use the system selected by the family and educational system (cued speech, auditory-verbal training). Although not the primary therapist with the acquisition of language skills, the occupational therapist can supplement and complement speech development in their therapy sessions encouraging use of language by the child just as with children with normal hearing (e.g., naming toys, selecting activities, and talking about actions, feelings, and tasks). As with learning sign, the occupational profile of the child and family can be appropriately ascertained and used to obtain information on the language that is most meaningful to the child and family.

The occupational therapist may also be involved in the initial stages of hearing aid use. Often a history shows that the child had a hearing aid but rejected it. This sometimes can be traced to the lack of professional support for the parents and child during the adjustment period, or it can be traced to the professional's lack of familiarity with the aid. The occupational therapy perspective on sensory processing, modulation, and integration can be useful in addressing these issues in the wearing of hearing aids if rejection is attributed to significant sensory-based difficulties.

Hearing aids can be of great assistance to children with hearing impairment, depending on the type and severity of hearing loss. They are of great help in auditory learning and can assist the child in sound and speech awareness, localization, recognition, identification, and comprehension. Most hearing aids are now digital, which provide noise cancellation systems, but distance and noise are still problems for hearing aid wearers, as they are for people with normal hearing. Speaking close to the child's hearing aid, in a conversational volume, is the most effective for communication, particularly in large therapy rooms which tend to have walls that reverberate auditory signals.

Because the head is one of the most sensitive parts of the body, one of the main problems found in children with new aids is tactile sensitivity. However, the child must learn to think of the aid as a piece of clothing that is put on automatically in the morning, along with shoes and socks. The earlier an aid is programmed appropriately for a child and put into use, the better the chances for language development.[66]

Children who use hearing aids need to adjust to the feel of the aid and recognize its importance. It usually is best for the child to begin wearing the aid during a quiet activity that involves just one person speaking. The maximum benefit from an aid is obtained in relatively quiet settings. The child progresses in the amount of time the hearing aid is worn each day, until, usually by at least 1 month after initial fitting, the child wears the hearing aid during all waking hours.

The hearing aid is a sensitive piece of equipment with several parts, and it can often need repair. It is estimated that as many as 50% of hearing aids used by school-age children are not working properly.[93] Everyone involved with the child should be aware of some of the common problems because an improperly working aid is useless to the child. Four common problems are (1) dead batteries, (2) improperly placed or corroded batteries, (3) squeal or feedback (check for looseness of the earmold), and (4) impaction of the earmold with wax, which must be cleared.

The type of hearing aid prescribed for a particular child depends on the degree and configuration of the loss.[78] Two types of hearing aids are widely used, the *in-the-ear* type and the *behind-the-ear* type. The in-the-ear aid has no external components and, although it can provide more power than those worn behind the ear, is more quickly outgrown in children, thus causing trouble with feedback; the smaller size also is more easily lost. The behind-the-ear aid is used for mild to profound losses and is the most appropriate type of aid for children. It is a small unit, made up of a microphone, amplifiers, and receiver. These components are located together behind the ear and are connected by a short tube to a silicone earmold that has been custom formed to the shape of the child's external auditory canal. The earmold is seated directly in the ear (Figure 25-6, *A*). The microphone picks up the sound waves and converts them to electric signals. The amplifiers then increase the strength of the signal, and the receiver changes the electrical signals back to sound waves that are sent to the earmold. A *monaural aid* refers to the use of just one

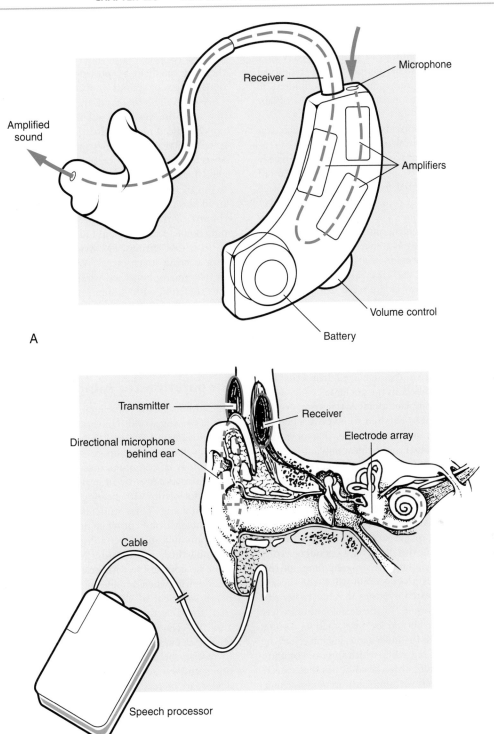

FIGURE 25-6   A, Diagram of a behind-the-ear hearing aid. **B,** Diagram of a cochlear implant.

aid, and *binaural aid* refers to the use of two separate aids. Binaural fitting is the standard of practice, whenever possible, since it gives the child localization and better hearing in noise, and keeping the auditory nerve stimulated.

Cochlear implants (Figure 25-6, *B*) are devices that can be surgically implanted in the cochlea of individuals with severe to profound hearing losses.[45,76] They have been used in young children since the early 1980s and are becoming very common in this age group. Cochlear implants create possibilities for auditory input for those who could not benefit from traditional hearing aids. These devices provide the sensation of sound by acting as substitutes for hair cells in the organ of

Corti; they provide direct stimulation to the auditory nerve, providing access to all speech sounds. Cochlear implants can now be fitted in children as young as 12 months, usually after the child has gone through a trial period with a traditional hearing aid. It is now strongly recommended that children be implanted under the age of 4 to maximize the window of language acquisition.

The implant has five components: (1) a receiver seated in the temporal bone, (2) a transmitter, (3) an external microphone, (4) a speech processor that records and electronically codes incoming sounds, and (5) an electrode array implanted in the cochlea itself. The external transmitter is held in place on the head by a magnet that attracts a magnet in the receiver embedded in the temporal bone. The receiver is attached to the electrode array in the cochlea, and a cord connects the transmitter and microphone to the speech processor. If the child wears a body-worn processor, the cord is usually run under the child's clothing, and the speech processor is contained in a fanny pack worn at the waist. Most children, however, now wear behind-the-ear speech processors.

Sound flows from the microphone to the speech processor, where it is converted into an electrical signal. The coded signal is sent back to the transmitter and then to the receiver, where it is decoded and delivered to the actual electrodes in the cochlea. The electrodes bypass the damaged hair cells and directly stimulate the nerve fibers in the cochlea.

Like a hearing aid, the implant does not restore normal hearing, but it does allow many children to perceive open-set speech (i.e., speech without context). Factors that positively influence the child's benefit from the cochlear implant include: later age at onset of hearing loss, shorter duration of deafness, no other disabilities, a high level of parent support, and exclusively auditory-oral educational program.[22] As with the hearing aid, the best results are achieved if the device is worn consistently. When the child has tactile defensiveness, the occupational therapist can provide strategies to improve the child's comfort when wearing the device and encourage consistent use of the device. Mapping, or programming, of the speech processor is a complex process upon which the success of the implant depends. Research indicates that the earlier the implantation, the better the results.[18] The deaf community has debated whether the device should be implanted in young children before they are able to understand and take part in the decision- making process regarding which form of communication they will use. Research, however, indicates that speech perception abilities in children with implants are approaching levels of performance similar to those in normal-hearing controls, even in test contexts of competing noise.[24]

Therapists must be aware of the external equipment and its location during motor activities with the child. The equipment is expensive, and components worn on the child's body can be damaged by water, rough physical activity, or electrostatic discharge (ESD). ESD is of special concern to the occupational therapist because various pieces of therapy equipment such as plastic therapy balls and mats can interfere with the mapping of the speech processor and damage the implant. The therapist should discuss these concerns with the parent, who may decide that the external components should be removed before engaging with such therapy equipment or activities.

Like hearing aids, cochlear implants have external components and may cause problems related to tactile defensiveness;

therefore desensitization can be an appropriate goal for therapists working with children who have been fitted with these devices. As part of the intervention team, the occupational therapist can help by providing feedback to the audiologist on the types of sounds or speech the child appears to hear.

As with the hearing aid, the key to success with the cochlear implant is use during all waking hours. All adults working with the child need to check that the equipment is in good working order and that the child is spoken to throughout the session. Speech volume should be the same as that used with any other child during therapy activities. The therapist should speak as close to the microphone as possible to make speech clearer to the child. In addition, language should be kept at age level and within the context of the situation. Directions should be given in short but complete sentences, not just using single words.

In school settings, FM systems are often used with children with hearing impairments. With an FM system, the teacher wears a microphone and wireless transmitter to speak directly into the child's FM system, hearing aid, or cochlear implant. This device helps control the level of background noise in the classroom because the teacher's voice can be amplified for the students who have hearing loss without disturbing other students in the classroom.

Preparation for Adulthood

The adolescent with hearing impairment may struggle to blend into a hearing world. Universal recognition of the importance of inclusion and required accommodations in school and work settings has afforded more opportunities, and the growing technology of communication has improved future prospects. For most adolescents, an important task is learning to drive a car. Adolescents with hearing impairment can receive special driver training. These students are taught to constantly visually scan the environment while driving.

Communication over a distance has become more possible for individuals with hearing impairment. Telephones, by law, must be compatible with hearing aids and cochlear implants. In addition, when amplification with the aid or implant alone is not sufficient to allow the wearer to understand conversation, the Telecommunication Device for the Deaf (TDD) is available. The TDD is a communication device that uses the telephone lines with a keyboard to "talk" and a printout device to receive the conversation, which is read on a screen at the other end by someone who has similar equipment. These devices are increasingly being required by law in various public places such as airports. The telephone ring is replaced with a flashing light or a fan that moves back and forth to indicate an incoming call. The obvious disadvantage of the TDD is that both ends of the line must be equipped with this system.

The telephone itself, however, has been eclipsed by the advent of a dazzling array of distance communications, from e-mailing, video telephones, and IM-ing (instant messaging) on the Internet to text messaging on cell phones. These technologies have opened up the world of wireless communications to hearing-impaired individuals, who can easily communicate with anyone through these devices. These are rapidly becoming methods of communication replacing the need for TDD devices and have the definitive advantage of being used and well accepted by all segments of the population, thus adding to the mainstreaming process for individuals with hearing loss.

Watching television provides another aspect of daily life. The frequency of closed-captioned programs has increased, and all televisions manufactured after 1995 are required to have a built-in decoding device. The individual with hearing impairment uses this decoding device to view captioned versions of programs.

Occupational choice has always been difficult for young adults with hearing impairment. Fortunately, today many universities offer programs designed to integrate students with hearing loss into the general student population by providing special services, such as interpreters, computer-assisted real-time translation (CART), and note takers. The Americans with Disabilities Act (ADA) Amendments Act of 2009 (P.L. 110-325) requires that all public education programs provide interpreters, CART, or note takers for individuals with hearing impairment when it is determined that they are required.

When an individual with hearing impairment enters a work environment, he or she is likely to miss a great deal of information transmitted in conversation, along with environmental sounds.[45] Other factors that historically have adversely affected occupational choice for individuals with hearing loss include (1) differences that affect self-perception and perception of others, (2) a restricted life space, which adversely affects knowledge of areas other than the immediate social or geographic area, and (3) limited sociocultural understanding.[48,101] A recent qualitative study by Murray, Klinger, and McKinnon indicates that these issues continue to exist and that community participation in competitive employment and social activities can be severely limited.[75] Adolescents with a hearing impairment may lack work-related experiences, role models, exploration of their talents and interests, effective interpersonal skills, and knowledge of work behaviors needed for vocational success.[98]

Occupational therapists are aware of how important meaningful and purposeful activity is in the life and health of an individual. As part of an interdisciplinary team, therapists can help address many of these issues and prepare the child with hearing impairment for transition to work and fuller participation in work.

MULTISENSORY IMPAIRMENT

It is not uncommon for an occupational therapist to provide services to a child who has multiple disabilities that include both visual and hearing deficits. Sometimes a child's visual impairment or hearing impairment may be the primary focus of intervention and education, and other sensory or learning impairments may go undetected; conversely, a child with obvious multiple disabilities may have visual or hearing impairments that are not identified.[112] Children who have concomitant visual and hearing impairments are often identified as deaf-blind (i.e., to be identified as a student with a disability who is eligible for special education services under IDEA) and have unique developmental and learning needs.[46,47]

Diagnostic Information

Children with multiple disabilities comprise a majority of young children with visual impairment who receive services.[84] Whenever a developing brain incurs injuries, the chances of

multiple impairments are significantly greater. For instance, visual impairment is common in children with cerebral palsy, and about 30% have some form of hearing, speech, or language impairment.[82] The incidence of visual and hearing deficits is also high for children with intellectual disabilities. About one half to two thirds of children with developmental disabilities have visual problems.[71] When both visual and hearing impairments are present, accurate assessment of acuity, awareness, and perception is often difficult because these children do not always give the examiner reliable feedback.

Embryologic studies show that the timetables for development of the eye and ear are similar[51]; therefore, a number of diagnoses involve both systems (e.g., cytomegalovirus infection, maternal rubella, toxoplasmosis, congenital syphilis, Hurler syndrome, Waardenburg syndrome, and Goldenhar syndrome). Meningitis is a leading cause of noncongenital hearing and visual impairment in children.

Other Services

As mentioned earlier, a team of professionals may be involved with children who have multisensory impairment. Orthopedists, neurologists, and cardiologists are a few of the medical specialists whose expertise is often needed. Given the multiple needs of these children, it is highly likely that the occupational therapist will become involved. He or she may be a major team member, especially for the physically impaired child who has visual deficits, or for the child who is both visually and hearing impaired. Often the occupational therapist's first encounter with visual and/or hearing impairment is through providing service to a child with multiple disabilities.

Occupational Therapy Evaluation and Intervention

A primary consideration and focus in the care and management of visual impairment in children with multiple disabilities is to provide individualized plans for helping the child to use his or her functional vision.[124] Many of the behaviors and occupational performance concerns discussed previously also apply to children with multisensory impairment. Children with both visual and hearing impairments may show extreme tactile defensiveness. The therapist should consider how frightening it may be for a child who has two sensory channels that are unavailable or that provide information that is out of focus or indistinct. These children may not like anything new or different, and changes of any type often are not well accepted. Oral hypersensitivity may also be present, and the transition from smooth to textured foods may be a difficult process. Neuromotor function often is affected by hypotonicity and hypermobility of the joints or by spasticity. Some children learn to walk, but they may remain cautious about giving up support.

Children who have visual and hearing impairments often experience significant difficulties in infancy, such as negative reactions to parental handling during caregiving activities, which can lead to less parental handling and thus reduce the infant-caregiver interactions needed to build attachment and relationship. Environmental stimuli may not make sense to children with multisensory impairment so they may ignore the stimulus or respond in a defensive manner.[16]

Stereotypical behaviors may be observed, and these may be confused with signs of autistic spectrum disorder (as described previously). It bears repeating that the presence of stereotypic behaviors does not automatically indicate a diagnosis of autism (although some studies suggest it may be more likely in children with multiple disabilities), and conversely, it cannot be assumed that atypical or stereotypical behaviors in children with multiple disabilities are primarily attributable to their sensory impairment.

With the child who has visual and/or hearing impairment, and physical or intellectual disabilities, it is important for occupational therapists to remember that consistent repetition often is needed for the child to learn skills in everyday contexts and situations, and that progress can be made, but may occur slowly and in smaller increments. For example, a simple task such as learning the hand-to-mouth sequence necessary for self-feeding with utensils may require months of practice with multiple cues and strategies used on a consistent basis. Hand-over-hand guidance is often used during activities with children with multiple and severe disabilities. However, this approach takes control away from the child and may actually lead to passivity or overreliance on the adult. An alternative approach is hand-*under*-hand guidance, with the child's hand on top of the adult's. Although facilitating movement from underneath the hand can be a more difficult maneuver for the occupational therapist, it affords the child a better feel for the action and it is easier for the adult to decrease or remove support subtly to promote the child's independence in the activity.

Campbell, McInerney, and Cooper found that functional patterns of movement were achieved at faster rates when children with multiple disabilities were able to practice the desired movement patterns more frequently.[12] Other studies have found that orientation and mobility training for infants and toddlers with visual and other impairments is beneficial and that parents can effectively implement premobility programs to help them develop the necessary skills.[53] Training of caregivers and school staff, therefore, becomes extremely important. The orientation and mobility specialist and the occupational therapist should evaluate the child and identify specific tasks or movements to be targeted, determine the appropriate intervention strategies, and instruct others in how to carry out the task or movement with accuracy.

With this population, the role of the occupational therapist often is that of the consultant. Consultation and monitoring to promote self-care skills, such as dressing, require that the occupational therapist develop rapport with those carrying out the activities and strategies, and develop the ability to encourage and provide feedback that support the caregivers' participation. Diagrams or pictures with clearly written directions can be helpful guides for caregivers who are carrying out the recommended program. The occupational therapist monitors the program by observing others implement a technique or strategy and also by directly implementing the technique with the child to receive direct feedback about the child's performance.

Evaluation

The occupational therapist can be a key member of the intervention team, assisting in the diagnostic process through evaluation and description of the child's occupational performance in relation to age, developmental level, and severity of impairment. The occupational therapist also can interpret behaviors and can offer hypotheses that could help tease out whether, for example, sensory processing or modulation difficulties, or other underlying factors, are contributing to the behaviors.

The use of standardized assessment tools is particularly difficult with children who have multiple disabilities because adaptations that can be made for children who are singly impaired are usually not applicable.[46] If such assessments are administered, caution must be used in interpreting any scores or age equivalents that may be obtained in light of reliability and validity concerns, even though a profile of the child's abilities and skills may be presented. Alternate methods and assessment tools for evaluation may be used that will provide information that can be considered for planning intervention. Of particular interest are the child's prehension and tactile processing abilities because almost everything has to be taught using manual guidance strategies. Play- and occupation-based assessment tools, along with skilled observations, are useful and can provide a comprehensive description of the child's skills, occupational performance, behaviors, and challenges. The occupational therapist typically observes and evaluates social skills, fine motor and manipulative skills, activities of daily living, and participation in different contexts (e.g., home, school, community).

The child with multisensory impairment should be observed in familiar and unfamiliar settings, and in structured and unstructured situations, and significant others should be consulted about the child's skills. In addition, all evaluation team members should be aware of the child's interests, major methods of communication, postural and positioning needs, and movement status.[26] The occupational therapist, along with other members of the team, analyzes the findings and observations, arrives at hypotheses about the degree to which functional limitations can be attributed to various factors, and designs appropriate interventions. The occupational therapist's holistic perspective is valuable in identifying and addressing the child's and family's ability to engage in meaningful occupations. The focus is on identifying the skills needed to perform age- or developmentally appropriate life tasks rather than on sequential skill acquisition.

Intervention Goals and Methods

It is particularly important for the child with visual and hearing impairments to experience meaningful activities in natural settings during everyday routines[46,47] with systematic behavioral observations, and incorporation of educational opportunities and communication strategies. Intervention goals depend on the individual evaluation of the child and his or her identified levels of functioning, but interventions should build on all the skills and remaining sensory channels available to the child.[86] Although goals can vary from child to child, some typical goals of occupational therapy intervention include the following:

- *Promote or establish self-feeding skills.* Feeding is often a problem for children with multisensory impairment. They frequently have several medical problems that require long periods of nonoral feeding. Hypersensitivities and resistance to change are two major difficulties that can be intensified with the presence of increased tone and reflex patterns. Strategies need to be developed for the child who remains on a bottle or frequently drinks a high-calorie food supplement. The transition from bottle-feeding to drinking from a glass or cup and eating table foods may require several years to achieve. To increase independence, adaptive equipment often is required (e.g., adapted seating and positioning; a wheelchair tray with raised edges; a scoop bowl with suction cup; adapted utensils). Chapter 15 further describes feeding interventions.

- *Promote or establish self-care skills.* Achieving as much independence in self-care skills (including self-feeding) often is a goal that is important for the child's family (but it is also important to be aware of and take into consideration cultural, religious, and other factors that may influence the family's values and practices that may be different from those of the dominant culture or the occupational therapist). Toileting is often a challenge because of resistance to the task and difficulty understanding what is required. For the child who has physical disabilities in addition to visual and hearing impairments, adapted toilet seats and scheduling techniques may be needed. Dressing, hygiene, and grooming activities may also be difficult for the child with visual and hearing impairments to perform and the occupational therapist may incorporate physical guidance or assistance, adaptations and modifications, and other strategies to promote participation in these activities. Discussion and collaboration with the caregivers, and possibly with the child, are critical to determine what is most meaningful and to what extent the child should expend effort, energy, and time at the expense of engagement in other activities (e.g., focusing on and taking a long time for self-feeding at the expense of social interaction with peers or family at mealtime).

- *Promote or establish play skills.* It is important that children with multisensory impairment be provided a variety of experiences and opportunities to engage in play with objects, toys, and with other children so that they can learn about their world and how to interact with objects and people. Because they have multiple impairments that affect their ability to engage in interactions, these children are at risk of becoming isolated, and therefore, they need many opportunities to participate in daily play activities, with targeted facilitation of specific skills and interactions and promoting the joy and pleasure of play. Occupational therapists may provide interventions that address the underlying performance and process skills needed to engage in play (and learning and self-care activities).

- *Promote tactile awareness, enhance tactile processing, and promote adequate sensory modulation of tactile experiences.* Because acceptance of touch is basic to any interaction, integration of the tactile system often is an initial goal. Gradual introduction to a variety of tactile experiences in the context of everyday activities is beneficial for the child with multisensory impairment, along with encouragement to reach out and explore within the level of his or her capability and interest. Use of vibration and proprioceptive input in preparation or during intervention activities may also be helpful.

- *Promote postural alignment and postural control.* The child with multisensory impairment often is fearful of moving through space independently. In addition, habitual postural patterns may develop that could affect the alignment of the body. For these reasons, adequate positioning of the child to allow interaction with the environment and to prevent contractures and deformities is extremely important. Engaging the children in vestibular-proprioceptive activities at the level they can tolerate often is helpful to influence arousal, muscle tone, and posture. The occupational therapist may use facilitation and handling techniques to promote postural control and movement with a child with multisensory impairment.

- *Develop a sense of mastery or competence.* Children with multisensory impairment need to be able to experience control and mastery at whatever level they are functioning in a variety of contexts and situations. Young children need to learn about cause-and-effect relationships and that the actions have an effect on others and the environment. Many switch-activated toys (e.g., toys that have a switch the child can press to activate a movement, music, vibration) provide sensory input and feedback that is pleasurable and motivating to these children and can help them learn that they can make something work or happen. This sense of mastery and competence should be promoted continually as the child grows older, and the occupational therapist can help to establish a balance between providing the "just right" challenge and providing supports or assistance.

- *Develop socially acceptable behaviors.* Children with multisensory impairment who have stereotypical behaviors need to be taught more acceptable and functional strategies for meeting their sensory needs (e.g., the behaviors may serve a sensation-seeking purpose) or communicative needs (e.g., the child does not have a means to convey wants or needs). If the behavior is simply extinguished, without addressing the underlying intent of the behavior or providing an acceptable alternative, the child may find another, still unacceptable way to fulfill the need. Rather than viewing the child as a "behavior problem," the occupational therapist should evaluate the behaviors in the context in which they occur and arrive at possible hypotheses for why they occur, which can then lead to developing strategies or alternatives that are meaningful to the child. In addition, the child with multisensory impairment needs consistency and continuity in routines with clear expectations. Whatever cues, prompts, or strategies are used, they should be simple and applied consistently from one person to the next across settings. Small group activities and engagement in social play activities are meaningful contexts to facilitate interpersonal and communication skills.

- *Provide family members with support and education.* Family members need information about appropriate levels of stimulation and effective strategies for interaction with the child with multisensory impairment. Information about and referrals to support groups, Internet resources, agencies, and other parents of children with similar disabilities can go a long way to helping families learn about the child's disabilities; sharing and learning about strategies that help them cope with the demands and challenges that every family faces and those unique to them; obtaining resources and services; and developing a social network with other families.

Special Techniques and Strategies

Special techniques and strategies used with children with multisensory impairment often address promoting or supporting functioning in the areas of self-care, communication, and mobility. Children with visual and hearing impairments can learn sign language through use of their residual vision, or can be taught using a hand-over-hand approach when visual access is too limited. Cochlear implants are also available to children with visual and hearing impairments, allowing auditory connection with the world around them, auditory scanning of the environment, and access to spoken language strategies to develop communication. Other technologies are available to provide academic access, such as large computer screens for reading activities, and other low vision aids.

Task analysis and breaking down a task into its smallest component parts can be useful in setting realistic goals for therapy and in establishing objectives for the IFSP or IEP. Task analysis can be especially helpful in setting realistic goals for therapy and establishing objectives in daily living and vocational activities. For example, in teaching a child with multiple sensory disabilities to butter a piece of bread, the total task can be broken down into steps, which then can be repeated in a backward or forward order (i.e., chaining). In *backward chaining*, all steps are performed for the child except the last step, which is the first taught, then the next to last, and so on. In *forward chaining*, the first step is taught until it is mastered, then the second, and so on. Regardless of the instructional direction used, it is important to fade out assistance but still give as much support as is needed to help the child master the task in its entirety. Other techniques may include modeling and demonstration (for those children with some vision), use of routines, and reinforcement.

Another useful approach with children who have multisensory impairment is *behavior modification*. This is a systematic approach to alter the child's behavior through environmental programming. In behavior modification, reinforcement is often used and detailed records of the child's responses are kept. Often a positive or desired behavior (e.g., urinating when placed on the toilet) needs to be reinforced, or a negative or undesirable behavior (e.g., eye poking, uncontrollable tantrums) is ignored, discouraged, shaped, or extinguished, depending on the intensity and potential for harm to self or others and other factors. The occupational therapist charts the frequency of target behaviors. Although being ignored is negative reinforcement for many children, it may not be effective with some children with multisensory impairment who may prefer to be left alone.

For the child with multisensory impairment and severe physical and intellectual challenges, the occupational therapist often focuses on safety, survival, or self-care skills. These skills may be learned in a rote manner and require extremely specific environmental cues to elicit, but are important to the child's ability to participate in activities at whatever level he or she is able in different settings. Family members and other individuals involved with the child should be encouraged to reinforce the strategies.

Assistive technology and adapted devices can be incorporated to provide a means of communication or mobility. These may include a range of options from communication boards to sophisticated augmentative communication devices. Touch cues (e.g., a touch to the child's shoulder or arm) can be used to signal to the child that a person is approaching or that an event is about to happen, and objects can also be used to indicate the initiation of routine activities (e.g., a clean diaper touched to the child's cheek for changing).[29] Sign language can also be introduced, first with more common and simple signs such as for "more" or "eat." Depending on the child's ability, it can progress to increasing the vocabulary and use of sentences. Mobility equipment such as wheelchairs may be necessary for those children with multisensory impairments and physical disabilities, but those children who are ambulatory may be able to use some travel skills and techniques (e.g., human guide, trailing) that were described previously, and adapted playground equipment can provide safe opportunities for physical play experiences.

Preparation for Adulthood

The occupational therapist's focus with an adolescent with multisensory impairment and severe physical or intellectual disabilities is preparing him or her to function in supported living settings or residential settings and supported employment. Several key behaviors and skills that the adolescent needs to develop for more self-sufficient living are (1) ability to use some means of communication using basic emergency and survival words such as "stop," "eat," "more," "no," and "finish;" (2) social skills; (3) self-care skills; (4) telling time; (5) cooking and shopping skills; (6) home management; (7) travel and community mobility; and (8) housekeeping. Supported living and group home settings with supervision available are possible options for some individuals with multiple disabilities. If the child has remained at home with the family through school, adolescence often is when a move to a residential setting may be considered. Both the family members and the adolescent with multisensory impairment must be prepared for this change. Also the adolescent's emerging sexuality must be dealt with at the level of his or her understanding.

For the most part, supported employment activities may be repetitive and involve manipulative skills; they can include folding, stamping, collating, counting, gluing, bending, sorting, assembling, wrapping, stuffing, filing, measuring, stapling, and clipping. If the individual has abilities that can be supported through the use of a job coach in a work setting, the occupational therapist can assist with evaluating the skills that can be matched to the job, and recommend any accommodations or modifications that may be needed in the work place.

SUMMARY

This chapter provided an overview of occupational therapy services with the child with visual and/or hearing impairment. Occupational therapy evaluation emphasizes how the child's development and functioning are affected by the loss of one or both of these senses. General intervention goals have been presented, stressing provision of activities and experiences that allow the child to develop adaptive behaviors. Brief explanations of specialized techniques used with these children have also been provided including the use of hearing aids, cochlear implants, sign language, Braille, basic skills for travel such as human guide, trailing, and protective techniques, and low vision aids. Occupational therapists use their knowledge of adaptation, task and activity analysis, and development to help children who have visual and/or hearing impairments engage in meaningful and purposeful occupations in different contexts.

REFERENCES

1. American Foundation for the Blind. (2008). *Statistics and sources for professionals.* Retrieved August 18, 2008 from http://www.afb.org/section.asp?SectionIE=154DocumentID=1367#prev

2. Anderson, S., Boigon, S., & Davis, K. (1986). *Oregon project skills inventory* (5th ed.). Medford, OR: Jackson Education Service District.

3. Angeli, S. (2003). Value of vestibular testing in young children with sensorineural hearing loss. *Archives of Otolaryngology-Head & Neck Surgery, 129,* 478–482.

4. Anthony, T. L., Bleier, H., Fazzi, D. L., Kish, D., & Pogrund, R. L. (2002). Mobility focus. Developing early skills for orientation and mobility. In R. L. Pogrund & D. L. Fazzi (Eds.), *Early focus: Working with young children who are blind or visually impaired and their families* (2nd ed., pp. 326–404). New York: AFB Press.

5. Ayvazoglu, N. R., Oh, H., & Kozub, F. M. (2006). Explaining physical activity in children with visual impairments: A family systems approach. *Exceptional Children, 72,* 248–255.

6. Baird, S., Mayfield, P., & Baker, P. (1997). Mothers' interpretations of the behavior of their infants with visual and other impairments during interactions. *Journal of Visual Impairment and Blindness, 91,* 467–483.

7. Baker-Nobles, A., & Rutherford, A. (1995). Understanding cortical visual impairment in children. *American Journal of Occupational Therapy, 49,* 899–911.

8. Baker-Nobles, L. (2005). Ocular pathology and cortical visual impairment in pediatric low vision. In M. Gentile (Ed.), *Functional visual behavior in children. An occupational therapy guide to evaluation and treatment options* (2nd ed., pp. 315–338). Bethesda, MD: AOTA Press.

9. Bayley, N. (2006). *Bayley scales of infant and toddler development administration manual* (3rd ed.). San Antonio, TX: Harcourt Assessment.

10. Bornstein, H., Saulnier, K., & Hamilton, L. (1983). *A comprehensive signed English dictionary.* Washington, DC: Gallaudet College Press.

11. Caballo, C., & Verdugo, M. A. (2007). Social skills assessment of children and adolescents with visual impairment: Identifying relevant skills to improve quality of social relationships. *Psychological Reports, 100,* 1101–1106.

12. Campbell, P. H., McInerney, W. F., & Cooper, M. A. (1984). Therapeutic programming for students with severe handicaps. *American Journal of Occupational Therapy, 38,* 594–602.

13. Celeste, M. (2002). A survey of motor development for infants and young children with visual impairment. *Journal of Visual Impairment and Blindness, 96,* 169–174.

14. Chaikin, L. E., & Downing-Baum, S. (2005). Optometry and occupational therapy collaboration in vision therapy. In M. Gentile (Ed.), *Functional visual behavior in children. An occupational therapy guide to evaluation and treatment options* (2nd ed., pp. 229–250). Bethesda, MD: AOTA Press.

15. Chamberlain, C., Morford, J. P., & Mayberry, R. I. (2000). *Language acquisition by eye.* Mahwah, NJ: Lawrence Erlbaum.

16. Chen, D. (1999). Interactions between infants and caregivers: The context for early intervention. In D. Chen (Ed.), *Essential elements in early intervention: Visual impairment and multiple disabilities* (pp. 22–54). New York: AFB Press.

17. Chomsky, H. (1993). *Language and thought.* Wakefield, RI: Moyer Bell.

18. Christiansen, J. G., & Leigh, I. W. (2002). *Cochlear implants in children.* Washington, DC: Gallaudet University Press.

19. Cochrane, G., Lamoureux, E. L., & Keeffe, J. (2008). Defining the content for a new quality of life questionnaire for students with low vision. (The impact of vision impairment on children: IVI_C). *Ophthalmic Epidemiology, 15,* 114–120.

20. Coplan, J. (1999). Voice, speech and language disorders. In F. D. Burg, E. R. Wald, J. R. Ingelfinger, & R. A. Polini (Eds.), *Gellis and Kagan's current pediatric therapy* (16th ed., pp. 425–429). Philadelphia: W.B. Saunders.

21. Correa, V. I., Fazzi, D. L., & Pogrund, R. L. (2002). Team focus. Current trends, service delivery, and advocacy. In R. L. Pogrund & D. L. Fazzi (Eds.), *Early focus: Working with young children who are blind or visually impaired and their families* (2nd ed., pp. 405–441). New York: AFB Press.

22. Dowell, R. C., Dettman, S. J., Blarney, P. J., Barker, E. J., Clark, G. M. (2006). Speech perception in children using cochlear implants: Predictions of long-term outcomes [Electronic version]. *Cochlear Implants International, 3*(1), 1–18.

23. Easterbrooks, S. R., & Baker, S. (2002). *Language learning in children who are deaf and hard of hearing.* Boston: Allyn & Bacon.

24. Eisenberg, L. S., Johnson, K. C., Martinez, A. S., Cokely, C. G., Tobey, E. A., Quittner, S. L., et al. (2006). Speech recognition at 1-year follow-up in the childhood development after cochlear implant study: Methods and preliminary findings. *Audiology & Neurology, 11,* 259–268.

25. Ek, U., Fernell, E., Jacobson, L., & Gillberg, C. (1998). Relation between blindness due to retinopathy of prematurity and autistic spectrum disorders: A population-based study. *Developmental Medicine & Child Neurology, 40,* 297–301.

26. Erin, J. N., Fazzi, D. L., Gordon, R. L., Isenberg, S. J., & Paysse, E. A. (2002). Vision focus. Understanding the medical and functional implications of vision loss. In R. L. Pogrund & D. L. Fazzi (Eds.), *Early focus: Working with young children who are blind or visually impaired and their families* (2nd ed., pp. 52–106). New York: AFB Press.

27. Estabrooks, W. (2006). *Auditory-verbal therapy and practice.* Washington, DC: AG Bell.

28. Fazzi, D. L. (2002). Social focus. Developing social skills and promoting positive interactions. In R. L. Pogrund & D. L. Fazzi (Eds.), *Early focus: Working with young children who are blind or visually impaired and their families* (2nd ed., pp. 188–217). New York: AFB Press.

29. Fazzi, D. L., & Klein, D. (2002). Cognitive focus. Developing cognition, concepts, and language. In R. L. Pogrund & D. L. Fazzi (Eds.), *Early focus: Working with young children who are blind or visually impaired and their families* (2nd ed., pp. 107–153). New York: AFB Press.

30. Fazzi, E., Rossi, J., Signorini, S., Rossi, G., Bianchi, P. E., & Lanzi, G. (2007). Leber's congenital amaurosis: Is there an autistic component? *Developmental Medicine & Child Neurology, 49,* 502–507.

31. Fazzi, E., Zaccagnino, M., Gahagan, S., Capsoni, C., Signorini, S. E., & Ariaudo, et al (2008). Sleep disturbances in visual impaired toddlers *Brain & Development, 30,* 572–578.

32. Ferrell, K. A. (1998). *Project PRISM: A longitudinal study of developmental patterns of children who are visually impaired. Executive summary (CFDA 84.0203C—Field-initiated research H025C10188).* Washington, DC: Office of Special Education Programs, Office of Special Education and Rehabilitative Services, U.S. Department of Education.

33. Fischer, J. L., & Rosenthal, B. P. (2005). Optometric assessment and treatment of low vision in children and adults. In M. Gentile (Ed.), *Functional visual behavior in children* (2nd ed., pp. 291–314). Bethesda, MD: AOTA Press.

34. Folio, M. R., & Fewell, R. R. (2000). *Peabody Developmental Motor Scales* (2nd ed.) [PDMS-2]. Austin, TX: Pro-Ed.

35. Freeman, K., Salt, A., Prusa, A., Malm, G., Ferret, N., & Buffolano, W., et al. (2005). Association between congenital toxoplasmosis and parent-reported developmental outcomes, concerns, and impairment in 3 year old children. *BMC Pediatrics, 5,* 25. Retrieved from http://www.biomedcentral.com/1471-2431/5/25

36. Freeman, P. B. (2002). Low vision: Overview and review of low vision evaluation and treatment. In M. Gentile (Ed.), *Functional visual behavior in children. An occupational therapy guide to evaluation and treatment options* (2nd ed., pp. 265–289). Bethesda, MD: AOTA Press.

37. Gallaudet Research Institute. (2006). *Regional and national summary report of data from the 2006–2007 Annual Survey of Deaf and Hard of Hearing Children and Youth.* Washington, DC: GRI, Gallaudet University Press.

38. Gitlin-Weiner, K., Sandgrund, A., & Schaefer, C. (2000). Introduction, emergence, and evaluation of children's play as a focus of study. In K. Gitlin-Weiner, A. Sandgrund, & C. Schaefer (Eds.), *Play diagnosis and assessment* (2nd ed., pp. 1–12). New York: John Wiley & Sons.

39. Glass, P. (1995). Development of visual function in preterm infants: Implications for early intervention. *Infants & Young Children, 6,* 11–20.

40. Glass, P. (2002). Development of the visual system and implications for early intervention. *Infants & Young Children, 15*(1), 1–10.

41. Goldstand, S., Koslowe, K. D., & Parush, S. (2005). Vision, visual-information processing, and academic performance among seventh-grade school children: A more significant relationship than we thought? *American Journal of Occupational Therapy, 59,* 377–389.

42. Goodman, R., & Ashby, L. (1990). Delayed visual maturation and autism. *Developmental Medicine & Child Neurology, 32,* 808–819.

43. Gustafson, G., & Zawalkow, E. (1990). *Signing exact English.* Los Alamitos, CA: Modern Signs Press.

44. Hatton, D. D., Bailey, D. G., Burchinal, M. R., & Ferrell, K. A. (1997). Developmental growth curves of preschool children with vision impairments. *Child Development, 58,* 788–806.

45. Herrer, G. A., Knightly, C. A., & Steinberg, A. G. (2007). Hearing: Sounds and silences. In M. L. Batshaw, L. Pellegrino, & N. J. Roizen (Eds.), *Children with disabilities* (6th ed., pp. 157–183). Baltimore: Brookes.

46. Holte, L., Prickett, J. G., Van Dyke, D. G., Olson, R. J., Lubrica, P., Knutson, C. L., et al. (2006). Issues in the evaluation of infants and young children who are suspected of or who are deaf-blind. *Infants & Young Children, 19,* 213–227.

47. Holte, L., Prickett, J. G., Van Dyke, D. G., Olson, R. J., Lubrica, P., Knutson, C. L., et al. (2006). Issues in the management of infants and young children who are deaf-blind. *Infants & Young Children, 19,* 325–337.

48. Hull, R. H. (1997). *Aural rehabilitation: Serving children and adults* (3rd ed.). San Diego, CA: Singular.

49. Humphries, T., & Padden, D. (2004). *Learning American sign language.* Boston: Pearson.

50. Joint Committee on Infant Hearing. (2007). *Year 2007 position statement: Principles and guidelines for early hearing detection and intervention.* Retrieved from http://www.asha.org/policy

51. Jones, K. L. (1997). *Smith's recognizable patterns of human malformation* (5th ed.). Philadelphia: W.B. Saunders.

52. Kawar, M. (2005). A sensory integration context for vision. In M. Gentile (Ed.), *Functional visual behavior in children. An occupational therapy guide to evaluation and treatment options* (2nd ed., pp. 87–144). Bethesda, MD: AOTA Press.

53. Kelley, P. A., Sanspree, M. J., & Davidson, R. C. (2000). Vision impairment in children and youth. In B. Silverstone, M.

A. Lang, B. P. Rosenthal, & E. E. Faye (Eds.), *The Lighthouse handbook on vision impairment and vision rehabilitation*: Vol. 2. Vision rehabilitation (pp. 1137–1151). New York: Oxford University Press.

54. Kenna, M. A. (1999). Hearing loss. In F. D. Burg, E. R. Wald, J. R. Ingelfinger, & R. A. Polini (Eds.), *Gellis and Kagan's current pediatric therapy* (16th ed., pp. 1019–1021). Philadelphia: W.B. Saunders.

55. Kern, T., & Barbier, A. C. (2005). Treatment options and collaborative interventions for vision impairment in children ages 3 through 12. In M. Gentile (Ed.), *Functional visual behavior in children. An occupational therapy guide to evaluation and treatment options* (2nd ed., pp. 339–389). Bethesda, MD: AOTA Press.

56. Kochkin, S., Luxford, W., Northern, J. L., Mason, P., & Tharpe, M. (2007). Are 1 million dependents with hearing loss in America being left behind? *Hearing Review,* 2–11.

57. Koenig, A. J., & Holbrook, M. C. (2002). Literacy focus. Developing skills and motivation for reading and writing. In R. L. Pogrund & D. L. Fazzi (Eds.), *Early focus: Working with young children who are blind or visually impaired and their families* (2nd ed., pp. 154–187). New York: AFB Press.

58. Kramer, S. J., & Williams, D. R. (1993). The hearing-impaired infant and toddler: Identification, assessment, and intervention. *Infants & Young Children, 61,* 35–39.

59. Kuhl, P. K. (1988). Auditory perceptions and the evolution of speech. *Human Evolution, 3,* 19–43.

60. Kutzbach, B. R., Summers, C. G., Holleschau, A. M., & MacDonald, J. T. (2008). Neurodevelopment in children with albinism. *Ophthalmology, 115,* 1805–1808.

61. Lamoureux, E. L., Pallant, J. F., Pesudovs, K., Hassell, J. B., & Keeffe, J. E. (2006). The impact of vision impairment questionnaire: An evaluation of its measurement properties using Rasch analysis. *Investigative Ophthalmology & Visual Science, 47,* 4732–4741.

62. Lamoureux, E. L., Pallant, J. F., Pesudovs, K., Rees, G., Hassell, J. B., & Keeffe, J. E. (2007). The impact of vision impairment questionnaire: An assessment of its domain structure using confirmatory factor analysis and Rasch analysis. *Investigative Ophthalmology & Visual Science, 48,* 1001–1006.

63. Lampert, J. L. (1998). Working with students with visual impairment. In J. Case-Smith (Ed.), *Occupational therapy: Making a difference in school system practice.* Bethesda, MD: American Occupational Therapy Association.

64. Lederberg, A. R. (1993). The impact of deafness on mother-child and peer relationships. In M. Marschark & M. D. Clark (Eds.), *Psychological perspectives on deafness* (pp. 93–119). Hillsdale, NJ: Lawrence Erlbaum.

65. Linder, T. W. (2008). *Transdisciplinary play-based assessment* (2nd ed.) (TPBA-2). Baltimore: Brookes.

66. Ling, D. (1989). *Foundations of spoken language for hearing impaired children.* Washington, DC: A. G. Bell Association.

67. Marschark, M. (1993). Origins and interactions in social, cognitive, and language development of deaf children. In M. Marschark & M. D. Clark (Eds.), *Psychological perspectives on deafness* (pp. 7–26). Hillsdale, NJ: Lawrence Erlbaum.

68. Meadow, P. M. (1980). *Deafness and child development.* Berkeley, CA: University of California Press.

69. Meadow-Orlans, P. M. (1990). Research on developmental aspects of deafness. In D. F. Moores & K. P. Meadow-Orlans (Eds.), *Educational and developmental aspects of deafness* (pp. 283–320). Washington, DC: Gallaudet University Press.

70. Michelman, S. (1971). The importance of creative play. *American Journal of Occupational Therapy, 25,* 285–290.

71. Miller, M. M., & Menacker, S. J. (2007). Vision: Our window to the world. In M. L. Batshaw, L. Pellegrino, & N. Roizen (Eds.), *Children with disabilities* (6th ed., pp. 137–155). Baltimore: Brookes.

72. Mohay, H. (2000). Language in sight: Mothers' strategies for making language visually accessible to deaf children. In P. E.

Spencer, C. J. Erling, & M. Marschark (Eds.), *The deaf child in the family and at school. Essays in honor of Kathryn P. Meadow-Orlans* (pp. 151–166). Mahwah, NJ: Lawrence Erlbaum.

73. Moores, D. F. (2001). *Educational and developmental aspects of deafness*. Boston: Houghton Mifflin.

74. Mukaddes, N. M., Kilincaslan, A., Kucukyazici, G., Seveketoglu, T., & Tuncer, S. (2007). Autism in visually impaired individuals. *Psychiatry and Clinical Neurosciences, 61*, 39–44.

75. Murray, J. B., Klinger, L., & McKinnon, C. C. (2007). The deaf: An exploration of their participation in community life. *Occupational Therapy Journal of Research: Occupation, Participation and Health, 27*, 113–120.

76. Nevins, M. E., & Chase, P. M. (1996). *Children with cochlear implants in educational settings*. San Diego, CA: Singular.

77. Newborg, J. (2005). *Battelle Developmental Inventory* (2nd ed.). Chicago: Riverside.

78. Northern, J. L., & Downs, M. P. (2002). *Hearing in children* (5th ed.). Baltimore: Lippincott Williams & Wilkins.

79. Parham, L. D. (2008). Play and occupational therapy. In L. D. Parham & L. S. Fazio (Eds.), *Play in occupational therapy for children* (2nd ed. pp. 3–39). St. Louis: Mosby.

80. Parks, S. (1999). *Inside HELP: Administration and reference manual for the Hawaii early learning profile (birth-3)*. Palo Alto, CA: VORT.

81. Paul, P. V. (2001). *Language and deafness* (3rd ed.). San Diego, CA: Singular.

82. Pellegrino, L. (2007). Cerebral palsy. In M. L. Batshaw, L. Pellegrino, & N. J. Roizen (Eds.), *Children with disabilities* (6th ed., pp. 387–408). Baltimore: Brookes.

83. Pinker, S. (1994). *The language instinct*. New York: Morrow.

84. Pogrund, R. (2002). Refocus. Setting the stage for working with children who are blind or visually impaired. In R. L. Pogrund & D. L. Fazzi (Eds.), *Early focus: Working with young children who are blind or visually impaired and their families* (2nd ed., pp. 1–15). New York: AFB Press.

85. Pogrund, R. (2002). Independence focus. Promoting independence in daily living and recreational skills. In R. L. Pogrund & D. L. Fazzi (Eds.), *Early focus: Working with young children who are blind or visually impaired and their families* (2nd ed., pp. 218–249). New York: AFB Press.

86. Porr, S. M. (1999). The visual and auditory systems. In S. M. Porr & E. B. Rainville (Eds.), *Pediatric therapy: A systems approach* (pp. 241–266). Philadelphia: F.A. Davis.

87. Recchia, S. (1997). Play and concept development in infants and young children with severe visual impairments: A constructionist view. *Journal of Visual Impairment and Blindness, 91*, 401–406.

88. Rogers, S. J., & Newhart-Larson, S. (1989). Characteristics of infantile autism in five children with Leber's congenital amaurosis. *Developmental Medicine & Child Neurology, 31*, 598–608.

89. Roid, G. H., & Miller, L. J. (1997). *General instructions for the revised Leiter international performance scales*. Wood Dale, IL: Stoelting.

90. Roizen, N., Kasza, K., Karrison, T., Mets, M., Noble, A. G., Boyer, K., et al. (2008). Impact of visual impairment on measures of cognitive function for children with congenital toxoplasmosis: Implications for compensatory intervention strategies [Electronic version]. *Pediatrics, 118*, e379–e390. Retrieved from www.pediatrics.org/cgi/content/full/118/2/e379

91. Roman-Lantzy, C. (2007). *Cortical visual impairment. An approach to assessment and intervention*. New York: AFB Press.

92. Ross, G., Lipper, E. G., Abramson, D., & Preiser, L. (2001). The development of young children with retinoblastoma. *Archives of Pediatric and Adolescent Medicine, 155*, 80–83.

93. Ross, M., Brackett, D., & Maxon, A. (1991). *Assessment and management of mainstreamed hearing impaired children*. Austin, TX: Pro-Ed.

94. Ross, S., & Tobin, M. J. (1997). Object permanence, reaching, and locomotion n infants who are blind. *Journal of Visual Impairment and Blindness, 91*, 25–32.

95. Sameroff, A. J., & Fiese, B. H. (2000). Transactional regulation: The developmental ecology of early intervention. In J. P. Shonkoff & S. J. Meisels (Eds.), *Handbook of early childhood intervention* (2nd ed., pp. 135–159). Cambridge, MA: Cambridge University Press.

96. Sanspree, M. J. (2000). Pathways to habilitation: Best practices. In B. Silverstone, M. A. Lang, B. P. Rosenthal, & E. E. Faye (Eds.), *The Lighthouse handbook on vision impairment and vision rehabilitation: Vol. 2. Vision rehabilitation* (pp. 1167–1182). New York: Oxford University Press.

97. Schaaf, R. C., & Smith Roley, S. (2006). Sensory integration for children with visual impairments, including blindness. In R. C. Schaaf & S. Smith Roley (Eds.), *SI: Applying clinical reasoning to practice with diverse populations* (pp. 149–169). San Antonio, TX: Harcourt Assessment.

98. Scheetz, N. A. (2001). *Orientation to deafness*. Boston: Allyn & Bacon.

99. Scheiman, M. (2002). Optometric model of vision, parts one, two and three. In *Understanding and managing vision deficits: A guide for occupational therapists* (2nd ed., pp. 17–84). Thorofare, NJ: Slack.

100. Scheiman, M. (2002). Management of refractive, visual efficiency, and visual information processing disorders. In *Understanding and managing vision deficits: A guide for occupational therapists* (2nd ed., pp. 117–164). Thorofare, NJ: Slack.

101. Schein, J. D., & Delk, M. T. (1975). *The deaf population in the United States*. Silver Spring, MD: National Association for the Deaf.

102. Schiarti, V., Matsuba, C., Houbé, J. S., & Synnes, A. R. (2008). Severe retinopathy of prematurity and visual outcomes in British Columbia: A 10-year analysis. *Journal of Perinatology, 28*, 1–7.

103. Schlumberger, E., Narbona, J., & Manrique, M. (2004). Nonverbal development of children with deafness with and without cochlear implants. *Developmental Medicine and Child Neurology, 46*, 599–606.

104. Shapiro, D. R., Moffett, A., Lieberman, L., & Dummer, G. M. (2005). Perceived competence of children with visual impairments. *Journal of Visual Impairment and Blindness, 99*, 15–25.

105. Sharma, A., Dorman, M., Spahr, A., & Todd, N. W. (2002). Early cochlear implantation in children allows normal development of central auditory pathways. *Annals of Otology, Rhinology, & Laryngology, 111*, 38–41.

106. Smith Roley, S., & Schneck, C. (2001). Sensory integration and visual deficits, including blindness. In S. Smith Roley, E. I. Blanche, & R. C. Schaaf (Eds.), *Understanding the nature of sensory integration with diverse populations* (pp. 313–344). San Antonio, TX: Therapy Skill Builders.

107. Spencer, R. (2006). Long-term visual outcomes in extremely low-birth-weight children. (An American Ophthalmological Society thesis.) *Transactions of the American Ophthalmological Society, 104*, 493–516.

108. Sternberg, M. L. (1998). *American sign language dictionary*. New York: Harper Collins,

109. Stoel-Gammon, C., & Otomo, K. (1986). Babbling development of hearing-impaired and normally hearing subjects. *Journal of Speech and Hearing Disorders, 51*, 33–41.

110. Strickling, C. A. (1998). *Impact of vision loss on motor development. Information for occupational and physical therapists working with students with visual impairments*. Austin, TX: Texas School for the Blind and Visually Impaired.

111. Strickling, C. A., & Pogrund, R. L. (2002). Motor focus. Promoting movement experiences and motor development. In R. L. Pogrund & D. L. Fazzi (Eds.), *Early focus: Working with young children who are blind or visually impaired and their families* (2nd ed., pp. 287–325). New York: AFB Press.

112. Teplin, S. W. (1995). Visual impairment in infants and young children. *Infants & Young Children, 8*(1), 18–41.

113. Titcomb, R. E., & Okoye, R. (2005). Functional vision. A developmental, dynamic, and integrated process. In M. Gentile (Ed.), *Functional visual behavior in children. An occupational therapy guide to evaluation and treatment options* (2nd ed., pp. 1–40). Bethesda, MD: AOTA Press.

114. U.S. Department of Education. (2007). *27th annual report to Congress on the implementation of the Individuals with Disabilities Education Act, 2005* (Vol. 2). Washington, DC: Office of Special Education Programs, U.S. Department of Education. Retrieved from www.ed.gov/offices/OSERS/OSEP

115. Vernon, M. C., & Andrews, J. F. (1990). *The psychology of deafness: Understanding deaf and hard-of-hearing people.* New York: Longman.

116. VORT. (1995–1999). *HELP for Preschoolers. Assessment & curriculum guide.* Palo Alto, CA: Author.

117. Warren, D. (1994). *Blindness in children: An individual differences approach.* New York: Cambridge University Press.

118. Warren, D. (2000). Developmental perspectives. In B. Silverstone, M. A. Lang, B. P. Rosenthal, & E. E. Faye (Eds.), *The Lighthouse handbook on vision impairment and vision rehabilitation: Vol. 1. Vision impairment* (pp. 325–337). New York: Oxford University Press.

119. Weib, L. M., Hassell, J. B., & Keeffe, J. (2002). Assessment of the impact of vision impairment. *Investigative Ophthalmology & Visual Science, 43,* 927–935.

120. Wilbur, R. (1987). *American sign language: Linguistics and applied dimensions* (2nd ed.). Boston: Little Brown.

121. Wiley, S., & Moeller, M. P. (2007). Red flags for disabilities in children who are deaf/hard of hearing. *The ASHS Leader, 8–9,* 28–29.

122. Yeargin-Allsopp, M., Drews-Botsch, C., & Van Naarden Braun, K. (2007). Epidemiology of developmental disabilities. In M. L. Batshaw, L. Pellegrino, & N. J. Roizen (Eds.), *Children with disabilities* (6th ed., pp. 215–243). Baltimore: Brookes.

123. Yucel, E., & Derim, D. (2008). The effect of implantation age on visual attention skills. *International Journal of Pediatric Otorhinolaryngology, 72,* 869–877.

124. Zambone, A. M., Ciner, E., Appel, S., & Garboyes, M. (2000). Children with multiple impairments. In B. Silverstone, M. A. Lang, B. P. Rosenthal, & E. E. Faye (Eds.), *The Lighthouse handbook on vision impairment and vision rehabilitation: Vol. 1. Vision impairment* (pp. 325–337). New York: Oxford University Press.

Hospital and Pediatric Rehabilitation Services

Brian J. Dudgeon • Laura Crooks*

OBJECTIVES

1. Understand the characteristics that accompany hospitalization of children.
2. Explain the roles and functions of occupational therapists in pediatric hospitals.
3. Describe occupational therapy intervention in various types of medical and rehabilitation units.
4. Describe the types of children who are commonly treated within hospital-based pediatric rehabilitation units and those who typically receive specialized outpatient clinic and therapy services.
5. Discuss existing research of pediatric rehabilitation programs and of specific interventions for children with common diagnoses.
6. Identify and describe collaborative relationships with other providers in interdisciplinary and transdisciplinary practice settings.
7. Propose and apply a prioritization system for assessment and intervention planning that guides the selection of therapy goals and intervention approaches.
8. Emphasize teaching strategies as an integral component of therapy designed to optimize occupational performance.
9. Describe intervention approaches commonly used in pediatric rehabilitation and apply them in a complementary manner in intervention planning.
10. Recognize opportunities for family involvement and explain levels of family participation.
11. Discuss the elements of a plan for transition of care from the hospital setting to home and the community.

HOSPITALIZATION

Children receive care at a hospital for a wide variety of diagnostic and treatment reasons. Most commonly children are admitted for respiratory and gastrointestinal problems,[29,33] and while these disorders may warrant referral to therapy services, those children with neurologic and musculoskeletal disorders may be more likely to receive attention from rehabilitation services, including occupational therapy. For children who need hospitalization, issues of safety for the child and concerns about the influence of hospitalization on the child's life experiences often arise.[15] Historically, a strong reluctance to hospitalize children was often expressed owing to the potential for psychological reactions accompanying separation from home and family. But needs for careful and ongoing medical monitoring, specialized equipment, and environments for diagnosis and treatments lead to the inevitability of hospitalization for many kinds of pediatric conditions. Chronic disease and disorders appear to be on the rise among children in developed countries.[97] Physicians are being alerted to these problems, which are often viewed as stemming from children's challenges with weight gain, inactivity, and other lifestyle habits.

With the unique specialized care needs of children, hospitals developed to exclusively care for and manage children's health challenges. The first children's hospitals in America were established in the 1850s in Philadelphia, and others soon followed. Today there are more than 150 such institutions. These community and regional efforts often led to programs that addressed not only health but also special education needs of children. While modern hospitals are almost exclusively for medical concerns, educational needs are still paramount in children's lives, and not surprisingly, school-based programs are often a part of children's experience with hospitalization. In addition to addressing needs for education, children's hospitals often create special environments that can be designed

*I wish to thank the children and families involved with Seattle Children's Hospital, Seattle, for their willingness to share their experiences. I also want to acknowledge the advice and help of colleagues from the same institution in preparation of this chapter.

to cater to children and families.[92] Positive aspects of hospitals for children include environmental features such as art, colors, and spaces that are friendly, warm and inviting, allow space for play and enable families to group and communicate. Volunteers are frequently present to assist with child and family services and active fund-raising to support costs and offset expenses for children's care. Also unique to these settings are child life specialists, who attend to the child's emotional and developmental needs and help to reduce the stresses of the hospital stay by assisting families to cope with the hospital experience by providing information about play, child development, and adjustment to illness.

Interventions with children in hospitals present the occupational therapist with a unique set of challenges. The demands of the evolving health care system, the varied medical conditions of the children, family dynamics, and the hospital's milieu all impact occupational therapy practice. This chapter describes occupational therapy services to pediatric clients within the children's hospital setting. It illustrates varied models of service delivery and explains the roles and function of hospital-based occupational therapy practitioners.

In the past, children who required pediatric rehabilitation often experienced long-term hospital stays or frequent hospitalizations. These environments addressed medical care and rehabilitative intervention and often branched into programs addressing socialization, education, and vocation.[9,27] In modern times, the major portion of pediatric therapy is delivered through school systems. This shift in policy, along with advances in medical care and rehabilitation practice, has changed the role of hospital-based pediatric rehabilitation. In general, most hospital-based programs now focus on acute-onset problems and provision of specialized services for children and adolescents with disabilities that are of low occurrence but of high complexity. Hospital-based programs continue to evolve, aiming to address known and newly identified health threats in a way that emphasizes a partnership with the child and family and resources in their local community.

Characteristics of Children's Hospitals

Hospital-based services may include either or both inpatient and outpatient care for the ill and injured, in addition to prevention or wellness programs designed to reduce the need for future hospitalizations and treatments. Hospitals in which pediatric clients are served generally fall into three categories: general hospitals, trauma centers, and children's hospitals. *General hospitals* strive to serve the needs of the community in which they are located. Given specific local populations, a wide variety of clients can be served in this type of hospital and this typically includes the entire lifespan from infants to geriatrics. The therapist working in the general hospital setting may serve both pediatric and adult clients. Hospitals that offer labor and delivery services often have neonatal intensive care services in which therapy services may be called upon. Some general hospitals may also have special units dedicated to serving the needs of pediatric populations; however, children with more involved or complex needs are often referred to children's hospitals.

Trauma centers are hospitals certified to treat patients with more acute life-threatening injuries. Such centers most often are situated in large metropolitan areas. Patients taken to trauma centers may have extensive musculoskeletal, neurologic, skin, and internal organ injuries requiring multiple specialists. As in the general hospital setting, the occupational therapist working in the trauma center may serve patients of a various ages and with a variety of injuries or illnesses. Metropolitan areas often have burn units and other special trauma unit or programs that are organized to handle the evaluations and treatments initially directed toward life saving and sustaining procedures and to prevent unnecessary complications (e.g., splinting, positioning, and evaluating oral motor skills for initial feeding). As a child in such settings becomes more stable, additional types of interventions, such as activities of daily living (ADLs) training and age appropriate play, can be implemented. In addition to the stress on the family of having their child in the trauma center, there may be additional family members receiving care, or families may be some distance from their homes. Therapists need to be sensitive to the stress that the families experience when their children are in these centers. Once patients are stabilized and treatment has been established, patients in the trauma centers may receive ongoing care in that particular hospital, or they may be transferred to a children's hospital or a general hospital in their community.

Children's hospitals are specialty hospitals that offer a full range of inpatient and outpatient services organized for infants, children, and adolescents with a wide range of diagnoses. The therapist working with children in such a hospital may have exposure to children with diseases rarely seen, and sometimes having limited information on treatment protocols or outcomes. For this reason, the therapist working in these settings must have good communication skills to obtain information from medical team members of various specialties, and she or he must have a solid medical treatment foundation as a basis for making intervention decisions.

Region (Locations) Served

Children's hospitals, as specialized health care institutions, tend to serve a broader geographic region than general hospitals. This may result in a child being hospitalized a significant distance from home, increasing the sense of separation from family, peers, and familiar environment. The distance between the home and the hospital may affect the family's ability to visit the child and remain in contact with the health personnel caring for the child. Frequently only one family member may be available to remain with the child. This can pose additional challenges for the family—not only the financial burden and psychological strains of having a child in the hospital, but also the distance among family members that may produce additional pressures. The size of the service area, and the part of the country in which it is located, may also mean greater cultural diversity and socioeconomic variation among those served by the hospital. Diversity in clientele requires the medical team to be sensitive to the cultural beliefs and practices of the patient and family.[94] The broader geographic region served by most children's hospitals usually requires hospital personnel to interact with a great number of organizations and programs in the varied communities serviced by the children's hospital.[41] This distance can pose challenges for the hospital-based occupational therapist to communicate with community-based therapists regarding the child's care programs and community functioning. Hospital-based and community-based therapists should oordinate the child's transition to home, accessing local community resources and outpatient or school-based programs.

Missions of Children's Hospitals

Goals of such children's hospitals often include effective advocacy for child health, conducting leading-edge pediatric research to improve upon clinical outcomes, and creating and implementing a model for family-centered care. These and other program specific missions do influence day-to-day operations of such facilities and programs and provide guidance to how clinical care is approached and conducted. Promotion of child health may be seen in local outreach programs where children's hospital personnel educate others in public schools and other community programs regarding a wide range of children's health and safety issues. At the national level, advocacy for policies and programs to promote public health, and health care reforms that would enable pediatric health care coverage and the conducting of research to prevent and address pediatric health conditions, are often cited (see National Association for Children's Hospitals and Related Institutions [NACHRI]).[69]

Although most hospital services are directed toward providing medical care to the ill or injured, many hospitals also include teaching and research as a component of their mission. The hospital, as a teaching institution, provides clinical education experiences for medical students, interns, residents, nursing students, and students from other health-related professions. As a research institution, the hospital often provides resources and opportunities for clinical research to advance medical knowledge and practice. In training and research hospitals, occupational therapists can access many different educational opportunities, including access to many different health care professionals. Continuing education and teaching within these settings, not only for the occupational therapy student, but also for students of other health professions, generally have high priority. Another benefit to the occupational therapist working in a teaching institution is access to the latest intervention strategies and clinical trials to facilitate new medical options. The therapist may participate in research or provide information to a researcher conducting a study, making it important for that therapist to understand the hospital's policies on informed consent, confidentiality, and protection of research participants.

Research Regarding Systems and Care Outcomes

Research missions of children's hospitals and research conducted as part of clinical care can be both broad and specific, and are generally motivated by a local facility's particular interests and needs. Specialization is inherent in research programs and a specific review of a particular program's research activities may be warranted. These may be stand-alone efforts based in a hospital setting, affiliated with local research universities or affiliated with regional, national, or international research programs.

Two prominent types of research conducted at children's hospitals are addressing and reducing risks of care so as to reduce iatrogenic causes of ill health, and exploring best practices and evidence for effective outcomes in specific clinical services. NACHRI recognizes safety as a major concern within hospitals and that such environments may pose risks for infection and a variety of other medical and behavioral consequences of care.[69] Research on efforts to reduce and eliminate such threats is both wide-ranging and specific. Children's hospitals, like other health care facilities, recognize that infections are sometimes transmitted by hand contact. Transmission of germs thus occurs from one patient to another. Effective hand-washing habits have been difficult to implement, with most hospitals striving to enable and monitor such habits by reminding everyone, providing cleaning opportunities, and enforcing routines by monitoring and creating a culture of peer to peer feedback (see NACHRI).[69] Other safety measures relate to body substance isolation through conditional uses of gloves, masks, and gowns with proper disposal of at-risk materials. Departments of risk management and infectious diseases work to identify potential risks and to institute measures that prevent new and ongoing hazards.

Occupational therapists may participate in research of clinical services and outcomes. For example, ADL and IADL status, discharge placement, health-related quality of life, and well-being are some of the typical measures used to document rehabilitation outcomes.[35,36] During the past few decades, increasing emphasis has been placed on outcomes and ways to use research outcomes in evidence-based decision making.[10,62] Occupational therapy practitioners use research studies that describe medical and functional sequelae, validity of assessment tools related to diagnostic problem solving, and effectiveness of specific treatment strategies or techniques.[88] O'Donnell and Roxborough recognize the challenge for therapists to find current research relevant to their practices.[70] They offer guidelines on seeking evidence in pediatric rehabilitation. Researchers can now find systematic reviews (e.g., The Cochrane Library), seek topical reviews (e.g., *Bandolier Journal*), or pursue a precise search for research literature through electronic information sources (e.g., PubMed, CINAHL).

Whereas adult inpatient rehabilitation programs have received considerable attention, comparable benefits of similar programs designed for children have been more lacking. So far, most research about inpatient pediatric rehabilitation outcomes has described residual disability.[48] Particular attention is usually paid to the most common diagnostic groups treated in these settings. For example, Dumas, Haley, Ludlow, and Rabin have reported functional gains demonstrated by children with traumatic brain injury (TBI) undergoing inpatient pediatric rehabilitation.[25] The greatest gains were made in mobility, but also in social function and self-care for all ages of children. But after TBI, an extended period of recovery is expected. Boyer and Edwards reviewed outcomes for 220 children and adolescents with TBI who were admitted to a comprehensive pediatric rehabilitation program.[8] They reported continued progress in mobility, ADLs, and education and cognition for up to 3 years after the injury. Physical recovery was greatest in the first year, with cognitive and language gains generally occurring later. Researchers have also recommended following and studying complications from TBI by following children identified in trauma registries.[16,51] Jaffe and others conducted a thorough follow-up of children with head injury.[31,52–54] In this series, researchers developed an age-matched cohort to provide a careful appraisal and monitoring of sequelae from mild, moderate, and severe classifications of TBI. Among these children, who were 6 to 15 years of age at the time of injury, many with moderate and most with severe injury evidenced persisting and widespread cognitive, language, academic, behavioral, and functional deficits.

Evidence regarding efficacy of specific intervention strategies is known to be lacking because it is tremendously difficult and costly to conduct research that analyzes the application of particular techniques or rehabilitation strategies. Experimental research of rehabilitation effectiveness is particularly difficult to conduct because of the heterogeneity of participants and ethical conflicts encountered by suspending or withholding services to specific children. Randomized clinical trials are particularly problematic and alternate research strategies have been proposed,[71] with an emphasis on humanistic elements as part of therapeutic practice[49] and client's views about process and outcomes.[2,61] However, a specific analysis of different priorities within pediatric rehabilitation, mixtures of service providers, or contrasts with less intensive subacute or outpatient services have generally not been reported. Chen, Heineman, Gode, Granger, and Mallinson reported on a review of hospital-based pediatric rehabilitation programs, services, and outcomes.[13] Among 12 programs reporting on 814 admissions, they found that the intensity of specific service delivery seemed to relate to outcomes. Those receiving greater occupational therapy services made the most gains in ADLs, greater PT services made more mobility gains, and more speech language services showed greater communication and cognitive gains.

Family and Child-Centered Care

Family-centered care of hospitalized children is a hallmark of most Children's Hospitals and has lead to new insights and directions for care.[26] To implement family-centered care, families are valued as a member of the health care team and take an active part in the decision making required to develop a treatment plan for the child. The occupational therapist working in the hospital setting where family-centered care has been adopted for the pediatric clientele must use clear descriptions to communicate evaluation results to the family, seek input from the family on which intervention outcomes for the child have priority, and come to a mutually agreed upon treatment plan. As evaluations are completed and team meetings established, family caregivers become an integral part of the health care decision-making team.

The occupational therapist's knowledge of age-appropriate developmental tasks and understanding of the importance of purposeful activity can help the child achieve a sense of control in the foreign environment of the hospital. The occupational therapist can also help other members of medical teams understand developmental issues of concern, suggesting strategies to caregivers, family members, and others to support typical development that may help the child better cope with hospitalization.

Accrediting and Regulatory Agencies

Pediatric rehabilitation advocates and service providers have both influenced and been shaped by accreditation processes. For example, the Centers for Medicare and Medicaid Services (CMS) designates requirements for services that are organized and paid to provide "medical rehabilitation." To meet CMS guidelines for rehabilitation, rules are placed on such systems that mandate specific program emphasis, dedicated space and personnel, admission and discharge procedures, service intensity, goal setting, and monitoring of progress toward goals. Most rehabilitation programs also pursue voluntary accreditation by groups such as The Joint Commission (formerly the Joint Commission on Accreditation of Healthcare Organizations [JCAHO]) and the Commission on Accreditation of Rehabilitation Facilities (CARF), and government agencies such as the Occupational Safety and Health Administration (OSHA), which have set standards regarding hospital operations. These organizations assign additional mandates that also shape program characteristics. Such guidelines may include integrated planning with community-based services and continuous quality improvement procedures. Every few years accreditation standards and procedures based on The Joint Commission and CARF recommendations shift emphasis and specification of essential requirements. Generally, after initial accreditation, reaccreditation reports or visits are scheduled every 3 years, and programs may be subject to periodic interim review and reporting about their overall performance.

Employee education regarding safety practices (when there is risk of exposure to patient blood or body fluids) or to hazardous materials is also mandated (Occupational Exposure to Blood-Borne Pathogens, 56 *Fed. Reg.* 64175-64182). Of particular importance in working with pediatric populations in the hospital setting is the inclusion that occupational therapists are mandated reporters of child abuse. They are required to report any suspicion of abuse to designated personnel within the hospital setting, who, when appropriate, contact community support services such as law enforcement or child protective services (CPS) personnel. Specific training in each institution regarding reporting protocols must be established and provided to the therapists in these settings. These accrediting bodies also promote strategic planning and systematic program evaluation.

One trend among hospitals has been the affiliation with similar institutions, offering opportunities for consolidation of information and equipment, achievement of common goals, and program development. Hospitals are generally part of medical systems directed by a single administration and linking facilities that share certain resources and specialized personnel. One such system offers patients a spectrum of care options including acute and subacute rehabilitation, satellite outpatient clinics and programs, and home health care.[14,42,57]

Reimbursement for Services

Inpatient services are typically funded by a combination of private insurance carriers, Medicaid, or special programs within a state, and under some circumstances by Medicare. Preadmission review and authorization are generally required. For adults, as part of the Balanced Budget Act of 1997, inpatient rehabilitation units are now required to use a prospective payment funding system.[17] Implementation of similar funding approaches with children's hospitals has been more controversial and has been put on indefinite hold.

Occupational therapy has typically been recognized as a service that is reimbursed within inpatient hospitals and medical rehabilitation units, home health care, and less commonly in outpatient services. Medicare guidelines are generally universal across different states. However, each state's Medicaid rules and regulations and local insurance companies have differing provisions related to funding of occupational therapy services and supplies or assistive devices that may be suggested. Local regulations must be reviewed to ensure that appropriate levels of reimbursement are available and that families are informed about service options.

Lengths of stay within children's hospitals are varied, from as short as a few days, to weeks, or perhaps months. As in other hospitals, third-party payers and other regulators strive to control costs by seeking shortened lengths of stay and by transferring patients more quickly to less costly skilled nursing facilities or home care, outpatient, or school-based services. Changes within and across treatment settings can be problematic, often creating confusion within families about entitlements and expectations for services. Clearly stated goals and time frames for outcomes in each care setting are desirable. Case managers who are familiar with funding rules and regulations work with families and service teams to coordinate care and prepare the family for transitions among care settings.

An issue of concern facing hospitals that provide service to children is the cost of health care. In recent years, heath maintenance organizations (HMOs) and preferred provider organizations (PPOs) have proliferated, and between 75% and 90% of all those insured are in a managed care plan.[38,58] Prospective payment systems, created within Medicare to better estimate and contain costs, have a strong impact on reimbursement for services. This system uses preestablished rates of reimbursement for almost 1900 diagnostic groups and using more than 8000 current procedural terminology (CPT) codes.[46] Although this does not have as great an implication for the pediatric population as for the adult patient, payers do take these guidelines into consideration when authorizing care for inpatient stays. The therapist should be aware of payment limitations when providing care and clearly communicate with families when establishing an intervention program.

Occupational Therapy Services Within Children's Hospitals

Organization of occupational therapy and other rehabilitation services within a hospital can be varied. Programs in this chapter focus on four broad types of services: consultation, rehabilitation, and outpatient clinics. Each of these services is described in more detail with case examples later in the chapter. In brief, consultation services are those wherein therapy services are ordered directly from a medical service or unit not always staffed by a therapist or other rehabilitation providers. Intensive care, acute care, and other units or programs are most likely to order consultation therapy services. These may include medical services such as neurology and neurosurgery, oncology or cancer care, general surgery, orthopedics, heart and pulmonary services, and, in many children's hospitals, transplantation services. Reasons for referral to consultation services commonly include therapist's appraisal, interventions for immediate needs, and assistance in planning transition to other services or discharge to home. In the case of secondary sensory motor impairment, occupational therapy consultation services may be requested to evaluate and make recommendations specific to those issues. Pediatric rehabilitation services are often located within a specific location within the children's hospital, and this may include special facilities with bedrooms and bathrooms to enable effective independence training with lifts, mobility devices, and other durable medical equipment. Spaces for individual and group sessions, socialization, and group engagements are often available as well. Outpatient services include both regularly scheduled hospital-based specialty clinics that address children and families' long-term needs, and individual child services in community-based satellite clinics.

Issues to be addressed in each service area are unique, and are described later in this chapter with case examples. This chapter applies a systematic approach to hospital service areas that includes prioritization of care, evaluation strategies used, goal-setting guidelines, and selection of interventions. This framework is applied to each service area (e.g., consultation, rehabilitation, and outpatient clinics) to exemplify the breadth of diagnoses and clinical approaches that may be encountered within children's hospitals.

Functions of Occupational Therapists

The primary focus of the occupational therapy practitioner within children's hospitals is on ADLs and other instrumental tasks associated with independent living, education, and community participation. Therapists use many frames of reference to develop insights about the child's function, establish priorities for treatment, and guide the organization of intervention goals with the child, family, and local care providers. In most forms of hospital care, the therapist follows a prioritization system that focuses first on prevention of problems associated with illness, trauma, or disability; then, resumption of the able self and finally on restoration of lost skills and functions. A key concept in care is the recognition that many therapeutic outcomes relate to learning principles.[84] Thus therapists employ behavioral and cognitive learning principles and attend to the teacher-pupil relationship. The therapist blends his or her technical competency with personal caring. Goals and activities are jointly planned with children and families.

Task, activity, and occupation analyses are universal strategies that therapists use to determine the skill requirements of functional tasks and the therapeutic uses of occupation to improve skills. These analyses break down tasks into performance skills and factors, such as demands placed on body structures and functions, motor, process, and communication and interaction strategies used in functioning. The therapist can reorganize or adapt activities so that certain skills are substituted for or emphasized over those that are missing or in deficit. Specific intervention techniques used to achieve priority goals combine biomechanical, sensorimotor, perceptual-cognitive, and rehabilitative treatment approaches (discussed in detail in Chapters 9 to 21).

Prevention

Primary prevention is a term used to denote efforts that decrease the likelihood of accidents, violence, or disease for everyone. *Secondary prevention* and *tertiary prevention* refer to specific interventions, arrangement of care systems, and environmental modifications to prevent the onset of problems among at-risk populations. Children admitted to the hospital are typically at risk for developing a number of secondary disabilities. The therapist, along with other team members, has a responsibility to be familiar with such risks. Included are concerns for safety in positioning and movement, risks of aspiration in swallowing, and lack of orientation to time and place stresses experienced in an unfamiliar environment. Therapists must be aware of risks and avoid involving the child in activities that would be harmful or would perpetuate behaviors that could hamper recovery. Complications from immobilization, abnormal muscle tone, and other neuromuscular abnormalities often necessitate careful attention to maintaining range of

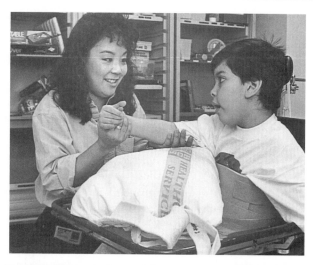

FIGURE 26-1 Active assistive range of motion exercises are performed several times each day to prevent joint and muscle contractures with this boy who sustained a severe closed head injury. Stretch is also applied to existing contractures, along with other joint mobilization techniques.

motion, strength, and general fitness (Figure 26-1). Concern for wound healing and protection of neurogenic skin are also essential to the early planning and ongoing achievement of goals, interventions, and education of the child and his or her family.

Resumption

The second level of priority for occupational therapy is a focus on resuming the use of available skills and independence in easily accomplished tasks. Emphasizing the able self provides the child with an opportunity to resume doing tasks on his or her own, or at least to have a say about how he or she is assisted. Such an approach may be important in preventing the child or adolescent from developing dependent behaviors or learned helplessness. Efficiency demands placed on nursing may often result in the child's becoming a passive recipient of care. The therapist should provide the child with sufficient time to perform activities on his or her own. Early emphasis on providing children with opportunities to make choices about the types of assistance they receive or activities they pursue should help them develop confidence in their skills and returning abilities.

Restoration

Lost skills and function follow in priority with efforts to restore abilities. The therapist uses biomechanical, sensorimotor, perceptual-cognitive, and rehabilitative approaches in various combinations to restore function. Time available to address restoration of abilities may be quite limited within hospital settings. Rehabilitation units and outpatient or other community-based programs most often address restoration of skills more directly. Such approaches may include extensive retraining or complex adaptations.

Each prioritization level may capitalize on intervention approaches that directly address performance skills and factors. For example, biomechanical and sensorimotor techniques are designed to improve skills and factors such as strength, range of motion, postural control, skilled movements, and coordination. Such approaches include the use of therapeutic activities

and exercise, splinting and positioning, facilitation of movement, and the use of biomedical interventions such as functional electrical stimulation. Other physical agent modalities such as superficial heat or cold may also be used, whereas deep-heating techniques such as with ultrasound are often avoided because children's bone epiphyseal (growth plates) areas may be damaged.[66]

The occupational therapist often helps the child or youth practice activities that selectively challenge individual skills or factors with the expectation that gains will then transfer or generalize to occupational performance areas. Rehabilitative approaches contrast with biomechanical and sensorimotor techniques, which are designed to address underlying performance skills and factors. In the rehabilitative approach, therapists teach clients compensatory techniques that use existing skills to maintain or restore occupational performance. In rehabilitative approaches, therapists teach clients to use adapted routines and assistive technology (AT) devices and modify environments to promote optimal function. Initial training and the use of AT devices to enable manipulation, mobility, cognition, and communication are part of restoration. Client outcomes are optimal when occupational therapy practitioners use complementary strategies to improve the child's skills, adapt functional activities, and modify environmental contexts.

Evaluation

In nearly all instances, occupational therapy services in hospital-based care are initiated through physician's orders. Often required by law or regulatory guidelines, therapists respond to initial orders and negotiate as necessary with the physician to add specific elements to assessment and intervention activities. Most commonly, initial orders for occupational therapy involve a focus on ADLs and specific performance skills related to functional capacities.

Multiple sources for data acquisition are available within the children's hospital setting. Review of medical records and discussions with other providers may form the initial basis for evaluation. In general, evaluation consists of asking (e.g., clinical interview), looking (e.g., clinical observation), touching (e.g., physical examination), and testing (e.g., using standardized assessments). Most often, the therapist uses clinical interview and observation to initiate the assessment process. Observed areas of concern may necessitate a more thorough evaluation through physical examination and direct observation with the use of standardized tests. Such measures help in the diagnostic process. Generally, performance is limited by body structure or body function impairments. Once the therapist makes hypotheses about the impairments and initiates intervention plans, the repeated use of clinical examination and standardized tests serves as an objective measure of skill improvement. For diagnostic purposes, the therapist judges the child's performance against normed scores, but for evaluative purposes, the therapist most often judges the child's scores on reassessment against his or her previous performance. Selection of a specific measure should be based on its reliability, sensitivity, and appropriateness for the child's age and diagnosis.

Evaluation of ADL and IADL skills helps prioritize which performance skills and factors may be impaired and require the use of more specific assessments. After the child's ability to participate in functional activities has been evaluated, the therapist analyzes performance skills and factors to determine those to be targeted in intervention and the types of adaptations that may be warranted. The child's home, school, and community contexts affect occupational performance and may require careful analysis and modification.

The therapist may organize assessment of ADL and IADL status around checklists or other reporting tools that specify activities and methods of rating the individual's level of skill. For example, the Functional Independence Measure (FIM) was developed as part of a Uniform Data System for Medical Rehabilitation for use in client-specific and program monitoring and outcome evaluation systems.[59] The FIM is generally for individuals 7 years of age and older. A pediatric version of this tool, called the Wee-FIM, has been developed for children of developmental age 6 months to 7 years,[68] and validity studies have been completed.[72] Eighteen specific ADL tasks, including communication and social cognition, are rated for dependence based on the individual's need for adaptation and assistance from a helper.

Another tool that the therapist can use for rating and describing function in children is the Pediatric Evaluation of Disability Inventory (PEDI).[47] Based on a combination of interview and observation, the PEDI specifies discrete levels of skills in domains of self-care, mobility, and social function. A description of needs for care provider assistance and reliance on AT devices is included with the measure. Both the FIM and PEDI are used for individualized assessment and planning, and both can also be used as part of program evaluation. The PEDI and Wee-FIM have been shown to measure similar constructs.[99] Although these tools focus directly on daily functional tasks, additional broad-based measures that assess play- and school-related performance can also be used.

Following these functional assessments, the therapist has specific needs to pursue an analysis of performance. Tools and methods to evaluate performance skills and factors are described in Chapters 7 and 8. Careful appraisal of motor, process, and communication skills helps to identify intervention goals and plans. Performance contexts can enable or hinder function. Cultural, spiritual, and social contextual factors influence the selection of intervention strategies and styles of communicating and interacting with both children and family members.

Determining Intervention Goals

A critical component of all intervention planning is also the occupational therapist's attention to goal setting.[60] A collaborative process with families is essential in specifying goals, although the goals must also relate to the particular therapeutic techniques being used.[7]

As stated throughout this text, goals for services must be explicitly stated, measurable, and functionally relevant. A goal to "increase ADL skills" is not adequate. For the child, family, and third-party payers, the therapist must specify clearer targets for functional outcomes. The therapist should write long-term goals to reflect the outcomes expected during the child's length of stay (e.g., acute care versus rehabilitation). The therapist specifies short-term goals as interim steps toward reaching long-term goals. Goals describe specific tasks that the child will perform, conditions of performance, and the type and frequency of assistance needed. Component skills that are emphasized by the therapist may be described as goals if

they are appropriately linked to meaningful functional outcomes (e.g., achieve eye-hand coordination and manipulation skills sufficient for desktop activities and writing at school).

Functional goals must include specification of skills and the level of independence that is being sought. Levels of *independence* describe various degrees of dependence on personal assistance, adaptive environments, and the use of AT devices. In cases of a more involved youth, ADL goals may describe how he or she will manage personal care attendants to achieve a self-managed dependence. On most ADL scales, level of independence is rated as the amount of physical and cognitive assistance needed as a proportion of the task (e.g., moderate assist = 50+% assistance for the amount of time required for partial task, whole task, and task transition assistance by a care provider). However, when concerned with the integration of an individual back into his or her home, the concept of *interdependence* among family members may be a more important consideration. Given the negative value associated with dependence in the Anglo-American culture, a more positive term to express shared needs between family members may be termed *interreliance*. Such language is suggested to focus on the shared duties within households.

Selection of specific goals is influenced by various factors. Goals based on the family's priorities are likely to garner the best participation and support. Priorities for function are individualized and may differ from those presumed by therapists. The child or adolescent's ability to regain skills in personal ADLs and important everyday occupations typically helps restore a sense of well-being. However, institutional and insurance directives also influence the selection of goals. A reduction of dependence makes care possible in progressively less restrictive and less costly environments. Intervention goals most often focus on functional skill acquisition that enables the child to be discharged from inpatient hospital settings to services provided within long-term care, home health care, outpatient care, and eventually to use of nonmedical community support systems.

Interventions

For most children who are referred, services are provided in a relatively brief period, requiring the occupational therapist to be highly efficient. This brief period requires the therapist to establish realistic intervention priorities appropriate for the patient's projected length of stay in the hospital. To do this, the evaluation process must be streamlined, and occupational therapists must prioritize treatment goals as they are identified. Discharge plans may often be proposed at the start of the admission and initial evaluation. In a children's hospital, the broad range of diagnoses requires that occupational therapists have expertise in a wide range of assessment, modalities, and interventions. However, the need for a broad range of skills does not mean a lack of specialization.

Preventing Secondary Disability and Restoring Performance Skills

The prevention of secondary disability and the reduction of existing complications are of the highest priority in a treatment plan. The therapist typically addresses neuromuscular and musculoskeletal complications by using programs designed to help the client maintain or regain normal range of motion. Through the use of special handling techniques, the occupational and physical therapists carry out daily programs that can involve slow stretch and joint mobilization. The therapist can correct existing limitations by using a combination of these techniques and specialized positioning and splinting. The therapist may also apply splints for various purposes, including maintaining positions (e.g., resting hand splint), increasing range of motion (e.g., drop-out splints, dynamic splints with spring tension forces, or serial casting), or promoting function (e.g., wrist cock-up, tenodesis splints) (Figure 26-2).

The therapist facilitates improved movement and strength by using activities and exercises that are most often incorporated into play. For children and adolescents with musculoskeletal and lower motor neuron or motor unit disorders, the use of progressive exercise and activity routines may be appropriate. For those with brain injury that causes upper motor neuron dysfunction, muscle tone and voluntary motor control are addressed. The therapist can use various sensorimotor techniques to promote postural stability, balance, visual motor skills, and fine motor performance (see Chapters 9 and 10).

A second major concern is skin care. Pressure areas from bed positioning, static sitting, and the use of orthosis and splints call for routine skin monitoring. The child must often develop a tolerance to new positioning strategies and splint applications over several days, with skin tolerance being a critical issue in decisions to change bed positions, increase sitting time, and use splints or other orthotic devices.

Individuals often experience perceptual, cognitive, and behavioral impairments after traumatic brain injury (TBI). With a prevention emphasis, programs to ensure safety with physical activities and with manipulation of objects are critical. Environmental modifications are often made to ensure the child's safety. The therapist implements methods to help the child compensate for disorientation and memory loss, although restricted environments and restraints may be necessary initially. The placement of family pictures and other familiar items from home may create a stimulating and more comforting environment. When the child is more alert and aware of his or her surroundings, the therapist may use an educational approach coupled with behavioral interventions. The therapist should inform the child of unit rules, post such rules, and emphasize strict adherence to them. The therapist may carry

out reinforcement programs structured through a team and family approach to shape behaviors.[86] The therapist can also use daily orientation programs and memory books to ease the burden of confusion. It is important to teach the family about the child's perceptual and cognitive impairments and programs in place to ensure safety and comfort.

Resuming and Restoring Occupational Performance

After negotiating goals for ADL performance, the occupational therapist determines what the child needs to learn, how such learning will take place, and how training can best be organized within the clinical care setting. Through natural learning, the child or adolescent may discover, in one or more sessions, simple strategies to resume activity performance. If these techniques are safe and efficient, the therapist need only guide the child in determining appropriate means to achieve consistent performance. However, many times the child is unable to make natural adaptations to achieve performance. Therapists can then guide new learning by instructing the child or adolescent and other care providers in the principles of adaptation and engage them in joint problem solving to determine the most effective methods of performance.

Once it has been established what the child needs to learn, the therapist organizes specific and desired routines for learning. In guided learning, some form of instruction takes place through a combination of directions and the use of instructional aids. For initial instruction of new or adapted tasks, the therapist may demonstrate the task to be learned and have the child copy that demonstration. The therapist may also use verbal or manual guidance cues to assist learning (Figure 26-3). For some tasks, predetermined scripts or learning materials are available.[73,75]

After determining a particular task sequence, the therapist selects methods to achieve repetition, generalization, and development of new skills (Figure 26-4). For example, the therapist may help the child memorize a routine so that the child can guide his or her own performance using verbal, visual, or tactile feedback. If the child cannot memorize a routine, the therapist can use other training tools. A therapist can prepare written instructions, pictorial step cues, and audiotapes with specific directions. Whole-task instruction and the use of forward- or reverse-step sequence training are common methods. The therapist can implement training over several sessions that capitalize on the times when tasks are routinely performed (e.g., dressing in the morning and at night or before and after swimming). As training progresses, the therapist gradually reduces the extent of external cueing from a person or instructional aids so that only a minimal amount of such support is required for safe and efficient performance. Often the team and family plan for the gradual withdrawal of aides and assistance after the child is discharged from the inpatient hospital setting. Strategies that will continue to promote the child's participation in daily activities, including school, form the basis of family or care provider training.

The environment used for ADL therapy sessions is also important. Most therapists agree that children prefer familiar environments. However, except in home health care service delivery, environments must be simulated in hospital rooms or clinics. Generalization of performance from one setting to another can be difficult because familiar settings may provide unrecognized prompts that are not present in simulated settings. Sometimes as part of pediatric rehabilitation care, home

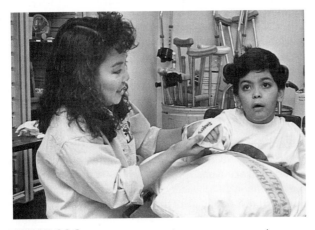

FIGURE 26-2 Splints are used to prevent or reduce contractures. The use of serial static splints requires regular monitoring and clear instructions for use by family members and other care providers.

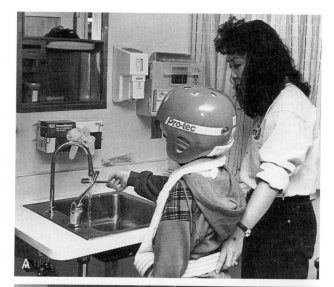

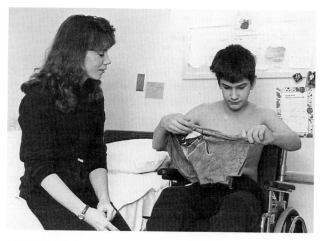

FIGURE 26-4   Adapted dressing routines are developed to achieve success and ease learning. For this boy, who has perceptual and cognitive deficits after brain injury, the occupational therapist cues him in a repetitive sequence of steps that accomplish the task.

Adaptations for ADL Skills

Basic principles apply to adapted performance of ADL skills, and these are described in Box 26-1. New learning is generally more difficult and more energy-consuming than old habit patterns, but change is often necessary. Safety in performance and the avoidance of abnormal or unsafe movements are essential. Principles of joint protection and work simplification are commonly used, and performance is geared toward functioning in a barrier-free environment with the use of familiar conveniences. Adaptations of a routine are aimed at reducing complexity, ensuring safety, and minimizing complications if errors occur.

Adaptive methods of ADL and IADL skills may include the use of different strategies and devices (see Box 26-1). A client's reliance on AT devices may be temporary or permanent. The early use of devices can increase safety or immediate function during recovery. The permanent use of devices is also common when the individual exhibits residual difficulties that necessitate adaptation. When selecting devices, therapists often choose to adapt existing equipment that is already familiar to them. If such adaptation is not desirable or practical, the therapist may direct the family toward purchase of items with features that are more compatible with the child's or adolescent's special needs through standard shopping sources. If needs cannot be met, specialized rehabilitation devices are purchased through medical and rehabilitation equipment vendors. AT devices are generally designed to accommodate or substitute for skill limitations in gross movement, reach, prehension and manipulation, sensation, or perception and cognition. The use of devices should reduce task difficulty and complexity, even though initial learning and use may seem awkward.

Documentation of Occupational Therapy Services

Documentation of patient care is an essential component of occupational therapy service provision in hospitals. Occupational therapy evaluation reports, treatment plans, patient

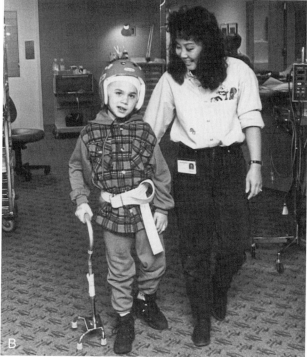

FIGURE 26-3   **A,** The occupational therapist provides the child with cues and performance feedback while he carries out an adapted personal ADL sequence. A helmet is required to protect the head because of an open skull fracture. **B,** Mobility is a fundamental part of ADL routines. After completing a morning care routine, this child walks to breakfast with assistance from the occupational therapist for safety and technique.

visits take place with the child and family to survey and collaborate in planning for organizational changes, equipment needs, and architectural modifications that may enable transition to home. Day or weekend home passes for the child are desirable when possible. The therapist often develops specific goals, and feedback from the family about the time at home can be important to prioritizing goals, obtaining equipment, and addressing family educational needs.

BOX 26-1 Basic Rehabilitation Strategies

Occupational therapists use several strategies for specific types of dysfunctions to adapt activities for children with functional limitations. In addition to these suggestions, ADL and IADL adaptations have been described (see Chapter 17) along with the uses of assistive technology (AT), which should be reviewed (see Chapters 20 and 21).

MOTOR LIMITATIONS

Limited Range of Motion

Reduced range of motion in the neck, trunk, and proximal and intermediate joints of the limbs limits ability to reach all parts of the body and objects within the immediate environment. Limitations of hand motion can reduce holding and handling of objects. To substitute for reach, the child should use extended and specially angled handles (e.g., long-handled spoon or fork, bath brush, dressing stick, or shoe horn) or devices that are more specialized, such as reachers. If a child is unable to use devices that extend reach, the therapist employs other strategies to permit function. Mounting objects on the floor, wall, or table and bringing the body part to the device (e.g., boot tree for removing shoes, friction pad on floor for socks, hook on the wall to pull pants up or down, or sponges mounted in the shower to wash) prove useful. For some tasks, devices may replace any reach requirement, such as the use of a bidet for hygiene after toileting or manual or electric feeders operated by microswitches to bring food to the mouth.

When motion of the hand is limited, the therapist can assist holding and manipulating of objects by providing enlarged or differently styled handles that reduce the grasp requirement (e.g., T-handled cup). The therapist can replace holding functions by the use of universal cuff or C-shaped handles. High-friction surfaces may provide more secure grasp. When forearm rotation is limited, swivel spoons or angled utensils may assist bringing food to the mouth.

Limited range of motion also reduces gross motor movements, such as in bed mobility and elevation changes (moving from sitting to standing and performing transfers in bathing and toileting). The therapist typically changes surface levels (i.e., raised or lowered) to limit the extent of elevation change required. The therapist may lower the bed height to allow ease in wheelchair transfers or raise it for ease in coming up to standing from sitting. Raised chairs, toilet seats, and bath benches reduce extreme changes in elevation required in transfers.

Decreased Strength and Endurance

Strength and endurance limitations are common among children who are acutely ill or injured. The goals of adaptation are to reduce the effects of gravity by the use of lightweight objects, movements in the horizontal plane, reduced friction, and, when possible, the use of body mechanics for leverage and gravity to assist movement. Electrically powered devices may meet goals of work simplification. Efficiency of movement is essential. Similar to limited range of motion, weakness can cause inability to reach body parts or make elevation changes. Extended handles may be necessary; however, increased weight and the forces required to handle and apply leverage can increase difficulty.

A major goal with activity adaptation for decreased strength is to limit the need to sustain static postures and prolonged holding. The therapist can use surfaces to support posture and proximal limb positions in various ways (e.g., bed positioning, seating adaptations, the use of armrests and table surfaces). The therapist reduces the need for sustained holding by

mounting devices or stabilizing devices with friction (e.g., Dycem or spike board) or using an enlarged lightweight object. Universal cuffs or C-cuffs are also commonly used to limit demands for grasp. Manipulation may be impaired and necessitate the use of hooks and loops on clothing and adaptation of fasteners by the use of Velcro, zippers, enlarged buttons, or elastic shoelaces. Less complex movement and reduced force are required to manipulate lever handles on faucets, doors, and appliances. The therapist helps the child reduce movement against gravity in transfers by changing the heights of surfaces and using devices such as sliding boards, springs, or hydraulic lifts to aid movement.

For children with cardiac or pulmonary disorders, progression of ADL performance may be based on estimated metabolic equivalent levels or by direct monitoring. The therapist should schedule and pace tasks, simplify work, and use rest breaks within tasks.

Incoordination

Incoordination primarily causes difficulty with manipulation skills. Incoordination can influence performance in different ways. These may include the range of movement required, weight and resistance of objects being handled, and positioning of the body in relation to objects. A primary concern is to achieve proximal stability when executing movements. Stabilizing the trunk and head while making movements of the arm and hand can improve skilled movements. Likewise, the therapist should stabilize the proximal segments of the limb while manipulating the hand (e.g., resting the elbow and forearm on the table while using the wrist and fingers to manipulate objects). High-friction surfaces and containers that hold objects being manipulated may also be suggested for stabilization of the limb (e.g., friction pad plate or nonslip cup).

Another common strategy is to determine if increased weight dampens exaggerated movements and tremor. The therapist may select heavier objects or add weight to objects. The therapist can attach a weight to the arm or apply resistance to movement by placing devices across joints (e.g., elastic sleeves, friction feeder) to determine if more precise movements can be achieved. When such methods are inadequate, other techniques employed are similar to those for reduced range of motion and strength, including mounting devices on stable surfaces and bringing the body to these devices using gross movements.

One-Handed Techniques

When a child has to perform most activities with one hand, the barriers to be overcome typically involve replacing the stabilization function of the other limb, improving the skills of the hand being used, and adapting tasks that require alternating movements of two hands. Generally, the child can accomplish many tasks easily with the use of one hand. If the hand being used was not previously the preferred or dominant hand, skilled movements may take a greater amount of time to develop. For those with perceptual and cognitive impairments, learning to use one hand may be particularly difficult. For children with hemiplegia, various dressing routines have been scripted that follow the rules of dressing the affected limb first and avoiding the use of abnormal postures. The stabilization function of the impaired limb may not be entirely lost, although the child may need to learn how to assist movement in placing or positioning the limb to effectively stabilize objects. To entirely replace the stabilization function of the impaired or lost upper limb, the therapist may use mounting or high-friction surfaces.

Continued

BOX 26-1 Basic Rehabilitation Strategies—cont'd

Some two-handed tasks require the use of specially designed devices or methods. For example, the therapist can provide the child with a rocker-knife or cutting-edged fork to help him or her cut with a knife and fork, a button hook to aid in buttoning, a special lacing technique to aid in shoe tying, and a one-handed keyboard arrangement and training program to aid in typing.

PERCEPTUAL AND COGNITIVE LIMITATIONS

Sensory, perceptual, and cognitive impairments alone pose various challenges to ADL performance but are most often associated with other physical disorders previously described. If retraining of performance skills is ineffective and dysfunction continues, the therapist should consider substitution for impaired skills by using more intact sensory, perceptual, or cognitive skills (e.g., using a bell on the hemiplegic arm to draw attention if being neglected tactually or visually). Compensation techniques may also be planned that modify the activity sequence and environment to enable the child to accomplish the challenging task.

Perceptual and Cognitive Deficits

Perceptual and cognitive deficits affect ADL skill routines and school performance. To compensate for perceptual or cognitive deficits, the therapist can design step-by-step routines with cueing systems and repeat them in training. The therapist employs work simplification principles and uses substitution strategies. Children with these deficits may rely on memorizing and reciting a verbal routine or follow audio-taped instruction. They may also rely on written instructions or pictorial cues. With impaired visual perception, the child may need to learn reliance on tactile feedback cues. At times, the therapist specially selects materials used in ADL tasks to compensate for impairments. The therapist may use color-contrasted clothing, texture, or color-coding cues with objects. Sometimes the therapist can encourage the use of mirrors to give the child feedback about his or her performance.

Visual Impairment

Blindness or severe visual impairment requires that the therapist employ strategies to substitute for vision by the use of other sensory skills and cognitive routines. Consistent organization of the environment and storage of items is necessary. The therapist may use tactile identifiers on objects such as raised letters and locations of more transient items described by a companion or a standard technique such as analog clock location. The therapist can build sound feedback into some items to aid in orientation or search. Mobility specialists instruct individuals to use techniques such as long canes or guide dogs for ambulation or wheelchair guidance and to use a leader's arm for guidance in walking.

---

progress notes, and discharge summaries are used to communicate occupational therapy intervention to the physician, other members of the medical team, the patient and family, and reimbursement age. Format and frequency of documentation are determined by the policies and procedures of the hospital and the occupational therapy department. Accreditation guidelines regarding documentation are provided to institutions by agencies such as the Joint Commission and the CARF. Agencies that reimburse services, such as Medicaid or private insurance, also have requirements for documentation with which occupational therapists must comply.

Documentation of services to hospitalized children through evaluation reports with accompanying treatment plans, progress notes, and discharge summaries occurs in the patient's medical chart. Because the medical chart remains on the unit or accompanies the patient when he or she receives services elsewhere in the hospital, information is readily available to other health professionals. The increasing use of information technology such as online charting has also facilitated access of information and documentation that is readily available to all providers. Documentation of occupational therapy intervention with outpatients may take a different form because reports are often sent to referring physicians or other agencies in the community. Copies of these outpatient reports are also retained in the child's hospital medical record. Documentation of services in clinics may follow a different format because each clinic may have a medical chart for the patient. However, regardless of the format, documentation of services must meet the criteria established by accrediting and reimbursement agencies.[56]

Scope of Occupational Therapy Services

Children are admitted to the hospital setting for several different reasons, and they can move through these categories as symptoms stabilize or effects become more apparent. Referrals to occupational therapy may be made at admission, during a stay, or near the end of a hospitalization. Responding in a timely manner to physician orders, addressing what has been requested, and asking for greater involvement to address needs may be necessary.

Children may be admitted for acute care for their illness. The therapist must perform an initial assessment and provide caregivers and the child with instructions, home programs, or follow-up outpatient services. The occupational therapist may also contribute to the diagnostic evaluation for a child specifically admitted for a comprehensive evaluation who is then transitioned to outpatient services. The child may initially be admitted for acute care reasons, then require more extensive and comprehensive therapy interventions in rehabilitation. In this case, the therapist must evaluate the level of functioning of the child, develop an intervention plan, and involve the family in implementation of the goals and objectives that lead to increased function and independence and the child's discharge from the hospital. In each case, occupational therapy intervention may differ according to the child's needs and the length of stay. In some instances, level of service may be affected by staff shortages, which results in prioritizing which patients receive occupational therapy services.[76] Payers may also dictate length of stay for the patient, and shortened stays necessitate streamlined service delivery.

The client with a single injury (e.g., a hand injury) or a single episode of illness tends to have a short hospital stay with a predictable course of treatment. Some clients admitted for an acute illness or injury may require extended rehabilitation, depending on the severity of the injury and resulting complications. TBI and spinal cord injury (SCI) are two examples of injuries that require both initial acute treatment and long-term rehabilitation. The length of the hospital stay for this type of patient during the acute phase of illness or injury tends to vary because the potential for complications is greater and these patients need to be relatively stable medically before transferring to the rehabilitative service.

The chronically ill client is hospitalized periodically for acute episodes of an illness or complications of an illness. Children with diabetes, cancer, or cardiac conditions fall into this category. The length of hospital stay for these clients is variable. Children hospitalized for diagnostic testing or adjustment of medications experience a comparatively short hospital stay. Consequently, the occupational therapist should focus on evaluation and treatment planning that is likely to transfer to community providers. Occupational therapy evaluation in acute-care services focuses on the child's developmental or functional status within the context of the illness or injury that has resulted in hospitalization. Completion of the assessment may present a challenge for the occupational therapist because the length of hospital stay is often short and other hospital services are competing for the child's time. Evaluations completed by the occupational therapist may also be used as a screen to rule out other illnesses or processes (e.g., in a child with pneumonia, an evaluation for aspiration can lead to an eventual diagnosis of reflux).

Organization of Hospital-Based Services

Most patient-care activity in hospitals is acute care. Acute care refers to short-term medical care provided during the acute phase of an illness or injury, when the symptoms are generally the most severe. The degrees of severity that categorize illnesses and injuries are matched to levels of acute care designed to meet these varied needs. The occupational therapist providing services to children during this phase must consider the long-term implications of the illness or injury while addressing the acute needs of the client. Families may experience increased stress during this phase and therefore may require that the information be repeated or may need more time to process the results from testing. The therapist should involve the family in intervention planning, including discharge planning. Because hospital stays tend to be short, available outpatient treatment options need to be considered early and caregivers given this information to facilitate continuity of services from inpatient to outpatient settings.

Critically ill clients who require continuous monitoring and frequent medical attention, and patients who often need special equipment to maintain or monitor vital functions, are admitted to *intensive care units (ICUs)* or *critical care units (CCUs)*. Hospitals may have various levels of ICUs, each of which is designated for a specific patient population or purpose. These can include *neonatal intensive care units (NICUs)*, *pediatric intensive care units (PICUs)* for older children, and post *surgical intensive care units (SICUs)*. Personnel who provide care for children in ICUs receive special training to enable them to respond quickly and effectively to meet the needs of medically unstable patients in this challenging environment (see examples in Chapter 22).

A child whose illness or injury results in hospitalization, but who does not need the continuous attention, high technology, and specialized care of an ICU, may be admitted to a *medical* or *surgical acute care unit*. Medical and surgical units also tend to be designated for specific types of clients. For example, children requiring neurosurgical services may be cared for on one unit, whereas children requiring orthopedic-related treatment

may be served on another. Within the designation of these units, children may also be grouped according to age. Placing children of similar ages together can facilitate developmentally appropriate care and allow for environments that are well designed to match children and youth's age-based interests.

Children with infectious conditions may have a variety of diagnoses that require treatment under isolation conditions. If this is the case, these patients are often placed in *special care units*. Three conditions that require a child to be treated in a special care unit are (1) *acute burns*, (2) *infectious diseases*, and (3) *bone marrow transplantation*.

Medical intervention for chronically ill children may also be provided in hospitals that emphasize acute care. Often, chronically ill patients are admitted for an acute exacerbation of their illnesses or for treatment of complications. Diabetes, asthma, cystic fibrosis, and cancer are examples of chronic illnesses occurring in children that may require periodic hospitalization. Children who have progressive illness may also be seen for acute issues relating to the next stage of the disease process. For example, a youth diagnosed with Duchenne muscular dystrophy may experience a decrease in oral motor skills and subsequently be admitted for aspiration pneumonia.

Rehabilitation Services

A primary concept in the practice of pediatric rehabilitation is the differentiation of *habilitation* from *rehabilitation*. For children, *habilitation* is the term most often used to denote attention to the child's acquisition of expected age-level skill and function. *Rehabilitation* is the term used to reflect the process of an individual working to regain skills and functions that had been established but subsequently lost. For most practitioners in pediatrics, the term *rehabilitation* is used to encompass both concepts. This is true because disability, whether new or chronic, creates ongoing challenges to current function and future demands that evolve as part of growth and development. In this chapter, the term *rehabilitation* is used to express both concepts. A specific focus on a sampling of such services and a case-based example of clinical reasoning and approaches taken as part of therapy services is listed in Box 26-2.

BOX 26-2 Examples of Rehabilitation Services

ACUTE MEDICAL CARE UNITS
- Necrotizing fasciitis with sepsis
- Failure to thrive

SPECIALTY UNITS (E.G., ORTHOPEDICS, CARDIAC AND PULMONARY SERVICES, AND ONCOLOGY AMONG OTHERS)

ONCOLOGY AND BONE MARROW TRANSPLANT
- Neuroblastoma

REHABILITATION SERVICES
- Head injury
- Developmental delay/cerebral palsy

OUTPATIENT SERVICES
- Spina bifida clinic

Rehabilitation Team

Hospital-based rehabilitation permits the child and family to benefit from a wide range of medical care specialists and services that they can access as needed. Pediatric rehabilitation teams also include various providers with differing expertise. Such teams are most often led by physicians who are trained as pediatricians and in other arenas of practice, such as neurology, orthopedics, or developmental medicine. Leadership and commitment in pediatric rehabilitation have come primarily from pediatricians who also are certified in the practice of physiatry (rehabilitation medicine).[87]

The rehabilitation team places an emphasis on interdisciplinary teamwork, with each discipline having particular capabilities or areas of focus. Sometimes the team uses a transdisciplinary model so that only one or two professionals work directly with a particular child or family. Specific roles for each discipline within acute rehabilitation have been described for teams consisting of physicians, nurses, occupational therapists, physical therapists, speech-language pathologists, therapeutic recreational specialists, psychologists, social workers, educators, and other specialists.[6,28,39] In larger programs, specialty teams may develop so that the same personnel treat children grouped by diagnosis (e.g., TBI or SCI).

Team Interaction

Interdisciplinary care within pediatric rehabilitation is common and mandated by most institutions' regulatory mechanisms. The success of such collaboration often depends on a shared mission that focuses the team's energy and creativity. Team conferences that involve the family are typical. The team holds family conferences on admission, at key decision points during the hospitalization, and at discharge to ensure communication and clarification of care recommendations with the family and local care providers. In addition, the team conducts weekly rounds to review the progress of each child and discuss any changes in treatment plans that are designed for each problem.

The occupational therapy practitioner's holistic concerns related to health, function, and participation necessitate and are enriched by the collaborative relationships among team members of multiple disciplines. Partnerships between occupational therapists and occupational therapy assistants can broaden the scope and timeliness of services. Need for frequent reevaluation and trials with new strategies necessitate dynamic and shared interventions. Team efforts are the rule rather than the exception in pediatric rehabilitation. For example, occupational and physical therapists often take a joint interest in addressing a child's gross and fine motor skills related to positioning, transfers, wheelchair seating, and functional mobility. Occupational therapists can evaluate and plan interventions for feeding, swallowing, and augmentative communication in cooperation with speech-language pathologists. Nursing and occupational therapy personnel typically have collaborative roles dealing with skills such as grooming, dressing, and bathing and training in special care routines of toileting and skin care. Occupational therapists may work together with therapeutic recreation specialists to provide adaptive play and socialization through activity and community outings.

A primary goal with children is to improve their participation and performance in educational programs. Acute rehabilitation programs and children's hospitals typically have teachers on staff. In conjunction with occupational therapists and other team members, these educators and developmental specialists can address skills and special needs that the child will have upon returning to school. Psychologists and those who specialize in neuropsychology also provide suggestions for school placement and may work with occupational therapists to adapt learning strategies for the child as he or she returns to the classroom. Social workers typically address issues of adjustment and coping with the child and family. All team members strive to be sensitive and supportive when educating family members to assume new duties as care providers. Recommendations should seek a realistic balance among the family culture, established roles, and new responsibilities for care.

Families

The therapist must recognize that many families are dealing with traumatic events or at least unexpected complications that seriously affect their life processes. The children and adolescents are also challenged to deal with changes, and this process can be further complicated by their own cognitive or behavioral impairments.[22] An educational model may provide a helpful perspective. Recognizing that family members have a short amount of time to learn a great deal about caring for their family member who is faced with new disabilities, rehabilitation team members also need to devote their time and attention to understanding the family's priorities and learning preferences. In all cases, the normal routines of the family are severely altered by hospitalization and residual disability.[77] This often creates worry, grief, and financial hardships that necessitate a transformation of relationships.[45] Families function in different ways, and variations in styles appear to have a lot to do with effective coping.[78] Healthy and resilient families may show exceptional caring, open communication, balancing of family needs, and positive problem-solving abilities. Families with limited coping skills may need increased support and help in identifying resources to meet immediate needs and in coping with problems that they will face in managing the child at home. In either case, the needs of families often change during the rehabilitation process, requiring ongoing attention to maintain a collaborative partnership that can achieve the best outcomes for the child.

Transition from Rehabilitation to the Community

To facilitate continuity of care when the child is discharged from a pediatric rehabilitation hospitalization, the team and the family should develop a comprehensive plan of transition. For example, a child with brain injury often requires special education services after discharge from the medical center, and readiness to return to school may be particularly problematic owing to social-behavioral challenges.[3] Team and family activities and communication need to focus on the transition from rehabilitation to school and community as soon as discharge is considered. Transition activities include interagency team meetings at which school and rehabilitation team members are represented. Ideally, at least one interagency meeting occurs in the rehabilitation unit and at least one in the school. By sharing where the meeting is hosted, team members get a realistic picture of the child's environments. When the meeting is at the team's home site, most, if not all, team members who worked with the child can be involved. By meeting the child and family before discharge and learning about the child's condition and needs, the school personnel can begin to plan and prepare an educational program. Visits by the medical team to the school at which the child will receive follow-up services can promote continuity of care.

In a visit to the school, the therapist from the hospital should share information with the school-based therapists related to concerns, priorities, and results of intervention approaches (what worked and what did not). The child's rehabilitation team can help problem-solve issues in the school's accessibility and possible modifications to the classroom and curriculum. Visits to the child's classroom can help identify accommodations that need to be in place. During these visits, the rehabilitation team can present information to the other students in the class about the child's disability, the rehabilitation process, and the types of changes that they may expect in their peer. An in-service presentation about the injury is most important when a child returns to his or her preinjury classroom because the student's peers have preset expectations about his or her behavior and personality or, in the case of severe burns, about the student's appearance. In addition, before discharge the child should visit his or her home, school, and other important environments to determine what accommodations will need to be made. Visits followed by a return to the hospital can allow both school and hospital teams to address the issues proactively.

The rehabilitation team often monitors the child's progress during the first few months after discharge. The child may continue with outpatient services while initiating school-based services. Duplicate services can be beneficial during the period of transition as the child continues to make rapid progress while struggling to adapt to new environments. The consistent individuals in the transition are the family members, who ultimately support the child through the transition to the home. In support of this, the teams involved should provide the parents with comprehensive information about the special education system in their community, their rights as parents of a child who newly qualifies for special education services, and other community programs, supports, and resources that they can access.

Medical Model and Team Interaction

In most medical systems, the physician is considered the leader of the medical team for a given child, although leadership may shift to other team members during the course of the child's stay.[12] The child's *care manager* is often a registered nurse or other medical professional whose services have been formally requested by the physician. The parents, who are also members of the team, are also responsible for the child's care.

Three factors that often affect the parents' participation in the child's care are (1) the distance between the family's home and the hospital, (2) the parents' other obligations including work and child care, and (3) cultural values. These factors may limit the parents' ability to visit the hospital and may limit their ability to interact with the professionals caring for their child. This is particularly true when the child is experiencing a prolonged hospital stay. When parents are limited in their ability to participate, the therapist must find alternative ways to facilitate communication regarding evaluations and treatment plans. Cultural implications may also influence family participation including experiential influences. Family members may have beliefs or experienced previous situations that lead to preconceived ideas of what will happen during the

hospital stay. This can lead to a feeling of discomfort with medical personnel and situations. The therapist must reflect on his or her own belief systems and attitudes and refrain from passing judgment on parents who have different obligations, attitudes, or beliefs, in order to foster open communication and thus enhance the therapy intervention process.

Another significant characteristic of medical teams is their dynamic nature. Because the health care disciplines represented in a specific case depend on the child's needs, the medical team is continually changing. For example, a child with a feeding disorder who is failing to grow and gain weight may have a physician, nurses, an occupational therapist, a dietitian, and a social worker as members of his or her medical team. However, a child hospitalized with multiple injuries resulting from a motor vehicle accident may have several physicians, nurses, an occupational therapist, a physical therapist, a speech-language pathologist, a dietitian, a respiratory therapist, and a social worker as members of his or her medical team. In addition, the team within one child's hospitalization may change. For example, the child admitted to the hospital for pneumonia may initially be seen by the pulmonary physician and perhaps the social worker, along with nursing personnel, later to have the occupational therapist and the speech-language pathologist involved when aspiration is suspected and later a physician from gastroenterology involved when it is discovered reflux is the culprit. As a potential member of multiple medical teams within one hospital, the occupational therapist must communicate and collaborate with professionals from many different health-related fields. The therapist may be required to continually redefine or explain the role of the occupational therapist to other team members, and to develop an understanding of the ways in which different team members' roles complement each other in the provision of services to children. With the trend toward "hospital systems," described previously, occupational therapists employed by hospitals may face the more complex challenges of defining their roles in several different settings within one integrated system of care and participating in interdisciplinary medical teams across the spectrum of care.[91]

Communication among hospital team members is dependent on a number of factors. One significant factor is the limited availability of team members for scheduled meetings. Communication tends to occur *formally* through documentation in the patient's chart and *informally* during telephone calls or chance meetings throughout the day.

Communication with the patient or parent occurs at separate times for most team members. Regular team meetings, although ideal, are often not feasible in a hospital setting because of the multiple demands on hospital personnel and the likelihood of schedule changes.

CONSULTATION SERVICES

Intensive Care Unit Services

In the ICU, the child is often evaluated and treated at bedside because of the critical nature of the illness or injury and the need for constant monitoring of the child's physiologic status. Occupational therapy intervention in ICUs supports medical priorities and goals for the child. It is essential that the therapist be knowledgeable about the child's diagnoses and potential precautions and the implications of medical procedures, the use of life support or monitoring equipment, and contraindications to certain activities or positions. Continuous monitoring of the child's status during the time with them, makes it imperative for the therapist to understand the significance of changes in the child's vital signs, respiratory function, appearance, or symptoms as a result of the assessments or intervention being completed.

Prolonged bed rest and immobility often occur as a result of ICU stays, where medical technology and equipment, or the need for restraints for the child's safety and care, are in use. The average length of stay for a child in the ICU may be just a few days; however, it may be extended if the illness or injury is severe. The potential impact of extended immobility includes potential for contractures, generalized weakness with decreased endurance, and cardiopulmonary compromise. Occupational therapists provide services to prevent such secondary problems by using graded activities and soliciting the child's participation to maintain strength and to enhance functional capacities. Although the therapist may have goals of increasing participation, independence, and endurance for the child, the nurse or family may feel that rest is required. Discussing the basis for treatment intentions includes consideration of medical precautions to facilitate the team's desired outcome. Establishment of a routine, including regular therapy times within the constraints of the intensive care unit, can also help with orientation for the patient and help facilitate regular participation. Family members or other caregivers may also be involved in carrying out treatments, such as range of motion, throughout the day. This provides them the opportunity to become more involved in the care of their child during this portion of their hospitalization.[89,90]

Occupational therapy interventions often include positioning recommendations and uses of splints to preserve range of motion and prevent deformity, and assistive devices to enable function. A plan for wear or use should be established and communicated with the family and other care providers to ensure follow through. Caregivers should also be instructed on any potential side effects, such as pressure areas with splints, so that interventions can be modified as needed (see Figure 26-2).

Sensory deprivation and stress resulting from the intensive care environment may also complicate a child's medical status and recovery. The lack of privacy, immobility, and the continuous sounds and lights of the intensive care unit provide the child with an atypical sensory experience. Over a prolonged period, ICU psychoses have been reported in which the child may have an altered mental status.[43,50] Within the ICU setting, there are few indicators to orient the child to changes in time and day. Occupational therapy intervention may help counteract the effects of this disorientation and sensory deprivation by fostering the establishment of a routine for the child and providing purposeful activities to facilitate cognitive, psychosocial, and motor functions (Case Study 26-1).[1] Positive social interaction and the use of entertainment and play activities may be especially helpful for reducing stress and promoting engagements of young children in the ICU.

General Acute Care Unit

General acute care units tend to be designated by medical specialty. Children of various ages, with different types of conditions and treatments, may be served in the same acute care unit. Similarly, children requiring different types of surgery may be admitted to the same general surgical unit for preoperative and postoperative care. Designating units in this manner enables physicians and other members of the medical team to use their client care time and equipment more efficiently.

In acute care units, children tend to be more medically stable and less dependent on life-sustaining equipment as part of their care. A lesser need for medical monitoring may enable them to receive greater involvement by rehabilitation specialists, including the occupational therapist, who may provide services at bedside or in the hospital's therapy clinic. Occupational therapists may be responsible for children in a variety of acute care units, requiring them to be familiar with the procedures of each unit, the types of children admitted to the different units, and the nurses and other hospital personnel who provide services.

Failure to Thrive

Failure to thrive (FTT) is a diagnosis given to children, frequently infants and young children, who fail to grow or gain weight. FTT may be designated as *organic,* arising from a diagnosable physical cause, or as *nonorganic,* which denotes impaired growth without apparent physical cause.[34] Children with FTT often require hospitalization for acute care and can have additional complications including immune deficiencies, generalized weakness, and developmental delay due to their malnutrition and behavioral difficulties.

Although organic FTT can be attributed to a specific physical disorder, nonorganic FTT is primarily (but not exclusively) associated with psychosocial factors. Disturbances in parent-child interaction and development of attachment early in life, difficult infant temperament and behavior, maternal social isolation, and financial difficulties within the family are some of the variables associated with nonorganic FTT.[5,64,74]

In some instances, FTT may be attributed to both organic and nonorganic factors. Frank suggested that children with nonorganic FTT also have biologic risks.[34] She identified three categories of risk: (1) *perinatal,* (2) *toxic and immunologic,* and (3) *neurodevelopmental.*

Perinatal risk refers to the potential for FTT in infants who are considered low-birth-weight, possibly as a result of prematurity or intrauterine growth retardation. Toxic and immunologic risks arise from significant nutritional deficiency, which has the potential to increase vulnerability to infection and increase susceptibility to lead toxicity. Neurodevelopmental risk results from effects of inadequate nutrition on the developing nervous system. Although toxic and immunologic risks are generally reversible through medical treatment, treatment may not fully reverse the neurodevelopmental consequences.

The complexity of factors implicated in FTT emphasizes the need for a coordinated team approach that offers medical, nutritional, developmental, and psychosocial intervention. As a member of the hospital-based team, the occupational therapist may contribute to both the diagnosis and the treatment of the child with FTT. A comprehensive occupational therapy assessment provides the medical team with information regarding the infant's developmental status, feeding behaviors, infant-caregiver interactions during play and feeding, and infant interactions with unfamiliar adults. Children may require enteral nutrition or a nasogastric tube for nutritional support during the initial phases of evaluation and treatment.

CASE STUDY 26-1 Michael

PRESENTING INFORMATION

Michael is a 6-year-old boy admitted to the intensive care unit with a diagnosis of necrotizing fasciitis with sepsis. He was initially seen at the general hospital in his community, approximately 2 hours distance from the children's hospital in the area. On initial examination, Michael was found to have decreased sensation with decreased circulation to both fingers and toes. He had a high fever (104.7 °F) and was lethargic. He was airlifted to the children's hospital, and en route he began experiencing organ failure, including a cardiac arrest. His mother was able to accompany him in the airlift, but his father had to drive due to space constraints.

BACKGROUND INFORMATION

Before his hospitalization, Michael was a typically developing young boy. He resided on a Native American reservation with both of his parents. He attended first grade at the local elementary school, achieving average grades for his age. He also took pride in participating in the Native American dance troupe associated with his tribe and had been participating in exhibits nationally with his troupe since age 3.

Michael had been playing in the park near his home with friends when he fell out of a tree and was deeply scratched by a branch. With little bleeding he did not return home right away, but once he did return, his mother noted that the area was red and slightly warm. She cleaned the area with soap and water and placed Band-Aids on the cut. The next day, Michael was noted to have a slight fever and was complaining of generalized discomfort. By the second day, he was increasing in his complaints, would not let anyone touch his arm, and his fever had increased, even with medication and home remedies. He was taken to his family physician. By the time he was seen in the physician's office, Michael had increased lethargy, was in and out of consciousness, and had a high fever. He was subsequently airlifted to the local pediatric hospital owing to his rapidly worsening condition.

MEDICAL AND OCCUPATIONAL THERAPY INTERVENTION

Upon arrival at the children's hospital, Michael had required a respirator for ventilation support, and his medical status continued to deteriorate. Evaluation revealed staphylococcal sepsis with intravascular coagulopathy and he was admitted to the intensive care unit. During the first 48 hours, Michael continued to decline and showed evidence of organ failure. He required continuous medical interventions including dialysis, ventilation support, and surgical intervention for increasing necrotizing digits including amputation of several toes and fingers.

With a focus on prevention, occupational therapy was consulted early in his care to provide positioning and maintain range of motion affected and unaffected joints and soft tissues. The occupational therapists fabricated splints for both his hands and feet, and he was placed on a schedule that required him to wear them at all times except during dressing changes. His parents were also instructed to carry out range of motion routines to maintain his range and to participate in his care.

Although Michael's condition initially continued to deteriorate, necessitating amputation of one leg above knee, the other at the ankle, and all but two fingers, his family held out hope that he would come through this devastating illness. The parents pulled in the assistance of their tribal leaders to provide guidance and use tribal medicine to enhance Western medicine techniques. Leaders were granted permission to visit Michael within the intensive care unit, with clear guidelines about acceptable procedures that could be used.

During this time, the occupational therapist continued to monitor positioning and range of motion. The therapist collaborated with nursing personnel to help with positioning both Michael and his medical devices to enable his mom to rock him in a chair at bedside. As his medical condition stabilized, Michael was weaned from ventilator support and could engage in strengthening and endurance activities. Occupational therapy also began to facilitate Michael in resuming his personal ADL tasks by introducing adaptive devices to enable his independence. Michael was provided with an appropriately sized wheelchair, and gloves were adapted to ease the use of his upper limbs so the he could propel the chair around the hospital unit. As he continued to increase his strength and function, he was eventually discharged from the intensive care unit and transferred to pediatric rehabilitation services where his functional performance challenges were further addressed by prosthetic fitting and the learning of adaptive methods and other compensatory strategies to restore capacities in personal care, and home and school functioning.

A more permanent gastric tube for feeding may be required if it is suspected that additional nutritional support may be needed for an extended period.

Denton differentiated between FTT in infants and children around 2 years of age, suggesting that 2-year-old children who fail to thrive can have poor feeding skills, which may be the result of behavioral issues.[20] Infant assessment emphasizes interactional issues with the caregivers, while the assessment of older children focuses more on behaviors in the feeding situation and attempts to differentiate between environmental factors and neuromotor difficulties that may be affecting feeding. A developmental and feeding history obtained from the parent is a valuable component of the occupational therapy assessment of all children with FTT.

Occupational therapy intervention goals with a child who has FTT may include ensuring effective oral motor and feeding skills and facilitating development (Case Study 26-2). Promoting positive parent-child interaction may also be emphasized, using strategies that help the parent understand the infant or child's behavioral cues and engage them with positive, developmentally appropriate play experiences. This emphasis on positive parent-child interaction also encourages parents to develop behavioral expectations consistent with the child's level of functioning. Ongoing outpatient therapy is often necessary following discharge to support goals established during the inpatient stay and to foster effective feeding behaviors.

CASE STUDY 26-2   Kevin

PRESENTING INFORMATION

Kevin was a 3-month, 7-day-old boy brought to the emergency department by his parents due to his unresponsive behavior and concern regarding possible seizure activity. Initial diagnoses included rule out abuse, severe nonorganic failure to thrive (FTT), anemia, rule out sepsis and bacteremia, hyponatremia, dehydration, and seizure risk. Kevin was noted to have bruising above both knees and over his right buttocks. He was also observed to have diaper rash and muscular wasting around the left hip and extremities. He demonstrated poor oral feeding and was subsequently admitted to the hospital for observation and monitoring. An attending physician referred Kevin to occupational therapy on the third day of hospitalization to address oral feeding skills.

BACKGROUND INFORMATION

Kevin's parents brought him to the hospital's emergency department after a home visit by a child protective services worker. Upon his hospital admission, his parents left and did not visit during his week-long stay at the children's hospital. His maternal great aunt visited occasionally, and she expressed interest in adopting him.

Kevin was born at term and weighed 5 pounds 12 ounces. He went home after a 48-hour hospital stay. He was hospitalized at 2 months of age for FTT, upper respiratory tract infection, and otitis media. He was discharged to his parents with home health nursing, a child protective services referral, and pediatrician follow-up. Kevin's parents had missed all follow-up appointments until they brought him to the emergency department.

MEDICAL AND OCCUPATIONAL THERAPY INTERVENTION

A pH probe showed severe gastroesophageal reflux. An upper gastrointestinal series was performed and ruled out anatomic abnormality. Stool samples were analyzed and showed malabsorption, reducing substances, increased fatty acids, and *Giardia lamblia,* all of which combined to reduce his level of nutrient absorption and increase fluid loss. As a result, Kevin was severely underweight and lethargic. Treatment for the reflux included positioning on an elevated wedge and the use of thickened feeds.

Kevin was evaluated by occupational therapy using clinical observations of his oral motor, feeding, and developmental skills. He demonstrated intact oral structures and sensation, with functional oral skills for safe oral feeding. He had small sucking pads with a weak suck and fair coordination of suck-swallow-breathe. His suck and coordination improved with support at his jaw and cheeks. Kevin's developmental skills were delayed, and he demonstrated poor state control with high irritability.

It was the therapist's impression that Kevin's weak suck, poor feeding, and irritability were from overall weakness, malnutrition, and recent intubation, rather than from a neurologic deficit. The occupational therapist developed a bedside plan of specific facilitation techniques to be used during feeding. These included jaw and cheek support, external tongue stimulation, flexion swaddling, decreasing external stimulation, upright and well-aligned feeding positioning, limiting oral feeding to 30 minutes, and turning off the continuous pump that fed Kevin through a nasal gastric tube.

After implementation of occupational therapy recommendations by nursing staff, Kevin's oral intake increased dramatically over the next 3 days, with the occupational therapist feeding him once daily to monitor progress. Once the acute feeding issues were resolved, occupational therapy emphasis switched to interaction skills, with the focus on developmental activities to improve self-calming, visual tracking, and social interactions.

Kevin was referred for outpatient occupational therapy and early intervention services before discharge. Children's protective services assumed custody of Kevin, and he was discharged to a foster home with a weight increase of 2.4 pounds (follow-up weekly weight checks were scheduled with his pediatrician). The occupational therapist provided the foster parents with a home program, including positioning, feeding, and activities to promote Kevin's play development.

SPECIALTY UNITS

Children's hospital units are also often designated for specialty care. These may include a focus on orthopedics, cardiac and pulmonary services, oncology, and other hospital-specific organization of units. Consultation services to these units may have a wide range of issues to be addressed and necessitates specific orientation and training to address care needs. As an example of such services, oncology care with children may involve a variety of strategies with both assessments and interventions.

Oncology and Bone Marrow Transplant Units

A highly specialized acute care service is the *oncology unit,* which may also include bone marrow transplant services. Children served on these units may include those diagnosed with various types of cancer, immunodeficiency disorders, hemophilia, and aplastic anemia. These units and services may be housed close together and share some resources including staff or may be located in separate areas within the hospital setting.

The staff on the oncology unit provides care for those children who are newly diagnosed with cancer and undergoing induction chemotherapy; are receiving chemotherapy courses that require close monitoring; may have complications from their treatments, such as fever with neutropenia; or may have undergone high-dose radiation and surgical tumor resection. The occupational therapist working with these children may encounter clients and families in different stages of the diagnostic and treatment continuum. Because of the chronic nature of illness for patients on this unit, the therapist may have time to develop relationships with the child and family. Children may come into and out of the hospital throughout their treatment, and the therapist may see the child for both inpatient and outpatient therapy or may coordinate with outpatient therapists to continue care while the patient experiences an extended inpatient stay. Children may also vary greatly in their ability to participate in treatments throughout the day or during the week. Coordinating therapy with other medical interventions may enhance therapy benefits by providing interventions when the child's energy is highest.

A bone marrow transplant unit has certain similarities to the oncology unit, with intensified therapies and additional toxic agents used as life-saving treatments. Bone marrow transplants are used as part of a medical treatment protocol for a number of life-threatening childhood illnesses, including leukemia, aplastic anemia, immunodeficiency syndromes, and tumors.[37,95,96] Because of the complications of the treatment, the therapist must be aware of the stages the child is in during the transplant process and must strictly adhere to any precautions required.[21,80,85]

Oncology Treatment

During the initial phase of treatment for cancer, children undergo a series of evaluations to determine cancer type and staging, which includes determining if the cancer has metastasized. Clients generally receive a permanent line placement through which they receive their chemotherapy. They are often hospitalized for their induction chemotherapy, which is the initial course, which may be quite intense for some children. Hospitalization is required initially to assess effects of chemotherapy and to watch for any complications. Children frequently decrease their oral intake during treatment, so nutrition and hydration need to be carefully monitored as well.

As treatment progresses, children are often discharged from the inpatient setting and are monitored between chemotherapy sessions in outpatient visits. If the child does not have a negative reaction, or if the agents given do not have high levels of toxicity, the child may receive chemotherapy on an outpatient basis. Children receiving chemotherapy are often at high risk for infections and are susceptible to contagious diseases; therefore, they need to take precautions, particularly if they are neutropenic, which affects their ability to fight off disease. This is a frequent cause for hospital admissions between chemotherapy sessions and can mean patients are readmitted multiple times throughout their treatment.

The occupational therapist working with these children should be aware of the cancer types and have general knowledge of chemotherapy drugs and their complications, radiation therapy effects, and surgical approaches that may be taken. All personnel must adhere to infection control procedures. Therapists may focus on prevention of secondary complications by implementing strengthening, range of motion, and endurance activities, and helping patients resume ADLs, feeding, or play activities, depending on their needs. Children and families frequently develop a close relationship with care providers because of the physical aspects of treatment, along with the normalcy and expectation of survival that families can perceive with everyday activities.

Occasionally, cure is not an option for the child and family, and focus of treatment may change to be palliative in nature. The therapist working with the dying child and his or her family must respect the cultural beliefs of the family, along with grief processes. The occupational therapist can assist with suggesting energy conservation techniques to enable the child to continue to play and interact with family members. Positioning becomes particularly important as the child develops increased weakness, difficulty with breath support, or pain, and the therapist can help families problem-solve alternative positioning to be close to their child when comfort is of utmost importance.[23] It is also important the therapist respect family and child's wishes for withdrawal or continuation of services. Certain families may wish to discontinue therapy intervention, choosing to narrow the circle of support; others develop a closeness with the therapist throughout the treatment and want to continue contact. The therapist needs to look at his or her own support systems, beliefs, and feelings about end-of-life issues to assist the child and family during this difficult time.[93]

Transplant Procedures, Complications, and Interventions

The procedure for bone marrow transplant involves chemotherapy, radiation, or both before the transplant. This is followed by intravenous infusion of the bone marrow taken from a compatible donor or from the patient before the pretransplant regimen of chemotherapy and radiation. Those children who are undergoing treatment for disease processes that do not invade the bone marrow may be eligible to undergo stem cell transplant.[82] This involves the harvest of stem cells throughout their initial chemotherapy treatment while in the remission stage. Although bone marrow and stem cell transplants both involve intense chemotherapy and radiation, individuals who receive a stem cell transplant experience lower rejection rates and fewer complications from graft versus host disease (GVHD). The intense chemotherapy or radiation before the transplant and the underlying disease processes cause severe immunosuppression in patients, making them highly susceptible to life-threatening infections until the new bone marrow is established and the child's immunohematopoietic system is once again functioning effectively.[63,98] Continued long-term effects are also a complication of transplant. Chronic GVHD, abnormal neuroendocrine function, secondary malignancies, and avascular necrosis are a few of the complications seen in pediatric clients.[81] Stretching, extremity weight bearing, and general endurance exercises improve function in children experiencing these GVHD complications.[4]

Because these children have significant compromise of their immune systems, the hospital environment is carefully designed to significantly reduce the risk of infection. Common strategies to protect bone marrow transplant recipients include room isolation, reverse isolation, and laminar airflow in a clean or sterile environment.[63] Additionally, persons having access to the unit may be limited. Those staff and visitors who have flu- or virus-related symptoms may not be allowed onto units serving these severely compromised patients.

Intervention by occupational therapists may include pretransplant assessment of the child's development and functional abilities, and identification of limitations or problems caused by the underlying disease process. After the transplant, the occupational therapist's goals may be to (1) promote age-appropriate play, daily living, and social participation occupations; (2) enhance coping and interaction skills; and (3) develop a plan for follow-up in the community. Case Study 26-3 describes a child from initial diagnosis and chemotherapy through the transplant process and posttransplant intervention.

CASE STUDY 26-3   Danielle

PRESENTING INFORMATION

Danielle was a 21-month-old girl who was initially seen at a general hospital near her home when she experienced a decrease in standing and sitting balance and was subsequently admitted to a pediatric tertiary care center approximately 400 miles from her community. Initial examination and imaging revealed a neuroblastoma in her spinal cord. Danielle was immediately placed on the pediatric oncology unit, a peripherally inserted central catheter (PICC) line was placed, and chemotherapy induction was initiated. At initial presentation, both parents flew in with Danielle, although they had been separated just before diagnosis.

BACKGROUND INFORMATION

Danielle was a typically developing girl before diagnosis, initially described as a reserved, cautious child. She resided with her mother, and her father had moved out just 1 month before her diagnosis. They lived in a small town, with many community friends available for support. Her parents had moved from a large city before conceiving Danielle to "obtain a simpler lifestyle." Upon hearing the diagnosis, the mother revealed that her grandfather had died of a glioblastoma just 1 year previously.

MEDICAL AND OCCUPATIONAL THERAPY INTERVENTION: ONCOLOGY PHASE OF TREATMENT

Danielle was initially referred for occupational therapy immediately after diagnosis. She was having initial complications coping with the increased noise and the number of caregivers, along with decreased performance. She was also seen by a child life specialist for developmentally appropriate coping strategies such as creating a calming environment and play to facilitate release of emotions. Danielle was not able to sit independently on initiation of treatment and her arm strength was diminished.

Danielle was given chemotherapy to reduce the size of the tumor and keep it from spreading. Because of its location, tumor resection was not possible. Stem cell transplant was discussed at initiation of treatment as the best course of possible cure for her cancer. Thus the medical plan was to reduce her tumor size, obtain remission, harvest stem cells, and prepare Danielle for transplant. She was placed on a chemotherapy protocol recommended for her tumor type, and the family was informed of all complications, side effects, and likely outcome possibilities.

In an initial assessment, the occupational therapist evaluated Danielle's performance skills and strength. She also completed family interviews to learn about the child's previous skill levels, occupations, and particular interests. A plan was made in conjunction with the parents and the nurse for a daily schedule, including times when Danielle could receive therapy. She was moved to a corner room to decrease noise, and times were posted when curtains were to be drawn to allow the family private time. Pictures of caregivers, including therapists, primary nurses, and physicians, were posted for reference for both Danielle and her parents.

Ongoing communication was established among all team members through the use of progress notes, team rounds, and a care book placed at Danielle's bedside where information and questions could be posted to further facilitate communication between both parents and medical personnel. In addition, care conferences were held weekly at which all team members, including parents, could get together to discuss ongoing treatments.

Occupational therapy treatments consisted of age-appropriate activities and play opportunities to facilitate strengthening and continued motor skill development. Personal ADLs were also encouraged and supported. Family members, along with the nurses, were instructed on position strategies to increase Danielle's function and enable participation. Her medical treatment made Danielle's ability to participate in regular sessions difficult, not only owing to nausea but also owing to neutropenic compromise resulting in additional weakness and lethargy. During particularly difficult periods, treatment sessions were limited to gentle range of motion or were sometimes canceled for the day.

As medical intervention, including chemotherapy, progressed, Danielle experienced an increase in function. Her occupational therapy treatment plan was continually revised to reflect increased strength and independence. In response to chemotherapy, Danielle began to have reduced oral food intake. Strategies were implemented to help maintain oral motor skills and optimizing self-feeding.

Danielle was eventually transitioned to outpatient care, where both her oncology treatment and her occupational therapy continued. Because of behavior challenges, family requests, and training expertise, direct physical therapy was discontinued. Instead, a collaborative approach of consultation with the occupational therapist at regular intervals to facilitate ambulatory and lower extremity skills was established. Her parents also divided care, with one parent returning to their home community, and alternating times when parents would be present.

Before transplant, Danielle regained her motor skills, and 2 days before the transplant she was able to walk again. She resumed doing and completing age-appropriate ADL tasks and participating in developmentally appropriate play activities. Medications were given between chemotherapy courses to facilitate production of stem cells, which were then harvested.

Once the transplant regimen was initiated, Danielle was hospitalized for an extended stay. She underwent intensive chemotherapy and radiation to ablate her current marrow and subsequently receive a stem cell transplant. During her initial stages, Danielle experienced a significant decrease in her strength and developmental skills. She had toxicity-related complications including sloughing of her skin and mouth sores, which made participation in activities difficult. As an added complication, Danielle also experienced life-threatening pulmonary complications that required ventilation support and necessitated a 2-week stay in the intensive care unit.

Family stresses throughout this portion of her treatment were enormous, and Danielle's mother asked Danielle's maternal grandmother to come for support. Once she arrived, interpreters translated necessary information as the parents desired. Danielle eventually achieved slow engraftment, and transplant-related complications diminished.

As engraftment progressed, Danielle began to regain her play and daily living skills, including ambulation. She was transferred to outpatient services and continued to receive occupational therapy intervention to address decreased strength and delayed motor skills. She was discharged back to her community once she had completed her 90-day posttransplant evaluation and engraftment was clear. She continued to receive ongoing occupational therapy in her community to help facilitate progress in her development.

REHABILTATION SERVICES: LEVELS OF REHABILITATION SERVICE

Levels of rehabilitation services can be subacute, acute, and outpatient or ongoing care. Subacute rehabilitation services are typically organized within skilled nursing facilities (SNFs) or other long-term care settings. Such programs are designed for children and adolescents who are too medically fragile or dependent to be cared for at home, but who are not yet able to engage in or benefit from the intensive efforts of acute rehabilitation.[44] Such settings can also address later stages of care that may involve palliative care or extended stays. After initial hospitalization, children and adolescents with moderate to severe head injury, multitrauma, or other systemic illnesses may be admitted to an SNF with subacute rehabilitation services. In these settings, they may receive daily therapy to prevent secondary complications and work toward goals of greater independent function. This interdisciplinary care may culminate in admission to an acute rehabilitation program or a planned discharge to an organized home- and community-based service system of care.

Acute rehabilitation is characterized by inpatient hospital units and services. Most common are dedicated rehabilitation units within a children's hospital. Another form of organization is the specification of beds and services for pediatric patients within a large rehabilitation hospital. Adolescents 15 years of age or older may be admitted to rehabilitation units that commonly serve adults. Children and adolescents are admitted to acute rehabilitation from other acute or transitional care medical services within the hospital, other local hospitals, or subacute rehabilitation settings. Overall, admission to pediatric rehabilitation and length of inpatient stay are largely based on the child's or youth's level of function and services needed.[19]

Essential to acute rehabilitation programs is the presence of a broad range of services, including occupational therapy. The mixture and intensity of services are planned to meet systematically developed goals. Such programs are characterized as meeting three types of needs:

1. Organize and implement a planned approach for the management of recovery and rehabilitation of children with rapid-onset disorders.
2. Redirect care after onset of complications in children with chronic disorders.
3. Provide an environment for specialized medical or surgical procedures that involves specific care regimens and protocols.

Children and adolescents who sustain a sudden illness or injury are the most common type of admission in acute rehabilitation. Table 26-1 indicates the common problems that affect a typically developing child who experiences injury from accidents, violence, or rapid-onset disease. Acquired injuries or diseases represent a substantial health threat to children.[67,79,100] Injuries are the leading cause of death and disability among children older than 1 year of age.[30] Traumatic brain injuries (TBIs), including closed head injury, skull fracture, and penetrating brain injuries, are an ongoing concern for children and adolescents as a result of transportation-related crashes, falls, recreational injury, and violence.[65,83] These traumas are also associated with children who sustain spinal cord injury (SCI) and multitrauma. Environmental hazards, accidents, and abuse are also implicated among children who experience burns, near drowning, smoke inhalation, carbon monoxide poisoning, or drug overdose.

TABLE 26-1 Rapid Onset Conditions

Type of Onset	Examples
Accidental injury	Traumatic brain injury (e.g., closed head injury)
	Skull fracture or penetrating head injury
	Burns and smoke inhalation
	Multitrauma
	Near drowning
	Spinal cord injury
Violence	Multitrauma
	Traumatic brain injury (e.g., gunshot wound)
	Burns (e.g., iron burns, cigarette burns, scalding)
Disease processes	Central nervous system infection (e.g., encephalitis, meningitis)
	Transverse myelitis
	Guillain-Barré syndrome
	Cancer
	Organ transplant

Aside from known hazards, children may also develop infections that involve the central nervous system (CNS); they may sustain cerebrovascular accidents or develop other neurologic disorders such as transverse myelitis or Guillain-Barré syndrome. Cancer and its treatment may cause children and adolescents to develop problems that necessitate acute rehabilitation. All of these disorders are characterized by typical development until an acute health crisis causes a severe loss of function, a likelihood of prolonged recovery with residual disability, and potential chronic health complications associated with disability. For such children and their families, the purpose of rehabilitation is to prevent further deterioration or the development of complications, and to organize and implement an approach to initial and long-term management that optimizes function in family and community life.

Children with congenital or chronic disorders may also require acute rehabilitation (Table 26-2). Many with genetic disorders or other congenital abnormalities, or those who experience chronic disease, often have delayed or atypical patterns of functional skill development. These children are also at risk for complications that can create a gradual or critical loss of function. Episodes of respiratory complications, bony fractures and dislocations, skin breakdown, or other systemic complications may be associated with functional deterioration. Children with cerebral palsy, spina bifida, or other types of

TABLE 26-2 Complications in Children with Chronic Disorders

Type of Onset	Examples
Neurologic	Spina bifida
	Cerebral palsy
	Neurogenetic disorders
Orthopedic	Juvenile rheumatoid arthritis
	Congenital amelia and dwarfism
	Arthrogryposis multiplex congenita
Muscular	Muscular dystrophy
Pulmonary	Bronchopulmonary dysplasia

ongenital defects are included in this at-risk group. Likewise, those with congenital limb deficiency or arthrogryposis multiplex congenital syndrome may have reconstructive surgery necessitating acute rehabilitation. Children with osteogenesis imperfecta can have episodes of curtailed functional gains after injury and children with juvenile rheumatoid arthritis and systemic disorders can be associated with periods of rapid decline in function. For these children, the goals of rehabilitation are to limit or prevent further losses and facilitate reacquisition of skills consistent with the pattern of functional progression that was previously shown.

A third major group of children who receive acute rehabilitation services are those who are hospitalized for treatment with special medical, surgical, or technological procedures (Table 26-3). For children with cerebral palsy, casting procedures and uses of new medical interventions such as selective dorsal rhizotomy, continuous intrathecal baclofen, or other

TABLE 26-3 Special Medical Procedures

Type of Procedure	Examples
Clinical procedure	Selective dorsal rhizotomy
	Continuous intrathecal baclofen
	Ilizarov, distraction osteogenesis
	Organ transplant
Medical technology	Ventilator dependence

neurosurgical techniques to reduce spasticity may involve admission to acute rehabilitation.[32] Children with severe pulmonary complications or those who become ventilator dependent may be admitted for acute rehabilitation to assist families in learning how to perform care procedures and use medical technology,[11] for which long-term outcomes can be positive.[40] More and more children are also receiving organ transplants that may necessitate the teaching of special care procedures and redeveloping fitness following prolonged disease processes. These interventions often involve the therapists in following specific evaluation and treatment protocols designed to optimize functional outcomes (Case Study 26-4).

Outpatient Services

Another major component of pediatric rehabilitation exists within specialized outpatient services and clinics that provide ongoing care. Typically, as part of children's hospitals or rehabilitation hospitals, interdisciplinary outpatient clinics are organized to provide monitoring and interventions with children who experience particular types of chronic health risks and disabilities. Occupational therapists often provide follow-up and follow-along attention to children and families after hospitalization, but many of these children are never hospitalized. Therapists who work at these clinics most often focus on the child or adolescent's health status and development, emphasizing functional progress and participation in home, school, and community activities.

CASE STUDY 26-4 Stephen

PRESENTING INFORMATION

Stephen is an 8-year-old boy with mild R hemiplegia 2° traumatic brain injury and skull fracture. Precautions include dysphagia, aphasia, and risks for falls. Treatment objectives are to evaluate and train ADL skills, passive range of motion (PROM) with right upper extremity (RUE), facilitate the use of RUE, and evaluate and intervene for visual-perceptual and cognitive skill deficits.

REFERRAL HISTORY

Stephen is from a two-parent, three-sibling home in a small coastal town. Family members describe Stephen as being energetic and well-liked. In October, he was a passenger in an all-terrain vehicle crash. Stephen was not wearing a helmet and was reported to have struck his head. He was initially alert but soon experienced diminished wakefulness and was unresponsive when paramedics arrived. At the trauma center, Stephen was found to have a left basilar skull fracture, and a computed tomography (CT) scan showed bilateral frontal punctate lesions and an apparent left temporal-parietal focal lesion. Three days after the injury, Stephen became more responsive, but he demonstrated minimal movement of his right arm and leg, no vocalizations, and dysphagia. He continued to show gradual improvement in his level of consciousness and was evaluated for transfer to acute rehabilitation. His injury was classified as moderate. Twelve days after the accident, Stephen was transferred to the local children's hospital.

CLINICAL FINDINGS

On admission to rehabilitation, Stephen was following simple one-step commands and attempting to verbalize, but word finding was difficult. He was noted to be fatigued and difficult to engage for more than a few minutes at a time. He was also regarded as quiet, reserved, and fearful of being separated from his mother, who stayed with him nearly full-time during the day and evenings. Diminished alertness, easy distraction, and disorientation to place and time were also noted. These dysfunctions caused Stephen to become anxious during evaluation and treatments. Swallowing was judged safe from aspiration, although one-to-one supervision was recommended because of Stephen's tendency to over-stuff food and poorly sequence his intake of fluids and solids.

During grooming and dressing tasks, Stephen was observed as being disorganized. In part because of his age, he showed poor ability to make natural adaptations to hemiplegia. Continual verbal cues were needed to initiate, set up, and proceed with grooming, dressing, and bathing tasks. Physical demonstration and cues were needed to teach adapted sequences. No perceptual deficits were found by observation or by the use of standardized tests.

Further observations showed mild right hemiplegia, characterized by effortful movements of both upper and lower limbs. Little spontaneous use of his right arm was seen, and Stephen showed characteristic synergy patterns and increased muscle tone when he attempted to grasp objects on command. Passive

Continued

CASE STUDY 26-4 Stephen—cont'd

range of motion was normal. In sensory testing, Stephen showed impaired proprioception and localization to touch in distal portions of the arm and leg. Stephen did not ambulate but had partial weight bearing in stance with foot drop when he tried to walk. The physical therapist initiated the use of a right ankle-foot orthosis (R-AFO) and a cane.

INTERVENTION ACTIVITIES

The therapist initiated the use of an orientation board in Stephen's room, regular reminders provided by staff and his mother, written schedules, and a memory book that Stephen completed after each treatment session. The therapist planned consistent routines for personal ADLs, sequenced daily therapies, and structured play activities. The therapist used familiar play items, pictures of family, his own clothes, his favorite music, and art supplies to enhance comfort and provide memory cues and prompts for orientation. The therapist organized visits by other family members and friends from school and included them as part of scheduling and memory book entries.

The therapist scheduled Stephen for one-to-one therapy sessions twice each day and planned morning personal ADL training and afternoon therapeutic activities. In addition to structured ADL routines and orientation-memory programs, the therapist also engaged Stephen in selected activities to facilitate the use of his right arm and provide cognitive challenge in organizing steps, following sequences, and sustaining engagement in both familiar and novel tasks (Figure 26-5, A). The therapist taught Stephen daily range-of-motion exercises and whole-body stretches to maintain normal range and facilitate symmetric trunk and limb use.

Spontaneous use of his right arm improved, but poor recovery of his right hand resulted in Stephen's attempting to perform activities using his nondominant left hand. Such attempts proved to be awkward and unsuccessful. The therapist trained Stephen and cued him to use both hands together (Figure 26-5, B), using the right hand as an assist to the left

hand. This strategy improved his personal ADL performance so that the therapist discontinued use of adaptive devices such as a button-aid and a rocker knife after 2 weeks. Handwriting with either the right or left hand was not satisfactory for schoolwork because of language disorders, illegibility, and slow speed. The therapist introduced a computer keyboard and initiated supplementary handwriting activities to facilitate movement and augment function. The therapist judged Stephen's physical management of other school-related tasks to be adequate, although communication and cognitive impairments posed major challenges to his return to school. Three weeks after admission, Stephen was ambulatory with the use of an AFO. He continued to show evidence of topographic disorientation, getting lost between the hospital room and the clinic, but otherwise he was thought to be a safe ambulator, even on uneven surfaces and stairs. He groomed, dressed, and bathed with supervision for initiation and safety. Stephen appropriately initiated toileting, and his mother judged his hygiene after bowel movements to be adequate.

DISCHARGE FOLLOW-UP PLAN

Discharge planning included home program suggestions for Stephen and his family. In addition to organizing ADL routines for Stephen to use at home, the therapist wrote activities to promote fine motor skills and reviewed them with Stephen's mother. The team held meetings with school personnel to address academic program needs and potential benefits from school-based therapy services. The team attempted to determine eligibility for special education and used age/gender-normed tests that the school system would accept in its review. The team scheduled interim school visits by the hospital neuropsychologist to occur after Stephen's return to a half-day school program 2 weeks after discharge. The team scheduled a rehabilitation medicine outpatient clinic follow-up visit to include occupational therapy in 6 weeks, with a plan for regular follow-along clinic visits at 2-month intervals during the next 6 months.

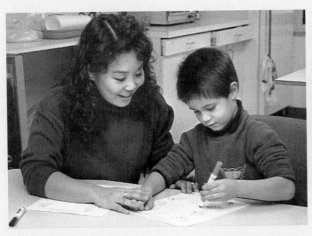
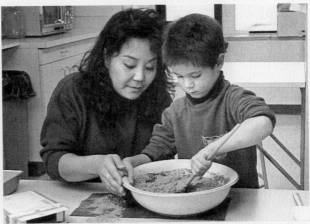

FIGURE 26-5 **A,** The occupational therapist promotes the use of the hemiparetic arm to hold the paper while the child carries out a drawing and writing activity. **B,** The therapist provides guidance in using both arms while participating in a cookie-baking activity.

TABLE 26-4 Outpatient Clinics and Programs Often Served by Occupational Therapists

Clinic Title	Example of Clients or Services
Congenital disorders	Spina bifida
Neuromuscular disorders	Cerebral palsy
Developmental disabilities	Down syndrome
	Fetal alcohol syndrome
Rheumatology	Juvenile rheumatoid arthritis
	Systemic lupus erythematosus
Adolescent medicine	Reflex Neurovascular Dystrophy
Craniofacial abnormality	Cleft lip and palate
Orthopedic	Traumatic hand injury
	Congenital limb deficiency
Rehabilitation	Traumatic brain injury
	Spinal cord injury
	Constraint Induced Therapy Program
Muscular dystrophy	Duchenne muscular dystrophy
	Spinal muscle atrophy
Limb deficiency	Congenital amelia
	Traumatic amputation
Cystic fibrosis	Cystic fibrosis
Assistive technology	Seating and positioning
	Wheelchair control
	Augmentative communication
	Computers and information technology
	Environmental controls

Clinic programs that most commonly involve occupational therapists are displayed in Table 26-4. Such clinic programs may be scheduled weekly, monthly, quarterly, or even annually as needed. Sometimes these programs are conducted away from the hospital facility at community sites such as schools. Often the therapists offer consultation and recommendations to the family and local therapists who know the particular child well but have limited experience with a specific disorder or type of specialized intervention. For example, school personnel may have limited experience with children who have arthrogryposis, brachial plexus and limb deficiency, or various forms of muscular dystrophy, whereas the hospital clinic therapists would have regular experience with these disabling conditions. Rapid developments in AT may also limit the likelihood that all schools or local programs can remain current and effective in applying new systems and approaches. Therapists who work in specialized hospital programs are provided with unique exposure to otherwise uncommon diagnoses and clinical procedures and can pass this experience on to other families and therapists as a conduit of information and new ideas. Specific study and preparation for consultation are suggested for entry-level therapists and can be an important skill for the therapist to develop as part of pediatric rehabilitation.[24]

Therapists also provide outpatient services in the form of individualized assessment and therapy trials at the hospital, home-based programs, or in free-standing outpatient clinics. Outpatient services often occur concurrently with the child's return to school and school-based therapy; the former is organized around medical needs, whereas the latter addresses educational performance.

Efforts to augment function beyond the child's current development are also represented by efforts to apply AT (see Chapters 20 and 21). The therapist may plan outpatient services to permit intensive evaluation and trials in the use of aided and augmentative communication systems, computer access and use of information technologies, therapeutic seating, powered mobility, or other technologies that enable environmental access and control. These applications of special procedures or AT devices are characterized by preplanned and often short trials leading to prescription of devices. Efforts culminate in intensive family training and transition to follow-up in the community, often in partnership with local providers in the environments in which AT devices are used.

Residential or intensive day-treatment programs constitute another form of outpatient pediatric rehabilitation service. Interdisciplinary services are most often organized for children and adolescents with brain injury. These extended care programs are geared toward direct assistance with community reentry and participation. Simulated or actual environments become the training site for skills that enable community participation and effective performance toward goals of independent living, education, and work activities.

Outpatient services are important components of the total spectrum of hospital care and may be provided at the hospital, at a hospital satellite center, or as part of an interdisciplinary hospital-based clinic (e.g., rheumatology clinic, neurodevelopmental palsy clinic, or special feeding clinics). Outpatient occupational therapy is generally provided for one of three purposes: (1) as part of a diagnostic assessment, (2) to provide needed intervention after hospital discharge, or (3) to provide occupational therapy intervention for individuals with disabilities or other medical conditions not requiring hospitalization.

Provision of inpatient occupational therapy services differs from provision of outpatient services in a number of ways. Services are usually provided to outpatients less frequently (e.g., one to three times per week) and may continue for weeks or months. The longer duration provides a greater opportunity for the occupational therapist to get to know the child's family and develop a collaborative relationship. In addition, it may provide the therapist a chance to observe the natural progression of some conditions, including healing progression, to better predict outcomes and to write realistic goals. Children seen on an outpatient basis are medically stable, as opposed to children who are hospitalized for an acute or transient illness.

One disadvantage of outpatient therapy is the limited opportunity for collaboration and communication with other professionals who provide services to the child. In most cases, the child served as an outpatient does not have a medical team with members who meet to discuss and coordinate services. If the therapist is part of a larger hospital therapy department, he or she may draw on the experience of fellow therapists within the working group to help guide practice. The therapist must also take the initiative to collaborate with other community professionals by participating in the care of the child when appropriate. These may include the primary care provider, school physical or occupational therapists, or educators. The occupational therapist must be diligent in obtaining consents for the sharing or releasing of information according to the

CASE STUDY 26-5 — Stacie

Stacie is an 8-year-old girl with midlumbar myelodysplasia. She ambulates with AFOs and uses Lofstrand crutches for longer distances at this time. Although she is functional for mobility in her home and at school, her future mobility demands may necessitate use of a wheelchair as she grows older and her independent mobility needs grow and change. Poor hand coordination skills with less than age-expected quality and speed in hand writing tasks is evident through developmental and skill-based assessment. Stacie has been introduced to using a keyboard for writing and some computer skills. She is using a computer to complete some school work in her third grade integrated classroom.

Stacie is assisted at home with some dressing challenges, most notably with clothing fasteners, but is otherwise independent with her morning and evening ADLs. With a neurogenic bowel and bladder, she is on a clean intermittent catheterization (CIC) program and daily bowel program. Her mother has traditionally done her catheterization and is trying to transition to have her perform more of it on her own. At school, a nurse assists with her two-times-per-day catheter schedule. She is somewhat successful with her bowel program, typically having bowel movements in the morning or during the evenings at home. Timed programs include uses of diet and suppositories. Occasional bowel accidents are acknowledged, and she uses pull-ups to contend with such problems.

Although many of the activity and participation concerns with Stacie are addressed as part of school therapy and reflected in her IEP, the role of the specialty clinic follow-up has two major purposes. One of these is to carefully monitor her motor skill development and status. Children with spina bifida often have shunts neurosurgically placed early in life to reduce hydrocephalus. Such shunts can become obstructed, and families and service providers are vigilant in attending to signs of shunt failure. Worsening of coordination and visual-perception skills can be one or more of these signs and the specialty clinic therapist often performs normative hand function assessment to determine stability of performance over time. In this clinic the therapist measures grip and pinch strength and coordination testing using the Jebsen-Taylor Hand Function Test, which has norms for children, adolescents, and adults of both sexes. Developmental visual-perceptual tests may also be used. In her most recent visit, Stacie's scores were similar to prior year's findings, with her scoring about 1.5 SD below the mean on most tasks. Her grip and pinch strength were also around the 40th percentile for her age and gender.

Another role of the clinical specialist is to facilitate growth in children's ADL and IADL skill independence. Children with spina bifida have different timing and patterns of skill development that often needs specific advising and uses of adaptive methods and devices.[18,55] For example, this may include how orthotic devices are being managed, how wheelchair skills and device management are proceeding, and how participation and eventual independence in bladder and bowel care programs are promoted. Stacie, as indicated, was doing well with managing most of her personal care and was participating in a few chores at home. Suggested to her and her family was to select clothes to be worn to school the night before and to focus on purchasing of clothes without need for fasteners, or with a preference for zippers and snaps. Clinical follow-up may occur more often than annually, with exchange of information with school-based therapy programs to promote health monitoring and encourage effective participation and performance.

standard established by the Health Insurance Portability and Accountability Act of 1996, Privacy Rule (HIPAA).

Outpatient services provided as part of an interdisciplinary specialty medical clinic usually have a specific focus (e.g., feeding clinic, behavioral disorders clinic). Occupational therapy services in specialty clinics are limited because children typically attend only one to two times a year (Case Study 26-5). In some instances, the occupational therapist functions as a consultant, completing an assessment, then making recommendations to the physician. In other cases, the occupational therapist is an integral part of the decision-making team and may be involved in child assessment, treatment or equipment recommendations, or the provision of splints and adaptive equipment.

SUMMARY

The provision of occupational therapy services to children in hospitals is a specialized and challenging area of practice. Occupational therapists in hospitals must have a thorough understanding of the characteristics of health care systems; the numerous factors and trends that affect hospitals, including legal and accreditation requirements; and the specialized needs of hospitalized children and their families. The occupational therapist must also understand the roles of others involved in the care for children to accomplish both medical and functional goals. Occupational therapists who are employed in hospitals have the opportunity to gain expertise in assessment and treatment of children of various ages with many different diagnoses, often within a dynamic, fast-paced environment. As hospitals broaden their range of services in response to a changing health care system, hospital-based occupational therapists will have opportunities to broaden their areas of expertise, apply different models of service delivery, and develop new practitioner roles.

Hospital-based pediatric rehabilitation services play a unique role in the overall management of children and adolescents with a new or chronic disability. In addressing acute and chronic problems, the emphasis of practice is nearly always on function and participation in life's events at home, at school, and in the community. Both new and established impairments and disabilities pose risks for further complications, which necessitate a prevention prioritization through subacute, acute, and outpatient or ongoing rehabilitation interventions. Services are medically oriented and delivered within constraints imposed by accreditation and regulatory agencies and third-party payers. Collaboration with school- and community-based services is critical to effective intervention and transition. The challenge of hospitalization and pediatric rehabilitation is to address the acute problems while considering the overall development of the individual and the priorities of the family.

REFERENCES

1. Affleck, A. T., Lieberman, S., Polon, J., & Rohrkemper, K. (1986). Providing occupational therapy in an intensive care unit. *American Journal of Occupational Therapy, 40*, 323–332.

2. Armstrong, K., & Kerns, K. A. (2002). The assessment of parent needs following paediatric traumatic brain injury. *Pediatric Rehabilitation, 5*, 149–160.

3. Bedell, G. M., Haley, S. M., Coster, W. J., & Smith, K. W. (2002). Participation readiness at discharge from inpatient rehabilitation in children and adolescents with acquired brain injuries. *Pediatric Rehabilitation, 5*, 107–116.

4. Beredjiklian, P. K., Drummond, D. S., Dormans, J. P., Davidson, R. S., Brock, G. T., & August, C. (1998). Orthopaedic manifestations of chronic graft-versus-host disease. *Journal of Pediatric Orthopeadics, 18*(5), 572–575.

5. Bithoney, W. G., & Newberger, E. H. (1987). Child and family attributes of failure-to-thrive. *Developmental and Behavioral Pediatrics, 8*, 32–36.

6. Blatzheim, L. L., Edberg, A., & Lacy, L. (1987). Operationalizing primary nursing in the pediatric rehabilitation setting. *Journal of Pediatric Nursing, 2*, 434–437.

7. Bower, E., McLellan, D. L., Arney, J., & Campbell, M. J. (1996). A randomised controlled trial of different intensities of physiotherapy and different goal-setting procedures in 44 children with cerebral palsy. *Developmental Medicine and Child Neurology, 38*, 226–237.

8. Boyer, M. G., & Edwards, P. (1991). Outcome 1 to 3 years after severe traumatic brain injury in children and adolescents. *Injury, 22*, 315–320.

9. Burkett, K. W. (1989). Trends in pediatric rehabilitation. *Nursing Clinics of North America, 24*, 239–255.

10. Bury, T., & Mead, J. (1998). *Evidence-based healthcare: A practical guide for therapists.* Boston: Butterworth-Heinemann.

11. Buschbacher, R. (1995). Outcomes and problems in pediatric pulmonary rehabilitation. *American Journal of Physical Medicine and Rehabilitation, 74*, 287–293.

12. Case-Smith, J., & Wavrek, B. B. (1998). Models of service delivery and team interaction. In J. Case-Smith (Ed.), *Pediatric occupational therapy and early intervention* (2nd ed., pp. 83–107). Boston: Butterworth-Heinemann.

13. Chen, C. C., Heinemann, A. W., Bode, R. K., Granger, C. V., & Mallinson, T. (2004). Impact of pediatric rehabilitation services on children's functional outcomes. *American Journal of Occupational Therapy, 58*, 44–53.

14. Cheng, T. L., Greenberg, L., Loeser, H., & Keller, D. (2000). Teaching prevention in pediatrics. *Academic Medicine. 75*, S66–S71.

15. Colville, G. (2008). The psychologic impact on children of admission to intensive care. *Pediatric Clinics of North America, 55*, 605–616.

16. Coster, W. J., Haley, S., & Baryza, M. J. (1994). Functional performance of young children after traumatic brain injury: A 6-month follow-up study. *American Journal of Occupational Therapy, 48*, 211–218.

17. Cotterill, P. G., & Gage, B. J. (2002). Overview: Medicare postacute care since the Balanced Budget Act of 1997. *Health Care Financing Review, 24*(2), 1–6.

18. Davis, B. E., Shurtleff, D. B., Walker, W. O., Seidel, K. D., & Duguay, S. (2006). Acquisition of autonomy in adolescents with myelomeningocele. *Developmental Medicine and Child Neurology, 48*, 253–258.

19. DeNise-Annunziata, D. K., & Scharf, A. A. (1998). Functional status as an important predictor of length of stay in a pediatric rehabilitation hospital. *Journal of Rehabilitation Outcomes Measurement, 2*, 12–21.

20. Denton, R. (1986). An occupational therapy protocol for assessing infants and toddlers who fail to thrive. *American Journal of Occupational Therapy, 40*, 352–358.

21. Diaz de Heredia, C., Moreno, A., Olive, T., Iglesias, J., & Ortega, J. J. (1999). Role of the intensive care unit in children undergoing bone marrow transplantation with life-threatening complications. *Bone Marrow Transplantation, 24*, 163–168.

22. Donders, J. (1993). Bereavement and mourning in pediatric rehabilitation settings. *Death Studies, 17*, 517–527.

23. Drake, R., Frost, J., & Collins, J. J. (2003). The symptoms of dying children. *Journal of Pain & Symptom Management, 26*, 594–603.

24. Dudgeon, B. J., & Greenberg, S. L. (1998). Preparing students for consultation roles and systems. *American Journal of Occupational Therapy, 52*, 801–809.

25. Dumas, H. M., Haley, S. M., Ludlow, L. H., & Rabin, J. P. (2002). Functional recovery in pediatric traumatic brain injury during inpatient rehabilitation. *American Journal of Physical Medicine and Rehabilitation, 81*, 661–669.

26. Eckle, N., & MacLean, S. L. (2001). Assessment of family-centered care policies and practices for pediatric patients in nine US emergency departments. *Journal of Emergency Nursing, 27*, 238–245.

27. Edwards, P. A. (1992). The evolution of rehabilitation facilities for children. *Rehabilitation Nursing, 17*, 191–195.

28. Eigsti, H., Aretz, M., & Shannon, L. (1990). Pediatric physical therapy in a rehabilitation setting. *Pediatrician, 17*, 267–277.

29. Elixhauser, A. (2008). *Hospital stays for children, 2006.* Rockville, MD: HCUP Statistical Brief #56, Agency for Healthcare Research and Quality, Retrieved from http://www.hcup-us.ahrq.gov/reports/statbriefs56.pdf

30. Falesi, M., Berni, S., & Strambi, M. (2008). Causes of accidents in pediatric patients: What has changed through the ages. *Minerva Pediatrics, 60*, 169–176.

31. Fay, G. C., Jaffe, K. M., Polissar, N. L., Liao, S., Rivara, J. B., & Martin, K. M. (1994). Outcome of pediatric traumatic brain injury at three years: A cohort study. *Archives of Physical Medicine and Rehabilitation, 75*, 733–741.

32. Fleet, P. J. (2003). Rehabilitation of spasticity and related problems in childhood cerebral palsy. *Journal of Paediatrics and Child Health, 39*, 6–14.

33. Flores, G., Abreau, M., Claisson, C. E., & Sun, D. (2003). Keeping children out of hospital: Parents' and physicians' perspectives on how pediatric hospitalizations for ambulatory care-sensitive conditions can be avoided. *Pediatrics, 112*, 1021–1030.

34. Frank, D. A. (1985). Biologic risks in "nonorganic" failure to thrive: Diagnostic and therapeutic implications. In D. Drotar (Ed.), *New directions in failure to thrive* (pp. 17–26). New York: Plenum Press.

35. Fuhrer, M. J. (1987). *Rehabilitation outcomes, analysis and measurement.* Baltimore: Brookes.

36. Fuhrer, M. J. (2000). Subjectifying quality of life as a medical rehabilitation outcome. *Disability Rehabilitation, 22*, 481–489.

37. Furman, W. L., & Feldman, S. (1990). Infectious complications. In F. L. Johnson & C. Pochedly (Eds.), *Bone marrow transplantation in children* (pp. 427–450). New York: Raven Press.

38. Gabel, I., Levitt, L., Holve, E., Pickreign, J., Whitmore, H., & Dhoni, K., et al. (2002). Job-based health benefits in 2002: Some important trends. *Health Affairs, 21*(5), 143–151.

39. Gardner, J., & Workinger, M. S. (1990). The changing role of the speech-language pathologist in pediatric rehabilitation/habilitation. *Pediatrician, 17*, 283–286.

40. Gilgoff, R. L., & Gilgoff, I. S. (2003). Long-term follow-up of home mechanical ventilation in young children with spinal cord injury and neuromuscular conditions. *Journal of Pediatrics, 142*, 476–480.

41. Gilkerson, L., Gorski, P., & Panitz, P. (1990). Hospital-based intervention for preterm infants and their families. In S. Meisels & J. Shonkoff (Eds.), *Handbook of early childhood intervention* (pp. 445–468). Cambridge, MA: Cambridge University Press.

42. Gipe, B. T. (2000). The cost and quality of hospitalists. *Cost & Quality, 6,* 20–23.

43. Granberg, A., Engberg, I. B., & Lundberg, D. (1999). Acute confusion and unreal experiences in intensive care patients in relation to the ICU syndrome, part II. *Intensive & Critical Care Nursing, 15,* 19–33.

44. Grebin, B., & Kaplan, S. C. (1995). Toward a pediatric subacute care model: Clinical and administrative features. *Archives of Physical Medicine and Rehabilitation, 76*(Suppl. 12), SC16–SC20.

45. Guerriere, D., & McKeever, P. (1997). Mothering children who survive brain injuries: Playing the hand you're dealt. *Journal of the Society of Pediatric Nurses, 2,* 105–115.

46. Guske, P. (2003). Follow the codes. *Rehabilitation Management, 16,* 58–60.

47. Haley, S. M., Coster, W. J., Ludlow, L. H., Haltiwanger, J. T., & Andrellos, P. J. (1992). *Pediatric Evaluation of Disability Inventory.* San Antonio, TX: Psychological Corp.

48. Haley, S. M., Dumas, H. M., & Ludlow, L. H. (2001). Variation by diagnostic and practice pattern groups in the mobility outcomes of inpatient rehabilitation programs for children and youth. *Physical Therapy, 81,* 1425–1436.

49. Halstead, L. S. (2001). The John Stanley Coulter lecture. The power of compassion and caring in rehabilitation healing. *Archives of Physical Medicine and Rehabilitation, 82,* 149–154.

50. Hewitt-Taylor, J. (1999). Children in intensive care: Physiological considerations. *Nursing in Critical Care, 4,* 40–45.

51. Jaffe, K. M. (2008). Pediatric trauma rehabilitation: A value-added safety net. *Journal of Trauma, 64,* 819–823.

52. Jaffe, K. M., Fay, G. C., Polissar, N. L., Martin, K. M., Shurtleff, H. A., & Rivara, J. B., et al. (1993). Severity of pediatric traumatic brain injury and neurobehavioral recovery at one year—A cohort study. *Archives of Physical Medicine and Rehabilitation, 74,* 587–595.

53. Jaffe, K. M., Massagli, T. L., Martin, K. M., Rivara, J. B., Fay, G. C., & Polissar, N. L. (1993). Pediatric traumatic brain injury: Acute and rehabilitation costs. *Archives of Physical Medicine and Rehabilitation, 74,* 681–686.

54. Jaffe, K. M., Polissar, N. L., Fay, G. C., & Liao, S. (1995). Recovery trends over three years following pediatric traumatic brain injury. *Archives of Physical Medicine and Rehabilitation, 76,* 17–26.

55. Johnson, K. L., Dudgeon, B., Kuehn, C., & Walker, W. (2007). Assistive technology use among adolescents and young adults with spina bifida. *American Journal of Public Health, 97,* 330–336.

56. Jongbloed, L., & Wendland, T. (2002). The impact of reimbursement systems on occupational therapy practice in Canada and the United States of America. *Canadian Journal of Occupational Therapy, 69,* 143–152.

57. Jordan, W. J. (2001). An early view of the impact of deregulation and managed care on hospital profitability and net worth. *Journal of Healthcare Management, 46,* 161–171.

58. Keisler, C. A. (2000). The next wave of change for psychology and mental health services in the health care revolution. *American Psychologist, 55,* 481–487.

59. Keith, R. A., Granger, C. V., Hamilton, B. B., & Sherwin, F. S. (1987). The functional independence measure: A new tool for rehabilitation. *Advances in Clinical Rehabilitation, 1,* 6–18.

60. Kielhofner, G., & Barrett, L. (1998). Meaning and misunderstanding in occupational forms: A study of therapeutic goal setting. *American Journal of Occupational Therapy, 52,* 345–353.

61. Kramer, A. M. (1997). Rehabilitation care and outcomes from the patient's perspective. *Medical Care, 35*(6 Suppl.), JS48–JS57.

62. Law, M., & MacDermid, J. (Eds.). (2008). *Evidence-based rehabilitation: A guide to practice.* Thorofare, NJ: Slack.

63. Lenarsky, C. (1990). Technique of bone marrow transplantation. In F. L. Johnson & C. Pochedly (Eds.), *Bone marrow transplantation in children* (pp. 53–67). New York: Raven Press.

64. Mantymaa, M., Puura, K., Luoma, I., Salmelin, R., Davis, H. J., & Tsiantis, J., et al. (2003). Infant-mother interaction as a predictor of child's chronic health problems. *Child: Care, Health & Development, 29,* 181–191.

65. Mazzola, C. A., & Adelson, P. D. (2002). Critical care management of head trauma in children. *Critical Care Medicine, 30* (Suppl. 11), S393–S401.

66. Michlovitz, S. L. (1996). *Thermal agents in rehabilitation* (3rd ed.). Philadelphia: F.A. Davis.

67. Moront, M., & Eichelberger, M. R. (1994). Pediatric trauma. *Pediatrics Annals, 23,* 186–191.

68. Msall, M. E., DiGaudio, K. M., & Duffy, L. C. (1993). Use of functional assessment in children with developmental disabilities. *Physical Medicine and Rehabilitation Clinics of North America, 4,* 517–527.

69. National Association for Children's Hospitals and Related Institutions (NACHRI). (2009). Home page. Retrieved August 2009 from http://www.childrenshospitals.net.

70. O'Donnell, M. E., & Roxborough, L. (2002). Evidence-based practice in rehabilitation. *Physical Medicine and Rehabilitation Clinics of North America, 13,* 991–1005.

71. Ottenbacher, K. J., & Hinderer, S. R. (2001). Evidence-based practice: Methods to evaluate individual patient improvement. *American Journal of Physical Medicine and Rehabilitation, 80,* 786–796.

72. Ottenbacher, K. J., Msall, M. E., Lyon, N., Duffy, L. C., Ziviani, J., & Granger, C. V., et al. (2000). Functional assessment and care of children with neurodevelopmental disabilities. *American Journal of Physical Medicine and Rehabilitation, 79,* 114–123.

73. Pendleton, H. M., & Schultz-Krohn, W. (Eds.). (2006). *Pedretti's occupational therapy: Practice skills for physical dysfunction* (6th ed.). St. Louis: Mosby.

74. Piazza, C. C., Fisher, W. W., Brown, K. A., Shore, B. A., Patel, M. R., & Katz, R. M., et al. (2003). Functional analysis of inappropriate mealtime behaviors. *Journal of Applied Behavior Analysis, 36,* 187–204.

75. Radomski, M. V., & Trombly, C. A. T. (Eds.). (2008). *Occupational therapy for physical dysfunction* (6th ed.). Baltimore: Lippincott Williams & Wilkins.

76. Rausch, G., & Melvin, J. L. (1986). Nationally speaking: A new era in acute care. *American Journal of Occupational Therapy, 40,* 319–322.

77. Rivara, J. B. (1993). Family functioning following pediatric traumatic brain injury. *Pediatric Annals, 23,* 38–43.

78. Rivara, J. B., Jaffe, K. M., Polissar, N. L., Fay, G. C., Liao, S., & Martin, K. M. (1996). Predictors of family functioning and change 3 years after traumatic brain injury in children. *Archives of Physical Medicine and Rehabilitation, 77,* 754–764.

79. Rodriguez, J. G., & Brown, S. T. (1990). Childhood injuries in the United States. *American Journal of Diseases of Children, 144,* 627–646.

80. Rogers, M., Weinstock, D. M., Eagan, J., Kiehn, T., Armstrong, D., & Sepkowitz, K. A. (2000). Rotavirus outbreak on a pediatric oncology floor: Possible association with toys. *American Journal of Infection Control, 28,* 378–380.

81. Sanders, J. E. (1991). Long term effects of bone marrow transplantation. *Pediatrician, 18,* 76–81.

82. Sanders, J. E. (1997). Bone marrow transplantation for pediatric malignancies. *Pediatric Oncology, 44*(4), 1005–1020.

83. Schneier, A. J., Shields, B. J., Hostetler, S. G., Xiang, H., Smith, G. A. (2006). Incidence of pediatric traumatic brain injury and associated hospital resource utilization in the United States. *Pediatrics, 118,* 483–492.

84. Schwartz, R. K. (1991). Educational and training strategies, therapy as learning. In C. Christiansen & C. Baum (Eds.), *Occupational therapy: Overcoming human performance deficits* (pp. 664–698). Thorofare, NJ: Slack.

85. Shaw, P. J. (2002). Suspected infection in children with cancer. *Journal of Antimicrobial Chemotherapy, 49,* 63–67.

86. Silver, B. V., Boake, C., & Cavazos, D. I. (1994). Improving functional skills using behavioral procedures in a child with anoxic brain injury. *Archives of Physical Medicine and Rehabilitation, 75,* 742–745.

87. Sneed, R. C., May, W. L., Stencel, C., & Paul, S. M. (2002). Pediatric physiatry in 2000: A survey of practitioners and training programs. *Archives of Physical Medicine and Rehabilitation, 83,* 416–422.

88. Tickle-Degnen, L. (2000). Gathering current research evidence to enhance clinical reasoning. *American Journal of Occupational Therapy, 54,* 102–105.

89. Tomlinson, P. S., Swiggum, P., & Harbaugh, B. L. (1999). Identification of nurse-family intervention sites to decrease health-related family boundary ambiguity in PICU. *Issues in Comprehensive Pediatric Nursing, 22,* 27–47.

90. Tomlinson, P. S., Thomlinson, E., Peden-McAlping, C., & Kirschbaum, M. (2002). Clinical innovation for promoting family care in pediatric intensive care: Demonstration, role modeling and reflective practice. *Journal of Advanced Nursing, 38,* 161–170.

91. Treloar, C., & Graham, I. D. (2003). Multidisciplinary cross-national studies: A commentary on issues of collaboration methodology, analysis, and publication. *Qualitative Health Research, 13,* 924–932.

92. Vavili, F. (2000). Children in hospital: a design question. *World Hospital Health Services, 36,* 31–39, 45–46.

93. Vincent, J. L. (2001). Cultural differences in end-of-life care. *Critical Care Medicine, 29,* N52–N55.

94. Watkins, P. (2003). Ethnicity and clinical practice. *Clinical Medicine, 3,* 197–198.

95. Williams, T. E. (1990). Ethical and psychosocial issues in bone marrow transplantation in children. In F. L. Johnson & C. Pochedly (Eds.), *Bone marrow transplantation in children* (pp. 497–504). New York: Raven Press.

96. Williams, T. E., & Safarimaryaki, S. (1990). Bone marrow transplantation for treatment of solid tumors. In F. L. Johnson & C. Pochedly (Eds.), *Bone marrow transplantation in children* (pp. 221–242). New York: Raven Press.

97. Wise, P. (2004). The transformation of child health in the United States. *Health Affairs, 23*(5), 9–25.

98. Zander, A. R., & Aksamit, I. A. (1990). Immune recovery following bone marrow transplantation. In F. L. Johnson & C. Pochedly (Eds.), *Bone marrow transplantation in children* (pp. 87–110). New York: Raven Press.

99. Ziviani, J., Ottenbacher, K. J., Shepard, K., Foreman, S., Astbury, W., & Ireland, P. (2001). Concurrent validity of the functional independence measure for children (WeeFIM) and the pediatric evaluation of disabilities inventory in children with developmental disabilities and acquired brain injuries. *Physical and Occupational Therapy in Pediatrics, 21,* 91–101.

100. Zuckerbraun, N. S., Powell, E. C., Sheehan, K. M., Uyeda, A., Rehm, K. P., & Barlow, B. (2004). Community childhood injury surveillance: An emergency department-based mode. *Pediatric Emergency Care, 20,* 361–366.

SUGGESTED READINGS

Molnar, G. E., & Alexander, M. A. (Eds.). (1999). *Pediatric rehabilitation* (3rd ed.). Philadelphia: Hanley & Belfus.

Perkin, R. M., Swift, J. D., & Newton, A. (Eds.). (2007). *Pediatric hospital medicine: Textbook of inpatient management* (2nd ed.). Philadelphia: Lippincott Williams & Wilkins.

27 Transition Services: From School to Adult Life

Karen C. Spencer

Individuals with disabilities may spend up to 21 years receiving a public education. Education is viewed as a way for these young people to develop the knowledge, skills, and experiences necessary to make the critical transition from school into a variety of adult roles and activities. Upon exiting high school, young adults with and without disabilities can face a dizzying array of options, including postsecondary education, paid employment, volunteer work, establishing a home, and participating in meaningful and healthy relationships. When a person has a disability, this transition can become more complex and often requires timely planning plus access to variety of supports and services that begin during and extend after high school.

The requirement to provide school-to-adult life transition services was established in 1990 by the Individuals with Disabilities Education Act (IDEA) (P.L. 101–476). The more recently amended version of the IDEA (P.L. 108–446) states that transition-related planning must begin for students with disabilities when they are 16 years old or earlier based on individual student needs (§614 (d)(1)(A)(i)(VII)). Students receiving transition-related planning and services may graduate or complete high school around the age of 18 with their age peers who do not have disabilities. Others may continue to receive school-funded education and transition services through the age of 21. The high school exit point differs for different students. Ideally students either graduate or complete their schooling and do not drop out. High school exit decisions (before age 22) are based on individual student needs and goals as determined by the transition team.

Transition team is a term that is used throughout this chapter. It refers to the interdisciplinary and interagency team required by IDEA and that is assembled by the school. The transition team is responsible for the development of the student's individualized education program (IEP) and subsequent transition services (§614 (d)). In some school districts, the transition team goes by other names such as IEP team or individualized transition team. Regardless of the team's name, the role remains the same and all team members share responsibility for the student's achievement of positive post–high school outcomes.

The student is the most critical and central member of his or her transition team and is joined by an array of school and community professionals. When appropriate, the student's parent or guardian joins the team as an essential partner. It is the student's parents or other family members who most often accompany the student during the entire journey into adult life by providing essential support along the way. In contrast, professional members of the transition team are involved for only portions of the student's journey. When considered in this way, e need for professional members of the transition team to rtner with family members becomes evident.

Students who receive transition services must have a disabil- that fits one or more of the disability categories recognized IDEA: mental retardation; hearing impairment including afness, speech, or language impairments; visual impairments ncluding blindness); serious emotional disturbance; orthope- c impairments; autism; traumatic brain injury; other health npairments; or specific learning disabilities (§602 (3)(A)(ii)). urthermore, students with identified disabilities who receive ecialized instruction (special education) are automatically igible for related services such as occupational therapy.

OCCUPATIONAL THERAPY CONTRIBUTIONS TO TRANSITION

ccupational therapy is included as a transition service when ae transition team determines that occupational therapy can elp the student access, participate in, and benefit from his r her specialized education and transition services. Regardless f the student's disability label, the occupational therapist's ivolvement with a particular student is based on that stu-ent's demonstrated or anticipated problem(s) in performance nd participation in education and transition-related activities nd contexts. These contexts may include the high school lassroom, a variety of in-school environments, public trans-ortation systems, the general community, home, internship lacements, community job sites, and more.

Occupational therapists and occupational therapy assistants re highly qualified to serve as transition team members. Occu-ational therapy personnel working in schools understand the ducational performance and participation demands, opportu-ities, and challenges experienced by children and youth with lisabilities. Of importance, they use conditional reasoning[56] o understand and, to some extent, anticipate how a student's lisability may affect his or her transition to post–high school ctivities and roles including postsecondary or vocational edu-ation, employment, and community living. Occupational herapists' positive, future-oriented view of students combines commitment to student-centered services, collaborative team work, and achievement of performance and participation out-omes, making them a valuable addition to a student's transi-ion team.

Transition service follows the major steps outlined in the Occupational Therapy Framework: Domain and Process.[4] Student-focused evaluation, intervention, and outcome achieve-ment characterize the occupational therapy process and are read-ly integrated and coordinated with the work of other transition team members. For instance, a transition-focused student *evalu-ation* completed by the therapist considers the student in his or her actual performance contexts and all *evaluation* findings are shared with the team to guide subsequent planning and services (*intervention*). Occupational therapy *intervention* may then occur directly with the student, indirectly through other mem-bers of the team, or at a system level. For instance, a transition-focused *intervention* recommended by the occupational therapist to promote student self-determination can be carried out by the therapist by working directly with the student and can be imple-mented by other team members after training and with support provided by the occupational therapist. In another context, the

therapist *intervenes* on behalf of the student by working at the system level to expand the high school's work-study or internship program to better include students with disabilities.[3,28,34] Dur-ing the intervention process, the occupational therapist may establish a system for the student's job coach to consistently gather data on the student's job performance. Systematic data collection and monitoring of student performance allow the entire team to understand student progress and to modify ser-vices as needed. The third and final step of the occupational ther-apy process focuses on the extent to which the student has achieved targeted performance and participation outcomes. Occupational therapy's outcome focus is absolutely consistent with the intent of transition services as mandated by IDEA. Occupational therapists who are already familiar with the need to help students make tangible progress toward desired perfor-mance outcomes will be an asset to any transition team. It is this critical focus on performance and participation outcomes that drives evaluation and intervention activities and that justifies occupational therapy involvement with transition-age students.

When the occupational therapy process is examined at a dee-per level, occupational therapists will recognize that their ser-vices can occur at multiple levels and can address student performance skills and patterns, performance contexts, and activity demands. Transition-focused occupational therapists will find themselves helping students establish new skills, transfer skills to new contexts and activities, modify contexts and activ-ities to better support performance and participation, and, at times, use approaches to prevent new performance problems.[4] Given the age of the students being served and the positive focus of transition services on student ability versus disability, rarely will the therapist work to remediate underlying student variables tied to body structure or function. Alternatively, com-pensation and adaptation play a very prominent role in the design and delivery of transition services provided by the occu-pational therapist and other members of the transition team.[68]

This chapter connects transition policy and research-supported practices in a way that allows occupational therapy personnel to see, understand, and articulate their role in the transition process and as members of a collaborative, interdisci-plinary, and interagency transition team. A variety of student stories and examples are included throughout to further illustrate how occupational therapy personnel work with transition-age youth. Occupational therapy, when added to the mix of transition services, can make a real difference in the lives of young people, whose goals and dreams include some combination of post–high school employment, commu-nity living, further education or training, economic self-sufficiency, and social connections.[35]

THE INTERSECTION OF POLICY AND SCIENTIFIC EVIDENCE

The federal mandate for comprehensive school-to-adult life transition services was issued in 1990 following years of study by the Office of Special Education Programs in the U.S. Department of Education.[42,68] While laws guaranteeing all chil-dren a free and appropriate public education have been in place since 1975 after passage of the Education of all Handicapped Children Act (P.L. 94–142), outcome-focused research during 1980s and 1990s revealed that educational results for youth with disabilities were disappointing at best. The extensive public investment in specialized education and related services was not consistently producing competent, well-adjusted, and self-sufficient adults. High rates of unemployment or underemployment, dependency, and social isolation characterized post–high school years for students with disabilities.[29,44,64,65]

While very important in the shaping of federal transition policy, early outcome-focused research did little to help education and related service professionals identify which specific transition practices were most likely to produce the best results for youth. Transition policy as stated in IDEA (P.L. 105-17) specified system level processes and expected post high school outcomes, but does not specify practices to promote those outcomes.

In the absence of research-supported practices, responsibility for the early design and implementation of transition services landed squarely on the shoulders of local and state education agencies, teachers and related service professionals, and others who worked directly with youth. At the same time, the U.S. Department of Education began to invest in transition-related research, model demonstration projects, and personnel preparation efforts to build the knowledge and skill base of transition-focused education and related service professionals.[42] This effort continues today through the "What Works" and other research programs sponsored by the U.S. Department of Education's Institute for Education Sciences. Research findings from a variety of federally funded projects are constantly growing and are presented in understandable and usable formats through the U.S. Department of Education website.

Unlike the transition pioneers of the 1990s, special education and related service professionals in the twenty-first century can now draw upon a growing body of practice-focused research, which takes much of the guesswork out of transition service design and delivery. Furthermore, research-demonstrated relationships between particular transition practices and positive student outcomes provide local school districts with greater confidence that they can meet both the intent and letter of the transition provisions laid out in IDEA. It will be the ongoing interaction between policy and research that will add needed detail to the transition services "road map" used by education and related service professionals working to prepare youth to reach their adult life destinations.

IDEA initially established transition policy and outcome-focused transition services. It is not, however, the only federal law that addresses the transition needs of youth. Other federal laws with particular relevance include Section 504 of the Rehabilitation Act (P.L. 93-516), the Americans with Disabilities Act (ADA) (i.e., PL 101-336), and Ticket to Work Incentive Improvement Act (P.L. 106-170). Beginning with the IDEA, these four federal laws are introduced here because of their central importance in the overall transition landscape.

Transition Policy

Individuals with Disabilities Education Act

The Individuals with Disabilities Education Improvement Act of 2004 (P.L. 108-446), still known as IDEA, is the federal law most responsible for ensuring that children and youth with disabilities have access to publicly funded, individualized

education including school-to-adult life transition services. Initially passed in 1975, IDEA is the law responsible for the strong presence of occupational therapists in public schools. Foundational to IDEA are the following core beliefs expressed by the U.S. Congress and written into the law:

> Disability is a natural part of the human experience and in no way diminishes the right of individuals to participate in or contribute to society. Improving educational results for children with disabilities is an essential element of our national policy of ensuring equality of opportunity, full participation, independent living, and economic self-sufficiency for individuals with disabilities (§601(d)(1)(A)).

Beginning with the 1997 amendments to IDEA, participation of all students within the general education context became a central focus. Specifically, students with disabilities receiving specialized instruction (special education) were expected to participate and show progress in the general curriculum alongside their same-age peers without disabilities. This means that for students with and without disabilities, the general education standards provide educational achievement and performance targets.

With specialized support, many students with disabilities can and will achieve general education targets. For other students with disabilities, steady and individualized progress towards general education standards is the expectation. IDEA's focus on student participation in general education has significantly raised the educational bar for the nation's children and youth who have disabilities. The general education focus of IDEA challenges previously held views and practices of separate special and general education programs, staff, and curricula.[20,42]

Accompanying the shift toward a single general education system, special educators and related service personnel including occupational therapists are similarly shifting their roles and activities to better support students and their teachers within a variety of general education and transition-related contexts. Collaboration with teachers and others characterizes the evolving role of transition-focused occupational therapists, who are expected to help students achieve postsecondary education, vocational training, employment, and/or community living outcomes.

Occupational therapists working under the auspices of IDEA must understand the overarching purpose of the law and its key provisions. The full text of the IDEA law and a variety of interpretive resources are readily available at the U.S. Department of Education website (http://www.ed.gov) and are essential reading for school-based occupational therapy personnel. As a starting point, familiarity with the following IDEA purpose statement and definitions will be helpful:

- The purpose of IDEA is "to ensure that all children with disabilities have available to them a free appropriate public education that emphasizes special education and related services designed to meet their unique needs and prepare them for further education, employment, and independent living" (§601(d)).
- Special education is defined as "specially designed instruction, at no cost to parents, to meet the unique needs of a child with a disability" (§602(29)).

- Related services are defined as "transportation, and such developmental, corrective, and other supportive services (including speech-language pathology and audiology services, interpreting services, psychological services, physical and occupational therapy, recreation, including therapeutic recreation, social work services, school nurse services designed to enable a child with a disability to receive a free appropriate public education as described in the individualized education program of the child, counseling services, including rehabilitation counseling, orientation and mobility services, and medical services, except that such medical services shall be for diagnostic and evaluation purposes only) as may be required to assist a child with a disability to benefit from special education, and includes the early identification and assessment of disabling conditions in children" (§602 (26)).

- Transition services are defined as a coordinated set of activities for a child with a disability that "(A) is designed to be within a results-oriented process, that is focused on improving the academic and functional achievement of the child with a disability to facilitate the child's movement from school to post-school activities, including post-secondary education, vocational education, integrated employment (including supported employment), continuing and adult education, adult services, independent living, or community participation; (B) is based on the individual child's needs, taking into account the child's strengths, preferences, and interests; and (C) includes instruction, related services, community experiences, the development of employment and other post-school adult living objectives, and, when appropriate, acquisition of daily living skills and functional vocational evaluation" (§602(26)).

Section 504 of the Rehabilitation Act

A second federal law that impacts public education and the school-to-adult life transition process is Section 504 of the Rehabilitation Act (as amended in 1998 by P.L. 93–516). Initially signed into law in 1973, Section 504 was among the first civil rights laws prohibiting discrimination on the basis of disability by any program or agency receiving federal funding and defines individuals with disabilities as "persons with a physical or mental impairment which substantially limits one or more major life activities" (34 C.F.R. §104.3 (j)(2)(i)). Subparts of the law address specific areas in which discrimination is prohibited, including employment, building and program accessibility, schooling (preschool through secondary education), and postsecondary education (colleges, universities, community colleges, vocational programs).

The concept of "reasonable accommodation" first appeared in Section 504 and is tied to the law's employment protections. Reasonable accommodation means that an employer (or educational institution) must take reasonable steps to accommodate an individual's disability. This may mean installing grab bars in work or learning areas, purchasing assistive technology to support job or school performance, ramping an entrance, or providing specific job-related training (refer to the U.S. Department of Health and Human Services Office for Civil Rights' Web page at http://www.hhs.gov/ocr/504.html). The term "reasonable," while somewhat vague, is used in the law to protect employers from "undue hardship" when accommodations are needed or requested. The law recognizes that for some employers, the resources needed to provide accommodations for an individual employee who has a disability may exceed employer resources. Most accommodations, however, are in fact low cost, which is outweighed by the benefit of having a motivated and reliable worker who happens to have a disability.

As transition-age students begin to explore the realm of work and careers (Figure 27-1), it is important to recognize that organizations receiving federal funding have a history of Section 504 compliance. Furthermore, these organizations

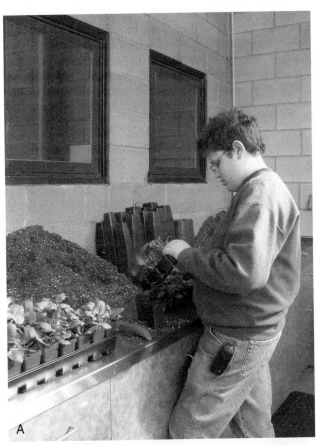

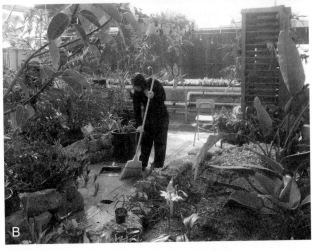

FIGURE 27-1 Career exploration through community volunteer opportunities.

may be very receptive to hiring high school students or recent high school completers who have disabilities. Similarly, post-secondary education programs (e.g., community colleges, vocational schools, universities) that receive federal funding must comply with Section 504 and are often well equipped to accommodate students who have disabilities as they pursue their career-focused education and training.

While Section 504 prohibits discrimination against individuals on the basis of disability, these individuals must still meet all employment and education-related qualifications or admission criteria. Section 504 does not provide the same specialized education and related services that are available under IDEA.

Prevention of disability-related discrimination is at the core of the Rehabilitation Act and Section 504; however, the law also created a nationwide network of vocational rehabilitation (VR) services to enable potential workers with disabilities to ultimately enter and be successful in the workforce. VR is supported by a blend of federal and state resources and provides needed employment and independent living support for adults with disabilities. An individual who is eligible for VR services works with a VR counselor, who can serve as an important member of school-based transition team. The VR counselor is expected to work in concert with school personnel to plan for the student's future job-related education/training, job placement, and independent living. VR can provide qualified individuals with needed financial support for job training, job placement services, job coaching, postsecondary education, and independent living. In all cases, VR-supported services are outcome oriented, with community employment and improved self-sufficiency as the end goal. School-based occupational therapists may work closely with VR counselors on behalf of young adults with disabilities, to optimize the match between the individual and available job or postsecondary education opportunities, to recommend needed accommodations, and to address community and independent living needs.

Americans with Disabilities Act

The Americans with Disabilities Act (ADA) of 1990 (amended in 2008) (P.L. 110–325) is a civil rights law and, like Section 504 of the Rehabilitation Act, focuses on accessibility and non-discrimination. Unlike Section 504, ADA protections extend beyond programs and services that receive federal funding. The ADA addresses access and discrimination in public and private schools, business establishments, and public buildings. The law also establishes clear accessibility standards for new building construction and public facilities. Occupational therapists working with transition-age youth are advised to become familiar with the ADA and its many provisions so they can assist employers and public facilities to eliminate barriers and provide reasonable accommodations for young adults with disabilities.

Ticket to Work and Work Incentive Improvement Act

Ticket to Work and Work Incentive Improvement Act (P.L. 106-170) was initially passed in 1999. It allows workers who have disabilities and who receive Medicare or Medicaid insurance to keep their needed health care benefits after they obtain paid employment. Before the Ticket to Work program, workers with disabilities faced the potential loss of needed medical insurance and health care when they became employed. Among individuals with disabilities who can and want to work, the possibility of losing needed health care benefits can create a powerful disincentive for employment and self-sufficiency. Ticket to Work now provides a safety net for workers who do not have access to private or employer-provided health insurance. Income earned by workers enrolled in Ticket to Work offsets federal or state disability income. The result is a more self-sufficient worker who has access to needed health care and who has reduced his or her need for publicly funded disability income.

Given the critical nature of health care for many individuals who have disabilities, high-quality transition services must address the student's future health care needs and available health care insurance. For students whose future employment or postsecondary education opportunities are unlikely to include health care benefits, applying for Ticket to Work benefits is a particularly important component of the transition planning process.

Evidence-Based Practice

Federal education policy and our nation's commitment to civil rights and equal educational opportunity mobilized initial school-to-adult life transition efforts in the United States. Policies specify expected education outcomes plus procedures and processes that must be followed by state and local education agencies to ensure that all children have access to a free and appropriate education. Policies, however, do not specify which research-supported practices are most likely to produce the desired outcomes. Added to the challenge of identifying the most effective practices is the challenge of generating high-quality research evidence that can be widely applied to diverse students who are enrolled in many different types of educational contexts and activities.[49] Despite challenges, promising transition practices have emerged from the ongoing work of education and related service professionals and, increasingly, research (Box 27-1).

Using scientifically based transition practices is an expectation of IDEA, which states that services must be based on "peer-reviewed research to the extent practicable" (§614 (d) (1)(A)(i)(IV)). Like special education, the occupational

---

BOX 27-1 The Complexities of Special Education Research

Special education research, because of its complexity, may be the hardest of the hardest-to-do science. One feature of special education research that makes it more complex is the variability of the participants...A second dimension of complexity is the educational context. Special education extends beyond the traditional conceptualization of 'schooling' for typical students... or adolescents and youth adults with disabilities, special education may take place in community living or vocational settings in preparation for the transition out of high school and into the workplace.

From Odom, S., Brantlinger, E., Horner, R., Thompson, B., & Harris, K. (2005). Research in special education: Scientific methods and evidence-based practices. *Exceptional Children, 71*, 139.

therapy profession is also dedicated to the principles of evidence-based practice and the continuous expansion of high-quality, peer-reviewed research to improve services and results for the individuals, groups, and organizations served.[41]

The school-to-adult life transition needs of youth with disabilities can be met by blending policy, a growing body of peer-reviewed research, and the accumulated experience of thoughtful transition service providers. The following set of four recommended practices provide critical direction for transition-focused programs and are based on scientific studies presented in the peer-reviewed literature. Though widely used, these practices are effective only when accompanied by another type of scientific evidence: the systematic monitoring of individual student progress and performance in relevant contexts.[55] This second type of evidence is student and context specific; it is not generally reported in peer-reviewed research journals. For the purposes of this chapter, it is be termed "practice-based evidence."[4,18,19,37,55,61]

Recommended transition practices from the peer-reviewed scientific literature include the following:

1. Collaborative, interdisciplinary, and interagency teamwork that is outcome-oriented, student-centered, and that enlists family members as transition partners[5,46,48,68]
2. Application of ecologic assessment and intervention to include the use of accommodation strategies linked to the student's actual performance context[5,46,68]
3. Self-determination, self-regulation, and social competence training[2,5,15,45,46,67]
4. Paid work experience during high school[5,46,68]

The preceding practices are supported by research, and none exists in isolation from the others. For example, the recommended practice of evaluating student performance in a variety of actual work or community contexts (ecologic assessment) can be helpful only if it leads to student placement in meaningful community-based work opportunities (paid work experience). Similarly, seeking partnerships with families and then failing to address each family's unique time and resource constraints can undermine the family's ability to support and participate as valued team members during transition planning and services (collaborative teamwork). Teams that provide meaningful and real opportunities for students to participate in and influence the future course of their lives (self-determination) can accept student input even when this leads to employment or postsecondary education decisions that do not match the preferences or values of individual team members. Teams that respectfully invite and honor the contributions of students will find that even students with very limited abilities can demonstrate self-determined actions.[2,45]

Transition-related research appears primarily in the special education literature and relies on multiple research methodologies. Much of this research may be termed "emergent" or "preliminary" in that it offers strong beginning evidence for the use of certain transition practices that are linked with specific student outcomes such as employment, postsecondary education, or community living. Occupational therapy has also been termed a "research emergent" field, which indicates that the body of knowledge linking specific interventions or practices with occupational performance and participation outcomes is still growing.[33] Over time and with additional high-quality research, the evidence linking specific transition practices with student outcomes will come into sharper focus.[16,41,49] This

chapter considers transition practices that are based on multiple scientific studies and reported in the peer-reviewed research literature as evidence-based practice.

Collaborative Interdisciplinary and Interagency Teamwork

Outcome-oriented, student-centered planning and services based on collaborative teamwork are at the center of high-quality transition services.[67] For transition-age students, this teamwork is accomplished by the individualized education program (IEP) team. *IEP team* is synonymous with *transition team*, the term used throughout this chapter because it conveys an essential transition focus for IEP processes and documentation. As students with disabilities move toward the end of their high school careers, all IEP planning and services must converge around the student's postsecondary goals and activities.[38]

Membership on the transition team is determined in part by IDEA policy and in part by the unique interests and needs of the student. At a minimum, the team must include the student, a special education teacher, a general education teacher, and a school district representative (§614 (d)(1) (B)). Transition teams are strongly advised in IDEA and through research to include the student's parent or family representative and selected representatives from community agencies or programs that are currently providing services to the student or that are likely to provide support or service at a future date (Box 27-2).[46]

When the student, family members, teachers, and related service personnel are joined on the transition team by representatives from nonschool agencies, the interdisciplinary team becomes an interagency team. Congress, when crafting the IDEA, did not intend for schools to have sole responsibility for transition processes and outcomes. Interagency linkages became a part of IDEA in 1990, indicating the expectation for shared responsibility across local education agencies and adult or community programs. Establishing interagency linkages, while challenging, can be of enormous benefit to students with disabilities who are preparing to exit the public education system.[60]

Upon graduation or completion of public education programs, a student's IDEA-based entitlement to school-sponsored

---

BOX 27-2 Family-Professional Partnerships

Common sense and ordinary human decency are at the heart of positive partnerships between families and professionals serving children with disabilities....Discussion between parents and professionals in each community or school setting is important because it provides...an opportunity for parent and professionals to understand each other's points of view. Professionals need to hear directly from families their stories about how various actions or inactions have impacted their family, and about how well-intentioned actions or comments did or did not have their intended effect. On the other side, parents need to hear and experience professional's perspectives about who and why certain actions were taken, and what the limitation of their own lives might be (p. 181).

From Blue-Banning, M., Summers, J., Frankland, H. C., Nelson, L., & Beegle, G. (2004). Dimensions of family and professional partnerships: Constructive guidelines for collaboration. *Exceptional Children, 70,* 167-184.

educational, vocational, and other services ends. In the place of one lead agency (the school system), a confusing assortment of service providers fills the landscape (e.g., the state vocational rehabilitation agency, the state departments of mental health and developmental disabilities, state brain injury programs, postsecondary education or training programs). Individuals who are no longer eligible for the school's transition-focused special education or related services become responsible for identifying where to obtain the ongoing services they need and for demonstrating their eligibility to receive those services.

Interagency responsibilities and linkages should be clearly stated in IEP documents developed by the transition team. Failure to initiate and formalize these connections during high school can result in the student's being left out of services, sitting for extended periods on waiting lists, or losing skills and motivation because of lost opportunities to participate in employment, community living, or postsecondary education. The importance of strong interagency linkages cannot be overstated.

As important as having the right mix of team members is consideration for how the team works together. *Collaboration* has long been considered an essential quality of effective education and transition teams.[23,24,28,50,58] Rainforth and York-Barr provided an enduring description of collaboration within educational contexts: "an interactive process in which individuals with varied life perspectives and experiences can join together in a spirit of willingness to share resources, responsibility, and rewards in creating inclusive and effective educational programs and environments for students with unique learning capacities and needs" (p. 18).[51]

For transition-age students, collaboration is viewed as an effective way for a team to come together to help them plan for and achieve desired transition outcomes in the areas of postsecondary education, community living and recreation, and employment. Collaborative teams have a shared sense of purpose with shared responsibility for student outcomes.[28,58] An effective transition team is not simply a collection of individuals, each with a different set of skills or degrees. In the language of Hanft and Shepherd, transition teams cannot function if the members behave as "lone rangers."[28] Collaboration should be evident during the planning of individualized transition services, which is captured in the student's IEP document and can also be observed during the implementation of transition services by multiple members of the team in a variety of school and community contexts (Box 27-3).

Essential for collaborative teamwork is the creation of a shared, positive vision for student outcomes that drives all subsequent team decisions. To illustrate, a transition-related evaluation to guide service planning for a student who plans to attend college, live in a dorm, and study culinary arts will be significantly different from the transition-related evaluation completed for a student who plans to live at home and work in a private, home-based childcare setting directly out of high school (Figure 27-2). By remaining focused on desired student outcomes and targeted performance contexts, the evaluation process can help team members get "on board" while also building team momentum towards desired results.

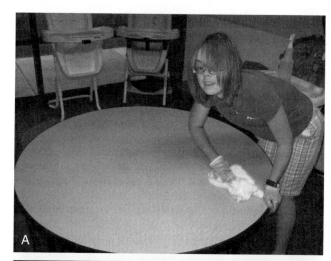

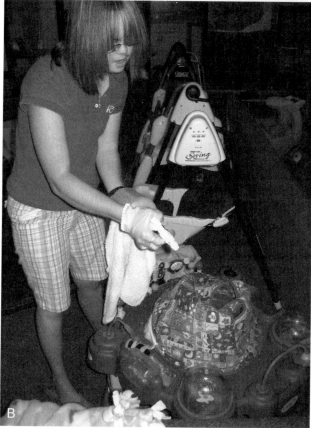

FIGURE 27-2 A real job in a daycare setting.

BOX 27-3 Collaboration: What Is It?

School-based collaboration is an interactive team process that focuses student, family, education, and related services partners on enhancing the academic achievement and functional performance of all students in school (p. 3).

  Key collaboration ingredients include the following:
  A group of people working towards a shared goal
  An interactive group process characterized by a true
    desire to share resources, responsibility, and rewards
  More than cooperation and compromise; requires shared
    meaning, decision making, and accountability

From Hanft, B., & Shepherd, J. (2008). *Collaborating for student success: A guide for school-based occupational therapy.* Bethesda, MD: AOTA Press.

Numerous formats exist to help the team move through the critical "vision" process to identify potential transition outcomes.[47,57] For example, the student and the team may discuss a future that includes living in an apartment or a home with others who are identified or chosen by the student, use of community services (e.g., transportation, shopping, banking) and amenities (e.g., joining a health club, attending public concerts), employment (full- or part-time employment or other productive volunteer work), postsecondary education (vocational training or university enrollment), and relationships. Not surprisingly, these are goals that most people, with or without disabilities, envision for themselves or their loved ones.

While establishing a positive vision for the student's future, the team also begins to consider the student's anticipated long-term needs for resources and support that will allow the vision to become reality. For example, a young adult with significant disabilities may require long-term job support in the form of a job coach, who provides on-the-job training and other support needed to maintain employment. Another individual with high-functioning autism may require social and academic support or accommodations to be in place and operational at the selected university before the start of the school year.

This type of planning is often termed person-centered[47] and involves a group of individuals who know the student well and who have come together to engage in positive, facilitated discussion focused on the student's future. Emerging from this discussion is a comprehensive understanding of the student's unique strengths and interests, effective support and accommodations, and potential resources and opportunities that can be incorporated into the student's transition services. Collaborative, group-oriented planning processes have been shown to be a reliable and valid approach to student evaluation and transition planning.[31]

Depending on the student's age, anticipated exit point from high school, and the complexity of student needs, the future being envisioned may be 1 to 5 years into the future. To help the team consider all aspects of transition, including desired outcomes and needed support or services, Wehman recommends that transition teams address eight areas[67]: Many of these can be directly supported by occupational therapy personnel serving as collaborative members of the transition team.[67]

1. Employment opportunities
2. Postsecondary education opportunities
3. Living opportunities
4. Financial and income needs
5. Friendship and socialization needs
6. Transportation needs
7. Health and medical needs
8. Legal and advocacy needs

Transition outcomes that emerge from a collaborative team process help establish a set of transition goals that all members of the team work toward.[28,34] Not needed are discipline-specific goals (e.g., "occupational therapy goals" or "special education goals") established by individual members of the team. Collaboratively developed transition goals help the team unify efforts and share responsibility for services and the ultimate achievement of targeted outcomes (Box 27-4). The collaborative nature of teamwork is illustrated in Case Study 27-1 concerning Mike, a 16-year-old student with emotional, behavioral, and mild cognitive disabilities.

BOX 27-4   Examples of Outcome-Oriented Transition Goals

Goal: By the start of her senior year, Marybeth will secure a paid, part-time horticulture job that is accessible by public bus.

Goal: By the end of the spring semester and in preparation for apartment living, Travis will independently prepare nutritious lunches for himself on 10 consecutive school days using a picture-based meal plan.

Goal: By the end of her senior year, Anna will be registered as a part-time community college student in courses of her choice that can accommodate her use of adapted computing technology to access information, communicate, and complete assignments.

CASE STUDY 27-1   Mike

Following the establishment of a shared vision for Mike's future, members of the team were asked to work together to address Mike's interests and needs in the area of employment. The occupational therapist, teacher, paraprofessional, and vocational rehabilitation counselor began working with Mike toward his interest in a job involving automobiles. Mike's father confirmed Mike's long-time interest in cars and referred the team to a local automotive shop operated by a family friend. Follow-up by the occupational therapist secured two job trials for Mike: one through the family friend and another through a separate contact. Job trials provided essential opportunities for the occupational therapist to conduct observational evaluations of Mike's job-related performance during actual job tasks. Of importance was Mike's ability to take directions from others, ask questions, work steadily to complete assigned tasks, monitor the quality of his own performance, and interact socially with other workers and customers. During the job trials, the occupational therapist identified supports that improved Mike's work performance (e.g., a watch to self-manage time, a visual schedule of job tasks with a prompt for Mike to turn off his cell phone, job instructions provided via demonstration). A first-hand understanding of Mike's work-related performance and promising accommodation strategies allowed the occupational therapist and Mike to collaborate with the special education teacher and vocational rehabilitation counselor to seek a part-time job. Of importance would be finding a job that "matched" Mike's interests and abilities.

When a job opportunity was identified, the occupational therapist collaborated with the prospective employer, Mike, and the paraprofessional who was to serve as Mike's "job coach." Occupational therapy services focused on preparing the job coach to support Mike's initial orientation and training on the job while also facilitating Mike's independent performance. The therapist directly instructed the job coach how to use subtle and nonstigmatizing strategies to support and teach Mike while also monitoring Mike's job performance and job-related needs. Periodic job site "checks" by the special education teacher were arranged to ensure Mike's ongoing success and to support the employer's and the job coach's efforts to increase Mike's independence and competence.

Mike's story illustrates the benefits of collaborative teamwork and the involvement of different team member perspectives and knowledge that come together to create effective, individualized services. In addition to the benefits realized by the student, collaboration can benefit team members. Collaborative practices promote cooperative and caring relationships among members of the team, which is characterized by open communication, shared responsibility, and mutual support.[28]

Ecologic Approaches

Ecologically focused curricula for student learners with disabilities were first recommended in the 1970s.[13] In the education literature, the ecologic approach is also referred to as community-referenced or environmentally referenced teaching and learning.[46] Viewed as highly functional, relevant, and contextual, ecologic approaches are considered an essential feature of effective transition practices.[23,51,68] An ecologic approach supports the identification of student performance needs and abilities in the environments that he or she currently uses or is expected to use as an adult. For example, if the team seeks to identify the student's interests, needs, and abilities as they relate to future community living, an ecologic assessment would take place, to a large extent, in the community and the home. Systematic and careful observation of the student's performance during home chores, food shopping, banking, using transportation, and bill paying may be completed to identify discrepancies between the demands of the task or context and the student's current performance level. Services are subsequently designed to reduce these discrepancies by directly teaching the student needed living skills or by modifying tasks and providing accommodations.

Occupational therapy personnel will recognize the ecologic approach; it is deeply ingrained in the field's view of individuals, groups, and populations who desire participation in all areas of human occupation.[4] Ecologic approaches consider the characteristics of the individual and the physical, social, cultural, and temporal demands being placed on that individual by his or her performance context. Similarly, the occupational therapy field has long recognized that human performance and participation can be influenced by strategic changes in features within the environment (e.g., adaptive equipment, addition of social support, task modification).

Occupational therapists can help transition teams adopt ecologic evaluation and intervention approaches. Ecologic thinking contrasts with approaches that emphasize the remediation of a student's underlying deficits (e.g., physical, cognitive, or psychological) as a precondition for performance and participation in targeted transition-related activities. Ecologic approaches accept and value the student's current level of performance, which provides the starting point for improving or refining that performance to better match specific environmental demands or opportunities. This is accomplished by pairing context and task-specific training for the student with any needed adjustments to the performance environment.[46]

Parallels may be drawn between ecologic approaches and dynamic systems theory, which has begun to replace hierarchical and linear explanations of human development and learning.[53] Dynamic systems theory offers, in part, an explanation of human behavior and learning tied directly to the opportunities and demands present within that individual's performance context.[26] Extended to the transition process, students with disabilities may be viewed as complex and dynamic systems that change over time based in large part on their direct interactions with opportunities and challenges present in everyday activities and environments. The opportunities or challenges afforded by the environment may, in fact, be inseparable from an individual's learning and the resulting performance.

Ecologic approaches, as recommended in the transition literature, emphasize ability (versus deficit) thinking. A student's lack of performance is viewed as a mismatch between the student's current abilities or interests and the demands or expectations present in the environment (e.g., completing a school assignment, using the telephone, asking for assistance). Student evaluation by members of the transition team, therefore, requires a balanced look at the student as he or she operates within everyday contexts and activities, followed by services that target both the student's identified learning needs and the environmental demands. The goal is to optimize the match between the student and the demands of a particular context.[5,46]

Occupational therapists and others on the team can contribute to a transition-focused, ecologic assessment by doing the following:

1. **Specify the environments** in which the student will likely participate (e.g., home, postsecondary education, vocational, community, leisure).
2. **Prioritize the performance environments** considered to be most essential in the short term and those that will become more important over time.
3. **Identify the activities** that occur naturally in the selected, prioritized environments (because of validity concerns, team members are strongly discouraged from using contrived activities or artificial or simulated environments for assessment purposes).
4. **Divide responsibility** for conducting different parts of the assessment among members of the educational team. Family members and professionals may share responsibilities during the assessment process.
5. **Conduct assessments** by actually observing student performance during activities in the selected environments. Based on careful observation, discrepancies between the environment and activity demands and the student's ability to perform can be noted. This type of *discrepancy analysis* forms the heart of the assessment and guides later planning and decision making.
6. **Record the evaluation findings** for the purposes of communicating with all members of the educational team, including the student and his or her parents.
7. **Share findings** with the team to facilitate goal setting and the planning of transition services based on an ecologic model.

Table 27-1 contrasts an ecologic assessment (left column) with a more conventional assessment (right column) for a student named Amelia.

Self-Determination, Self-Regulation, and Social Competence Training

A student's active involvement in planning and decision making is considered an important aspect of effective transition services.[2,5,15,45,46,68] To effect self-determination, students need to become positive agents of change in their own lives, who have goals, and who are active (versus passive) in the pursuit of those goals. Such students will realize multiple benefits in the form of positive relationships, community engagement, and quality of

TABLE 27-1 Transition-Focused Evaluations and Services

Amelia is an 18-year-old student who plans to complete high school in approximately 1 year. Her transition goals include sharing an apartment with her sister, having responsibility for some of the household chores, and working part time at her uncle's business stocking supplies and implementing the company's recycling program. Amelia's sister is a student at the local university and her apartment is within walking distance of her uncle's business and a local grocery store. Because of Amelia's diagnosis of autism, her communication and social skills are limited, as is her ability to learn new skills. With an established routine and minimal cuing, Amelia is independent with self-care at home and at school.

	Transition-Focused Evaluation		Transition Services	
	Ecologic Evaluation	**Nonecologic Evaluation**	**Ecologic Services**	**Nonecologic Services**
Home and community living	Observational assessment of meal preparation at sister's apartment (completed by sister with structure provided by OT)	Use of formal assessments within school contexts to evaluate Amelia's level of language development, social skills, compared with peers (completed by special education teacher, speech-language pathologist); observation of Amelia's meal preparation during home arts classes at school (completed by home arts teacher)	An overnight per week at sister's apartment to include meal preparation and selected household chores (OT collaboration with sister, parent, and paraprofessional)	Meal preparation with a small group of students one afternoon per week using the home arts classroom (home arts teacher and paraprofessional)
Community mobility	Observational assessment (completed by OT) of community mobility (travel from apartment to/from workplace, local stores); observational assessment of grocery shopping (completed by speech language pathologist)	Observation of Amelia's mobility and independence within the high school (completed by special education teacher)	Weekly grocery shopping including walking travel between sister's apartment and the local grocery store (OT collaboration with paraprofessional)	Weekly grocery shopping at the store nearest the high school, with a small group of students using the school van for transportation to and from the school (special education teacher and paraprofessional)
Work interests and abilities/employment	Observational assessment of work environment, work demands, and Amelia's performance during work-related tasks at her uncle's business (completed by special education teacher and supported by the OT)	Observation of Amelia's work skills while collecting recyclable materials from school offices and classrooms (completed by special education teacher)	Job trial at uncle's business three afternoons per week (teacher and OT collaboration with employer and school-supported job coach)	Job trial with the janitorial staff at the high school 3 days per week (teacher and OT collaboration with janitorial staff and paraprofessional)

life.[2,15,66,71] Promoting self-determined student engagement in the transition process permeates all transition services and must be supported by all members of the transition team.

Regardless of the type or severity of the student's disability, it is incumbent upon the team to enlist the active involvement of the student to the maximum extent possible. Research indicates that the transition planning meeting or IEP provides an important opportunity for positive and proactive student involvement.[15,45,70] For example, the student (with or without support) may prepare the agenda, introduce team members, or chair the meeting. To assume these functions, students need direct support and preparation from a member of the transition team to consider possible transition goals, activities, and timetables. During the transition-focused IEP meeting, attending professionals and parents must be willing to relinquish "expert control" and support the student's lead while maintaining a focus on the student's strengths and abilities versus deficits (Box 27-5).

To help transition team members prepare students to be self-determined, a number of curricula are available.[69] With or without a specific curriculum, it is critical that all members of the transition team, including the occupational therapist, have knowledge about self-determined student participation and its relationship to positive transition outcomes. Furthermore, all members of the team must collaborate to implement strategies that promote student self-determination across multiple school and community contexts including engagement in planning and decision making. This means that promoting self-determination cannot be assigned to a single team member and cannot occur within a single context.

Among the critical ingredients needed for students to become self-determined and self-directed agents in their own future are social competencies[67] and the ability to self-regulate.[1,73] Transition team members must consistently provide students with opportunities to learn and practice

---

BOX 27-5   Self-Determination and Student-Directed Planning Meetings

IDEA calls for students to be actively involved in planning their individualized education programs (IEPs) and transition-related services. Student involvement in planning provides an opportunity to learn and practice critical self-determination skills and is considered essential preparation for postschool decision making and success. A number of self-directed IEP approaches, when used by students with disabilities, have been linked to positive changes in student self-determination. These approaches have been demonstrated to be effective with students who are often unengaged in their own future planning, including students who have emotional and behavioral disabilities, significant learning disabilities, and moderate to severe developmental disabilities.

Data from Carter, E. W., Lane, K. L., Pierson, M. R., & Glaeser, B. (2006). Self-determination skills and opportunities of transition-age youth with emotional and learning disabilities. *Exceptional Children, 72* (3), 333-346; and Martin, J. E., Van Dycke, J. L., Christensen, W. R., Greene, B. A., Gardener, J. E., & Lovett, D. L. (2006). Increasing student participation in IEP meetings: Establishing the self-directed IEP as an evidence-based practice. *Exceptional Children, 72* (3), 299-316.

self-monitoring and regulation strategies in a variety of contexts while receiving support and constructive feedback (Box 27-6).

Incidents of widely publicized youth violence in schools magnify the importance of building and supporting social competence and self-regulation among transition-age youth. Furthermore, promoting a school climate that skillfully recognizes and addresses bullying and other forms of violence is now considered

---

BOX 27-6   Social Competence and Job Performance for Adolescents with Emotional and Behavioral Disabilities

For students with emotional and behavioral disabilities, completing high school poses a significant challenge, with more than half of these students dropping out. When compared with their age peers who do not have disabilities, these students experience substantial difficulty obtaining and maintaining community employment owing in part to a lack of essential workplace social skills and behaviors.

Compounding these concerns is the lack of adolescent awareness and insight regarding their own job performance. These youth view their own performance significantly more favorably than their employers do.

Implications for practice:

Explicit training and programming must be offered during secondary school to address social and work skills deemed critical for job success.

Because of the variable expectations for workers in different job settings, social skill training must be context specific, with immediate supervisors (not school personnel) evaluating the adolescent's work skills and behaviors.

Job-related social skills training, practice, and feedback must be provided during a variety of actual work experiences in a respectful and supportive manner to minimize the stigma associated with having an emotional or behavioral disability.

Data from Carter, E.W. & Wehby, J.H. (2003). Job performance of transition-age youth with emotional and behavioral disorders. *Exceptional Children, 69,* 449-465.

BOX 27-7   Youth Violence: Considerations for Transition Planning

Youth violence is a leading cause of death in injury among youth. It includes bullying, verbal threats, physical assault, domestic abuse, and gunfire. Youth violence is associated with multiple risk factors that reside within the individual (e.g., mental illness) and the environment (e.g., history of being abused, addiction, poverty). It can lead to school failure, disability, and premature death.

From an occupational therapy perspective, youth violence and its causes can restrict engagement in meaningful occupations and severely compromise an individual's future opportunities. Occupational therapists can support change by helping youth make positive occupational choices during the school-to-adult life transition process.

essential.[7,36] School-based transition teams must take seriously the opportunity provided by transition policy and individualized transition services to help youth who are at risk for school or postschool failure or involvement in violence. These students must learn how to set goals, make positive plans, take responsibility, work well with others, and handle challenges or frustration. For youth with significant emotional or behavioral disabilities, this is particularly important and requires early and ongoing attention by the transition team in cooperation with other school-based or community-based professionals (Box 27-7).[15]

Because social competence is such an important part of self-determined engagement in the school-to-work transition process, students who have autism may have a significant disadvantage in this area (Box 27-8). Self-determination generally requires some level of interaction with others and with a

---

BOX 27-8   Social Competence for Students with Autism As They Make the Transition to Postsecondary Education

Students with autism who are entering postsecondary education programs can experience difficulties with socialization and social competence. These students risk social isolation, social exploitation, and high levels of social stress.

The following supports are recommended for students with autism spectrum disorders involved in the transition from high school to college life:

Explicit teaching, coaching and support to develop needed self-advocacy skills (e.g., when and how to disclose a disability, how to approach instructors for needed accommodations, how to approach classmates)

Establishment of a liaison or "point person" the student can access with questions or when feeling overwhelmed or confused by social or academic demands

Establishment of a peer mentor (a supportive and knowledgeable college student) who can provide social translation and support

Identification of a safe place to go or relax

Identification of people to contact if hazing or exploitation occur

---

Data from Adreon, D. & Durocher, J.S. (2007). Evaluating the college transition needs of individuals with high-functioning autism spectrum disorders. *Intervention in School and Clinics, 42,* 271-279.

BOX 27-9   Transitioning from High School to Postsecondary Education and Training Programs

While students are enrolled in high school and as they begin the transition to postsecondary education, direct and facilitated opportunities must be provided for students to develop and practice the following skills:

- Self-advocacy (e.g., communicating needs to instructors, asking questions, requesting reasonable accommodations, initiate study groups)
- Self-regulation (e.g., goal setting and attainment, self-observation and evaluation, problem identification and problem solving, persistence)
- Internal locus of control (e.g., self-confidence and change agent, expectation for positive results)
- Self-knowledge (e.g., understanding of own learning style and needs, awareness and timely use of alternative learning and performance strategies)

Having and using these skills will allow students to be empowered and to take responsibility for their own learning.

Data from Hong, B., Ivy, W. F., Gonzalez, H. R., & Ehrensberger, W. (2007). Preparing students for postsecondary education. *Teaching Exceptional Children, 40,* 32-38.

variety of "systems" (e.g., employers, postsecondary education institutions, roommates). Well-planned and timely academic, social, and vocational support can greatly facilitate meaningful participation in adult roles and activities by students who have autism (Box 27-9).

Case Study 27-2 illustrates how transition-related services can support self-determined student participation in transition planning and the ongoing practice of social and self-regulation skills.

Recommended Practice: Paid work experience during high school

According to the National Longitudinal Transition Study 2 commissioned by the Institute for Education Sciences of the U.S. Department of Education, student engagement in paid work before his or her exit from high school is strongly associated with post high school employment.[14,44] Even for students who plan to pursue postsecondary education, the ability to obtain and hold down a job is considered a critical life skill that cannot be delayed until all formal education is complete. Furthermore, parallels may be drawn between inclusive educational practices that occur in elementary and secondary school and community-based employment for transition-age youth who have disabilities. Perhaps student employment in the community during the transition from school to adult life is simply an extension of inclusive school practices.[59] The importance of paid employment for youth with disabilities cannot be overstated; such employment is often at the center of many school-to-adult life transition programs.

Although there are many ways in which individuals may go about securing paid work,[9] students who have disabilities may lack the ability to effectively access or use conventional job search strategies. For these students, supported employment provides an excellent alternative that has strong research support.[39,43,52] Simply defined, supported employment is real work that is paid and that occurs in community businesses and organizations with on-the-job training and support

provided as needed by a job coach. Robert Lawhead, a parent and supported employment professional from Colorado, described supported employment in the following way during his testimony before the U.S. Senate on Oct. 20, 2005:

> In the late seventies and early eighties, professionals developed a process for employing people with very significant disabilities within the regular workforce. The process has been refined over the past 25 years and is referred to as "supported employment" which is defined as integrated paid work, within businesses and industry, with ongoing support. Presently it is estimated that nearly 200,000 people with severe disabilities are employed within our business communities through supported employment and similar strategies such as supported self-employment and customized employment.
>
> Evidence-based research completed over the last 25 years shows that employment programs placing people into business and industry represents a good tax-payer investment. When one public dollar is spent on supported employment service costs, tax-payers earn more than a dollar in benefits through increased taxes paid, decreased government subsidies, and foregone program costs. Further, this positive cost-benefit relationship for community employment holds true for people with the most significant disabilities and is stronger when people are employed individually as opposed to within group models of employment (e.g., sheltered employment).[40]

Many variations on supported employment exist to meet unique individual or contextual needs. Occupational therapy personnel can be instrumental in helping the transition team apply different supported employment strategies such as job carving or job customization.

According to Griffin and Targett, *job carving* is defined as "determining the job seeker's skills, interests, and contributions and matching these to a set of duties found in the local workplace. Because such job descriptions rarely appear as a perfect match, carving involves creating a new list of duties that meet both employer and employee needs and which complement the common interests of both." (p. 290).[27] For example, a student may obtain an office job with one primary duty carved out of the typical list of office worker duties: paper shredding. In this case, paper shredding matches the abilities, interests, and needs of the student worker *and* the employer (Figure 27-3).

Customized employment, according to the U.S. Department of Labor, "may include employment developed through job carving, self-employment, or entrepreneurial initiatives, or other job development or restructuring strategies that result in job responsibilities being customized and individually negotiated to fit the needs of individuals with a disability." For example, a student who cannot handle the noise and distractions associated with working in a busy warehouse may work with her transition team to arrange an "after hours" shift to break down, stack, and bundle cardboard boxes for recycling.

Enabling youth who have disabilities to secure community employment that is individually matched to their interests is among the most important achievements of transition-focused teams. It is primarily around employment that local VR agencies become involved and can apply state VR resources to either support the student's job search and placement process or to fund postsecondary education at a university, community college, or vocational training program as long as a career/job path is evident.[5,46] Case Study 27-3 demonstrates how supported employment can work for a young woman who sustained a brain injury.

CASE STUDY 27-2 Brian

Brian is 17 years old and receives special education and related services at his local high school. Staying in school has been a challenge for Brian, who is making limited progress in his academic subjects. He reports, "I'm not very smart—just look at my grades. What's the point of trying, I never get anywhere." School staff who have reached out to Brian have discovered that he is very interested in art and music, is a self-taught electric bass player, and likes to hang out in the music room at school, where he helps the teacher with a variety of tasks. Brian particularly enjoys searching on the computer for music-related images and cartoons that the teacher can use when creating concert posters and class handouts. The music teacher has a very positive and open relationship with Brian even though Brian is not enrolled in any of his classes. When asked who Brian would like to include on his transition team, he identified the music teacher, who has since joined the team along with his special education teacher, the occupational therapist, his school counselor, the school social worker, and Brian's mother.

Brian has a history of depression and specific learning disabilities that affect reading, writing, and organization. He is being raised by his mother, who works multiple jobs to make ends meet for herself and her two children (Brian has a younger brother). Brian has few friends at school and is often seen alone in the hallways and at lunch. A recent stretch of absences revealed that he was ditching school and hanging out with a group of former students known for drug use and petty crime.

The occupational therapist on the team recognized Brian's "hands-on" drawing, music, and computer skills. She also understood Brian's sensitivity about having an identified disability and his long history of less-than-stellar academic performance. The therapist was aware of Brian's tendency to use verbal confrontations with teachers and other adults, which had earned him a negative reputation at his high school. The school social worker contacted Brian's mother, who revealed that she was struggling to interact with Brian in a positive manner.

To address these challenges, the occupational therapist suggested that Brian convene his transition team to make some plans. Brian replied, "OK, if that will get some of these people off my back." She and the music teacher then met with Brian to develop an agenda for the upcoming transition meeting and to discuss Brian's ideas about what he might do after high school. As expected, music was an interest, although Brian could not describe what he would actually do other than "jam with friends." To help Brian envision a

variety of ways in which he could be engaged with music, the music teacher, the occupational therapist, and Brian brainstormed ideas and discussed local resources and opportunities. Discussion of potential music-related activities drew heavily from the experience of the music teacher and his own music-related contacts. The therapist served as the "recorder" for this meeting using a computer so she could send Brian electronic notes he could review later using screen-reading software available in the school's computer center.

When the transition team met, Brian (with the help of the occupational therapist) had prepared an agenda on the white board in the meeting room. The agenda was complete with illustrations and artwork depicting what is important to Brian and arrows pointing toward possible music-related activities. Brian chaired the meeting and asked the team for help to meet the following goal he had set for himself: "to host a contemporary rock show at a local radio station."

With Brian's goal in mind, members of the transition team discussed resources and strategies. Brian then agreed to work with the music teacher on a 1-hour audition CD that could be shared with local radio station managers. Brian also agreed to accompany the occupational therapist on an individualized tour of two different radio stations to include some hands-on time at the controls. Brian's mother agreed to help with Brian's transportation home after each radio station visit.

With Brian's permission, the counselor agreed to rearrange Brian's course schedule so he could receive independent study credit for his work with the music teacher and also enroll in a community college music appreciation class being taught by a popular local musician. The occupational therapist and the social worker offered (and Brian accepted) to work with Brian on time management strategies and the use of a hand-held personal digital assistant (PDA) combined with regular check-ins with the social worker to ensure that school work was being completed and problems were being identified early enough to allow for prompt resolution and prevention of unpleasant confrontations with teachers and others.

When issues related to future independent living and postsecondary education came up at the meeting, Brian decided to postpone discussion, saying, "I have enough to work on for now." The team accepted this and offered Brian positive feedback for his ability to set priorities and make a plan.

Education policy and research are focused on improving the quality of education for all students. Special education research relies on multiple research methodologies that identify effective practices that align with IDEA.[25] The preceding evidence-based transition practices have been reported in peer-reviewed journals. As with all areas of special education research, the addition of new studies to the literature will help build needed scientific evidence and refine transition practices. Future research will be increasingly scrutinized for quality and

the extent to which it answers important and relevant questions. According to Odom and colleagues, "Researchers cannot just address simple questions about whether a practice in special education is effective; they must specify clearly for whom the practice is effective and in what contexts" (p. 41).[49]

Similar to the emphasis on high-quality research evidence in occupational therapy,[41,54,61] special education scholars are developing and debating research guidelines and quality indicators for evidence-based practices.[8,49]

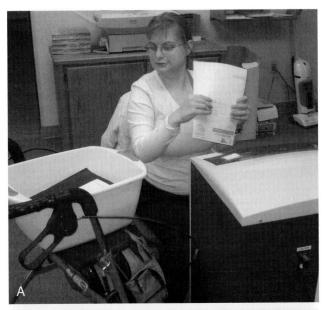

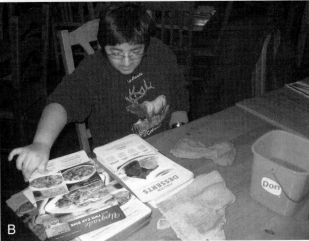

FIGURE 27-3   Job carving. **A,** Creating a job focused on shredding office paper. **B,** Creating a job focused on cleaning menus.

The long history of research in occupational therapy and special education has relied on many different research methodologies that are being increasingly scrutinized for rigor. Special education has seen the widespread use of four research methodologies, all of which have the potential to add to the evidence base for transition: qualitative,[12] correlational,[62] single-subject,[32] and finally, group and quasi-experimental designs.[22] Connected with each of these approaches are proposed quality indicators to help researchers and practitioners evaluate the extent to which the research actually provides evidence for a particular practice.[49] As in occupational therapy, special education has not reached consensus on a single standard for evidence or a single set of quality indicators. What is important, however, is the commitment and dedication of special education and related service scientists to continuously meet rigorous research standards regardless of the research approach taken.[16,49] To this end, the U.S. Department of Education's Institute for Education Sciences is actively moving high-quality special education research forward by only

---

CASE STUDY 27-3   Renee

Renee is a 20-year-old student participating in a transition-focused program at her high school. Renee sustained a severe brain injury when she was a sophomore as a result of an automobile accident. Her injuries resulted in hemiparesis and limitations in expressive communication. With the support of a job developer who is on staff at the school's transition program, Renee is now applying for a part-time job stocking and cleaning shelves at a local sporting goods store and has completed her application and interview. Renee really wants this job since it is within walking distance of her home and has good hours. If she gets the job, Renee hopes to keep it after she completes high school with ongoing support provided by the state vocational rehabilitation agency. Renee's prospective employer has indicated to the job developer that while he liked Renee, he is uncertain about having a person with a disability working at his store. Furthermore, he indicated that he is uncertain about what Renee could do, if she and his customers would be safe, and if she would be a productive employee.

Wanting to preserve this job opportunity for Renee, the job developer contacted the occupational therapist who regularly consults with the transition program staff. The occupational therapist knows Renee because she helped the team evaluate Renee's job-related interests and skills, and she is also familiar with the job site and the potential job demands Renee will encounter. With Renee's hoped-for job offer hanging by a thread, the occupational therapist decided to once again visit the job site, this time to meet directly with the employer. Following permission from Renee and her parents, the occupational therapist sat down with the employer over a cup of coffee to share information about brain injury and how a brain injury can affect a person's performance of everyday activities. The occupational therapist also shared examples of effective strategies used by other employers who had employees with disabilities similar to Renee's.

While meeting with the employer, the occupational therapist also took the opportunity to educate the employer about supported employment—a service that would be available to Renee and her employer. After a half-hour meeting, the occupational therapist thanked the employer, provided him with her business card, and encouraged him to call with any further questions or concerns. The next day, Renee received a phone call from the employer offering her the position.

In this situation, the occupational therapist's well-timed sharing of information and resources helped reassure a prospective employer. The employer's knowledge of brain injury and supported employment were expanded, allowing him to ultimately make the decision to hire Renee. The occupational therapist also used an educational approach to positively reframe the employer's perception of Renee's disability by sharing positive contributions made by people with disabilities and job support strategies that are realistic and effective.

---

funding studies that that will generate research evidence and that meet one of five different research goals[63]:

1. Identify programs, practices, and policies that may have an impact on student outcomes, and factors that may mediate or moderate the effects of these programs, practices, and policies.

2. Develop programs, practices, and policies that are theoretically and empirically based.
3. Establish the efficacy of fully developed program, practices, and policies.
4. Evaluate the impact of programs, practices, and policies implemented at scale.
5. Develop and/or validate data and measurement systems and tools.

Occupational therapy personnel and special educators working together on transition teams are expected to apply findings from high-quality, peer-reviewed research to the design of transition programs and services for youth (evidence-based practice). Transition services, guided by scientific evidence, are expected by IDEA and the professional and regulatory bodies that oversee teaching and related service professionals. Accompanying peer-reviewed research evidence is the need for systematic progress monitoring and data-based decision making at the individual student and context level.[55] This type of practice-based evidence requires attention to the growing body of peer-reviewed research and the systematic monitoring of individual student performance in response to transition services using valid and reliable measures administered with high fidelity.[11,21] The following section further explains practice-based evidence.

Practice-Based Evidence

High-quality peer-reviewed research evidence sets the stage for the systematic monitoring of individual student performance during everyday school activities and contexts.[21,55] It is the intersection between peer-reviewed research and individual progress monitoring that ensures scientifically based transition practice. The term *practice-based evidence*[18] describes the gathering and interpreting of individual student or client performance data as the basis for intervention planning and actions. Sometimes termed effective practice,[61] practice scholarship,[19,37] or intervention review,[4] practice-based evidence is concerned with the systematic examination of student performance associated with specific education or related service interventions over time (Box 27-10). It is a form of individual progress monitoring called for by IDEA and documented in each student's IEP (Box 27-11).[4,30,72]

All members of a student's transition team engage in the generation and use of practice-based evidence. Unlike research-based evidence derived from peer-reviewed studies,

---

BOX 27-10 **Practice-Based Evidence**

Practice-based evidence (PBE) is a term being used by interdisciplinary rehabilitation teams at the Craig Hospital and other rehabilitation hospitals in the Denver region. PBE represents a practice-centered process of examining client performance outcomes resulting from specific rehabilitative interventions. Systematic, intervention-centered PBE research seeks to address questions regarding intervention effectiveness and efficiency. Over time, knowledge generated from PBE is expected to shed light on "best practices" for specific diagnostic groups within specific service contexts.

From Craig Hospital. (2009). *Improving spinal cord injury rehabilitation outcomes.* Retrieved January 16, 2009, http://www.craighospital.org/Research/Abstracts/SCIRehab.asp.

BOX 27-11 Effective Practice in a Research Emergent Profession: Occupational Therapy

The competent school-based occupational therapist must think about 'effective practice' and engage in systematic data collection related to desired student outcomes. At all times, the therapist must utilize student/client evaluation and intervention activities to collect and document student performance (outcomes) that justify ongoing decisions about occupational therapy service continuation, modification, or discontinuation (p. 27).

From Swinth, Y., Spencer, K. C., & Jackson L. L. (2007). *Occupational therapy: Effective school-based practices within a policy context. (COPSSE Document Number OP-3).* Gainesville, FL: University of Florida, Center on Personnel Studies in Special Education.

---

practice-based evidence is specific to a student. This means that data-gathering strategies and performance findings cannot be readily generalized or transferred to other students, groups, or contexts. Data are gathered during student engagement in a variety of transition-related activities and in a variety of contexts.

The occupational therapist's ability to observe and record student performance and performance patterns while simultaneously considering the demands of the activity and environment can yield important information for the team. This type of performance analysis[4] tied to activities at school, in the community, at home, on the job, or during a student visit to a university campus can yield needed data for individualized transition planning and help the team evaluate the relative effectiveness of individualized interventions. A well-executed performance analysis can identify what a student is doing well and where performance breaks down. *Performance analysis*, which is "the analysis of occupational performance focuses on collecting and interpreting information using assessment tools designed to observe, measure, and inquire about factors that support or hinder occupational performance" (p. 649),[4] also allows the evaluator to examine the amount and type of assistance, adaptation, or accommodation needed to support effective student performance.[17]

Performance analysis can be paired with an activity analysis to pinpoint activity-specific factors that limit or support student participation. *Activity analysis* is "an important process used by occupational therapy practitioners to understand the demands that a specific desired activity places on a client.... When activity analysis is completed and the demands of a specific activity that the client needs or wants to do are understood, the client's specific skills and abilities are then compared with the selected activity's demands" (p. 651).[4] Activity analysis (further defined in Box 28-13) focuses on the context-specific demands of a specific activity.

Case Study 27-4 illustrates the concept of practice-based evidence while also demonstrating how performance and activity analysis can contribute to this critical aspect of transition service planning, intervention, and outcome monitoring. Case Study 27-5 further illustrates the concept of practice-based evidence through combined performance and activity analysis.

Occupational therapists are well acquainted with progress monitoring and documentation. In many occupational therapy contexts, this process is driven by insurance reimbursement policies. In school contexts, progress monitoring is driven by the IDEA's accountability expectations and the need for data to guide service planning and intervention.

Both education and related service professionals are expected to contribute to the ongoing data collection for monitoring of individual student learning, performance, and achievement over time.[10,55,74] Anyone who has participated in publicly supported education within the United States is familiar with the central role that student evaluation plays in education. Some classroom assignments and tests are informal, whereas others impact decisions about a student's course grade, school placement, or which education or related services will be provided. Beyond individual student assessment, educational progress is monitored at the school and district levels by states and the federal government (No Child Left Behind Act, P.L. 107–110).

Response to intervention (RTI) is another form of practice-based evidence that is addressed by the IDEA and widespread in U.S. schools (§613 (f)). RTI is the strategic application of educational interventions and the subsequent monitoring of student performance based on those interventions.[6] RTI can target any student (including those involved with transition services), who is demonstrating learning difficulty. Initially intended for students with specific learning disabilities, RTI has potential applications to a broader population of learners who are struggling.[34] The timely application of strategic,

scientifically based educational interventions accompanied by systematic data collection and progress monitoring (practice-based evidence) characterizes RTI. Considered preventive, the RTI model seeks to meet a variety of student learning needs within the general curriculum and through high-quality instruction. When done well, RTI is expected to prevent the overidentification of disability and the inappropriate referral of students for special education and related services.

RTI begins with the least amount of intervention. Simply stated, this means strong general education instruction for all children based on universal design principles (Box 27-12) that can address a variety of student learning styles. Termed *Tier 1* intervention, this strong general instruction is accompanied by systematic evaluation of the student's response to the instruction (practice-based evidence). When good general instruction does not sufficiently boost student performance, more individualized instruction can be implemented for specific students within the context of the general curriculum (Tier 2). Finally, when progress monitoring and systematic data collection reveal that a student has not responded to Tier 1 and 2 intervention and the student continues to lag educationally or behaviorally, intensive and individualized interventions become necessary (Tier 3). Tier 3 intervention can include specialized education and related services. All tiers in the RTI process require continuous student performance evaluation based on measures that are reliable and valid. RTI is an

CASE STUDY 27-4   Todd

Todd is a 17-year-old student who is learning to use public transportation so he can travel independently to and from his internship site at a local greenhouse (Figure 27-4). Todd has significant developmental disabilities that limit his cognition, communication, and mobility. The occupational therapist on Todd's team plays a major role in matching students like Todd to appropriate community learning opportunities including internships. The occupational therapy (OT) assistant assigned has been scheduled to work with Todd on bus travel. Specifically, the OT assistant helps Todd learn to travel safely and independently to and from his internship site. Among the skills Todd must master are identifying and boarding the correct bus, interacting politely with the driver and other passengers, and exiting at the correct stop. Systematic data collection by the OT assistant on the type and amount of assistance provided at each major step in the bus travel sequence (activity analysis) allows the OT assistant and other members of the team to evaluate changes in Todd's performance (performance analysis) linked to specific types of intervention.

In Todd's situation, the team recommended that the OT assistant use specific prompting strategies and an individualized bus card created just for Todd. The bus card identified the correct bus and provided a means for Todd to communicate with his bus drivers. Performance data (practice-based evidence) gathered consistently by the OT assistant during multiple bus trips and presented to the transition team painted an accurate picture of Todd's progress. With data in

hand, the team can determine which types of cuing, accommodations, and support are working and areas in which Todd still has learning and support needs. Similarly, sustained changes in Todd's performance and independence are clearly documented. The easy-to-use data collection format shown in Figure 27-5 illustrates how the OT assistant in Todd's scenario can systematically gather data that can later be summarized (practice-based evidence) and shared with the team.

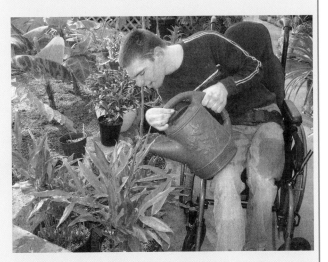

FIGURE 27-4   Real work in the community depends on being able to get to and from the job site.

Continued

CASE STUDY 27-4   Todd—cont'd

Student: Todd Adams

Teacher: Ms. Garcia, special education

Consultants: Ms. Patterson, occupational therapist

Primary supporter/trainer for this activity: Mr. Friedman, OT assistant

Activity: Riding the public bus from the high school to community work setting then back to the high school at the end of the work shift.

Transition goal supported by this activity: Todd will complete a semester-long internship at a community job site that matches his interests and that is accessible by public transportation.

Activity Setting/Context: City bus #4, bus stops at school and at community job site.

Activity Steps	Accommodation or Support strategy	Student Performance				
		Date:	Date:	Date:	Date:	Date:
1. Board appropriate bus	Match bus # with the # on pocket-sized bus card created for this student					
2. Greet, then notify driver of desired stop	Model greeting; show driver laminated bus card with the desired stop identified					
3. Take seat close to drive—quiet conversation						
4. Pull cord to notify driver of stop	Verbal or gestural prompts to identify landmarks matched to bus card					
5. Disembark bus with all belongings	Verbal or gestural prompt to gather items and scan area					
6. Go directly to destination	Gestural prompt					
Performance KEY : (Performance target: achieve "I" for each step)		I = Independent P = Prompt (verbal, gestural, touch) D = Direct instruction NC = Not completed				

FIGURE 27-5   Individual progress monitoring/performance analysis.

CASE STUDY 27-5   Amanda

Amanda, an 18-year-old student, plans to attend college and must complete multiple college applications including personal essays. Because of Amanda's learning disability and subsequent difficulty with organization and writing, the occupational therapist on the transition team arranges for Amanda to use specialized software that has a number of built-in grammatical, spelling, word finding, and editing features. Amanda is delighted to discover software-based accommodations, knowing that she will need multiple tools and strategies to meet the future demands of college-level writing.

With initial support and training provided by the occupational therapist, Amanda learned to use the software for her high school writing assignments. Effectiveness of the software-based intervention was monitored by the student, the teacher, and the occupational therapist. The English teacher and Amanda reviewed drafts of each assignment, correcting each and recording the number and nature of any errors using a table format. This process allowed her to monitor her own performance over time and identify a persistent problem area: overall essay organization and transitions between topics.

Continued

CASE STUDY 27-5 Amanda—cont'd

Armed with data on the student's performance, the occupational therapist decided that the next step was to help Amanda learn how to use a graphic outlining feature that was previously unexplored in the software package. Following documented improvements in the student's writing performance, the teacher shifted her focus to help Amanda prepare her college-level essay using all the software tools previously identified. By the end of the semester, Amanda had prepared and submitted her college application essay and she had become proficient using software-based writing accommodations (Figure 27-6.)

Student: Amanda Allen

Teacher: Ms. Haley, English

Consultants: Ms. Clark, occupational therapy; Mr. Hanneman, history teacher

Primary supporter/trainer for this activity: Ms. Haley, English

Activity: Writing multi-paragraph essays as assigned for English and history

Transition goal supported by this activity: Amanda will complete and submit 4 college applications including personal essays by the end of the semester.

Activity Setting/Context: In-class or homework essay writing (as assigned for English and history classes) using a laptop computer with adapted software

Expected Performance (identified by teacher)	Accommodation or Support strategy (identified by teachers and OT)	Student Performance (evaluated jointly by Ms. Haley and Amanda)				
		Paper topic: Date:	Paper topic: Date:	Paper topic: Date:	Paper topic: Date:	Paper topic: Date:
1. Create outline	Adapted software: Diagrammatic outline/topic web created on computer					
2. Introduction	Convert diagrammatic outline into a document outline (adapted software)					
3. Organization and flow of ideas, conclusions	Re-read aloud (screen reading feature)					
4. Transitions between ideas or topics	Refer to list of alternative wording prompts created by student and teacher					
5. Use of "active voice"	Re-read, edit					
6. Spelling	Computer spell check					
7. Word choice	Re-read aloud, "word prediction" feature					
8. Conclusion	Re-read with original diagrammatic outline					
9. References	Refer to teacher's guide					
Performance KEY: (Performance target "++" or "+" for each item)	++ excellent + good o OK, average - needs improvement in several areas – absent or many errors					

FIGURE 27-6 Individual progress monitoring/performance analysis.

BOX 27-12 Universal Design for Learning

Universal Design for Learning [UDL] helps meet the challenge of diversity by suggesting flexible instructional materials, techniques, and strategies that empower educators to meet these varied needs. A universally designed curriculum is designed from the outset to meet the needs of the greatest number of users, making costly, time-consuming, and after-the-fact changes to curriculum unnecessary. Three principles guide UDL:

Provide multiple means of representation

Provide multiple means of action and expression

Provide multiple means of engagement

From CAST. (2008). Universal design for learning guidelines version 1.0, p. 4. Wakefield, MA: CAST.

example of how practice-based evidence is used to guide educational decision making. Occupational therapists can support the design and implementation of RTIs at all tier levels and carry responsibility with other team members to monitor the student's response to the intervention and to adjust services and supports accordingly.

SUMMARY

The transition from school to adult life represents a major life step for young adults. When a disability is present, this transition can be challenging and requires comprehensive and timely planning and service from an interdisciplinary and interagency transition team. Transition teams must have a deep understanding of transition-related policy, research-supported transition practices as presented in the peer-reviewed literature and the ability to systematically gather and use practice-based evidence during the day-to-day delivery of transition services. Occupational therapy personnel on the team are expected to collaborate with other team members during all phases of the transition process: establishing a vision for the student's future, evaluation of student performance and participation in relevant contexts and activities, outcome-oriented planning, service delivery, and ongoing progress and outcome monitoring. The success of the student and therefore the transition team may be measured by the extent to which students actually achieve postsecondary education, employment, community living, and/or involvement in meaningful and enduring relationships.

Although exciting and absolutely essential, providing effective transition services may feel messy or complicated. How true! Consider the number of players involved along with the number and variety of educational and community contexts needed for valid student evaluation and services, plus the constantly emerging research evidence for specific practices. Occupational therapy personnel are reminded that transition services, even when planned and delivered well, always include an element of uncertainty and unpredictability. However, by holding high expectations for student performance combined with a spirit of flexibility and creativity, occupational therapists and other members of the transition team will be amazed at what students can and do achieve during the school-to-adult life transition process.

REFERENCES

1. Agran, M., Sinclair, T., Alper, S., Cavin, M., Wehmeyer, M., & Hughes, C. (2005). Using self-monitoring to increase following direction skills of students with moderate to severe disabilities in general education. *Education and Training in Developmental Disabilities, 40,* (1), 3–13.
2. Agran, M., Wehmeyer, M. L., Cavin, M., & Palmer, S. (2008). Promoting student active classroom participation skills through instruction to promote self-regulated learning and self-determination. *Career Development for Exceptional Individuals, 31*(2), 106–114.
3. American Occupational Therapy Association. (2006). *Transforming caseload to workload in school-based and early intervention occupational therapy services.* Retrieved May 29, 2008 from www.aota.org
4. American Occupational Therapy Association. (2008). Occupational therapy practice framework: Domain and process (2nd ed.). *American Journal of Occupational Therapy, 62,* 625–683.
5. Bambara, L. M., Wilson, B. A., & McKenzie, M. (2007). Transition and quality of life. In S. M. Odom, R. H. Horner, M. E. Snell, & J. Blacher (Eds.), *Handbook of developmental disabilities* (pp. 371–389). New York: Guilford Press.
6. Batsche, G., Elliott, J., Graden, J. L., Grimes, J., Kovaleski, J., & Prasse, D. (2005). *Response to intervention: Policy consideration and implementation.* Alexandria, VA: National Association of State Directors of Special Education.
7. Baugh, T. (2003). *Bystander focus groups: Bullying—roles, rules and coping tools to break the cycle.* Washington, DC: George Washington University.
8. Berliner, D. C. (2002). Educational research: The hardest science of all. *Educational Researchers, 31*(8), 18–20.
9. Bolles, R. N. (2008). *What color is your parachute?* Berkeley, CA: Ten Speed Press.
10. Bradley, R., Danielson, L., & Doolittle, J. (2007). Responsiveness to intervention: 1997–2007. *Teaching Exceptional Children, 39,* 8–12.
11. Bradley, R., Danielson, L., & Hallahan, D. P. (2002). *Identification of learning disabilities: Research to practice.* Mahway, NJ: Lawrence Erlbaum.
12. Brantlinger, E., Jimenez, R., Klingner, J., Pugach, M., & Richardson, V. (2005). Qualitative studies in special education. *Exceptional Children, 71*(2), 195–207.
13. Brown, L., Branston-McLean, M. B., Baumgart, D., Vincent, L., Falvey, M., & Schroeder, J. (1979). Using the characteristics of current and future least restrictive environments in the development of curricular content for severely handicapped students. *American Association for Education of the Severe and Profound Handicapped Review, 4*(4), 407–424.
14. Cameto, R. (2005). Employment of youth with disabilities after high school. In M. Wagner, L. Newman, R. Cameto, N. Garza, & P. Levine (Eds.), *After high school: A first look at the postschool experiences of youth with disabilities. A report from the national longitudinal transition study-2 (NLTS2)* (pp. 5.1–5.21). Menlo Park, CA: SRI International. Available at http://www.nlts2.org/reports/2005_04/nlts2_report_2005_04_ch5.pdf
15. Carter, E. W., Lane, K. L., Pierson, M. R., & Glaeser, B. (2006). Self-determination skills and opportunities of transition-age youth with emotional and learning disabilities. *Exceptional Children, 72*(3), 333–346.
16. Cook, B. G., Tankersley, M., Cook, L., & Landrum, T. J. (2008). Evidence-based practices in special education: Some practical considerations. *Intervention in School and Clinic, 44*(2), 69–75.
17. Coster, W., Deeney, T., Haltiwanger, J., & Haley, S. (1998). *School function assessment.* San Antonio, TX: Psychological Corp./Therapy Skill Builders.
18. Craig Hospital. (2009). *Improving spinal cord injury rehabilitation outcomes.* Retrieved January 16, 2009 from http://www.craighospital.org/Research/Abstracts/SCIRehab.asp

19. Crist, P., Munoz, J. P., Hansen, A. M. W., Bensen, J., & Provident, I. (2005). The practice-scholar program; An academic-practice partnership to promote the scholarship of "best practices." *Occupational Therapy in Health Care, 19*(1/2), 71–93.

20. Falvey, M. A., Rosenberg, R. L., Monson, D., & Eshilian, L. (2006). Facilitating and supporting transition: Secondary school restructuring and the implementation of transition services and programs. In P. Wehman (Ed.), *Life beyond the classroom: Transition strategies for young people with disabilities* (pp. 165–182). Baltimore: Brookes.

21. Fuchs, L. S., & Fuchs, D. (2002). *What is scientifically-based research on progress monitoring? (Technical report).* Nashville, TN: Vanderbilt University.

22. Gersten, R., Fuchs, L. S., Compton, D., Coyne, M., Greenwood, C., & Innocenti, M. S. (2005). Quality indicators for group experimental and quasi-experimental research in special education. *Exceptional Children, 71*(2), 149–164.

23. Giangreco, M. (1996). *Vermont interdependent services team approach: A guide to coordinating educational support services (VISTA).* Baltimore: Brookes.

24. Giangreco, M. F., Cloninger, C. J., & Iverson, V. S. (1998). *Choosing outcomes and accommodations for children (COACH): A guide to educational planning for students with disabilities* (2nd ed.). Baltimore: Brookes.

25. Graham, S. (2005). Preview. *Exceptional Children, 71*(135).

26. Gray, J. M., Kennedy, B. L., & Zemke, R. (1996). Application of dynamic systems theory to occupation. In R. Zemke & F. Clark (Eds.), *Occupational science: The evolving discipline.* Philadelphia: F.A. Davis.

27. Griffin, C., & Targett, P. S. (2006). Job carving and customized employment. In P. Wehman (Ed.), *Life beyond the classroom: Transition strategies for young people with disabilities* (pp. 289–308). Baltimore: Brookes.

28. Hanft, B., & Shepherd, J. (2008). *Collaborating for student success: A guide for school-based occupational therapy.* Bethesda, MD: American Occupational Therapy Association.

29. Hasazi, S., Hock, M., & Cravedi-Cheng, L. (1992). Vermont's post-school indicators: Using satisfaction and post-school outcome data for program improvement. In F. Rusch, L. Destefano, J. Chadsey-Rusch, L. A. Phelps, & E. Szymanski (Eds.), *Transition from school to adult life: Models, linkages, and policy* (pp. 485–506). Pacific Grove, CA: Brooks/Cole.

30. Heaton, J., & Bamford, C. (2001). Assessing the outcomes of equipment and adaptations: Issues and approaches. *British Journal of Occupational Therapy, 64*(7), 346–356.

31. Holburn, S., & Vietze, P. M. (2002). *Person-centered planning: Research, practice, and future directions.* Baltimore: Brookes.

32. Horner, R. H., Carr, E. G., Halle, J., McGee, G., Odom, S., & Wolery, M. (2005). The use of single-subject research to identify evidence-based practice in special education. *Exceptional Children, 71*(2), 165–180.

33. Ilott, I. (2004). Challenges and strategic solutions for a research emergent profession. *American Journal of Occupational Therapy, 58*(3), 347–352.

34. Jackson, L. L. (Ed.). (2008). *Occupational therapy services for children and youth under IDEA* (3rd ed.). Bethesda, MD: AOTA Press.

35. Kardos, M., & White, B. P. (2005). The role of the school-based occupational therapist in secondary education transition planning: A pilot survey study. *American Journal of Occupational Therapy, 59*, 173–180.

36. Keenan, S. (2004). Bullying: A culture of fear and disrespect. *The Council for Children with Behavioral Disorders, 18*(2), 1–2, 4.

37. Kielhofner, G. (2005). A scholarship of practice: Creating discourse between theory, research and practice. *Occupational Therapy in Health Care, 19*, 7–16.

38. Kohler, P. D., & Field, S. (2003). Transition-focused education: Foundation for the future. *Journal of Special Education, 37*(3), 174–183.

39. Kregel, J., & Dean, D. H. (2002). Sheltered work vs. supported employment: A direct comparison of long-term earnings outcomes for individuals with cognitive disabilities. In J. Dregel, D. H. Dean, & P. Wehman (Eds.), *Achievements and challenges in employment services for people with disabilities: The longitudinal impact of workplace supports.* Richmond, VA: Virginia Commonwealth University, Rehabilitation Research and Training Center on Workplace Supports.

40. Lawhead, R. A. (2005). *Hearing on opportunity for too few? Oversight of federal employment programs for people with disabilities.* U.S. Senate: Testimony before the Health, Education, Labor, & Pensions Committee, October 20, 2005.

41. Lieberman, D., & Scheer, J. (2002). AOTA's evidence-based literature review project: An overview. *The American Journal of Occupational Therapy, 56*, 344–349.

42. Lipsky, D. K., & Gartner, A. (1997). *Inclusion and school reform: Transforming America's classrooms.* Baltimore: Brookes.

43. Mank, D., O'Neill, C., & Jansen, R. (1998). Quality in supported employment: A new demonstration of the capabilities of people with severe disabilities. *Journal of Vocational Rehabilitation, 11*(1), 83–95.

44. Marder, C., Cardoso, D., & Wagner, M. (2003). Employment among youth with disabilities. In M. Wagner, T. Cadwallader, & C. Marder (Eds.), *Life outside the classroom for youth with disabilities. A report from the national longitudinal transition study-2 (NLTS2)* (pp. 5.1–5.11). Menlo Park, CA: SRI International. Retrieved from www.nlts2.org/reports/2003_04-2/nlts2_report_2003_04-2_complete.pdf

45. Martin, J. E., Van Dycke, J. L., Christensen, W. R., Greene, B. A., Gardener, J. E., & Lovett, D. L. (2006). Increasing student participation in IEP meetings: Establishing the self-directed IEP as an evidence-based practice. *Exceptional Children, 72*(3), 299–316.

46. McMahan, R., & Baer, R. (2001). IDEA transition policy compliance and best practice: Perceptions of transition stakeholders. *Career Development for Exceptional Individuals, 24*, 169–184.

47. Mount, B. (1997). *Person-centered planning: Finding direction for change using personal futures planning* (2nd ed.). New York: Graphic Features.

48. National Center for School Engagement (NCSE). (2005). *What research says about family-school-community partnerships.* Retrieved November 2008 from http://www.schoolengagement.org.

49. Odom, S., Brantlinger, E., Horner, R., Thompson, B., & Harris, K. (2005). Research in special education: Scientific methods and evidence-based practices. *Exceptional Children, 71*, 137–148.

50. Pugach, M. C., & Johnson, L. J. (1995). *Collaborative practitioners, collaborative schools.* Denver CO: Love Publishing.

51. Rainforth, B., & York-Barr, J. (1997). *Collaborative teams for students with severe disabilities: Integrating therapy with educational services* (2nd ed.). Baltimore: Brookes.

52. Revell, G., Wehman, P., Kregel, J., West, M., & Rayfield, R. (1994). Funding supported employment: Are there better ways? In P. Wehman, J. Kregel, & M. West (Eds), *Supported employment research: Expanding competitive employment opportunities for persons with significant disabilities.* Richmond, VA: Virginia Commonwealth University Rehabilitation Research and Training Center on Supported Employment.

53. Roberton, M. A. (1993). New ways to think about old questions. In L. Smith & E. Thelen (Eds.), *A dynamic systems approach to development: Applications.* Cambridge, MA: MIT Press.

54. Sackett, D., Rosenburg, W., Gray, J., Haynes, R., & Richardson, W. (1996). Evidence-based medicine: What it is and what it isn't. *British Medical Journal, 31*, 71–72.

55. Safer, N., & Fleischman, S. (2005). Research matters/How student progress monitoring improves instruction. *Educational Leadership, 62*(5), 81–83.

56. Schell, B., & Schell, J. (2008). *Clinical and professional reasoning in occupational therapy.* Philadelphia: Lippincott Williams & Wilkins.

57. Smull, M. W., & Harrison, S. (1992). *Supporting people with severe reputations in the community.* Alexandria, VA: National Association of State Mental Retardation Program.

58. Snell, M. E., & Janney, R. E. (2005). *Collaborative teaming* (2nd ed.). Baltimore: Brookes.

59. Spence-Cochran, K., & Pearl, C. E. (2006). Moving toward full inclusion. In P. Wehman (Ed.), *Life beyond the classroom: Strategies for young people with disabilities* (4th ed., pp. 133–164). Baltimore: Brookes.

60. Stodden, R. A., Brown, S. E., Galloway, L. M., Mrazek, S., & Noy, L. (2004). *Essential tools: Interagency transition team development and facilitation.* Minneapolis, MN: University of Minnesota, Institute on Community Integration, National Center on Secondary Education and Transition.

61. Swinth, Y., Spencer, K. C., & Jackson, L. L. (2007). *Occupational therapy: Effective school-based practices within a policy context (COPSSE Document No. OP-3).* Gainesville, FL: University of Florida, Center on Personnel Studies in Special Education.

62. Thompson, B., Kiamond, K. D., McWilliam, R., Snyder, P., & Snyder, S. W. (2005). Evaluating the quality of evidence from correlational research for evidence-based practice. *Exceptional Children, 71*(2), 181–194.

63. U.S. Department of Education. Institute for Education Services. Home page. Retrieved February 29, 2008 from http://ies.ed.gov.

64. Wagner, M., Newman, L., Cameto, R., Levine, P., & Garza, N. (2006). *An overview of findings from wave 2 of the National Longitudinal Transition Study-2 (NLTS2).* Menlo Park, CA: SRI International, Retrieved from www.nlts2.org/reports/2006_08/nlts2_report_2006_08_complete.pdf.

65. Ward, M. (1992). Introduction to secondary special education and transition issues. In F. Rusch, L. Destefano, J. Chadsey-Rusch, I. A. Phelps, & E. Szymanski (Eds.), *Transition from school to adult life: Models, linkages, and policy* (pp. 387–389). Pacific Grove, CA: Brooks/Cole.

66. Ward, M. J., & Kohler, P. D. (1996). Promoting self-determination for individuals with disabilities: Content and process. In L. E. Powers, G. H. S. Singer, & J. Sowers (Eds.), *On the road to autonomy: Promoting self-competence in children and youth with disabilities* (pp. 275–290). Baltimore: Brookes.

67. Wehman, P. (2006). Individualized transition planning: Putting self determination into action. In P. Wehman (Ed.), *Life beyond the classroom: Transition strategies for young people with disabilities* (pp. 71–96). Baltimore: Brookes.

68. Wehman, P. (2006). *Life beyond the classroom: Transition strategies for young people with disabilities* (4th ed.). Baltimore: Brookes.

69. Wehmeyer, M. L., Gragoudas, S., & Shogren, K. A. (2006). Self-determination, student involvement, and leadership development. In P. Wehman (Ed.), *Life beyond the classroom: Transition strategies for young people with disabilities* (pp. 41–70). Baltimore: Brookes.

70. Wehmeyer, M. L., & Sands, D. J. (1998). *Making it happen: Student involvement in education planning, decision making, and instruction.* Baltimore: Brookes.

71. Wehmeyer, M. L., & Schwartz, M. (1997). Self-determination and positive adult outcomes: A follow-up study of youth with mental retardation or learning disabilities. *Exceptional Children, 63,* 245–255.

72. Welch, A. (2002). The challenge of evidence-based practice to occupational therapy: A literature review. *Journal of Clinical Governance, 10*(4), 169–176.

73. Woods, L. L., & Martin, J. E. (2004). Improving supervisor evaluations through the use of self-determination contracts. *Career Development for Exceptional Individuals, 27,* 207–220.

74. Ysseldyke, J. (2002). Response to "Learning disabilities: Historical perspectives." In R. Bradley, L. Danielson, & D. P. Hallahan (Eds.), *Identification of learning disabilities: Research to practice* (pp. 89–98). Mahwah, NJ: Lawrence Erlbaum.

Index